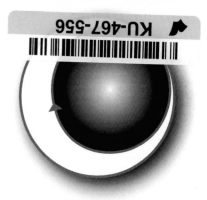

# Core
# Clinical
## Cases in

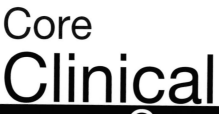

# Medicine
# and Medical
# Specialties

## Second edition

Edited by

**Steve Bain** MA MD FRCP
Professor of Medicine (Diabetes), Institute of Life
Sciences, Swansea University, Swansea
Honorary Consultant Physician, ABM University Health
Board, Singleton Hospital, Swansea

**Jeffrey W Stephens** BSc MBBS PhD FRCP
Professor of Medicine (Diabetes and Metabolism),
Institute of Life Sciences, Swansea University, Swansea
Consultant Physician, Morriston Hospital, ABM University
Health Board, Swansea

Core Clinical Cases series edited by

**Janesh K Gupta** MSc MD FRCOG
Professor in Obstetrics and Gynaecology, University
of Birmingham, Birmingham Women's Hospital,
Birmingham, UK

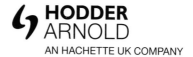

## HODDER
ARNOLD
AN HACHETTE UK COMPANY

First published in Great Britain in 2006 by Hodder Arnold
This second edition published in 2012 by
Hodder Arnold, an imprint of Hodder Education, a division of Hachette UK

338 Euston Road, London NW1 3BH

http://www.hodderarnold.com

Hachette UK's policy is to use papers that are natural, renewable and recyclable products and made from wood grown in sustainable forests. The logging and manufacturing processes are expected to conform to the environmental regulations of the country of origin.

Whilst the advice and information in this book are believed to be true and accurate at the date of going to press, neither the authors nor the publisher can accept any legal responsibility or liability for any errors or omissions that may be made. In particular (but without limiting the generality of the preceding disclaimer) every effort has been made to check drug dosages; however it is still possible that errors have been missed. Furthermore, dosage schedules are constantly being revised and new side effects recognized. For these reasons the reader is strongly urged to consult the drug companies' printed instructions before administering any of the drugs recommended in this book.

*British Library Cataloguing in Publication Data*
A catalogue record for this book is available from the British Library

*Library of Congress Cataloging-in-Publication Data*
A catalog record for this book is available from the Library of Congress

ISBN: 978-1-4441-4542-7

1 2 3 4 5 6 7 8 9 10

Commissioning Editor: Joanna Koster
Project Editor: Stephen Clausard
Production Controller: Joanna Walker
Cover Design: Amina Dudhia
Indexer: Lisa Footitt

Typeset in 9 on 11pt Frutiger by Phoenix Photosetting, Chatham, Kent
Printed and bound by CPI Group (UK) Ltd., Croydon, CR0 4YY.

What do you think about this book? Or any other Hodder Arnold title?
Please visit our website: www.hodderarnold.com

# Contents

# Contributors

Steve Bain MA MD FRCP
Professor of Medicine (Diabetes), Institute of Life Sciences, Swansea University, Swansea
Honorary Consultant Physician, ABM University Health Board, Singleton Hospital, Swansea

Morgan Cadman-Davies MBChB
ST1 General Practice Trainee, Hereford County Hospital, Hereford

Indranil Dasgupta MBBS MD DM FRCP
Consultant Nephrologist and Honorary Senior Lecturer, Birmingham Heartlands Hospital, Birmingham

Chris Ellis MB FRCP DTM&H
Consultant in Infectious Diseases, Birmingham Heartlands Hospital, Birmingham

Christopher Fegan MBBS MD FRCP FRCPath
Consultant Haematologist, Llandough Hospital, Cardiff

Andrew Levy PhD FRCP
Professor of Medicine, Bristol University, Bristol
Honorary Consultant Physician, Bristol Royal Infirmary, Bristol

Neeraj Prasad MD FRCP
Consultant Cardiologist, Hereford County Hospital, Hereford

C.S. Probert MD FRCP FHEA
Professor of Gastroenterology, Department of Gastroenterology, Institute of Translational Medicine, University of Liverpool, Liverpool

Mark Pugh DTM DCH MD FRCPI
Consultant Rheumatologist and Clinical Tutor, Department of Rheumatology, St Mary's Hospital, Newport, Isle of Wight

Daniel Rea MBBS BSc PhD FRCP
Senior Lecturer in Medical Oncology, University of Birmingham, Birmingham

Malcolm Shepherd MBChB MRCP PhD
Balmforth Intermediate Clinical Scientist Research Fellow, University of Glasgow, Glasgow

Nevianna Tomson MBChB MRCP
Consultant Dermatologist, West Suffolk Hospital, Bury St Edmunds

Peter Wallis MBBS FRCP
Consultant Geriatrician and Honorary Senior Clinical Lecturer, University of Birmingham, Department of Elderly Medicine, Birmingham Heartlands Hospital, Birmingham

Stuart Weatherby MBChB MRCP MD
Consultant Neurologist, Derriford Hospital, Plymouth
Honorary University Fellow to the Peninsula Medical School, Plymouth

# Series preface

## 'A history lesson'

Between about 1916 and 1927 a puzzling illness appeared and swept around the world. Dr von Economo first described encephalitis lethargica (EL), which simply meant 'inflammation of the brain that makes you tired'. Younger people, especially women, seemed to be more vulnerable, but the disease affected people of all ages. People with EL developed a 'sleep disorder', fever, headache and weakness, which led to a prolonged state of unconsciousness. The EL epidemic occurred during the same period as the 1918 influenza pandemic, and the two outbreaks have been linked ever since in the medical literature. Some people confused it with the epidemic of Spanish flu at that time, while others blamed weapons used in the First World War.

Encephalitis lethargica was dramatized by the film *Awakenings*, based on the book written by Oliver Sacks, an eminent neurologist from New York, and starring Robin Williams and Robert De Niro. Professor Sacks treated his patients with l-dopa, which temporarily awoke his patients, giving rise to the belief that the condition was related to Parkinson's disease.

Since the 1916–1927 epidemic, only sporadic cases of EL have been described. Pathological studies have revealed an encephalitis of the midbrain and basal ganglia, with lymphocyte (predominantly plasma cell) infiltration. Recent examination of archived EL brain material has failed to demonstrate influenza RNA, adding to the evidence that EL was not an invasive influenza encephalitis. Further investigations found no evidence of viral encephalitis or other recognized causes of rapid-onset parkinsonism. Magnetic resonance imaging of the brain was normal in 60 per cent but showed inflammatory changes localized to the deep grey matter in 40 per cent.

As late as the end of the twentieth century, it seemed that the possible answers lay in the clinical presentation of the patients in the 1916–1927 epidemic. It had been noted by the clinicians at that time that the central nervous system (CNS) disorder had presented with pharyngitis. This led to the possibility of a post-infectious autoimmune CNS disorder similar to Sydenham's chorea, in which group A beta-haemolytic streptococcal antibodies cross-react with the basal ganglia and result in abnormal behaviour and involuntary movements. Anti-streptolysin-O titres have subsequently been found to be elevated in the majority of these patients. It seemed possible that autoimmune antibodies may cause remitting parkinsonian signs subsequent to streptococcal tonsillitis as part of the spectrum of post-streptococcal CNS disease.

Could it be that the 80-year-old mystery of EL has been solved by relying on the patient's clinical history of presentation rather than focusing on expensive investigations? More research in this area will give us the definitive answer. This scenario is not dissimilar to the controversy about the idea that streptococcal infections were aetiologically related to rheumatic fever.

With this example of a truly fascinating history lesson, we hope you will endeavour to use the patient's clinical history as your most powerful diagnostic tool to make the correct diagnosis. If you do, you are likely to be right 80–90 per cent of the time. This is the basis of the Core Clinical Cases series, which will make you systematically explore clinical problems through the clinical history of presentation, followed by examination and then the performance of appropriate investigations. Never break those rules!

Janesh Gupta

# Abbreviations

| | |
|---|---|
| **AAFB** | acid- and alcohol-fast bacilli |
| **ABGs** | arterial blood gases |
| **ACE** | angiotensin-converting enzyme |
| **ACh** | acetylcholine |
| **ACTH** | adrenocorticotrophic hormone |
| **A&E** | accident and emergency |
| **AED** | anti-epileptic drug |
| **AF** | atrial fibrillation |
| **AIDP** | acute inflammatory demyelinating polyneuropathy |
| **AIDS** | acquired immunodeficiency syndrome |
| **AKI** | acute kidney injury |
| **ALP** | alkaline phosphatase |
| **ALS** | advanced life support |
| **ANA** | antinuclear antibody |
| **ANCA** | anti-neutrophil cytoplasmic antigen |
| **ARDS** | adult respiratory distress syndrome |
| **ARF** | acute renal failure |
| **5-ASA** | 5-acetylsalicylic acid |
| **AST** | aspartate aminotransferase |
| **ATN** | acute tubular necrosis |
| **AV** | atrioventricular |
| **BCC** | basal cell carcinoma |
| **BMI** | body mass index |
| **cANCA** | cytoplasmic anti-neutrophil cytoplasmic antigen |
| **CEA** | carcinoembryonic antigen |
| **CFA** | cryptogenic fibrosing alveolitis |
| **CIDP** | chronic inflammatory demyelinating polyneuropathy |
| **CKD** | chronic kidney disease |
| **CMV** | cytomegalovirus |
| **CNS** | central nervous system |
| **CO** | carbon monoxide |
| **COPD** | chronic obstructive pulmonary disease |

| | |
|---|---|
| **CPAP** | continuous positive airway pressure |
| **CPK** | creatine phosphokinase |
| **CPR** | cardiopulmonary resuscitation |
| **CRH** | corticotrophin-releasing hormone |
| **CRP** | C-reactive protein |
| **CSF** | cerebrospinal fluid |
| **CT** | computed tomography |
| **CTPA** | computed tomography pulmonary angiogram |
| **CVP** | central venous pressure |
| **CVVH** | continuous veno-venous haemofiltration |
| **DC** | direct current |
| **DEXA** | dual-energy X-ray absorptiometry |
| **DIC** | disseminated intravascular coagulation |
| **DKA** | diabetic ketoacidosis |
| **DMARD** | disease-modifying anti-rheumatoid drug |
| **DOT** | directly observed therapy |
| **dsDNA** | double-stranded DNA |
| **DVLA** | Driver and Vehicle Licensing Agency |
| **DVT** | deep vein thrombosis |
| **EAA** | extrinsic allergic alveolitis |
| **ECG** | electrocardiogram |
| **eGFR** | estimated glomerular filtration rate |
| **EGFR** | epidermal growth factor receptor |
| **EL** | encephalitis lethargica |
| **ENA** | extractable nuclear antigen |
| **ENT** | ear, nose and throat |
| **ERCP** | endoscopic retrograde cholangiopancreatography |
| **ESR** | erythrocyte sedimentation rate |
| **ESRF** | end-stage renal failure |
| **FBC** | full blood count |
| **FEV$_1$** | forced expiratory volume in 1 s |
| **FSGS** | focal segmental glomerulosclerosis |
| **FSH** | follicle-stimulating hormone |
| **FT4** | free thyroxine |
| **5FU** | 5-fluorouracil |

| | |
|---|---|
| **FVC** | forced vital capacity |
| **GAD** | glutamate decarboxylase |
| **GBM** | glomerular basement membrane |
| **GCS** | Glasgow coma score |
| **G-CSF** | granulocyte colony-stimulating factor |
| **GH** | growth hormone |
| **GI** | gastrointestinal |
| **GLP-1** | glucagon-like peptide 1 |
| **GP** | general practitioner |
| **GTN** | glyceryl trinitrate |
| **Hb** | haemoglobin |
| **HbA1c** | glycated haemoglobin |
| **HBGM** | home blood glucose monitoring |
| **HbS** | haemoglobin S |
| **HIV** | human immunodeficiency virus |
| **HLA** | human leucocyte antigen |
| **HONK** | hyperosmolar non-ketotic pre-coma or coma |
| **HPLC** | high-performance liquid chromatography |
| **HRT** | hormone replacement therapy |
| **IBD** | inflammatory bowel disease |
| **IBS** | irritable bowel syndrome |
| **ICD** | implantable cardioverter defibrillation |
| **IFG** | impaired fasting glycaemia |
| **IgA** | immunoglobulin A |
| **IgE** | immunoglobulin E |
| **IGF-I** | insulin-like growth factor I |
| **IGT** | impaired glucose tolerance |
| **IHD** | ischaemic heart disease |
| **IUCD** | intrauterine contraceptive device |
| **IV** | intravenous |
| **IVIG** | intravenous immunoglobulin |
| **JVP** | jugular venous pressure |
| **LDH** | lactate dehydrogenase |
| **LDL** | low-density lipoprotein |
| **LEMS** | Lambert–Eaton myasthenic syndrome |

| | |
|---|---|
| **LFTs** | liver function tests |
| **LGV** | large goods vehicle |
| **LH** | luteinizing hormone |
| **LHRH** | luteinizing hormone-releasing hormone |
| **LMW** | low molecular weight |
| **LV** | left ventricular |
| **LVEF** | left ventricular ejection fraction |
| **MAOI-B** | monoamine oxidase type B |
| **MCH** | mean cell haemoglobin |
| **MCV** | mean cell volume |
| **MEN-1** | multiple endocrine neoplasia type 1 |
| **MI** | myocardial infarction |
| **MMSE** | Mini-Mental State Examination |
| **MND** | motor neuron disease |
| **MRA** | magnetic resonance angiography |
| **MRCP** | magnetic resonance cholangiopancreatography |
| **MRI** | magnetic resonance imaging |
| **MRSA** | methicillin-resistant *Staphylococcus aureus* |
| **MS** | multiple sclerosis |
| **MSH** | melanocyte-stimulating hormone |
| **MSU** | midstream urine specimen |
| **NASH** | non-alcoholic steatohepatitis |
| **NICE** | National Institute of Health and Clinical Excellence |
| **NSAID** | non-steroidal anti-inflammatory drug |
| **NYHA** | New York Heart Association |
| **OGTT** | oral glucose tolerance test |
| **pANCA** | perinuclear anti-neutrophil cytoplasmic antigen |
| **PaO$_2$** | partial pressure of oxygen in arterial blood |
| **PCI** | percutaneous coronary angioplasty |
| **PCV** | passenger-carrying vehicle |
| **PE** | pulmonary embolism |
| **PEF** | peak expiratory flow |
| **PPI** | proton pump inhibitor |
| **PRV** | polycythaemia rubra vera |
| **PSA** | prostate-specific antigen |

| | |
|---|---|
| **PT** | prothrombin time |
| **PTE** | pulmonary thromboembolism |
| **PTH** | parathyroid hormone |
| **PUVA** | psoralen and ultraviolet A |
| **QCT** | qualitative computed tomography |
| **RAS** | renal arterial stenosis |
| **RAST** | radioallergosorbent |
| **RF** | rheumatoid factor |
| **RRT** | renal replacement therapy |
| **rTPA** | recombinant tissue plasminogen activator |
| **RV** | right ventricular |
| **RVH** | right ventricular hypertrophy |
| **SCC** | squamous cell carcinoma |
| **SIADH** | syndrome of inappropriate antidiuretic hormone secretion |
| **SIRS** | systemic inflammatory response syndrome |
| **SLE** | systemic lupus erythematosus |
| **SUDEP** | sudden unexplained death in epilepsy |
| **SVCO** | superior vena cava obstruction |
| **SVT** | supraventricular tachycardia |
| **TB** | tuberculosis |
| **TIA** | transient ischaemic attack |
| **TNF** | tumour necrosis factor |
| **TSH** | thyroid-stimulating hormone |
| **TSS** | toxic shock syndrome |
| **TTP** | thrombotic thrombocytopenic purpura |
| **U&Es** | urea and electrolytes |
| **UKPDS** | UK Prospective Diabetes Study |
| **UTI** | urinary tract infection |
| **VF** | ventricular fibrillation |
| **VT** | ventricular tachycardia |
| **VTE** | venous thromboembolism |
| **WBC** | white blood cell |
| **WCC** | white cell count |
| **WHO** | World Health Organization |

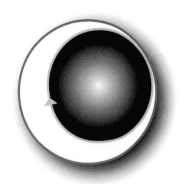

# 1 Diabetes

*Steve Bain*

# DIAGNOSIS

## Questions

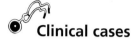
### Clinical cases

## For each of the case scenarios given, consider the following:

> **Q1**: What specific questions would you ask the patient?
> **Q2**: What investigations would you request to confirm a diagnosis?
> **Q3**: What examination would you perform?
> **Q4**: What would be the initial management?
> **Q5**: What are the long-term sequelae?
> **Q6**: What issues need to be addressed apart from blood glucose control?

### CASE 1.1 – A 73-year-old man with glycosuria and a finger-prick glucose of 11.4 mmol/L.

A 73-year-old man is found to have glycosuria on urine testing as part of a new patient assessment. A random finger-prick test by the practice nurse using a modern calibrated glucose meter gives a level of 11.4 mmol/L. Arrangements are made for a repeat blood test after an overnight fast; this plasma glucose level is analysed by the local hospital clinical chemistry department and is reported at 6.7 mmol/L.

### CASE 1.2 – A 57-year-old woman with lethargy and thrush and a fasting plasma glucose of 8.2 mmol/L.

A 57-year-old woman presents to the surgery with lethargy. She has a long history of recurrent episodes of vaginal irritation, which had been formally diagnosed as candidal thrush on one occasion. Treatment with clotrimazole leads to a short amelioration of symptoms. A fasting plasma glucose level has been reported by the laboratory to be 8.2 mmol/L.

### CASE 1.3 – A 21-year-old woman with a random finger-prick glucose of 18.9 mmol/L and urinary ketones.

A 21-year-old woman who has always been fit and well visits you shortly after her honeymoon. She has been profoundly thirsty and noticing blurring of her vision. A finger-prick test in the surgery shows a blood glucose level of 18.9 mmol/L and a fresh urine specimen has both glycosuria and heavy ketones (+++).

## 👥 OSCE counselling cases

## OSCE COUNSELLING CASE 1.1 – 'Will I always have diabetes?'

A 53-year-old man is diagnosed with type 2 diabetes mellitus. He is treated with diet and subsequently oral agents. A couple of years after diagnosis, he begins to take his diet more seriously and takes up regular exercise. He loses weight and his glucose levels fall to such an extent that he is experiencing frequent hypoglycaemia. He is keen to reduce his medication and wants to know if the diabetes is disappearing.

## OSCE COUNSELLING CASE 1.2 – 'Does having diabetes affect my driving licence?'

A 48-year-old man is admitted to hospital with newly diagnosed diabetes. He is discharged on twice-daily insulin and after 6 weeks has established reasonable diabetic control with no hypoglycaemia. He has previously driven heavy goods vehicles and is keen to return to work. He asks your advice about driving.

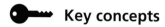

## Key concepts

To work through the core clinical cases in this chapter, you will need to understand the following key concepts.

### DIAGNOSTIC CRITERIA FOR TYPE 2 DIABETES PUBLISHED BY THE WORLD HEALTH ORGANIZATION (WHO) AND RECOMMENDED BY DIABETES UK (2000)

Diagnostic tests should use plasma glucose measurements from a venous sample and performed in an accredited laboratory. Diagnosis should never be made on the basis of glycosuria or stick testing of a finger-prick blood glucose alone (although these may be useful for screening).

If symptoms are present (i.e. polyuria, polydipsia, unexplained weight loss), the diagnosis can be made on the basis of a single:

- random plasma glucose ≥11.1 mmol/L
- fasting plasma glucose ≥7.0 mmol/L.

If symptoms are not present, two abnormal results (as above) on separate days are needed.

A fasting plasma glucose of 6.1–6.9 mmol/L is termed *impaired fasting glycaemia* (IFG) and should be followed up by a formal glucose tolerance test to exclude diabetes.

*Impaired glucose tolerance* (IGT) is defined by a formal glucose tolerance test as a 2-h plasma glucose of 7.8–11.0 mmol/L. This should lead to assessment of vascular risk factors and yearly screening of fasting plasma glucose.

More recently, the WHO (2011) has updated its criteria to include glycated haemoglobin (HbA1c) testing, a value >6.5% being diagnostic of diabetes in the presence of symptoms (two values are required in asymptomatic patients). Although this has been widely welcomed in the UK, there has not been a formal adoption at the time of printing, largely because of the uncertainty surrounding a lower cut-off for the diagnosis of impaired glucose tolerance ('pre-diabetes').

## Answers

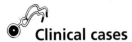
### Clinical cases

### CASE 1.1 – A 73-year-old man with glycosuria and a finger-prick glucose of 11.4 mmol/L.

#### A1: What specific questions would you ask the patient?

The detection of glycosuria has led to two tests to investigate the possibility of diabetes. The random glucose is elevated (≥11.1 mmol/L) but, as a single test, is diagnostic only when it satisfies two criteria: it must be a venous sample (not finger-prick) analysed in an accredited laboratory, and it must be in association with symptoms of hyperglycaemia. The patient should be quizzed about typical symptoms, which will include lethargy, weight changes (gain or loss is possible), polydipsia, polyuria, visual disturbance and infections (e.g. thrush, balanitis, boils). Even in the presence of symptoms, a diagnosis of diabetes would not be made because this has not been confirmed by the fasting plasma glucose, which is <7.0 mmol/L.

#### A2: What investigations would you request to confirm a diagnosis?

This patient has IFG because his fasting plasma glucose is in the range 6.1–6.9 mmol/L. The guidelines suggest that IFG should be followed up by a formal oral glucose tolerance test (OGTT). This may confirm a diagnosis of: IFG, if the 2-h glucose is <7.8 mmol/L; IGT, if the 2-h level is 7.8–11.0 mmol/L; or diabetes, if the 2-h glucose is ≥11.1 mmol/L.

#### A3: What examination would you perform?

Given the provisional diagnosis of IFG, there should be no evidence of diabetes-specific small vessel complications (retinopathy, neuropathy, nephropathy); however, large vessel complications are possible and indeed likely. The cardiovascular system should be examined for evidence of large vessel disease (e.g. carotid auscultation, palpation of peripheral pulses).

#### A4: What would be the initial management?

Assuming that diabetes is not subsequently diagnosed by an OGTT, the patient would receive general health-care advice about diet and exercise. The advice on diet is also appropriate for the treatment of diabetes (i.e. high carbohydrate, high fibre, low saturated fat, low refined carbohydrate), with weight reduction if appropriate. A target body mass index (BMI) of 25 kg/m² is generally quoted. Recommended levels of exercise are regular moderate physical activity for sedentary individuals and 30 min on 5 days a week for people who already take some moderate activity. Patients with IGT would be followed annually by means of a fasting plasma glucose level.

#### A5: What are the long-term sequelae?

Neither IFG nor IGT imparts any risk of specific small vessel complications and glycosuria related to a low renal threshold for glucose is a benign condition. A diagnosis of IGT increases the future risk of type 2 diabetes, however, and is associated with significant cardiovascular risk (in some studies, equivalent to the diagnosis of diabetes itself). It is assumed that IFG carries similar prognoses.

## A6: What issues need to be addressed apart from blood glucose control?

Cardiovascular risk factors need to be addressed, specifically smoking, lipid levels, blood pressure, exercise and obesity. Aspirin is not currently considered appropriate in this scenario.

## CASE 1.2 – **A 57-year-old woman with lethargy and thrush and a fasting plasma glucose of 8.2 mmol/L.**

### A1: What specific questions would you ask the patient?

In this case, the presence of symptoms (lethargy, recurrent thrush) and the elevated fasting plasma glucose (≥7.0 mmol/L) are sufficient to make the diagnosis of diabetes, which, given her age, is almost certain to be type 2. She should be questioned for other symptoms of hyperglycaemia (polyuria, polydipsia, visual disturbance, weight change) and symptoms relating to small vessel disease (tingling, burning of the feet) and large vessel disease (e.g. angina, claudication). A family history should be elicited along with a drug history to exclude the use of diabetogenic drugs (e.g. steroids, beta-blockers, thiazide diuretics).

### A2: What investigations would you request to confirm a diagnosis?

The diagnosis is already confirmed and additional tests are not necessary. Most clinicians would request a measure of long-term glycaemic control (e.g. HbA1c) as a baseline for future comparison.

### A3: What examination would you perform?

The UK Prospective Diabetes Study (UKPDS) showed that 40 per cent of patients with type 2 diabetes have evidence of complications at diagnosis; examination should, therefore, focus on small and large vessel diabetic complications. For small vessel complications, this would involve examination of the ocular fundi through dilated pupils (or arrangement for this to be performed via a formal screening programme), and examination of the feet for evidence of peripheral neuropathy, in addition to their general condition and the presence of pulses. There should also be a thorough examination of the cardiovascular system. The patient should be weighed and a BMI calculated (weight (kg)/[height (m)]²).

### A4: What would be the initial management?

In the UK most patients with type 2 diabetes are given a period of non-pharmacological management. Dietary advice, preferably from a state-registered dietitian, should promote a diet high in complex carbohydrates but low in fat and refined sugars. If the patient is overweight (BMI >27 kg/m²), calorific reduction should also be advised. The benefits of regular exercise should be stressed where appropriate. The patient should be taught how to monitor the impact of these changes by testing their blood (finger-prick testing), although the long-term value of this type of monitoring is uncertain.

These conservative measures are usually continued for at least 3 months, unless the patient becomes more symptomatic, in which case oral medication should be started. Current advice in the United States would lead to the immediate use of metformin alongside these lifestyle modifications.

### A5: What are the long-term sequelae?

The patient is at risk of both small vessel and large vessel disease. Regular screening (at least yearly) should be performed for diabetic retinopathy, diabetic neuropathy and diabetic nephropathy. Blood pressure and lipids should be monitored and treated if necessary.

### A6: What issues need to be addressed apart from blood glucose control?

Other cardiovascular risk factors include the following.
- *Smoking:* advise complete cessation.

- *Lipid levels:* in a patient over 40 years of age with type 2 diabetes, the target lipid levels according to the National Institute of Health and Clinical Excellence (NICE; Clinical Guideline 66, 2008) are total cholesterol <4.0 mmol/L and low-density lipoprotein (LDL) cholesterol <2.0 mmol/L ('<4&2'), with the use of simvastatin recommended as first-line therapy in patients above these targets.
- *Blood pressure:* treat initially with an angiotensin-converting enzyme (ACE) inhibitor or an angiotensin receptor blocker when over 140/80 mmHg.

## CASE 1.3 – **A 21-year-old woman with a random finger-prick glucose of 18.9 mmol/L and urinary ketones (+++).**

### A1: What specific questions would you ask the patient?

In this case, the diagnosis is type 1 (insulin-dependent) diabetes until proved otherwise. This diagnosis is based on the age of the patient and the presence of ketones in the urine. Answers to further questions will probably support this view but should not dissuade you from it. One might expect there to have been a short duration of symptoms (days to weeks), such as profound weight loss, polyuria, nocturia, lethargy and recurrent infection.

In the absence of ketonuria, especially in obese Asian people, there is the possibility of early-onset type 2 diabetes, although this is by no means the 'epidemic' suggested by the medical journals. A strong family history of early-onset type 2 diabetes (affecting siblings, parents and grandparents) may also point to one of the rare autosomal dominant forms of diabetes (maturity-onset diabetes of the young), but again ketonuria effectively excludes this.

### A2: What investigations would you request to confirm a diagnosis?

No laboratory confirmation is necessary. Blood should be taken for a laboratory plasma glucose, but this must not delay initial treatment. A baseline level of glycaemic control would usually be requested (HbA1c) and a screen for associated autoimmune disease (especially thyroid function) may be checked. Autoantibodies (e.g. islet cell, anti-insulin, antibodies to glutamate decarboxylase [GAD]) are negative in 20–30 per cent of newly diagnosed patients and so are of little clinical use (they will also take some time to be reported). Insulin levels, likewise, are of little help and are rarely performed.

### A3: What examination would you perform?

In a typical case of type 1 diabetes, there will be no evidence of diabetic complications at diagnosis because the duration of hyperglycaemia will have been short. Assessment should focus on the conscious level and circulatory state of the patient because she could easily be acidotic, despite the relatively modest level of hyperglycaemia. Near-patient plasma ketone testing is now available and should be performed to exclude diabetic ketoacidosis (DKA) and to inform the patient of this possibility as part of their initial education.

### A4: What would be the initial management?

The patient needs to be treated with insulin and so should be in a setting where the necessary expertise is available (in the UK, typically a hospital). If the patient is fit, insulin can be started without the need for admission. Patients will need to be taught how to monitor blood glucose using finger-prick tests and to understand the concepts of hypo- and hyperglycaemia. They will also need to be shown how to test blood or urine for ketones and understand the significance of these. Dietary advice will be needed and appropriate targets for blood glucose levels agreed. Frequent contact over the early days and weeks after diagnosis will be essential, ideally with an experienced diabetes nurse specialist.

## A5: What are the long-term sequelae?

By virtue of her younger age at onset, this patient is at particular risk of the small vessel complications of diabetes, specifically diabetic retinopathy, diabetic neuropathy and diabetic nephropathy. The minority of patients who go on to develop diabetic nephropathy (which usually manifests clinically after 15–25 years of disease) are prone to premature cardiovascular disease and are more susceptible to the other small vessel complications.

## A6: What issues need to be addressed apart from blood glucose control?

The risks of specific diabetic complications and large vessel disease can be dealt with over the following months and years. Of a higher priority are matters that may have an immediate impact. The first of these is hypoglycaemia, which can occur from the moment that insulin injections are commenced. Patients need to be able to recognize the symptoms of 'hypos' and take appropriate action (see Case 1.15 and OSCE counselling case 1.10). Patients should also be aware that rapid lowering of blood glucose level can induce these symptoms, even when the blood glucose levels are within the 'normal' range. This patient should be given counselling about future pregnancy (exemplary diabetic control is necessary in the periconception period to reduce the risk of fetal abnormality) and driving.

## 👥 OSCE counselling cases

## OSCE COUNSELLING CASE 1.1 – 'Will I always have diabetes?'

The answer is, unfortunately, 'yes'. This is certainly the case as far as medical and insurance matters are concerned. By strict adherence to diet and regular exercise, however, it may be possible to reduce or even eliminate the need for medication. This applies to both oral agents and insulin in patients with type 2 diabetes. In the case presented, medication should be decreased or withheld to reduce the risk of hypoglycaemia.

Glucose levels tend to rise with age, and so patients with type 2 diabetes who control their diabetes with diet alone will ultimately need oral medication (often labelled 'diet failures') and patients on tablets may well need to go on to insulin.

People with type 1 diabetes may go through a period in the weeks to months after diagnosis where insulin can be withheld. This is labelled the 'honeymoon period' and is thought to reflect the removal of the influence of hyperglycaemia, which depresses β-cell function (so-called 'glucose toxicity'). The continued (autoimmune) β-cell destruction ultimately means that insulin will be required.

The prospect for a cure of diabetes is some way off in type 2 diabetes but may be possible for type 1 diabetes. Pancreas transplantation is becoming a feasible option in type 1 diabetes but is typically limited to patients with advanced complications, such as patients who will need to take anti-rejection drugs for a renal transplant or patients with hypoglycaemia unawareness. Recent advances in islet cell transplantation have allowed patients to become independent of insulin for more than 2 years, but long-term independence from insulin is uncommon. Unfortunately, problems surrounding islet availability and preparation mean that this therapy is limited to small numbers of patients.

## OSCE COUNSELLING CASE 1.2 – 'Does having diabetes affect my driving licence?'

The answer in this case is currently 'yes'. The Driver and Vehicle Licensing Agency (DVLA) issues regular guidance on the medical standards of fitness to drive. Licences are split into two groups (groups 1 and 2), with group 2 including heavy goods vehicles, now termed large goods vehicles (LGVs), and passenger-carrying vehicles (PCVs). This patient should be advised to notify the DVLA that he is taking insulin and that, while he does so, he is barred in law from driving LGVs. If the use of insulin is temporary, he may reapply for a licence when he has been transferred to another treatment.

Regarding his group 1 (motor car and motor cycle) licence, he must notify the DVLA but he can retain his licence as long as he can recognize the warning symptoms of hypoglycaemia and is not experiencing disabling hypos. He should also advise his insurance company of his change in health status.

Note that regulations are changing at the time of going to print and readers are advised to avail themselves of the most recent DVLA guidance from its website. These may allow for patients treated with insulin to drive LGVs but with frequent monitoring and regular specialist review.

### Notes about group 1 entitlement (motor cars and motor cycles) in the UK

- Patients with type 2 diabetes managed on diet alone need not notify the DVLA unless they develop relevant complications (e.g. retinopathy affecting visual acuity or visual fields).
- Patients with type 2 diabetes treated with oral hypoglycaemic medication should notify the DVLA but will be allowed to retain their licence until the age of 70 years, unless complications cause disability (such as vision loss).
- Patients on insulin should notify the DVLA and must be able to recognize the warning symptoms of hypoglycaemia. There are the same provisos regarding visual complications. Licences are granted for 1-, 2- or 3-year periods.

# GLUCOSE CONTROL FOR PATIENTS WITH DIABETES MELLITUS

## Questions

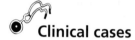

### Clinical cases

## For each of the case scenarios given, consider the following:

**Q1**: What are the treatment options?
**Q2**: What factors influence the choice of therapy?
**Q3**: What would be the preferred choice of treatment?
**Q4**: How would the impact of treatment be assessed?
**Q5**: What are the potential complications?
**Q6**: What issues need to be addressed when the patient has fully recovered?

### CASE 1.4 – **A 72-year-old man with newly diagnosed type 2 diabetes.**

A 72-year-old man has recently been diagnosed with type 2 diabetes. He is mildly symptomatic with lethargy, thirst and polyuria. A random blood glucose level is 13 mmol/L and dipstick urine testing revealed +++ glucose but no ketones. He is known to have hypertension and takes bendroflumethiazide 5 mg once a day. His weight is stable at 94 kg (BMI 32 kg/m²). On examination, there is no evidence of large or small vessel complications.

### CASE 1.5 – **An 84-year-old woman with type 2 diabetes has been treated with gliclazide for 4 years.**

A fit 84-year-old woman with type 2 diabetes had been started on metformin after strict dietary adherence failed to control her symptoms. She now presents with persistently high glucose levels (home blood glucose monitoring [HBGM] 12–15 mmol/L) and has an elevated HbA1c level (9.0%, 73 mmol/mol) despite taking metformin 1 g twice a day. She is symptomatic with lethargy, frequency and dysuria. Random finger-prick glucose is 15 mmol/L and urine dipstick shows ++++ glucose, ++ albumin and + haematuria. Her blood pressure is normal, her weight is 67 kg (BMI 24 kg/m²) and she has no evidence of retinopathy. There is early peripheral neuropathy and foot pulses are absent.

### CASE 1.6 – **A 57-year-old man treated with gliclazide 160 mg twice a day and metformin 500 mg three times a day, who has suboptimal glycaemic control.**

A 57-year-old man with type 2 diabetes is currently treated with gliclazide 160 mg twice a day and metformin 500 mg three times a day, but his glycaemic control is suboptimal. He reports blood glucose levels between 12 mmol/L and 20 mmol/L and has an elevated HbA1c level (11.0%, 97 mmol/mol). He claims good dietary adherence but is overweight (110 kg, BMI 33 kg/m²). He denies any symptoms and has previously refused to consider insulin. He has normal visual acuity but fundal photography shows hard exudates encroaching on the left macula.

## 👥 OSCE counselling cases

OSCE COUNSELLING CASE 1.3 – **'I have been diagnosed as having maturity-onset diabetes. Does this mean that I will never need go on to injections?'**

OSCE COUNSELLING CASE 1.4 – **'I hate doing injections and painful blood tests for my diabetes. Can I try an insulin pump instead?'**

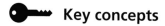 **Key concepts**

To work through the core clinical cases in this chapter, you will need to understand the following key concepts.

## GLUCOSE CONTROL FOR PATIENTS WITH DIABETES MELLITUS

Type 2 diabetes is a condition caused by a combination of resistance to the action of circulating insulin (insulin resistance) and β-cell failure (lack of insulin). The loss of β-cell function is a progressive disorder and is not modified by commonly used hypoglycaemic therapies (although more modern agents may have this benefit). This means that diet and then tablet and injectable therapies will ultimately fail and, if the patient lives for long enough, rising blood glucose levels will eventually require insulin therapy.

In the UK, the usual approach to glycaemic management is to start with modification of diet and exercise, often in the hope of achieving weight reduction (obesity is associated with insulin resistance). Unless the patient is very symptomatic or glucose levels are particularly high, this would be tried for at least 3 months. The target would be a HbA1c level below 7.0%, 53 mmol/mol, although some people would advocate lower levels (e.g. NICE suggests an initial target below 6.5%, 48 mmol/mol). If the target is not achieved, oral medication is added. Metformin is the first-line agent, especially in obese people, because it does not promote weight gain and in monotherapy should not render patients hypoglycaemic. Unfortunately, metformin has significant side effects, including anorexia, nausea, abdominal discomfort, constipation and diarrhoea. These side effects are less pronounced if the dose is increased slowly, so 500 mg once a day is commonly prescribed, building up to 1 g twice a day with meals, with weekly dose increases of 500 mg.

If metformin is ineffective or not tolerated, sulphonylureas are used. Gliclazide is the most commonly prescribed sulphonylurea in the UK, starting at 80 mg once a day with breakfast and increasing to a maximum of 320 mg, usually in two divided doses. More modern preparations of this and other sulphonylureas allow for single daily dosing. As sulphonylureas act by increasing endogenous insulin secretion, they can promote both hypoglycaemia and weight gain as side effects.

In patients who do not achieve target with metformin and a sulphonylurea, triple oral therapy may be initiated. The options include pioglitazone, a thiazolidinedione, which reduces insulin resistance, or a gliptin (e.g. saxagliptin, linagliptin), which enhances insulin secretion in a glucose-dependent way. These third-line agents do not induce hypoglycaemia but their side effects differ. Pioglitazone often induces weight gain and can cause oedema, leading to heart failure. Pioglitazone also increases the risk of bone fracture and may be associated with a small increase in bladder cancer. The gliptins are weight-neutral and have a placebo-like side-effect profile.

Before the initiation of insulin, use of injectable glucagon-like peptide 1 (GLP-1) therapies may be considered. Like the gliptins, these drugs have a glucose-dependent mechanism of action (i.e. they lower glucose only when levels are high) and so do not cause hypoglycaemia. They also induce weight loss in a significant number of patients. Their major side effect is nausea, occasionally with vomiting, but this tends to diminish over time.

There are various ways of starting insulin in type 2 diabetes. Insulin can be added to oral therapy, usually as a single dose of long-acting insulin (either isophane insulin or analogues such as glargine or detemir). This regimen has the advantages of simplicity but is ultimately doomed to fail with patients needing fast-acting insulin to prevent postprandial hyperglycaemia. This can either involve the addition of three pre-meal injections (a standard basal bolus regimen) or a change to two pre-meal injections of premixed insulin. As far as reaching HbA1c targets is concerned (NICE suggests 7.5%, 58 mmol/mol), the twice-daily and add-on regimens are equally (in)effective and one can argue there is less activity going straight to twice-daily insulin when tablets fail. This also has the advantage that patients can stop taking many tablets, although metformin is often continued to try to reduce the weight gain that can be associated with insulin use. Gliptins can be used with insulin but GLP-1 injections are currently unlicensed for this combination, a situation that is likely to change soon.

## Answers

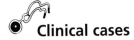

### Clinical cases

## CASE 1.4 – A 72-year-old man with newly diagnosed type 2 diabetes.

### A1: What are the treatment options?

The treatment options are wide and include the following:

- dietary review and manipulation
- exercise
- weight loss (achieved by diet and exercise)
- change of antihypertensive agent
- oral hypoglycaemic agents (metformin).

### A2: What factors influence the choice of therapy?

The choice of therapy is influenced by factors including the level of symptoms, the degree of hyperglycaemia, the patient's weight and the fact that there has been no weight loss, and the patient's age. This patient is said to have type 2 diabetes, and this fits with his age, symptoms, obesity and hypertension. His symptoms are mild, his glucose level is moderately elevated, and there are no ketones in the urine. He currently takes a high-dose thiazide diuretic, which in some cases can cause glucose intolerance, and so the dose should be reduced or the drug should be replaced by an ACE inhibitor.

### A3: What would be the preferred choice of treatment?

A reasonable course of action would be to advise on diet (see answer A4 to Case 1.1), with the aim of reducing daily calorie intake and increasing exercise. The bendroflumethiazide could be stopped and replaced with an ACE inhibitor. Assuming that he does not become more symptomatic, this regimen could be followed for 3 months, at which point oral hypoglycaemic agents may be considered. The first-line agent would be metformin, based on his obesity.

### A4: How would the impact of treatment be assessed?

The patient should be made aware of the symptoms of hyperglycaemia and should make contact if these worsen, especially if weight loss is marked. The technical options to assess the glycaemic response are near-patient (usually self-) testing of blood glucose and laboratory testing (HbA1c levels).

Home blood glucose monitoring is commonly taught to patients in this scenario, but critics argue that it is of little value and is very expensive. Unless a patient or the clinician is going to manipulate therapy based only on the results of HBGM (and this is unlikely to be the case here), one can argue that it should not be routine practice. On the other hand, HBGM will provide immediate feedback to the patient on which aspects of the diet worsen his glucose levels and can be seen to be an essential aspect of patient empowerment. HbA1c levels provide a long-term indication of glycaemic control (typically quoted to be 2–3 months) and, if compared with a baseline value, will give a good indication as to whether conservative measures are being effective. HbA1c also allows for targets to be set, initially aiming for a level below 6.5%, 48 mmol/mol.

Do not forget that a change in blood pressure therapy means that blood pressure monitoring will need to be performed on a monthly basis and, if an ACE inhibitor is used, electrolytes will need to be checked before treatment and after 7–14 days of treatment.

## CASE 1.5 – **An 84-year-old woman with type 2 diabetes has been treated with gliclazide for 4 years.**

### A1: What are the treatment options?

The treatment options include:

- further dietary review and manipulation
- add another oral hypoglycaemic agent (sulphonylurea, pioglitazone, gliptin)
- add insulin
- exclude urinary tract infection (UTI) or treat if this is confirmed.

### A2: What factors influence the choice of therapy?

The choice of therapy is influenced by the natural history of the patient's condition, her weight, her current therapy and her age. Type 2 diabetes is a progressive disease and so failure of diet and then oral monotherapy to control her symptoms should be anticipated (and not attributed to failure on the part of the patient). Although a dietary assessment is reasonable (and should be performed as part of the annual diabetes review), she has previously been strict and is not currently overweight. In this setting, it is unlikely that dietary change will make a significant impact. Her current dose of metformin is not at the maximum recommended; however, the dose–response curve tends to be flattened at higher doses (and a further increase is likely to induce side effects), and so additional therapy would be instituted. UK guidelines suggest a sulphonylurea as second-line, but many clinicians prefer to add a gliptin, as the combination with metformin will not put the patient at risk of hypoglycaemia. Given her age, tight glycaemic control is not a priority and symptomatic relief with low risk of hypoglycaemia is the main aim of therapy. Note that the possibility of diabetic foot complications does not influence the treatment choices.

Although hyperglycaemia causes lethargy and frequency, dysuria with proteinuria and haematuria on dipstick testing suggest the possibility of a UTI (common in hyperglycaemia and a cause of worsened diabetic control). If UTI is confirmed by urine culture, a course of antibiotics would be indicated.

### A3: What would be the preferred choice of treatment?

Add a second oral agent to the patient's current dose of metformin. Options include a gliptin, pioglitazone and a sulphonylurea. The reduction achieved with any of these therapies is likely to be the same; side effects, especially the risk of hypoglycaemia, are the major reason for opting for a gliptin rather than a sulphonylurea. If the patient remains symptomatic and her HbA1c remains very high, then insulin (in combination with metformin) may have to be considered, but again this would increase the risk of hypoglycaemia.

### A4: How would the impact of treatment be assessed?

Given that the patient is already performing HBGM, it is not unreasonable for her to continue this practice. Fasting, pre-meal and pre-bed glucose testing is the norm, with targets below 10 mmol/L without hypoglycaemia being reasonable in this case. HbA1c testing could also be performed for comparison with the pretreatment level. Symptomatic improvement is the main aim of therapy, and the HbA1c target needs to be individualized since the benefits of tight control in this age group are unproven and the side effects of treatment (especially hypoglycaemia) are dangerous.

## CASE 1.6 – **A 57-year-old man treated with gliclazide 160 mg twice a day and metformin 500 mg three times a day, who has suboptimal glycaemic control.**

### A1: What are the treatment options?

The treatment options include:

- further dietary review and manipulation
- increasing the dose of metformin
- adding another oral hypoglycaemic agent (pioglitazone or a gliptin)
- add a GLP-1 injectable therapy
- add insulin.

### A2: What factors influence the choice of therapy?

The choice of therapy is influenced by the natural history of the condition, the patient's current therapy, age and weight, and the presence of retinopathy. The progressive nature of type 2 diabetes is such that almost all patients will end up on insulin if they survive for long enough. Although he is not on maximal doses of metformin, further increases are unlikely to achieve glycaemic targets. Addition of pioglitazone or a gliptin (triple therapy) is an alternative but is often a disappointing combination in this type of scenario. Use of a GLP-1 injectable therapy would now be a popular option in the UK, although current NICE guidelines suggest that this should be offered to patients only where the BMI is over 35 kg/m². Insulin thus becomes a leading option, especially given the patient's young age and the development of diabetic retinopathy. Clearly the patient is not keen to go on insulin and the reasons for this need to be explored, because many patients are pleasantly surprised at how painless insulin injections are (compared with HBGM) and feel much better when their glycaemic control improves. A dietary assessment is reasonable because weight gain is highly likely with insulin; for this reason, metformin should be continued (while the sulphonylurea may be withheld).

### A3: What would be the preferred choice of treatment?

Suggest to the patient that he tries insulin for a period. This will allow him to see how simple the procedure can be and if, like many patients, he feels better on insulin, he may well wish to stay on it. Twice-daily insulin using fixed mixtures before breakfast and evening meal is a simple regimen that may seem less daunting than basal bolus (where the patient injects fast-acting insulin before each meal and a night-time injection of long-acting insulin). Given the risk of weight gain, the patient should continue on metformin but can cease taking his sulphonylurea.

If a GLP-1 receptor agonist is preferred by the patient (many people hate the idea of insulin, not because of the injections but due to a bad family experience or to fears of hypoglycaemia), then the current options are exenatide or liraglutide. Exenatide can be prescribed as a twice-daily or once-weekly preparation, and liraglutide is given once a day. Both can cause nausea and vomiting. UK guidelines suggest their impact on glycaemic control and weight should be assessed after 6 months, with treatment failure (HbA1c reduction of less than 1% and weight loss of less than 3%) leading to drug withdrawal.

### A4: How would the impact of treatment be assessed?

Symptomatic improvement (he may recognize and admit to symptoms in retrospect, especially lethargy) and HBGM will provide feedback on the patient's progress. He should also monitor his weight. HbA1c will be the ultimate assessment with a lower target (7.0–7.5%, 53–58 mmol/mol) given his young age.

**OSCE counselling cases**

## OSCE COUNSELLING CASE 1.3 – 'I have been diagnosed as having maturity-onset diabetes. Does this mean that I will never need go on to injections?'

The short answer is 'no'. Maturity-onset diabetes is the old term for non-insulin-dependent diabetes, now called type 2 diabetes mellitus. The natural history of this condition has been convincingly demonstrated and is one of progressive deterioration in blood glucose control. This is felt to reflect progressive loss of β-cell function over time. Insulin resistance, the other contributing metabolic abnormality, appears to deteriorate before the diagnosis of type 2 diabetes but then remains relatively fixed.

As a result of β-cell failure, dietary change is likely to have a limited and temporary impact, leading to the introduction of oral hypoglycaemic agents and GLP-1 receptor agonists. Ultimately these agents will fail and the patient may need insulin to achieve reasonable glycaemic control. One can argue that if an individual with type 2 diabetes lives for long enough, then insulin is inevitable. This can be used as a justification for early exposure to the use of insulin (handling injection devices, experiencing the injection) so that, when insulin is needed, it is not delayed by unjustified anxieties.

The exception to this rule of progressive glycaemic deterioration may be patients who are obese at diagnosis and manage to lose vast amounts of weight, thereby restoring insulin sensitivity. There are also preliminary data that gliptins and GLP-1 agents can slow the progression of β-cell dysfunction, but these data need to be confirmed.

### Learning points

- Type 2 diabetes is the modern name for maturity-onset (non-insulin-dependent) diabetes.
- The natural history of this condition is for blood glucose control to deteriorate over time as a result of β-cell failure.
- If survival is prolonged, insulin treatment will be needed in most cases of type 2 diabetes.
- It is the treatment, not the patient, that fails; this should be expected and anticipated. Patients can be introduced to the concept of insulin at an early stage and should not be 'threatened' with its introduction.

## OSCE COUNSELLING CASE 1.4 – 'I hate doing injections and painful blood tests for my diabetes. Can I try an insulin pump instead?'

Insulin pumps (also known as continuous subcutaneous insulin infusions, CSII) are available in the UK but this is not a good reason for using one because the amount of finger-prick testing is typically increased.

The use of an insulin pump involves the insertion of a cannula into the subcutaneous tissue, through which small amounts of insulin are continuously delivered. In addition, bolus doses can be administered by the same equipment, to coincide with meals. The pump is a small device and can easily be carried in a belt or holster.

NICE has advised that pump therapy can be made available to people with type 1 diabetes where multiple insulin dose therapy has failed to achieve good glycaemic control. Type 2 diabetes is not currently regarded as an indication for pump use. Patients should be able to maintain 'a high order of personal hygiene' (to avoid catheter site infection) and test finger-prick blood glucose four times a day. In addition, patients should be capable of estimating carbohydrate and calorie consumption, programming the pump and changing the cannula site every 2–3 days.

## Learning points

- Insulin pumps are available for therapy of type 1 diabetes in the UK.
- Insulin pumps are indicated where control remains poor despite multiple insulin injection regimens.
- Patients need to be motivated and technically competent.

# DIABETIC SMALL VESSEL COMPLICATIONS

## Questions

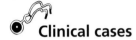
### Clinical cases

### For each of the case scenarios given, consider the following:

> **Q1**: What questions would you ask the patient and why?
> **Q2**: What investigations would you request?
> **Q3**: What examination would you perform?
> **Q4**: What are the differential diagnoses related to diabetes?
> **Q5**: What are the potential complications?
> **Q6**: What issues need to be addressed when the patient has fully recovered?

### CASE 1.7 – A 75-year-old man with long-standing type 2 diabetes complains of difficulty in seeing television programmes.

A 75-year-old man with diabetes of 15 years' standing complains of difficulty in seeing programmes on the television. There has been no pain or redness affecting his eyes and he has not had headaches. His diabetic control is poor but stable.

### CASE 1.8 – A 31-year-old man with type 1 diabetes has albuminuria on urine dipstick testing.

A 31-year-old man with type 1 diabetes has joined your practice. He was diagnosed at age 12 years. Having attended the clinic regularly as a child, he defaulted from the adult clinic, attending only when he needed replacement equipment (e.g. injection devices). He takes no other medication and has had no treatment for complications. Blood pressure is 160/80 mmHg. Dipstick urine testing shows +++ glucose, ++ albumin and + blood, but no ketones. Visual acuity is 6/6 in both eyes.

### CASE 1.9 – A 56-year-old man with newly diagnosed type 2 diabetes complains of pins and needles in his feet.

A 56-year-old man is diagnosed with type 2 diabetes by his local optometrist. He attends your practice and during diabetic review complains of 'pins and needles' affecting both of his feet and his right hand. The symptoms are worse at night when he is in bed. Discomfort in his hand often disturbs his sleep. There is no discomfort in his feet during the day and his exercise tolerance has been unaffected.

## 👫 OSCE counselling cases

OSCE COUNSELLING CASE 1.5 – **'Do all people with diabetes end up on kidney dialysis treatment?'**

OSCE COUNSELLING CASE 1.6 – **'My friend has diabetes and she says that all people with diabetes should go to a chiropodist. Is this true?'**

**Key concepts**

To work through the core clinical cases in this chapter, you will need to understand the following key concepts.

Long-term complications of diabetes are traditionally divided into diabetes-specific small vessel complications (meaning that only patients with diabetes are at risk) and diabetes-non-specific large vessel complications (increased risk in diabetes but not limited to patients with diabetes). The small vessel complications are:

- *eye disease:* diabetic retinopathy – the most common cause of blindness in the working population of the UK
- *nerve disease:* diabetic neuropathy – usually a progressive peripheral neuropathy that presents with tingling and burning affecting the feet and progresses to complete sensory loss
- *kidney disease:* diabetic nephropathy – the most common cause of end-stage renal failure in western countries.

There is crossover between the small and large vessel complications – e.g. patients with diabetic nephropathy have a greatly increased risk of ischaemic heart disease, and most will succumb to this rather than end-stage renal failure.

The diabetes annual review aims to detect diabetes complications at an early stage and institute therapy before there has been irreversible damage (e.g. laser treatment for retinopathy to prevent loss of visual acuity).

# Answers

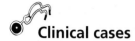 **Clinical cases**

## CASE 1.7 – A 75-year-old man with long-standing type 2 diabetes complains of difficulty in seeing television programmes.

### A1: What questions would you ask the patient and why?

Symptoms of cataract progression include halos around bright lights, such as car headlights. The symptoms are usually slow in progression but patients may report abrupt changes. Maculopathy may give either a slow or a sudden loss of vision in one eye, whereas a bleed related to proliferative diabetic retinopathy classically causes sudden painless visual loss in one eye. Note that patients may be unaware of the extent of loss of vision if the good eye compensates. Changes in vision related to poor glycaemic control (usually enhanced long vision and difficulty reading) may affect both eyes and can be variable over short periods. During periods of poor glycaemic control (e.g. at diagnosis), patients should be advised against changing their lens prescription.

### A2: What investigations would you request?

In the vast majority of cases, the history and examination will be sufficient.

### A3: What examination would you perform?

Visual acuity should be tested, with correction with spectacles if the patient normally uses these for distance vision. Pinhole correction should be performed if the visual acuity is 6/9 or less. Examination of the fundi through dilated pupils (1% tropicamide) is mandatory. This will allow detection of a cataract by examination of the red reflex and also detection of retinal abnormalities by direct visualization, including those concerning diabetes and related medical disorders. Ideally, binocular stereomicroscopy should be performed (usually in the setting of an ophthalmic clinic), which facilitates the detection of macular oedema. Digital images may also be requested.

### A4: What are the differential diagnoses related to diabetes?

The major possibilities related to the patient's diabetes are:

- cataract
- diabetic retinopathy (more likely maculopathy than proliferative diabetic retinopathy)
- change in blood glucose levels leading to alteration in lens shape
- related retinal disorders such as central retinal vein or artery occlusion.

## CASE 1.8 – A 31-year-old man with type 1 diabetes has albuminuria on urine dipstick testing.

### A1: What questions would you ask the patient and why?

He should be asked about symptoms of UTI (e.g. frequency, dysuria, nocturia, haematuria). Although his attendance at clinic has been sporadic, he should have had urine testing previously, so he should be quizzed as to whether he had been told about urinary abnormalities (especially albuminuria) before. Previous blood pressure assessments would also be of value because this one-off reading may reflect anxiety-induced ('white-coat') hypertension. A family history of hypertension and ischaemic heart disease are also more common in patients at risk of diabetic nephropathy.

## A2: What investigations would you request?

A midstream urine specimen should be sent for culture to exclude a UTI. If UTI is excluded, formal assessment of the albumin excretion is needed; this can be by one of the following, depending on the patient's expected compliance: 24-h urine collection for albumin; timed overnight urine collection for albumin excretion rate; first voided urine for albumin/creatinine ratio. Blood should be sent for HbA1c to assess glycaemic control, lipids should be checked (total and high-density lipoprotein [HDL]-cholesterol), and creatinine should be checked to estimate the glomerular filtration rate (eGFR). Haematuria is not typical of diabetic nephropathy and so renal ultrasonography should be arranged to exclude other causes (rare in this setting).

## A3: What examination would you perform?

People with type 1 diabetes and diabetic nephropathy are at high risk of other complications. The feet should be examined for evidence of peripheral neuropathy and reduced circulation. Coexisting diabetic retinopathy is almost inevitable and so arrangements for dilated fundoscopy should be made. Blood pressure should be repeated after a period of rest and then follow-up arrangements for more blood pressure checks over the next 2–3 months to establish whether there is a persistent elevation. If diabetic nephropathy is confirmed, a target systolic pressure of 130 mmHg is recommended.

## A4: What are the differential diagnoses related to diabetes?

The following major possibilities are related to the patient's diabetes.

- Diabetic nephropathy: the duration of disease (19 years) is typical, and it is likely that his control has been poor, given the poor clinic attendance. In addition to the albuminuria, he has a raised blood pressure, which is part of the syndrome.
- UTI (in view of the + blood).

## CASE 1.9 – **A 56-year-old man with newly diagnosed type 2 diabetes complains of pins and needles in his feet.**

### A1: What questions would you ask the patient and why?

Peripheral neuropathy symptoms (to which burning dysaesthesiae may be added) are of gradual onset, typically worse at rest and in bed, when bedclothes can be particularly irritating. Autonomic neuropathy (rare) may also be present, with symptoms including gustatory sweating (facial sweating after meals) and postural hypotension.

Carpal tunnel syndrome is common at night, patients often being awoken with discomfort and typically shaking the hand to relieve symptoms. Excessive use of the hands (e.g. in painting) may also induce symptoms. It may be associated with loss or change of sensation in the hand, and symptoms may be referred to the whole forearm. Again, gradual onset of symptoms would be expected and the other hand may also be affected.

Given the association of carpal tunnel syndrome with myxoedema, acromegaly, rheumatoid arthritis and osteoarthritis, symptoms of these conditions may be elicited.

### A2: What investigations would you request?

Nerve conduction studies will confirm a diagnosis of both peripheral diabetic neuropathy and carpal tunnel syndrome. They are most useful in the latter, where surgical intervention can be considered when entrapment is confirmed. Bloods to exclude hypothyroidism and vitamin B12 deficiency (more common with metformin treatment) should also be requested.

## A3: What examination would you perform?

Examination of the feet for abnormal sensation using monofilaments and vibration sensation as screening tools can be done. Ulceration (painless) should be excluded and skin care assessed. Peripheral pulses should be examined, which may be enhanced ('bounding') in the neuropathic foot.

In carpal tunnel syndrome there may be sensory loss over the palmar aspects of the first three and a half fingers and wasting of the thenar eminence. In advanced cases, there can be weakness of abduction, flexion and apposition of the thumb. Symptoms can be worsened by various manoeuvres such as percussion of the carpal tunnel (Tinel's sign), flexion of the wrist (Phalen's sign) and hyperextension of the wrist.

Given the association of carpal tunnel syndrome with myxoedema, acromegaly, rheumatoid arthritis and osteoarthritis, signs of these conditions may be looked for.

## A4: What are the differential diagnoses related to diabetes?

The major possibilities related to the patient's diabetes are:

- peripheral diabetic neuropathy affecting the feet and possibly the right hand – although diagnosed only recently, the patient has clearly had diabetes for some time to manifest retinal changes. Hence other long-term complications of diabetes may also be present
- carpal tunnel syndrome affecting the right hand
- mononeuropathy affecting the right hand
- vascular insufficiency is an *unlikely* cause of symptoms given the absence of claudication.

**OSCE counselling cases**

### OSCE COUNSELLING CASE 1.5 – 'Do all people with diabetes end up on kidney dialysis treatment?'

No. There may appear to be a paradox in that diabetes is now the most common cause of end-stage renal failure in the western world and renal dialysis as a result of diabetes is becoming more frequent. This relates, however, to the massive increase in the number of people diagnosed with type 2 diabetes, and the vast majority will never need dialysis treatment.

Taking the example of type 1 diabetes, studies from the 1960s and 1970s show that only a minority (at most, 40 per cent) of patients will develop diabetic nephropathy, irrespective of their glycaemic control. This is likely to represent a genetic predisposition to diabetic nephropathy, which means that most patients are protected from this complication (contrast with diabetic retinopathy, where all patients continue to be at risk). Continued improvements in blood pressure, lipids and glucose control will inevitably reduce this proportion.

In type 2 diabetes, the major risk associated with abnormal albumin excretion is cardiovascular disease, which tends to cause premature death long before renal dialysis becomes a possibility.

### Learning points

- Diabetes is the most common cause of end-stage renal disease in the western world.
- The number of people with diabetes going on to renal dialysis programmes is likely to increase as a result of the rise in prevalence of diabetes.
- Susceptibility to diabetic nephropathy is partly genetically determined, with most patients protected from this complication.
- With advances in blood pressure, lipid and glucose management, the proportion of people with diabetes, especially type 1, needing renal replacement therapy is likely to fall.
- Diabetic nephropathy greatly increases the risk of other diabetic complications, including premature coronary heart disease.

### OSCE COUNSELLING CASE 1.6 – 'My friend has diabetes and she says that all people with diabetes should go to a chiropodist. Is this true?'

No. The level of resource directed towards diabetic foot care should be dictated by the individual needs. This has led to a risk categorization with varying levels of input.

*Normal feet (low risk)* – all newly diagnosed patients should receive basic foot health advice and subsequently be reviewed on an annual basis. This assessment can be carried out by a doctor, diabetes nurse specialist or practice nurse (with the appropriate level of training). If at any stage the patient is found to be 'at risk' or to have active foot disease, then referral should be made as follows.

- *At risk:* patients with reduced sensation or reduced pedal pulses or unable to perform nail chiropody (or have it provided by a responsible carer) should be seen every 3–6 months for review by a chiropodist. Foot care advice should be given and the need for vascular assessment reviewed.
- *High risk:* patients with a risk factor for foot disease and either foot deformity or a previous ulcer should be seen every 1–3 months by a senior podiatrist. Specialist foot care treatment and advice should be given, as per the published guidelines. There should be easy access to a shoe-fitter, surgical appliances and, where necessary, a limb-fitting centre.
- *Active foot disease:* patients with active ulceration, cellulitis, osteomyelitis, a Charcot joint or foot discoloration should be seen urgently in a multidisciplinary diabetic foot clinic.

## Learning points

- All people with diabetes need foot assessment and advice at diagnosis and at least yearly thereafter.
- This can be performed by different health-care professionals, so long as they have been adequately trained.
- The intensity of clinical input depends on the risk categorization of each individual case.

# DIABETIC LARGE VESSEL COMPLICATIONS

## Questions

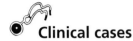
### Clinical cases

### For each of the case scenarios given, consider the following:

> **Q1**: Are further assessments required before the italicized finding provokes a drug intervention?
>
> **Q2**: If drug therapy were indicated, which would be the most appropriate choice of agent?
>
> **Q3**: What sort of follow-up is indicated?
>
> **Q4**: What other issues need to be addressed with regard to cardiovascular risk?
>
> **Q5**: What are the potential complications?
>
> **Q6**: What issues need to be addressed when the patient has fully recovered?

### CASE 1.10 – **A 68-year-old man with type 2 diabetes and *a total cholesterol of 5.6 mmol/L*.**

A 68-year-old man with type 2 diabetes has a new person check in primary care. He has no significant medical history apart from diabetes and he does not smoke. His BMI is 32 kg/m² and he has no evidence of diabetic retinopathy or foot complications. His blood pressure is 170/96 mmHg and urinalysis shows glycosuria ++ but no protein. A random total cholesterol is 5.6 mmol/L and triglycerides 2.3 mmol/L. He takes metformin 1 g twice a day and has an HbA1c level of 7.5%, 58 mmol/mol.

### CASE 1.11 – **A 76-year-old woman with type 2 diabetes and *a stable blood pressure of 166/70 mmHg*.**

A 76-year-old woman with type 2 diabetes is under regular review. She has a history of angina, which is well controlled, and does not smoke. Her BMI is 28 kg/m² and she has background diabetic retinopathy and absent foot pulses. Her blood pressure is 166/70 mmHg and urinalysis shows persistent + albuminuria in the absence of infection. Blood pressure recordings over the previous 6 months have shown similar levels. She takes gliclazide 80 mg twice a day, and isosorbide mononitrate 60 mg, simvastatin 10 mg and aspirin 75 mg once a day. A random total cholesterol is 4.8 mmol/L, triglycerides 2.3 mmol/L and HbA1c 7.8%, 62 mmol/mol.

### CASE 1.12 – **A 21-year-old woman with type 1 diabetes and *microalbuminuria (urinary albumin/creatinine ratio 3.7)*.**

A 21-year-old woman with type 1 diabetes of 15 years' standing has an annual review of her diabetes. She injects insulin using a basal bolus regimen and does not smoke. Her BMI is 22 kg/m², her blood pressure is 120/60 mmHg and she has good pedal pulses. She has minimal background diabetic retinopathy and slightly diminished sensation in her feet. Random total cholesterol is 5.7 mmol/L, triglycerides 1.1 mmol/L and HbA1c 6.5%, 48 mmol/mol. Analysis of a random urine shows an albumin/creatinine ratio of 2.7, which is reported as 'microalbuminuria'. Previously, urinalysis had been negative for dipstick proteinuria.

## 👥 OSCE counselling cases

OSCE COUNSELLING CASE 1.7 – **'As someone with diabetes, should I be taking aspirin?'**

OSCE COUNSELLING CASE 1.8 – **'Why is my blood pressure so difficult to control?'**

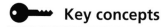 **Key concepts**

To work through the core clinical cases in this chapter, you will need to understand the following key concepts.

People with diabetes get the same large vessel disease as people who do not have diabetes, but they get it earlier and it is more widespread.

- *Cardiovascular disease:* 75 per cent of people with type 2 diabetes will die as a result of ischaemic heart disease. Some studies suggest that IGT carries a similar cardiovascular prognosis to overt type 2 diabetes. This implies that glucose control is not the dominant issue and is consistent with the limited impact of glycaemic control in many studies. This is in stark contrast to the major impact of blood pressure and lipid control on cardiovascular outcomes in patients with type 2 diabetes.
- *Peripheral vascular disease:* diabetes is the most common cause of non-traumatic lower limb amputation in the UK.
- *Cerebrovascular disease:* stroke is two to four times more common in diabetic cohorts.

There is a focus on coronary heart disease prevention (both primary and secondary) in diabetes management, with attention to lipids, blood pressure control (and, to a lesser extent, aspirin) and a sound evidence base. Microalbuminuria screening is also recommended in this context (as a marker of early vascular disease), but the rationale for this is less convincing.

# Answers

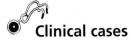

## Clinical cases

### CASE 1.10 – **A 68-year-old man with type 2 diabetes and a** *total cholesterol of 5.6 mmol/L.*

**A1:** Are further assessments required before the italicized finding provokes a drug intervention?

The total cholesterol warrants consideration in terms of primary prevention of cardiovascular disease. Issues include whether fasting lipids are required, the potential impact of diet, and what level of cholesterol justifies drug treatment.

Total cholesterol is not altered by recent food intake (unlike triglycerides), and so a fasting sample is not mandatory. Most clinicians would, however, repeat the lipids to include an HDL-cholesterol, allowing for calculation of the LDL-cholesterol. This allows for assessment of the patient's 10-year coronary heart disease risk using the Framingham or similar calculation. For most patients, diet has little impact on total cholesterol levels; this is borne out by the large statin trials, which show a reduction of only 2–4 per cent in diet-treated patients.

The generally quoted targets for lipids in patients with type 2 diabetes are total cholesterol <4.0 mmol/L and LDL-cholesterol <2.0 mmol/L.

**A2:** If drug therapy were indicated, which would be the most appropriate choice of agent?

Simvastatin should be prescribed, aiming for a daily dose of 40 mg. If the lipid targets are not achieved with this dose, then a more potent statin should be introduced and consideration given to the co-prescription of ezetimibe (although the evidence base supporting this agent is much less). There is currently no evidence that fibrates produce cardiovascular benefits in patients with diabetes.

**A3:** What sort of follow-up is indicated?

Liver function tests (LFTs) and creatine kinase should be checked before initiation of statin treatment but probably do not need to be checked again. At the same time, thyroid function tests could be requested to exclude underlying hypothyroidism, which can raise cholesterol levels. Patients should be aware of the risk of muscle pains, which are rarely the result of myositis; creatine kinase should be checked if the patient experiences this symptom. Lipids should be repeated after 3 months of treatment and, if targets have been hit, checked on a yearly basis thereafter.

**A4:** What other issues need to be addressed with regard to cardiovascular risk?

One needs to give consideration to glycaemic control, smoking, BMI, blood pressure and drug therapy, although not necessarily in that order. The evidence that improving blood glucose control and reducing weight would have a major impact on coronary heart disease risk in this case is weak. In contrast, blood pressure control is crucial; however, one needs to know that the reading taken on this visit is representative and not anxiety induced (so-called 'white coat hypertension'). An electrocardiogram (ECG) may be helpful because evidence of left ventricular hypertrophy would imply long-standing hypertension; however, if this were normal, then repeated blood pressure checks should be arranged. A minimum of three recordings over a 3-month period would be appropriate, with consideration of drug therapy if the level remains above 140/80 mmHg. Aspirin is not currently recommended at this stage.

## CASE 1.11 – **A 76-year-old woman with type 2 diabetes and a stable blood pressure of 166/70 mmHg.**

### A1:  Are further assessments required before the italicized finding provokes a drug intervention?

This patient with diabetes, ischaemic heart disease and peripheral vascular disease has isolated systolic hypertension confirmed by multiple assessments over time. The literature strongly supports reduction of her systolic pressure using drugs to a target of less than 130 mmHg. Further attention to weight, exercise and glycaemic control would be beneficial, but these will have minimal impact on her blood pressure. Apart from baseline urea and electrolytes (U&Es), no further investigations are required at this point.

### A2:  If drug therapy were indicated, which would be the most appropriate choice of agent?

The first-line antihypertensive agent in a person with diabetes and proteinuria should be an inhibitor of the renin–angiotensin system. This would typically be an ACE inhibitor, with consideration of an angiotensin II receptor blocker if side effects (most often cough) are experienced. In either case, check that U&Es have been performed before initiation and 7–10 days thereafter. For a substantial proportion of people with diabetes, monotherapy is not sufficient to achieve blood pressure targets, and additional classes of blood pressure medication will be needed. A typical second-line agent in this case would be a calcium channel blocker or a low-dose diuretic.

### A3:  What sort of follow-up is indicated?

The effect of drug therapy may take 2 months to become apparent. An interim target blood pressure of 160 mmHg is appropriate; if the patient feels well having achieved this, further increases in medication should be made, aiming for systolic blood pressure below 130 mmHg. Once stabilized, blood pressure can be checked every 3–6 months. Patients on ACE inhibitors and angiotensin II receptor blocker should have renal function and electrolytes checked at regular intervals (every 6 months) because renal function can deteriorate at any time. Additional tests are required if the dose of ACE inhibitor or angiotensin II receptor blocker is increased, additional medication is added, or there is intercurrent illness.

### A4:  What other issues need to be addressed with regard to cardiovascular risk?

Attention to glycaemic control, weight and exercise is justified but unlikely to have a significant impact on the risk of coronary heart disease. The patient's other medications should be reviewed: the simvastatin dose should be increased to 40 mg once a day (the dose on which most of the evidence for this agent is based), and the dose of aspirin should be increased to 150 mg once a day, given her known ischaemic heart disease (i.e. secondary prevention).

## CASE 1.12 – **A 21-year-old woman with type 1 diabetes and microalbuminuria (urinary albumin/creatinine ratio 3.7).**

### A1:  Are further assessments required before the italicized finding provokes a drug intervention?

Screening for microalbuminuria in patients with type 1 diabetes is part of the diabetes annual review. It aims to detect the early stage of diabetic nephropathy before the onset of dipstick-positive proteinuria (so-called macroalbuminuria). Diabetic nephropathy is a clinical syndrome of persistent proteinuria, hypertension and declining renal function. Patients with this complication have increased premature morbidity and mortality as a result of end-stage renal failure, cardiovascular disease and other diabetes complications, which cluster in this cohort. In well-controlled patients, the discovery of microalbuminuria after 15 years of diabetes would be typical of the natural history of this complication.

The issue surrounds the validity of this screening result. Urinary albumin excretion rates are highly variable, being affected by infection, posture and exercise, and this means that sampling procedures are very important. The test should be performed on a first-voided urine sample and, if positive, infection should be excluded by culture. If microalbuminuria is confirmed, then a timed overnight collection should be arranged for assessment of the albumin excretion rate; if this is also positive, a further two overnight collections should be organized. No treatment should be instituted on the basis of this one-off finding.

## A2: If drug therapy were indicated, which would be the most appropriate choice of agent?

Evidence supports the use of ACE inhibitors to delay the progression of microalbuminuria towards diabetic nephropathy, even in the presence of normal blood pressure. A further consideration in this case, however, is that ACE inhibitors should not be used in pregnancy and so appropriate contraceptive measures should be instituted before prescription is considered.

## A3: What sort of follow-up is indicated?

Once a definitive diagnosis has been made, annual screening is probably satisfactory. This is definitely the case if the repeat urine tests are negative. If a diagnosis of persistent microalbuminuria is made and the patient opted to take an ACE inhibitor, sequential urine testing is unlikely to alter management – hence, yearly screening as part of the annual review would be appropriate.

## A4: What other issues need to be addressed with regard to cardiovascular risk?

This person has no evidence of coronary heart disease and she is currently normotensive, non-smoking and lean. In this age group there is no evidence to support the use of long-term lipid-lowering therapy or aspirin, and she has good glycaemic control. Apart from advice on keeping her weight under control and taking regular exercise, no other issues need to be addressed.

**OSCE counselling cases**

## OSCE COUNSELLING CASE 1.7 – 'As someone with late-onset diabetes, should I be taking aspirin?'

'Late-onset diabetes' is an old term for non-insulin-dependent diabetes, now termed type 2 diabetes mellitus. The short answer to the question is 'probably no'. This advice, however, is based more on consensus expert opinion than on trial evidence.

Patients with known coronary heart disease should receive secondary prevention with aspirin prescribed at a dose of 150 mg once daily. For patients with no evidence of coronary heart disease, primary prevention with aspirin 75 mg once daily used to be the norm but the risk of bleeding is now thought to outweigh the benefits. The outcome of a large trial (called ASCEND) assessing the use of aspirin in 'low-risk' type 2 diabetes is awaited.

## OSCE COUNSELLING CASE 1.8 – 'Why is my blood pressure so difficult to control?'

Hypertension is commonly associated with type 2 diabetes but is difficult to treat to target. This difficulty is made worse by the lowering of target levels, based on results of large clinical trials. In the UKPDS, blood pressure targets were less stringent than those that are now advocated for routine primary care (140/80 mmHg in type 2 diabetes); nevertheless, more than one-third of patients required three or more antihypertensive drugs. Added to this is the tendency for blood pressure to rise with age and obesity.

All of the major classes of antihypertensive agent can be used in patients with diabetes and raised blood pressure, and all classes produce an equivalent antihypertensive action and achieve target levels in a similar proportion of patients. Current guidelines support the use of ACE inhibitors as first-line in diabetes, followed by calcium channel blockers and low-dose diuretics.

## DIABETES EMERGENCIES

## Questions

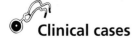

## Clinical cases

## For each of the case scenarios given, consider the following:

**Q1**: What is the likely diagnosis?
**Q2**: What investigations would be performed?
**Q3**: How would the diagnosis be confirmed?
**Q4**: What would be the initial management?
**Q5**: What are the potential complications?
**Q6**: What issues need to be addressed when the patient has fully recovered?

### CASE 1.13 – A 77-year-old man who is drowsy and dehydrated and with a plasma glucose of 84 mmol/L.

A 77-year-old man has been found collapsed at home by a care assistant. He was previously independent but known to have hypertension, angina and osteoarthritis. His regular medication is bendroflumethiazide 5 mg once a day, atenolol 50 mg once a day and aspirin. He had been noted to be lethargic over the previous few weeks and had been incontinent of urine on a couple of occasions. On arrival in the accident and emergency (A&E) department he is drowsy but oriented. Vital signs are normal but he is clinically dehydrated. Urinalysis shows ++++ glucose, ++ protein and + ketones. Plasma glucose is 84 mmol/L.

### CASE 1.14 – A 32-year-old woman with abdominal pain and vomiting and a plasma glucose of 22 mmol/L and urinary ketones.

A previously well 32-year-old woman presents to the general practice surgery with a 24-h history of abdominal pain and vomiting. On direct questioning, she admits to weight loss over the previous 2 weeks, associated with thirst, polydipsia and polyuria. A finger-prick glucose is 22 mmol/L and urine dipstick testing shows +++ ketones.

### CASE 1.15 – A 18-year-old man, known to have type 1 diabetes, who is unconscious.

An 18-year-old man who is known to have type 1 diabetes is found unconscious in his front garden. He had been playing football earlier in the day but had not complained of symptoms at that time. The diabetes is treated with four injections of insulin a day and his control is regarded as excellent.

## 👥 OSCE counselling cases

OSCE COUNSELLING CASE 1.9 – **'What should I do with my insulin if I develop a vomiting illness that stops me eating?'**

OSCE COUNSELLING CASE 1.10 – **'What advice do I give to my partner if they witness me having a "hypo" reaction?'**

## Key concepts

To work through the core clinical cases in this chapter, you will need to understand the following key concepts.

### HYPOGLYCAEMIA

Hypoglycaemia in diabetes is caused by an imbalance of insulin (too much), exercise (too much) and glucose (too little). Patients usually experience warning symptoms and signs of hypoglycaemia, which prompt them to take treatment in the form of glucose. These are often listed as adrenergic (related to autonomic nervous system) and neuroglycopenic (brain hypoglycaemia); however, in reality patients will have warnings that are a combination of the two.

- *Adrenergic:* sweating, palpitations, hunger, tachycardia.
- *Neuroglycopenic:* dizzy, faint, confused, abnormal behaviour, unconsciousness.

### HYPERGLYCAEMIA

Hyperglycaemia in type 1 diabetes may develop into diabetic ketoacidosis (DKA), while in type 2 diabetes it may develop into hyperosmolar non-ketotic pre-coma or coma (HONK).

Hyperglycaemic coma may be a presenting feature of diabetes or the result of intercurrent illness, manipulation of insulin (usually DKA) or concomitant medication (HONK). In many cases, the cause remains unknown.

Symptoms include lethargy, thirst, polydipsia, polyuria, nocturia, blurred vision and diminished conscious level, although unconsciousness is uncommon (below 5 per cent). Patients with DKA hyperventilate (as a result of the acidosis) and have sweet-smelling ketones on their breath. They may also have mildly raised plasma glucose levels, so the severity of their condition should not be judged on this measure. Abdominal pain, masquerading as an acute abdomen, is frequently present.

In HONK, patients are severely dehydrated and glucose levels are always very high. The prognosis in HONK is poor as a result of the concomitant illnesses (coronary heart disease, renal disease, cardiovascular disease) seen in this usually elderly cohort.

# Answers

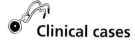

## Clinical cases

### CASE 1.13 – **A 77-year-old man who is drowsy and dehydrated with a plasma glucose of 84 mmol/L.**

#### A1: What is the likely diagnosis?

The likely diagnosis is hyperosmolar non-ketotic coma, which usually affects older people with type 2 diabetes and can be the presenting feature (as in this case). Precipitating causes include concurrent medication, including thiazide diuretics, and intercurrent illness (a UTI being possible in this scenario). Although termed 'coma', it is unusual for patients to be unconscious. Although this patient has + ketones, this is unlikely to represent acidosis, where more than ++ urinary ketones would be expected. Extremely high plasma glucose levels may be seen, as in this case.

#### A2: What investigations would be performed?

- venous blood for plasma glucose, U&Es, osmolality, bicarbonate, amylase and full blood count (FBC)
- arterial blood gases (ABGs)
- culture of urine and venous blood (and sputum if available)
- chest radiograph
- ECG.

#### A3: How would the diagnosis be confirmed?

Hyperglycaemia has already been demonstrated. Hyperosmolality can be confirmed after U&Es results are available using the formula $[2(Na^+ + K^+) + urea + glucose] > 350\,mmol/L$. Plasma ketones should be within normal limits, and there should be no acidosis confirmed by ABGs or venous bicarbonate.

#### A4: What would be the initial management?

- Attention to airways, breathing and circulation, as necessary.
- Gain intravenous access and set up an intravenous infusion.
- Cardiac monitor.
- Treatment should then be given with intravenous insulin and intravenous fluids while monitoring electrolytes (Box 1.1).
- A nasogastric tube should be inserted and the patient should be fully anticoagulated with heparin.
- Consideration should be given to central venous pressure monitoring, urinary catheterization and broad-spectrum antibiotics.

#### A5: What are the potential complications?

The prognosis for HONK remains poor (20–30 per cent). Patients are at high risk of thromboembolism and congestive cardiac failure as a result of the fluid regimen. As a result of age and comorbidity, ischaemic heart disease, renal failure and stroke are common. Aspiration of gastric contents may occur in the setting of reduced consciousness.

---

**Box 1.1   Hyperosmolar non-ketotic coma (HONK)**

*Insulin management of HONK*

- Insulin 3 units/h via intravenous (IV) pump.
- Monitor glucose every hour using meter and laboratory testing.
- Aim for fall in glucose level of 3–6 mmol/h.
- At plasma glucose <12 mmol/L, reduce to 1.5 units/h.
- Continue insulin infusion for at least 2 h.

*Fluid management of HONK guided by central venous pressure line*

- IV 0.9% saline if $Na^+$ <160 mmol/L:
  - 1 L in 1 h      hour 1: 1 L
  - 1 L in 2 h      hour 3: 2 L
  - 1 L in 2 h      hour 5: 3 L
  - 1 L in 4 h      hour 9: 4 L
- Then every 4 h.
- Change to 5% dextrose when plasma glucose <12 mmol/L.

*Electrolyte ($K^+$) management of HONK*

- No $K^+$ in litre 1, pending laboratory reading:
  - usually $K^+$ 3.5–5.5 mmol/L: add 20 mmol/L
  - recheck every 2 h and then every 4 h
  - if $K^+$ >5.5 mmol/L: no $K^+$ and then recheck in 1 h
  - if $K^+$ <3.5 mmol/L: add 40 mmol/L and then recheck in 1 h.
- If $Na^+$ >160 mmol/L, use half 0.9% saline.

---

## A6: What issues need to be addressed when the patient has fully recovered?

Despite the level of presenting glycaemia, management of the diabetes often does not involve insulin and some patients manage on diet only. The patient needs to be given dietary advice and specific diabetes education on issues such as monitoring and foot care. This would usually involve the specialist diabetes nurse and a dietitian. Other aspects of cardiovascular risk need to be assessed and, in this case, blood pressure medication may be changed from a high-dose thiazide to an ACE inhibitor.

## CASE 1.14 – A 32-year-old woman with abdominal pain and vomiting and a plasma glucose of 22 mmol/L and urinary ketones.

### A1: What is the likely diagnosis?

The likely diagnosis is diabetic ketoacidosis. This is an emergency complication of type 1 diabetes and can be the presenting feature, as in this scenario. Precipitating causes include intercurrent illness (e.g. UTI) and withholding insulin (in an established case of type 1 diabetes). Abdominal pain and vomiting are common and can lead to the erroneous diagnosis of an acute abdomen.

### A2: What investigations would be performed?

- Venous blood for plasma glucose (to confirm the finger-prick test), U&Es, osmolality, bicarbonate, amylase and FBC.
- Plasma ketones may become a more widely used test with the arrival of near-patient analyses.
- ABGs (will be performed less frequently as plasma ketone testing becomes available).

- Culture of urine and venous blood.
- Chest radiograph.
- ECG.

## A3: How would the diagnosis be confirmed?

Confirmation of hyperglycaemia with ketonuria and acidosis (pH <7.2, H⁺ >63 mmol/L). Note that the hyperglycaemia is often not pronounced.

## A4: What would be the initial management?

A4: The patient should be admitted to hospital. Intravenous access should be established for blood tests and infusion, and a cardiac monitor attached. Treatment should then be given with intravenous insulin and intravenous fluids while monitoring electrolytes (Box 1.2).

## A5: What are the potential complications?

The prognosis for DKA should be good, given that it affects young people who rarely have other significant comorbidities. Cerebral oedema may occur during treatment, although the cause of this complication is unknown. Aspiration of gastric contents may occur in the setting of reduced consciousness.

## A6: What issues need to be addressed when the patient has fully recovered?

The diagnosis of DKA implies that the patient has type 1 diabetes and will require life-long insulin. She will therefore need to be educated about the condition, and taught to inject insulin and how to

---

**Box 1.2   Diabetic ketoacidosis (DKA)**

*Insulin management of DKA*

- Insulin: 6 units/h via intravenous (IV) pump.
- Monitor glucose every hour using meter and laboratory testing.
- Aim for fall in glucose level of 3–6 mmol/h.
- At plasma glucose <12 mmol/L, reduce to 2–3 units/h.
- Continue insulin infusion for at least 24 h and no urinary ketones.

*Fluid management of DKA*

- IV 0.9% saline:
  - 1 L in 1 h     hour 1: 1 L
  - 1 L in 1 h     hour 2: 2 L
  - 1 L in 2 h     hour 4: 3 L
  - 1 L in 2 h     hour 6: 4 L
  - 1 L in 4 h     hour 10: 5 L.
- Then every 4 h.
- Change to 5% dextrose when plasma glucose <12 mmol/L.

*Electrolyte (K⁺) management of DKA*

- No K⁺ in litre 1, pending laboratory reading:
  - if K⁺ >5.5 mmol/L: no K⁺ and recheck in 1 h
  - if K⁺ <3.5 mmol/L: add 40 mmol/L and recheck in 1 h
  - if K⁺ 3.5–5.5 mmol/L: add 20 mmol/L and recheck every 2 and then every 4 h.

self-monitor using finger-prick testing. She will need to be given information about the immediate complications of her condition (hypoglycaemia, DKA) and advised to avoid pregnancy until good glycaemic control is achieved. Ultimately she will need to understand the long-term risks of small and large vessel disease. These issues are best addressed by a diabetes nurse specialist and a formal education programme.

## CASE 1.15 – **A 18-year-old man, known to have type 1 diabetes, who is unconscious.**

### A1: What is the likely diagnosis?

The likely diagnosis is hypoglycaemia. As a general rule, an unconscious person with diabetes is hypoglycaemic until proved otherwise. This diagnosis is very likely in an otherwise fit young person who takes insulin. Precipitating factors in this case may be the exercise earlier in the day (the effects of exercise can last for many hours) and tight glycaemic control, which may provoke hypoglycaemia unawareness.

### A2: What investigations would be performed?

See the answer to A3.

### A3: How would the diagnosis be confirmed?

Treatment can be initiated without any investigation and before the hypoglycaemia has been confirmed (indeed, a satisfactory response to treatment will itself confirm the diagnosis). Finger-prick blood glucose testing will confirm a low blood glucose level.

### A4: What would be the initial management?

In an unconscious patient the two main options are administration of glucagon or intravenous dextrose. Glucagon may be available because patients with type 1 diabetes are encouraged to keep a supply for this type of emergency. It comes as a powder that must be dissolved in water (a vial of sterile water is part of the kit). One vial = 1 mg = 1 unit, which is the standard injection, usually into muscle (but it can be subcutaneous or intravenous).

Intravenous dextrose is given by diluting 50% dextrose to half-strength and injecting 50 mL via a cannula. An infusion of 5% dextrose is then set up to reduce the risk of phlebitis.

### A5: What are the potential complications?

Patients can suffer injury if they have lost their warnings of hypoglycaemia. In older patients, hypoglycaemia may present with neurological signs typical of stroke. Death is thought to be uncommon in this setting, although hypoglycaemia has been implicated in the higher incidence of the 'dead-in-bed' syndrome seen in type 1 diabetes. There is increasing evidence to implicate frequent hypoglycaemia as a risk factor for cardiovascular disease. With regard to the treatments, intravenous dextrose can cause phlebitis and glucagon is associated with nausea and vomiting.

### A6: What issues need to be addressed when the patient has fully recovered?

You need to find out the cause of the event (too much insulin, too much exercise or too little food) and then provide education to prevent future recurrence. In this case, the active issues would be manipulation of the treatment regimen to be able to cope with exercise and possibly a relaxing of glycaemic control to reduce the risk of hypoglycaemia and decrease hypoglycaemia unawareness.

## ᴧᴧ OSCE counselling cases

## OSCE COUNSELLING CASE 1.9 – 'What should I do with my insulin if I develop a vomiting illness that stops me eating?'

The issue here is what most people with diabetes refer to as 'sick day rules'. Patients will understandably be concerned that they may become hypoglycaemic by taking insulin without food. Any intercurrent illness can cause blood glucose levels to rise, however, probably by increasing insulin resistance – hence the advice that *'You should never stop insulin!'*.

The patient should perform more frequent finger-prick testing, at least every 4 hours. This will allow detection of hypoglycaemia; if, as is likely, glucose levels rise, additional insulin (rapid acting) may then be needed.

For patients with type 1 diabetes, vomiting should raise the possibility of DKA and urine ketones should be checked at least twice a day. If these are positive to +++ or more, medical advice, and probably admission to hospital, must be sought. Near-patient plasma ketone testing is now more frequently performed by patients with type 1 diabetes, and they should be educated on the levels that may need medical intervention. In young people with type 1 diabetes, dehydration can develop very quickly and a low threshold for seeking medical advice should be promoted.

Patients should be aware of the actions to take during illness and how to access appropriate advice (probably not NHS Direct). This will mean telephone numbers of the diabetes specialist nurse team and agreed guidelines for out-of-hours management of diabetes emergencies

## OSCE COUNSELLING CASE 1.10 – 'What advice do I give to my partner if they witness me having a "hypo" reaction?'

Symptoms of hypoglycaemia include lack of concentration, bad temper, change in behaviour, confusion and pallor, all of which are easily (perhaps more easily) recognized by a third party. It is vital that the partner of a person with diabetes is aware of the symptoms and signs of hypoglycaemia and is able to take appropriate action.

If the person's partner suspects hypoglycaemia, ideally he or she should encourage the patient to check a finger-prick glucose level. There is little to be lost by instituting treatment without confirmation of the diagnosis, however. Assuming the patient is alert, this involves taking food by mouth, usually in the form of glucose tablets: 10 g glucose is equivalent to three sugar lumps or one Dextrosol tablet. Patients with diabetes should always carry some form of glucose replacement; Dextrosol tablets are recommended because they are less palatable than sweets (and so less likely to be consumed as treats). Alternatives include 200 mL milk or 100 mL Coca-Cola (not Diet Coke). A longer-acting carbohydrate such as bread or biscuits should then be consumed.

If the patient is semiconscious, a glucose gel can be administered via the buccal membrane. Glucostop is a glucose gel supplied in a plastic bottle with a nozzle. The gel can be squeezed into the mouth between the teeth and cheek and is absorbed into the circulation without the need for swallowing.

If the patient is unconscious, he or she should be placed into the recovery position. If the person's partner has been trained, glucagon can be administered (see above), otherwise medical aid should be summoned.

Perhaps the most important advice to the partner is not to panic and to be reassured that the normal outcome of a 'hypo' is that blood glucose levels rise in response to the body's natural adrenergic response.

## REVISION PANEL

- Diagnostic guidelines for diabetes are revised every 10 years or so and are based on consensus opinion rather than absolute cut-offs for symptoms or complications. These typically apply to type 2 diabetes. The diagnosis of type 1 diabetes, if suspected, should never be delayed by requesting investigations such as a glucose tolerance test or HbA1c, which may take days to be reported.
- A diagnosis of diabetes should never be casually applied to a patient, since it is likely that this can never be erased from their medical record and will have a major impact on their insurance premiums (e.g. life assurance, travel insurance). This shows the importance of laboratory testing rather than near-patient testing in type 2 diabetes.
- Diabetes has major implications for driving, the authorities being particularly interested in hypoglycaemia and the presence of complications such as retinopathy and peripheral neuropathy. The regulations are constantly changing, and readers should refer to the relevant website for the latest situation for their country.
- Targets for glycaemic control, typically measured by HbA1c, should be tailored according to the circumstances of the individual, bearing in mind the downsides of treatment (hypoglycaemia, weight gain).
- There are several therapeutic options that may be used to lower blood glucose (currently seven classes). The choice will be guided by considerations of cost, safety, efficacy and patient preference. Cost pressures have had a major impact on national guidelines, such as those of NICE.
- Small vessel, diabetes-specific complications affect the eyes, feet and kidneys. Screening for these complications forms part of the diabetes review, with prevention being far more effective than 'cure'.
- Large vessel complications, affecting the coronary, cerebral and peripheral arteries, are more common in people with diabetes, and hence there are aggressive blood pressure and lipid targets. The impact of tight glycaemic control, especially in people with established large vessel disease, is a controversial topic.
- An unconscious person with diabetes should always be suspected of being hypoglycaemic. In a person with diabetes who has abdominal pain and vomiting, diabetic ketoacidosis should be excluded.

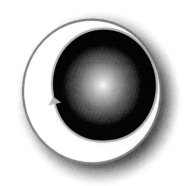

# 2 Endocrinology

*Andrew Levy*

## HYPERTHYROIDISM

## ADDISON'S DISEASE (AUTOIMMUNE ADRENAL FAILURE)

## CUSHING'S DISEASE

## Answers

# ACROMEGALY

## Questions

## Answers

# HYPERTHYROIDISM

## Questions

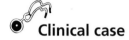
### Clinical case

### For the case scenario given, consider the following:

**Q1**: What do you think the likely diagnosis is?
**Q2**: What tests could you do to confirm this?
**Q3**: What tests would help establish the cause?
**Q4**: What is the initial management?
**Q5**: What are the long-term complications/sequelae?

### CASE 2.1 – **A 26 year-old-receptionist presents with palpitations and weight loss.**

Although pleased about the weight loss, the patient is concerned that her menstrual periods have stopped and it is the anxiety related to this, she believes, that is responsible for disturbing her sleep. Her partner has insisted that she seek a medical opinion.

## 👥 OSCE counselling cases

OSCE COUNSELLING CASE 2.1 – **'Do I have to have surgery?'**

OSCE COUNSELLING CASE 2.2 – **'Will I be able to have children after radioiodine treatment?'**

# Key concepts

To work through the core clinical cases in this section, you will need to understand the following key concepts.

Graves' disease is an autoimmune condition characterized by thyroid overactivity, eye changes (Graves' infiltrative ophthalmopathy or, more specifically, 'orbitopathy') and skin changes (pretibial myxoedema and finger clubbing, known as thyroid acropachy). The three components may occur in isolation, in any combination or not at all. Their clinical courses are usually independent and unpredictable. Skin changes are rare. Note that 'myxoedema' was an old term for thyroid underactivity but is now reserved for the skin changes that sometimes occur in Graves' disease.

In all patients with hyperthyroidism (even if iatrogenic), sympathetic overactivity leads to retraction of the upper lid, with widening of the gap between the upper and lower lids when the eyes are open (the palpebral fissure). Increased exposure of the cornea and conjunctiva leads to grittiness and soreness of the eyes.

In Graves' orbitopathy, which can occur without hyperthyroidism, autoimmune-mediated infiltration of the contents of the orbit and periorbital tissue leads to non-pitting and boggy soft tissue swelling, with increased volume of extraocular muscles, connective tissue and fat. This pushes the globe of the eye forward and can interfere with the function of the extraocular muscles, optic nerves and eyelids, reducing protection afforded by the tear film and leading to double vision and even blindness.

People with hyperthyroidism tend to be sweaty, tremulous, anxious and sometimes rather aggressive. Proximal myopathy (weakness of the thigh and arm muscles) makes their muscles ache and, although tired, sleeping is often difficult. Appetite is increased, weight tends to decrease and stools are often softened but not frankly diarrhoeal. Fertility is reduced, and menstrual periods become lighter or stop altogether. Patients often find that their short-term memory is impaired, and it may become difficult for them to make rational decisions.

In addition to sore eyes, the patient may complain of fast palpitations. If present, a thyroid bruit (the sound of blood rushing through the highly vascular overactive gland) is a useful sign because it excludes thyroiditis and exogenous thyroid hormone as causes of hyperthyroidism.

# Answers

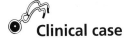

## Clinical case

### CASE 2.1 – **A 26-year-old receptionist presents with palpitations and weight loss.**

### A1: What do you think the likely diagnosis is?

Hyperthyroidism would fit all of the symptoms here and, as it is very common, it is certainly an important diagnosis to confirm or refute. There are differential diagnoses: panic attacks, agitated depression, tachyarrhythmias (e.g. paroxysmal supraventricular tachycardia, atrial fibrillation or flutter) and excessive caffeine or other stimulant ingestion could be responsible for some, if not all, of the symptoms. Anyone taking thyroxine surreptitiously or being prescribed an excessive dose for the treatment of hypothyroidism may also present in this way. Much rarer endocrine conditions such as phaeochromocytoma should also be kept in mind.

### A2: What tests could you do to confirm this?

Laboratories vary in the thyroid function tests that they are willing to run for screening, but all provide a measure of thyroid-stimulating hormone (TSH), which is suppressed by most causes of thyrotoxicosis. A free thyroxine (FT4) is also useful and will be raised above the upper limit of normal in hyperthyroidism. Unusually for tests of endocrine function, the TSH and FT4 are very reliable, and single samples taken at any time of day will be representative of thyroid function.

### A3: What tests would help establish the cause?

Clinically, the presence of Graves' eye disease establishes the diagnosis in a patient presenting with thyrotoxicosis, and no further investigations need to be done. Similarly, if a thyroid bruit is present, this is unequivocal evidence of primary hyperthyroidism and excludes thyroiditis and the effects of exogenous thyroid hormones. Thyroid autoantibodies (antimicrosomal antibodies) are usually present, but this test is not often particularly helpful.

Imaging the thyroid using ultrasonography or isotope scans is not often required in patients presenting with hyperthyroidism. Confirming the presence of a solitary 'hot nodule', however, can be useful because radioiodine is a more appropriate treatment than anti-thyroid medication, which, although effective, would have to be continued in the long term to maintain euthyroidism.

### A4: What is the initial management?

In this case, after suitable explanation of the various options, treatment with carbimazole 40 mg daily, to which thyroxine (100 µg daily) is added after a couple of weeks, is probably the most secure route to rapid restoration of euthyroidism. The patient must be warned that carbimazole can cause dangerous neutropenia idiosyncratically, and that the first sign of this is a sore throat. If this symptom occurs, the patient must be advised to stop the drug immediately and seek medical advice.

An alternative to the block and replace regimen described above is to treat with carbimazole alone and repeat thyroid function tests every 3–4 weeks, and to reduce the dose of carbimazole as the condition comes under control, aiming for a dose of 5–10 mg daily after 2–3 months.

## A5: What are the long-term complications/sequelae?

Abnormalities of thyroid function are very common and highly amenable to treatment. We often forget, however, just how uncomfortable these conditions can be for the patient. Graves' eye disease, for example, can produce major cosmetic problems, even if vision remains entirely unaffected. Primary hyperthyroidism often takes well over a year or longer to treat effectively, and during this time the patient's ambient thyroid hormone levels, symptoms and mood often fluctuate uncomfortably.

Persistent hyperthyroidism is associated with osteoporosis, proximal myopathy and cardiomyopathy, manifesting as atrial fibrillation and its associated increase in thromboembolic risk.

## ⛷ OSCE counselling cases

### OSCE COUNSELLING CASE 2.1 – 'Do I have to have surgery?'

In the past, subtotal thyroidectomy was extensively used to treat hyperthyroidism. Radioiodine is a very effective treatment and anti-thyroid drugs are also safe to use as a long-term therapy if the patient objects to radioiodine or if there is concern that radioiodine might worsen Graves' orbitopathy. Thyroid surgery is reserved for patients in whom very rapid and permanent control of hyperthyroidism is required, or in whom a goitre is causing compressive or cosmetic problems.

It is hoped that early and aggressive immunosuppressive treatment, principally with prednisolone, will reduce the frequency and extent of surgery required to correct problems associated with Graves' orbitopathy.

### OSCE COUNSELLING CASE 2.2 – 'Will I be able to have children after radioiodine treatment?'

It is a commonly held misconception that radioiodine has an adverse effect on fertility or that having children is inadvisable after radioiodine treatment. Neither is true. The only caveats to radioiodine use in this respect are that radioiodine has exactly the same effect on the thyroid of the developing fetus as it does on the mother. It is therefore vital that radioiodine is not inadvertently given to a woman who is pregnant. Health and safety regulations also seek to limit third-party exposure to irradiation and, for that reason, it is not an ideal treatment for anyone who cannot at least temporarily escape spending a great deal of time in close proximity to young children.

# ADDISON'S DISEASE (AUTOIMMUNE ADRENAL FAILURE)

## Questions

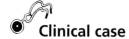 **Clinical case**

### For the case scenario given, consider the following:

> **Q1**: What do you think the likely diagnosis is?
> **Q2**: What tests could you do to confirm this?
> **Q3**: What tests would help establish the cause?
> **Q4**: What is the initial management?
> **Q5**: What are the long-term complications/sequelae?

### CASE 2.2 – A 19-year-old student presents with an 18-month history of progressive tiredness, weight loss and lethargy.

One year before presentation she had a common cold that forced her to stay away from lectures for 2 days. Three months before presentation, another common cold laid her low for almost 2 weeks, during which time she lost 3 kg in weight. The local student health doctors assured her that the symptoms were the result of either being pregnant or taking drugs. On examination, she was noted to have darker skin than her mother and pigmented palmar creases.

## ᴀᴀ OSCE counselling cases

OSCE COUNSELLING CASE 2.3 – **'Why did this happen to me?'**

OSCE COUNSELLING CASE 2.4 – **'How will it affect my life?'**

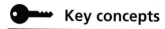 **Key concepts**

To work through the core clinical cases in this section, you will need to understand the following key concepts.

Before steroids (glucocorticoids) became available, autoimmune destruction of both adrenal glands invariably led to death from circulatory collapse. In much the same way that the autoimmune destruction of pancreatic islets, which characterizes type 1 diabetes mellitus, does not become apparent until many months after it starts, autoimmune destruction of the adrenal glands has usually been advancing for many months by the time it is recognized. In retrospect, the patient may have noticed progressive impairment of the ability to respond appropriately to acute stress and that it is taking longer to recover from trivial illnesses such as the common cold.

Both adrenal glands, including the zona glomerulosa, the aldosterone-producing and the angiotensin II responsive layer, are entirely destroyed in primary adrenal failure. Consequently, the patient becomes critically deficient in both glucocorticoids (cortisol) and mineralocorticoids (aldosterone), resulting terminally in profound hyperkalaemia and hyponatraemia. Lack of glucocorticoid feedback at the level of the hypothalamus and pituitary leads to a marked increase in adrenocorticotrophic hormone (ACTH) and associated melanocyte-stimulating hormone (MSH), which stimulates skin melanocytes. By making the patient look suntanned, the increase in skin pigmentation (including parts that are not exposed to the sun and new scars) tends to disguise the fact that the patient is gravely ill, and it can be surprisingly easy to overlook or ascribe the associated history of weakness, weight loss and intermittent vomiting to other causes.

In secondary adrenal failure (i.e. resulting from pituitary failure), lack of glucocorticoids is not as absolute, and catastrophic inability to respond to stress is rare. In addition, as ACTH levels are low rather than high, pigmentation does not occur and mineralocorticoid production is impaired only modestly because it is controlled by the renin–angiotensin–aldosterone pathway rather than the pituitary. As secondary adrenal failure is often associated with hypogonadotrophic hypogonadism, adrenal pre-androgens and gonadal testosterone are both low and secondary sexual hair is often lost.

# Answers

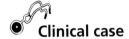

## Clinical case

### CASE 2.2 – **A 19-year-old student presents with an 18-month history of progressive tiredness, weight loss and lethargy.**

#### A1: What do you think the likely diagnosis is?

This is a fairly classic presentation of Addison's disease. It is relatively easy in retrospect to put together the symptoms and signs of Addison's disease, but it can be very difficult to recognize, particularly in its early stages, when adrenal function is only suboptimal under stress. Delay in diagnosis is therefore very understandable.

#### A2: What tests could you do to confirm this?

The characteristic biochemical changes of hyperkalaemia and hyponatraemia tend to occur relatively late and, if the diagnosis is suspected, it is perfectly acceptable to start treatment with glucocorticoids immediately, pending an opportunity to carry out a diagnostic test. The confirmatory test (Synacthen) is described below in OSCE counselling case 2.3.

#### A3: What tests would help establish the cause?

In the developed world at least 80 per cent of cases of Addison's disease are caused by autoimmune destruction of the adrenal glands. Tuberculosis (TB) remains a relatively common cause of Addison's disease in the absence of autoimmune disease and is suggested by the presence of enlarged adrenal glands with necrotic areas and often dots of calcification visible on computed tomography (CT). In boys under 16 years of age, X-linked adrenoleukodystrophy, diagnosed by measuring an increase in circulating very-long-chain fatty acids, is an important cause of adrenal failure. In older patients, measurement of anti-cardiolipin antibodies, a marker of primary antiphospholipid syndrome, is useful if features such as recurrent venous thrombosis suggest that the condition is not idiopathic.

In primary adrenal failure, a random plasma ACTH will be high. In secondary adrenal failure, the symptoms and signs related to the condition are usually much more subtle and the biochemical signs do not appear. ACTH will be low or low-normal and the cortisol response to exogenous ACTH will be suboptimal.

#### A4: What is the initial management?

Glucocorticoid replacement (usually with 10–15 mg hydrocortisone first thing in the morning and another 5 mg hydrocortisone at around 4pm) is required immediately. In primary Addison's disease, mineralocorticoid replacement with fludrocortisone 50–100 µg/day is also required. As Addison's disease is often disclosed by an episode of acute stress, it is not uncommon for glucocorticoid treatment to be given parenterally and at a higher dose at least initially.

#### A5: What are the long-term complications/sequelae?

Patients with autoimmune Addison's disease are more likely to have other autoimmune diseases, and a proportion of them claim to 'not feel right' despite what appears to be adequate replacement therapy. Under conditions of stress, patients should be asked to step up their glucocorticoid dose two- or threefold for a few days; they are asked to wear a MedicAlert bracelet or necklace and carry an injectable form of glucocorticoid to use if they find themselves unable to take oral steroids. For some patients, a longer-acting glucocorticoid such as prednisolone seems to be more comfortable than the short-acting hydrocortisone.

OSCE counselling cases

## OSCE COUNSELLING CASE 2.3 – 'Why did this happen to me?'

All patients with autoimmune Addison's disease have detectable adrenal cortex or steroid 21-hydroxylase autoantibodies. The specific human leucocyte antigen (HLA) subtypes HLA-A1, HLA-B8 and HLA-DR3 predispose to developing the condition. It is not clear, however, why some patients develop the condition and others do not. The risk of developing other autoimmune conditions such as type 1 diabetes mellitus, primary gonadal failure, hypoparathyroidism, Hashimoto's thyroiditis, vitiligo and pernicious anaemia is modestly increased in patients with Addison's disease.

If the diagnosis is suspected in an ill patient, formal diagnosis can wait and immediate treatment with glucocorticoids is usually appropriate. A high plasma ACTH in the presence of low random cortisol is often sufficient to confirm the diagnosis. If doubt remains, a cortisol response of less than 495 nmol/L 1 h after a 250 µg intravenous bolus of synthetic ACTH (Synacthen) confirms the diagnosis.

## OSCE COUNSELLING CASE 2.4 – 'How will it affect my life?'

For most patients the diagnosis of Addison's disease has no adverse long-term effects on life or lifestyle. Some patients, however, claim not to feel as well as they did before the onset of overt disease, despite optimized glucocorticoid and mineralocorticoid replacement. For some of these patients, additional replacement of adrenal pre-androgens has been advocated, but there is little good evidence to support this at the present time.

The long-term outlook for Addison's disease is good, provided that the patient is fully aware of the implications of the condition and the need to respond to stressful situations by temporarily increasing the glucocorticoid dose.

# CUSHING'S DISEASE

## Questions

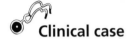

### Clinical case

### For the case scenario given, consider the following:

**Q1**: What do you think the likely diagnosis is?
**Q2**: What tests could you do to confirm this?
**Q3**: What tests would help establish the cause?
**Q4**: What is the initial management?
**Q5**: What are the long-term complications/sequelae?

### CASE 2.3 – A 56-year-old woman presents with depression, hirsutism, weight gain and muscle weakness.

On examination, her general practitioner found her to be hypertensive and to have wide purple striae on her abdomen and thighs. Her visual fields were full to confrontation and there was no bruising.

## **👥 OSCE counselling cases**

OSCE COUNSELLING CASE 2.5 – **'Will "the tumour" spread to other parts of my body?'**

OSCE COUNSELLING CASE 2.6 – **'Can I have tablets instead of an operation?'**

## Key concepts

To work through the core clinical cases in this section, you will need to understand the following key concepts.

Hypercortisolaemia (Cushing's syndrome) is in most cases iatrogenic, an unavoidable side effect of the high-dose glucocorticoid treatment required for many immune and autoimmune conditions. Rarely, hypercortisolaemia is pituitary dependent (Cushing's disease) and is the result of a pituitary adenoma secreting ACTH. Cushing's syndrome can also result from other sources of ACTH such as carcinoid tumours of the lung or gut or from adrenal adenomas and carcinomas secreting inappropriate amounts of cortisol. It is often surprisingly difficult to identify the source of the problem with certainty and to treat it adequately, because even the most careful battery of well-organized investigations can be misleading. The first task is to confirm the presence of hypercortisolaemia and, if that can be confirmed, investigations are redirected to identify the source.

In hypercortisolaemia of malignancy, there may be insufficient time for the typical phenotype to develop. In more chronic cases, patients characteristically gain weight, develop neuropsychiatric problems (often accentuation of premorbid personality – miserable people become more miserable and vice versa), proximal myopathy (difficulty standing from sitting without using the arms), muscle wasting, central accumulation of fat (filling in the temporal fossae and development of the characteristic 'moon face' and 'buffalo hump'), and weakening of the skin leading to the formation of wide purple stretch marks (striae) and easy bruisability (although bruises are not often evident in the clinic). Hypertension, hirsutism (caused by increased ACTH drive to adrenal androgen production) and glucose intolerance are also common. In Cushing's disease the ACTH-induced increase in production of adrenal pre-androgens (responsible for the hirsutism) tends to protect against steroid-induced thinning of the skin.

# Answers

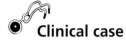
## Clinical case

## CASE 2.3 – A 56-year-old woman presents with depression, hirsutism, weight gain and muscle weakness.

### A1: What do you think the likely diagnosis is?

Although Cushing's syndrome is suggested by the combination of mental and physical changes listed, the only one that is specific in the circumstances is the presence of wide purple striae rather than pale striae. Simple gross obesity could be responsible for everything else. Obese people are often depressed about their inability to lose weight, and the sheer mass of tissue to carry around can make them feel weak, even though they tend to be much stronger than an equivalent patient with hypercortisolaemia. The fat tissue can aromatize pre-androgens to androgens and oestrogens, leading to hirsutism, and there is an association between obesity and hypertension, both of which are extremely common. Cushing's syndrome is an important diagnosis to make, but it is as well to remember that Cushing's disease is extremely rare compared with simple obesity.

### A2: What tests could you do to confirm this?

If hypercortisolaemia is suspected, one of the most reliable screening tests currently available in the UK is to measure 24-h urinary free cortisol, three samples of which should be assayed along with creatinine clearance to ensure that the patient has managed to produce complete collections. Pregnancy, pain, heavy alcohol ingestion or alcohol withdrawal and vigorous exercise, particularly if the patient gets up very early every morning to run, will increase urinary free cortisol to above the normal range. As cortisol is metabolized by the kidneys during filtration, if the patient drinks more than 5 L of fluid daily, urinary free cortisol will be high. In addition, some drugs unexpectedly increase urinary free cortisol (e.g. statins) or interfere with analytical methods, such as co-eluting with cortisol on high-performance liquid chromatography (HPLC) (e.g. carbamazepine). The best test to distinguish Cushing's from pseudo-Cushing's is the dexamethasone suppressed corticotrophin-releasing hormone (CRH) test. Eight 0.5 mg doses of dexamethasone are given orally at strict 6-h intervals from midday, ending at 6am on the morning of the test. Two hours later, the patient is given 100 µg CRH (strictly 1 µg/kg); 15 min later a single cortisol above 38 nmol/L suggests hypercortisolaemia.

### A3: What tests would help establish the cause?

Establishing the cause of Cushing's syndrome can be difficult. Delays associated with various investigations can make it difficult to carry them out in a logical order without taking an excessive time to reach a conclusion. A peripheral ACTH measurement is useful because a very high level suggests ectopic ACTH syndrome and a very low level suggests adrenal disease. Pituitary magnetic resonance imaging (MRI) may show a macroadenoma (a tumour greater than 10 mm in diameter or distorting the sella turcica), in which case it is very likely to be responsible for the Cushing's syndrome. Conversely, as the prevalence of incidental pituitary adenomas under 4 mm in diameter in the general population is very high (probably around 10 per cent), an MRI scan is insufficient evidence to send a neurosurgeon in after it. Computed tomography or MRI of the adrenal glands showing a unilateral nodule with contralateral atrophy suggests a primary adrenal lesion. For many patients, petrosal sinus sampling, i.e. sampling the venous outflow of the pituitary, is necessary to confirm or refute a pituitary source of excess ACTH. The level of ACTH should be at least double the level found in peripheral samples taken simultaneously and should increase further (to at least three times peripheral levels) in response to CRH.

## A4:  What is the initial management?

The initial management of Cushing's disease (i.e. pituitary-dependent Cushing's syndrome) is trans-sphenoidal microadenomectomy by a skilled neurosurgeon. If the problem is a carcinoid tumour of the lungs secreting ACTH, or an adrenocortical tumour producing too much cortisol, the respective tumours should be removed by an appropriate specialist.

## A5:  What are the long-term complications/sequelae?

Unfortunately, cure of Cushing's disease is difficult to achieve and a large minority of patients relapse at some time or have only a partial remission and end up with persistent hypercortisolaemia. Improvements in trans-sphenoidal surgery and endoscopic adrenal surgery should allow a higher percentage of 'long-term remissions' in the future and a reduction in the prevalence of patients suffering the consequences of persistent hypercortisolaemia, principally osteoporosis and the risks associated with impaired glucose tolerance or frank diabetes mellitus, hypertension and obesity.

## ii OSCE counselling cases

### OSCE COUNSELLING CASE 2.5 – 'Will "the tumour" spread to other parts of my body?'

Metastatic spread of pituitary tumours has been documented but is extremely rare. The word 'benign' is, however, a little misleading in that some corticotrophic adenomas can infiltrate locally, particularly after bilateral adrenalectomy, which removes endogenous feedback inhibition of tumour growth (Nelson's syndrome). It is not unusual for corticotrophic adenomas to be so small that, despite causing dramatic symptoms and signs, they are not visible on pituitary MRI. Even stranger is the relatively high remission rate when unaffected pituitary tissue is excised at surgery.

Cushing's disease has such a high risk of recurrence or failure of initial treatment that the word 'remission' rather than 'cure' is used.

Standard fractionated linear accelerator pituitary radiotherapy to the remnant reduces recurrence rate about fivefold but is associated with a small increased risk of other tumour formation in the radiation field and an increase in the risk of stroke. It is an important treatment, particularly if the patient has had bilateral adrenalectomy as part of the management of the condition.

Appropriate treatment of the primary disease does result in weight loss, but many patients find that it is difficult to shed all of the extra weight they accumulated before effective treatment was instigated.

### OSCE COUNSELLING CASE 2.6 – 'Can I have tablets instead of an operation?'

Tablets tend not to be used first-line because surgery offers the chance of immediate remission, confirmation of the diagnosis histologically, and an opportunity to debulk an adenoma that may subsequently be associated with space-occupying problems if allowed to continue to grow in situ. Drugs are sometimes used in preparation for surgery or if the patient has very aggressive disease causing severe neuropsychiatric symptoms, but they are often not very well tolerated. In the UK, metyrapone is used to inhibit adrenal hormone synthesis competitively. Ketoconazole, an imidazole antifungal agent, is also a useful adrenocortical hormone synthesis inhibitor. Etomidate at low dose is useful if rapid intravenous control of excessive glucocorticoid levels is required, as is sometimes the case in Cushing's syndrome secondary to malignant disease.

# ACROMEGALY

## Questions

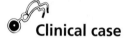 **Clinical case**

### For the case scenario given, consider the following:

**Q1**: What do you think the likely diagnosis is?
**Q2**: What tests could you do to confirm this?
**Q3**: What tests would help establish the cause?
**Q4**: What is the initial management?
**Q5**: What are the long-term complications/sequelae?

### CASE 2.4 – A 44-year-old woman presents with excessive sweating and an increase in hat size over a 3-year period.

She comments that her face and hands just seem 'bigger' than before.

**Key concepts**

To work through the core clinical cases in this section, you will need to understand the following key concepts.

Acromegaly is caused by the presence of a growth hormone (GH)-secreting tumour of the anterior pituitary (somatotroph adenoma) that develops after puberty. Coarsening of the facial features, headaches, drenching sweats and a progressive increase in jaw, glove, ring and shoe sizes are well-known features of excess GH. The most common and troublesome symptoms are, however, carpal tunnel syndrome, obstructive sleep apnoea and osteoarthritis, caused by persistent growth of soft tissue and cartilage. These changes can be partially reversed in some patients when the condition is treated, but unfortunately many of the changes remain and widespread arthritis, caused by disruption of joint cartilage, can be disabling.

If a somatotroph adenoma occurs before increased sex hormones cause the epiphyses of long bones to fuse at puberty, the patient has the potential to become a giant. In true gigantism, the somatotroph adenoma not only arises early in life but also impairs the function of pituitary gonadotrophs, giving rise to hypogonadotrophic hypogonadism. Without gonadotrophins (follicle-stimulating hormone [FSH], luteinizing hormone [LH]), puberty cannot proceed, and if the epiphyses remain open persistent growth of long bones can continue throughout life, leading in exceptional cases to remarkably tall stature.

As GH is involved primarily in the growth of the long bones, whereas sex hormones are responsible for growth of the axial skeleton, patients with gigantism tend to have very long limbs but relatively short backs. These so-called 'eunuchoid' proportions, where span exceeds standing height, also tend to be found in other conditions associated with low sex hormone levels such as Klinefelter's syndrome (XXY).

Thickening of the tissues of the nasopharynx predisposes to severe snoring and frequent episodes of complete obstruction of the airways during the night. This leads to arterial blood oxygen desaturation and increasing respiratory efforts, causing partial wakefulness until eventually airflow resumes. Consequently, patients frequently complain of tiredness in the morning. Obstructive sleep apnoea has also been implicated in the pathogenesis of hypertension, which affects over one-third of people with acromegaly.

Treatment of acromegaly involves trans-sphenoidal debulking of the tumour and in some cases pituitary radiotherapy. Drug treatment is also used, with long-acting parenteral somatostatin (GH-release inhibiting hormone) analogues such as octreotide LAR or lanreotide, dopamine (D2) analogues such as cabergoline or bromocriptine, which reduce GH and insulin-like growth factor I (IGF-I) levels in about 10 per cent of patients, and GH-receptor blockers (pegvisomant). Surgery to relieve arthritis, nerve compression syndromes, snoring and facial deformity is also sometimes required. It is believed that acromegaly is associated with an increased incidence of bowel tumours, and patients in some centres are offered a routine colonoscopic screening when first diagnosed and at the age of 60 years.

## Answers

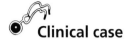
### Clinical case

### CASE 2.4 – **A 44-year-old woman presents with excessive sweating and an increase in hat size over a 3-year period.**

### A1: What do you think the likely diagnosis is?

Acromegaly is likely. It should be remembered that there can be large discrepancies between circulating GH levels and the phenotypic changes that result. Some patients with very high levels of GH do not seem to develop many of the phenotypic features of acromegaly. Other patients with only modestly elevated GH levels sometimes continue to grow. Growth of the hands and feet is relatively pronounced because of the multiple cartilaginous interfaces between the many small bones. Growth of the skull is minimal and is a feature that is more characteristic of Paget's disease of bone. In acromegaly, increased hat size is the result of facial soft tissue growth rather than bony growth, although on radiograph and CT some skull thickening does occur.

Excessive sweating is also a feature of oestrogen withdrawal and thyrotoxicosis, both of which should be considered because they are much more prevalent problems, even though neither would explain the rest of this patient's symptoms.

### A2: What tests could you do to confirm this?

In many cases, the phenotypic changes of acromegaly are so obvious that little needs to be done to confirm the diagnosis. The condition might be 'burnt out', however, and, as persistent disease is an indication for surgery, it is important to measure a few random GH levels (three samples 20–30 min apart) and an IGF-I, and to request an MRI scan of the pituitary. The pulsatile nature of GH release means that a single measure of GH is not useful. If doubt remains about the diagnosis (and usually it does not), failure to suppress GH to <2 mU/L (0.6 mg/L) after 75 g glucose orally confirms the diagnosis.

### A3: What tests would help establish the cause?

Rarely, acromegaly is part of the multiple endocrine neoplasia type 1 (MEN-1) syndrome, Carney complex or the isolated familial acromegaly syndrome. Somatotrophic adenomas have been described in association with GH-releasing hormone-secreting gangliocytomas in the region of the pituitary. The cause of acromegaly, however, is *always* a somatotrophic adenoma secreting too much GH.

### A4: What is the initial management?

In an elderly patient with comorbidity, in whom somatotroph adenoma is unlikely to cause local space-occupying problems, it is perfectly reasonable to do nothing. In a younger patient, trans-sphenoidal microadenomectomy or debulking of a macroadenoma is still first-line treatment. In terms of GH reduction, drug treatment with somatostatin analogues or the new GH-receptor blockers has a higher chance of success than surgery, but both are prohibitively expensive and, as far as we know at the moment, necessitate long-term treatment.

### A5: What are the long-term complications/sequelae?

Complications of acromegaly and its treatment are hypopituitarism, local space-occupying issues (such as visual field changes) and the effects of excessive GH levels on somatic growth and metabolism. Growth hormone is diabetogenic, and acromegaly is associated with hypertension and an enhanced risk of cardiomyopathy (which might be specific to acromegaly), and respiratory complications related to altered chest shape and movements.

## REVISION PANEL

- Thyrotoxicosis is a common endocrine condition resulting from excess thyroid hormone as part of Graves' disease, a multinodular goitre or a solitary toxic nodule.
- Thyrotoxicosis can be treated medically with anti-thyroid medication (e.g. carbimazole), radioactive iodine or surgery.
- Addison's disease results in glucocorticoid and mineralocorticoid deficiency from autoimmune primary adrenal insufficiency, but secondary glucocorticoid deficiency may result from pituitary disease and lack of ACTH.
- Addison's disease requires life-long hormone replacement with glucocorticoids (e.g. hydrocortisone) and mineralocorticoids (e.g. fludrocortisone).
- Hypercortisolaemia (Cushing's syndrome) may result from either excess adrenal glucocorticoid synthesis (adrenal tumour), excessive steroid therapy, or secondary to excess ACTH production from a pituitary adenoma, carcinoid tumour or rarely other ACTH-secreting tumours (e.g. lung).
- The optimal treatment of Cushing's syndrome is surgery to remove the source of excessive ACTH.
- Acromegaly results from excessive GH production from a pituitary tumour. If the tumour is active before sex hormone production, then this will result in gigantism.
- The optimal treatment of acromegaly and gigantism is to remove the tumour responsible for excess growth hormone production.

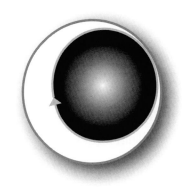

# 3 Rheumatology

*Mark Pugh*

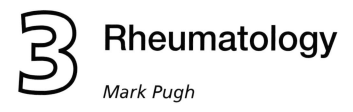

## POLYARTHRITIS

## MONOARTHRITIS

## SYSTEMIC RHEUMATOLOGICAL ILLNESSES

## Answers

# BACK PAIN

## Questions

## Answers

# POLYARTHRITIS

## Questions

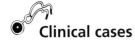 **Clinical cases**

## For each of the case scenarios given, consider the following:

> **Q1**: What is the likely differential diagnosis?
> **Q2**: How would you investigate this patient?
> **Q3**: How would you confirm the likely diagnosis?
> **Q4**: How would you initially manage the patient?
> **Q5**: What are the principles of long-term management?
> **Q6**: What is the prognosis?

### CASE 3.1 – **A 38-year-old man develops painful and swollen hand joints.**

A 38-year-old man presents with a 4-month history of pain and swelling of the knuckles, wrists, knees, ankles and toes. He has no significant past history and the general practitioner confirms the swelling of the joints and notes a history of more than an hour's stiffness of the joints in the morning. Initial blood tests reveal a microcytic anaemia of 11.8 g/dL and a C-reactive protein (CRP) of 9.6 g/dL.

### CASE 3.2 – **Pain in the hands, knees and feet in a 46-year-old woman.**

A recently postmenopausal woman presents with a 6-month history of pain and swelling in her hands, knees, neck and feet. The pain limits her ability to use her hands, and the knee and foot pain limits her mobility. Apart from her joint pain she is otherwise well and there is no contributory past medical history. Examination demonstrates tender double bumps over the ends of her fingers, especially the index and middle finger, tenderness around the base of the thumb, limited neck movement, crunching knees with swelling, and bilateral early bunions.

### CASE 3.3 – **Knee pain in a schoolgirl.**

A 16-year-old girl has a 6-year history of intermittent knee pain. She presented previously at the age of 10 years also for knee pain, which was attributed to growing pains. Now she describes pain in the knees worse at the end of the day and especially bad after exercise. Her knees are often sore after sitting, and difficult pain on ascending stairs has adversely affected her school attendance. Knee swelling occurs sometimes. She also has pain in her hands, elbows and tops of her legs. Her joints often click so loudly that other people pass remarks. She seems well in other respects and, apart from the previous assessment for knee pain, there is no past medical history. Her general practitioner detected no obvious joint problem and the full blood count (FBC), erythrocyte sedimentation rate (ESR) and rheumatoid factor (RF) were reported as normal.

##  OSCE counselling case

OSCE COUNSELLING CASE 3.1 – **'What can be done if I get a flare-up of my rheumatoid arthritis?'**

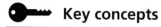 **Key concepts**

To work through the core clinical cases in this section, you will need to understand the following key concepts.

Patients generally describe any pain around a joint as 'arthritis'. Arthritis, by definition, means inflammation of the joint and therefore in the absence of confirmatory signs should not be diagnosed. Arthralgia is the name for a painful joint without signs of inflammation. Pain can also be referred as well as originating from ligaments, tendons, muscles, nerves, arteries and skin around the joint.

There are a wide number of causes of arthritis, including:

- degenerative: osteoarthritis
- trauma
- infective: viral, septic, reactive, parasitic, fungal
- endocrine: hypothyroid, hyperthyroid, hyperparathyroid
- malignancy: paraneoplastic, secondary or primary malignancy
- allergic: erythema nodosum, drug-induced
- autoimmune: connective tissue disease, seronegative arthritis, vasculitis
- crystal arthritis: gout, pseudo-gout
- congenital: Stickler's syndrome.

## Answers

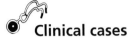

### Clinical cases

---

## CASE 3.1 – A 38-year-old man develops painful and swollen hand joints.

### A1: What is the likely differential diagnosis?

With a history of multiple, small joint swelling, more than 60 min of morning stiffness and a raised ESR, rheumatoid arthritis is a likely diagnosis. Other causes of arthritis also need to be considered, such as other connective tissue disorders, seronegative arthritis, infection, endocrine disorders, drugs and malignancy.

### A2: How would you investigate this patient?

A full history and examination are important. Examination should confirm the presence of inflammation of the joints characterized by pain and swelling. All the joints and other systems should be examined, looking for evidence of systemic involvement and other possible causes of the arthritis apart from rheumatoid arthritis. Ultrasound or magnetic resonance imaging (MRI) could be used where the signs of synovitis are equivocal.

### A3: How would you confirm the likely diagnosis?

The diagnosis is clinical, with the presence of inflammation in the characteristic joints being sufficient to indicate arthritis. The American College of Rheumatology diagnostic criteria are often quoted, but the inclusion of erosions and rheumatoid nodules means that these criteria have low sensitivity in early disease. A high CRP or positive RF, although not always present in early disease, suggests a likelihood of progression to early erosions.

### A4: How would you initially manage the patient?

The initial management should be clinically to confirm the diagnosis, followed by baseline investigations including FBC, CRP (or similar measurement of inflammation), urea and electrolytes (U&Es), liver function tests (LFTs), and screening for RF and antinuclear factors. These tests should be consistent with rheumatoid arthritis and should not suggest an alternative diagnosis. The tests are also useful because many of the drugs used to treat rheumatoid arthritis are toxic. Radiographs of the hands and feet, any other involved joints and the chest will often not demonstrate change early in the disease course but will be useful to monitor disease progression. If the presentation is sufficiently characteristic, the patient should be referred for specialist assessment immediately to maximize the chances of commencing treatment early in the disease course, which has been shown to improve the prognosis. The use of analgesics and anti-inflammatory drugs may provide some symptom relief while baseline investigations are undertaken. When rheumatoid arthritis is confirmed, the patient should be offered disease-modifying anti-rheumatoid drugs (DMARDs), usually in combinations including methotrexate, without delay to prevent the development of joint damage.

### A5: What are the principles of long-term management?

The ongoing management of rheumatoid arthritis involves ensuring complete control of inflammation, monitoring joint damage, checking for other systemic manifestations, and screening for the development of treatment side effects. As with the development of any chronic illness, patient education about the illness and its treatment is important to allay fears and promote treatment compliance. Patients with autoimmune arthritis are at significant risk of the development of cardiovascular disease and should be screened for this.

## A6: What is the prognosis?

Extra-articular manifestations of rheumatoid arthritis include:

- *skin:* ulcers and nodules
- *lung:* fibrosis, effusions and nodules
- *neurological:* myopathies and neuropathies
- *eye:* secondary Sjögren's syndrome and inflammation
- *systemic:* anaemia, weight loss and fevers
- *skeletal:* osteoporosis
- *cardiovascular:* high incidence of cardiovascular disease and rare muscle, valve or pericardial involvement.

The progress for joint damage is as follows: 5–10 per cent of patients do not develop damage; the remainder of patients do develop damage, with 40–70 per cent after a chronic disease course developing significant levels of damage and disability, and 20–40 per cent after a relapsing and remitting course associated with lesser levels of damage. Aggressive early treatment is believed to hold the key to improving the long-term prognosis in rheumatoid arthritis.

## CASE 3.2 – **Pain in the hands, knees and feet in a 46-year-old woman.**

### A1: What is the likely differential diagnosis?

There is a wide differential, but the presence of Heberden's nodes in the hands, a characteristic pattern of joint involvement and the absence of synovitis point to a diagnosis of osteoarthritis.

### A2: How would you investigate this patient?

Blood tests are not essential but will help rule out alternative diagnoses. Radiographs of the symptomatic joints may demonstrate the typical changes of joint space narrowing, subchondral sclerosis, bone cysts and osteophytes.

### A3: How would you confirm the likely diagnosis?

A history and examination should be sufficient to rule out alternative diagnoses and confirm the diagnosis. A radiograph is probably the most useful diagnostic test, but early changes can be subtle and it is possible to have osteoarthritis coexisting with gout or an inflammatory arthritis.

### A4: How would you initially manage the patient?

Conservative measures should be addressed, including weight control, the use of padded footwear such as trainers, and regular exercise. A walking stick can help knee symptoms, and orthoses will help foot symptoms. Physiotherapy can alleviate local symptoms. Topical non-steroidal anti-inflammatory drugs (NSAIDs) or capsaicin cream provide some relief. Intra-articular steroids are safer than NSAIDs and may be appropriate to relieve joint symptoms. Patients should always be encouraged to use analgesics other than NSAIDs as first-line drugs, e.g. paracetamol. Although scientific data are sparse, there is some evidence that complementary therapies may provide some symptom relief, and they are popular with patients.

### A5: What are the principles of long-term management?

The complications of osteoarthritis relate to the development of disability secondary to joint involvement. Patients can be reassured that, although activity may produce increased symptoms, only heavy manual work or professional-level sports activity will probably accelerate joint damage. Treatment may produce complications that require treatment, of which NSAID-induced gastrointestinal damage is probably the most common. Surgery, especially of the knee and hip, is very successful for patients with significant pain and disability associated with significant radiological damage.

## A6: What is the prognosis?

Most patients are concerned about the development of future disability but can be reassured that this is unlikely The key to successful management is to ensure that the patient self-manages the problem because cure is not possible and medical disease modification remains unachievable.

## CASE 3.3 – **Knee pain in a schoolgirl.**

### A1: What is the likely differential diagnosis?

Benign hypermobility is the most likely diagnosis. An underlying inflammatory arthritis is unlikely because of the length of the history, the normal-looking joints and the absence of inflammatory markers in the blood, but it needs to be ruled out.

### A2: How would you investigate this patient?

A history looking for pointers to alternative diagnoses, such as psoriasis, or systemic features of a connective tissue disorder or juvenile idiopathic arthritis, is important. A family history of joint pains in childhood is often present, highlighting a familial link in this disorder. Examination of the joints, looking for the absence of joint deformity or ongoing synovitis, would virtually rule out an underlying inflammatory arthritis. Radiographs and blood tests would be helpful to rule out alternative diagnoses.

### A3: How would you confirm the likely diagnosis?

Generalized benign hypermobility is diagnosed by demonstrating hypermobility in classic sites, including bending the little finger to a right angle, bending the thumb back to touch the forearm, hyperextension of the elbow, and bending forwards and placing the palms of the hands flat on the floor. Although normal on initial examination, retropatellar pain can often be elicited by Clarke's test (compression of the patella with restricted knee extension). Flat feet are usually present. More unusual causes of hypermobility, such as Marfan's and Ehlers–Danlos syndromes, should be considered.

### A4: How would you initially manage the patient?

Reassurance that this is not the start of a deforming arthritis is usually very important. Anti-inflammatory and analgesic drugs offer some relief and can be important if the pain is severe enough to disrupt sleep or limit activities. Physiotherapy can improve pain by limiting joint movement through muscle development. Orthoses to correct flat feet and raise the heel can improve not only foot and ankle symptoms but also those from the knee, hip and back.

### A5: What are the principles of long-term management?

Occasionally these patients can have recurrent dislocations of the shoulder, hip or knee. This may require joint-stabilizing surgery but if possible this should be avoided. On a day-to-day basis, most of the problems relate to maintaining normal functions such as school attendance and physical activity.

### A6: What is the prognosis?

Symptoms typically improve with age, but improvement is not universal. Benign hypermobility does not appear to be associated with the development of early osteoarthritis.

**OSCE counselling case**

## OSCE COUNSELLING CASE 3.1 – 'What can be done if I get a flare-up of my rheumatoid arthritis?'

Patients can find the psychological impact of flare-ups difficult and need to be reassured that, even with a background of good control, flare-ups can occur. Sometimes no identifiable reason can be found to explain the flare-up; otherwise a waning of the effect of current medication, intercurrent infection or stress may be involved. Single joint flare-ups are usually easier to deal with than multiple joint problems. Patients should be advised to maximize their analgesic and anti-inflammatory medication, rest the affected joint and use ice packs. With no more intervention, the flare-up may settle. If it does not, intra-articular steroid for a localized problem, or intramuscular, oral or intravenous steroid for a more generalised flare-up, may be necessary. A change in disease-modifying therapy or stepping up to biological therapy may be indicated if the flare-up signals a loss of effect of the patient's current therapy.

# MONOARTHRITIS

## Questions

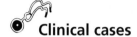 **Clinical cases**

### For each of the case scenarios given, consider the following:

**Q1**: What is the likely differential diagnosis?
**Q2**: How would you investigate this patient?
**Q3**: How would you confirm the likely diagnosis?
**Q4**: How would you initially manage the patient?
**Q5**: What are the principles of long-term management?
**Q6**: What is the prognosis?

### CASE 3.4 – **An elderly man presents with a reddened, very painful and swollen ankle of short duration.**

A 73-year-old man requires an urgent appointment for assessment of a painful left ankle. This started suddenly 2 days ago and is now so painful that he cannot put his foot to the floor. On examination, the ankle is red and significantly swollen, but the rest of his joints are unremarkable. He has a history of two episodes of pain, redness and swelling of his right big toe, which settled over 2–3 weeks with NSAIDs and rest. Currently, he is on bendroflumethiazide for treatment of hypertension but is otherwise fit and well.

### CASE 3.5 – **'It all started when my second toe swelled like a red sausage.'**

A 32-year-old woman describes a painful swelling of the second toe. This came on spontaneously 7 weeks ago. Examination of her other joints, including her back, reveals no abnormality of joint shape or function. While examining her joints, you notice scaling patches of skin with underlying erythema over her elbows and knees. She has had these for 3–4 years and has treated it as dermatitis with simple cream. More recently, she has noticed some flaking of her toenail on the end of the painful toe. The rest of the general physical examination is normal.

### CASE 3.6 – **A 50-year-old man with a painful knee.**

A 50-year-old travelling salesman presents with difficult pain in his right knee after he has been driving for more than an hour. This has been coming on for the past 3 years. He describes discomfort while walking up stairs and occasional pain in his knee in bed at night. Typically he has few symptoms earlier in the day, but his knee aches by the end of the day. On review of his musculoskeletal system, he has a history of low back pain, and pain in the ends of his fingers, the base of the thumb and big toe. He had a cartilage operation on his right knee at the age of 29 years after a football injury.

## OSCE counselling case

OSCE COUNSELLING CASE 3.2 – **'I am not keen on taking medication every day. Is there anything else I can do to help my osteoarthritis?'**

## Key concepts

To work through the core clinical cases in this section, you will need to understand the following key concepts.

Monoarthritis is usually caused by a different diagnosis from polyarthritis, although there is some overlap. Septic arthritis is typically monoarticular and therefore joint aspiration is a more important investigation in this group of patients than in patients with polyarthritis. Aspiration can both aid diagnosis and be of therapeutic value.

Septic arthritis requires prolonged antibiotic treatment, and every effort should be made to confirm the diagnosis before treatment is started. Most peripheral joints can be aspirated at the bedside; however, hip joint aspiration is usually best done with ultrasonic guidance.

Other causes of monoarthritis include osteoarthritis, crystal arthritis (e.g. gout), sarcoidosis and seronegative arthritis.

## Answers

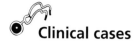
### Clinical cases

### CASE 3.4 – **An elderly man presents with a reddened, very painful and swollen ankle of short duration.**

#### A1: What is the likely differential diagnosis?

With a similar history of self-limiting arthritis in the toe and a risk factor for hyperuricaemia with diuretic therapy, the most likely diagnosis is gout. The diagnosis not to miss is septic arthritis. This could also represent an alternative crystal arthropathy or an intermittent seronegative rheumatoid arthritis.

#### A2: How would you investigate this patient?

At the time of the attack, there is typically a very high ESR or CRP, with a raised white blood cell (WBC) and platelet count. The serum urate is sometimes decreased during an acute attack, producing a falsely normal-looking serum urate level. Hyperuricaemia is common in gout but not essential, and a normal urate level does not exclude the diagnosis. Factors associated with gout include alcohol, warfarin therapy, low-dose aspirin, myeloproliferative disorders, tumour lysis, psoriasis and renal function. Tophi show up on radiographs, and gout can produce a typical pattern of joint damage, although radiological findings are not always present.

#### A3: How would you confirm the likely diagnosis?

The definitive diagnostic test would be joint aspiration of the affected joint, with demonstration of urate crystals under a polarizing microscope; appropriate microbiological assessment should also rule out sepsis. Identification of urate crystals from another larger and possibly easier to aspirate joint, tophus or bursa would be virtually diagnostic. A raised serum urate level is usual but not inevitable.

#### A4: How would you initially manage the patient?

The initial management of gout attempts to control pain and promote resolution of the acute attack. Rest is advised and patients should be well hydrated. If gout is secondary to an underlying medical problem such as renal failure, this may need addressing. Provided that there are no contraindications, medical options include NSAIDs, colchicine, and intramuscular or intra-articular steroids. If nothing else, the attack should settle spontaneously in 4 weeks.

#### A5: What are the principles of long-term management?

Prophylactic treatment should not be started until 2–3 weeks after the acute event (due to the risk of exacerbation). Once the patient has recovered from the acute attack it, may be necessary to start prophylactic treatment. The most commonly used drug is allopurinol, which is started at a low dose and titrated upwards, balanced against normalization of the hyperuricaemia. The drug is usually well tolerated but, in the event of problems such as rash and occasional leucopenia, alternatives include the uricosurics probenecid and sulfinpyrazone, febuxostat or low-dose daily colchicine. Sometimes it is necessary to use combination therapy to ensure the treatment goal of a low normal serum urate level.

### A6: What is the prognosis?

Repeated attacks of gout can damage the underlying joint. The associated hyperuricaemia may produce a nephropathy or renal stones. Provided the hyperuricaemia can be controlled by correcting the cause or using specific therapy, however, the outlook for this condition is very good.

## CASE 3.5 – 'It all started when my second toe swelled like a red sausage.'

### A1: What is the likely differential diagnosis?

The rash is likely to be psoriasis and the dactylitis is most probably associated psoriatic arthritis. Infection and gout can also produce dactylitis.

### A2: How would you investigate this patient?

Examination of the flexures and scalp may reveal additional psoriasis. Further examination of the fingernails may reveal characteristic nail pitting. A radiograph of the toe will most probably reveal little of diagnostic value but, as psoriatic arthritis is typically a chronic problem, a radiograph should be done for baseline assessment to allow future mapping of possible damage. Routine blood testing will usually reveal a raised inflammatory response.

### A3: How would you confirm the likely diagnosis?

The diagnosis is clinical, based on a picture of a distal small joint and predominantly lower limb large joint arthritis in association with, or with a history of, psoriasis. Routine testing should not point to another diagnosis. Family history is often helpful, revealing arthritis, psoriasis or inflammatory bowel disease.

### A4: How would you initially manage the patient?

The first aim should be to control the patient's pain. Anti-inflammatory medication may settle the attack; intra-articular steroid injection may also help. Some patients need to start taking DMARDs to control the problem. Anti-tumour necrosis factor (TNF) therapy can be used in patients with resistant disease.

### A5: What are the principles of long-term management?

This may represent the start of a chronic and possibly more widespread problem requiring long-term therapy. It should always be borne in mind that in the future the patient may develop associated ankylosing spondylitis, iritis, inflammatory bowel disease and genitourinary tract inflammation.

### A6: What is the prognosis?

The prognosis depends on the number of joints involved. Limited joint involvement has an excellent long-term outlook, whereas multiple joint involvement has a prognosis similar to that of chronic progressive rheumatoid arthritis.

## CASE 3.6 – A 50-year-old man with a painful knee.

### A1: What is the likely differential diagnosis?

Based on the history of previous cartilage surgery and pain on exercise at the end of the day, as well as pain in typical sites, osteoarthritis is the most likely diagnosis.

### A2: How would you investigate this patient?

The most useful single investigation would be a weight-bearing radiograph of the knee. Radiographs of the other sites may also reveal degenerative changes. Blood tests looking for alternative diagnoses may be helpful.

### A3: How would you confirm the likely diagnosis?

The absence of any other cause of arthritis and the presence of the typical radiological changes of osteoarthritis, including joint space narrowing, subchondral sclerosis, subchondral bone cysts and osteophytes, should be sufficient. Examination of the knee may demonstrate a joint effusion, decreased joint movement with discomfort, and possible crepitus.

### A4: How would you initially manage the patient?

Aspiration of the knee may ease symptoms, especially when combined with intra-articular steroid injection. Physiotherapy may relieve symptoms. Simple analgesics or NSAIDs may provide additional relief.

### A5: What are the principles of long-term management?

Osteoarthritis is not associated primarily with systemic complications but drug treatment is and therefore should be used in the lowest dose and for the shortest period possible.

### A6: What is the prognosis?

Full recovery is unlikely, and the chronic nature of the problem may threaten this man's livelihood. Consideration should be given to advice about an automatic car or possibly a change in position in his company if his symptoms cannot be helped. Surgical treatment may be necessary in the longer term but is not inevitable.

## 👥 OSCE counselling case

### OSCE COUNSELLING CASE 3.2 – 'I am not keen on taking medication every day. Is there anything else I can do to help my osteoarthritis?'

The patient's concerns about medication can sometimes be allayed by discussion about the risks and benefits of medication. Education about the nature of the condition will promote independence. Reducing obesity, minimizing traumatic activity and using padded footwear will improve the prognosis. Orthoses can improve the symptoms of foot osteoarthritis, and a walking stick can help mobility in patients with knee and hip osteoarthritis. Regular exercise aimed at improving aerobic fitness, muscle strength and proprioception will also improve mobility. Other forms of physiotherapy can be used to treat local symptoms. Many patients who dislike the idea of taking oral medication are happy to consider topical treatment in the form of NSAIDs or capsaicin. Intra-articular steroids or hyaluronic acid derivatives can also help symptoms.

# SYSTEMIC RHEUMATOLOGICAL ILLNESSES

## Questions

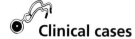

### Clinical cases

## For each of the case scenarios given, consider the following:

> **Q1**: What is the likely differential diagnosis?
> **Q2**: How would you investigate this patient?
> **Q3**: How would you confirm the likely diagnosis?
> **Q4**: How would you initially manage the patient?
> **Q5**: What are the principles of long-term management?
> **Q6**: What is the prognosis?

### CASE 3.7 – A young woman with joint pains and feeling unwell.

A 29-year-old woman presents with a 6-month history of pain and swelling, which started in the fingers and wrists and then spread to her shoulders, knees and ankles. She was treated for pleurisy twice 4 and 3 months ago, and since then says she has felt unwell. Most recently, she says that she has developed a rash on her cheeks and forehead.

### CASE 3.8 – 'You've seen me before with sinusitis. Now I feel terrible, my eye is sore and I think I coughed up blood today.'

A 49-year-old man feels unwell with temperatures, myalgia, and pain in his wrists, knees and ankles. He is losing weight and cannot work. His left eye has become increasingly sore and red. For some time he has had a cough productive of yellow/white sputum, but today he coughed up red blood. Investigations reveal a haemoglobin (Hb) of 10.8 g/dL, white cell count (WCC) of $14.8 \times 10^9$/L and ESR of 98 mm/h. Urinalysis demonstrated blood +++ and protein ++. Apart from a 3-year history of sinusitis requiring antibiotics and nasal spray, there is no significant past medical history.

### CASE 3.9 – An elderly woman with aching shoulders and thighs, a painful temporal headache and a sudden onset of sight loss in her right eye.

A 73-year-old woman describes a 3-week history of stiffness in her proximal arms and thighs, which have become increasingly painful. The pain is especially bad at night and first thing in the morning. In the past 2 days she has noticed tenderness in the scalp when combing her hair and headache over the same site. Today she awoke to realize that she had no sight in her right eye.

## 👥 OSCE counselling case

OSCE COUNSELLING CASE 3.3 – **'Will having lupus give me problems if I want to become pregnant?'**

# Key concepts

To work through the core clinical cases in this section, you will need to understand the following key concepts.

The multisystem involvement of this group of conditions, although rare in routine practice, requires all clinicians to maintain awareness of them. Involvement of systems such as the kidneys and lungs can often be silent in the early stages, requiring active screening. Many of the differential diagnoses in this group will have similar investigation findings such as a high CRP and a positive antinuclear antibody (ANA), which can be found in infection and malignancy.

The connective tissue disorders are a group of conditions including rheumatoid arthritis, systemic lupus erythematosus (SLE), Sjögren's syndrome, myositis/dermatomyositis, scleroderma and undifferentiated connective tissue disease. Although recognizably different, they share many features and should be screened for as a group.

The vasculitides are a diverse group of conditions that can be primary or secondary in nature. The primary, or systemic, vasculitides are usually classified on the basis of the size of the arteries involved:

- *large vessel:* temporal and Takayasu's vasculitis
- *medium-sized:* polyarteritis nodosa, Kawasaki's disease
- *small vessel:* Wegener's granulomatosis, Churg–Strauss syndrome, microscopic polyarteritis, Henoch–Schönlein purpura, essential cryoglobulinaemic vasculitis, leucocytoclastic vasculitis.

Secondary causes include the connective tissue diseases, infection, malignancy and allergy, e.g. drug induced.

# Answers

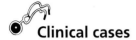

## Clinical cases

### CASE 3.7 – **A young woman with joint pains and feeling unwell.**

#### A1: What is the likely differential diagnosis?

With a symmetrical small and large joint arthritis, a systemic illness including pleurisy and a facial rash in a woman, SLE (lupus) is a possible diagnosis. Consider infection, sarcoid, vasculitis and malignancy.

#### A2: How would you investigate this patient?

A routine blood screen including FBC, ESR, U&Es and LFTs should be ordered, as well as ANA, double-stranded DNA (dsDNA) and antibodies to extractable nuclear antigen (ENA). Urinalysis looking for blood or protein should be checked. In view of the previous chest symptoms, a chest radiograph should be ordered.

#### A3: How would you confirm the likely diagnosis?

Finding a positive ANA rarely leads to a diagnosis of lupus. The diagnosis, like much of rheumatology, is clinical, and a specialist opinion usually needs to be sought to confirm it. Often the American College of Rheumatology revised diagnostic criteria are used as a basis to establish the diagnosis, which requires having four of a list of 11 typical features of the condition. Lupus is also diagnosed by demonstrating typical histological features, especially when patients do not fulfil the College diagnostic criteria.

#### A4: How would you initially manage the patient?

Once the diagnosis has been confirmed, the management depends on the extent of systemic involvement – e.g. a patient with active lupus nephritis will require more aggressive management initially than a patient who has mild arthritis and a rash. Isolated rash and arthritis can be managed with NSAIDs, hydroxychloroquine and sunblock. Systemically ill patients often require prednisolone, usually combined with immunosuppressive drugs to control their disease.

#### A5: What are the principles of long-term management?

The management of lupus requires a broad range of clinical skills and may require input from several disciplines. Patients with complex disease are best managed by clinicians with experience of the condition. Lupus can affect any system in the body, and any new symptoms should be investigated to check for possible lupus involvement. Renal, lung and cardiovascular involvement need to be screened for regularly. The use of toxic therapies can complicate matters with side effects. There is also an increased risk of infection as a result of the immunosuppressing nature of SLE and its treatments. In a young woman, future pregnancies may well need careful planning because the disease and drugs may adversely affect fertility. Pregnancy can impose additional strains on already damaged organs such as the lungs or kidneys.

## A6: What is the prognosis?

Spontaneous remission or cure is unlikely. The prognosis of lupus depends on the severity of the condition and is particularly influenced by the presence or absence of renal disease, with only 70 per cent of patients with renal disease being alive after 15 years.

## CASE 3.8 – 'You've seen me before with sinusitis. Now I feel terrible, my eye is sore and I think I coughed up blood today.'

### A1: What is the likely differential diagnosis?

With renal and upper and lower respiratory symptoms, eye inflammation, myalgia and arthralgia, and blood evidence of inflammation, systemic vasculitis is probable, and in this case Wegener's granulomatosis is the most likely subtype. Alternative diagnoses such as malignancy need to be positively ruled out.

### A2: How would you investigate this patient?

Tests should aim to assess the cause, extent and severity of the involvement. Full blood count, ESR, U&Es and LFTs may all demonstrate abnormal results. A sinus radiograph, possibly including CT, chest radiograph, 24-h urine protein loss and urine microscopy should also be performed. Testing for ANA, complements C3 and C4 and anti-neutrophil cytoplasmic antigen (ANCA) will help establish the diagnosis. Specialist ophthalmological and ear, nose and throat (ENT) assessment and treatment may be helpful. Renal or lung investigation may require specialist input.

### A3: How would you confirm the likely diagnosis?

Treatment of vasculitis is long term and typically requires long-term toxic therapy; therefore biopsy is regarded as the gold standard for diagnosis. The nasal mucosa, lung and kidney are possible sites for biopsy. A positive cytoplasmic ANCA/PR3 result is highly specific and sensitive for Wegener's granulomatosis.

### A4: How would you initially manage the patient?

Having assessed the extent of involvement, treatment typically involves an induction phase designed to arrest inflammation and a longer-term treatment phase aimed at maintaining disease suppression. Drugs commonly used are steroids, immunosuppressants and cytotoxics. Co-trimoxazole is prescribed for patients with *Staphylococcus aureus* in the nose because it is believed to reduce relapses of the condition when used in combination with other immunosuppressants.

### A5: What are the principles of long-term management?

In this patient with renal involvement, potential renal failure needs to be assessed. The lung involvement can progress to fibrosis. Involvement of the upper airways can produce aggressive local damage, even eroding through the floor of the anterior skull. Untreated eye involvement can lead to blindness. Secondary infection is a constant threat as a result of the condition or treatment. Flare-ups are not uncommon, often requiring temporary increases in treatment.

### A6: What is the prognosis?

A medical cure is not possible. Long-term follow-up with careful multisystem assessment is essential to maximize the success of treatment. The prognosis is adversely affected by renal involvement; overall, the 10-year survival rate is about 80 per cent.

## CASE 3.9 – **An elderly woman with aching shoulders and thighs, a painful temporal headache and a sudden onset of sight loss in her right eye.**

### A1:  What is the likely differential diagnosis?

The history of polymyalgic symptoms, temporal headache and sudden onset of blindness strongly suggests a diagnosis of temporal arteritis.

### A2:  How would you investigate this patient?

This is a rare example of a rheumatological emergency. Consideration should be given to whether ordering tests will delay the introduction of prednisolone. After just 48 h of prednisolone therapy, the typical blood findings of a highly raised ESR and the characteristic biopsy evidence will disappear. Prompt initiation of steroids, however, may promote return of vision in the affected eye and should preserve vision in the non-affected eye.

### A3:  How would you confirm the likely diagnosis?

The definitive test is biopsy of an affected temporal artery. As a result of the irregular pattern of vessel involvement, single biopsy may be falsely negative in up to 30 per cent of patients.

### A4:  How would you initially manage the patient?

The initial management involves high-dose prednisolone, typically 40 mg/day or more. As treatment will last for more than 3 months, the patient should be commenced on bone protection therapy with a bisphosphonate and calcium and vitamin D3.

### A5:  What are the principles of long-term management?

The longer-term management involves reducing the steroids, balancing them against the recurrence of symptoms such as headache and proximal myalgia and a raised ESR. Most patients will eventually be able to come off steroids. If it is not possible to reduce the maintenance steroid dose, it may be necessary to commence steroid-sparing drugs such as azathioprine or methotrexate.

### A6:  What is the prognosis?

Blindness occurs in up to 15 per cent of patients with this condition. The mortality is not raised compared with a matched population, even though aortic aneurysm and cerebral and myocardial infarction are rare complications of the condition.

**OSCE counselling case**

## OSCE COUNSELLING CASE 3.3 – 'Will having lupus give me problems if I want to become pregnant?'

Having lupus can affect pregnancy in a number of ways. Overall, lupus increases the risk of a conception not progressing to term from the normal 10 per cent to 25 per cent. Antiphospholipid antibody syndrome increases the risk of miscarriage. Women who have Ro and La antibody-associated lupus have an approximately 5 per cent chance of transplacental spread of antibodies, producing neonatal lupus, which can include neonatal heart block. Renal and pulmonary disease can be complicated by pregnancy. Finally, many of the drugs used to treat lupus may adversely affect fertility.

# BACK PAIN

## Questions

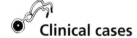

### Clinical cases

## For each of the case scenarios given, consider the following:

> **Q1**: What is the likely differential diagnosis?
> **Q2**: How would you investigate this patient?
> **Q3**: How would you confirm the likely diagnosis?
> **Q4**: How would you initially manage the patient?
> **Q5**: What are the principles of long-term management?
> **Q6**: What is the prognosis?

### CASE 3.10 – **A sudden onset of back pain in an elderly woman.**

A 72-year-old woman describes an acute onset of mid-back pain. She has not had anything like this before and presents to the accident and emergency (A&E) department. There was no obvious precipitant for her back problem. A radiograph reveals a wedge fracture of T8.

### CASE 3.11 – **A stiff painful back and a red eye.**

An ophthalmologist recommends a 26-year-old man to seek an opinion about his long history of back pain and stiffness after developing a red and painful left eye.

**OSCE counselling case**

OSCE COUNSELLING CASE 3.4 – **'What can I do to prevent osteoporotic fractures in the future?'**

## 🔑 Key concepts

To work through the core clinical cases in this section, you will need to understand the following key concepts.

Most adults will suffer back pain at some stage, but for many people it is a chronic problem. For this group of patients, reassurance, active support and advice to mobilize early and not expect a complete cure are important if disability is to be avoided. Patients under the age of 25 years or over the age of 55 years who present with constant back pain of longer than 6 weeks' duration usually require radiological assessment. A history of malignancy, pain that wakes the patient, demonstrable motor weakness, bowel or bladder involvement and associated systemic involvement suggest significant pathology that may require more than just a simple radiograph.

## Answers

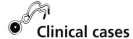 **Clinical cases**

### CASE 3.10 – **A sudden onset of back pain in an elderly woman.**

#### A1: What is the likely differential diagnosis?

A spontaneous osteoporotic fracture of the spine is the probable diagnosis. Other causes of a fracture include trauma, infection and malignancy. Women generally have a lower bone stock than men and with increasing age are prone to develop osteoporosis. The condition can be secondary to a number of medical conditions, including chronic obstructive pulmonary disease (COPD), malabsorption, inflammatory arthritis, steroid use, premature menopause, hyperparathyroidism, hyperthyroidism, chronic renal failure, immobility and autoimmune arthritis.

#### A2: How would you investigate this patient?

A history should be taken to look for the above risk factors, and for a past history of other low trauma fractures. Blood testing should be normal in primary osteoporosis, but it is important to rule out secondary causes of osteoporosis and alternative diagnoses. Family history is a very important risk factor for osteoporosis.

#### A3: How would you confirm the likely diagnosis?

The gold standard for diagnosis is a dual-energy X-ray absorptiometry (DEXA) scan of the lumbar spine and hip. Other techniques exist, including qualitative computed tomography (QCT), peripheral DEXA scan and ultrasonography of the heel. A DEXA scan of the spine and hip is best at predicting hip fracture and is sensitive and specific enough to allow monitoring of therapy. In this case, provided that no alternative diagnoses are present, it is not necessary to scan the woman to justify starting medication.

#### A4: How would you initially manage the patient?

Pain control is the first goal of management. Typically this will require opiate-based treatment and advice about rest. The pain normally settles progressively over 12 weeks. Calcitonin injections or nasal spray can be used in the first week after a fracture to augment pain control. The use of transcutaneous electronerve stimulation can augment pain control. Surgery, although still at an early stage of development, can be used to reform the vertebrae and reduce pain.

#### A5: What are the principles of long-term management?

The fracture, although painful, rarely produces neurological deficit. The principal risk is that having one osteoporotic fracture is a strong risk for future fractures. Further vertebral fracture can produce a fixed kyphosis. Fracture of the hip is the most serious of the osteoporosis-associated fractures; up to one-third of patients may die and only one-third of patients will return to an independent existence after the fracture. Treatment involves bisphosphonates and usually calcium and vitamin D3. Further fractures despite appropriate treatment with bisphosphonates may require treatment with a parathyroid hormone (PTH) analogue or denosumab, a monoclonal antibody treatment.

#### A6: What is the prognosis?

Treatment of osteoporosis needs to be linked to a fall-prevention strategy to maximize the longer-term outlook. Successful treatment reduces the risk of future fracture by half.

## CASE 3.11 – **A stiff painful back and a red eye.**

### A1: What is the likely differential diagnosis?

The connection to make is iritis and ankylosing spondylitis. It is possible that no connection exists, in which case in a young person the cause of the back pain could be mechanical, post-traumatic, associated with disc disease or developmental.

### A2: How would you investigate this patient?

A blood screen may demonstrate raised inflammatory markers. A radiograph may demonstrate sclerosis and erosion of the sacroiliac joint and squaring of the vertebrae, with calcification of the intervertebral ligaments. Magnetic resonance imaging can demonstrate changes not visible on a radiograph. An isotope bone scan can detect inflammation in the sacroiliac joint or lower back.

### A3: How would you confirm the likely diagnosis?

Demonstration of the typical radiological changes, although not present in every case, is diagnostic. The presence of the human leucocyte antigen HLA-B27 gene is not diagnostic because it is found in at least 7 per cent of the general population. Its absence, however, virtually rules out ankylosing spondylitis.

### A4: How would you initially manage the patient?

The principal mode of treatment of mild to moderate forms of the disease is physiotherapy. This can be augmented by NSAIDs; phenylbutazone, banned from general use, still has a place for pain relief in this condition. Methotrexate and sulfasalazine, although helpful for peripheral disease, do not influence axial disease significantly. More aggressive ankylosing spondylitis not responding to the above measures can be treated with anti-TNF therapies.

### A5: What are the principles of long-term management?

The more the spine is involved in ankylosis, the more complications can occur, including the mechanical effects of kyphosis or ankylosis of the ribs producing respiratory restriction, and a risk of fracture as a result of associated osteoporosis and the altered mechanics of the stiff spine. It is possible to develop an associated peripheral arthritis, psoriasis, iritis, colitis and inflammation of the genitourinary tract. Rarely, associated cardiac and pulmonary complications can occur.

### A6: What is the prognosis?

Long-term surveillance aims to detect the complications of this chronic illness early. An essential part of follow-up also involves the monitoring of compliance with physiotherapy. The prognosis is adversely affected by age of onset before 16 years, early hip involvement, raised CRP and peripheral joint involvement.

#  OSCE counselling case

## OSCE COUNSELLING CASE 3.4 – 'What can I do to prevent osteoporotic fractures in the future?'

About 70 per cent of the risk of developing osteoporosis is genetic, but a number of factors are important. Lifestyle measures such as refraining from smoking, keeping alcohol consumption within recommended limits and maintaining a healthy body mass index (BMI) are beneficial. Calcium intake equivalent to 800 mg/day is important throughout adult life. The use of vitamin D3 supplementation in frail elderly people is associated with a reduced incidence of hip fractures. Levels of exercise in childhood and adolescence are one of the determining factors of peak bone mass. In later life, regular exercise reduces bone loss and decreases the incidence of falls. In elderly people who are at risk, the use of hip protectors may reduce the incidence of hip fractures. Premature menopause is a risk factor for osteoporosis, and the use of hormone replacement therapy (HRT) delays the onset of menopausal bone loss until therapy is stopped. This translates into a lifetime fracture reduction risk of about 3 per cent. In people with risk factors, a DEXA scan can be used to assess bone density, and appropriate therapy can reduce the risk of future fracture.

## REVISION PANEL

- Rapid diagnosis and early commencement of combination therapy and possibly biological drugs improve the prognosis in rheumatoid arthritis.
- Blood tests and X-rays are typically normal in early osteoarthritis.
- Hypermobility is a common cause of recurrent intermittent joint pain in young teenagers.
- Flare-ups of underlying autoimmune arthritis often signal the need to increase treatment.
- Gout presents with intermittent severe arthritis, often affecting the big toe joint, and is usually associated with a raised serum urate level.
- Dactylitis, a swollen digit, is classically associated with psoriatic arthritis or gout, but rarely it may be a sign of infection.
- An isolated positive ANA result is rarely associated with lupus (SLE). The diagnosis is based on characteristic clinical and investigational results.
- Systemic vasculitis is rare, but recognition and appropriate treatment are important to reduce mortality. Most patients are systemically unwell and have signs that can be confused with infection. Early major organ involvement can be silent and needs active screening to detect.
- Giant cell arteritis requires urgent diagnosis and commencement of high-dose steroids to reduce the risk of blindness.
- Osteoporosis is generally asymptomatic until a patient fractures something. Pre-fracture diagnosis is most frequently made with a DEXA scan. Treatment can significantly reduce the future risk of fracture.
- Ankylosing spondylitis usually develops in young males who nearly always possess the HLA-B27 gene. Be aware, however, that this gene is relatively common and having it only rarely leads to ankylosing spondylitis.

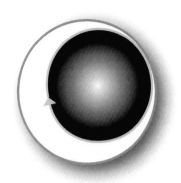

# 4 Renal medicine

*Indranil Dasgupta*

## RENAL EMERGENCIES

## RENAL CASE STUDIES

## CHRONIC KIDNEY DISEASE

# RENAL EMERGENCIES

## Questions

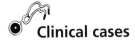

### Clinical cases

## For each of the case scenarios given, consider the following:

**Q1**: What is the likely diagnosis?
**Q2**: What investigations would be performed?
**Q3**: What would be the initial management?
**Q4**: What would be the long-term management?

### CASE 4.1 – A 60-year-old man presenting with diarrhoea, vomiting and renal impairment.

A 60-year-old man, previously fit and well, presents to the accident and emergency (A&E) department with a 1-week history of diarrhoea and vomiting. He is unwell, clammy, his skin turgor is poor, his pulse is 120/min and his blood pressure is 80/60 mmHg. Initial investigations show serum sodium of 126 mmol/L, potassium of 3.0 mmol/L, urea of 28 mmol/L and creatinine of 306 μmol/L (estimated glomerular filtration rate [eGFR] 19 mL/min/1.73 m$^2$).

### CASE 4.2 – A 72-year-old man presenting with hyperkalaemia.

A 72-year-old man has been referred by his general practitioner (GP) to the emergency assessment unit with a history of being non-specifically unwell for 2 days. He has a past history of ischaemic heart disease, atrial fibrillation, congestive cardiac failure and stable chronic kidney disease (CKD). His regular medications include isosorbide mononitrate, digoxin, furosemide, spironolactone and an angiotensin-converting enzyme (ACE) inhibitor. On examination, the patient is mildly confused, dehydrated, peripherally cold, bradycardic and hypotensive (blood pressure 96/60 mmHg). His initial blood tests show a sodium of 130 mmol/L, potassium of 7.2 mmol/L, urea of 42 mmol/L and creatinine of 412 μmol/L (eGFR 14 mL/min/1.73 m$^2$).

### CASE 4.3 – A 68-year-old woman with chronic kidney disease (CKD) presenting with shortness of breath.

A 68-year-old woman, known to have CKD, has presented to the A&E department with acute shortness of breath. Computer records suggest that her most recent serum creatinine from about a month earlier was 256 μmol/L (eGFR 21 mL/min) and her regular medication includes furosemide 80 mg daily. She has recently been commenced on a non-steroidal anti-inflammatory drug (NSAID) for arthritis. On examination, she has oedema up to the mid-thighs, jugular venous pressure (JVP) is raised at 6 cm, and there are crackles in both lung bases up to the mid-zones. Her admission electrocardiogram (ECG) does not show any ischaemic changes. Her urea and electrolytes (U&Es) results show: sodium 138 mmol/L, potassium 5.6 mmol/L, urea 38 mmol/L and creatinine 446 μmol/L (eGFR 12 mL/min/1.73 m$^2$).

## CASE 4.4 – **A 34-year-old man presenting with severe hypertension and renal impairment.**

A 34-year-old man of African Caribbean origin has been referred by his GP for severe hypertension. On examination, his blood pressure is 240/140 mmHg, he is slightly confused, there is mild pedal oedema, there are a few basal crackles, and neurological examination is normal except for bilateral papilloedema. Urine analysis shows blood ++ and protein ++. His haemoglobin is 10.2 g/dL and U&Es show sodium 136 mmol/L, potassium 3.0 mmol/L, urea 14 mmol/L and creatinine 206 μmol/L (eGFR 54 mL/min/1.73 m²).

# Key concepts

## COMMON CAUSES OF ACUTE KIDNEY INJURY (AKI)

- *Pre-renal* – due to ineffective perfusion of kidneys that are structurally normal:
  - hypovolaemia – blood loss, gastrointestinal loss, burns
  - low cardiac output states
  - shock
  - certain drugs – NSAIDs, ACE inhibitors.
- *Renal* – structural damage to glomeruli and tubules:
  - acute tubular necrosis (ATN) – most common cause (45 per cent), results from prolonged hypoperfusion (as above)
  - acute glomerulonephritis and vasculitis
  - acute interstitial nephritis – idiopathic, drugs, infection
  - vascular disease.
- *Post-renal* – due to urinary tract obstruction:

  - prostatic hypertrophy
  - bladder tumour
  - gynaecological malignancy
  - neuropathic bladder.

## INVESTIGATIONS TO ORGANIZE IN AKI

- *Urine:*
  - dipstick (blood and protein suggest acute glomerulonephritis)
  - microscopy (red blood cell [RBC] casts diagnostic of acute glomerulonephritis)
  - urine electrolytes (to distinguish pre-renal failure from ATN).
- *Blood:*
  - FBC, clotting (for disseminated intravascular coagulation [DIC], rarely haemolytic uraemic syndrome/thrombotic thrombocytopenic purpura [TTP])
  - U&Es, calcium and $PO_4$, glucose, creatine kinase (for rhabdomyolysis), CRP (for vasculitis, sepsis)
  - immunology – autoantibodies (for systemic lupus erythematosus, [SLE]), anti-neutrophil cytoplasmic antigen (ANCA; for vasculitis), anti-glomerular basement membrane (GBM) antibodies (for Goodpasture's disease), complements (low in SLE and infective endocarditis), immunoglobulins (for immunoglobulin A [IgA] nephropathy, myeloma)
  - blood cultures (sepsis, infective endocarditis), hepatitis B and C (in preparation for dialysis).
- *ECG* – for hyperkalaemic changes.
- *Chest X-ray* – for pulmonary oedema, pneumonia.
- *Abdominal ultrasound* – to exclude urinary obstruction.

## INDICATIONS FOR URGENT DIALYSIS IN AKI

- severe hyperkalaemia (>6.5 mmol/L or less with ECG changes, despite medical treatment)
- pulmonary oedema
- severe acidosis (pH <7.1)
- severe uraemia (vomiting, encephalopathy)
- uraemic pericarditis.

Overall mortality in AKI is about 50 per cent (up to 80 per cent in patients who require dialysis).

## Answers

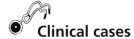

### Clinical cases

### CASE 4.1 – **A 60-year-old man presenting with diarrhoea, vomiting and renal impairment.**

#### A1: What is the likely diagnosis?

The likely diagnosis is pre-renal failure or ATN due to reduced circulatory blood volume secondary to diarrhoea and vomiting. Loss of circulatory volume, due to either salt and water depletion or haemorrhage, leads to reduced renal blood supply. This results in selective cortical vasoconstriction and oliguria (urine output <400 mL/day). Initially this is reversible, but when prolonged it leads to ATN (ischaemic injury to the proximal tubular epithelial cells) and rarely to acute cortical necrosis.

#### A2: What investigations would be performed?

Urinalysis (dipstick test for blood and protein), urine microscopy, urine electrolytes, FBC, and serum bicarbonate, calcium and phosphate levels need to be done. The presence of a significant amount of blood and protein (++ or more) would raise a suspicion of acute glomerulonephritis. Urine sodium below 20 mmol/L would suggest reversible pre-renal failure, while urine sodium above 40 mmol/L would suggest ATN has set in. Low haemoglobin or a raised serum phosphate may indicate the presence of pre-existing CKD.

#### A3: What would be the initial management?

Intravenous (IV) access and an IV infusion should be set up immediately. The ideal fluid replacement in this setting would be normal saline with potassium supplementation. In the presence of severe metabolic acidosis, sodium bicarbonate (1.26%) infusion should be considered. It is preferable to transfer the patient to a high-dependency unit with a view to establishing central venous access to monitor central venous pressure (CVP). Pulse, blood pressure and urine output should be monitored hourly. In the absence of CVP monitoring, lung bases should be auscultated frequently to prevent overhydration leading to pulmonary oedema. Urea and electrolytes should be repeated in 4–6 h to review progress.

#### A4: What would be the long-term management?

Pre-renal failure is a rapidly reversible condition. In established AKI (formerly known as acute renal failure [ARF]) due to ATN, it may take as long as 6 weeks for renal function to return to normal; the patient will require dialysis treatment for this period (1 per cent of patients require long-term dialysis). If the patient is haemodynamically compromised, an initial period of continuous veno-venous haemofiltration (CVVH) may be necessary (generally in the intensive care unit). If renal function does not improve within 24 h, an ultrasound scan should be requested to exclude urinary tract obstruction. Small shrunken kidneys on ultrasound scan would suggest that the patient suffers from CKD.

### CASE 4.2 – **A 72-year-old man presenting with hyperkalaemia.**

#### A1: What is the likely diagnosis?

The likely diagnosis is severe hyperkalaemia due to a combination of a potassium-sparing diuretic and an ACE inhibitor in the setting of chronic renal impairment. There is also a possible acute-on-chronic renal impairment due to over-diuresis, as evidenced by a disproportionately high blood urea level and low sodium.

## A2: What investigations would be performed?

A 12-lead ECG should be done to see if there are any changes of hyperkalaemia – tall-peaked T-waves, widening of QRS, reduction in height of P- (may disappear) and R-waves, and sine wave pattern (pre-cardiac arrest).

## A3: What would be the initial management?

Severe hyperkalaemia (>6.5 mmol/L) and the presence of ECG changes in this scenario warrant urgent treatment of hyperkalaemia, as follows:

- calcium gluconate – 10 mL of 10% IV over 5 min to counteract the adverse effect of hyperkalaemia on the cardiac conduction system (through central line or large cannula in a big vein to avoid delay)
- infusion of 10 u insulin in 50 mL of 50% glucose IV through a pump over 30 min to drive $K^+$ into intracellular space
- nebulized salbutamol – 5 mg to help $K^+$ enter intracellular space
- sodium bicarbonate – 50 mL of 8.4% IV over 30 min should be considered, especially if acidotic (*caution:* may precipitate tetany if the serum calcium is low)
- Calcium Resonium® – 30 g by rectum or 15 g orally to help exchange $K^+$ for $Ca^{2+}$ in the gut
- check U&Es in 2 h and repeat glucose and insulin infusion and nebulized salbutamol if serum potassium remains dangerously high (>6.5 mmol/L) or ECG changes persist
- if serum potassium remains above 6.5 mmol/mL or ECG changes persist despite treatment, haemodialysis may be required
- IV infusion of normal saline to correct dehydration.

## A4: What would be the long-term management?

The ACE inhibitor and spironolactone must be stopped. Refer the patient to a nephrologist for long-term management. If renal function returns to near baseline, the ACE inhibitor may be restarted cautiously in the future if clinically indicated, i.e. poor left ventricular function on echocardiography. The patient should be followed up closely, preferably in the renal clinic.

## CASE 4.3 – **A 68-year-old woman with chronic kidney disease (CKD) presenting with shortness of breath.**

### A1: What is the likely diagnosis?

This patient's severe shortness of breath is likely to be due to pulmonary oedema secondary to severe fluid retention. Acute deterioration in renal function has probably been precipitated by the recent introduction of an NSAID. Non-steroidal anti-inflammatory drugs reduce renal blood flow in patients with pre-existing renal disease and thereby cause deterioration of renal function. They can also cause acute interstitial nephritis, leading to acute renal impairment.

### A2: What investigations would be performed?

A chest X-ray should be done to confirm the diagnosis of pulmonary oedema (Figure 4.1). Arterial blood gas analysis should be done to assess the degree of hypoxia, to ascertain whether there is any evidence of $CO_2$ retention, and to assess the degree of metabolic acidosis associated with renal failure.

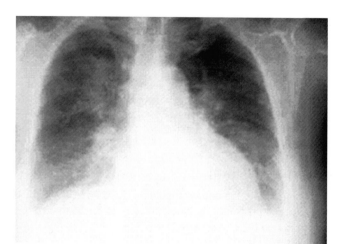

**Figure 4.1** Chest radiograph for Case 4.3.

## A3: What would be the initial management?

The initial management is furosemide 80 mg IV. If there is no significant diuresis, furosemide should be repeated using a higher dose (up to 250 mg IV). High-concentration oxygen should be given with a facemask. It may be necessary to use continuous positive airway pressure (CPAP) or even to ventilate the patient in intensive care if she is severely hypoxic or gets tired. If the patient remains severely short of breath and oligoanuric despite high-dose IV furosemide, she will need to be referred for urgent haemodialysis or haemofiltration.

## A4: What would be the long-term management?

Long-term management will depend on whether the patient's renal function returns to or near baseline after stopping the NSAID. If her renal function improves, long-term management will consist of salt and fluid restriction, high-dose oral diuretic therapy, and avoidance of nephrotoxic agents. The patient will need to be prepared for dialysis treatment. If her renal function fails to improve, she will require acute dialysis, leading to long-term dialysis treatment.

## CASE 4.4 – **A 34-year-old man presenting with severe hypertension and renal impairment.**

### A1: What is the likely diagnosis?

The likely diagnosis is malignant hypertension. Malignant hypertension is defined as severe hypertension, often above 200/140 mmHg, which is associated with papilloedema, usually accompanied by retinal haemorrhage and exudates, with or without renal impairment or neurological symptoms. It most commonly occurs in patients with long-standing uncontrolled hypertension. Differential diagnosis of this patient would be acute glomerulonephritis with severe hypertension.

### A2: What investigations would be performed?

A chest X-ray must be done to confirm or exclude pulmonary oedema. If confusion persists or deteriorates (deteriorating Glasgow coma score, [GCS]), an urgent computed tomography (CT) scan of the brain should be done to exclude infarction or haemorrhage.

## A3: What would be the initial management?

Controlled lowering of blood pressure should be attempted with IV infusion of labetalol (a combined alpha- and beta-adrenergic blocker) or sodium nitroprusside (a combined arteriolar and venous dilator). The goal is to lower blood pressure by 10 per cent in the first hour and by 10–15 per cent in the next 2–6 hours (to around 160/100 mmHg at 6h). Rapid lowering of blood pressure may lead to cerebral vasospasm, resulting in cerebral infarction. The patient should, ideally, be treated in a high-dependency unit. If parenteral antihypertensive agents are not available, oral agents may be used, but their use (especially sublingual nifedipine) is associated with the risk of rapid lowering of blood pressure, leading to stroke or myocardial infarction.

## A4: What would be the long-term management?

Once the blood pressure is controlled, the patient should be switched to oral antihypertensive therapy after 6–12 h, with gradual reduction of diastolic blood pressure to 85–90 mmHg over a few weeks. The patient should be investigated for a secondary cause of hypertension. Renal biopsy is indicated if renal function fails to stabilize with blood pressure control. Long-term follow-up is needed for careful monitoring of renal function and strict control of blood pressure, as renal function may deteriorate progressively to end-stage renal failure (ESRF).

# RENAL CASE STUDIES

## Questions

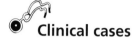

### Clinical cases

## For each of the case scenarios given, consider the following:

> **Q1**: What is the likely diagnosis?
> **Q2**: How would you investigate this patient?
> **Q3**: How would you manage this patient?
> **Q4**: What is the prognosis?

### CASE 4.5 – A 22-year-old woman presenting with progressive swelling of the legs.

A 22-year-old white European woman presents to her GP with progressive swelling of her legs of 2 weeks' duration. She is otherwise asymptomatic. On examination, she has oedema up to both knees and her blood pressure is 120/70 mmHg. Urinalysis reveals +++ proteins but no blood, serum creatinine is 92 µmol/L and serum albumin is 18 g/L.

### CASE 4.6 – A 34-year-old man presenting with microscopic haematuria.

A 34-year-old man is found to have microscopic haematuria on an insurance medical examination. He is asymptomatic. His blood pressure is 124/80 mmHg and his serum creatinine is 102 µmol/L.

### CASE 4.7 – A 62-year-old woman presenting with raised serum creatinine, microscopic haematuria and proteinuria.

A 62-year-old woman presents to her GP with symptoms of tiredness, lethargy, aching joints, poor appetite and nausea of 4–6 weeks' duration. Physical examination is unremarkable, except for pallor and a blood pressure of 160/100 mmHg. Routine blood tests reveal a haemoglobin of 10 g/dL, blood urea of 26 mmol/L and serum creatinine of 386 µmol/L (eGFR 14 mL/min/1.73 m²). The patient is referred to the local hospital. Further examination reveals purpuric spots on both legs and +++ blood and +++ protein on urinalysis.

### CASE 4.8 – A 76-year-old man presenting with dysuria and nocturia.

A 76-year-old man presents to his GP with a history of difficulty in passing urine in the form of hesitancy, poor stream and occasional pain of 3 months' duration. He also has nocturia. Physical examination is unremarkable. Urinalysis shows the presence of + blood and + protein. Blood testing shows a raised serum creatinine of 560 µmol/L (eGFR 11 mL/min/1.73 m²). The patient is urgently referred to the nearby district general hospital. Further examination in the hospital reveals a palpable bladder and a smoothly enlarged prostate on rectal examination.

## CASE 4.9 – **A 58-year-old man with raised serum creatinine.**

A 58-year-old South Asian man is found to have a raised serum creatinine of 156 μmol/L (reference range 60–120 μmol/L). He has been on antihypertensive treatment for 10 years and a smoker for 40 years. He is on nifedipine, atenolol and simvastatin. His serum creatinine was 121 μmol/L a year ago.

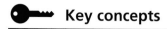

## Key concepts

To work through the core clinical cases in this section, you will need to understand the following.

### RELATIONSHIP BETWEEN SERUM CREATININE AND GLOMERULAR FILTRATION RATE
See Figure 4.2.

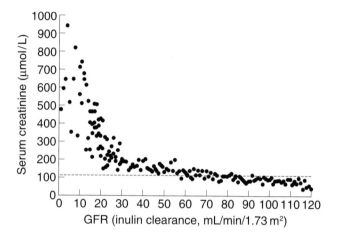

**Figure 4.2** Relationship between serum creatinine and glomerular filtration rate (GFR). Serum creatinine remains normal until GFR is about 60 mL/min.

### FORMULAE FOR CALCULATING CREATININE CLEARANCE AND GFR
### Cockroft–Gault formula – creatinine clearance (mL/min)
*Males:* creatinine clearance = [1.23×(140−age)×weight]/[creatinine]
*Females:* creatinine clearance = [1.04×(140−age)×weight]/[creatinine]

### MDRD formula – GFR (mL/min/1.73 m$^2$)
*Males:* GFR = 186×([creatinine]/88.4)$^{-1.154}$×age$^{-0.203}$
*Females:* GFR = 138×([creatinine]/88.4)$^{-1.154}$×age$^{-0.203}$
Multiply by 1.21 if the patient is African Caribbean.

### STAGES OF CHRONIC KIDNEY DISEASE
See Table 4.1.

**Table 4.1** Stages of chronic kidney disease – updated classification

| Stage* | GFR (mL/min/1.73m$^2$) | Description |
| --- | --- | --- |
| 1 | ≥90 | Kidney damage with normal or high GFR |
| 2 | 60–89 | Mild |
| 3A | 59–45 | Moderate |
| 3B | 44–30 | Moderate |
| 4 | 29–15 | Severe |
| 5 | <15 | End-stage kidney failure or on dialysis |

*Add the suffix p to denote significant proteinuria.
Adapted from the National Institute for Health and Clinical Excellence CKD Guidelines (2008).

## COMMON CAUSES OF END-STAGE RENAL FAILURE

Diabetes is the most common cause of ESRF, accounting for about 24 per cent of cases in England and Wales (nearly 50 per cent in the USA). The other main causes are glomerulonephritis (12 per cent), pyelonephritis (8 per cent), renovascular disease (7 per cent), hypertension (6 per cent) and adult polycystic kidney disease (7 per cent) (UK Renal Registry, 2009). In a fifth of patients in England and Wales, the aetiology is uncertain because these patients present late, when it is difficult to establish a primary renal diagnosis.

## Answers

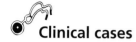

### Clinical cases

### CASE 4.5 – **A 22-year-old woman presenting with progressive swelling of the legs.**

#### A1: What is the diagnosis?

The diagnosis is nephrotic syndrome, defined as the presence of oedema, heavy proteinuria (>3 g/day) and hypoalbuminaemia with or without hypercholesterolaemia and hypertension.

The most common cause of nephrotic syndrome is minimal-change nephropathy, especially in children. In adults, membranous nephropathy and focal segmental glomerulosclerosis (FSGS) are also common causes of nephrotic syndrome. In as many as 30 per cent of patients, nephrotic syndrome is due to a systemic disease such as diabetes mellitus, SLE, amyloidosis or multiple myeloma.

#### A2: What further investigations would you do?

The patient should be referred to a nephrologist for a renal biopsy. Blood sugar and lipids should be checked. Blood should be sent off for immunological tests such as antinuclear antibodies (ANA), complements, serum immunoglobulins and cryoglobulins.

#### A3: How would you manage this patient?

Management depends on the findings of the renal biopsy. Minimal-change disease is treated with high-dose prednisolone (1 mg/kg, maximum 80 mg/day). This is continued until 1 week after remission (which may take up to 16 weeks). The dose is then reduced gradually, with a view to stopping between 8 and 12 weeks. Sometimes FSGS responds to a prolonged course of corticosteroids. Patients with resistant and relapsing disease are treated with ciclosporin. Membranous nephropathy with deteriorating kidney function is often treated with ciclosporin or a chemotherapeutic agent such as cyclophosphamide or chlorambucil. Oedema is treated with salt restriction and loop diuretics. Severely nephrotic patients are treated with heparin and admitted to hospital to prevent venous thromboembolism. An ACE inhibitor is often used to treat hypertension and reduce proteinuria. Hypercholesterolaemia should be treated with a statin.

#### A4: What is the prognosis?

Minimal-change nephrotic syndrome in children responds promptly to high-dose corticosteroid therapy. In adults, it does not always respond to corticosteroids as quickly and often relapses. Membranous nephropathy spontaneously remits in up to 25 per cent of patients but progresses to ESRF in about 40 per cent of patients at 15 years. In about 50 per cent of patients, FSGS leads to ESRF and often recurs in transplanted kidney.

### CASE 4.6 – **A 34-year-old man presenting with microscopic haematuria.**

#### A1: What is the diagnosis?

The diagnosis is isolated microscopic haematuria. The most common causes of this in young people are IgA nephropathy and thin basement membrane disease. IgA nephropathy is the most common form of glomerulonephritis and is characterized by deposition of IgA in the mesangium. Thin basement membrane disease is a familial condition characterized by uniform thinning of the glomerular basement membrane. The other causes of microscopic haematuria are stones, cystic diseases of the kidney, tumour and inflammatory diseases of the urinary tract. Urological causes predominate in older patients.

## A2: What further investigations would you do?

Urinalysis needs to be repeated, as transient microscopic haematuria may not be significant. The presence of significant proteinuria (++ or more) may signify a more aggressive from of glomerulonephritis. Ideally, urine should be sent for microscopy to ensure there are two or more RBCs per high-power field. Dipsticks are very sensitive and often detect less significant haematuria, haemoglobin and myoglobin. An ultrasound scan of the kidneys and urinary tracts should be done to exclude a macroscopic pathology. Serum immunoglobulins, complements, autoantibodies and ANCA should be checked. A raised serum IgA level will support a diagnosis of IgA nephropathy. Normal autoantibody, complement and ANCA tests suggest that an underlying autoimmune disease or vasculitis is unlikely. If there is significant proteinuria (>1 g/day), renal biopsy is indicated to exclude acute glomerulonephritis. In older patients with microscopic haematuria, a flexible cystoscopy should be carried out to exclude bladder pathology.

## A3: How would you manage this patient?

No specific treatment is indicated. The patient should be followed up on a regular basis – perhaps annually – for measurement of blood pressure, urinalysis and serum creatinine. Should the patient develop significant proteinuria or there is a rise in serum creatinine, renal biopsy should be considered. If the patient develops hypertension, it should be treated, preferably with an ACE inhibitor.

## A4: What is the prognosis?

Prognosis is usually good. IgA nephropathy rarely progresses to advanced renal failure in the absence of significant proteinuria, hypertension or raised serum creatinine at presentation. Thin basement membrane disease rarely causes proteinuria, renal impairment or hypertension.

## CASE 4.7 – A 62-year-old woman presenting with raised serum creatinine, microscopic haematuria and proteinuria.

### A1: What is the diagnosis?

The diagnosis is acute glomerulonephritis possibly associated with systemic vasculitis.

### A2: What further investigations would you do?

Urine microscopy should be done – the presence of RBC casts will support the diagnosis of acute glomerulonephritis. Blood should be sent off for immunological tests including ANCA, anti-GBM antibodies, ANA, immunoglobulins and complements. A positive ANCA test will support a diagnosis of systemic vasculitis (cytoplasmic ANCA [cANCA] is associated with Wagener's granulomatosis; perinuclear ANCA [pANCA] is associated with microscopic polyangiitis). A positive ANA (especially anti-double-stranded DNA [dsDNA]) with low complements supports a diagnosis of lupus nephritis. Raised ant-GBM antibody titre suggests Goodpasture's disease. Chest X-ray should be requested to look for consolidation, cavitation or pulmonary haemorrhage, supporting a diagnosis of either systemic vasculitis or anti-GBM disease. An ultrasound scan of the kidneys should be done. Renal biopsy will confirm the diagnosis of acute glomerulonephritis.

[This 'real' patient had a positive cANCA test, and renal biopsy showed the presence of acute necrotizing crescentic glomerulonephritis.]

### A3: How would you manage this patient?

Immunosuppressive treatment is initiated after confirmation of diagnosis by a renal biopsy. If the patient is too ill to biopsy, a presumptive diagnosis is made based on clinical features and a positive ANCA test. The standard immunosuppressive regime consists of oral prednisolone (1 mg/kg/day, maximum 80 mg/day) and cyclophosphamide (2 mg/kg/day). Intravenous pulsed methyl prednisolone or plasma exchange is used for induction of remission in patients with aggressive (life- or organ-threatening) disease. After 2 weeks, the dose of prednisolone is reduced gradually to 15 mg at 3 months and 10 mg at 6 months. To minimize the side effects with prolonged use, cyclophosphamide is changed after 3 months to azathioprine for maintenance treatment. Because of the risk of relapse (30–50 per cent at 3–5 years), long-term maintenance treatment using small doses of prednisolone and azathioprine is often continued.

### A4: What is the prognosis?

Untreated systemic vasculitis is associated with high mortality (90 per cent at 2 years). Immunosuppressive treatment, as described above, leads to control of the disease in 80–90 per cent of patients. Pulmonary haemorrhage and dialysis dependence at presentation are poor prognostic features. As a rule, patients who require dialysis treatment at presentation are less likely to have significant improvement in their kidney function.

## CASE 4.8 – **A 76-year-old man presenting with dysuria and nocturia.**

### A1: What is the diagnosis?

The diagnosis is acute or acute-on-chronic renal impairment due to bladder neck obstruction by an enlarged prostate.

### A2: What investigations would you do?

Urinary catheterization should be done – a large residual volume of urine confirms the diagnosis of urinary retention due to bladder neck obstruction. Ultrasound scan of the abdomen and pelvis reveals bilateral hydronephrosis, hydroureter and an enlarged prostate. Bilateral small kidneys or cortical thinning would suggest that the obstruction is long-standing (chronic retention). Serum prostate-specific antigen (PSA) assay should be done – a high serum concentration suggests possible prostatic malignancy (*caution:* a sample taken after rectal examination or catheterization may show a spuriously high serum level).

### A3: How would you manage this patient?

Immediate bladder catheterization should be done to relieve obstruction. If catheterization is difficult, the urology team should be informed, as suprapubic catheterization may be required. Fluid balance (intake and output) should be monitored, as the patient is likely to have a large diuresis. Urea and electrolytes should be monitored daily. If the patient is unable to drink a large amount of fluid to keep up with the urine output, IV fluid (normal saline with or without potassium chloride, depending on the serum potassium level) should be infused. When renal function stabilizes, the urology team should be involved for long-term management of prostatic enlargement. Occasionally, bilateral nephrostomy drainage is required if there is no significant diuresis after bladder catheterization or no significant improvement in hydronephrosis on repeat ultrasound scanning.

### A4: What is the prognosis?

The prognosis depends on the chronicity of urinary obstruction. In most cases, renal function improves significantly and remains stable for many years. In patients with long-standing chronic obstruction, especially those who have very thin renal cortex on ultrasound scan, renal function may not improve at all. These patients go on to need dialysis treatment.

## CASE 4.9 – **A 58-year-old man with raised serum creatinine.**

### A1: What is the diagnosis?

The likely diagnosis is CKD. Although this patient's serum creatinine was just outside the normal range a year ago, his eGFR using the Modification in Diet in Renal Disease Study (MDRD) formula was 57 mL/min/1.73 m$^2$ and his current eGFR is 40 mL/min/1.73 m$^2$. Serum creatinine is not a reliable test to assess renal function, as it is influenced by a number of factors, including age, muscle mass, renal tubular secretion and extra-renal loss of creatinine. A number of regression equations that can predict GFR and creatinine clearance are available, of which the MDRD and Cockroft–Gault are most commonly used.

The cause of chronic renal failure in this case is uncertain pending further investigations, although hypertensive nephrosclerosis is a possibility.

### A2: How would you investigate this patient?

Urinalysis, FBC, serum calcium and phosphate, immunology and renal ultrasound would be the initial investigations. A low haemoglobin, high serum phosphate and bilateral small kidneys on ultrasound scan will support the diagnosis. Normal-sized kidneys with significant microscopic haematuria and proteinuria, with or without a positive immunological test, will indicate the need for a renal biopsy to establish an underlying cause of CKD.

### A3: How would you manage this patient?

This patient has moderate CKD (stage 3). Hypertension and proteinuria are the two most important progression promoters. Aggressive blood pressure control is the most important measure to prevent or slow down progression of renal disease to ESRF. The target blood pressure should be 130/80 mmHg. The ACE inhibitors and angiotensin receptor blockers reduce proteinuria and have been shown to retard progression of renal disease. These patients also have very high cardiovascular risk and should be urged to stop smoking, lose weight if obese and be treated for hyperlipidaemia. The patient should be advised to avoid NSAIDs and other nephrotoxic drugs.

### A4: What is the prognosis?

Chronic kidney disease in this patient is likely to progress to ESRF requiring dialysis or renal transplantation. Patients with CKD stage 3 have a significantly increased risk of cardiovascular morbidity and mortality.

# CHRONIC KIDNEY DISEASE

## Questions

 **OSCE counselling cases**

OSCE COUNSELLING CASE 4.1 – **'I have recently been diagnosed with chronic kidney disease. What problems can I expect to have?'**

OSCE COUNSELLING CASE 4.2 – **'As a patient with chronic kidney disease, do I have a higher risk of heart disease?'**

OSCE COUNSELLING CASE 4.3 – **'As a patient with kidney failure, do I need to stick to a special diet?'**

OSCE COUNSELLING CASE 4.4 – **'As a patient with chronic kidney disease, do I need to avoid any drugs?'**

OSCE COUNSELLING CASE 4.5 – **'I have chronic kidney disease. When will I need to go on dialysis treatment, and what are the treatment options?'**

## Answers

### 👥 OSCE counselling cases

#### OSCE COUNSELLING CASE 4.1 – 'I have recently been diagnosed with chronic kidney disease. What problems can I expect to have?'

Mild or moderate chronic kidney disease (GFR >30 mL/min/1.73 m²) does not generally cause any symptoms. In severe CKD (GFR <30 mL/min/1.73 m²), common symptoms are tiredness and generalized itching. As dialysis approaches, patients develop anorexia, nausea and vomiting. These 'uraemic symptoms' are due to progressive accumulation of waste products (uraemic toxins) and anaemia.

The common complications of CKD are as follows.

- *Anaemia:* this results mainly from a low concentration of erythropoietin. The other factors that contribute to anaemia in CKD are functional iron deficiency, anaemia of chronic disease, upper gastrointestinal blood loss, and direct suppression of bone marrow by the waste products. Anaemia is investigated and erythropoietin treatment considered when haemoglobin drops below 11 g/dL.
- *Salt and fluid retention:* this leads to oedema, hypertension and, in severe cases, pulmonary oedema. The patient is advised to restrict salt and fluid intake and is treated with loop diuretics.
- *Hypertension:* this is common, and strict blood pressure control is needed to slow down or prevent deterioration of kidney function. The target blood pressure is 130/80 mmHg. The ACE inhibitors and angiotensin receptor blockers are particularly beneficial in terms of protection of renal function.
- *Renal bone disease or osteodystrophy:* this is not a single entity but comprises secondary hyperparathyroidism, adynamic bone disease (due to low bone turnover), osteomalacia or a combination of these. Phosphate retention and diminished production of active vitamin D (due to impaired 1-alpha hydroxylation) are the initiating events. The patient is advised to follow a low phosphate diet from an early stage and is put on phosphate binders such as calcium carbonate and acetate. The patient is also treated with alpha-hydroxylated vitamin D (alphacalcidol) or calcitriol if the serum parathyroid hormone (PTH) concentration is high.
- *Cardiovascular disease:* patients with chronic kidney disease have a very high risk of heart disease and strokes.
- *Malnutrition:* this occurs due to a combination of anorexia with nausea and vomiting in the later stages of CKD, and dietary restrictions imposed to tackle high serum phosphate and potassium. Most renal units employ dietitians who advise these patients regularly.
- *Infections:* these are common because of reduced immunity due to a combination of impaired T-cell and neutrophil functions. The patient is immunized with hepatitis B vaccination at an early stage. It is also recommended that the patient has influenza vaccination annually and pneumococcal vaccination every 5 years.

#### OSCE COUNSELLING CASE 4.2 – 'As a patient with chronic kidney disease, do I have a higher risk of heart disease?'

Chronic kidney disease is associated with high cardiovascular risk. There is a graded relationship between reduced eGFR and the risk of death, cardiovascular events and hospitalization – the lower the eGFR, the higher the risk. One study showed that the hazard ratios for cardiovascular events were 1.4, 2, 2.8 and 3.4, and those for death were 1.2, 1.8, 3.2 and 5.9, in patients with CKD stages 3a, 3b, 4 and 5, respectively, compared with patients with stage 2 CKD.

Patients with ESRF who are on dialysis have an even higher cardiovascular risk. Death due to cardiovascular disease is 10–20 times higher in patients on dialysis compared with the general population.

Apart from the classic risk factors such as hypertension, hyperlipidaemia and smoking, these patients also have left ventricular hypertrophy, chronic anaemia, abnormal apolipoproteins, raised serum phosphate (with or without a high Ca×P product), arterial calcification, elevated plasma homocysteine level, enhanced coagulability, chronic inflammation and abnormal endothelial function. All of these probably contribute towards the extremely high cardiovascular morbidity and mortality in these patients. It is, therefore, important to treat blood pressure aggressively, urge the patient to stop smoking, and put the patient on statin. Serum phosphate level is generally controlled with dietary restriction and the use of phosphate binders. Anaemia should be treated early and effectively with erythropoietin.

## OSCE COUNSELLING CASE 4.3 – 'As a patient with kidney failure, do I need to stick to a special diet?'

Most renal units have specialist renal dietitians who advise patients regularly regarding their dietary and fluid restrictions. Patients with chronic renal failure need to restrict their phosphate intake at an early stage; recent guidelines suggest phosphate restriction should be instigated when GFR drops below 60 mL/min. Phosphate is found in almost all foods but is especially high in milk and milk products, liver, dried beans and nuts. Dialysis does not clear phosphate very effectively, and therefore the patient needs to continue on a low phosphate diet even when on dialysis. Patients are also asked to restrict their potassium intake. Major sources of potassium are fruits (especially citrus fruits and banana), vegetables, chocolate, coffee and salt substitutes. Salt restriction is recommended to help blood pressure control and fluid retention, even when the patient is on dialysis. Patients are advised to restrict their total fluid intake to about a litre a day unless they have a significant urine output.

## OSCE COUNSELLING CASE 4.4 – 'As a patient with chronic kidney disease, do I need to avoid any drugs?'

A variety of insults that would have little impact on healthy kidneys may cause significant loss of renal function in patients with pre-existing kidney damage. When more than one nephrotoxic factor is present, the risk of worsening renal function is much increased. Apart from renal disease itself, important predisposing factors include the following:

- old age – GFR falls by 50 per cent by 80 years of age due to normal ageing processes
- diabetes
- atherosclerosis – peripheral vascular disease often involves the renal arteries
- cardiac failure – low cardiac output leads to 'pre-renal' uraemia
- hypovolaemia
- hepatic failure – associated with renal vasoconstriction and 'pre-renal' uraemia
- myeloma – with or without hypercalcaemia or hyperuricaemia
- transplant kidney – vulnerable even with a normal creatinine.

Common nephrotoxic agents include the following:

- ACE inhibitors and angiotensin receptor blockers – reduce GFR in renal arterial stenosis (RAS) and sometimes in chronic renal failure; do not use if RAS is likely. Captopril is shorter-acting and so more quickly reversible. Beware a major drop in blood pressure in volume-depleted patients. Check creatinine before and 7 days after starting treatment. Watch potassium levels
- NSAIDs – reduce the vasodilatory effect of prostaglandins and lead to unopposed vasoconstriction
- aminoglycosides – trough and peak levels should be measured. The nephrotoxic effect may also be related to the total cumulative dose received
- ciclosporin – has a dose-related NSAID-like effect
- X-ray contrast – protection of GFR with adequate hydration pre-study is essential

- tetracyclines – doxycycline is metabolized in the liver and is the only safe tetracycline for use in renal disease.

## OSCE COUNSELLING CASE 4.5 – ' I have chronic kidney disease. When will I need to go on dialysis treatment, and what are the treatment options?'

Renal replacement therapy (RRT) is generally required when the GFR is around 10–15 mL/min/1.73m$^2$ (end-stage kidney failure). Most patients with CKD are symptomatic (with anorexia, nausea and vomiting) at this stage. Some people advocate starting RRT earlier, but there is no convincing evidence to suggest a survival benefit of early commencement of dialysis. Patients with diabetes often become symptomatic at an earlier stage and start dialysis with a higher GFR compared with patients without diabetes. Some patients with CKD start dialysis as an emergency because of intractable hyperkalaemia or severe pulmonary oedema.

There are three modalities of RRT:

- haemodialysis
- peritoneal dialysis – either continuous ambulatory or automated
- renal transplantation.

The optimal choice of modality of RRT depends on the patient's age, functional capacity, comorbidities, family support and choice. Some patients receive all three modalities of RRT at various stages of their illness. Some patients, who choose not to have dialysis treatment or are deemed unlikely to benefit from dialysis, are treated conservatively with full supportive treatment, including erythropoietin therapy.

The annual acceptance rate and prevalence of RRT in the UK are, respectively, 108 and 774 per 1 million population. Forty seven per cent of prevalent patients have a functioning transplant, and 43 per cent of patients are on haemodialysis.

## REVISION PANEL

- Acute kidney injury may be: (i) *pre-renal*, due to ineffective perfusion of kidneys that are structurally normal, (ii) *renal*, due to structural damage to the glomeruli and tubules, or (iii) *post-renal*, due to urinary tract obstruction.
- Indications for urgent renal dialysis include severe hyperkalaemia (>6.5 mmol/L or less with ECG changes, despite medical treatment), pulmonary oedema, severe acidosis (pH <7.1), severe uraemia (vomiting, encephalopathy) and uraemic pericarditis.
- ECG findings of hyperkalaemia include tall-peaked T-waves, widening of QRS, reduction in the height of P- (may disappear) and R-waves, and a sine wave pattern (pre-cardiac arrest).
- Nephrotic syndrome is defined as the presence of oedema, heavy proteinuria (>3 g/day) and hypoalbuminaemia, with or without hypercholesterolaemia and hypertension.
- The most common causes of microscopic haematuria in young people are IgA nephropathy and thin basement membrane disease. Other causes are stones, cystic diseases of the kidney, tumour and inflammatory diseases of the urinary tract. Urological causes predominate in older patients.
- Systemic vasculitis (such as Wagener's granulomatosis) may present with raised serum creatinine, microscopic haematuria and proteinuria and requires urgent immunosuppressive therapy.
- The common complications of CKD are anaemia, salt and fluid retention, hypertension, renal bone disease or osteodystrophy, cardiovascular disease, malnutrition and infections.
- Patients with CKD require long-term dietary phosphate and potassium restriction.

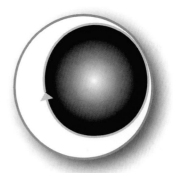

 # Cardiology

*Morgan Cadman-Davies, Nevianna Tomson and
Neeraj Prasad*

## Questions

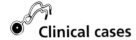

### Clinical cases

## For each of the case scenarios given, consider the following:

> **Q1**: What specific questions would you ask the patient?
> **Q2**: What is the likely diagnosis?
> **Q3**: What examination would you perform?
> **Q4**: What would be the initial management?
> **Q5**: What investigations would you request to confirm a diagnosis?
> **Q6**: What other issues should be addressed?

## CASE 5.1 – **A 34-year-old woman with palpitations.**

A 34-year-old woman presents with a 3-h history of palpitations. She is mildly dyspnoeic and has some chest pain. She has been feeling anxious and had insomnia for the past few weeks. On direct questioning, she admits to a 10-day history of diarrhoea. On examination, she has a tachycardia and her pulse is irregular.

## CASE 5.2 – **A 53-year-old man with sudden onset of chest pain.**

A 53-year-old man is brought into the accident and emergency (A&E) department by ambulance complaining of sudden onset of severe central chest pain. He is cold and clammy and appears breathless.

## CASE 5.3 – **An 80-year-old woman collapses, requiring cardiopulmonary resuscitation (CPR).**

A 80-year-old woman collapsed at home and has been brought into A&E unconscious. She was given basic life support at home by her daughter, who works as a ward sister on coronary care. The paramedics are performing CPR as the patient is wheeled into A&E accompanied by her tearful daughter.

## CASE 5.4 – **A 65-year-old man with tearing chest pain.**

A 65-year-old man is brought into A&E complaining of severe tearing pain between the shoulder blades. Initially the pain was extremely severe, but it has now mildly subsided to a dull ache in the chest. He is normally fit and well, apart from hypertension, for which he has been seeing his general practitioner (GP).

## CASE 5.5 – **A 25-year-old man with a heart murmur.**

A 25-year-old man recently attended a medical in the process of joining the police force. He has been told that he has a heart murmur.

# 👫 OSCE counselling cases

## OSCE COUNSELLING CASE 5.1 – 'Can I stop my warfarin?'

A 24-year-old woman had a metal prosthetic heart valve inserted 4 years ago after a severe episode of bacterial endocarditis that degenerated her mitral valve. She has done very well since the surgery and has been on warfarin, regularly attending an anticoagulation clinic. She has come to see you today because she wants to have a family but has read on the Internet that warfarin can damage the baby. Can she stop her warfarin?

## OSCE COUNSELLING CASE 5.2 – 'I'm on various medicines for my angina. How should I take them and what side effects do they have?'

A 73-year-old man has recently been diagnosed with angina. He is able to walk 300 m before experiencing chest tightness but considerably less distance when there is an incline. His recent exercise stress test has indicated ischaemic heart disease (IHD) and he has been prescribed sublingual glyceryl trinitrate (GTN) tablets and a beta-blocker. Advise him on how to use the medication and explain any side effects of which he should be aware.

## OSCE COUNSELLING CASE 5.3 – 'I have heart failure. Do I need to take my medications for life?'

A 65-year-old man with known IHD, hypertension and diabetes mellitus has recently been complaining of shortness of breath. An echocardiogram has confirmed left ventricular (LV) systolic dysfunction, which is moderately severe, and he has been started on ramipril 10 mg once a day, bisoprolol 2.5 mg once a day and spironolactone 25 mg once a day. He is very concerned about the number of medications that he is now on because these are additional to his other therapies. Explain the importance of his diagnosis and treatments to him.

## 🔑 Key concepts

To work through the core clinical cases in this chapter, you will need to understand the following key concepts.

### BENEFITS OF DRUG MANAGEMENT IN CHRONIC HEART FAILURE

- *Diuretics:* loop diuretics and thiazide diuretics improve symptoms of congestion.
- *Spironolactone 25–50 mg once a day:* improves survival in severe (New York Heart Association [NYHA] stage III/IV) heart failure.
- *Angiotensin-converting enzyme (ACE) inhibitors:* improve symptoms, exercise capacity and survival in patients with asymptomatic and symptomatic systolic dysfunction:
  - lisinopril 2.5 mg initial dose, 20 mg once a day target dose, sometimes up to 30 mg once a day
  - ramipril 1.25–2.5 mg initial dose, 10 mg once a day target dose
  - captopril* 6.25 mg initial dose, 50 mg three times a day target dose (now used infrequently).
- *Angiotensin II antagonists:* treatment of symptomatic heart failure in patients intolerant to ACE inhibitors*:
  - losartan and valsartan.
- *Beta-blockers:* improve symptoms and survival in stable patients who are already receiving an ACE inhibitor with LV systolic dysfunction:
  - bisoprolol 1.25 mg once a day titrated with close monitoring to 10 mg once a day
  - carvedilol 3.125 mg twice a day, increasing with close monitoring to 25–50 mg twice a day.
- *Digoxin:* improves symptoms and exercise capacity and reduces admissions to hospital.
- *Nitrates and hydralazine:* improve survival in symptomatic patients who are intolerant to ACE inhibitors or angiotensin II receptor antagonists*.
- *Amiodarone:* prevents arrhythmias in patients with symptomatic ventricular arrhythmias.
- *Ivabradine:* can be used to reduce heart rate if rate <60 bpm on beta blockers or if intolerant to beta blockers.

*Prefer long-acting drugs such as ramipril, which can be used in a twice a day dosing regime if the blood pressure is low.

### BENEFITS OF INTERVENTIONS IN CHRONIC HEART FAILURE

Some patients fail to respond to maximal pharmacological therapy and remain symptomatic.

If there is poor contractile function with prolongation of QRS duration (i.e. reduced cardiac output measured by left ventricular ejection fraction [LVEF] on echocardiography), the patient may get symptomatic benefit from a biventricular pacing system designed to improve contractility ± correction of life-threatening arrhythmias if also fitted with an internal defibrillator. Indications for insertion of a biventricular pacemaker ± a defibrillator are:

- stage III/IV NYHA heart failure
- either QRS >150 ms or QRS 120–149 ms with mechanical dyssynchrony on echocardiography
- LVEF <35 per cent, non-sustained ventricular tachycardia (VT) on Holter monitoring and inducible VT on electrophysiology studies
- already on optimal pharmacological therapy.

### CARDIAC ARRHYTHMIAS

See Table 5.1 and Figures 5.1 and 5.2.

Table 5.1 Arrhythmias

| Arrhythmia | Basic pathology | Medical management | Intervention or surgical management |
| --- | --- | --- | --- |
| **Non-myocardial infarction (MI)-related** | | | |
| AF or atrial flutter | Increasing prevalence with age<br><br>Look for possible underlying causes: *cardiac* – mitral valve disease, IHD, pericarditis, cardiomyopathy, endo-/myocarditis, post-cardiac surgery; *atrial myxoma*; *lung pathology* – pneumonia, pulmonary embolic malignancy, trauma/surgery; *metabolic* – thyrotoxicosis, excessive alcohol, electrolyte imbalance/acidosis | Control rate with digoxin/beta-blocker/amiodarone and restore to sinus rhythm by chemical (flecainide/amiodarone)/electrical cardioversion<br><br>Heparin or warfarin should be considered<br><br>If hypotensive, consider immediate DC cardioversion<br><br>Acute AF/flutter often reverts spontaneously within 24 h<br><br>Correct underlying cause if possible | Persistent AF/flutter needs anticoagulation with warfarin and consideration for DC cardioversion, depending on underlying pathology<br><br>Electrophysiological ablation should be considered<br><br>Occasionally AV node ablation and permanent pacemaker are needed to control heart rate in patients not responsive to other medical therapy |
| SVT | Accessory pathway between atria and ventricles causing re-entrant circuit, e.g. Wolff–Parkinson–White syndrome, AV node re-entrant tachycardia, ectopic atrial focus or AF/atrial flutter | DC cardioversion if hypotensive<br><br>Vagal manoeuvres, e.g. carotid massage/Valsalva manoeuvre<br><br>IV adenosine (3–12 mg)<br><br>Consider intravenous or oral verapamil or beta-blocker (but not in Wolff–Parkinson–White syndrome, where flecainide can be considered) | Rarely atrial overdrive pacing<br><br>Electrophysiology studies and ablation if medical treatment not adequate |
| VT | Associated with IHD, hypertensive heart disease, cardiomyopathy<br><br>Can be precipitated by bradycardia, hypokalaemia, hypomagnesaemia, MI or long QT interval | Synchronized DC cardioversion if hypotensive; if stable give IV lidocaine<br><br>Correct metabolic abnormalities<br><br>Amiodarone may be necessary to stabilize patient | Consider electrophysiological studies/ablation or implantable defibrillator |

*Continued*

| Arrhythmia | Basic pathology | Medical management | Intervention or surgical management |
|---|---|---|---|
| Ventricular premature beats | Ectopic focus within ventricle | Treatment offers no benefit to survival<br>Give antiarrhythmic if symptomatic (beta-blocker) | Rarely electrophysiological ablation for very frequent unifocal ventricular ectopic beats |
| Torsades de pointes | Associated with inherited or acquired prolongation of QT interval, e.g. drugs, hypokalaemia, hypomagnesaemia, hypocalcaemia, IHD | Correct electrolyte imbalance<br>Stop drugs prolonging QT interval<br>Intravenous magnesium<br>Consider beta-blocker in hereditary QT interval | Consider temporary pacing<br>Discuss with EP team |
| VF | See Case 5.4 | | |
| **Post-MI arrhythmias** | | | |
| AF/atrial flutter | AF often transient post-MI | Rate control; usually reverts spontaneously; treat as above if present | |
| VF | Acute MI is common cause of VF | As non-MI treatment<br>Note that antiarrhythmic drug treatment is not necessary after VF within first 24 h of acute MI | Recurrent or late VF (>48 h) indicates risk of subsequent sudden death; these patients should be considered for coronary angiography for possible revascularization and ICD |
| VT | Associated with IHD, especially acutely post-MI | Treatment as above<br>Note that antiarrhythmic drug treatment is not necessary after VF within first 24 h of acute MI | Recurrent or late VT (>48 h) indicates risk of subsequent sudden death; these patients should be considered for coronary angiography for possible revascularization and ICD |
| Ventricular premature beats | Common acutely post-MI/post-thrombolysis | Often no treatment required | |
| Sinus bradycardia | Commonly complicates RV infarction/inferior infarction | If heart rate <60 beats/min with hypotension or cardiac failure, give IV atropine 0.6 mg | Temporary or permanent pacing may be needed |

*Continued*

| AV block | Commonly complicates RV infarction/ inferior infarction | First-degree heart block requires no treatment | Temporary or permanent pacing may be needed |
|---|---|---|---|
| | | Second-/third-degree heart block with inferior infarction requires treatment only if associated with hypotension, syncope, cardiac failure or 'escape' ventricular arrhythmias. Atropine 0.6 mg IV bolus up to 3 mg IV can be given | Second-/third-degree heart block associated with anterior infarction should always be considered for temporary pacing because may lead to ventricular standstill |

AF, atrial fibrillation; AV, atrioventricular; DC, direct current; ICD, implantable cardioverter defibrillation; IHD, ischaemic heart disease; IV, intravenous; MI, myocardial infarction; RV, right ventricular; SVT, supraventricular tachycardia; VF, ventricular fibrillation; VT, ventricular tachycardia.

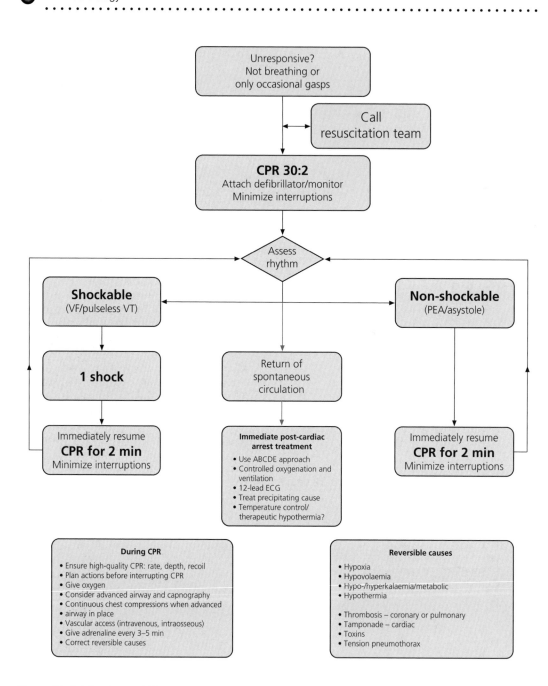

**Figure 5.1** Adult advanced life support.

CPR, cardiopulmonary resuscitation; ECG, electrocardiogram; PEA, pulseless electrical activity; VF, ventricular fibrillation; VT, ventricular tachycardia.

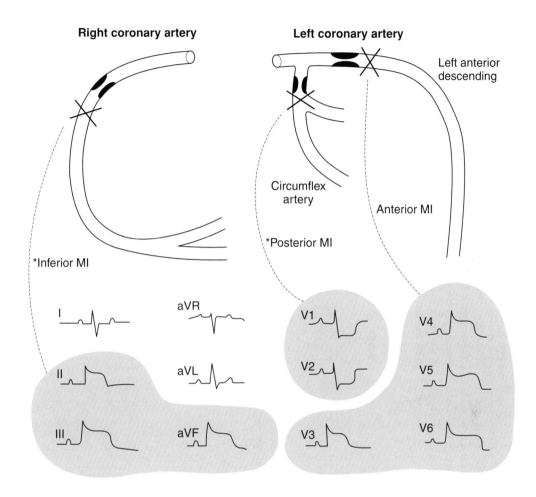

**Figure 5.2** Chest pain.

*There is an overlap between inferior and posterior, depending on the patient's anatomy, i.e. where the right coronary artery or circumflex artery is dominant.

MI, myocardial infarction.

## VALVULAR HEART DISEASE

See Table 5.2.

**Table 5.2** Valvular heart disease

| | Cause | Symptoms | Signs | Management |
|---|---|---|---|---|
| Aortic stenosis | Degenerative (± calcification), calcification of congenital bicuspid valve, occasionally rheumatic fever | Symptoms usually occur only when aortic orifice is reduced to a third of its normal size: angina, dyspnoea and exercise-induced syncope | Slow-rising pulse and narrow pulse pressure; thrusting non-displaced or displaced apex; an ejection click may precede harsh ejection systolic murmur, which is loudest over right upper sternal edge and radiates to carotids | Valve replacement if symptomatic and high valve gradient on echocardiogram <br><br> Valvuloplasty in young patients (rarely) <br><br> Transcatheter aortic valve insertion for patients with high surgical risk; decision taken by multidisciplinary team, with interventional cardiologists, cardiac surgeons and cardiac anaesthetist |
| Aortic regurgitation | Damage of aortic valve cusps: bicuspid aortic valve (congenital), infective endocarditis, rheumatic fever; dilation of aortic root/valve ring: arthritides, e.g. Reiter's syndrome, ankylosing spondylitis, severe hypertension, aortic dissection, rare causes e.g. Marfan's syndrome, syphilis | Usually asymptomatic unless severe; exertional dyspnoea and fatigue | Collapsing pulse and wide pulse pressure; nail-bed capillary pulsations (Quinke's sign), head nodding (de Musset's sign), and pistol shot sounding femoral arteries are sometimes seen; apex is laterally displaced and thrusting; early diastolic murmur at lower left sternal edge heard best with the patient sitting forward in full expiration | Regular dental visits and good dental hygiene <br><br> Diuretics and vasodilators for mild symptoms <br><br> Valve replacement after patient is symptomatic or left ventricle or aortic root is dilating |

| | Causes | Symptoms | Signs | Management |
|---|---|---|---|---|
| Mitral stenosis | Rheumatic fever | Exertional dyspnoea, cough ± haemoptysis, palpitations | AF, malar flush, palpable first heart sound ('tapping' apex); loud first heart sound, opening snap in early diastole, followed by rumbling mid-diastolic murmur at apex with presystolic accentuation; pulmonary hypertension, RVH and eventually right heart failure | Valvuloplasty if valve not calcified and no significant mitral regurgitation<br>Valve replacement |
| Mitral regurgitation | MVP, rheumatic fever, papillary muscle dysfunction/rupture post-MI, LV dilation, endocarditis; rare causes – SLE, Marfan's syndrome | Exertional dyspnoea and lethargy; pulmonary oedema if acute regurgitation | Laterally displaced apex; soft first heart sound; pansystolic murmur loudest at apex and radiating to axilla and throughout precordium; third heart sound often present | Regular dental visits and good dental hygiene<br>Diuretics and ACE inhibitors<br>Valve repair or replacement if symptomatic or progressive LV dilation or dysfunction (i.e. reducing LVEF) |
| Mitral valve prolapse | Unknown cause (more common in women); associated with Marfan's syndrome/IHD | Usually asymptomatic; can present with atypical chest pain or palpitations | Midsystolic click ± murmur; mitral regurgitation may occur | Beta-blockers if symptomatic<br>If severe MR, as above |
| Tricuspid stenosis | Rheumatic fever, carcinoid | Usually associated with mitral and aortic valve disease, which dominate symptoms and signs | | Valvuloplasty or valve replacement |

Continued

| | Cause | Symptoms | Signs | Management |
|---|---|---|---|---|
| Tricuspid regurgitation | Raised pulmonary pressure (look for causes, e.g. pulmonary embolism, lung disease, left heart causes [mitral valve disease, LV dysfunction]); can be physiological; rare causes – rheumatic heart disease, infective endocarditis, carcinoid | Symptoms and signs of underlying lung pathology and right heart failure may be present | Raised JVP and giant 'v' waves, pulsatile liver and pansystolic murmur at left lower sternal edge, accentuated with inspiration; peripheral oedema and ascites may be present | If functional, signs usually improve with diuretic therapy<br><br>Annuloplasty or replacement very rarely required |
| Pulmonary stenosis | Congenital (usually with other defects, e.g. Fallot's tetralogy) | Fatigue, syncope, RV failure | Systolic murmur at left sternal edge; signs of right heart failure | Valvuloplasty, valve replacement |
| Pulmonary regurgitation | Pulmonary hypertension, endocarditis (in people who misuse IV drugs) | Usually asymptomatic | Early diastolic murmur at upper left sternal edge | Treatment rarely needed |
| Ventricular septal defect | Congenital, post-MI (ventricular septal rupture) | May be asymptomatic; Eisenmenger's syndrome occurs later in life when pulmonary vascular disease develops | Pansystolic murmur loudest at third or fourth intercostal space; pulmonary hypertension signs may be present | Repair defect surgically or consider percutaneous approach |
| Atrial septal defect | Congenital | Arrhythmias and heart failure | Wide fixed splitting of S2; pulmonary ejection systolic murmur as result of increased flow; pulmonary hypertension with tricuspid or pulmonary regurgitation may occur | Surgical or percutaneous closure if symptomatic or developing Eisenmenger's syndrome |

ACE, angiotensin-converting enzyme; AF, atrial fibrillation; IHD, ischaemic heart disease; JVP, jugular venous pressure; LV, left ventricular; LVEF, left ventricular ejection fraction; MI, myocardial infarction; MVP, mitral valve prolapse; RVH, right ventricular hypertrophy; SLE, systemic lupus erythematosus

## Answers

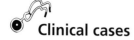

### Clinical cases

### CASE 5.1 – **A 34-year-old woman with palpitations.**

#### A1: What specific questions would you ask the patient?

Elicit from the history the onset of symptoms and any associated features (e.g. chest pain, dyspnoea, nausea, tremor). The patient's symptoms may be related to the arrhythmia, or an ischaemic event might have caused it. The patient may be able to identify whether the rhythm is regular or irregular or to tap out the arrhythmia. Determine whether the palpitations have occurred in the past. Ask specifically for precipitating or relieving factors and for any medical conditions that the patient has that predispose to arrhythmias, e.g. thyrotoxicosis or valvular heart disease. A drug history is very important because some drugs may precipitate arrhythmias or influence the management of the arrhythmia (e.g. verapamil must not be given to patients who are on beta-blockers because it may result in circulatory collapse).

#### A2: What is the likely diagnosis?

The likely diagnosis is atrial fibrillation (AF) secondary to thyrotoxicosis as a result of the history of diarrhoea and insomnia that are features in this condition. Other causes of arrhythmia to consider are described in the key concepts.

#### A3: What examination would you perform?

A full physical examination is necessary. Determine the rate, character and volume of the pulse. Note if the patient is haemodynamically stable: record the blood pressure and examine for signs of heart failure. Auscultate for heart murmurs. Examine for thyroid status if appropriate.

#### A4: What would be the initial management?

This depends on the cause of the palpitations. If the patient has a tachycardia and is haemodynamically unstable (systolic blood pressure <80 mmHg, reduced level of consciousness, severe pulmonary oedema), consider immediate direct current (DC) cardioversion. If the patient has a bradycardia and is haemodynamically compromised, give atropine 0.6–1.2 mg IV. If there is persistent bradycardia, consider external pacing while organizing transvenous pacing wire insertion. See Key concepts.

#### A5: What investigations would you request to confirm a diagnosis?

Record a 12-lead electrocardiogram (ECG) to determine the nature of the arrhythmia (regular versus irregular, narrow versus broad QRS complex). Take blood for routine haematology, biochemistry, calcium, magnesium, cardiac enzymes, thyroid function tests and glucose. A chest radiograph is useful to estimate heart size and look for signs of pulmonary oedema.

#### A6: What other issues should be addressed?

This depends on the arrhythmia and its underlying cause (see Key concepts).

## CASE 5.2 – **A 53-year-old man with sudden onset of chest pain.**

### A1: What specific questions would you ask the patient?

There is a wide range of differential diagnoses for chest pain and it is thus very important to establish the exact nature of the pain. A constricting central chest pain that occurs on exertion and is relieved by rest or GTN suggests angina. A similar crushing central chest pain when more prolonged and of greater severity indicates myocardial infarction (MI); unlike angina, the pain of MI is not relieved by rest or GTN and is typically associated with extreme distress, sweating, nausea/vomiting and dyspnoea. Cardiac pain can radiate to one or both arms and up the neck to the jaw. Risk factors for IHD to seek are diabetes mellitus, hypertension, hyperlipidaemia, smoking and any family history of IHD. Male sex, increasing age and obesity are also risk factors. Other causes of chest pain to consider include pericarditis, dissecting aortic aneurysm, pulmonary embolus, pleurisy, gastro-oesophageal reflux, perforated peptic ulcer, pancreatitis and cholecystitis.

### A2: What is the likely diagnosis?

The most likely diagnosis is MI. This is usually caused by rupture of an atherosclerotic plaque with formation of thrombus and complete occlusion of a coronary artery.

### A3: What examination would you perform?

A full physical examination is needed. The patient is usually very distressed and appears pale, grey and sweating. The pulse must be noted because arrhythmias are common, particularly if the MI is of the right coronary artery, which supplies the sinoatrial node. Hypotension may also occur; blood pressure is often measured in both arms to look for any significant difference (>15 mmHg) that may indicate aortic dissection. The jugular venous pressure (JVP), if raised, indicates right heart failure and right ventricular (RV) infarction must be considered. Listen for any murmurs and then examine for pulmonary oedema. Cardiogenic shock can be recognized from the following: systolic blood pressure <90 mmHg, heart rate >100 beats/min or <40 beats/min, pulmonary oedema (oxygen saturation <90 per cent), cold peripheries, agitation/confusion and oliguria.

### A4: What would be the initial management?

Immediate treatment is aimed at relief of pain, limitation of infarct size and management of complications if they arise. Oxygen is administered via a facemask (28% if history of chronic bronchitis/emphysema) and the patient is attached to an ECG monitor. Intravenous access is obtained and 5 mg diamorphine is given with 10 mg metoclopramide as an antiemetic. Further 2.5 mg boluses of diamorphine should be given until the patient is pain-free. Soluble aspirin 300 mg and sublingual GTN (provided that the patient is not hypotensive) must also be given if not already administered by the ambulance paramedics. A 12-lead ECG is done as a priority to decide whether primary percutaneous coronary angioplasty (PCI) or thrombolysis is appropriate. Patients who have a ST elevation MI should have primary PCI with or without stenting of vessel occlusion as early as possible, which improves the clinical outcome. If the time to primary PCI is over 2 h (or 90 min for patients under 75 years of age), immediate thrombolysis should be administered (streptokinase or recombinant tissue plasminogen activator [rTPA] and intravenous heparin) and the patient should be transferred for rescue PCI within 3–24 h. Patients with a non-ST elevation MI should also have PCI. High-risk patients should have PCI within 24 h and lower-risk patients within 72 h. G2b3a inhibitors can be considered with dynamic ECG changes or ongoing ischaemia if an interventional option is delayed. See Key concepts.

### A5: What investigations would you request to confirm a diagnosis?

The diagnosis is usually made on the basis of a history and 12-lead ECG, and confirmed later with a rise in cardiac enzymes. ST-segment elevation on the ECG occurs within minutes and is followed by T-wave inversion that persists after the ST segment returns to baseline. The indication of transmural infarction is the development of Q-waves, usually hours or days later. The infarct site may be determined by the location of ECG changes. Other ischaemic changes on the ECG that may occur are new left bundle-branch block, right bundle-branch block, tachy- or bradyarrhythmias, left or right axis deviation or atrioventricular (AV) block. Troponin-T myofibrillar protein and high-resolution troponin-T are routinely measured, rising within 4 h and remaining elevated for 2 weeks. This is a specific marker of myocardial disease and important diagnostically. Creatine phosphokinase (CPK) (and more specifically the isoenzyme CK-MB) and lactate dehydrogenase (LDH) can be used as markers of disease severity or to indicate reinfarction. CK-MB rises at 4–8 h, peaks at 24 h and returns to normal in 3–4 days. A chest radiograph to determine cardiac size and look for pulmonary oedema must be performed. Blood must be taken for routine haematology and biochemistry investigations, and for random glucose and cholesterol measurement.

## A6: What other issues should be addressed?

The patient should be admitted to the coronary care unit if possible and have bedrest for 24–36 h. Subcutaneous heparin is used as prophylaxis against deep venous thrombosis. Patients with uncomplicated MI can be discharged home after 5 days. Complications that may occur include cardiogenic shock, reinfarction, dysrhythmias, pericarditis, acute mitral regurgitation, ventricular septal defect and myocardial rupture. If pain persists or there is no resolution of ST elevation, the patient is considered for repeat thrombolysis or referred for urgent angiography, with the aim of revascularization, usually by coronary angioplasty. Secondary prevention post-MI is important; each patient is prescribed aspirin, a beta-blocker, an ACE inhibitor and a lipid-lowering statin (atorvastatin 80 mg daily if tolerated), unless specific contraindications are present. The patient should be on clopidogrel or prasugrel for 1 year if a coronary stent is implanted. On discharge, patients should be advised to inform the Driver and Vehicle Licensing Authority (DVLA) of their admission; they can usually resume driving in 6 weeks and return to work in 3 months. Every patient should be entered into a cardiac rehabilitation programme and have active follow-up.

## CASE 5.3 – An 80-year-old woman collapses, requiring CPR.

### A1: What specific questions would you ask the patient?

Obtain as much history as possible from the daughter and paramedics. Events immediately preceding the arrest are particularly important because they may indicate the cause. Enquire specifically about any illness that the patient may have had and obtain a past medical history, such as IHD, diabetes mellitus (consider hypoglycaemia) and depression (consider drug overdose). Establish the medication that the patient is on and enquire about illicit drug use if appropriate (especially in a young patient, where examination may yield evidence of IV drug misuse). It is also important to identify the length of time before resuscitation and the duration of resuscitation before admission. Without CPR, permanent cerebral dysfunction occurs after 3–4 min of cardiopulmonary arrest. The longer the period of arrest, the less likely it is that resuscitation will be successful and the patient restored to a healthy life.

### A2: What is the likely diagnosis?

The most common cause of a cardiac arrest is ventricular fibrillation (VF). Other causes include other dysrhythmias (pulseless VT, bradydysrhythmia), sudden pump failure (MI), circulatory obstruction (pulmonary embolus) and cardiovascular rupture (myocardial rupture/dissecting aortic aneurysm).

### A3: What examination would you perform?

The initial assessment of the airway, breathing and circulation would have already been performed by the paramedics. Examine the patient briefly to check that CPR is effective: palpate for a pulse and check that both lungs are ventilated. Look for any signs of bleeding such as haematemesis or melaena that may suggest hypovolaemia as the cause of the arrest. If the abdomen is distended, an intra-abdominal catastrophe such as a ruptured abdominal aortic aneurysm may be suspected.

## A4: What would be the initial management?

Effective basic life support and early defibrillation are the most vital elements of successful resuscitation. The patient is already being resuscitated by the paramedics, and IV access has usually been established. The patient should be attached to a defibrillator via ECG leads to determine whether the cardiac rhythm is 'shockable' (VF/pulseless VT) or not shockable (asystole/electromechanical dissociation). If the patient is in a shockable rhythm, DC cardioversion should be given without delay. Advanced CPR should be continued according to the algorithm determined by the patient's cardiac rhythm each time it is assessed (see Key concepts). The patient should be intubated if this has not already been done. Adrenaline (1 mg IV) should be given every 3 min; if the patient is in asystole, 3 mg atropine should be given once only. In refractory VF/VT (after four cycles of advanced life support [ALS]), amiodarone is recommended. An arterial blood gas (ABG) is taken during ALS; if hyperkalaemia is present, calcium chloride is administered. Bicarbonate can be given in severe acidosis (pH <7.0) and in hyperkalaemia. Treatable causes must be considered (see Figure 5.1) and where possible an attempt made to correct them.

## A5: What investigations would you request to confirm a diagnosis?

In the event of successful resuscitation, a 12-lead ECG must be done to look for evidence of MI that may have precipitated the arrest. A chest radiograph may show pulmonary oedema or identify rib fractures secondary to vigorous CPR and is useful to check the position of the endotracheal tube. Routine blood biochemistry, haematology, cardiac enzymes, glucose and group and save are taken, and blood is cross-matched if a bleed is suspected. An ABG will indicate whether ventilation is adequate.

## A6: What other issues should be addressed?

Most patients need admission to intensive care post-arrest and may require ventilation and support with inotropes such as adrenaline. The patient may require a central line and therapeutic hypothermia. A member of the medical team must speak with the family and inform them of the future management and likely prognosis.

## CASE 5.4 – **A 65-year-old man with tearing chest pain.**

### A1: What specific questions would you ask the patient?

Establish the nature of the pain. Aortic dissection pain can mimic MI, and caution must be taken to distinguish the two because treatment is different. Abrupt onset of tearing chest pain that radiates to the back and abdomen indicates dissection. Patients may present with symptoms and signs of occlusion of one or more of the branches of the aorta as the dissection progresses: stroke, limb ischaemia, paraplegia, MI. Risk factors to enquire about include hypertension, arteriosclerosis (IHD/peripheral vascular disease), pregnancy, history of trauma and rarely Marfan's syndrome.

### A2: What is the likely diagnosis?

The most likely diagnosis is aortic dissection. This may be proximal (type I starts in the ascending aorta but progresses down the aorta; type II is localized to the ascending aorta) or distal (type III starts in the descending aorta after the arch), involving the descending aorta only.

### A3: What examination would you perform?

A full examination is necessary. A blood pressure difference between the right and left arms (>15 mmHg) occurs in 10 per cent of patients with a dissection. There may be a difference in pulse between the right and left arms or radial and femoral pulses. An elevated JVP and pulsus paradox indicate cardiac tamponade caused by rupture of the aortic wall into the pericardium. Aortic regurgitation may be heard when the aortic root is involved. The patient should be examined for any neurological deficit.

### A4: What would be the initial management?

Resuscitation is the initial management. Oxygen must be given via a facemask. Intravenous access is established and pain relief with diamorphine given. Systolic blood pressure must be reduced to 100–120 mmHg using drugs that decrease the inotropic force of the heart, e.g. labetalol infusion.

### A5: What investigation would you request to confirm a diagnosis?

The diagnosis of aortic dissection can be made in several ways. The diagnosis is often suspected from the chest radiograph, which may demonstrate a widened mediastinum. This is an unreliable sign, however, and chest computed tomography (CT) with contrast or magnetic resonance imaging (MRI) is usually preferred to make the diagnosis non-invasively. An echocardiogram is also useful to look at the aortic root in detail in type I or II dissection, but a transoesophageal echocardiogram is preferred if possible to obtain detailed views of the descending thoracic aorta. Cardiac catheterization will aid planning of surgical repair.

### A6: What other issues should be addressed?

Over 50 per cent of patients die in the first 24 h of presentation. Urgent surgical repair is needed in type I or II dissection, and frequently in type III dissection, if the patient is to have a chance of survival.

## CASE 5.5 – **A 25-year-old man with a heart murmur.**

### A1: What specific questions would you ask the patient?

Elicit from the history whether the patient has any symptoms suggestive of valvular stenosis or regurgitation: dyspnoea, oedema, dizziness, syncope, palpitations or chest pain. Haemoptysis or recurrent bronchitis may indicate pulmonary hypertension. A past medical history may suggest a cause, such as rheumatic heart disease or MI causing papillary muscle rupture. Consider underlying conditions and family history that may predispose to valvular abnormalities, such as dilated or hypertrophic cardiomyopathy, Marfan's syndrome or ankylosing spondylitis. Ask about any symptoms that may suggest endocarditis (rash, fevers) or predisposing factors such as IV drug misuse.

### A2: What is the likely diagnosis?

A heart murmur is heard when there is turbulent blood flow, the cause usually being an abnormal heart valve that may be incompetent (regurgitant), stenotic or both. An 'innocent murmur' produced by a normal heart valve tends to occur in the setting of a hyperdynamic circulation, such as anaemia, thyrotoxicosis or pregnancy. See Key concepts for causes of each murmur.

### A3: What examination would you perform?

A full physical examination is necessary. Determine the characteristics of the pulse and blood pressure. Look for signs of right heart failure (raised JVP, ankle oedema, enlarged liver) and for pulmonary oedema indicating LV failure. Determine whether the murmur is systolic or diastolic. The character of the murmur (e.g. pansystolic in mitral regurgitation) and the location and radiation of the murmur will give further clues to the diagnosis (see Key concepts). Bear in mind that a soft midsystolic murmur that varies with posture and is not associated with signs of heart disease is usually benign.

## A4: What would be the initial management?

Medical therapy is aimed mainly at treatment of complications (AF, heart failure). Surgical treatment may be valve repair, valve replacement or valvotomy (see Key concepts). Surgery must be performed before irreversible LV dysfunction and pulmonary oedema become established.

## A5: What investigations would you request to confirm a diagnosis?

Valve dysfunction is confirmed with trans-thoracic echocardiography, trans-oesophageal echocardiogram or cardiac MRI. An ECG may show LV hypertrophy and confirm AF or, if the patient is in sinus rhythm, show the bifid P-wave ('P mitrale') of left atrial hypertrophy in mitral stenosis or the tall P-wave ('P pulmonale') of pulmonary hypertension. A chest radiograph may indicate cardiomegaly.

## A6: What other issues should be addressed?

Prosthetic valves are either mechanical (e.g. Starr–Edwards ball-and-cage valve (old type of valve), Björk–Shiley tilting disc valve) or bioprosthetic valves (porcine xenograft). Bioprosthetic pig valves typically degenerate after about 10 years and hence are preferably used in elderly people. Mechanical valves last longer but need life-long anticoagulation. All prosthetic valves and native abnormal valves are susceptible to infection. Patients should always be advised that antibiotic prophylaxis is no longer required for routine surgical or dental procedures under new guidance, but good dental hygiene is important.

##  OSCE counselling cases

### OSCE COUNSELLING CASE 5.1 – 'Can I stop my warfarin?'

The answer is *definitely not!* Anticoagulation must never be stopped in a patient with a metal heart valve without a specialist cardiology consultation and a robust alternative plan.

If the patient stops anticoagulation, there is a significant risk of thrombosis, especially in the hypercoagulable state of pregnancy. A clot may obstruct the valve, causing sudden stenosis, or embolize and cause a stroke.

Her worries are genuine, however. Warfarin does indeed have teratogenic effects, particularly if the patient requires high doses, and it can also cause intracerebral haemorrhage in the fetus. Women who continue warfarin throughout pregnancy have approximately a 7 per cent chance of having a baby with a congenital abnormality and a further 16 per cent risk of stillbirth or spontaneous abortion. There are also increased complications after delivery.

The answer is to advise the patient to change to heparin (subcutaneous) for the first 3 months of the pregnancy, restart warfarin at 3 months and change again to heparin 2–4 weeks before the expected delivery date. Heparin is not teratogenic, but it is associated with a higher risk of abortion and a higher incidence of bleeding. This can be monitored and the dose adjusted. This requires a tertiary cardiology review/plan; some centres will use subcutaneous heparin throughout pregnancy.

Another point of note is that warfarin is excreted in breast milk (in small amounts), and it is advisable that mothers on warfarin should not breastfeed.

### OSCE COUNSELLING CASE 5.2 – 'I'm on various medicines for my angina. How should I take them and what side effects do they have?'

#### GTN

Nitrates are potent vasodilators, but the main benefit in angina is by causing a reduction in venous return, which reduces LV work. Sublingual GTN is used to treat symptoms in angina on an as-required basis. It comes in spray or tablet form, with the advantage of the spray having a longer storage life once opened. The onset of action is 1–2 min and effects last for up to 20 min. Sublingual GTN can be taken repeatedly, but the patient should be advised to seek medical attention if they do not get any relief after repeated use.

Headaches are common, especially in the first few days after starting treatment. The patient should be advised that if the headache is severe, they can spit out or swallow the tablet to deactivate it. Flushing and postural hypotension causing syncopal attacks are also reported and may limit therapy.

#### Beta-blockers

Beta-blockers decrease myocardial oxygen demand by causing a fall in heart rate and blood pressure and decreasing myocardial contractility. They are contraindicated in asthma and chronic obstructive pulmonary disease, however, and are relatively contraindicated in diabetes mellitus, peripheral vascular disease and severe LV dysfunction.

Lethargy is a common side effect of beta-blockers; interference with exercise capacity may cause patients to discontinue their medication. Coldness of extremities and sleep disturbances may also lead to non-compliance. Bradycardia and other conduction disorders may also occur.

## OSCE COUNSELLING CASE 5.3 – 'I have heart failure. Do I need to take my medications for life?'

Unfortunately, a diagnosis of heart failure (in this case, moderate to severe on echocardiogram assessment) is associated with a worse prognosis than most cancers (50 per cent 5-year mortality rate if untreated). With correct therapeutic management, the patient's symptoms will improve and his annual risk of death will be cut by half.

It is very important to use medications that have been shown in large randomized trials to be effective (see Key concepts).

Ask the patient whether he is having any particular problem with the drugs prescribed, particularly symptoms of hypotension. Advise the patient that, if possible, the dose of bisoprolol may be increased to try to reach the target dose of 10 mg once a day. Advise the patient that he will require regular blood checks (initially every 1–2 weeks and then every 3 months, watching for hyperkalaemia and rising creatinine) because of the potential interaction between ACE inhibitors and spironolactone.

The patient should be advised to monitor his weight regularly and to seek advice if his weight rises, because this may be a sign of fluid overload.

## REVISION PANEL

- Cardiac arrhythmias may occur due to IHD, valvular heart disease and thyrotoxicosis. In a young person, thyrotoxicosis should be excluded.
- If the patient has a tachycardia and is haemodynamically unstable (systolic blood pressure <80 mmHg, reduced level of consciousness, severe pulmonary oedema), consider immediate DC cardioversion.
- If the patient has a bradycardia and is haemodynamically compromised, give atropine 0.6–1.2 mg IV. If there is persistent bradycardia, consider external pacing while organizing transvenous pacing wire insertion.
- Risk factors for IHD include diabetes mellitus, hypertension, hyperlipidaemia, smoking, family history, male sex, increasing age and obesity.
- Apart from coronary ischaemia, other causes of chest pain to consider include pericarditis, dissecting aortic aneurysm, pulmonary embolus, pleurisy, gastro-oesophageal reflux, perforated peptic ulcer, pancreatitis and cholecystitis.
- A heart murmur is heard when there is turbulent blood flow, the cause usually being an abnormal heart valve that may be incompetent (regurgitant), stenotic or both.
- An 'innocent murmur' produced by a normal heart valve tends to occur in the setting of a hyperdynamic circulation, such as anaemia, thyrotoxicosis or pregnancy.
- Always exclude bacterial endocarditis if a patient is acutely unwell with a cardiac murmur.
- Anticoagulation should never be stopped in a patient with a prosthetic metal heart valve without careful consideration.

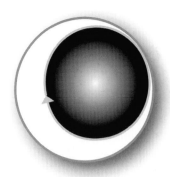

# ⑥ Care of elderly people

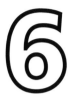

*Peter Wallis*

## FALLS

## IMMOBILITY

## ACUTE CONFUSIONAL STATES

# FALLS

## Questions

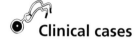

### Clinical cases

**For each of the case scenarios given, consider the following:**

**Q1**: What is the differential diagnosis?
**Q2**: What features in the history support the diagnosis?
**Q3**: What additional features in the history would you seek to support the potential diagnoses?
**Q4**: What other features would you look for on clinical examination?
**Q5**: What investigations would you perform?
**Q6**: What treatment options are available?

### CASE 6.1 – A 71-year-old man has been brought to the accident and emergency (A&E) department after a fall while shopping.

He lost consciousness momentarily and has little recollection of the event. He describes previous episodes of dizziness, sometimes on exertion and often associated with shortness of breath. His past history includes a hiatus hernia, diverticular disease, and osteoarthritis of his neck and knees. He is taking regular omeprazole, a dietary fibre supplement and a compound analgesic containing paracetamol and codeine (co-codamol). Examination discloses a regular pulse and blood pressure of 114/76 mmHg. There is an ejection systolic cardiac murmur radiating to the neck. The lung fields are clear. Neurological examination is normal.

### CASE 6.2 – An 82-year-old woman presents with recurrent falls.

The patient is housebound. Her most recent fall occurred while getting up to go to the toilet at night. She has arthritis, heart failure and poor vision as a result of macular degeneration, and she has had a previous hip replacement. She receives treatment with furosemide, ramipril, co-codamol, amitriptyline and temazepam. She is very frail. The main findings on examination are: abbreviated mental test 6/10, vision – large print only, kyphotic spine, brisk reflexes bilaterally, peripheral oedema, clear lung fields and normal jugular venous pressure (JVP), heart rate 112/min, atrial fibrillation (AF), blood pressure sitting 114/62 mmHg, mitral regurgitation.

### CASE 6.3 – A 78-year-old man who lives alone is brought to A&E after being found on the floor at home by his neighbour.

The patient is confused and disoriented. His head is bruised and he appears unkempt. He is immobile and there is cog-wheel rigidity in all his limbs. There are no focal neurological signs. Reflexes are hard to elicit as a result of the muscle stiffness. Plantar responses are down-going. There are signs of a lower respiratory tract infection. Temperature is 38.2 °C, blood pressure is 102/60 mmHg and heart rate is 94/min.

The investigation discloses: normal plasma glucose and electrolytes; urea 24 mmol/L; creatinine 142 μmol/L; haemoglobin (Hb) 15.5 g/dL; white cell count (WCC) $14.3 \times 10^9$/L; platelets $342 \times 10^9$/L; chest radiograph – consolidation right lower lobe; electrocardiogram (ECG) – sinus tachycardia.

##  OSCE counselling cases

### OSCE COUNSELLING CASE 6.1 – **What advice would you give the following patient?**

An elderly housebound woman has fallen at home on several occasions and has recently attended A&E with a Colles' (wrist) fracture. Her daughter is concerned about the presence of osteoporosis and seeks your advice at the surgery about the need for calcium tablets to prevent further fractures.

### OSCE COUNSELLING CASE 6.2 – **'What is the underlying condition, and how has it come about?'**

A housebound 94-year-old woman who has epilepsy (controlled with phenytoin) presents with falls, weakness and generalized aches and pains. Biochemical tests reveal calcium (corrected) 1.85 mmol/L (normal range 2.05–2.60 mmol/L); phosphate 0.68 mmol/L (normal range 0.8–1.45 mmol/L); albumin 32 g/L (normal range 35–48 g/L); alkaline phosphatase (ALP) 458 U/L (normal range 30–200 U/L).

What is the likely diagnosis? What factors might have precipitated this condition? What signs would you look for on examination? How would you treat the condition?

## 🔑 Key concepts

To work through the core clinical cases in this section, you will need to understand the following key concepts.

Older people are at much greater risk of falling compared with younger people. Most falls occur at home. The risk of falling is much higher in older people who reside in an institutional environment such as a residential or nursing home or hospital, as a result of the increased frailty of this group of patients. One-third of people aged over 65 years will fall in a year, often repeatedly. Falls resulting in injury are a leading cause of death in older people, accounting for two-thirds of injury-related deaths in people aged 85 years and over. Most falls do not result in death, but they can give rise to substantial morbidity. The fear of falling often leads to loss of confidence, increased dependence on others and restriction of activity.

Most patients fall because of age-related or disease-associated damage to one or more systems essential for the maintenance of balance and posture. Vision, vestibular, sensory, locomotor, cardiovascular and central processing mechanisms are all important in this regard. A careful history detailing the circumstances surrounding the fall is essential. Often there is little recollection of the prodromal events, and so corroborative information from a witness is invaluable. Patients will often provide their own explanation – 'I must have tripped, doctor' – but be cautious about accepting such well-meaning accounts of events without further enquiry. Accurate diagnosis, treatment of predisposing illness, and amelioration of risk factors such as impaired vision, polypharmacy, inadequate footwear and environmental hazards are all important. Multidisciplinary falls clinics (with physiotherapy and occupational therapy support) and exercise programmes (including activities that promote balance and strength) can reduce the risk of falling.

Many falls result in bone fractures such as wrist, pelvis, neck of humerus or, most feared of all, hip. Such fragility fractures should prompt an assessment for osteoporosis, which can be assumed to be present in patients over 75 years old. Treatments for osteoporosis include bisphosphonates, calcium and vitamin D supplements. The latter are particularly indicated for older people who are housebound or cared for in a residential or nursing home setting. Hip protectors can reduce the risk of femoral neck fractures in selected frail older people when worn.

# Answers

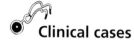

## Clinical cases

### CASE 6.1 – **A 71-year-old man has been brought to A&E after a fall while shopping.**

**A1:** What is the differential diagnosis?

- aortic stenosis
- cardiac arrhythmia
- silent myocardial infarction (MI)
- postural hypotension
- vasovagal episode
- hindbrain transient ischaemic attack (TIA).

### A2: What features in the history support the diagnosis?

The syncopal event occurred on exertion, and this is consistent with significant aortic stenosis. In this situation, syncope can be precipitated by impaired cardiac output or a transient arrhythmia such as ventricular tachycardia. The history of previous exertional dizziness and breathlessness lends support to this diagnosis.

Silent MI or cardiac arrhythmia must be considered too. Myocardial infarction can present without chest pain, particularly in older patients.

Postural hypotension – postural dizziness when standing (e.g. arising from bed at night) – might be volunteered. Enquire about medications with hypotensive properties (e.g. diuretics, antihypertensives, antidepressants). Co-codamol is not usually a cause of postural hypotension, but the opiate component (codeine) can reduce alertness and impair balance.

Vasovagal episodes are a common cause of syncopal events, particularly in younger patients. In this case, the lack of any precipitating event (e.g. prolonged standing) or prodromal symptoms (e.g. faintness, nausea) and the presence of other cardiac symptoms and signs make the diagnosis unlikely.

Finally, the patient has an arthritic neck. When severe, this can compromise the vertebrobasilar circulation, especially if there is significant atheroma affecting the vertebrobasilar system and circle of Willis. The apparent absence of sudden neck movement before syncope and the lack of other features such as dizziness, vertigo, nausea or sudden loss of tone in the legs ('drop attack') make this diagnosis less likely.

### A3: What additional features in the history would you seek to support the potential diagnoses?

The presence of exertional chest pain (angina) and dyspnoea supports the diagnosis of aortic stenosis (syncope, angina, dyspnoea = SAD).

### A4: What other features would you look for on clinical examination?

In aortic stenosis, the following might be present:

- ejection systolic murmur radiating to the neck
- slow rising pulse
- low pulse pressure

- ejection click sometimes heard
- early diastolic murmur if there is also aortic regurgitation
- quiet second heart sound.

In silent MI, the following might be present:

- signs of heart failure
- cool, clammy peripheries resulting from low cardiac output.

In postural hypotension, there is a fall in standing blood pressure <20 mmHg associated with symptoms of dizziness or faintness. In hindbrain ischaemia, symptoms are sometimes precipitated by head movement.

### A5: What investigations would you perform?

ECG, chest radiograph, cardiac enzymes or troponin testing, echocardiography and ECG (Holter) monitoring should be done.

### A6: What treatment options are available?

A precise diagnosis is essential first. If aortic stenosis is severe, the patient should be referred to a cardiologist for consideration of valve replacement. Transaortic valve implantation has extended the option of valvular repair to include patients not previously considered robust enough for open heart surgery. The patient should be advised to avoid sudden strenuous exertion in the meantime.

Admission is necessary if MI or arrhythmia is suspected. If there is postural hypotension, consider discontinuing or reducing the dose of any offending medication. The patient should be educated regarding avoidance of precipitating events. Compression hosiery should be used.

Aspirin and statin should be given for hindbrain TIA.

## CASE 6.2 – An 82-year-old woman presents with recurrent falls.

### A1: What is the differential diagnosis?

There are multiple causes, including:

- poor vision
- postural hypotension
- polypharmacy
- neurological dysfunction – previous stroke, cervical myelopathy, vitamin B12 deficiency
- arthritis/osteomalacia
- arrhythmia – AF.

### A2: What features in the history support the diagnosis?

- *Poor vision:* the fall occurred at night when environmental hazards are more difficult to see and avoid.
- *Postural hypotension:* the fall occurred as the patient was getting out of bed to go to the toilet. She is on a lot of medications that can impair postural blood pressure control – a diuretic, an angiotensin-converting enzyme (ACE) inhibitor and amitriptyline (a tricyclic antidepressant with anticholinergic properties).
- *Polypharmacy:* postural hypotension:
  - impaired balance and cognition caused by temazepam, opiate analgesic and tricyclic antidepressant
  - muscle weakness; diuretic-induced hypokalaemia.
- *Neurological dysfunction:* brisk reflexes are suggestive of upper motor neuron dysfunction. Common causes at this age include stroke disease, cervical myelopathy and occasionally vitamin B12 deficiency.

As a result of the history of falls and the finding of cognitive impairment, a chronic subdural haematoma should also be considered.

- *Atrial fibrillation:* poorly controlled (rapid) ventricular rate on exertion causing syncope. AF might also be a manifestation of sick sinus syndrome, predisposing to supraventricular tachycardia or bradycardia.

## A3: What additional features in the history would you seek to support the potential diagnoses?

- *Poor vision:* access to spectacles, ability to read or identify objects, adequacy of lighting in the home.
- *Postural hypotension:* dizziness or falls when upright, with associated symptoms of faintness or syncope, and rapid recovery when recumbent.
- *Polypharmacy:* concordance with medication regimen and any potential to exceed the intended dosing schedule.
- *Neurological dysfunction:* history suggestive of previous stroke or TIA.
- *Neck arthritis:* giddiness on head movement and pain radiating to shoulders and upper limbs (cervical spondylitic radiculopathy) suggest cervical myelopathy as a potential cause of falling.
- *Enquire about* diet, previous gastric surgery, bowel (terminal ileal) disease or resection, anaemia and symptoms of sensory neuropathy in suspected vitamin B12 deficiency.
- *Fluctuating alertness:* confusion or consciousness with a history of falls and head injuries (even trivial) should highlight the possibility of subdural intracranial bleeding.
- *Bone pains and muscle weakness:* in a housebound patient with poor diet, these point to osteomalacia.
- *Cardiac arrhythmia:* recurrent episodes of dizziness or syncope unrelated to posture or activity with prompt recovery suggest an intermittent cardiac rhythm disturbance.

## A4: What other features would you look for on clinical examination?

- *Poor vision:* Snellen chart to assess visual acuity, examination of eyes for common causes of visual loss in older people (i.e. refractive disorder), cataracts, glaucoma, macular degeneration, diabetic retinopathy.
- *Postural hypotension:* lying and standing blood pressure.
- *Neurological disorders:* thorough central nervous system (CNS) examination essential. Focal upper motor neuron signs suggestive of stroke or subdural haematoma. Up-going plantar responses, consistent with cervical myelopathy; peripheral neuropathy and posterior column dysfunction (joint position/vibration sense) suggest vitamin B12 deficiency.
- *Arthritis/osteomalacia:* joint examination, back pain, muscle weakness.

## A5: What investigations would you perform?

The following tests are necessary:

- lying and standing blood pressure
- ECG
- plasma urea, creatinine and electrolytes (U&Es) and glucose
- full blood count (FBC) (and vitamin B12/folate levels if macrocytic anaemia present)
- radiograph of painful bones and significantly arthritic joints
- vitamin D, calcium, albumin and alkaline phosphatase (ALP; for osteomalacia).

Other tests might be indicated after preliminary assessment and investigation, including:

- cervical spine radiograph with option to proceed to magnetic resonance imaging (MRI) cervical spine if cervical myelopathy is probable and surgery is a realistic option

- computed tomography (CT) of the brain
- thyroid function.

## A6: What treatment options are available?

- *Vision:* occupational therapist home visit to remove environmental hazards and improve lighting. Assess for spectacles and ophthalmic referral as needed.
- *Postural hypotension and polypharmacy:* review the need for and doses of all medications.
- *Neurological dysfunction:* beyond the scope of this case scenario.
- *Osteomalacia:* calcium and vitamin D supplements.
- *Atrial fibrillation:* discuss the need for rhythm or rate control – options include cardioversion, digoxin, beta-blockers and amiodarone. If the patient has a bradyarrhythmia, they will require assessment for cardiac pacemaker. Owing to the risk of further falls, anticoagulation with warfarin is often not appropriate without very careful assessment of the ongoing risks. Always involve the patient, family and general practitioner (GP) in such discussions.

## CASE 6.3 – A 78-year-old man who lives alone is brought to A&E after being found on the floor at home by his neighbour.

### A1: What is the differential diagnosis?

- pneumonia
- dehydration
- parkinsonism
- head injury with intracranial bleed or contusion.

### A2: What features in the history support the diagnosis?

Hypostatic pneumonia and dehydration often complicate a long period of immobility after a fall. Aspiration pneumonia should also be considered.

The generalized muscle cog-wheel rigidity is suggestive of parkinsonism. Reflexes can be difficult to elicit in this situation. Spasticity caused by cerebrovascular disease would more usually be associated with hyperreflexia and up-going plantar responses. Parkinsonism might be a result of idiopathic Parkinson's disease or secondary to other causes such as medication (e.g. neuroleptics such as haloperidol or risperidone) or vascular (arteriosclerotic). The patient's unkempt state suggests a chronic insidious decline before this acute presentation. Parkinson's disease and parkinsonism can present in this way.

Head injury is obvious on examination, but the severity is difficult to assess. A subdural haematoma (acute or chronic) must be considered in this setting.

### A3: What additional features in the history would you seek to support the potential diagnoses?

Further history from family, neighbours and so on is essential to establish the time course and pattern of the patient's decline and any history of previous falls. An accurate medication history is required, from the GP's records if necessary. Any suggestion of alcohol abuse is important. As always, details of past medical history are essential, such as a history of stroke disease, vascular dementia, and previous psychiatric history requiring neuroleptic medication.

### A4: What other features would you look for on clinical examination?

Assessment of conscious level and airway is essential because the patient is at risk of airway obstruction and aspiration.

Signs of weight loss or lymphadenopathy (tuberculosis [TB]) and clubbing (bronchial carcinoma) should be looked for. The rigidity of parkinsonism is usually of lead-pipe or cog-wheel type. A pill-rolling resting tremor may also be present, but not invariably so.

Evidence should be sought of urinary outflow obstruction (enlarged bladder), faecal impaction (rectal examination), bony injuries (hip, skull) and pressure sores, which can be overlooked in this setting.

## A5:  What investigations would you perform?

Additional investigations include:

- arterial oxygen saturation/blood gases
- blood and sputum cultures (for pneumonia)
- calcium (confusion caused by hypercalcaemia)
- urea, creatinine, electrolytes and creatinine kinase (for dehydration, kidney failure, rhabdomyolysis)
- ECG (for arrhythmias)
- radiographs of skull and sites of other apparent bony injuries
- CT of head (for acute or chronic subdural haematoma).

## A6:  What treatment options are available?

The following treatment options are available:

- rehydration with monitoring of urine output
- oxygen therapy as directed by O$_2$ saturation or arterial blood gas (ABG) measurements
- broad-spectrum antibiotics for hypostatic/aspiration pneumonia (e.g. benzylpenicillin, levofloxacin and metronidazole  – but consult local antibiotic guidelines)
- discontinuation of any drugs likely to cause parkinsonism
- if idiopathic Parkinson's disease is suspected, gradual introduction of ʟ-dopa-based medication (e.g. co-careldopa) once resuscitation completed.

## ♟ OSCE counselling cases

### OSCE COUNSELLING CASE 6.1 – **What advice would you give the following patient?**

The daughter has a valid point, but you will need to explain that to prevent further fractures measures are needed to reduce the risk of falling in addition to a consideration of treatment for osteoporosis.

The patient would benefit from a multidisciplinary assessment to identify remediable medical illnesses that might precipitate falls (e.g. cardiovascular disease, medications, poor eyesight, Parkinson's disease). Advice from a physiotherapist or occupational therapist on measures to enhance fitness and safety at home, and to secure help if further falls supervene, is also essential.

If the patient is aged 75 years or older, osteoporosis can be assumed in the setting of a low trauma fracture. Having excluded secondary causes of osteoporosis (e.g. thyrotoxicosis, steroid therapy, multiple myeloma, hyperparathyroidism), treatment for age-associated osteoporosis should be considered. In this setting, calcium and vitamin D supplements are helpful and relatively safe, although it is prudent to measure the plasma calcium level before and 6–8 weeks after initiating treatment. A regular bisphosphonate is also indicated, providing the requirements for safe and effective oral dosing can be followed. Oesophageal and peptic ulcer disease and renal impairment will require caution with respect to bisphosphonate therapy. Thorough discussion with the patient is essential before initiating treatment.

### OSCE COUNSELLING CASE 6.2 – **'What is the underlying condition, and how has it come about?'**

The likely diagnosis is osteomalacia. Lack of exposure to sunlight, poor diet if socially isolated, poor health, and enhanced metabolism of vitamin D as a result of treatment with phenytoin (a liver enzyme inducer) may have precipitated the condition. Diseases causing malabsorption and chronic renal failure can also predispose to osteomalacia.

You need to look for proximal muscle weakness, bony tenderness (pseudo-fractures or Looser's zones on radiograph), and skeletal deformities such as kyphosis and bowing of the limbs. Significant hypocalcaemia can precipitate tetany with a positive Chvostek sign (spasm of the facial muscles on tapping over the branches of the facial nerve in front of the ear) and Trousseau's sign (spasm of the hand and forearm muscles after compression of the forearm).

The blood level should be checked for 25-hydroxy-vitamin D, and vitamin D supplements should be given either orally or intramuscularly. An adequate calcium intake should be provided, if necessary with oral calcium supplements (1 g/day). There should be a thorough discussion with the patient about the risks and benefits of changing to an alternative anticonvulsant such as sodium valproate.

# IMMOBILITY

## Questions

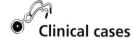

### Clinical cases

## For each of the case scenarios given, consider the following:

---

### CASE 6.4

**Q1**: What is the differential diagnosis?
**Q2**: What features in the history support the diagnosis?
**Q3**: What additional features in the history would you seek to support the potential diagnoses?
**Q4**: What other features would you look for on clinical examination?
**Q5**: What investigations would you perform?
**Q6**: What treatment options are available?

### CASE 6.5

**Q7**: What investigations would you perform?
**Q8**: What treatment options are available?
**Q9**: What are the likely causes of his immobility?
**Q10**: What can be done to improve the situation at home?

### CASE 6.6

**Q11**: What treatment options are available?
**Q12**: In addition to regular medical and nursing attention, which members of the multidisciplinary team ought to be involved with care?
**Q13**: What medical complications might supervene during the next 4–6 weeks?

---

## CASE 6.4 – **A 74-year-old man who has difficulty walking is referred to the elderly medicine day hospital.**

The patient is confined to his chair unless assisted to stand. He cannot get into bed at night. His past history includes neck surgery for cervical spondylosis. He has hypertension treated with nifedipine. He is obese, his legs are oedematous and he is incontinent of urine. He has ulceration and cellulitis affecting his lower legs. A CNS examination reveals normal cognition and cranial nerves, but weak arms and legs (power 4/5), brisk reflexes bilaterally and up-going plantar responses. His feet are warm but foot pulses are impossible to assess owing to oedema.

## CASE 6.5 – **You have been called to see a 72-year-old man who lives alone at home.**

The district nurse has become increasingly concerned about his health. The patient has been housebound for some time but is now unable to rise from his chair. He is a large man and his left hip is very painful. There is no history of a fall. He is unkempt and his clothes smell of urine. He is a heavy smoker, and he is breathless and wheezy with a chronic cough. His legs are swollen and blistered. Detailed examination is difficult but reveals signs of airflow obstruction, cyanosis, elevated JVP and peripheral oedema. Movement at the left hip is restricted and painful. He is very reluctant to leave his home.

## CASE 6.6 – **A 68-year-old previously active woman is unable to walk or stand having sustained a stroke (left middle cerebral artery territory infarction) 3 weeks previously.**

The patient has a dense right hemiparesis, homonymous hemianopia and sensory disturbance. She is also dysphasic and has difficulty swallowing. Recovery has been complicated by aspiration pneumonia. She has a urinary catheter and needs regular toileting. She is in AF, and her blood pressure is 142/78 mmHg. She is reluctant to engage with her programme of rehabilitation.

## 👥 OSCE counselling cases

OSCE COUNSELLING CASE 6.3 – **A 75-year-old man who lives in a nursing home is confined to his bed or chair as a result of a previous left-sided stroke.**

The patient is a large man and his care is made even more challenging as a result of the presence of dysphasia, dysphagia and mild cognitive impairment. The patient's GP visits the nursing home periodically to review his care and general condition. Give five important areas that the GP should enquire about or assess when visiting the patient. Give a brief explanation of why each of these areas needs review.

OSCE COUNSELLING CASE 6.4 – **A 65-year-old woman is reviewed in clinic following recent colonic surgery.**

Shortly after surgery the patient developed a hot swollen leg from a deep vein thrombosis (DVT), confirmed on duplex scanning. She has been started on anticoagulation therapy. She is upset that this developed and wants you to explain why it occurred and what was done to prevent it. How would you approach answering this patient?

OSCE COUNSELLING CASE 6.5 – **The wife of an elderly man is distressed because her husband's attendance at the local elderly care day hospital for physiotherapy has been discontinued. He had a severe stroke 3 months ago and is now confined to a wheelchair. He has difficulty speaking as a result of dysphasia. What advice would you give?**

## 🔑 Key concepts

To work through the core clinical cases in this section, you will need to understand the following key concepts.

Many chronic diseases in older people present with difficulty walking or transferring from chair to bed. Immobility itself is not a diagnosis but a symptom for which there are any number of causes. Common illnesses in older people that impair walking include:

- stroke disease
- osteoarthritis
- parkinsonism
- dementia
- visual impairment
- chronic cardiorespiratory disease
- injuries and complications of falling
- problems with feet and footwear.

Careful and accurate assessment is essential, with the aim of identifying treatable causes in order to focus the efforts of the multidisciplinary team. Remember that being immobile can lead to further disabling and potentially fatal complications such as pressure sores, hypostatic pneumonia, DVT, osteoporosis, limb contractures, urinary retention and faecal impaction. Depression often occurs in such situations.

## Answers

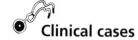 **Clinical cases**

---

### CASE 6.4 – **A 74-year-old man who has difficulty walking is referred to the elderly medicine day hospital.**

#### A1: What is the differential diagnosis?

- cervical myelopathy
- gravitational and calcium antagonist-induced lower limb oedema
- infected leg ulcers
- possible DVT.

#### A2: What features in the history support the diagnosis?

The history of neck surgery for arthritis and the finding of upper motor neuron signs in the arms and legs (with no evidence of neurological dysfunction above the neck) is highly suggestive of cervical myelopathy consequent to degenerative disease of the cervical spine.

Impaired mobility, obesity and dependency of the lower legs predispose to venous stasis, oedema and ulceration (and in due course infection). This is a potent setting for venous thrombosis. Calcium antagonists can exacerbate peripheral oedema.

Urinary incontinence is inevitable in this setting owing to immobility and impaired bladder control caused by compression of the cervical spinal cord.

#### A3: What additional features in the history would you seek to support the potential diagnoses?

- history of neck trauma or injury or arthritic symptoms – acute-on-chronic deterioration will require urgent neurosurgical opinion and possible intervention
- constipation – common in this setting and exacerbated by calcium antagonists
- history of previous venous thrombosis or peripheral vascular disease
- symptoms of breathlessness or chest pain (pulmonary embolism).

#### A4: What other features would you look for on clinical examination?

- signs of pulmonary embolism or heart failure
- pressure sores (buttocks, sacrum, heels)
- faecal impaction and urinary retention.

#### A5: What investigations would you perform?

- FBC (infection)
- renal function and plasma glucose (renal failure and diabetes mellitus)
- urinalysis:
  - heavy proteinuria if oedema caused by nephrotic syndrome
  - glycosuria
  - protein and blood consistent with urinary infection

- midstream urine specimen (MSU; infection)
- leg ulcer swab and blood cultures (to guide antibiotic therapy)
- venous and arterial Doppler studies of legs (detection of venous thrombosis and exclusion of ischaemic leg ulceration)
- cervical spine radiograph (cervical spondylosis/osteoarthritis)
- MRI cervical spine (to detect spinal cord compression)
- chest radiograph and ECG (heart failure and pulmonary embolism).

## A6: What treatment options are available?

Neck surgery for cervical myelopathy is unlikely to be successful in this setting as a result of chronicity of symptoms. Surgery could also be very hazardous as a result of significant comorbidity.

The following treatment options are available:

- elevation of legs to diminish oedema
- antibiotics for cellulitis
- compression bandaging or hosiery to control peripheral oedema once cellulitis has resolved and arterial ischaemia has been excluded
- pressure-relief mattress/cushion for areas at high risk of pressure sores
- anticoagulant therapy if venous thrombosis is confirmed (consider DVT prophylaxis if absent)
- discontinuation of calcium antagonist – consider an alternative antihypertensive agent such as a diuretic (might exacerbate incontinence), an ACE inhibitor (might impair renal function) or a beta-blocker (care if uncontrolled heart failure/diabetes present), or an alpha-blocker (watch for postural hypotension)
- treatment for heart failure if confirmed
- attention to bowel and bladder function
- referral to multidisciplinary team for rehabilitation and resettlement at home in due course.

## CASE 6.5 – You have been called to see a 72-year-old man who lives alone at home.

## A7: What investigations would you perform?

Basic investigations should include:

- hip radiograph (essential for osteoarthritis or avascular necrosis of femoral head or fractured neck of femur)
- FBC (secondary polycythaemia and infection)
- renal function tests (uraemia and electrolyte imbalance)
- measurement of ABGs should be considered because of the signs of respiratory failure and possible hypercapnia
- chest radiograph and ECG (to support the diagnosis of chronic obstructive pulmonary disease [COPD] and cor pulmonale)
- peak expiratory flow rate or spirometry before and after inhaled bronchodilator will confirm COPD and determine the degree of reversibility.

## A8: What treatment options are available?

Management will be difficult at home as a result of the need for radiographs and specialist tests, and the presence of respiratory failure. Brief hospital assessment (a rapid-access day hospital clinic or short-stay elderly care ward) is advisable to confirm the diagnoses and assess the degree of respiratory failure. Time will be needed for rehabilitation and adaptations to the home environment.

Treatment will be along the following lines:

- analgesia for osteoarthritis (avoiding opiates and non-steroidal anti-inflammatory drugs [NSAIDs] if possible – potential respiratory depression and fluid retention, respectively)
- bronchodilators, controlled oxygen and cautious use of diuretics for COPD and cor pulmonale
- laxatives and enemas for faecal impaction or constipation
- in due course, consideration of hip replacement if the patient is agreeable and cardiorespiratory status permits.

## A9: What are the likely causes of his immobility?

The likely causes are:

- osteoarthritic hip – a hip fracture is less likely as a result of the chronicity of the symptoms and absence of trauma
- COPD (chronic bronchitis and emphysema) and cor pulmonale
- urinary incontinence caused by immobility – almost inevitable in this situation, perhaps exacerbated by coexisting prostatism or faecal impaction.

## A10: What can be done to improve the situation at home?

Much depends on the patient's potential to improve and the feasibility of hip surgery. Adaptations to the home with appropriate seating and bedding, and a review of toilet and washing arrangements, will be necessary. The patient's ability to climb stairs safely will need to be assessed. He will need assistance with shopping and other household tasks. A multidisciplinary team approach is required to resolve these various issues, including physiotherapy, occupational therapy and social worker involvement. Early discharge from hospital can be achieved with forward planning and use of domiciliary rehabilitation services.

## CASE 6.6 – A 68-year-old previously active woman is unable to walk or stand, having sustained a stroke (right middle cerebral artery territory infarction) 3 weeks previously.

### A11: What treatment options are available?

Depression is common at this stage and can seriously interfere with rehabilitation. An antidepressant in conjunction with psychological support and a positive approach by the multidisciplinary team can help alleviate this.

- *Anticoagulants* – due to AF, there is a risk of further stroke (12–15 per cent per annum), which can be reduced by two-thirds after anticoagulation with warfarin (international normalized ratio [INR] 2.0–3.0).
- *Antiembolic stockings* – reduce the risk of DVT and lower limb oedema.
- *Laxative* – to prevent constipation.
- *Analgesia* – pain and stiffness are common in this situation.
- *ACE inhibitor* – if blood pressure persistently >140/80 mmHg (but be vigilant about the risk of precipitating symptomatic postural hypotension).

## A12: In addition to regular medical and nursing attention, which members of the multidisciplinary team ought to be involved with care?

- *physiotherapist* – to prevent contractures, maintain posture, avoid shoulder injury and improve function
- *occupational therapist* – to promote independence and overcome functional impairments caused by motor, sensory and visual impairments
- *speech and language therapist* – including assessment and therapy to improve swallowing
- *dietitian* – modification of diet to enhance safe swallowing and maintain adequate hydration and nutrition
- *stroke nurse specialist/psychologist* – specialist advice, support and counselling to patient and family
- *social worker* to explore any social issues relevant to a timely, safe and supported discharge from hospital.

## A13: What medical complications might supervene during the next 4–6 weeks?

- painful shoulder caused by joint subluxation or capsular/rotator cuff injury (correct manual handling essential to minimize this complication)
- DVT/pulmonary embolism
- pneumonia (aspiration or hypostatic)
- urinary tract infection (UTI)
- faecal impaction
- pressure sores
- limb contractures
- depression
- post-stroke epilepsy
- recurrent stroke (haemorrhage transformation or reinfarction).

**OSCE counselling cases**

## OSCE COUNSELLING CASE 6.3 – **A 75-year-old man who lives in a nursing home is confined to his bed or chair owing to a previous left-sided stroke.**

The GP should enquire about or assess the following.

- *Skin care and pressure areas:*
  - pressure sores (especially the sacrum, hips and heels)
  - intertrigo in skin folds such as the groins, axillae and perineum
  - leg ulcers complicating dependent oedema of the lower limbs
  - soft tissue infections.
- *Bladder and bowels:* urinary incontinence is inevitable in this situation and will necessitate regular toileting or containment by pads, sheath drainage or (as a last resort) urinary catheterization. Urinary catheter care will include regular catheter changes (every 3–4 months) to prevent encrustation, blockage and leakage. Bowel function will need review. Faecal incontinence, constipation and faecal impaction with overflow diarrhoea may all need appropriate management.
- *Nutrition:* obesity will exacerbate nursing difficulties. On the other hand, difficulty swallowing, resulting in poor nutrition, might cause weight loss. Provision of food and drink of the appropriate consistency and manoeuvres to improve swallowing will need discussion. Nutritional and vitamin supplementation may prove necessary. Liaison with the dietitian and speech and language therapist may be helpful.
- *Limb contractures/oedema:*
  - Flexion contractures of the limbs can develop over time and can be ameliorated to some extent by appropriate positioning of the hemiplegic limb, physiotherapy, and antispasticity drugs such as baclofen or botulinum toxin injections.
  - Dependent oedema and DVT can develop in an immobile lower limb. Elastic hosiery can help to prevent this.
  - Shoulder pain can develop as a result of incorrect handling/lifting techniques.
- *Respiratory complications:* aspiration or hypostatic pneumonia.
- *Medication review:* the need for laxatives, analgesics and hypnotics and the appropriateness of medication for secondary stroke prevention (aspirin, a statin, antihypertensives) will need periodic review.
- *Social and psychological wellbeing:* good-quality care should encompass this important area. Apathy and depression are common after a disabling stroke. Boredom and isolation can lead to difficult behaviour. Regular visits from friends and family should be facilitated. Interest in former hobbies and pursuits should be encouraged as far as is possible. Social activities and access to radio and television are important, being mindful of the patient's preferences and interests. Advice from a speech and language therapist will be helpful to maximize communication. Anticipatory care discussions should be broached so that the patient's wishes concerning potential future treatment interventions can be recorded. This will require assessment of his mental capacity and, if he is willing, discussion about advance care directives, lasting power of attorney and so on.

## OSCE COUNSELLING CASE 6.4 – **A 65-year-old woman is reviewed in clinic after recent colonic surgery.**

The essence of this case is to discuss risk reduction and distinguish this from prevention. Deep vein thrombosis is a well-recognized problem post-surgery. The risk is higher in people with prothrombotic states such as malignancy or a hypercoagulable syndrome (e.g. factor V Lieden mutation) and where venous return may be compromised (pelvic surgery, lower limbs raised intraoperatively, e.g. lithotomy position or with a pneumoperitoneum – laparoscopic surgery).

To reduce the risk, the patient is given a low-molecular-weight (LMW) heparin, is preoperatively well hydrated with intravenous (IV) fluids (especially if they have had preoperative bowel preparation), will be wearing thromboembolic deterrent stockings and may have been asked to stop any prothrombotic medication before surgery (e.g. tamoxifen). (LMW heparin works by activating anti-thrombin III; it inhibits platelet aggregation and decreases the availability of thrombin. It has a longer half-life than heparin and therefore requires only a single daily administration. The fact that its response is much easier to predict removes the need for monitoring.) During surgery the legs are slightly elevated to aid venous return and intermittent calf compression can be used. Post-surgery, early mobilization is encouraged.

Even with these precautions there is still a risk of a DVT developing. The importance of making the diagnosis and treating appropriately should be emphasized.

If there has been an aberration to the normal protocols, increasing the patient's risk, the aberration should be admitted and a reason sought. There is often a reason that can be explained (e.g. not giving heparin preoperatively if an epidural is to be inserted). Did the preoperative consent discuss the risk of DVT?

## OSCE COUNSELLING CASE 6.5 – **The wife of an elderly man is distressed because her husband's attendance at the local elderly care day hospital for physiotherapy has been discontinued.**

This is a difficult situation and the decision has probably been made because the patient is not making progress with rehabilitation. A feeling of abandonment heightens the wife's sense of distress at the withdrawal of therapy by the multidisciplinary team. This situation can be avoided or ameliorated in a number of ways:

- setting clear goals for rehabilitation with realistic timescales that are understood by the patient's family and carers and whenever possible the patient
- use of a graded reduction in therapy, transferring the emphasis of care into more socially oriented activities such as former hobbies and interests
- ongoing support from a stroke nurse or another member of the multidisciplinary team such as a social worker or home-care assistant
- recognition of the needs of the carer – attendance at the day hospital may have been a lifeline for the patient's wife in terms of providing regular respite from caring. Alternative arrangements such as a carer to sit with the patient at home or attendance at a local day centre or stroke club may be helpful.

## ACUTE CONFUSIONAL STATES

## Questions

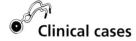

### Clinical cases

### For each of the case scenarios given, consider the following:

**Q1**: Give the most likely causes of the patient's confusional state.
**Q2**: What initial investigations should you perform?
**Q3**: What treatment would you consider appropriate?
**Q4**: [Case 6.9 only] The patient's niece is worried about her aunt returning home alone at the conclusion of the hospital admission. How would you address this concern?

### CASE 6.7 – **An 83-year-old man who has been brought to A&E.**

The patient lives in a residential home. For the past 2 days he has become confused. He is not eating or drinking and his walking has deteriorated. He has Parkinson's disease, a history of angina and type 2 diabetes mellitus. His medication includes co-beneldopa, selegiline, gliclazide, a nitrate preparation and aspirin.

On examination the significant findings are as follows:

- abbreviated mental test 4/10; he is agitated and restless
- dry tongue and superficial veins are empty
- blood pressure 108/62 mmHg
- heart rate 104/min, regular
- clear chest
- marked signs of parkinsonism (rigidity, tremor and bradykinesia)
- urinalysis: protein ++, blood +, glucose ++ and ketones negative.

### CASE 6.8 – **A 74-year-old man with a history of alcohol abuse admitted to hospital 24 h ago after two witnessed epileptic seizures.**

The patient recovered fully and was initially lucid, but he is now very restless and agitated. He seems to be hallucinating. Examination is difficult. He has a low-grade fever and is tremulous and sweating. There are no obvious focal neurological signs. He is not jaundiced or anaemic. His blood pressure is 178/84 mmHg and his heart rate is 106/min, with AF.

### CASE 6.9 – **An 84-year-old woman brought to hospital after being found wandering in the street at night by the neighbours.**

The patient is very disoriented and confused. She is alert but restless and agitated. She is convinced that she is late for work. A telephone call to her niece confirms that the patient has been somewhat confused and forgetful for the past 9 months or so. Further enquiry reveals that the patient needs help with her household and financial affairs. She has never wandered before.

Examination discloses AF (heart rate 126/min), cardiomegaly, mitral incompetence and peripheral oedema. Her feet are in a state of neglect and there is an infected bunion. Abbreviated mental test is 4/10. There are no focal neurological signs. The remainder of the examination is unremarkable.

## ⅈⅈ OSCE counselling cases

OSCE COUNSELLING CASE 6.6 – **What advice should be given to the matron of a local nursing home who telephones the local GP to report that one of her elderly residents, who has Alzheimer's disease, has become uncharacteristically agitated and restless?**

OSCE COUNSELLING CASE 6.7 – **An 84-year-old woman has been brought to A&E, having been found wandering at night.**

The patient is alert but confused (Mini-Mental State Examination [MMSE] 12/30 (normal 27+/30)). There are no focal neurological signs, but she is cold (core temperature 35.5 °C). She is unable to give a coherent history. You telephone the patient's daughter to gain more historical information. Give five key aspects of the history that you need to establish in discussion with the daughter.

# 🔑 Key concepts

To work through the core clinical cases in this section, you will need to understand the following key concepts.

Acute confusion or delirium is a syndrome rather than a diagnosis and can be the mode of presentation of almost any illness, especially in older people. The most important question is 'why?'. There is great danger (for lack of collateral history) in assuming that the patient has 'always been like this' or that only one factor is involved. Always search for multiple pathology.

Common precipitating factors include:

- infections
- metabolic disturbances (e.g. hypo-/hyperglycaemia, dehydration, electrolyte imbalance, uraemia, hypothermia)
- hypoxia or heart failure
- pain or injury
- surgery or anaesthesia
- drugs (especially anticholinergic, dopaminergic or opiate therapy and alcohol/tranquillizer withdrawal states)
- sensory overload (e.g. unfamiliar surroundings or situations)
- pre-existing cognitive impairment (often mild and previously unnoticed) or sensory impairment (deafness or poor vision), chronic diseases and polypharmacy are all common predisposing factors in older people. Pre-existing dementia will present an acute-on-chronic confusional state
- Delirium can present as a hyperactive (agitated) or hypoactive (drowsy) state. Delirium has a short period of onset (hours or a few days), fluctuates in severity and can alternate between hyper- and hypoactive states.

The cornerstone of management is to detect and correct the underlying causes and use general measures to reorientate and reassure the patient and prevent complications. Sedation should be considered only when agitation or confusion is preventing essential tests or treatment, the patient's behaviour poses a danger to him- or herself or others, or it is necessary to relieve severe distress in an agitated patient. The maxim 'start low and go slow' when prescribing for older patients is particularly germane in this setting.

## Answers

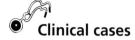
### Clinical cases

### CASE 6.7 – **An 83-year-old man who has been brought to A&E.**

#### A1: Give the most likely causes of the patient's confusional state.

His confusional state is multifactorial. Precipitating factors may include a UTI, dehydration and hyperglycaemia. Drugs prescribed for Parkinson's disease such as selegiline (a monoamine oxidase type B [MAOI-B] inhibitor) and levodopa can precipitate confusion, particularly in susceptible patients, e.g. those with pre-existing cognitive impairment. Other potential factors might include silent MI (hypotension and history of coronary artery disease) or stroke (symptoms and signs difficult to elicit owing to confusion and agitation). Enquiry about falls and head injury (even trivial) is important because of the potential for subdural haematoma. Hypoglycaemia must be quickly excluded by capillary blood glucose testing. Long-acting hypoglycaemic drugs carry particular risk in this setting (e.g. modified-release gliclazide, glibenclamide).

#### A2: What initial investigations should you perform?

- FBC – infection
- sepsis screen – urine and blood cultures and chest radiograph
- renal function tests – electrolyte imbalance and uraemia
- capillary/plasma glucose and glycated haemoglobin (HbA1c) – to assess diabetic control
- C-reactive protein (CRP) or erythrocyte sedimentation rate (ESR) – non-specific markers of an inflammatory process
- ECG – MI
- arterial oxygen saturation – to identify hypoxaemia caused by cardiopulmonary disease.

#### A3: What treatment would you consider appropriate?

- rehydration (IV) and correction of electrolyte disturbance
- sliding-scale insulin infusion for control of diabetes
- broad-spectrum antibiotic to cover UTI (after obtaining appropriate cultures)
- discontinue selegiline – this drug is more likely to precipitate confusion than L-dopa-based medications
- maintain co-beneldopa at minimum dose required to control parkinsonian symptoms
- general measures to reassure and reorient the patient
- prevention of falls and pressure sores
- avoid major tranquillizers (e.g. haloperidol), which, in the presence of Parkinson's disease, may precipitate a severe neuroleptic sensitivity reaction. Low-dose short-term quetiapine can be used in Parkinson's disease when necessary, but only after specialist advice and if other measures have failed to ameliorate the patient's agitation and distress.

## CASE 6.8 – **A 74-year-old man with a history of alcohol abuse admitted to hospital 24 h ago after two witnessed epileptic seizures.**

### A1: Give the most likely causes of the patient's confusional state.

Alcohol withdrawal causing delirium tremens is very likely, given the time course of the patient's confusional state. Hypoglycaemia may also be present, given the history of alcohol abuse and the potential for liver disease.

Occult head injury should also be considered. Patients who are inebriated or fitting are at great risk of injury and will have little, if any, recollection of the event. Older patients who misuse alcohol are particularly susceptible to subdural intracranial bleeding as a result of the combined effects of trauma, cerebral atrophy and coagulopathy.

The history of seizures raises the possibility of an intracranial space-occupying lesion (e.g. subdural haematoma, tumour), although alcohol excess and alcohol withdrawal can also precipitate seizures. Electrolyte imbalance, particularly hyponatraemia (syndrome of inappropriate antidiuretic hormone secretion, [SIADH]), must be considered in the setting of head injury or intracranial space-occupying lesion.

Pneumonia, meningitis and UTI are all possibilities in this setting. Liver encephalopathy is unlikely in the absence of jaundice.

A check for gastrointestinal bleeding (per rectal examination) is important (note sweating and tachycardia), although the elevated blood pressure militates against this.

### A2: What initial investigations should you perform?

- capillary glucose – hypoglycaemia
- plasma U&Es – SIADH
- liver function tests (LFTs) and INR – liver damage and synthetic liver function
- FBC – bleeding and infection
- blood cultures – urine dipstick and culture should be sent as soon as a sample can be obtained
- chest radiograph when feasible – pneumonia
- arterial oxygen saturation – hypoxia
- CT of head – space-occupying lesion/bleeding.

Lumbar puncture should be considered (meningitis?) if the above tests fail to identify a cause and there is no evidence of a space-occupying lesion, bleeding or raised intracranial pressure on CT of the brain and no coagulopathy.

### A3: What treatment would you consider appropriate?

Delirium tremens is very likely and should be treated with a benzodiazepine (e.g. IV diazepam followed by oral chlordiazepoxide) tapered over 3–4 days. IV thiamine is also advisable because malnourished individuals with alcohol problems are at risk of developing Wernicke's encephalopathy.

If hypoglycaemia is detected on capillary glucose reading (send plasma sample to laboratory for confirmation, but do not delay treatment while awaiting result), IV glucose (25 mL 50% dextrose IV) should be given.

Once the patient's agitation and confusion have been controlled, careful clinical examination is needed to assess for other causes of confusion, as outlined above.

## CASE 6.9 – An 84-year-old woman brought to hospital after being found wandering in the street at night by the neighbours.

### A1: Give the most likely causes of the patient's confusional state.

The history is very suggestive of an acute-on-chronic confusional state, the former precipitated by acute illness(es). Underlying cognitive impairment as a result of early Alzheimer's diseases is quite likely in this setting but must not be assumed. A search for acute illnesses such as infection (UTI, infected bunion, respiratory), side effects of medication, heart failure and metabolic disturbance (e.g. diabetes, uraemia) is essential. The patient was found wandering at night, so hypothermia must be considered.

In addition to an acute illness, causes of chronic confusion must be considered, such as dementia (Alzheimer's or vascular brain disease), thyroid dysfunction, vitamin B12 deficiency and hypercalcaemia. If there is a poorly maintained gas appliance at home, chronic carbon monoxide (CO) poisoning may need to be excluded.

### A2: What initial investigations should you perform?

- FBC – anaemia, infection
- urinalysis and MSU – infection, diabetes
- blood cultures and swab from infected bunion
- plasma electrolytes, glucose and renal function – metabolic disturbance and uraemia
- calcium – confusion caused by hypercalcaemia
- thyroid function tests – often difficult to interpret in acute illness, but in this case important to exclude thyroid dysfunction, particularly hyperthyroidism as a result of AF and heart failure
- chest radiograph – infection, heart failure
- ECG – to confirm AF
- arterial oxygen saturation (and spectrophotometry for carboxyhaemoglobin if CO poisoning suspected).

Once the acute illnesses have settled, and if chronic confusion persists, CT of the brain should be considered to exclude potentially treatable causes of chronic confusion such as hydrocephalus, meningioma and chronic subdural haematoma. Vitamin B12 and folate levels are needed if there is macrocytic anaemia.

### A4: The patient's niece is worried about her aunt returning home alone at the conclusion of the hospital admission. How would you address this concern?

This is a difficult issue and there is insufficient information provided to formulate a full answer to this question. Once acute confusion has settled, the patient's cognitive and functional status should be reassessed by the multidisciplinary team (in particular, the occupational therapist and social worker). An old-age psychiatry consultation may be required, particularly if a new or former diagnosis of dementia is confirmed, so that an assessment of the patient's mental capacity can be made. If the patient insists on returning home alone, a formal judgement as per the Mental Capacity Act 2005 concerning her capacity to assess the risk involved will be important. If the patient is judged to have capacity regarding discharge destination, the risks associated with returning home should be minimized by her family and the multidisciplinary team, including social services if required. Assessment of the patient's home environment will also be important before a decision about discharge is finalized. If the patient lacks capacity to make decisions about her discharge destination, a formal 'best interests meeting' as per the Mental Capacity Act will need to be convened. Discharge home may still be the preferred option after full assessment. Acetylcholinesterase inhibitor therapy (e.g. donepezil) to enhance cognition is contraindicated in this patient because of significant cardiac disease.

## ⅲ OSCE counselling cases

OSCE COUNSELLING CASE 6.6 – **What advice should be given to the matron of a local nursing home who telephones the local GP to report that one of her elderly residents, who has Alzheimer's disease, has become uncharacteristically agitated and restless?**

This is a common scenario, often referred to as an acute-on-chronic confusional state, i.e. delirium complicating underlying dementia. Older people with impaired cognitive reserve are at greater risk of delirium, and this is often precipitated by events such as intercurrent illness (commonly infection), an adverse reaction to medication, emotional distress or pain/discomfort. The first priority is to ensure the patient's safety while identifying and correcting the offending precipitant.

The nurses should check for symptoms and signs of common infections such as UTI (fever, dysuria, incontinence, abnormalities on urinalysis) and respiratory infection (cough, wheezing, dyspnoea). A check for dehydration is important; if identified, dehydration can be corrected by giving regular drinks under supervision. Capillary glucose should be checked, even if there is no history of diabetes – a new diagnosis is always possible in this setting. The patient's medication chart should be reviewed to see whether there are any new medications or amended dosages. Physical distress resulting from urinary retention, faecal impaction, pain from injury (any recent fall?) or emotional upset should be identified and corrected. If there is any suspicion of underlying medical illness, a prompt medical assessment will be needed.

In the interim, the nurses should be advised to monitor the patient unobtrusively, enhance her orientation by using adequate soft lighting in familiar surroundings, and ensure any hearing aid is operational and spectacles are worn. A calm, confident approach is needed; the reassurance of a close family member or friend is helpful.

The nurses should be asked to watch the patient closely to prevent accidents and injury, and to encourage her to drink fluids to correct or prevent dehydration.

It is likely that the patient's confusional state will settle if the offending precipitant is identified and corrected, although it may take a few days or sometimes longer for the older person to settle back to 'normal'. In many instances, hospital admission (with its attendant hazards to a frail older person) can be avoided, but this will require close cooperation of the doctor, nursing staff and family and carers.

OSCE COUNSELLING CASE 6.7 – **An 84-year-old woman has been brought to A&E, having been found wandering at night.**

In discussion with the patient's daughter, you need to establish the following key aspects of the history.

- *Duration of confusion:* is this an acute, acute-on-chronic or chronic confusional state? Acute and acute-on-chronic confusion suggest the presence of delirium and warrant a diligent search for intercurrent general medical conditions that may have precipitated the current delirious state (e.g. infection, CNS event such as head injury, metabolic disturbance, hypothyroidism). The presence of chronic confusion (duration >6 months) is suggestive of a dementing illness such as Alzheimer's disease.
- *Systems enquiry:* the patient cannot give a coherent account of events, but while lucid she may have previously reported important symptoms to a close relative or carer. Enquiry along these lines may reveal, for example, a description of a recent head injury (subdural haematoma), urinary symptoms

(infection), thirst and urinary frequency (diabetes mellitus), or cold intolerance (hypothyroidism). Any predisposing factors for hypothermia should be sought.

- *Previous medical history:* this may give important information relevant to the patient's current presentation – e.g. a history of liver disease, cerebrovascular disease, chronic renal impairment or cardiopulmonary disease may cause or predispose to an acute confusional state. You need to find out if there is a previous formal diagnosis of dementia or other psychiatric history.
- *Drug history:* medications commonly cause confusion in older patients. Offending agents include anticholinergics (e.g. trihexyphenidyl for Parkinson's disease), tricyclic antidepressants (e.g. amitriptyline), opiates, hypoglycaemic agents (e.g. glibenclamide) and dopaminergic drugs (e.g. L-dopa). Alcohol should also be considered. Polypharmacy (more than five medications) can be the cause of a confusional state when many drugs, each with weak anticholinergic properties, combine to produce appreciable central anticholinergic side effects (e.g. digoxin, nitrates, warfarin, furosemide, ranitidine, cyclizine).
- *Social history:* this information is essential to gain a proper understanding of the context of the patient's presenting illness, potential for rehabilitation and, in due course, discharge planning.

# INCONTINENCE

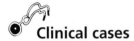

### Clinical cases

## For each of the case scenarios given, consider the following:

---

### CASES 6.10 AND 6.11

**Q1**: What are the likely causes of urinary incontinence in this patient?
**Q2**: How should the problem be investigated?
**Q3**: What can be done to help?

### CASE 6.12

**Q4**: What are the likely causes of urinary incontinence in this patient?
**Q5**: What treatments should be considered?
**Q6**: Suggest three reasons why the incontinence has gone unreported by the patient for so long.

---

### CASE 6.10 – **A 78-year-old woman disabled by stroke and cared for by her daughter.**

Care at home is proving difficult as a result of persistent urinary incontinence, such that a nursing home placement is now being considered. The patient has a right hemiparesis and dysphasia and needs help to stand, transfer and walk. She receives treatment with aspirin (for stroke), amlodipine (for hypertension) and furosemide (for swollen ankles).

The patient is alert and responsive, but she has difficulty communicating as a result of her dysphasia. Sometimes she is able to indicate that she needs to use the lavatory, but she is usually wet before toileting can be achieved.

In addition to the signs of stroke, examination shows an excoriated perineum. There is no palpable bladder. Rectal examination is normal. There is no uterovaginal prolapse.

### CASE 6.11 – **An 82-year-old man with advanced Parkinson's disease and dementia is cared for in a nursing home.**

His nursing needs are usually fairly predictable. Of late, he has become more agitated than usual. He seems uncomfortable and has started to shout and rattle the bedsides, and occasionally he hits out at the nurses. The on-call GP has prescribed a sedative to settle the patient at night. The patient is continuously wet with urine and, unusually for him, he is now incontinent of liquid faeces too. He has no fever and other vital signs are normal.

## CASE 6.12 – **A 90-year-old woman who lives alone has slipped and fallen in her bathroom at home.**

She has escaped serious injury. Subsequent visits by the district nurse to assess the situation reveal that the elderly woman's clothing is always soaked in urine and the house has a strong smell of urine. The patient is reluctant to discuss the situation but does admit to a swelling 'down below'. She is sensible and independent in her activities of daily living. She is reluctant to be examined by the nurse, but in due course assessment reveals a swelling at the vaginal introitus, which on further examination is shown to be the cervix. When the patient stands up she leaks urine. Her bowel function is normal.

There are no other abnormal findings. In particular, there is no palpable bladder, neurological examination is normal and urinalysis is negative.

## ** OSCE counselling cases

### OSCE COUNSELLING CASE 6.8 – **An elderly woman with hypertension is attending the surgery for regular assessment of her blood pressure.**

On this occasion her daughter attends as well and mentions that the family is very concerned about the patient's apparent incontinence of urine. The daughter goes on to say that her mother's house and clothing have now developed a constant smell of urine. On direct questioning, the patient makes light of this problem. She seems sensible. How would you proceed?

### OSCE COUNSELLING CASE 6.9 – **An 86-year-old woman is distressed by persistent incontinence of urine.**

Outline the key steps to establishing the cause of this problem in a primary care setting.

**Key concepts**

To work through the core clinical cases in this section, you will need to understand the following key concepts.

Urinary incontinence to some degree is common in older people, affecting about 12 per cent of men and 20 per cent of women aged 65 years and over, compared with 1 per cent of men and 6 per cent of women aged 15–64 years. Transient causes include confusional states, immobility, urine infection, diabetes, stroke, retention with overflow and drugs. Incontinence can persist if the above conditions remain unresolved. Established incontinence can also occur in many other chronic disorders – e.g. unstable bladder resulting from detrusor muscle instability (urge incontinence), pelvic floor incompetence (stress incontinence), neurogenic bladder (e.g. spinal cord lesions, cerebrovascular disease), incontinence associated with dementia, prostatism or bladder tumour or stone, and immobility from any cause.

Assessment must include a full history and examination, including per rectum and (if appropriate) per vagina examinations, and CNS and locomotor assessments. Investigations include urinalysis, MSU, U&Es, glucose, calcium, plain abdominal radiograph or ultrasonography and, in some patients, urodynamic studies.

Accurate diagnosis and treatment are essential. Effective treatments for urge incontinence include bladder retraining and drugs to stabilize the bladder (e.g. anticholinergics such as oxybutynin and solifenacin), but side effects can be problematic in elderly people. Stress incontinence can be helped by pelvic muscle exercises to strengthen the pelvic floor and surgical suspension procedures. Devices to ameliorate incontinence (pads, sheath drainage, urinals, intermittent self-catheterization) are effective to varying degrees and are appropriate steps to avoid permanent catheterization and its attendant hazards (e.g. infection, soreness, bypassing, embarrassment).

Faecal incontinence is less frequent than urinary incontinence but can be much more distressing to the patient and carers. Community-based studies reveal a 2 per cent prevalence of faecal incontinence in people aged over 65 years, rising to about 25 per cent in people aged over 85 years. Prevalence rates in nursing homes and hospital are even higher. In a British study, only half of people reporting faecal incontinence had discussed this with a health-care professional. Causes include underlying diseases in the rectum or anus (e.g. proctitis, tumour), faecal impaction with overflow diarrhoea (secondary to immobility caused by, for example, stroke or arthritis), neurological disorders affecting sphincter control (similar to those causing urinary incontinence), and cognitive disorders such as dementia or severe depression. Accurate diagnosis and treatment of remedial factors are essential (e.g. enemas for faecal impaction). When remedial measures fail or are inappropriate, faecal incontinence can be controlled by means of a drug-induced constipation regimen alternating with periodic planned bowel evacuation by enema or suppository.

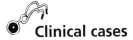

# Answers

## Clinical cases

### CASE 6.10 – A 78-year-old woman disabled by stroke and cared for by her daughter.

#### A1: What are the likely causes of urinary incontinence in this patient?

In this situation there are several factors responsible for the urinary incontinence.

- Damage to the CNS by a stroke will have impaired the central capacity to inhibit bladder (detrusor) contractions, resulting in frequency and urgency of micturition.
- Immobility and difficulty calling for help and perhaps cognitive dysfunction will precipitate urinary incontinence.
- Diuretic therapy will exacerbate the situation, as the patient will need to pass urine quickly.
- Immobility and incomplete bladder emptying both predispose to UTI, which can cause incontinence.

#### A2: How should the problem be investigated?

- urinalysis and MSU – to assess for infection, diabetes and occult renal disease
- U&Es – hypokalaemia, hyponatraemia and renal failure
- plasma glucose – polyuria caused by hyperglycaemia
- FBC – infection.

#### A3: What can be done to help?

- Discontinue the diuretic and observe. There are no history or signs of heart failure. Ankle swelling is a common side effect of calcium antagonist medication such as amlodipine. If this can be withdrawn, diuretic therapy may no longer be required. Persistent hypertension may be better managed by a beta-blocker, ACE inhibitor or angiotensin receptor blocker. In this situation, elastic hosiery is a more appropriate method for controlling dependent oedema.
- Assess communication and cognition with the help of a speech and language therapist. Try to improve the patient's ability to communicate the need to pass urine (e.g. bell, picture card, gestures).
- There should be an assessment of the patient's home environment and toilet facilities by an occupational therapist. Techniques to allow clothing to be removed quickly, assistance with transfers, and equipment to facilitate toileting (e.g. commode, grab-rails, raised toilet seat) will promote continence.
- The district nurse and carer need to work with the patient to establish a regular toileting regimen to anticipate and thus prevent incontinence. Pads and barrier cream are needed to protect the perineum.
- Antibiotics should be given if UTI is confirmed.
- If the above measures prove insufficient, consider stabilization of the bladder with anticholinergic medication, e.g. solifenacin or oxybutynin. Such treatment needs to be used with caution because of predictable anticholinergic side effects (e.g. confusion, glaucoma, constipation, dry mouth).
- The patient needs assistance with toileting and washing at home from the home-care service and regular monitoring of the situation by the district nursing team. Regular respite care should be considered to sustain the daughter in her caring role.

## CASE 6.11 – **An 82-year-old man with advanced Parkinson's disease and dementia is cared for in a nursing home.**

### A1:  What are the likely causes of urinary incontinence in this patient?

Urinary and faecal incontinence are not uncommon in the setting of dementia and relative immobility caused by conditions such as Parkinson's disease. Nevertheless, regular toileting and maintenance of a daily bowel habit by appropriate diet, simple laxatives and, when necessary, suppositories are usually sufficient to maintain control of the situation. In this scenario, it is very likely that faecal impaction has supervened, with overflow of liquid stool. This is a most uncomfortable situation for the elderly man, who is unable, as a result of confusion, to draw attention to his predicament. Urinary retention with overflow of urine is also very common in this setting, particularly if there is pre-existing urinary outflow obstruction as a result of prostatic enlargement. Anticholinergic drugs, sometimes used (inappropriately) in older patients with Parkinson's disease, and opiate-based analgesics can also precipitate this problem.

Urinary infection is not infrequent in this setting but would usually be associated with fever and offensive urine. Infective diarrhoea would tend to produce profuse liquid stool associated with fever, abdominal tenderness and dehydration, and there may also be other affected residents in the home. *Clostridium difficile* enteritis should be considered, especially if the patient has received a broad-spectrum antibiotic.

### A2:  How should the problem be investigated?

A careful clinical examination (even if difficult) is essential, with particular reference to fever, hydration, abdominal tenderness or distension, bladder enlargement (often non-tender in chronic retention) and rectal examination (prostatic enlargement or impaction with hard stool).

Urinalysis and, if appropriate, stool culture should be done for evidence of infection. A bladder scan should be done to assess for urinary retention. Plasma U&Es should be sent if obstructive uropathy or dehydration is suspected.

### A3:  What can be done to help?

Faecal impaction should be relieved by regular enemas, with attention to regular bowel care as outlined above. Once constipation is relieved, urinary retention may resolve spontaneously, especially if the patient is able to sit or stand to pass urine. Failing this, temporary urinary catheterization (with measurement of residual urine to confirm the diagnosis) should be performed until the bowel function has normalized. Anticholinergic and opiate-based medication should be withdrawn whenever possible. Treatment for UTI should be guided by antibiotic therapy. Infectious diarrhoea will require 'barrier nursing' precautions to prevent the spread of infection. *Clostridium difficile* enteritis will require oral metronidazole or vancomycin.

## CASE 6.12 – **A 90-year-old woman who lives alone has slipped and fallen in her bathroom at home.**

### A4:  What are the likely causes of urinary incontinence in this patient?

The patient has a third-degree uterine prolapse, resulting in stress incontinence as a result of pelvic floor (sphincter) incompetence. A history of leakage of urine when straining, coughing, laughing or standing is usual. There is a recognized relationship between stress incontinence and weakness of the pelvic floor musculature and sphincter tone. Ageing, oestrogen deficiency, previous multiparity and surgical interference at parturition are also predisposing factors.

## A5: What treatments should be considered?

Lesser degrees of pelvic floor incompetence can be treated to good effect by pelvic floor exercises taught by a physiotherapist, in conjunction with oestrogen replacement therapy. The situation described in this scenario requires gynaecological referral and control of uterine descent by pessary or surgery.

## A6: Suggest three reasons why the incontinence has gone unreported by the patient for so long.

Incontinence is often unreported by older patients. Embarrassment, social isolation, fear of investigation or treatment, and acceptance as a part of 'normal' ageing or that 'nothing can be done' are all factors to a greater or lesser degree.

## 👥 OSCE counselling cases

### OSCE COUNSELLING CASE 6.8 – **An elderly woman with hypertension is attending the surgery for regular assessment of her blood pressure.**

Urinary incontinence is a common problem in old age and is often unreported. The reasons for this reluctance to seek medical advice are multifactorial and include embarrassment and a belief that nothing can be done or that it is an inevitable consequence of ageing. Health-care professionals may fail to enquire about the symptom or, if it is mentioned, may feel unable to intervene in an effective manner.

The first step is to secure the patient's confidence and trust. An approach by the practice nurse may be a more successful first step to gain an initial history and preliminary assessment. It will be important for the nurse or doctor to emphasize that assessment is relatively simple and that an effective treatment is very likely. Even if cure is not feasible, improvement or containment of symptoms is certainly possible.

The initial assessment should include a thorough history and examination (note rectal and vaginal examinations), paying particular attention to medications and any gynaecological or neurological symptoms and signs. Urinalysis, urine culture and bladder scan (to assess bladder emptying and residual volume) are also essential steps in the assessment. Most assessments can be completed in a general practice setting, and measures can be instituted to improve the common conditions of urge and stress incontinence. The advice of a continence nurse specialist is useful for the treatment of complex cases and where a more detailed knowledge of containment devices and pads is required.

### OSCE COUNSELLING CASE 6.9 – **An 86-year-old woman is distressed by persistent incontinence of urine.**

The key steps include a full history focusing on:

- precipitating factors
- pattern of voiding, including assessment of frequency and volume
- previous and current medical and surgical illnesses, including obstetric procedures and problems
- drug history, especially diuretics, anticholinergics, sedatives and opiates
- assessment of functional status and toileting arrangements
- corroborative details from carer or relative.

A full examination should be done, focusing on:

- abdomen – retention of urine, pelvic masses
- rectal examination – constipation, tumour, anal tone
- vaginal examination – prolapse, tumour, atrophic changes
- full neurological assessment – search for evidence of cognitive dysfunction and other CNS diseases, e.g. stroke, Parkinson's disease, spinal cord disease, autonomic dysfunction
- locomotor examination.

Simple, focused investigations in response to the findings on history and examination include:

- urinalysis
- MSU
- measurement of residual volume (by bladder scan or catheterization)
- capillary glucose
- plasma urea, creatinine and electrolytes
- plain radiograph or ultrasound scan of kidneys, ureters and bladder (for renal/bladder stone)
- urodynamic assessment if the above investigations fail to elucidate the cause.

# IATROGENIC ILLNESS IN FRAIL OLDER PATIENTS

## Questions

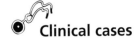

### Clinical cases

### For each of the case scenarios given, consider the following:

> **Q1**: What iatrogenic illness may result from the given intervention?
> **Q2**: What risk factors for iatrogenic illness are present in this case?
> **Q3**: Suggest some alternative management strategies.
> **Q4**: How can these complications be minimized?

### CASE 6.13 – An 84-year-old man is agitated and restless.

The patient is disturbing other residents in the residential care home. He has a history of cardiac and cerebrovascular disease with vascular dementia. The on-call doctor who attends prescribes haloperidol 2.5 mg stat and then 1 mg three times a day to follow.

### CASE 6.14 – An 86-year-old woman who is a nursing home resident has become more drowsy than usual.

The patient is immobile due to osteoarthritis and cerebrovascular disease. She also has cardiac failure and type 2 diabetes mellitus, with end-organ damage. She has an indwelling urinary catheter. The weather is hot and she is having difficulty drinking sufficient fluid. There is no fever. Her blood pressure is 106/52 mmHg and heart rate is 102/min. Urine dipstick testing shows positive + for protein, glucose and blood with nitrites present; there are no ketones. Several weeks ago the patient was unwell with a UTI, which was treated successfully with ciprofloxacin. The nurse in charge has suggested that you prescribe an antibiotic in case the patient has another UTI.

### CASE 6.15 – A 92-year-old woman is feeling dizzy and nauseated and is not her usual self.

She has AF with cardiac failure and is receiving treatment with furosemide, digoxin, aspirin, spironolactone and ramipril. The dose of furosemide was increased 3 weeks ago following outpatient department attendance. Examination shows AF rate 54/min, blood pressure 106/64 mmHg, JVP not visible and no oedema. Blood tests show sodium 135 mmol/L, potassium 6.0 mmol/L, urea 18 mmol/L and creatinine 270 μmol/L. ECG confirms slow AF.

### CASE 6.16 – An 84-year-old woman with dementia is admitted from a residential home because she has had some falls.

The patient is described as being frail. She is restless and agitated and has a respiratory infection. Her skin is fragile, with several small lacerations and bruises caused by her recent falls. The electronic prescribing process prompts the admitting medical team to assess for venous thromboembolism (VTE) risk. She is considered at risk because of her age, dehydration and infection. Should she be prescribed VTE prophylaxis with subcutaneous enoxaparin?

## CASE 6.17 – A frail 92-year-old woman has fallen at home. The ambulance service has conveyed her to the local A&E department for further assessment.

Further enquiry reveals the patient lives alone and has mild dementia and previous osteoporosis-related fragility fractures (wrist and thoracic vertebra). She has poor vision and hearing. She receives help from local family and the home-care service. She has not sustained any bone injury. Physiological parameters are stable. She is taking diuretics for ankle swelling. There are concerns about her safety at home. Should she be admitted to hospital?

## Key concepts

To work through the core clinical cases in this section, you will need to understand the following key concepts.

Illness in frail older people often presents in a non-specific way, e.g. falls, functional decline, confusion, anorexia and weight loss, or following an observation from a family member or carer that the patient is not their 'usual self'. The older person may also underreport illness owing to cognitive decline, depression, anxiety, sensory impairments, decreased expectations and stoicism. Symptoms that are modified by age-related physiological decline or coexisting chronic disease(s) further complicate the diagnostic process.

Frailty itself is a physiological syndrome characterized by decreased reserve, diminished resistance to stress, cumulative decline across multiple systems and vulnerability to adverse outcomes. Such frailty is a marker of poor outcome, especially in relation to hospital admission. Compared with more robust older patients, those with markers of frailty are more likely to experience a longer length of hospital stay, are at increased risk of institutional care or social isolation, and are more likely to experience adverse outcomes following health-care interventions. The mortality in this patient group is substantially increased.

The assessment and management of illness in frail older patients require comprehensive assessment, attention to detail and knowledge of the background social situation. It is important to understand why the patient has presented now and their current and previous functional status. In the presence of multiple impairments and chronic illness, it is important to identify any remediable factors or conditions. When there is no cure, the focus should turn to modification of the situation and amelioration of symptoms. Creating a problem list and prioritizing the actions is a useful way to proceed. Bearing in mind the increased risk of adverse outcomes in such patients, any intervention should be weighted for risks and benefits, allowing the patient (and, where relevant, the patient's advocate) to be part of the decision-making process. Outcomes viewed from the ninth or tenth decade are sometimes very different from those considered best by younger professionals or carers. The relevance of rehabilitation and limitation of disability will also require focus from the multidisciplinary team. End-of-life situations are not uncommon. At this time in particular, the emphasis of care must be on comfort and dignity.

# Answers

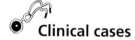

## Clinical cases

### CASE 6.13 – **An 84-year-old man is agitated and restless.**

#### A1: What iatrogenic illness may result from the given intervention?

Short-term side effects may include hypotension, sedation and immobility, increasing the risk of dehydration, poor nutrition and pressure sores. If continued for more than several days, there is a risk of drug-induced parkinsonism and falls. If continued long term, there is an increased risk of stroke, accelerated cognitive decline and continued parkinsonism. Mortality is increased when neuroleptics are continued long term in such situations.

#### A2: What risk factors for iatrogenic illness are present in this case?

Age, cardiac disease and vascular brain disease increase the risk of adverse events.

#### A3: Suggest some alternative management strategies.

If the agitation and restlessness are of recent onset, this is hyperactive delirium and there are underlying causes, such as infection, pain, discomfort or metabolic disturbance. Such precipitants should be carefully identified and treated as appropriate. Non-pharmacological means to settle the patient's agitation should be tried, including reorientation, the calming presence of a family member or familiar carer, encouraging the patient to wear his glasses and hearing aid if required, and hydration. Every opportunity to avoid pharmacological sedation should be considered.

#### A4: How can these complications be minimized?

If sedation is required, then the initial dose of haloperidol should be kept low (1 mg initially); if necessary, a further dose can be given 20–30 min later. Follow-on medication should be given only if necessary, and in this situation should be low dose (0.5 mg twice a day). Treatment should not be continued beyond 3 days and should never be continued indefinitely. If the patient has pre-existing parkinsonism, a small dose of lorazepam 0.5–1 mg can be considered as an alternative.

### CASE 6.14 – **An 86-year-old woman who is a nursing home resident has become more drowsy than usual.**

#### A1: What iatrogenic illness may result from the given intervention?

There is a high risk of C. difficile colitis if antibiotics are used in this setting. Bowel colonization with C. difficile is not uncommon in residents of care homes (around 25 per cent of residents). Further disturbance of the normal large bowel bacterial flora by broad-spectrum antibiotics (especially ciprofloxacin) carries a high risk of precipitating C. difficile infection.

#### A2: What risk factors for iatrogenic illness are present in this case?

Age, comorbid illnesses, care-home settings and recent use of broad-spectrum antibiotics all increase the risk of C. difficile infection.

## A3: Suggest some alternative management strategies.

In this scenario, there is no definite evidence of UTI. The abnormal urine dipstick result may be caused by (i) diabetic/hypertensive kidney disease, (ii) bladder irritation due to the urinary catheter or (iii) asymptomatic bacteriuria (present in up to 40–50 per cent of residents of care homes). The patient has hypoactive delirium, most likely caused by dehydration and hyperglycaemia. The dehydration should be corrected by giving regular oral fluids. Renal function, plasma electrolytes and capillary glucose should be checked and corrective action taken as necessary. The patient should be monitored regularly by the nursing staff, including charting of fluid balance and temperature. Resolution of the current symptoms and signs over the next 24 h will confirm that the management plan is working and that antibiotic treatment is not required.

## A4: How can these complications be minimized?

If fever develops and there is no likely source of infection other than urine, then treatment for UTI must be considered. An elevated plasma white cell count or CRP will provide further support for UTI. Keeping the antibiotic course short (3–5 days) and using a narrow-spectrum agent (trimethoprim v. ciprofloxacin) where possible will minimize the risk of *C. difficile* colitis. A discussion with the patient and the nursing staff regarding removal of the urinary catheter and managing continence by other means (e.g. regular toileting, pads) will substantially reduce the risk of UTI in this setting.

## CASE 6.15 – **A 92-year-old woman is feeling dizzy and nauseated and is not her usual self.**

### A1: What iatrogenic illness may result from the given intervention?

A1: Digoxin toxicity, hypotension and renal failure may all result. Hypotension and renal failure are related to treatment with diuretics and ramipril. Hyperkalaemia is related to treatment with spironolactone (an aldosterone antagonist) and ramipril. The dizziness is multifactorial – digoxin toxicity, cardiac arrhythmia and hypotension are all possible causes.

### A2: What risk factors for iatrogenic illness are present in this case?

Chronic renal failure – either disease- or age-associated – will cause digoxin accumulation as the drug is excreted via the kidneys and has a long half-life (36 h with normal renal function). A recent increase in diuretic dose can result in excessive diuresis, which will further compromise kidney function due to volume depletion. Nausea due to digoxin toxicity will reduce fluid intake and exacerbate the situation. Spironolactone is contraindicated in the presence of kidney disease because of the risk of hyperkalaemia, a situation aggravated by ACE inhibition.

### A3: Suggest some alternative management strategies.

Adjustments in diuretic dose require close monitoring in this situation, ideally with serial weight, blood pressure and kidney function tests. Regular home assessments by a nurse specialist in cardiac failure are a valuable means of monitoring such treatment in frail older patients, rather than relying on frequent visits to the surgery or outpatient department.

### A4: How can these complications be minimized?

Renal function declines progressively with age. The severity can be underestimated in frail older patients, as plasma creatinine is often lower than expected because of reduced muscle mass (estimated glomerular flow rate is a better guide to renal function in this situation). The digoxin dose should be reduced accordingly (62.5 µg/day or on alternate days in this scenario), and clinical effects and the digoxin level should be monitored carefully if events supervene that further compromise kidney function.

Spironolactone should be avoided in chronic kidney disease because hyperkalaemia is a predictable complication. ACE inhibition requires caution, as this medication can compromise renal perfusion.

## CASE 6.16 – **An 84-year-old woman with dementia is admitted from a residential home because she has had some falls.**

### A1: What iatrogenic illness may result from the given intervention?

Head injury and intracranial bleeding are a substantial risk because of the patient's frailty, confusion and risk of further falls. Low-dose enoxaparin will substantially increase this risk. The distress caused by subcutaneous injections may exacerbate the patient's delirium. There may be cutaneous bruising at injection sites and elsewhere due to the patient's restlessness and agitation and resulting minor trauma.

### A2: What risk factors for iatrogenic illness are present in this case?

Fall-related head injury carries a higher than normal risk of intracranial bleeding, particularly subdural haemorrhage, because of age- and dementia-associated cerebral atrophy.

### A3: Suggest some alternative management strategies.

The patient could be assessed for anti-thromboembolic stockings if peripheral circulation is satisfactory. Rehydration, treatment of respiratory infection and supervised mobilization will reduce the risk of VTE.

### A4: How can these complications be minimized?

The risk of VTE has to be balanced against the substantial risk (in this case) of harm from increased bleeding. A supportive nursing environment and medical management aiming to reverse treatable conditions and resolve delirium are important. If the patient is judged not to have capacity to participate in treatment-related decisions, then the medical team should act in her best interests. Timely involvement of family members or any legally appointed representative (lasting power of attorney) is imperative.

## CASE 6.17 – **A frail 92-year-old woman has fallen at home. The ambulance service has conveyed her to the local A&E department for further assessment.**

### A1: What iatrogenic illness may result from the given intervention?

This a common scenario. The patient is frail and will be at substantial risk from hospital admission-related complications such as delirium, further falls, health-care-associated infection, deconditioning due to reduced activity and loss of functional skills. Local support networks will be destabilized by her admission. These risks have to be balanced against the hazards of returning to a potentially unsafe environment and occult illness.

### A2: What risk factors for iatrogenic illness are present in this case?

The presence of frailty, cognitive impairment and sensory impairments substantially increases the risk of delirium and falls within the hospital environment. Any subsequent ward moves with unfamiliar routines and interventions will add to this risk.

### A3: Suggest some alternative management strategies.

Assessment by a rapid-response therapy and nursing team skilled in the assessment of frail older people is essential in this A&E setting. The patient should have a supported discharge home with reinstatement of her existing care plan, supplemented by short-term additional social and therapy support as necessary. There should be further early review at home or attendance at a community or day hospital-based falls clinic (depending on local availability of services) for further comprehensive geriatric assessment. This will identify modifiable conditions and implement treatment and support to enhance care at home and reduce risk of further falls.

## A4: How can these complications be minimized?

Safe alternatives to hospital admission should always be considered in frail older people. A working knowledge of local services and community teams is essential. Close liaison and reassurance to the patient's family and carers are also important. The medical role in A&E is to quickly exclude life-threatening or serious illness, and this will provide focus to the rapid-response nursing/therapy team to permit early supported discharge. Many such teams are supported by elderly-care physicians who are able to give further confidence with respect to medical stability, immediate changes to medication and follow-up plans.

## REVISION PANEL

- One-third of people aged over 65 years fall in a year, often repeatedly. Falls resulting in injury are a leading cause of death in older people, accounting for two-thirds of injury-related deaths in people aged 85 years and over.
- Falls in elderly people may be related to one or more underlying medical conditions, including aortic stenosis, cardiac arrhythmia, silent MI, postural hypotension, vasovagal episode, and hindbrain TIA.
- Osteomalacia (vitamin D deficiency) may occur due to lack of exposure to sunlight, poor diet if socially isolated or in poor health, and enhanced metabolism of vitamin D as a result of treatment with phenytoin (a liver enzyme inducer). Diseases causing malabsorption and chronic renal failure can also predispose to osteomalacia.
- There are many common causes of difficulty in walking in elderly people, including stroke, osteoarthritis, parkinsonism, dementia, visual impairment, chronic cardiorespiratory disease, injuries and complications of falling, and problems with feet and footwear.
- Acute confusion is more prevalent in elderly people. Common causes include metabolic and electrolyte problems, infection, medication and cerebrovascular disease.
- Drug toxicity (e.g. digoxin, phenytoin) is more common in elderly people due to polypharmacy and chronic renal and hepatic impairment.

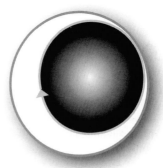

# 7 Respiratory medicine

*Malcolm Shepherd*

## DYSPNOEA

## PLEURITIC CHEST PAIN

## HAEMOPTYSIS

## Answers

# DYSPNOEA

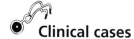

## Clinical cases

## For each of the case scenarios given, consider the following:

**Q1**: What is the likely differential diagnosis?
**Q2**: What issues in the given history support the diagnosis?
**Q3**: What additional features of the history would you seek to support a particular diagnosis?
**Q4**: What clinical examination would you perform, and why?
**Q5**: What investigations would be most helpful, and why?
**Q6**: What treatment options are appropriate?

## CASE 7.1 – **A 35-year-old woman with episodic breathlessness and wheeze.**

A 35-year-old mother attends the medical outpatient clinic complaining of breathlessness with wheeze. This can occur at rest and has been getting worse over the past 2 years. Between episodes of breathlessness she feels better but does not feel that she ever returns to 'normal'. Occasionally she wakes with shortness of breath and coughing in the early hours of the morning.

## CASE 7.2 – **A 66-year-old man with chronic dyspnoea and cough.**

A 66-year-old retired publican attends the respiratory outpatient clinic complaining of severe exercise limitation as a result of breathlessness. He has trouble moving about the house and rarely goes outside. He feels worse in the mornings and describes wheeze. His symptoms have developed over 3 years. His general practitioner (GP) has tried inhalers, but they have not helped. He has had a cough with sputum for more than 10 years. He has been a smoker for more than 40 years and has smoked five to ten cigarettes per day over this time.

## CASE 7.3 – **A 66-year-old man with progressive dyspnoea and weight loss.**

A 66-year-old man presents complaining of worsening exercise tolerance as a result of breathlessness. He can walk 200 m on a flat road, whereas a year ago he could manage at least a mile. He describes feeling short of breath at rest. He is severely restricted on hills and stairways. He denies cough, but he has lost 3 kg over the past 6 months. He is a lifelong non-smoker. He worked in the shipbuilding industry, where he was exposed to asbestos fibres. His GP describes inspiratory crackles at both lung bases.

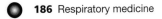
 ## OSCE counselling case

## OSCE COUNSELLING CASE 7.1 – 'Can I have oxygen at home? I'm sure it would help me'.

A 72-year-old man with cryptogenic fibrosing alveolitis (CFA) attends the clinic with his daughter. They both feel that he requires oxygen to help him with his daily activities. What criteria should you assess before prescribing oxygen? What advice would you give to him about the use of oxygen?

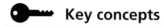 **Key concepts**

To work through the core clinical cases in this section, you will need to understand the following key concepts.

## SPIROMETRY

This is a useful test that is quick to perform and has good reproducibility. Spirometry measures the volume and velocity of a forced exhalation over approximately 5 s. Two important values are derived: the volume of air expired in the first second, known as the forced expiratory volume in 1 s ($FEV_1$), and the total volume exhaled in 5 s, known as the forced vital capacity (FVC). In the context of dyspnoea, two patterns are frequently found: if both values are lower than predicted for an individual's size, age and gender, then the pattern is described as 'restrictive'; if the $FEV_1$ is disproportionately smaller than the FVC ($FEV_1$/FVC $\leq 75$ per cent), then the pattern is described as 'obstructive'.

## Answers

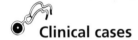

## Clinical cases

### CASE 7.1 – **A 35-year-old woman with episodic breathlessness and wheeze.**

### A1: What is the likely differential diagnosis?

The differential diagnoses are asthma, hyperventilation and recurrent pulmonary embolism (PE).

### A2: What issues in the given history support the diagnosis?

Episodic breathlessness, wheeze and cough with spontaneous resolution are typical of asthma. Symptoms tend to occur at night, first thing in the morning or after exercise, but none of these clinical features is specific for asthma. Progression over 2 years may suggest insufficient treatment of asthma.

### A3: What additional features of the history would you seek to support a particular diagnosis?

A smoking history should be taken. It would be useful to assess the likelihood of other associated atopic diseases by enquiring about allergic rhinitis and eczema. Any environmental or other factors that exacerbate the patient's breathlessness should be identified, such as occupational asthma. A chronic cough without wheeze, currently or in the past, may suggest cough variant asthma. A family or personal history of thromboembolic disease may suggest pulmonary thromboembolism (PTE).

### A4: What clinical examination would you perform, and why?

Examination is likely to be normal unless the patient is suffering from an exacerbation. General examination should look for evidence of eczema (dermatitis, ichthyoid skin). Respiratory examination may reveal wheeze or hyperinflated lung fields.

### A5: What investigations would be most helpful, and why?

The metacholine or histamine provocation test is the recommended test to diagnose asthma. A fall in $FEV_1$ of more than 20 per cent (PC20) after inhalation of 25 mg/mL or less of metacholine is considered a positive test. A negative test has a high negative predictive value.

A 2-week recording of the peak expiratory flow (PEF) measured twice a day can identify diurnal variation that is characteristic of asthma ($\geq$20 per cent from baseline). This is a specific but insensitive diagnostic test.

A single spirometry measurement may be normal or may demonstrate a low $FEV_1$/FVC ratio (an obstructive pattern). An improvement in $FEV_1$ of more than 15 per cent and 200 mL after inhalation of a bronchodilator or a 2-week course of corticosteroid therapy is highly suggestive of asthma.

Chest radiograph is unhelpful in diagnosing asthma but may rule out alternative diagnoses or pneumothorax. A full blood count (FBC) is not useful, although blood eosinophilia may occur occasionally in asthma.

Common allergen tests may identify specific agents to which the patient is sensitive that could trigger asthmatic reactions. Common allergens include cat and dog hair, house-dust mite and grass pollen.

## A6: What treatment options are appropriate?

- Assess asthma control – pattern and severity of symptoms and exacerbations, supplemented where appropriate with serial PEF recording. An oral steroid trial (as above) may be required to demonstrate the patient's best spirometry.
- Eliminate trigger factors.
- Patient education – ensure understanding of medications and how to alter treatment in the event of deterioration, and check inhaler technique. Provide a written asthma action plan.

Stepwise drug treatment is as follows.

1. Mild intermittent asthma – inhaled short-acting beta$_2$ agonist as required.
2. Regular preventer therapy – add inhaled steroid 200–800 µg daily for patients with recent exacerbations, nocturnal asthma or using short-acting beta$_2$ agonists more than once a day.
3. Add-on therapy – add inhaled long-acting beta$_2$ agonist twice a day.
4. Persistent poor control – increase inhaled steroid dose up to 2000 µg daily, or consider trial of leukotriene receptor antagonist, theophylline preparation or oral beta-agonist.
5. Continuous or frequent use of oral steroids – use daily steroid tablets in lowest dose tolerated. Consider anti-immunoglobulin E (IgE) therapy if appropriate, based on total and specific IgE.

## CASE 7.2 – **A 66-year-old man with chronic dyspnoea and cough.**

### A1: What is the likely differential diagnosis?

The differential diagnoses are chronic obstructive pulmonary disease (COPD), asthma and bronchiectasis.

### A2: What issues in the given history support the diagnosis?

Chronic progressive breathlessness on the background of a long smoking history suggests COPD. Typical features include lack of spontaneous improvement or response to inhaled therapy, relentless progression of symptoms, and a combination of productive cough and dyspnoea. Although the patient has only a 20 pack-year smoking history, his occupation and the variable effects of cigarette smoking make COPD the most likely diagnosis.

### A3: What additional features of the history would you seek to support a particular diagnosis?

A history of previous reversible wheeze and dyspnoea may suggest chronic asthma. Productive sputum can accompany bronchiectasis, and predisposing features such as childhood infections should be sought. Assessment of severity in terms of lifestyle and exercise impairment should be made. Chronic lung disease can precipitate depression, and the patient's mood should be assessed because antidepressants can help.

### A4: What clinical examination would you perform, and why?

Physical examination is rarely diagnostic in COPD. Look for signs of respiratory failure (central cyanosis), hypercapnia (bounding high-volume pulse, flapping tremor) and cor pulmonale (raised jugular venous pressure [JVP], ankle or sacral oedema). Physical signs of airflow obstruction usually occur only when severe airflow obstruction is present, such as pursed-lipped breathing, hyperinflated thorax, paradoxical in-drawing of the intercostal spaces, resonant percussion note, poor breath sounds and wheeze.

## A5: What investigations would be most helpful, and why?

- *Spirometry:* baseline spirometry with reversibility to bronchodilators should be performed in all patients suspected of having COPD. The $FEV_1$ is typically less than 80 per cent of the predicted value, and the $FEV_1/FVC$ ratio is less than 70 per cent; these values do not return to normal with a bronchodilator. A short course of oral steroids can be used to help distinguish chronic asthma from COPD. Post-bronchodilator $FEV_1$ is used to classify the severity of COPD.
- *Chest radiograph:* no specific features, but upper-zone emphysema, hyperinflation (more than six ribs anteriorly) and a flattened diaphragm would support the diagnosis. It is useful to exclude an alternative diagnosis such as bronchial carcinoma.
- *Arterial blood gases (ABGs)/pulse oximetry:* these should be measured in patients with severe disease. Oxygen saturation of 92 per cent or less should lead to ABG measurement.
- *FBC:* this is useful to exclude anaemia or polycythaemia.
- *Alpha$_1$-antitrypsin:* this may identify deficiency in rare cases; check in patients aged under 45 years.

## A6: What treatment options are appropriate?

The aims of management are to lessen dyspnoea, reduce exacerbations and improve exercise tolerance, with minimal side effects, normally using both pharmacological and behavioural components. Smoking cessation is the most effective way to reduce the risk of developing COPD and slow or halt its progression.

Although no objective improvement in spirometry is seen in response to bronchodilator therapy in COPD, patients may derive symptomatic benefit. The patient should therefore be provided with an inhaled bronchodilator, either a short-acting beta$_2$ agonist or anticholinergic therapy. Patients with more severe symptoms should be given a trial with an inhaled long-acting beta$_2$ agonist or anticholinergic agent. Other agents may be tried on a symptomatic trial basis, including oral theophyllines.

Inhaled steroids result in small reductions in the frequency of exacerbation in severe COPD. Combination therapy of an inhaled long-acting beta$_2$ agonist and an inhaled steroid may reduce the frequency of exacerbations more effectively than either drug alone.

Long-term oxygen therapy is recommended for patients who have stopped smoking and who have chronic respiratory failure ($PaO_2 < 7.3\,kPa$, where $PaO_2$ is the partial pressure of oxygen in arterial blood). Pulmonary rehabilitation is useful to maximize the patient's functional capacity.

The patient should be immunized against influenza yearly. A mood assessment should be made with intervention for depression where appropriate.

## CASE 7.3 – **A 66-year-old man with progressive dyspnoea and weight loss.**

### A1: What is the likely differential diagnosis?

The differential diagnoses are CFA, pulmonary asbestosis and cardiogenic pulmonary oedema.

### A2: What issues in the given history support the diagnosis?

Progressive dyspnoea in a non-smoker with no history of cough may suggest fibrotic (interstitial) lung disease. Dyspnoea is frequently first encountered on effort, but progression to dyspnoea at rest is common. The history of occupational exposure to asbestos may suggest an industrial component to this disease, but formal diagnosis requires further investigations. Crackles are typical of some forms of interstitial lung disease and are frequently confused with pulmonary oedema.

### A3:  What additional features of the history would you seek to support a particular diagnosis?

An attempt should be made to quantify the degree of functional impairment experienced by the patient. The degree of exposure to asbestos fibres should be enquired about. The history should also include information on any systemic disease, drug therapy, travel and environmental exposures, such as agents known to cause extrinsic allergic alveolitis (EAA; e.g. bird protein, mouldy hay). A history of ischaemic heart disease (IHD) or hypertension makes pulmonary oedema more likely.

### A4:  What clinical examination would you perform, and why?

General examination should look for evidence of respiratory or cardiac failure. Ankle oedema, cyanosis, tachycardia and respiratory rate should all be examined. Finger clubbing is frequently associated with CFA but is seen less often in asbestosis. Respiratory examination may reveal poor thoracic excursion, normal percussion note and widespread inspiratory crackles. Weight loss frequently accompanies interstitial lung disease, but assessment for bronchial carcinoma should be made.

### A5:  What investigations would be most helpful, and why?

- *chest radiograph* – may be normal or reveal shrunken lungs with coarse vascular markings (honeycomb lung) or patchy areas of consolidation; evidence of asbestos exposure may be found such as pleural calcification or plaques
- *high-resolution computed tomography (HRCT)* – may reveal long-standing changes of fibrosis (honeycombing) or the more acute changes associated with active inflammation (ground-glass intra-alveolar shadowing)
- *pulmonary function tests* – typically a restrictive pattern of spirometry would be expected ($FEV_1$/FVC ratio normal, but both values less than predicted); total lung volumes and static volumes are reduced and the CO diffusion gradient is also reduced
- *oxygen saturation/tension* – it is useful to assess the degree of hypoxaemia, because this helps to quantify the severity of disease and may indicate patients who will benefit from the administration of domiciliary oxygen therapy; a 6 min walk test with oxygen saturation measurements is a sensitive test of early interstitial lung disease
- *serum markers of EAA* – serum precipitins to avian proteins and other causes of EAA should be sought
- *FBC* – of little use, although an elevated haematocrit may develop in response to chronic hypoxia
- *autoimmune antibodies* – may reveal coexistence of connective tissue diseases that may present with interstitial lung disease such as rheumatoid arthritis, systemic lupus erythematosus (SLE) or systemic sclerosis.

### A6:  What treatment options are appropriate?

The patient should avoid any causal agents. Advice on seeking industrial compensation is appropriate in the case of pulmonary asbestosis.

Controlling the progression of pulmonary fibrosis may be achieved in CFA by systemic corticosteroid therapy or immunosuppressive treatment, although the response to treatment is often disappointing. Domiciliary oxygen may be prescribed for patients with end-stage disease.

## ÅÅ OSCE counselling case

## OSCE COUNSELLING CASE 7.1 – 'Can I have oxygen at home? I'm sure it would help me'.

There is concern over the use of oxygen supplementation in the context of possible exposure to naked flames. Oxygen can promote combustion and may make house fires more likely. It is recommended that patients who smoke are not prescribed oxygen and that oxygen is not used in homes heated by open-flame fires.

Patients with interstitial pulmonary disease may benefit from oxygen as a palliative measure at later stages of the disease. The degree of alveolar hypoxia should be estimated by ABG measurement, and the secondary consequences of hypoxaemia should be assessed. If $PaO_2$ is less than 8 kPa and symptoms of dyspnoea are disabling to the patient, oxygen may be prescribed on an as-required basis.

Oxygen is administered from either constant-flow cylinders or concentrators, both of which must be delivered to the patient's home. The patient's capacity to use the device should be assessed; where necessary, training or additional support from, for example, a specialist nursing service should be arranged.

There is concern over the safety of overreliance on domiciliary oxygen. Patients should be advised that oxygen is safe in stable respiratory disease but is not a substitute for medical intervention in the event of a sudden deterioration. Therefore, if dyspnoea gets worse despite normal use of oxygen, medical advice should be sought.

There is concern about excess oxygen in COPD. Patients who have COPD may become dependent on hypoxic drive to stimulate respiration, and COPD can complicate many respiratory conditions, including fibrosing alveolitis. Although supplementary oxygen is safe if assessed properly, increasing the supply of oxygen may depress the patient's respiratory drive. Patients are advised not to make changes to the flow settings on their concentrators or cylinders without seeking advice.

# PLEURITIC CHEST PAIN

## Questions

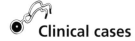
### Clinical cases

## For each of the case scenarios given, consider the following:

> **Q1**: What is the likely differential diagnosis?
> **Q2**: What issues in the given history support the diagnosis?
> **Q3**: What additional features of the history would you seek to support a particular diagnosis?
> **Q4**: What clinical examination would you perform, and why?
> **Q5**: What investigations would be most helpful, and why?
> **Q6**: What treatment options are appropriate?

### CASE 7.4 – A 35-year-old woman with sudden pleuritic chest pain and haemoptysis.

A 35-year-old woman is brought to the accident and emergency (A&E) department complaining of acute onset of chest pain the preceding evening and collapsing that afternoon. She is shocked and dyspnoeic. This pain is described as 'sharp', located posteriorly on the left hemi-thorax, and worse on inspiration and coughing. On the morning of admission there was some haemoptysis. She has recently been in hospital for treatment and investigation of recurrent miscarriage.

### CASE 7.5 – A 73-year-old man with gradual-onset pleuritic chest pain and haemoptysis.

A 73-year-old man attends his GP complaining of left-sided 'sharp' chest pain. The pain is worse on inspiration, does not radiate and has appeared in the past 2 days. He has not felt well for a week, with uncontrollable shivering bouts and sweats. He has had a cough with red-tinged sputum for 3 days. He smokes 20 cigarettes a day, and he has angina complicated by a myocardial infarction (MI) 2 years previously. He has recently felt increasingly short of breath with effort.

### CASE 7.6 – A 30-year-old man with sudden pleuritic chest pain and dyspnoea.

A 30-year-old man attends A&E complaining of chest pain and breathlessness. The pain developed suddenly, 16 hours before attendance, and he has gradually become increasingly short of breath since. The pain is described as 'sharp', worse on inspiration or coughing, and located on the right thoracic chest wall. He denies new cough or sputum production.

## 👥 OSCE counselling case

## OSCE COUNSELLING CASE 7.2 – 'Should I take oral contraceptives rather than risk a further pregnancy?'

This 35-year-old woman was finally diagnosed as having a life-threatening PE. Having received 6 months of anticoagulation therapy, she returns to her doctor for advice. Her main concerns surround whether she should now consider oral contraception rather than risk further pregnancy. What risks exist, and how should the GP advise her?

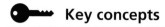 **Key concepts**

To work through the core clinical cases in this section, you will need to understand the following key concepts.

### PLEURITIC PAIN

Pleuritic pain is pain usually localized to the thoracic wall, whose severity varies with respiration. Typically the pain will be worse on inspiration and relieved by expiration. Commonly, coughing exacerbates this type of pain. The pain normally derives from inflamed layers of pleura moving over each other.

### THROMBOEMBOLISM

Thromboembolism is the passage of blood clots from a peripheral source to a more proximal vascular bed. Typically the origin of thromboembolism is the deep veins of the leg. Clots frequently lodge in the pulmonary arterial circulation.

### COMMUNITY-ACQUIRED PNEUMONIA

Community-acquired pneumonia is infective pneumonia that has developed in the community. It is distinguished from conditions that develop in a hospital setting, which are caused by different organisms and carry different prognoses.

### ADDITIONAL FACTORS ASSOCIATED WITH PULMONARY THROMBOEMBOLISM

Pre-test probability scores are designed to calculate the numerical risk of PE, based on clinical assessment, to guide the interpretation of more detailed investigation. The score includes the patient's age, history of thrombotic disease, predisposing condition such as malignancy, the presence of tachypnoea (respiratory rate >30/min), tachycardia, chest pain, clinical evidence of deep venous thrombosis (DVT), abnormal electrocardiogram (ECG; as a new finding) and abnormal chest radiograph. The presence of one or more clinical features plus one of the baseline investigations is said to have a sensitivity for PE of more than 80 per cent.

### ADDITIONAL FEATURES IN COMMUNITY-ACQUIRED PNEUMONIA

The British Thoracic Society guidelines for assessment of confusion score each of the following questions 1 mark, with a maximum score of 10 marks. A score of 8 or less indicates mental confusion:

- age
- date of birth
- time (nearest hour)
- year
- hospital name
- recall address (e.g. 24 West Street)
- date of First World War
- name of monarch
- count backwards from 20
- recognition of two people (e.g. doctor or nurse).

# Answers

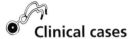

## Clinical cases

### CASE 7.4 – **A 35-year-old woman with sudden pleuritic chest pain and haemoptysis.**

#### A1: What is the likely differential diagnosis?

The differential diagnoses are PE, community-acquired pneumonia with septic shock, and tension pneumothorax.

#### A2: What issues in the given history support the diagnosis?

Pleuritic chest pain with dyspnoea and haemoptysis is typical of PE. A recent spell in hospital where the patient may have been relatively immobile, and the history of recurrent miscarriages, which may be associated with thrombophilia, are potential risk factors for PE. The sequence of a small embolic event followed by a more clinically significant episode with haemodynamic compromise is typical of PE.

#### A3: What additional features of the history would you seek to support a particular diagnosis?

Further enquiry should attempt to identify risk factors for DVT, such as smoking, history of DVT, PE or malignancy, recent long-haul airline flight, family history of DVT or PE, and recent surgical procedures and use of DVT prophylaxis. A history of leg swelling may indicate current DVT.

#### A4: What clinical examination would you perform, and why?

The clinical presentation demands urgent emergency assessment and should follow the standard advanced life support ABC (A – airway, B – breathing, C – circulation) protocol.

Further clinical assessment should be aimed at identifying the presence of DVT and assessing the severity of respiratory and haemodynamic compromise. The respiratory rate, pulse rate, blood pressure (typically low in PE) and presence of cyanosis should be recorded. Calves should be examined for swelling or tenderness, and any circumferential differences should be measured and documented. Detailed respiratory examination, including auscultation, which may reveal localized wheeze or a pleural rub or be normal, should be performed. A loud pulmonary second heart sound is rarely heard in acute PE.

#### A5: What investigations would be most helpful, and why?

- *chest radiograph* – may be normal or show oligaemia or pleural-based wedge-shaped shadowing
- *ECG* – tachycardia, atrial fibrillation, rarely S1, Q3, T3 pattern
- *oxygenation* – saturation or $PaO_2$ by arterial puncture is useful to assess severity
- *blood D-dimers* – have high negative predictive value; measure only when there is a reasonable suspicion of PE
- *computed tomography pulmonary angiogram (CTPA)* – replaced pulmonary angiogram as the imaging of choice
- *ventilation/perfusion isotope lung scan* – normal scans reliably exclude PTE; positive or negative scans are diagnostic in 30–50 per cent of cases, but rely on a normal chest radiograph appearance

- *thrombophilia screen* – important in this case, given the history of recurrent miscarriage; protein S, protein C, von Willebrand's factor, lupus anticoagulant and factor V Leiden should all be measured.

### A6: What treatment options are appropriate?

The initial management of this patient depends on the degree of haemodynamic compromise. Immediate steps should be made to stabilize her condition, including supplementary oxygen therapy, IV fluid resuscitation and transfer to a location where intensive monitoring can be performed.

If she remains haemodynamically unstable, thrombolytic therapy should be administered intravenously. Thrombolysis is the first-line treatment for massive PE.

If the patient is stable, a pre-test probability of PE should be made before investigation, and further management should be directed by the likelihood of PE based on this pre-test probability score and the appropriate investigations. If clinical suspicion of PTE is high, full-dose anticoagulation should be initiated with low-molecular-weight (LMW) heparin, while oral anticoagulant therapy (warfarin) is commenced at a loading regimen. Anticoagulation should be continued for a minimum of 6 months and discontinued if there are no obvious predisposing factors remaining. Consideration of life-long therapy should be made in the light of ongoing risk factors.

## CASE 7.5 – **A 73-year-old man with gradual-onset pleuritic chest pain and haemoptysis.**

### A1: What is the likely differential diagnosis?

The differential diagnoses are community-acquired streptococcal pneumonia, community-acquired pneumonia caused by 'atypical pathogen', PE and tuberculosis (TB).

### A2: What issues in the given history support the diagnosis?

Symptoms typical of infection (fevers or sweats) with pleuritic chest pain suggest pneumonia, but they can be associated with PE. Although there are no clinical features specific for a given pathogen, *Streptococcus pneumoniae* remains the most common cause of community-acquired pneumonia. The so-called 'atypical' pathogens such as *Mycoplasma* species, *Legionella pneumophila* and *Chlamydia* species represent a substantial minority. In this patient, the age, presence of pleuritic chest pain and cardiovascular comorbidity are all associated with streptococcal infections. The red-tinged or rusty sputum is said to typify streptococcal infections, but haemoptysis may occur with other pulmonary infections, especially TB.

### A3: What additional features of the history would you seek to support a particular diagnosis?

Comorbid conditions, associated with a poor outcome in community-acquired pneumonia, should be sought, such as diabetes mellitus, cystic fibrosis and chronic lung disease. If the patient has been bedridden or confused since the onset of symptoms, his prognosis is worse. It is very difficult to reliably determine the cause of pulmonary infections by history alone. Contact with TB should be enquired after.

### A4: What clinical examination would you perform, and why?

Clinical examination in community-acquired pneumonia is directed at confirming the diagnosis and measuring a severity score. The latter informs management decisions, including the best location for treatment (home, ward or intensive care unit) and the likely prognosis.

General examination should identify cachexia, pyrexia (absence of fever in community-acquired pneumonia carries a poor prognosis), cyanosis and peripheral lymphadenopathy, and the presence of labial herpes simplex. A Mini-Mental State Examination (MMSE) should be performed and recorded (a score below 8/10 is associated with a poor prognosis). Respiratory rate, pulse rate and blood pressure should be recorded. Respiratory examination should look for the typical features of consolidation, including dull percussion note, bronchial breathing, increased vocal fremitus and whispering pectoriloquy.

## A5: What investigations would be most helpful, and why?

Investigations are used to confirm the diagnosis and assess likely prognosis. Chest radiograph is the most useful investigation in confirming the diagnosis. Unfortunately, no single feature can identify the causative organism. Multilobar involvement or pleural effusions are more frequent in bacteriological pathogens, and cavitation is more common with *Staphylococcus aureus* or *Klebsiella pneumoniae* infections. Multilobar involvement carries a poor prognosis.

- *FBC* – high leucocytosis ($>20\times10^9$/L) or leucopenia ($<4\times10^9$/L) carries a poor prognosis
- *urea and electrolytes (U&Es)* – high urea has a worse prognosis, and renal failure suggests severe sepsis
- *liver function tests (LFTs) and creatine kinase* – commonly abnormal in *Legionella* infections
- *sputum culture* – unless previous antibiotics have been administered
- *blood cultures and sensitivities* – very sensitive marker for aetiology if positive
- *serum for serology* – paired samples for atypical serology
- *urine and blood samples* – for pathogen antigens.

## A6: What treatment options are appropriate?

Initial management decisions should be informed by a severity assessment score. The CURB-65 is commonly used. This score addresses confusion (MMSE <8/10), serum urea elevated >7 mmol/L, respiratory rate >30/min, abnormal blood pressure (systolic <90 mmHg, diastolic <60 mmHg) and age >65 years. Community treatment is likely to be safe if none or only one of these markers is present; the presence of two or more markers requires hospital assessment and may require admission to a ward or an intensive care setting.

Medical treatment should include supplementary oxygen if required, IV fluids and antibiotic therapy. Initially an empirical choice is required, but this should not be delayed because the time to first dose of antibiotic correlates with outcome. It is rare to have sufficient clues to the identity of the infecting organism to guide initial choice. In the UK, most streptococcal infections remain sensitive to beta-lactam antibiotics, whereas most atypical organisms are sensitive to macrolides. It is reasonable therefore to prescribe co-amoxiclav and clarithromycin in the first instance, and then to await sensitivities or treatment failure to guide further selection. In a hospital setting, an initial IV dose and a choice of IV or oral medication thereafter is frequently used. In the community, both penicillin and macrolide antibiotics are well absorbed orally.

## CASE 7.6 – A 30-year-old man with sudden pleuritic chest pain and dyspnoea.

### A1: What is the likely differential diagnosis?

The likely differential diagnoses are left-sided pneumothorax and PE.

### A2: What issues in the given history support the diagnosis?

Sudden onset of chest pain suggests either trauma or spontaneous pneumothorax. As no history of a precipitating event is given, spontaneous pneumothorax is the most likely diagnosis. Frequently the pneumothorax will enlarge over time, and thus dyspnoea may develop relatively late. Pulmonary embolus should always be considered; however, there is no supporting history given.

### A3: What additional features of the history would you seek to support a particular diagnosis?

The previous history of similar events is important because recurrent disease (even if not picked up clinically) is likely to lead to further episodes and will usually be treated by a definitive procedure. Employment history is important because professional diving and flying are banned after a pneumothorax. Recreational diving is also not recommended and should be enquired about.

### A4: What clinical examination would you perform, and why?

The patient should be assessed for severity: ABC (A – airway, B – breathing, C – circulation). Occasionally pneumothoraces may develop 'tension' and precipitate haemodynamic compromise. Cyanosis, tachycardia, hypotension and evidence of mediastinal shift (away from the side of the chest pain) are indications of severity. Respiratory examination may reveal tracheal shift (away from pneumothorax), hyperresonant percussion note on the side of the pneumothorax and normal on the opposite side; reduced or normal breath sounds may be present.

Assessment for predisposing conditions should be made, e.g. Marfan's syndrome may present with pneumothorax, and so it is worth examining arm span, palate and eyes for lens dislocation, and examining carefully for an ejection systolic murmur.

### A5: What investigations would be most helpful, and why?

- *chest radiograph* – if clinical suspicion of tension pneumothorax is high, treatment should not await radiological examination
- *oxygenation* – either saturation (if >93 per cent) or ABGs
- *FBC* – not useful in a pneumothorax
- *U&Es* – not useful in a pneumothorax
- *cardiac echocardiogram* – if clinical suspicion of aortic incompetence (in Marfan's syndrome).

### A6: What treatment options are appropriate?

If there is haemodynamic compromise, immediate puncture of the chest wall in the second intercostal space anteriorly with a large-bore Venflon should be done, releasing air from the pleural space. Attach a 50 mL syringe and a three-way tap after release of air and perform underwater-sealed aspiration of remaining air.

If there is no compromise and chest radiograph confirms the diagnosis, the first step is to perform aspiration under water seal. If there is no obvious predisposing lung disease, this should be sufficient to treat the pneumothorax. This procedure is less likely to be successful if there is underlying disease such as COPD or bullous disease (secondary pneumothorax).

For failed aspiration or secondary pneumothorax, a chest drain should be inserted and attached to an underwater seal to allow the gradual reinflation of the lung and removal of pleural gas. Administration of supplemental oxygen is said to hasten reabsorption of pleural gas.

If a second or recurrent pneumothorax is present, a pleural sealing procedure should be performed such as talc pleurodesis or video-assisted pleurectomy.

## ᎥᎥ OSCE counselling case

## OSCE COUNSELLING CASE 7.2 – 'Should I take oral contraceptives rather than risk a further pregnancy?'

Pulmonary embolus is a rare condition affecting 1–4/1000 people in the UK per year. This risk is increased in pregnant women tenfold over non-pregnant women. This risk is increased further if known risk factors coexist. Such risk factors include age >35 years, thrombophilia, obesity (body mass index >30 kg/m²), paraplegia and inflammatory bowel disease.

In this case, the history of life-threatening PE and recurrent miscarriage makes the presence of a thrombophilia more likely. The precise risk depends on the nature of each thrombophilia. This patient carries three risk factors: age, history and a likely thrombophilia.

Pre-pregnancy advice from a specialist should be sought. Extensive investigation of a thrombophilia is important. Treatment with LMW heparin can be instituted throughout pregnancy, so investigation before pregnancy is helpful.

The oestrogen content of the oral contraceptive pill is associated with a thrombotic risk. The history of life-threatening PE contraindicates the oral contraceptive in this case, and alternative methods of contraception should be used.

# HAEMOPTYSIS

## Questions

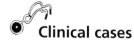

### Clinical cases

### For each of the case scenarios given, consider the following:

> **Q1**: What is the likely differential diagnosis?
> **Q2**: What issues in the given history support the diagnosis?
> **Q3**: What additional features of the history would you seek to support a particular diagnosis?
> **Q4**: What clinical examination would you perform, and why?
> **Q5**: What investigations would be most helpful, and why?
> **Q6**: What treatment options are appropriate?

### CASE 7.7 – A 60-year-old man with 2 weeks of trivial haemoptysis and weight loss.

A 60-year-old man attends the medical outpatient clinic complaining of 4 weeks of cough productive of white sputum and 2 weeks of haemoptysis. The haemoptysis is described as 'streaks of old blood through the spit' and is trivial in volume. It has remained constant throughout the 2-week period. There is no dyspnoea or chest pain, but the patient is a life-long smoker. He has noticed his clothes being looser over the previous 6 months and describes a loss of appetite, but he denies dysphagia or altered bowel habit. He is easily tired and notices his voice becoming hoarse in the evenings. He is a bookmaker and is married with two daughters, one of whom attends the clinic with him. She adds that her father appears slightly confused at times, particularly in the evenings.

### CASE 7.8 – A 45-year-old woman with chronic cough and massive haemoptysis.

A 45-year-old mother of two presents at A&E on a Sunday night, complaining of coughing large volumes of fresh red blood for the past 2 days. She estimates she has coughed up five mugs of fresh blood. She describes a cough with purulent sputum for the past month, but she cannot remember a time when she did not have a cough. She frequently receives antibiotics from her GP when the sputum turns green or increases in volume. She has been increasingly breathless for the past 2 weeks, although she has noticed increasing breathlessness for 3 years.

### CASE 7.9 – A 62-year-old man with 2 months of fevers and haemoptysis.

A 62-year-old man attends the respiratory clinic complaining of worsening cough, spit and haemoptysis. This has been of 2 months' duration and is associated with weight loss, anorexia, fevers, night sweats and purulent sputum. He denies chest discomfort or dyspnoea. He lives alone, smokes 20 cigarettes a day, and admits to drinking in excess of 40 units of alcohol a week. As a child he was treated for TB at the same time as his father. He was a welder in a shipyard before being made redundant.

## ii OSCE counselling case

### OSCE COUNSELLING CASE 7.3 – 'My father tends to drink too much and often forgets to take his tablets – is it important?'

The patient's daughter tells you that her father is an alcoholic and returns a large number of anti-TB tablets that he has not taken.

What are the risks of poor compliance with treatment in 'open TB'? What options are available to improve the patient's compliance?

## Answers

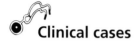
### Clinical cases

### CASE 7.7 – **A 60-year-old man with 2 weeks of trivial haemoptysis and weight loss.**

**A1:** What is the likely differential diagnosis?

The likely differential diagnoses are bronchial carcinoma, TB and upper respiratory tract infection.

### A2: What issues in the given history support the diagnosis?

Haemoptysis associated with weight loss suggests a systemic disease of uncertain duration. Bronchial carcinoma may present late with haemoptysis after a lengthy period of weight loss and cough. Smoking is associated with most cases of bronchial carcinoma, and a non-smoking history should suggest other causes. Associated features of fatigue are non-specific but frequently associated with pulmonary malignancy, whereas hoarseness and confusion should raise suspicions about complications of the disease, such as recurrent laryngeal nerve palsy or syndrome of inappropriate antidiuretic hormone secretion (SIADH).

### A3: What additional features of the history would you seek to support a particular diagnosis?

Employment with a history of asbestos exposure may support pulmonary malignancy. The cumulative lifetime amount of tobacco smoked should be noted, and the presence of constitutional features of fever and sweating may point towards an infective origin of haemoptysis. Pain is an important complication of bronchial carcinoma and can be effectively palliated. Thus, bone or chest wall pain (suggesting advanced disease) should specifically be addressed. An assessment of quality of life and the World Health Organization's 'performance status' is helpful to decide appropriate future management.

### A4: What clinical examination would you perform, and why?

Assessment of peripheral (hand–T1 root) muscle wasting, peripheral lymphadenopathy, hepatic enlargement and any unusual or new skin lesions helps to identify distant metastases. Finger clubbing is common but non-specific. Respiratory examination to identify lobar or lung collapse from a central obstructing tumour (tracheal deviation, apex beat, loss of breath sounds) or pleural metastases (signs of effusion) is helpful for baseline assessment of the extent of disease. An assessment of paraneoplastic syndromes can be helpful, e.g. blood pressure (autonomic neuropathy), skin rash (pigmentation [adrenocorticotrophic hormone] or dermatomyositis) or joint stiffness or discomfort (hypertrophic pulmonary osteoarthropathy).

### A5: What investigations would be most helpful, and why?

- *chest radiograph* – most important and may reveal diagnosis and complications
- *computed tomography (CT)* – may identify non-carcinoma causes of haemoptysis, and help staging and biopsy of peripheral lesions seen on chest radiograph; ideally performed before bronchoscopy to guide biopsy
- *bronchoscopy with lavage or biopsy* – important to provide histology, particularly in central tumours

- *sputum cytology* – generally unhelpful, with only 5 per cent sensitivity
- *U&Es* – helpful to exclude SIADH and assess fitness for treatment
- *serum calcium* – elevated in some cases of bronchial carcinoma
- *LFTs* – help exclude liver metastases
- *pulmonary function tests* – assess fitness for thoracic surgery.

## A6: What treatment options are appropriate?

Palliate the patient's symptoms, including haemoptysis, pain and anxiety. Then treat the underlying disease.

- *Small cell carcinoma:* chemotherapy-based treatment, either as palliation of symptoms (reduced dose) or with curative intent (full dose), may be given. Cisplatin-based regimens are now the usual treatment option.
- *Non-small cell carcinoma:* chemotherapy regimens are used only to downstage extensive disease and allow more definitive therapy to be instituted. Such options include surgical resection (pneumonectomy or lobectomy) and radiotherapy (radical or high-dose palliative).
- Fully palliative radiotherapy can be used for symptomatic control.

## CASE 7.8 – A 45-year-old woman with chronic cough and massive haemoptysis.

### A1: What is the likely differential diagnosis?

The likely differential diagnoses are bronchiectasis, PE and pulmonary TB.

### A2: What issues in the given history support the diagnosis?

Chronic productive cough is a feature of bronchiectasis, which occasionally presents with massive haemoptysis. Chest discomfort with haemoptysis may simply be associated with coughing-induced musculoskeletal discomfort, but PE should be considered. A change in the volume or purulence of sputum associated with the constitutional features suggests chest infection, which can herald haemoptysis in bronchiectasis.

### A3: What additional features of the history would you seek to support a particular diagnosis?

A history of a predisposing condition (childhood pneumonias, whooping cough, measles) should be sought, but its absence does not exclude bronchiectasis. Evidence of immunodeficiency may be suggested by recurrent infections outwith the chest. A history of fertility problems, such as assisted conception, and bowel irregularities throughout life may suggest cystic fibrosis.

### A4: What clinical examination would you perform, and why?

An initial cardiovascular examination should be performed to assess the degree of blood loss. Pulse rate, blood pressure and evidence of peripheral circulation should be measured to exclude shock.

A respiratory examination should be done, particularly searching for crackles in any region of the lungs. Palpation of the painful region should be done to confirm the musculoskeletal nature of the pain. Finger clubbing is not present in most cases of bronchiectasis. Wheeze occurs in 75 per cent and crackles in 60 per cent.

## A5: What investigations would be most helpful, and why?

- *chest radiograph* – very important; in one series 20 per cent of patients of haemoptysis with a normal chest radiograph had bronchiectasis
- *bronchoscopy* – only if haemodynamically significant volumes of blood or to exclude bronchial carcinoma
- *sputum* – helpful for microbiological identification, especially *Pseudomonas* species
- *HRCT* – diagnostic investigation of choice with 87–97 per cent sensitivity and 93–100 per cent specificity
- *bronchial angiography* – helpful if radiological treatment of haemoptysis is warranted
- *FBC* – for assessment of anaemia.

## A6: What treatment options are appropriate?

Resuscitation if required. Antitussives can be used if cough is severe. Sedation is sometimes used to control cough and anxiety. Treatment for infection should be guided by sputum sensitivities. Haemoptysis usually needs no specific treatment; if very severe and persistent, consider bronchial artery embolization or, as a last resort, surgical resection.

Bronchiectasis is a life-long condition that can result in chronic respiratory impairment. The patient should be warned that she may deteriorate over time and require frequent courses of antibiotics. Physiotherapy for lung hygiene may be helpful to reduce the frequency of infective exacerbations and preserve lung function. The evidence for the latter is currently lacking, but the patient should be taught the appropriate exercises tailored to her own specific capacity. The patient should be taught to look out for signs of infection, because prompt and appropriate antibiotic therapy may slow the decline in lung function often associated with bronchiectasis. Specialist therapies may be tried in individual patients, including nebulized antibiotic therapy or long-term rotational antibiotics (in which a series of antibiotics are taken chronically to keep bacterial levels to a minimum, with regular changes in the antibiotic to prevent drug resistance).

## CASE 7.9 – **A 62-year-old man with 2 months of fevers and haemoptysis.**

### A1: What is the likely differential diagnosis?

The likely differential diagnoses are TB, bronchial carcinoma, pneumonia, mycetoma and bronchiectasis.

### A2: What issues in the given history support the diagnosis?

A previous history of TB and the consumption of large quantities of alcohol suggest reactivation of old TB. The constitutional symptoms support this diagnosis, but bronchial carcinoma should also be excluded in a smoker with haemoptysis. Previous TB can give rise to mycetoma and bronchiectasis, both of which should be borne in mind. In case series where bronchial carcinoma is rare or excluded, bronchiectasis and TB represent the greatest cause of haemoptysis.

### A3: What additional features of the history would you seek to support a particular diagnosis?

Contact with other people with similar symptoms, and with close family members, should be ascertained. The type of therapy used for the historical TB may suggest inadequate treatment.

## A4: What clinical examination would you perform, and why?

Clinical examination should attempt to exclude TB. Respiratory examination may suggest focal signs of old TB, such as crackles in the upper lobes, but may be normal in active TB. Evidence of liver disease should be sought, given the patient's alcohol consumption and the possible need for anti-TB therapy.

## A5: What investigations would be most helpful, and why?

- *chest radiograph* – important
- *sputum* – three samples on different days for smears looking for acid- and alcohol-fast bacilli (AAFB) and culture of organisms (for up to 8 weeks)
- *bronchoscopy* – to exclude malignancy and allow bronchoalveolar lavage and biopsy
- *enzyme-linked immunosorbent spot assay* – lymphocyte activation testing has increased the rapidity of screening for TB
- *U&Es* – baseline
- *FBC* – assesses anaemia
- *LFTs* – baseline.

## A6: What treatment options are appropriate?

Assess infectivity and risk:

- sputum for AAFB – urgent consideration
- likely contact with children or others – if high risk of contact spread, admit patient for isolation until sputum is negative for organisms.

The patient should be assessed for likelihood of multidrug-resistant TB (human immunodeficiency virus [HIV], foreign contact). If the patient is at high risk, institute quadruple therapy; otherwise, start triple therapy with rifampicin, isoniazid and pyrazinamide (add ethambutol for quadruple therapy).

It is important in this case to include pyridoxine and multi-B vitamins to reduce the peripheral neuropathic complications of the anti-TB chemotherapy.

The patient's compliance with therapy should be assessed; if compliance is poor, consider starting directly observed therapy (DOT).

Try to find the trace, by contacting likely contacts, family members and regular contacts.

**OSCE counselling case**

## OSCE COUNSELLING CASE 7.3 – 'My father tends to drink too much and often forgets to take his tablets – is it important?'

Tuberculosis diagnosed by sputum examination is likely to be infectious. Although it may be safe to treat this man in the community if his contacts are known, screened and limited, incomplete or no treatment increases the risk to the general public of infectious spread. Before effective antibiotic treatment, TB was a fatal disease; failure to take appropriate anti-TB chemotherapy puts the patient's own health at risk. Incomplete or intermittent treatment increases the risk of developing drug-resistant TB. This can lead to chronic infection and the risk of community dissemination of multidrug-resistant TB.

Alcohol-related liver impairment may worsen the side-effect profile of some anti-TB drugs and may explain the patient's poor compliance. Such a problem should be sought and alternative drugs administered. Usually it is best to admit such a patient to a ward or clinic and reintroduce regular triple therapy in a stepwise manner until the problem can be identified. It is likely that this patient's lifestyle is 'chaotic', and therefore regular compliance with treatment is likely to be poor. In these circumstances, DOT may be instituted. Directly observed therapy requires that a trained health-care professional, e.g. TB specialist nurse or equivalent, visits the patient at a prearranged location, either daily or three times a week, and observes the treatment being taken. Such practice has been found to reduce the incidence of drug-resistant TB in areas with a relatively high prevalence. In very rare cases, compulsory admission can be arranged under public health law. This can be done only in the context of respiratory TB, where there is a considerable risk to public health. Compulsory administration of medications is not permissible, however, and it is therefore best to develop a concordant rather than a coercive relationship with the patient.

## REVISION PANEL

- The volume of air expired in the first second is known as the forced expiratory volume in 1 s ($FEV_1$). The total volume exhaled in 5 s is the forced vital capacity (FVC).
- Episodic breathlessness, wheeze and cough with spontaneous resolution are typical of asthma. Symptoms tend to occur at night, first thing in the morning or after exercise, but none of these clinical features is specific for asthma.
- Chronic progressive breathlessness on the background of a long smoking history suggests COPD. Typical features include lack of spontaneous improvement or response to inhaled therapy, relentless progression of symptoms, and a combination of productive cough and dyspnoea.
- Progressive dyspnoea in a non-smoker with no history of cough may suggest fibrotic (interstitial) lung disease.
- Pleuritic chest pain with dyspnoea and haemoptysis is typical of PE. Diagnosis can be confirmed by CTPA. Full-dose anticoagulation should be initiated with LMW heparin, while oral anticoagulant therapy (warfarin) is commenced at a loading regimen. Anticoagulation should be continued for a minimum of 6 months.
- Symptoms typical of infection (fevers or sweats) with pleuritic chest pain suggest pneumonia. *Streptococcus pneumoniae* remains the most common cause of community-acquired pneumonia. The so-called 'atypical' pathogens such as *Mycoplasma* species, *L. pneumophila* and *Chlamydia* species represent a substantial minority. The red-tinged or rusty sputum is said to typify streptococcal infections, but haemoptysis may occur with other pulmonary infections, especially TB.
- Sudden onset of chest pain suggests either trauma or spontaneous pneumothorax. Pulmonary embolus should always be considered.
- Bronchial carcinoma may present late with haemoptysis after a lengthy period of weight loss and cough. Smoking is associated with most cases of bronchial carcinoma, and a non-smoking history should suggest other causes.

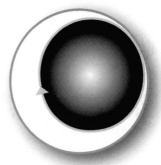

# 8 Gastroenterology

*C.S. Probert*

## GASTROENTEROLOGICAL EMERGENCIES

## PANCREATITIS

## INFLAMMATORY BOWEL DISEASE

# HEPATITIS

# IRRITABLE BOWEL SYNDROME

# COELIAC DISEASE

# GASTROENTEROLOGICAL EMERGENCIES

## Questions

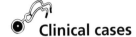

### Clinical cases

## For each of the case scenarios given, consider the following:

> **Q1**: What specific questions would you ask the patient?
> **Q2**: What is the most likely diagnosis?
> **Q3**: What examination would you perform?
> **Q4**: What would be the initial management?
> **Q5**: What investigations would you request to confirm a diagnosis?
> **Q6**: What other issues should be addressed?

### CASE 8.1 – A 73-year-old man with melaena.

A 73-year-old man presents with a 5-day history of passing black stools. On the fifth day he began to feel breathless and tired, particularly on climbing stairs.

### CASE 8.2 – A 26-year-old woman with bloody diarrhoea.

A 26-year-old woman presents with a 3-week history of bloody diarrhoea. The blood is fresh and mixed in the liquid stool. Initially, she thought she may have food poisoning, but she cannot recall eating anything unusual and has eaten the same food as her unaffected partner.

### CASE 8.3 – A 46-year-old man with alcohol problems and haematemesis.

A 46-year-old man with alcohol problems presents with haematemesis and shock.

OSCE counselling cases

## OSCE COUNSELLING CASE 8.1 – 'Are my symptoms caused by an infection, or is it all down to the colitis?'

You have determined that the woman in Case 8.2 has ulcerative colitis and tell her that you can treat it. She would like to know whether she could have passed it on to the children in the school where she is a catering assistant.

## OSCE COUNSELLING CASE 8.2 – 'Will my children get inflammatory bowel disease?'

The woman in Case 8.2 is worried that she may pass inflammatory bowel disease (IBD) on to her own children.

## Key concepts

To work through the core clinical cases in this section, you will need to understand the following key concepts.

- Initial assessment of the cause of gastrointestinal (GI) emergencies such as bleeding or severe diarrhoea should be carried out at the same time as resuscitation.
- Most patients with haematemesis or melaena will have bled from a peptic ulcer, most cases of which are painless.
- Initiating proton pump inhibitor (PPI) therapy before endoscopic assessment is not evidence based.
- Although stigmata of chronic liver disease may suggest varices as the cause of haematemesis, endoscopic assessment should be made before 'blind' treatment using a Sengstaken–Blakemore tube.
- Any form of colitis may be life-threatening.
- Infections should always be sought in parallel with treatment.

# Answers

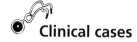

## Clinical cases

### CASE 8.1 – **A 73-year-old man with melaena.**

### A1: What specific questions would you ask the patient?

The presence of black stools indicates GI bleeding above the ligament of Trietz. The likely sources include benign and malignant ulceration of the stomach and peptic duodenal ulceration. The history should determine whether there are any symptoms suggestive of ulceration and risk factors and clues to whether the lesion is malignant. Postprandial and nocturnal burning epigastric pains are classic symptoms of peptic ulceration, particularly if the pain radiates to the back. These symptoms differentiate poorly between gastric and duodenal ulcers, however (20 per cent of patients with bleeding peptic ulcers have ulcer-like dyspepsia). Risk factors to seek include:

- past history of peptic ulceration or surgery for such disease
- recent ingestion of non-steroidal anti-inflammatory drug (NSAID) of any type, warfarin or antiplatelet drugs
- smoking
- alcohol use
- diabetes
- heart failure.

The last four of these are likely to relate to poor mucosal healing. Clues to malignancy include weight loss, anorexia and anaemia before the presenting gastrointestinal haemorrhage.

### A2: What is the most likely diagnosis?

The most likely diagnosis is a bleeding duodenal ulcer. It is unlikely that the patient is bleeding from an oesophageal lesion (carcinoma or oesophagitis) because, in most cases, haematemesis will occur at the same time. Of all patients with acute upper GI bleeding, 40 per cent have benign peptic ulcer disease. Duodenal ulcers appear to be more common than gastric ulcers.

### A3: What examination would you perform?

A full physical examination is necessary, with particular attention being paid to shock. In a patient of this age, however, a systolic blood pressure of 110 mmHg may be considered to be shock. Of secondary importance is the examination of the abdomen, during which an epigastric mass and palpable liver should be sought.

### A4: What would be the initial management?

The first step in the management is resuscitation. The patient should be laid flat and given oxygen via a facemask, while two large-bore cannulae are inserted, one of which ought to be a central line if the patient is shocked. As the cannulae are inserted, blood samples should be taken for full blood count (FBC), cross-match (4–6 units), and urea and electrolytes (U&Es) (urea is a marker of the amount of blood lost). Liver function tests (LFTs) are not of immediate importance. Clotting abnormalities need to be sought if the patient is taking warfarin or has jaundice. Fluid replacement should start as soon as the cannulae are in place. There is no advantage to using colloids. Blood transfusion should start as soon as possible if the patient is shocked or has a haemoglobin (Hb) level below 10 g/dL. A urinary catheter is desirable.

### A5: What investigations would you request to confirm a diagnosis?

Oesophagogastroduodenoscopy (endoscopy) should be performed within 24 h of admission. If the patient is shocked or has Hb ≤10 g/dL, this should be performed as soon as the patient has been resuscitated, or immediately if urgent surgery is contemplated (i.e. if resuscitation attempts are failing).

### A6: What other issues should be addressed?

The ulcer is likely to be *Helicobacter pylori*-related. Triple therapy should be instituted. This is typically a PPI with two antibiotics from amoxicillin, clarithromycin and metronidazole. If aspirin was being used, then clopidogrel may be substituted.

## CASE 8.2 – A 26-year-old woman with bloody diarrhoea.

### A1: What specific questions would you ask the patient?

The duration of the disease suggests that the cause is acute colitis. The differential diagnoses include microbial diarrhoea – *Clostridium difficile* (so a drug history is needed) or protozoa (a travel history should be taken) – side effects of medications such as NSAIDs, and familial adenomatous polyps (bleeding usually occurs in the context of normal stool, so a family history should be taken). Lifestyle and past medical history should be considered in case the patient is immunocompromised.

### A2: What is the most likely diagnosis?

The most likely diagnosis is acute colitis, most probably as a result of ulcerative colitis. Other forms of colitis caused by Crohn's colitis, drug side effects and *C. difficile* are possible. Cytomegalovirus (CMV) proctitis and amoebic dysentery are unlikely.

### A3: What examination would you perform?

A full physical examination is necessary, with particular attention to examination of the abdomen. Distension and tenderness are particularly worrying physical signs in such a patient. Shock caused by colitis is uncommon but critically important. Anaemia and a fever should be sought. Severe colitis is defined by the presence of tachycardia, fever and anaemia. Tenderness may indicate toxic dilation or perforation.

### A4: What would be the initial management?

The patient may require admission or at least discussion with a senior colleague. Assuming that the patient meets the criteria for admission (i.e. she has severe disease), the initial management includes bedrest, hydrocortisone 100 mg IV four times a day, transfusion to correct anaemia, and nutritional support (typically high-energy food cartons). Occasionally IV fluid replacement is required. Heparin is used in most centres: full anticoagulation may treat the disease, whereas prophylactic doses prevent thromboembolism, to which such patients are prone. It is important to confirm the diagnosis rapidly, however. At least three stool cultures should be taken. *Clostridium difficile* toxin must be sought if antibiotics have been consumed recently. Microscopy is often negative, but protozoa must be considered. A plain abdominal radiograph is necessary to assess the diameter of the transverse colon and to look for the distribution of faeces, which may be used to determine the extent of the disease.

### A5: What investigations would you request to confirm a diagnosis?

A limited sigmoidoscopy should be performed by a trained operator. This is a hazardous procedure in untrained hands, but assessment of the rectal mucosa often helps determine the aetiology of the colitis.

### A6: What other issues should be addressed?

The management of severe ulcerative colitis has two phases: control of the attack and maintenance of remission. If the patient does not respond to IV hydrocortisone by the fifth day, a surgical opinion should be sought, with a view to performing colectomy on day 7. An alternative approach is to initiate rescue therapy with IV ciclosporin or, in some situations, infliximab. Any patient who deteriorates despite IV hydrocortisone should also be considered for emergency colectomy. If hydrocortisone controls the attack, the patient should be weaned on to oral steroids and, probably, a 5-aminosalicylic acid (5-ASA) compound. Steroids should later be discontinued, with a view to controlling remission with the 5-ASA compound.

## CASE 8.3 – **A 46-year-old man with alcohol problems with haematemesis.**

### A1: What specific questions would you ask the patient?

This is bleeding oesophageal varices until proven otherwise. Although people with alcohol problems may bleed from all the same lesions as people who do not have this problem, a person with alcohol problems who has bled sufficiently to become shocked is most likely to have varices. If the patient is shocked, treatment must be started before a full history is obtained; indeed, the patient may be unable to give a history. If a history is available, ask for previous episodes of GI bleeding and treatment for varices.

### A2: What is the most likely diagnosis?

The most likely diagnosis is bleeding oesophageal varices.

### A3: What examination would you perform?

Shock should be evaluated quickly: blood pressure, heart rate and state of peripheral perfusion. Signs of portal hypertension would support the diagnosis: ascites, spider naevi, umbilical hernia. Other evidence of decompensated liver disease should be documented: Glasgow coma score (GCS), fetor, flapping tremor and bruising.

### A4: What would be the initial management?

The patient must be resuscitated as quickly as possible. The patient should be laid flat and given oxygen via a facemask while two large-bore cannulae are inserted, one of which should be a central line. As the cannulae are inserted, blood samples should be taken for FBC, cross-match (4–6 units) and U&Es (urea is a marker of the amount of blood lost). Albumin and clotting factors (prothrombin time, PT) can be measured to assess synthetic function; other tests, such as alanine transaminase and alkaline phosphatase, assess hepatocyte damage and biliary tract disease/cholestasis, respectively. Synthetic function is an important prognostic indicator. Fluid replacement should start as soon as the cannulae are in place. The central venous pressure (CVP) should be monitored and blood or albumin given to maintain a pressure of 10–12 cmH$_2$O. A urinary catheter is desirable. If the patient is in renal failure despite an adequate CVP, call for senior help. Vasopressin analogues are desirable, with senior guidance. If the patient remains shocked, a Sengstaken–Blakemore tube may be necessary.

## A5: What investigations would you request to confirm a diagnosis?

Urgent endoscopy is both diagnostic and therapeutic. This should be performed as soon as the patient is cardiovascularly stable. If such stability cannot be achieved, endoscopy may be performed while resuscitation is continued, provided that the airway is protected.

## A6: What other issues should be addressed?

Broad-spectrum antibiotics should be given because bacteraemia is common at the time of variceal haemorrhage. Anti-encephalopathy treatment (lactulose, metronidazole) should be started as soon as possible. Intravenous thiamine should be replaced before dextrose is given; without this, there is a risk of precipitating Wernicke's encephalopathy.

OSCE counselling cases

## OSCE COUNSELLING CASE 8.1 – 'Are my symptoms caused by an infection, or is it all down to the colitis?'

The answer is, fortunately, colitis. There are similarities in the symptoms between ulcerative colitis and infectious diarrhoea; this is because some infections damage the colon and cause a different kind of colitis. In this patient's case, however, infection has been ruled out by the stool tests. Furthermore, other tests (sigmoidoscopy ± biopsy) have shown that the patient's symptoms are caused by ulcerative colitis. In the acute phase, most forms of colitis are very similar. Infection should be ruled out in new patients with acute disease. Three sets of stool analysis are often necessary to exclude *C. difficile* with confidence. Campylobacter infection causes acute colitis with bloody diarrhoea, but myalgia and abdominal pain are conspicuous. Gastrointestinal infection may occur in patients with ulcerative colitis. Microbiological tests should be performed in patients with an established diagnosis if the attack is atypical or refractory to the usual treatment.

## OSCE COUNSELLING CASE 8.2 – 'Will my children get inflammatory bowel disease?'

The answer is, fortunately, 'no'. Although IBD can appear to run in families, the risk is comparatively small. The chances of the patient's children getting IBD are raised ten times, but the risk is still only 1 in 100 – i.e. their chances of getting IBD are less than their risk of getting diabetes or asthma. This is an important test of communication skills. The key is to explain relative and absolute risks. There is a genetic component to the risk of acquiring IBD. The risk to first-degree relatives is 10–20 times greater than that in unaffected families, but this raises the prevalence only from 1 in 1000 to 1 in 100. There is a wealth of literature describing genetic loci in IBD. Although few undergraduates will have read such literature, all should be aware that loci have been described, that the disease is not sporadic, and that there is not a simple mendelian inheritance.

## PANCREATITIS

## Questions

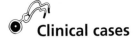

### Clinical cases

## For each of the case scenarios given, consider the following:

**Q1**: What specific questions would you ask the patient?
**Q2**: What is the most likely diagnosis?
**Q3**: What examination would you perform?
**Q4**: What would be the initial management?
**Q5**: What investigations would you request to confirm a diagnosis?
**Q6**: What other issues should be addressed?

### CASE 8.4 – A 67-year-old woman with pale stools and weight loss.

A 67-year-old woman presents with diarrhoea. She describes her stools as pale. You discover that she has lost weight and has nocturia and thirst.

### CASE 8.5 – A 26-year-old woman with abdominal pain and vomiting.

A 26-year-old woman presents with upper abdominal pain and vomiting. Previously she has experienced episodes of right upper quadrant colicky pain that had lasted several hours at a time. On one of these occasions she experienced a brief episode of jaundice accompanied by dark urine. The present episode is different, however. The pain has lasted for 2 days and appears to be worsening and, this time, it is non-colicky.

### CASE 8.6 – A 48-year-old man with alcohol problems with chronic abdominal pain.

A 48-year-old man with alcohol problems presents with upper abdominal pain with some radiation to the back.

## OSCE counselling cases

### OSCE COUNSELLING CASE 8.3 – 'Why have I got pancreatitis?'

A 26-year-old woman with pancreatitis secondary to gallstones asks 'Why have I got pancreatitis?'.

### OSCE COUNSELLING CASE 8.4 – 'Why should I stop drinking?'

A 46-year-old man with alcohol problems presents with chronic relapsing pancreatitis and asks 'Why should I stop drinking?'.

## 🔑 Key concepts

To work through the core clinical cases in this section, you will need to understand the following key concepts.

- Acute pancreatitis is a significant cause of mortality. It should be considered in the differential diagnosis of all cases of acute abdominal pain.
- The diagnosis can generally be confirmed by an elevated serum amylase.
- Risk factors for acute pancreatitis include alcohol abuse and gallstones.
- Chronic pancreatitis, in general, has an insidious onset.
- Presenting features arise from exocrine failure, later with endocrine failure, accompanied by epigastric pain that usually radiates to the back.
- Diagnosis is reached by assessment of exocrine function or imaging.

# Answers

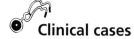
## Clinical cases

## CASE 8.4 – **A 67-year-old woman with pale stools and weight loss.**

### A1: What specific questions would you ask the patient?

The pale stool should prompt questions about malabsorption and obstructive jaundice. After asking about jaundice, itching and dark urine – which should all be absent – direct questions to the patient's stool. Look for fluffy, offensive, floating stools. Blood and mucus will be absent. The duration of the symptoms should be noted along with exacerbating and relieving factors. Abdominal pain should be sought, in particular epigastric pain. Such pain is unusual in coeliac disease (although bloating is curiously common) but common in patients with chronic pancreatitis. With regard to the nocturia, the volume should be assessed (small amounts suggest a urinary tract infection [UTI]; larger amounts suggest a diuresis – osmotic or drug-induced). Large-volume nocturia accompanied by thirst suggests diabetes or hypercalcaemia.

### A2: What is the most likely diagnosis?

The most likely diagnosis is chronic pancreatitis. The patient exhibits both exocrine and endocrine failure. Pain is absent in 50 per cent of older patients with chronic pancreatitis.

### A3: What examination would you perform?

A full physical examination is necessary, with particular attention being paid to the state of nutrition and the cause of the pancreatic failure. Alcoholism and haemochromatosis are associated with signs of liver disease and pigmentation, respectively. Most patients with alcohol problems, however, have either liver or pancreatic damage. Alcoholism and haemochromatosis are both associated with atrial fibrillation (AF) and cardiomyopathy. A per rectal examination should confirm the colour of the stool.

### A4: What would be the initial management?

The first step in the management is to corroborate the clinical diagnosis. Blood samples should be taken for calcium, glucose and urea. This will rapidly explain the source of the nocturia. Diabetes should be managed appropriately (see Chapter 1). Early dietetic input should be obtained.

### A5: What investigations would you request to confirm a diagnosis?

The pancreas should be imaged and its exocrine function assessed. Imaging modalities to consider include abdominal radiograph (to show calcification – present in 30 per cent of cases), ultrasonography and computed tomography (CT). The latter two have similar specificities (85–90 per cent), but CT is more sensitive than ultrasonography (75 per cent *v.* 65 per cent). Exocrine function is currently best tested by the pancreolauryl test, which is non-invasive, cheap and easy to perform. Faecal fats are no longer routinely available.

### A6: What other issues should be addressed?

After confirming the diagnosis, the diet should be modified – fats can be eaten and should not be avoided because the patient will continue to lose weight. Adequate pancreatic replacement therapy should be prescribed, along with acid-suppressing drugs. Pancreatic enzymes are usually buffered by bicarbonate secretion; however, in chronic pancreatitis, there may be too little bicarbonate and so acid suppression is essential.

## CASE 8.5 – **A 26-year-old woman with abdominal pain and vomiting.**

### A1: What specific questions would you ask the patient?

Earlier episodes of right upper quadrant pain suggest biliary colic. The episode accompanied by jaundice and dark urine suggests that a stone may have obstructed the common bile duct. The present problem suggests acute gallstone pancreatitis. As with any abdominal pain, the site, radiation, and exacerbating and relieving factors should be sought. Acute pancreatitis should always be considered in patients with acute abdominal pain.

### A2: What is the most likely diagnosis?

The most likely diagnosis is acute pancreatitis. The differential diagnosis for its aetiology is gallstone pancreatitis, hereditary hypertriglyceridaemia and drug-induced pancreatitis. The differential diagnosis of the pain is cholecystitis, peptic ulcer disease (perforation) and Crohn's disease.

### A3: What examination would you perform?

A full physical examination is necessary with particular attention being paid to the abdomen. Signs range from epigastric tenderness to a full-blown acute abdomen with distension and rigidity. The Grey–Turner and Cullen signs should be sought. An epigastric mass (pseudo-cyst) may be present. Shock may also be present.

### A4: What would be the initial management?

The first step in the management is to confirm the clinical diagnosis. Blood samples should be taken for amylase, calcium, glucose and blood gases. Amylase is elevated threefold in most cases of acute pancreatitis; occasionally, however, very shocked patients have a normal amylase. Acidosis, hyperglycaemia and hypocalcaemia are all poor prognostic indicators. The patient should receive analgesia (pethidine), an antiemetic, resuscitation with oxygen and IV fluids. Hyperglycaemia should be corrected with an insulin infusion. Early senior review of patients who are shocked or have other poor prognostic indicators is imperative.

### A5: What investigations would you request to confirm a diagnosis?

The pancreas should be imaged. Imaging modalities to consider include abdominal radiograph (to exclude a perforated viscus and possibly to show a sentinel loop). Ultrasonography and CT are preferable. Ultrasonography is useful because it can show gallstones and pancreatic necrosis; bowel gas may obscure the view, however. Computed tomography is more accurate than ultrasonography for grading the pancreatic damage (90 per cent v. 73 per cent). Endoscopic retrograde cholangiopancreatography (ERCP) has a role to play, primarily in treating the underlying pathology; magnetic resonance cholangiopancreatography (MRCP) is preferred for diagnosis, however, as ERCP can cause pancreatitis. Without intervention, 30–50 per cent of patients with gallstone pancreatitis have further episodes.

### A6: What other issues should be addressed?

After confirming the diagnosis, the patient should undergo supportive therapy. An underlying cause should be sought. Endoscopic retrograde cholangiopancreatography is recommended.

## CASE 8.6 – **A 48-year-old man with alcohol problems with chronic abdominal pain.**

### A1:  What specific questions would you ask the patient?

Epigastric pain may arise from pathology in three main sites: stomach/duodenum, gallbladder and pancreas. An accurate description of the pain may help to differentiate biliary colic from pancreatic and gastroduodenal pain, as the latter two are not colicky. Pancreatic pain tends to last for days or weeks rather than hours, as in the case of peptic ulceration. The relationship to food, lack of relief with antacids, and so on should be sought.

### A2:  What is the most likely diagnosis?

The most likely diagnosis is alcoholic chronic pancreatitis. Pain often precedes exocrine failure in people with alcohol problems.

### A3:  What examination would you perform?

A full physical examination is necessary, with particular attention being paid to the abdomen and the nutritional status.

### A4:  What would be the initial management?

The first step is to confirm the clinical diagnosis. This can be problematic in the absence of exo- and endocrine failure. The diagnosis is largely clinical, supported by anatomical changes when the pancreas is imaged and in the absence of other pathology such as duodenal ulcer disease.

### A5:  What investigations would you request to confirm the diagnosis?

The pancreas should be imaged. Imaging modalities to consider include abdominal radiograph (to show calcification – present in 30 per cent of cases), ultrasonography and CT. Ultrasonography and CT have similar specificities (85–90 per cent), although CT is more sensitive than ultrasonography (75 per cent v. 65 per cent). Exocrine failure is not clinically apparent until 90 per cent of the exocrine function has been lost. Faecal elastase may be measured to assess exocrine failure; the enzyme levels are lowered in patients with pancreatic insufficiency. Pancreolauryl test and faecal fats measurement are no longer routinely available.

### A6:  What other issues should be addressed?

After confirming the diagnosis, the patient should receive pain relief in line with the World Health Organization's (WHO's) 'pain ladder'. Most patients require opiates, and these should not be withheld because of concerns about their long-term use. Fifty per cent of patients respond to a nerve block. Surgery is seldom indicated.

# 👫 OSCE counselling cases

## OSCE COUNSELLING CASE 8.3 – 'Why have I got pancreatitis?'

An appropriate answer is: 'Unfortunately, your pancreas has become inflamed; this is called pancreatitis. The pancreas is an organ that lies beside the gallbladder. Stones have grown in your gallbladder. One (or some) of these stones has passed into the tube that links the gallbladder to the intestine. In this site, the same tube joins to the pancreas. As a result of the stone lying in these tubes, the pancreas has become inflamed. Pancreatitis may also be caused by alcohol and drugs; there is no suggestion that this is the case for you.'

This is an important test of communication skills. The key is to explain the anatomy of the biliary tree and how the gallstones lead to pancreatitis. It is important to explain that pancreatitis is a result of gallstones. As it can be a result of alcohol abuse, the patient should be reassured that you understand that her pancreatitis is not so caused. The explanation of diseases that may or may not be confused with those that are associated with social stigma requires particular skill and tact. Be prepared to discuss the management of any condition, the nature of which you have been asked to explain.

## OSCE COUNSELLING CASE 8.4 – 'Why should I stop drinking?'

An appropriate answer is: 'Your drinking has led to a serious disorder of your pancreas. This disorder may cause severe abdominal pain and failure to digest your food (resulting in weight loss); if severe, you may need surgery. In some patients it can be fatal. As alcohol is the cause, it is important that you stop drinking to reduce the risk of further severe attacks. If you continue to drink, the problem is likely to get worse. If you stop drinking, the disease may not progress.'

In answering this question, it is crucial to be honest and understanding. Patients may continue to have pain even if they do stop drinking. There is no place for blaming the patient if the pain continues. Supportive measures should be offered. Additional means of controlling the pain are likely to be called for, including long-term analgesics, nerve blocks and even surgery.

# INFLAMMATORY BOWEL DISEASE

## Questions

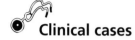

### Clinical cases

## For each of the case scenarios given, consider the following:

> **Q1**: What specific questions would you ask the patient?
> **Q2**: What is the most likely diagnosis?
> **Q3**: What examination would you perform?
> **Q4**: What would be the initial management?
> **Q5**: What investigations would you request to confirm a diagnosis?
> **Q6**: What other issues should be addressed?

### CASE 8.7 – **A 20-year-old woman with ulcerative colitis.**

A 20-year-old woman with ulcerative colitis has had symptoms for several weeks, so she presents to the accident and emergency (A&E) department.

### CASE 8.8 – **An 18-year-old man with colicky central abdominal pain and vomiting after meals.**

An 18-year-old male smoker presents with colicky central abdominal pain and vomiting 30–60 min after meals. He has been told that he may have IBD, but his mother is concerned because he has lost weight.

### CASE 8.9 – **A 21-year-old man with diarrhoea and a perianal abscess.**

A 21-year-old man has noted episodes of colicky lower abdominal pain over several months. It has been suggested that he may have IBD.

## ⋔⋔ OSCE counselling cases

### OSCE COUNSELLING CASE 8.5 – 'Will I get cancer?'

A 36-year-old man with established ulcerative colitis has heard that there is a risk of bowel cancer in patients with the condition.

### OSCE COUNSELLING CASE 8.6 – 'Will I need to have the bag?'

A 20-year-old woman with refractory ulcerative colitis is concerned that surgery is imminent.

## ⚷ Key concepts

To work through the core clinical cases in this section, you will need to understand the following key concepts.

Patients with IBD often present with symptoms that have been present for several weeks or months. Many will have been told that they have irritable bowel syndrome (IBS). A history and examination will often point to the correct diagnosis by the time the patient presents.

Patients should be counselled about the need for potentially embarrassing invasive investigations and the probable long-term nature of IBD. They should be encouraged to seek help from reputable sources such as Crohn's and Colitis UK (CCUK), formerly the National Association for Colitis and Crohn's Disease (NACC).

# Answers

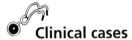

## Clinical cases

### CASE 8.7 – **A 20-year-old woman with ulcerative colitis.**

#### A1: What specific questions would you ask the patient?

The severity of the attack should be assessed. Specifically, the frequency and consistency of the stool should be assessed. The presence of blood should be sought. The presence, periodicity and site of abdominal pain, and any weight loss, should be assessed.

#### A2: What is the most likely diagnosis?

The most likely diagnosis is acute severe ulcerative colitis. The assessment of severity is based upon clinical observation. The differential diagnosis is infectious diarrhoea and hypersensitivity to her treatment.

#### A3: What examination would you perform?

A full physical examination is necessary, with particular attention being paid to the signs of disease severity (fever, anaemia, tachycardia) and to abdominal signs. Fever, anaemia and tachycardia define severe disease.

#### A4: What would be the initial management?

The first step is to corroborate the clinical diagnosis. Blood samples should be taken for FBC, C-reactive protein (CRP) and albumin. A plain abdominal radiograph should be performed to assess colonic diameter and to look for mucosal islands. Stool cultures should be performed. The patient should be admitted and commenced on IV hydrocortisone 100 mg four times a day and subcutaneous heparin 5000 U three times a day. A stool chart should be commenced, recording the frequency and amount of stool and the presence of blood. The patient's weight should be recorded.

#### A5: What investigations would you request to confirm a diagnosis?

Senior review should be sought, with a view to considering a cautious limited sigmoidoscopy. Sigmoidoscopy is potentially dangerous.

#### A6: What other issues should be addressed?

If after 3–5 days the CRP and stool frequency have not improved, a surgical opinion should be sought, with a view to colectomy on day 7. An alternative approach is to initiate rescue therapy on days 3–5 with IV ciclosporin or, in some situations, infliximab. Some centres recommend abdominal radiograph on alternate days. A deterioration in the abdominal radiograph or physical signs should prompt earlier surgical review.

### CASE 8.8 – **An 18-year-old man with colicky central abdominal pain and vomiting after meals.**

#### A1: What specific questions would you ask the patient?

The pain should be assessed, looking for site, radiation, exacerbating and relieving factors, and special precipitating factors, particularly foods. The frequency of the vomiting and its relationship to the pain and meals should be clarified. The amount of weight lost and the duration of this symptom should be documented. A family and travel history should be taken. Medication should be recorded.

## A2: What is the most likely diagnosis?

The symptoms suggest subacute obstruction. The differential diagnoses include adhesions, Crohn's disease and intussusception.

## A3: What examination would you perform?

A full physical examination is necessary, with particular attention being paid to the nutritional state, signs of inflammatory disease (fever, anaemia, tachycardia) and abdominal signs, specifically looking for a mass.

## A4: What would be the initial management?

The patient may warrant admission if he is malnourished, dehydrated or in pain, but subacute obstruction is often investigated in the outpatient setting. If the patient is admitted he will need analgesia, IV fluid replacement (2–3 L/day) and a nasogastric tube (to decompress the upper GI tract). Initial investigation of the admitted patient should include abdominal radiograph (for obstruction), U&Es, LFTs and FBC with CRP and plasma viscosity. If he is not admitted, he should be investigated as in A5 below.

## A5: What investigations would you request to confirm a diagnosis?

After resuscitation or in the outpatient setting, urgent barium follow-through (or small bowel enema) should be performed. Computed tomography or ultrasonography may be indicated if there is a mass. Computed tomography will show the 'pseudo-kidney sign' if intussusception is present. In general, magnetic resonance imaging (MRI) should not be used in this setting, as there is inadequate experience in interpreting this test.

## A6: What other issues should be addressed?

Subacute obstruction may be managed conservatively while the diagnosis is reached. Most cases come to surgery in the long term.

## CASE 8.9 – **A 21-year-old man with diarrhoea and a perianal abscess.**

### A1: What specific questions would you ask the patient?

The diarrhoea should be assessed with regard to frequency, duration, the presence of blood and mucus, and its relationship to the abdominal pain. Constitutional symptoms (fever, weight loss) should be sought. With regard to the patient's abscess, the duration of symptoms and the site and radiation of the pain should be determined. Previous episodes and their treatment should be recorded. Lifestyle, travel and a family history should be noted.

### A2: What is the most likely diagnosis?

The most likely diagnosis is Crohn's disease. Diarrhoea is not always accompanied by blood in patients with Crohn's disease. Perianal abscess may accompany ulcerative colitis.

### A3: What examination would you perform?

A full physical examination is necessary, with particular attention being paid to the abdomen, nutritional status, evidence of systemic illness (fever, tachycardia, anaemia) and the perineum. Per rectal examination is not indicated because the abscess encroaches on the anus. An examination under anaesthetic is preferred.

## A4: What would be the initial management?

The first steps in the management are to relieve suffering and confirm the clinical diagnosis. Pain should be relieved by analgesia while a prompt surgical opinion is sought. Investigations to support the diagnosis should be performed with FBC, LFTs, CRP and plasma viscosity as a prelude to a surgical review.

## A5: What investigations would you request to confirm a diagnosis?

Generally, an examination under anaesthetic is the preferred approach to such patients. During this procedure, the abscess may be drained, a sigmoidoscopy and rectal biopsy performed, and probing performed for a fistula. A stent may be placed if the fistula is found.

## A6: What other issues should be addressed?

After managing the abscess, the diagnosis of Crohn's disease should be confirmed. Imaging options include MRI and CT; MRI is the investigation of choice for imaging the soft tissues around the rectum and demonstrating fistulas, which usually underlie abscesses in Crohn's disease. Crohn's disease should be managed by draining the abscess, seeking out and treating other foci of infection, and treating the disease itself.

OSCE counselling cases

## OSCE COUNSELLING CASE 8.5 – 'Will I get cancer?'

An appropriate answer is: 'There is an increased risk of bowel cancer in some patients with ulcerative colitis. This risk does not apply to all patients. Young patients with extensive disease that has a grumbling course seem to be at greatest risk. The medication that is given for the treatment of colitis (mesalazine) appears to lower the risk of bowel cancer. We will assess your risk by plotting your disease extent. If the risk appears to be increased, we will discuss measures that may enable us to detect it at an early stage. We will check your bowel by performing a colonoscopy from time to time – perhaps as rarely as once every 5 years. Although the risk to patients with ulcerative colitis of getting bowel cancer is greater than that of people without colitis, the risk to an individual patient remains relatively small.'

It is important to be honest but to offer reassurance at the same time. Relative risk and absolute risk may be difficult concepts to explain to patients. It is worth planning your answer to such common questions.

## OSCE COUNSELLING CASE 8.6 – 'Will I need to have the bag?'

An appropriate answer is: 'Yes, at least in the short term'. Patients with refractory disease are often taking steroids at the time of surgery, and so the surgery is kept as simple as possible. The operation of choice is to remove as much diseased bowel as possible without operating deep in the pelvis (subtotal colectomy, oversewing the rectum). A stoma will be necessary. Most patients feel better very quickly, and many soon adapt to the stoma. These patients will later need a second operation to remove the rectum (proctectomy). Other patients may prefer an ileoanal pouch. The pouch brings about improved body image but is associated with the need to pass stool frequently (typically four to six times a day). Of patients, 15–20 per cent lose their bowel (undergo colectomy) in the long term. It is important to differentiate the emergency situation, in which the priority is to keep the patient alive and healthy, from the elective situation, where the aim is to restore quality of life. Ileoanal pouches are not a panacea. The quality of life of a patient with a pouch is only as good as that in a patient with mild ulcerative colitis. The stool of a patient with a pouch is likely to be loose and passed frequently. Pouchitis with bloody looser stools occurs in 5–20 per cent of patients; it can often be managed medically but may result in a reversal of the pouch and recreation of the stoma.

# PEPTIC ULCER DISEASE

## Questions

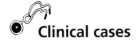
### Clinical cases

## For each of the case scenarios given, consider the following:

> **Q1**: What is the likely differential diagnosis?
> **Q2**: What in the given history supports the diagnosis?
> **Q3**: What additional features in the history would you seek to support a particular diagnosis?
> **Q4**: What clinical examination would you perform, and why?
> **Q5**: What investigations would be most helpful, and why?
> **Q6**: What treatment options are appropriate?

### CASE 8.10 – A 70-year-old man with indigestion.

A 70-year-old man with arthritis and ischaemic heart disease presents with indigestion. He has epigastric pain radiating to his back. He has been taking aspirin for his heart and ibuprofen for his arthritis.

### CASE 8.11 – A 35-year-old woman with indigestion and a feeling of discomfort after eating meals.

A 35-year-old woman presents with a feeling of discomfort after eating meals. She describes a fullness after eating a modest amount and can no longer finish the meal that she used to eat. The indigestion is also troublesome.

### CASE 8.12 – A 60-year-old man losing weight and vomiting.

A 60-year-old man is brought to see you accompanied by his wife. Together they describe that he has had progressively worsening vomiting for some months. He has lost a stone in weight. He finds that the vomiting is worse after a full meal, but liquids trouble him less than solid food. In the past he has suffered from indigestion and has taken over-the-counter remedies for this.

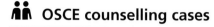 OSCE counselling cases

OSCE COUNSELLING CASE 8.7 – **'Can I take aspirin for my heart now that I have an ulcer?'**

OSCE COUNSELLING CASE 8.8 – **'The tablets for my ulcer were wonderful. Should I continue to take them?'**

## ⚷ Key concepts

To work through the core clinical cases in this section, you will need to understand the following key concepts.

*Helicobacter pylori* is found in more than 90 per cent of patients with duodenal ulcers and 70 per cent of patients with gastric ulcers. Non-steroidal anti-inflammatory drugs contribute to the aetiology of peptic ulcer disease. Smoking and alcohol are minor contributory factors.

The gold standard diagnosis is the demonstration of an ulcer by endoscopy or barium meal. Endoscopy is preferable because gastric ulcers can be biopsied, to look for malignancy, and *H. pylori* can be sought in the stomach of patients with peptic ulcers, whether gastric or duodenal.

As most ulcers are related to *H. pylori*, eradication of *H. pylori* should be prescribed. This consists of a PPI and two antibiotics from metronidazole, amoxicillin and clarithromycin.

## Answers

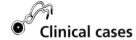
### Clinical cases

### CASE 8.10 – **A 70-year-old man with indigestion.**

#### A1: What is the likely differential diagnosis?

The differential diagnoses are peptic ulcer disease, carcinoma of the stomach and carcinoma of the pancreas.

#### A2: What in the given history supports the diagnosis?

Indigestion-like symptoms are usually a result of gastroduodenal disease. The diseases include mucosal inflammation (gastritis, duodenitis) and ulceration. Most duodenal ulcer disease is associated with *H. pylori*; NSAIDs, including aspirin and ibuprofen, enhance the risk of ulcer disease occurring in patients without *H. pylori* infection. This man is of an age where ulcer-complicating *H. pylori* is quite common. His consumption of NSAIDs increases his risk.

#### A3: What additional features in the history would you seek to support a particular diagnosis?

It is important to ask the patient about weight loss, because this may indicate that the patient has a carcinoma. His NSAID medication should be reviewed. Evidence from his history of earlier ulcer symptoms before the current episode should be sought.

#### A4: What clinical examination would you perform, and why?

A full physical examination should be performed, with particular attention being paid to lymphadenopathy in the neck, which may indicate metastatic disease from carcinoma of the stomach. The epigastrium should be examined with particular care for a mass. The liver edge should be identified. An irregular edge may indicate a carcinoma.

#### A5: What investigations would be most helpful, and why?

An endoscopy (oesophagogastroduodenoscopy) should be performed to look for peptic ulcer disease and to rule out carcinoma of the stomach. Histology should be obtained for *H. pylori*.

#### A6: What treatment options are appropriate?

If the patient has *H. pylori*, triple therapy should be prescribed, followed by a long-term PPI to protect him against future non-NSAID-associated risks. If he is *H. pylori*-negative, a PPI should be used alone. If the patient is found to have carcinoma of the stomach, it should be staged and surgery considered. Patients with a gastric ulcer should undergo repeat endoscopy after 6 weeks to ensure healing and to facilitate repeat biopsy to obtain further histological samples.

## CASE 8.11 – A 35-year-old woman with indigestion and a feeling of discomfort after eating meals.

### A1: What is the likely differential diagnosis?

The differential diagnoses are non-ulcer dyspepsia and peptic ulcer disease. Gastric cancer is very unlikely in a patient of this age. The role of *H. pylori* in the absence of ulceration in such patients is not clear.

Early satiety (feeling full before completing a meal) is associated with non-ulcer dyspepsia, but it may also occur in patients with gastric outlet obstruction and carcinoma of the stomach. The patient's age make these considerations unlikely.

### A2: What in the given history supports the diagnosis?

Non-ulcer dyspepsia is a functional disorder often exacerbated by stress. Stressors should be investigated. The early satiety means that non-ulcer dyspepsia is the most likely explanation, although if vomiting is present, carcinoma of the stomach or other sinister pathology should be considered.

### A3: What additional features in the history would you seek to support a particular diagnosis?

It is important, in the history, to look for the patient's ethnic background and family history, either of which may increase the risk of peptic ulcer disease. Exposure to NSAIDs should be sought in the history – these may be over-the-counter remedies. Consumption of alcohol and cigarettes should be investigated, although these are small contributory factors to peptic ulcer disease compared with *H. pylori*.

### A4: What clinical examination would you perform, and why?

A full examination should be performed, with consideration given to lymphadenopathy and epigastric mass. Such features are not expected in patients with non-ulcer dyspepsia.

### A5: What investigations would be most helpful, and why?

It is useful to look for *H. pylori* in young patients with dyspepsia. There are several ways in which this can be conducted: *H. pylori* can be identified by a urease breath test, necessitating a trip to the local hospital; *H. pylori* infection can also be sought using serology – most general practitioners (GPs) can perform this test and send the sample to a reference laboratory; or endoscopy may be used, although in a patient of this age, it is not usually indicated.

### A6: What treatment options are appropriate?

Triple therapy may be prescribed for the patient if she is *H. pylori*-positive: a PPI with two antibiotics from metronidazole, amoxicillin and clarithromycin (typically one is metronidazole). It is important to stop PPI therapy after *H. pylori* has been eradicated. Domperidone may also be prescribed to aid gastric emptying by increasing its motility.

## CASE 8.12 – A 60-year-old man losing weight and vomiting.

### A1: What is the likely differential diagnosis?

The likely differential diagnoses are pyloric stenosis secondary to *H. pylori*-associated peptic ulcer disease, carcinoma of the stomach, rare duodenal tumours, polyps, Crohn's disease and dysmotility syndrome.

### A2: What in the given history supports the diagnosis?

The clue to the diagnosis in this patient is previous use of over-the-counter remedies for indigestion, mainly in a patient with undertreated peptic ulcer. The vomiting suggests gastric outlet obstruction.

### A3: What additional features in the history would you seek to support a particular diagnosis?

Pyloric stenosis and carcinoma of the stomach may present in a similar manner. Duodenal Crohn's disease, polyps, and so on usually have a longer history. Dysmotility syndrome is unusual, except in patients with diabetes.

### A4: What clinical examination would you perform, and why?

On examination anaemia, lymphadenopathy, epigastric mass and irregular liver edge should be sought.

### A5: What investigations would be most helpful, and why?

Investigation is mandatory. Endoscopy or barium meal should be performed urgently. Computed tomography of the upper abdomen should be considered. If these investigations are negative, gastric emptying studies should be performed.

### A6: What treatment options are appropriate?

If the patient is found to have benign peptic stricture, endoscopic balloon dilation should be considered. Surgery is called for if balloon dilation fails. If the patient has carcinoma, staging should be performed and surgery considered. If the patient has duodenal obstruction, a gastroenterostomy should be performed. If the patient has dysmotility syndrome, domperidone or erythromycin should be prescribed.

## 👥 OSCE counselling cases

### OSCE COUNSELLING CASE 8.7 – 'Can I take aspirin for my heart now that I have an ulcer?'

In a patient who has a good indication for non-steroidal therapy such as coronary disease, transient ischaemic attack (TIA) or inflammatory arthritis, aspirin or non-steroidal therapy should be resumed after the ulcer has been treated appropriately, typically with triple therapy. A PPI should be co-prescribed with the non-steroidal drugs. Consider alternative use of clopidogrel, which may be safer.

### OSCE COUNSELLING CASE 8.8 – 'The tablets for my ulcer were wonderful. Should I continue to take them?'

The short answer to this patient is 'no'. He should be told that the *H. pylori* infection caused the ulcer. Eradicating infection will mean that the ulcer is unlikely to return. It is important to discontinue PPI therapy because of the problems of atrophic gastritis, achlorhydria and bacterial overgrowth.

# CIRRHOSIS

## Questions

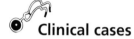

**Clinical cases**

### For each of the case scenarios given, consider the following:

> **Q1**: What is the likely differential diagnosis?
> **Q2**: What in the given history supports the diagnosis?
> **Q3**: What additional features in the history would you seek to support a particular diagnosis?
> **Q4**: What clinical examination would you perform, and why?
> **Q5**: What investigations would be most helpful, and why?
> **Q6**: What treatment options are appropriate?

## CASE 8.13 – A retired publican says he has 'turned yellow' and his 'stomach is swollen'.

A retired publican presents with progressive jaundice and abdominal swelling. He drinks more than 40 units of alcohol per week. Previously he has been admitted with fever and vomiting, which he was told was caused by alcohol.

## CASE 8.14 – The same patient has become confused.

After several days in hospital, the patient with jaundice and ascites becomes confused, disoriented and aggressive.

## CASE 8.15 – The same patient is vomiting blood.

A couple of days after showing evidence of encephalopathy, the patient with chronic liver disease has haematemesis.

**ᴀ̇ᴀ̇ OSCE counselling cases**

OSCE COUNSELLING CASE 8.9 – **'Should my husband have a transplant?'**

OSCE COUNSELLING CASE 8.10 – **'Why is my husband confused?'**

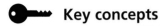 **Key concepts**

To work through the core clinical cases in this section, you will need to understand the following key concepts.

Decompensated liver disease is recognized from the following:

- *history* – jaundice, abdominal swelling, drowsiness, GI bleeding
- *examination* – jaundice, fetor, flapping tremor, ascites, oedema, impaired consciousness
- *laboratory investigations* – poor synthetic function – falling albumin and prolonging clotting times.

Bleeding varices are managed first by resuscitating with IV fluids (preferably blood products) and oxygen. Endoscopy is done with a view to injection sclerotherapy or band ligation. Finally, a Sengstaken tube may be placed or IV glypressin given.

Ascites caused by decompensated liver disease is managed first by analysing the ascitic fluid for spontaneous bacterial peritonitis. If the white cell count is >250/mL, spontaneous bacterial peritonitis is likely and should be treated with cephalosporins or ciprofloxacin. Therapy should be initiated:

- water restriction to <1.5 L/day or even <1 L/day with salt restriction
- spironolactone should be started at 50 mg, with a slow increase in dose
- therapeutic paracentesis should be considered with IV replacement – 100 mL 20% human albumin solution per 2–2.5 L ascites drained.

## Answers

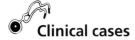

### Clinical cases

### CASE 8.13 – **A retired publican says he has 'turned yellow' and his 'stomach is swollen'.**

**A1: What is the likely differential diagnosis?**

The likely differential diagnoses are decompensated cirrhosis secondary to alcohol consumption or other causes of chronic liver disease, and carcinoma of the pancreas (or similar upper GI cancer with liver metastases) and peritoneal spread.

**A2: What in the given history supports the diagnosis?**

This man has a high-risk profession for alcoholic liver disease. His previous admission suggests that he may have had alcoholic hepatitis. He is still drinking. The abdominal swelling is likely to be the result of ascites. Together, the jaundice and ascites indicate that he has decompensated cirrhosis.

**A3: What additional features in the history would you seek to support a particular diagnosis?**

In the history it should be established whether he has been told that he has cirrhosis. Look for weight gain to support the diagnosis of ascites (weight loss may indicate a malignant process). Swelling of the ankles is common in cirrhosis at this stage. A history should be sought of previous ulcer disease, which may indicate gastric cancer. Previous bowel surgery may indicate a malignant process.

**A4: What clinical examination would you perform, and why?**

The signs of decompensated alcoholic liver disease should be sought, including Dupuytren's contracture, palmar erythema, spider naevi, gynaecomastia, hepatosplenomegaly and ascites.

**A5: What investigations would be most helpful, and why?**

Ultrasonography of the abdomen with liver biopsy should be performed at an early stage. Paracentesis should be carried out to look for a malignant process causing the ascites. The liver investigations should include hepatitis serology, autoimmune profile, serum ferritin, alpha-fetoprotein, anti-trypsin and caeruloplasmin.

**A6: What treatment options are appropriate?**

The ascites should be treated with fluid restriction and spironolactone. If these measures do not work, paracentesis with terlipressin and albumin (human albumin solution) cover should be instituted.

### CASE 8.14 – **The same patient has become confused.**

**A1: What is the likely differential diagnosis?**

The likely diagnosis is encephalopathy secondary to decompensation, sepsis, electrolyte disturbance or GI bleeding.

## A2: What in the given history supports the diagnosis?

Patients admitted with decompensated liver disease are at high risk of encephalopathy. The instrumentation for paracentesis may increase the risk of bacterial peritonitis. Venous access and urethral catheterization will increase the risk of sepsis in those sites. Treatment of ascites may precipitate encephalopathy as a result of electrolyte disturbance.

## A3: What additional features in the history would you seek to support a particular diagnosis?

From the patient's wife and the nurses, clues should be sought for the portal of entry of infection. The nurses should be asked whether the patient has had haematemesis or melaena. Charts should be checked for undue diuresis.

## A4: What clinical examination would you perform, and why?

A full physical examination with a view to finding a focus of infection should be carried out. This must include the chest and Venflon sites and careful abdominal palpation. Rectal examination may be necessary to rule out melaena.

## A5: What investigations would be most helpful, and why?

A full septic screen should be performed, with paracentesis, blood cultures, chest radiograph and urine cultures. Electrolytes should be assessed. Haemoglobin may be measured to look for evidence of sepsis (raised white cell count) and anaemia (indicating GI bleed).

## A6: What treatment options are appropriate?

The most likely explanation for the deterioration is sepsis. Cephalosporins or ciprofloxacin should be commenced. Consideration should be given to staphylococcal infection, which will require gentamicin or flucloxacillin. If methicillin-resistant *Staphylococcus aureus* (MRSA) is present, vancomycin may be used. Lactulose should be started immediately. Neomycin, or more probably metronidazole, should be used to suppress bacterial growth within the bowel. Electrolyte disturbance and hypoglycaemia should be corrected.

## CASE 8.15 – **The same patient is vomiting blood.**

### A1: What is the likely differential diagnosis?

The likely differential diagnoses are bleeding oesophageal varices and bleeding peptic ulcer disease.

### A2: What in the given history supports the diagnosis?

Patients with decompensated liver disease are at high risk of variceal bleeding, having demonstrated evidence of portal hypertension (through the ascites). Encephalopathy may have been precipitated by a GI bleed. Fifty per cent of patients with GI bleed on the background of cirrhosis actually bleed from non-variceal sources.

### A3: What additional features in the history would you seek to support a particular diagnosis?

No further features could be obtained in the history of this patient.

## A4: What clinical examination would you perform, and why?

Evidence of GI bleeding should be assessed, including observation of melaena and assessment of blood pressure and pulse, and sweating and anaemia should be sought.

## A5: What investigations would be most helpful, and why?

Urgent endoscopy should be performed, with a view to finding and treating the varices. Full blood count is likely to show anaemia. Clotting tests (international normalized ratio, [INR]) and a cross-match should be undertaken.

## A6: What treatment options are appropriate?

At endoscopy, banding or sclerotherapy should be used to stop variceal bleeding. Patients with peptic ulcer haemorrhage should receive the preferred treatment in the unit. In most hospitals this is adrenaline (epinephrine) injection; it is good practice to add a second measure such as applying a clip to the bleeding point or a heater probe. Resuscitation with blood or clotting factors is mandatory. The treatment for encephalopathy should be continued and possibly increased.

## OSCE counselling cases

### OSCE COUNSELLING CASE 8.9 – 'Should my husband have a transplant?'

Liver transplantation is not indicated in patients who are still drinking alcohol. The consensus of opinion is that patients should be abstinent from alcohol for 6 months before surgery. In the 6 months between stopping drinking and surgery, full liver support and psychological assessment should be offered.

### OSCE COUNSELLING CASE 8.10 – 'Why is my husband confused?'

Patients with liver disease become confused when the liver does not work properly. In this situation, the risk of infection is increased and chemical upsets now occur as part of the treatment. In addition, patients with this problem can bleed internally. All of these factors lead to a disturbance of brain chemical function; in most patients, however, this can be put right.

# CONSTIPATION

## Questions

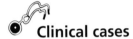
**Clinical cases**

### For each of the case scenarios given, consider the following:

**Q1**: What is the likely differential diagnosis?
**Q2**: What in the given history supports the diagnosis?
**Q3**: What additional features in the history would you seek to support a particular diagnosis?
**Q4**: What clinical examination would you perform, and why?
**Q5**: What investigations would be most helpful, and why?
**Q6**: What treatment options are appropriate?

### CASE 8.16 – A 50-year-old man with squamous carcinoma of the bronchus and bony metastases cannot open his bowels.

A 50-year-old man with squamous carcinoma of the bronchus and bony metastases is referred complaining of abdominal distension. He has not opened his bowels for 8 days. His abdominal pain has worsened and he has increased his morphine sulphate tablets, which previously he took only for bone pain.

### CASE 8.17 – A teenage girl who feels she does not empty her bowel.

A teenage girl presents with abdominal discomfort and a story of passing pellet-like stools. She experiences abdominal bloating before defaecation and after defaecation feels that she has not adequately emptied her bowels.

### CASE 8.18 – A 78-year-old man with faecal incontinence.

A 78-year-old man with Parkinson's disease is admitted from a nursing home with faecal incontinence. Previously he had been noted to have stubborn bowels. Both he and the nurses were surprised when he began staining his clothing.

## 👥 OSCE counselling cases

OSCE COUNSELLING CASE 8.11 – **'What can be done to stop my husband who needs to take painkillers becoming constipated again?'**

OSCE COUNSELLING CASE 8.12 – **'Why can't my daughter simply take senna when she has constipation?'**

## 🔑 Key concepts

To work through the core clinical cases in this section, you will need to understand the following key concepts.

Constipation is a consequence of slow or interrupted transit through the intestine, in particular the large bowel. In most patients it is a result of either drugs (anticholinergic side effects or opiates) or diet. Occasionally bowel motility is impaired by hormonal or colonic neuromuscular disorders.

A careful history should be obtained. Drugs causing constipation should be stopped or further drugs given to counter the side effects. Diet should be improved with the addition of fresh fruit and vegetables.

## Answers

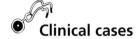

## Clinical cases

### CASE 8.16 – **A 50-year-old man with squamous carcinoma of the bronchus and bony metastases cannot open his bowels.**

#### A1: What is the likely differential diagnosis?

The likely differential diagnoses are opiate-induced constipation and hypercalcaemia-induced constipation secondary to squamous carcinoma or bony metastases.

#### A2: What in the given history supports the diagnosis?

Constipation is a symptom, not a disease. In this patient the risk factor for constipation is treatment with opiates. In addition, patients with bony metastases and squamous carcinoma are at risk of hypercalcaemia. This needs to be considered.

#### A3: What additional features in the history would you seek to support a particular diagnosis?

It is important to see whether the patient appears dehydrated or confused, which may suggest hypercalcaemia. In the history it should be determined whether the patient is taking laxatives while consuming morphine sulphate tablets.

#### A4: What clinical examination would you perform, and why?

Look for evidence of dehydration, which may accompany confusion, because this also indicates hypercalcaemia. This is an insidious problem and should be specifically looked for on examination. The abdomen should be palpated and a rectal examination performed.

#### A5: What investigations would be most helpful, and why?

The main investigations include biochemistry for hypercalcaemia and uraemia. Abdominal examination may be necessary to look for faecal loading if the patient has an empty rectum on physical examination.

#### A6: What treatment options are appropriate?

Most patients will respond to enemas and stimulant laxatives such as senna, accompanied by softeners such as docusate sodium. Co-danthramer is specifically indicated in patients with opiate-induced constipation in the terminal setting. A new preparation combining oxycodone and naloxone is useful as the patient will absorb the oxycodone while the naloxone will prevent the gastrointestinal side effects. If the patient has hypercalcaemia, fluids should be replaced intravenously and bisphosphonate treatment considered.

### CASE 8.17 – **A teenage girl who feels she does not empty her bowel.**

#### A1: What is the likely differential diagnosis?

The likely differential diagnoses are poor dietary habit, constipation-predominant IBS and dysmotility. Myxoedema, hypercalcaemia and Hirschsprung's disease are rare causes.

## A2: What in the given history supports the diagnosis?

This girl is a prime candidate for poor dietary intake. Girls of this age can have fickle diets. Breakfast is often avoided. The most likely explanation for her bowel disorder is poor dietary intake with an element of IBS.

## A3: What additional features in the history would you seek to support a particular diagnosis?

A full dietary history should be taken, with particular attention being paid to fruit, fibre and breakfast consumption. A history of stress should be sought. A history of sexual abuse should also be sought, which is more prevalent in girls with IBS than other patients. If the patient has vomiting or a family history, an underlying motility disorder may be the problem.

## A4: What clinical examination would you perform, and why?

On examination, look for evidence of hypothyroidism, demonstrated by dry skin and goitre, perhaps with a bradycardia. On examination of the abdomen, faecal loading should be sought. Rectal examination should be considered only after a history of sexual abuse has been sought.

## A5: What investigations would be most helpful, and why?

Thyroid-stimulating hormone (TSH) and calcium may be measured, but in most patients this is unnecessary. Consider transit time studies and full-thickness rectal biopsy.

## A6: What treatment options are appropriate?

Dietary advice should be given, with particular reference to fruit, fibre and breakfast consumption. It may be necessary to add linseed, kiwi or other dietary laxatives to her diet. Regular medication (laxatives) should not be prescribed.

Occasionally a barium enema can be therapeutic and provide reassurance.

## CASE 8.18 – A 78-year-old man with faecal incontinence.

### A1: What is the likely differential diagnosis?

The likely differential diagnoses are overflow diarrhoea (secondary to medication, immobility, depression or colonic dysmotility) and infection (e.g. norovirus, rotavirus, *C. difficile*).

### A2: What in the given history supports the diagnosis?

Parkinson's disease causes immobility but can also cause smooth muscle dysfunction of the GI tract. Dysphagia and constipation are common. The most common cause of faecal incontinence in this kind of patient is overflow diarrhoea.

### A3: What additional features in the history would you seek to support a particular diagnosis?

It is important to look for drugs that may contribute to constipation, including traditional anticholinergic medication for Parkinson's disease. The patient's immobility should be assessed. Patients who are bed- or chair-bound have a greater risk of constipation. Depression can also exacerbate immobility and is not uncommon in people with Parkinson's disease. A source of infectious diarrhoea should also be considered in a patient living in a nursing home.

### A4: What clinical examination would you perform, and why?

Signs of Parkinson's disease should be sought, along with signs of faecal loading on abdominal and rectal examinations.

### A5: What investigations would be most helpful, and why?

If the patient has a loaded colon on physical examination, no investigation is called for. If the patient has an empty rectum and no faecal loading on abdominal radiograph, an infection screen should be performed.

### A6: What treatment options are appropriate?

An enema followed by oral laxative should be prescribed. Consideration should be given to stopping anticholinergic drugs and dealing with any depression.

## ⚏ OSCE counselling cases

### OSCE COUNSELLING CASE 8.11 – 'What can be done to stop my husband who needs to take painkillers becoming constipated again?'

Stimulant laxatives should be prescribed in all patients receiving opiate medication. The frequency and strength of the laxative should match the strength of the opiate. A prescription with such laxatives should prevent further problems.

### OSCE COUNSELLING CASE 8.12 – 'Why can't my daughter simply take senna when she has constipation?'

It is important to treat the cause rather than the effect of the constipation. Senna is a stimulant laxative that can lead to problems later in life if started in such young patients. It is better to have a healthy mixed diet to help with normal GI function than to use laxatives.

# HEPATITIS

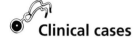

## Clinical cases

## For each of the case scenarios given, consider the following:

> **Q1**: What is the likely differential diagnosis?
> **Q2**: What in the given history supports the diagnosis?
> **Q3**: What additional features in the history would you seek to support a particular diagnosis?
> **Q4**: What clinical examination would you perform, and why?
> **Q5**: What investigations would be most helpful, and why?
> **Q6**: What treatment options are appropriate?

### CASE 8.19 – **An 18-year-old student returns from India with jaundice.**

An 18-year-old student has returned from a gap year spent in India with a short history of diarrhoea, abdominal discomfort and jaundice.

### CASE 8.20 – **A 30-year-old man who previously misused drugs presents with mildly abnormal LFTs.**

A 30-year-old who previously misused drugs presents with feeling vaguely unwell. His GP has obtained LFTs, which are mildly abnormal with an alanine aminotransferase of 50 IU/L (normal <40 IU/L).

## 👥 OSCE counselling cases

OSCE COUNSELLING CASE 8.13 – **'I have given up my drug habit, but I have hepatitis C. Do I need to be treated?'**

OSCE COUNSELLING CASE 8.14 – **'I have hepatitis A. Is there a risk I will pass it on?'**

## Key concepts

To work through the core clinical cases in this section, you will need to understand the following key concepts.

Hepatitis B and C may both become chronic.

Treatment is determined by the grade and stage of liver disease (activity and fibrosis). In addition, the patient must have no ongoing lifestyle risk factors (e.g. using IV drugs) for reinfection or other forms of liver disease (e.g. due to alcohol use).

For hepatitis B, therapy with interferon alpha or lamivudine is recommended. For hepatitis C, combination therapy with pegylated interferon alpha and ribavirin is recommended.

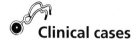

## Answers

### Clinical cases

---

## CASE 8.19 – **An 18-year-old student returns from India with jaundice.**

### A1: What is the likely differential diagnosis?

The likely differential diagnoses are hepatitis A or B, amoebic abscess, Weil's disease, side effects of medication and autoimmune hepatitis.

### A2: What in the given history supports the diagnosis?

The key to the diagnosis in this patient is the trip to India. Infectious (A) hepatitis is not uncommon in people returning from this part of the world. The pain and jaundice make a hepatobiliary problem most likely. The patient is too young to have gallstones unless she has a haemolytic disorder.

### A3: What additional features in the history would you seek to support a particular diagnosis?

In the history, attention should be paid to dark urine and pale stools, which may suggest cholestatic jaundice. If the patient has abdominal pain, its site should be elicited. It is expected that hepatobiliary pain will be epigastric and right upper quadrant in site. A history of dysentery should be sought, as this may predispose the patient to amoebic liver abscess. The patient's use of drugs (medical and recreational) should be considered.

### A4: What clinical examination would you perform, and why?

Full examination should be performed, including temperature, pulse, respiration and blood pressure. The degree of jaundice should be elicited. Anaemia should be sought. The size and texture of the liver should be found on examination. If the diaphragm appears to be raised on the right side, consideration should be given to amoebic abscess.

### A5: What investigations would be most helpful, and why?

Hepatitis serology should be performed urgently (hepatitis A and B). Amoebic serology may be considered. Ultrasonography of the liver should be performed to look for an abscess. Autoimmune profile should be obtained. Liver function tests, FBC, INR and a malaria screen should also be obtained.

### A6: What treatment options are appropriate?

The treatment of hepatitis A and B is supportive. Weil's disease is treated with penicillin-based antibiotics. Liver abscess requires drainage and treatment of the underlying infection. Autoimmune hepatitis should be treated with steroids.

## CASE 8.20 – **A 30-year-old man who previously misused drugs presents with mildly abnormal LFTs.**

### A1: What is the likely differential diagnosis?

The likely differential diagnoses are hepatitis C, non-alcoholic steatohepatitis (NASH) and hepatitis B.

## A2: What in the given history supports the diagnosis?

The patient's lifestyle predisposes him to hepatitis B and C, particularly hepatitis C. Modest elevation of alanine aminotransferase is more suggestive of hepatitis C than anything else, but NASH can give a similar picture.

## A3: What additional features in the history would you seek to support a particular diagnosis?

Previous jaundice should be sought in the history, which would suggest hepatitis B. If the patient is obese, NASH is a possibility. A history of alcohol consumption should be sought.

## A4: What clinical examination would you perform, and why?

On examination, stigmata of chronic liver disease should be sought for patients with hepatitis. If there are no signs other than simple obesity, NASH is likely.

## A5: What investigations would be most helpful, and why?

For hepatitis C, the investigations are serology (antibody to hepatitis C) and polymerase chain reaction for viral load, followed by liver biopsy, preferably guided by ultrasonography. Hepatitis B serology and liver biopsy are required. For NASH (patients negative for hepatitis B and C), an ultrasound-guided liver biopsy should be obtained.

## A6: What treatment options are appropriate?

If the patient is no longer taking drugs and the liver biopsy shows viral hepatitis of sufficient stage and grade, antiviral therapy should be undertaken: interferon and either ribavirin or lamivudine for hepatitis B and C, respectively. If the patient has NASH, weight reduction should be encouraged. If the patient appears to be drinking more alcohol than was apparent initially, abstinence should be encouraged.

## 👥 OSCE counselling cases

### OSCE COUNSELLING CASE 8.13 – 'I have given up my drug habit, but I have hepatitis C. Do I need to be treated?'

Treatment for hepatitis C is determined by the stage and grade of the disease (severity). This is determined by a liver biopsy. Any patients with active inflammation but no cirrhosis are candidates for antiviral therapy. Some patients require no therapy but need repeat biopsy instead.

### OSCE COUNSELLING CASE 8.14 – 'I have hepatitis A. Is there a risk I will pass it on?'

Hepatitis A is transmitted through poor hygiene. With good hand-washing, there is no chance of passing the virus. The virus appears only in faeces, and very good hygiene will prevent its transmission.

# IRRITABLE BOWEL SYNDROME

## Questions

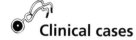

### Clinical cases

## For each of the case scenarios given, consider the following:

> **Q1**: What is the likely differential diagnosis?
> **Q2**: What in the given history supports the diagnosis?
> **Q3**: What additional features in the history would you seek to support a particular diagnosis?
> **Q4**: What clinical examination would you perform, and why?
> **Q5**: What investigations would be most helpful, and why?
> **Q6**: What treatment options are appropriate?

### CASE 8.21 – **A 24-year-old housewife with abdominal bloating.**

A 24-year-old housewife complains of abdominal bloating, which gets progressively worse during the day.

### CASE 8.22 – **After an elective period in India, a medical student returns to the UK with diarrhoea.**

The diarrhoea initially appeared to settle but has gradually worsened over the 2 months before coming to see you.

### CASE 8.23 – **A 42-year-old social worker presents with straining to pass stool.**

A 42-year-old social worker presents with a story of straining to pass stool, passage of mucus and perhaps blood on the tissue paper.

## 👥 OSCE counselling cases

OSCE COUNSELLING CASE 8.15 – **'I have severe bloating. Is it the result of food allergy?'**

OSCE COUNSELLING CASE 8.16 – **'I have been told that I have IBS. Should I take a fibre supplement?'**

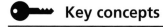

## Key concepts

To work through the core clinical cases in this section, you will need to understand the following key concepts.

The aetiology of IBS is largely unknown. Irritable bowel syndrome falls under the umbrella of 'functional illness'. Most research points to a role for stress – sexual abuse seems particularly important. Post-infectious IBS is well recognized following 'food poisoning'. Food intolerance is rarely the explanation.

Irritable bowel syndrome is diagnosed clinically, based on the Manning or Rome criteria. It is not a diagnosis of exclusion.

Stressors need to be identified and managed. Counselling may be necessary. Antidepressants are sometimes helpful. Specific drug therapy based on serotonin is not licensed.

# Answers

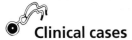

## Clinical cases

### CASE 8.21 – **A 24-year-old housewife with abdominal bloating.**

#### A1: What is the likely differential diagnosis?

The likely differential diagnoses are IBS, bacterial overgrowth, lactose intolerance and IBD.

#### A2: What in the given history supports the diagnosis?

Bacterial overgrowth, lactose intolerance and IBS can be difficult to separate from history alone. If the patient reports that certain foods (milk-based) exacerbate her symptoms and there is diarrhoea at the same time, then lactose intolerance is a possibility. Bacterial overgrowth can mimic this.

If the patient experiences relief of abdominal pain with passing flatus or faeces, it is likely to be IBS, particularly if the symptoms are episodic.

#### A3: What additional features in the history would you seek to support a particular diagnosis?

It is important to look for duration of the illness. Irritable bowel syndrome often has insidious onset for many months before patients seek help. Weight gain is often the case, although weight loss may be a consequence of stress. Weight loss is, however, more likely to indicate organic disorder such as IBD or coeliac disease. Abdominal pain that is worse on the day that the stool form is different suggests IBS. Straining to finish defaecation and mucus are often found in patients with IBS. No blood should be present.

#### A4: What clinical examination would you perform, and why?

On examination, there should be no abnormal findings. In IBD, tenderness, abdominal mass or perianal abnormalities may be found.

#### A5: What investigations would be most helpful, and why?

No investigations are needed if a clinical diagnosis of IBS is made. Normal CRP and plasma viscosity may be reassuring, however. NICE guidelines recommend a serological test to exclude coeliac disease.

#### A6: What treatment options are appropriate?

Irritable bowel syndrome is usually a consequence of stress. A careful social history should be obtained and attention paid to counselling around the issues described by the patient. Lactose exclusion may be helpful in some patients.

### CASE 8.22 – **After an elective period in India, a medical student returns to the UK with diarrhoea.**

#### A1: What is the likely differential diagnosis?

The likely differential diagnoses are post-infectious IBS and giardiasis.

### A2: What in the given history supports the diagnosis?

It is hard to distinguish between the differential diagnoses, but the history suggests that an infection was acquired in India, which has led to a subtle change in the bowel habit, giving chronic diarrhoea.

### A3: What additional features in the history would you seek to support a particular diagnosis?

Weight loss may suggest that the patient has ongoing giardiasis. Most patients with IBS have episodic symptoms, with some easing from time to time. If these symptoms do not wax and wane, it is likely that the patient has giardiasis rather than IBS.

### A4: What clinical examination would you perform, and why?

No abnormal findings are expected.

### A5: What investigations would be most helpful, and why?

Stool culture and duodenal biopsy should be undertaken to look for *Giardia lamblia*. A therapeutic trial of metronidazole may be considered.

### A6: What treatment options are appropriate?

If the patient has giardiasis, metronidazole will cure the problem. If *G. lamblia* is not present, it is likely that the problem is post-infectious IBS and the symptoms will gradually improve over time. Lactose avoidance may help ease the symptoms.

## CASE 8.23 – **A 42-year-old social worker presents with straining to pass stool.**

### A1: What is the likely differential diagnosis?

The likely differential diagnoses are IBS, mucosal prolapse, solitary rectal ulcer syndrome, gonorrhoea and haemorrhoids.

### A2: What in the given history supports the diagnosis?

The passage of mucus with an urge to strain suggests that the patient has rectal disease. Infrequent blood that is present only on the tissue paper makes it unlikely that the patient has proctitis, but this is not completely ruled out.

### A3: What additional features in the history would you seek to support a particular diagnosis?

It is important to determine whether there is an urge to strain at the start or the end of defaecation. Both are often present in IBS. If blood is present only on days when the patient strains, this suggests that the patient has haemorrhoids or solitary rectal ulcer syndrome. Proctitis tends to give rise to frequent passage of blood in the absence of the need to strain. Sexual practice should be investigated tactfully. Anal intercourse in either sex can cause local trauma and transmit a sexually transmitted infection. Some patients self-digitate when they feel they have inadequately emptied the bowel; this can traumatize the bowel.

## A4: What clinical examination would you perform, and why?

On examination, nothing is expected. Sigmoidoscopy should be performed. This may show proctitis or solitary rectal ulcer in the anterior wall of the rectum. Haemorrhoids may be seen prolapsing through the anus, but proctoscopy may be necessary to visualize them.

## A5: What investigations would be most helpful, and why?

Flexible sigmoidoscopy should be considered. Swabs should be considered if there has been anal intercourse. Physiological studies may be necessary in patients in whom tenesmus is severe.

## A6: What treatment options are appropriate?

Treatment is difficult. Stool softeners may help patients with haemorrhoids, but some patients require a surgical assessment with a view to band ligation or sclerotherapy. If proctitis is present, it should be treated with topical therapy (steroids or 5-ASA compound). Any local infection should be treated with appropriate antibiotics or antiviral agents.

Most patients will have IBS. This may respond to hypnotherapy and, in certain situations, biofeedback, which teaches the patient to respond differently to symptoms they perceive from their rectums and 'retrains' the manner in which they defaecate.

#  OSCE counselling cases

### OSCE COUNSELLING CASE 8.15 – 'I have severe bloating. Is it the result of food allergy?'

Bloating is unlikely to be caused by food allergy, although food intolerance (especially wheat) may aggravate bloating. Milk sugar (lactose) intolerance is a possibility; the patient should try avoiding all milk products (including goat's and sheep's milk) for 2 weeks and see whether this improves the symptoms.

### OSCE COUNSELLING CASE 8.16 – 'I have been told that I have IBS. Should I take a fibre supplement?'

The short answer is 'no'. High-fibre diets often worsen abdominal pain in IBS. The patient should eat a well-balanced diet including a mixture of fruit and vegetables.

# COELIAC DISEASE

## Questions

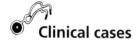

### Clinical cases

## For each of the case scenarios given, consider the following:

**Q1**: What is the likely differential diagnosis?
**Q2**: What in the given history supports the diagnosis?
**Q3**: What additional features in the history would you seek to support a particular diagnosis?
**Q4**: What clinical examination would you perform, and why?
**Q5**: What investigations would be most helpful, and why?
**Q6**: What treatment options are appropriate?

### CASE 8.24 – A 44-year-old woman with anaemia.

A 44-year-old woman presents with lethargy, breathlessness on exertion and a little chest tightness on walking uphill. She was turned down as a blood donor because of anaemia.

### CASE 8.25 – A 23-year-old woman with impaired fertility and loose stools.

She had loose stools throughout her teenage years. She is slightly built and has noted that it is difficult to increase her weight.

### CASE 8.26 – A man with coeliac disease who infrequently attends clinic but has weight loss and anaemia.

The patient presents with weight loss and anaemia at the insistence of his wife.

## 👫 OSCE counselling cases

OSCE COUNSELLING CASE 8.17 – **'I feel well. Why should I eat a gluten-free diet?'**

OSCE COUNSELLING CASE 8.18 – **'I have coeliac disease. Are my children at risk?'**

## 🔑 Key concepts

To work through the core clinical cases in this section, you will need to understand the following key concepts.

Coeliac disease is a true food allergy. An immune response to the alpha-gliadin component of gluten leads to an immune infiltrate in the mucosa of the proximal small intestine, with secondary crypt hyperplasia and villous atrophy.

Antibodies to gliadin, endomysium and tissue transglutaminase are often found in the serum of patients with coeliac disease, but these antibodies lack the sensitivity and specificity to be the gold standard for making the diagnosis. The gold standard remains the proximal small intestinal biopsy, typically obtained from the third part of the duodenum at endoscopy.

Untreated coeliac disease leads to complications associated with malabsorption, including anaemia (folate and iron deficiency), rickets, osteomalacia, bleeding disorders and subfertility.

Late complications include small bowel lymphoma and carcinomas arising in the small intestine, oesophagus, pharynx and colon.

## Answers

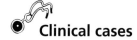

### Clinical cases

### CASE 8.24 – **A 44-year-old woman with anaemia.**

**A1: What is the likely differential diagnosis?**

The likely differential diagnoses are menorrhagia, dietary insufficiency (vegetarian) and coeliac disease.

**A2: What in the given history supports the diagnosis?**

The history is consistent with progressive iron-deficiency anaemia; lack of overt blood loss in the presenting complaint suggests malabsorption or menorrhagia as likely causes.

**A3: What additional features in the history would you seek to support a particular diagnosis?**

A dietary history should be obtained to exclude vegetarianism. Gynaecological history should be pursued to look for menorrhagia. A subtle change in the bowel habit should be sought that may suggest coeliac disease.

**A4: What clinical examination would you perform, and why?**

Nothing is expected on examination, except evidence of anaemia, perhaps with cheilosis or mouth ulcers.

**A5: What investigations would be most helpful, and why?**

Duodenal biopsy may be done; some clinicians use anti-endomysial or anti-tissue transglutaminase antibodies as a justification for duodenal biopsy. If the dietary history is non-contributory and the gynaecological history unremarkable, coeliac disease is the most likely explanation. Further investigations may be called for, however, if coeliac disease is not found.

**A6: What treatment options are appropriate?**

Treatment of coeliac disease is a gluten-free diet with possible mineral and vitamin supplements. The patient should be encouraged to join the Coeliac Society.

### CASE 8.25 – **A 23-year-old woman presents with impaired fertility and loose stools.**

**A1: What is the likely differential diagnosis?**

The likely differential diagnoses are coeliac disease, Crohn's disease, hormone disturbance (e.g. thyrotoxicosis) and anorexia nervosa.

**A2: What in the given history supports the diagnosis?**

The clue is the loose stool; without this, the differential diagnosis would be quite broad. People with anorexia rarely complain of inability to gain weight, so anorexia is unlikely. Crohn's disease, thyrotoxicosis and coeliac disease are all genuine differential diagnoses of diarrhoea and subfertility.

### A3: What additional features in the history would you seek to support a particular diagnosis?

The nature of the stool should be investigated: pale, bulky, floating stools suggest steatorrhoea, while bloody diarrhoea suggests Crohn's disease. Features of thyrotoxicosis (tremors and sweats) should be sought to rule out thyroid disease. Abdominal pain is unlikely in coeliac disease but common in Crohn's disease.

### A4: What clinical examination would you perform, and why?

On examination, little is expected in patients with coeliac disease, although clubbing and anaemia may be present. Mouth ulcers are also relatively common. A goitre would point to thyroid dysfunction, and proptosis would suggest Graves' disease.

### A5: What investigations would be most helpful, and why?

Anti-endomysial or anti-tissue transglutaminase antibodies or duodenal biopsy should be obtained. Duodenal biopsies are the standard investigation. Thyroid function should be assessed if the duodenal biopsy is normal. Consideration should be given to a barium follow-through.

### A6: What treatment options are appropriate?

The treatment for coeliac disease is a gluten-free diet. The treatment for thyrotoxicosis is carbimazole or radiotherapy with thyroxine replacement. Crohn's disease is treated according to symptoms; a 5-ASA compound may be used as maintenance medication.

### CASE 8.26 – A man with coeliac disease who infrequently attends clinic but has weight loss and anaemia.

### A1: What is the likely differential diagnosis?

The likely diagnosis is poor treatment compliance, with relapse of coeliac disease. Lymphoma or small bowel carcinoma complicating poorly controlled coeliac disease should also be considered.

### A2: What in the given history supports the diagnosis?

Poor clinic attendance suggests non-compliance. A history from the patient's wife would be useful to support this.

### A3: What additional features in the history would you seek to support a particular diagnosis?

The patient's diet should be reviewed, and barium follow-through and duodenal biopsy considered.

### A4: What clinical examination would you perform, and why?

Lymphadenopathy may be present, but often lymphoma in the GI tract does not present with lymphadenopathy.

### A5: What investigations would be most helpful, and why?

Duodenal biopsy, barium follow-through and CT scan of the abdomen would be most helpful.

### A6: What treatment options are appropriate?

The patient should be encouraged to reintroduce a gluten-free diet for coeliac disease. Oncological assessment with radiotherapy or chemotherapy is necessary if the patient has lymphoma.

## ⅈⅈ OSCE counselling cases

### OSCE COUNSELLING CASE 8.17 – 'I feel well. Why should I eat a gluten-free diet?'

Most patients with coeliac disease have insidious symptoms, gradually leading to presentation with diarrhoea or anaemia. Without control of coeliac disease, malabsorption as a consequence will occur in most patients. Untreated coeliac disease increases the risk of lymphoma and gastrointestinal malignancy.

### OSCE COUNSELLING CASE 8.18 – 'I have coeliac disease. Are my children at risk?'

There is a weak association. This is not simple inheritance such as that found in patients with haemophilia or cystic fibrosis. Although the risk to the children is small, a delay in weaning or prolonged breastfeeding is thought to be helpful. If the child fails to thrive, coeliac disease should be considered.

## REVISION PANEL

- Most patients with haematemesis or melaena will have bled from a peptic ulcer, most cases of which are painless.
- The differential diagnoses for acute bloody diarrhoea are acute colitis, microbial diarrhoea (C. difficile – a drug history is needed; protozoa – a travel history should be taken), side effects of medications such as NSAIDs, and familial adenomatous polyps (bleeding usually occurs in the context of normal stool, so a family history should be taken).
- Acute pancreatitis is a significant cause of mortality. It should be considered in the differential diagnosis of all cases of acute abdominal pain. The diagnosis can generally be confirmed by an elevated serum amylase. Risk factors for acute pancreatitis include alcohol abuse and gallstones.
- Patients with IBD often present with symptoms that have been present for several weeks or months. Many will have been told that they have IBS.
- *Helicobacter pylori* is found in over 90 per cent of patients with duodenal ulcers and 70 per cent of patients with gastric ulcers. Non-steroidal anti-inflammatory drugs contribute to the aetiology of peptic ulcer disease. Smoking and alcohol are minor contributory factors.
- Decompensation is recognized from jaundice, abdominal swelling, drowsiness, GI bleeding, fetor, flapping tremor, ascites, oedema, impaired consciousness, falling albumin and prolonged clotting times.
- Constipation may be related to poor dietary habit, IBS and dysmotility. Myxoedema, hypercalcaemia and Hirschsprung's disease are rare causes.
- Coeliac disease is a food allergy to gluten that leads to an immune infiltrate in the mucosa of the proximal small intestine, with secondary crypt hyperplasia and villous atrophy. Antibodies to gliadin, endomysium and tissue transglutaminase are often found in the serum of patients with coeliac disease. The gold standard diagnostic test remains the proximal small intestinal biopsy, typically obtained from the third part of the duodenum at endoscopy.

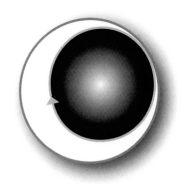

# 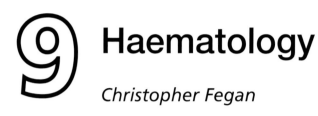 Haematology

*Christopher Fegan*

## ANAEMIA

## ABNORMAL FULL BLOOD COUNT

## HAEMOGLOBINOPATHIES

## Answers

# ANAEMIA

## Questions

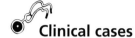

### Clinical cases

### For the case scenarios given, consider the following:

> **Q1**: What are the likely diagnosis and the possible differential diagnoses?
> **Q2**: What are the relevant points to elicit from the history?
> **Q3**: What are the possible clinical signs?
> **Q4**: What additional investigations are indicated?
> **Q5**: What is the treatment?
> **Q6**: What is the long-term outcome?

## CASE 9.1 – A 27-year-old woman is referred with palpitations and shortness of breath.

Her haemoglobin (Hb) is 8.2 g/dL (normal range 11.5–16 g/dL), white cell count (WCC) is 5.2×10⁹/L (normal range 4–11×10⁹/L) and platelets are 513×10⁹/L (normal range 150–400×10⁹/L). The mean cell volume (MCV) is 69 fL (normal range 80–100 fL) and the mean cell haemoglobin (MCH) is 23 pg (normal range 27–33 pg). She has a life-long history of menorrhagia but has declined therapeutic investigations and intervention. The serum ferritin is 3 ng/mL (normal range 6–81 ng/mL).

## CASE 9.2 – A 58-year-old woman is referred with a 12-month history of increasing difficulty in walking.

The patient has been relatively well throughout her life, and her only medication is thyroxine 150 µg once a day for hypothyroidism diagnosed many years earlier. Over recent months she has noticed increasing shortness of breath on exertion, although her decreased mobility has meant that this has not been a particular problem. She works as a clerical officer, smokes five cigarettes a day but drinks no alcohol.

On examination, the positive clinical signs elicited were pallor, tachycardia (100/min, regular), decreased sensation in both legs below the knee, absent ankle jerks and up-going plantar responses. Investigations reveal the following:

- Hb 8.2 g/dL (normal range 11.5–16 g/dL)
- MCV 124 fL (normal range 80–100 fL)
- WCC 2.4×10⁹/L (normal range 4–11×10⁹/L)
- platelets 102×10⁹/L (normal range 150–400×10⁹/L).
- urea and electrolytes (U&Es) are normal, as are the liver function tests (LFTs), apart from a slightly raised bilirubin of 45 µmol/L (normal <25 µmol/L) and a lactate dehydrogenase (LDH) level of 2374 U/L (normal range 200–500 U/L).

## CASE 9.3 – **A 78-year-old woman is referred with a 6-month history of general deterioration.**

On admission the patient is confused. Her daughter reports that she has been very thirsty for the past 4 weeks. Apart from back pain, there have been no other new symptoms. Clinical examination is unremarkable, except for signs of dehydration. Her full blood count (FBC) shows the following:

- Hb 9.5 g/dL (normal range 11.5–16 g/dL)
- WCC 4.2×10⁹/L (normal range 4–11×10⁹/L)
- platelet count 127×10⁹/L (normal range 150–400×10⁹/L).

The biochemistry profile reveals the following:

- sodium 126 mmol/L (normal range 133–147 mmol/L)
- potassium 4.8 mmol/L (normal range 3.5–5.0 mmol/L)
- urea 17 mmol/L (normal 2.5–7.5 mmol/L)
- creatinine 201 μmol/L (normal range 50–120 μmol/L)
- total protein 117 g/dL (normal range 60–80 g/dL)
- albumin 28 g/dL (normal range 35–48 g/dL)
- aspartate aminotransferase (AST) 39 U/L (normal <35 U/L)
- alkaline phosphatase (ALP) 214 U/L (normal range 90–430 U/L)
- calcium 3.4 mmol/L (normal range 2.05–2.6 mmol/L)
- glucose 4.0 mmol/L.

## ♟♟ OSCE counselling case

OSCE COUNSELLING CASE 9.1 – **A colleague phones asking whether or not to transfuse a 24-year-old Asian woman who is 34 weeks pregnant with a haemoglobin of 7.8 g/dL secondary to iron deficiency.**

What further information would you require, and what are the most salient points you would like to bring to your colleague's attention?

## 🔑 Key concepts

To work through the core clinical cases in this section, you will need to understand the following key concepts.

Anaemia is a very common topic because it impinges on all areas of medical care. A basic knowledge of the physiology of red cell production (erythropoiesis) is essential in understanding the causes of anaemia. There are several ways of classifying anaemia, the simplest of which is based on the red cell size: microcytic (MCV <80 fL), normocytic (MCV 80–100 fL) and macrocytic (MCV >100 fL). One can also consider anaemia as either a failure of red cell production or a reduction in red cell survival. The age at which anaemia develops, a good dietary and clinical history, and the knowledge of how to interpret the data given by the FBC are essential in narrowing down the differential diagnoses and requesting relevant investigations. The management of anaemia, and in particular the indications for blood transfusion, are a must-know area for any doctor.

# Answers

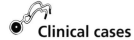

## Clinical cases

### CASE 9.1 – **A 27-year-old woman is referred with palpitations and shortness of breath.**

#### A1: What are the likely diagnosis and the possible differential diagnoses?

This woman presents with symptomatic, hypochromic (low MCH)/microcytic (low MCV) anaemia. There are only four conditions giving rise to hypochromic/microcytic anaemia: iron deficiency, thalassaemia, anaemia of chronic disease, and some rare (usually hereditary) types of sideroblastic anaemia. The low ferritin in this woman indicates that she has iron deficiency anaemia, probably secondary to excess menstrual blood loss.

#### A2: What are the relevant points to elicit from the history?

It is likely that the iron deficiency is secondary to the excess menstrual blood loss. It is important to ask about diet, however, to ensure that her oral iron intake is adequate and to check whether she is taking any non-steroidal anti-inflammatory drugs. Sufficient quantities of dietary iron are found in red meat (less in pork or chicken) and, therefore, iron deficiency is common in vegetarians. The patient should be asked about other routes of bleeding (especially gastrointestinal and urinary tract symptoms). The platelet count rises in any form of iron deficiency and is not necessarily a sign of blood loss. Oesophageal webs causing dysphagia are a rare associated feature.

#### A3: What are the possible clinical signs?

Clinical signs include pallor (difficult sign seen as pale conjunctivae), tachycardia, brittle hair and nails, koilonychia (spoon-shaped nails), smooth atrophic tongue and angular stomatitis.

#### A4: What additional investigations are indicated?

Depending on any symptoms elicited from the history, one might consider performing a rectal examination, upper and lower gastrointestinal endoscopy and faecal occult blood estimation. Coeliac disease is also possible, so anti-tissue transglutaminase or anti-endomysial antibodies should be requested. Given the long history of menorrhagia, thyroid function tests should be performed, together with consideration of referral to a gynaecologist for more specific tests and investigations.

#### A5: What is the treatment?

Treatment is with iron. Ideally patients should receive 6 months of ferrous sulphate 200 mg three times a day. Side effects, usually constipation or more rarely diarrhoea, can occur, in which case intravenous or more rarely intramuscular iron can be used; the latter is very painful, however. Intravenous iron can be given but may lead to severe anaphylactic reactions. In this patient, one could also consider using oral tranexamic acid or the combined oral contraceptive pill to reduce menstrual blood loss.

#### A6: What is the long-term outcome?

On the assumption that menstrual loss is the underlying cause of this anaemia, the outcome should be excellent.

## CASE 9.2 – A 58-year-old woman is referred with a 12-month history of increasing difficulty in walking.

### A1: What are the likely diagnosis and the possible differential diagnoses?

The patient's neurological examination reveals a combination of peripheral neuropathy and an upper motor neuron lesion in the lower limbs. In addition, there are symptoms and signs of anaemia, pancytopenia (all three cell lineages reduced) and macrocytosis. All these point to vitamin B12 deficiency and a diagnosis of pernicious anaemia with subacute combined degeneration of the spinal cord and peripheral neuropathy. Potentially reversible dementia can also occur. All dividing cells require vitamin B12; the bone marrow, as one of the tissues with the fastest turnover, is often affected first. The raised bilirubin and LDH are a result of ineffective erythropoiesis within the bone marrow (so-called intramedullary haemolysis). Folate deficiency can give rise to a similar blood and bone marrow picture, but neurological deficit does not occur.

### A2: What are the relevant points to elicit from the history?

Pernicious anaemia is an autoimmune disease, and so a personal and family history of other autoimmune diseases should be sought (e.g. type 1 diabetes, thyroid disease, Addison's disease, vitiligo). The patient should be asked if she has ever undergone any gastric surgery. Rarely, there is associated subfertility (but this would not apply in this age group) and visual loss. Vitamin B12 is present in foods of animal origin, including meat, eggs and milk products. Daily requirements of vitamin B12 are very low, and so it is very unusual for vegans to develop clinical vitamin B12 deficiency, but a dietary history should always be taken.

### A3: What are the possible clinical signs?

The tongue is said to be 'big and beefy' in contrast to the atrophic tongue seen in iron deficiency. The skin has a lemon tinge (caused by the mildly elevated bilirubin). Optic atrophy can also occur, and anecdotally patients are often said to be white-haired.

### A4: What additional investigations are indicated?

Measuring the serum vitamin B12 levels easily makes the diagnosis. Other useful tests are anti-parietal and intrinsic factor antibodies, which are present in 90 per cent and 60 per cent of patients, respectively. It may also be prudent to look for evidence of the other autoimmune disorders that are associated with pernicious anaemia. Historically, a Schilling test was performed to confirm vitamin B12 malabsorption, but this is rarely performed today because it exposes patients to radiation and does not usually alter the clinical management.

A bone marrow examination would confirm a megaloblastic anaemia but does not distinguish between vitamin B12 and folate deficiency and hence is not routinely performed.

### A5: What is the treatment?

Management is vitamin B12, usually given as 1 mg intramuscular injections for six doses over 2 weeks and then every 3 months for life. If required, the response to therapy can be assessed by the rise in reticulocytes and Hb and the fall in LDH.

### A6: What is the long-term outcome?

The blood and marrow changes will improve over the following few weeks, but the neurological deficit may take many, many months and if severe at diagnosis may not resolve completely.

## CASE 9.3 – **A 78-year-old woman is referred with a 6-month history of general deterioration.**

### A1: What are the likely diagnosis and the possible differential diagnoses?

The blood count shows mild pancytopenia; this, taken together with bony pain and hypercalcaemia, could indicate secondary cancer in the bone or possibly a primary haematological cancer of the bone marrow. The total protein is very high and the albumin low, meaning that the globulin level (total protein minus albumin) is very high. Supported by the presence of renal impairment, the diagnosis is likely to be multiple myeloma. When a very high globulin level occurs, a low sodium level is often seen (so-called pseudo-hyponatraemia).

### A2: What are the relevant points to elicit from the history?

Multiple myeloma is a disease of elderly people, and symptoms are often non-specific and attributed to old age. Symptoms caused by anaemia and bony pain (especially back) are typical, and myeloma should always be considered with this combination. There are relatively few causes of thirst, but the most common are diabetes (mellitus and insipidus), dehydration and hypercalcaemia. Hypercalcaemia also causes the confusion and polyuria that lead to dehydration (this will contribute to the raised creatinine in this patient). Renal impairment in myeloma is caused by dehydration, hypercalcaemia and paraprotein deposition in the kidney.

### A3: What are the possible clinical signs?

Back pain is common as a result of pressure on spinal nerve roots or pathological fractures. Vertebral collapse can lead to paraplegia. Note that there is usually no enlargement of the liver, spleen or lymph nodes, unless secondary amyloidosis has occurred.

### A4: What additional investigations are indicated?

Multiple myeloma is a cancer of the plasma cells. Immunoglobulins are normally produced by plasma cells, and therefore a malignant proliferation of plasma cells leads to uncontrolled production of a single type of immunoglobulin – so-called paraprotein. The plasma cells proliferate within the bone marrow, damaging normal bone marrow cells and bone and leading to anaemia and other blood cell cytopenias, hypercalcaemia and lytic lesions on radiographs.

The diagnosis of multiple myeloma depends on four tests:

- serum immunoglobulin estimation and protein electrophoresis
- urinary sample for Bence Jones protein (light chain) analysis
- skeletal survey looking for lytic lesions.
- bone marrow examination to assess malignant plasma cell infiltration.

### A5: What is the treatment?

In this case, treatment of the hypercalcaemia would be of most immediate priority because this may reduce the confusion and alleviate symptoms of dehydration. Local irradiation may be indicated for bony pain. The anaemia can be treated with blood transfusion in the short term, and possibly with erythropoietin therapy thereafter. Treatment for myeloma consists of chemotherapy with autologous stem cell transplantation for younger patients. Steroids and anti-angiogenic agents also have a role as upfront or palliative therapy. Regular bisphosphonate therapy reduces the risk of bony fracture and hypercalcaemia and has been shown to prolong overall survival.

### A6: What is the long-term outcome?

The prognosis is poor, with death usually within 2–3 years of diagnosis for patients not fit enough for autologous stem cell transplantation and around 5 years for those who are fit enough.

## ii OSCE counselling case

### OSCE COUNSELLING CASE 9.1 – **A colleague phones asking whether or not to transfuse a 24-year-old Asian woman who is 34 weeks pregnant with a haemoglobin of 7.8 g/dL secondary to iron deficiency.**

This is a common clinical scenario. It is imperative that you treat the patient and not the Hb level, and so first you need to know whether the patient is clinically compromised by her anaemia. You also need to know whether or not the patient has been taking iron supplements and if so what dose and for how long. It would also be helpful to know whether this is her first child or if there have been previous pregnancies, and the plans for delivery of this baby. In addition, it would be reassuring to be informed that this woman and her partner have been screened for thalassaemia and that she has no red cell antibodies that are likely to lead to haemolytic disease of the newborn.

In general terms, patients with iron deficiency anaemia should be treated with iron therapy and not blood transfusion. If the patient cannot tolerate oral iron, consideration should be given to parenteral iron. Adequate iron therapy raises the Hb by about 1 g/dL per week of therapy – within 3 weeks, therefore, the Hb should be >10 g/dL in this patient. Apart from the usual risks of blood transfusion (reactions, infections, fluid overload), this patient is of Asian origin and therefore blood transfusion has a much higher risk of leading to the development of alloantibodies, which may lead to future problems when cross-matching blood and can also predispose to haemolytic disease of the newborn (possibly in this pregnancy, but certainly in future pregnancies). Blood transfusion should be given only if the patient is clinically compromised by her anaemia and there is a need for 'urgent' delivery of the baby or if she is allergic to iron therapy, i.e. previous anaphylaxis with parenteral iron. It would be prudent to genotype the blood for cross-match to minimize the risk of alloantibody production. The patient should be counselled about the risks of blood transfusion and the fact that, although all reasonable steps have been taken to avoid alloantibodies, nothing can be guaranteed.

# ABNORMAL FULL BLOOD COUNT

## Questions

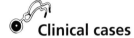

### Clinical cases

### For the case scenarios given, consider the following:

**Q1**: What are the likely diagnosis and the possible differential diagnoses?
**Q2**: What are the relevant points to elicit from the history?
**Q3**: What are the possible clinical signs?
**Q4**: What additional investigations are indicated?
**Q5**: What is the treatment?
**Q6**: What is the long-term outcome?

### CASE 9.4 – A 78-year-old retired mechanic is admitted with increasing left hypochondrial pain of a stabbing character over the previous 12 h.

The patient has not felt well for 3 months. He has lost 5 kg in weight and recently noticed night sweats. Clinical examination reveals hepatomegaly of 5 cm and splenomegaly of 15 cm. There is no lymphadenopathy.
    The FBC reveals the following:

- Hb 10.1 g/dL (normal range 13.0–16.5 g/dL)
- WCC 227×10⁹/L (normal range 4–11×10⁹/L) with prominent eosinophilia and basophilia
- platelets 741×10⁹/L (normal range 150–400×10⁹/L).

Urea and electrolytes and LFTs are normal, except for a uric acid level of 490 μmol/L (normal range 110–420 μmol/L).

### CASE 9.5 – A 63 year-old-man presents with a left-sided transient ischaemic attack (TIA).

The TIA follows on from a similar episode 1 week earlier that had been labelled a TIA. After the first TIA, the general practitioner (GP) performed some blood tests, the results of which are as follows:

- Hb 21.2 g/dL (normal range 13.0–16.5 g/dL)
- red cell count 6.7–10¹²/L (normal range 3.8–5.6–10¹²/L)
- haematocrit 0.61
- WCC 15.3×10⁹/L (normal range 4–10.5×10⁹/L)
- increased neutrophils and eosinophils
- platelets 897×10⁹/L (normal range 150–400×10⁹/L)
- sodium 142 mmol/L (normal range 135–145 mmol/L)
- potassium 4.8 mmol/L (normal range 3.4–5.0 mmol/L)
- urea 5.0 mmol/L (normal range 2.5–7.0 mmol/L)

- creatinine 79 µmol/L (normal range 50–100 µmol/L)
- total protein 71 g/dL (normal range 60–80 g/dL)
- albumin 43 g/dL (normal range 35–50 g/dL)
- bilirubin 8 µmol/L (normal range 1–22 µmol/L)
- AST 30 IU/L (normal range 19–48 IU/L)
- ALP 71 IU/L (normal range 30–115 IU/L)
- cholesterol 3.6 mmol/L (normal range 2.5–6.2 mmol/L)
- triglyceride 1.9 mmol/L (normal range 0.1–1.6 mmol/L).

## CASE 9.6 – **A 23-year-old man is brought into the accident and emergency (A&E) department having become acutely unwell while shopping.**

On admission the patient is barely rousable and unable to provide a history. His Glasgow coma score (GCS) is 12, with no obviously localizing signs. His temperature is 39.5 °C, his pulse is regular with a rate of 130/min and his blood pressure is 60/35 mmHg. His respiratory rate is 25/min, but on auscultation there are no added sounds. Abdominal examination is unremarkable, with no obvious tenderness, rigidity or guarding, and bowel sounds are present. An FBC was performed by his GP 2 days before this episode and shows the following:

- Hb 5.2 g/dL (normal range 13.0–16.5 g/dL)
- red cell count $1.9 \times 10^{12}$/L (normal range $3.8–5.6 \times 10^{12}$/L)
- WCC $93.3 \times 10^9$/L (normal range $4–10.5 \times 10^9$/L)
- neutrophils $0.1 \times 10^9$/L (normal range $2.0–8.0 \times 10^9$/L)
- platelets $7 \times 10^9$/L (normal range $150–400 \times 10^9$/L).

## 👥 OSCE counselling case

OSCE COUNSELLING CASE 9.2 – **What advice would you give a GP who writes to you about a 37-year-old African Caribbean woman with mild fluctuating neutropenia (0.8–1.5×10⁹/L; normal range 2.0–8.0×10⁹/L) over the past 4 years?**

# Key concepts

To work through the core clinical cases in this section, you will need to understand the following key concepts.

The FBC is basically a measure of the quantity and size of the blood cells circulating at that time. If a particular blood cell count is raised, the question is whether this is the result of something inherently wrong with the bone marrow or whether the bone marrow is simply reacting to something else going on within the body, such as inflammation, infection or malignancy. The answer may be obvious from the FBC but if it is not clear, a raised C-reactive protein (CRP) typically indicates a reactive process. An invaluable aid to diagnosis is a previous FBC, because this may show whether the changes are recent or old. A common scenario is a patient whose Hb rises over a few days during admission; assuming the patient has not received a red blood cell transfusion, a reduction in plasma volume (i.e. dehydration) is the usual cause. Likewise, a rapidly falling Hb does not necessarily indicate bleeding; one would expect the Hb to fall in a patient admitted with dehydration once rehydration is complete.

A blood film should be examined to ascertain the exact nature of any cells raised in the peripheral blood, such as leukaemia cells.

Low blood counts indicate either a failure of production by the bone marrow or reduced survival of that particular cell. In bone marrow failure, one would expect to see all normal blood cells eventually affected, i.e. falling white cells, red cells and platelets. Typically, the neutrophil count falls first because this has the shortest survival in the circulation – 24 h.

# Answers

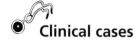

## Clinical cases

### CASE 9.4 – **A 78-year-old retired mechanic is admitted with increasing left hypochondrial pain of a stabbing character over the previous 12 h.**

#### A1: What are the likely diagnosis and the possible differential diagnoses?

This patient presents with hepatosplenomegaly, leucocytosis (with eosinophilia and basophilia) and thrombocytosis. This, taken together with the constitutional symptoms, indicates chronic myeloid leukaemia.

#### A2: What are the relevant points to elicit from the history?

During the history, direct evidence of hyperleucostasis should be sought, notably dizziness, headaches and visual loss.

#### A3: What are the possible clinical signs?

Splenic infarction leads to acute stabbing pain, and this may be elicited on examination. Infarction can occur during splenic enlargement, probably as a result of the very high WCC and hyperleucostasis. In the acute event, one may hear a splenic rub. Note that the gradual enlargement of the spleen is not, in itself, usually painful. Other signs of hyperleucostasis are retinal haemorrhages and retinal vein thrombosis.

#### A4: What additional investigations are indicated?

The diagnosis is easily confirmed by cytogenetic analysis of peripheral blood cells, where a translocation between chromosome 9 and 22 is found – the so-called Philadelphia chromosome.

#### A5: What is the treatment?

If there are symptoms or signs of hyperleucostasis, leucopheresis should be undertaken to lower the WCC. Immediate care should include analgesia, allopurinol or rasburicase (to prevent acute gout), hydration and chemotherapy. The WCC can be rapidly reduced using hydroxycarbamide (usually) or cytosine arabinoside (rarely required). Having reduced the WCC sufficiently, further therapy should be with the tyrosine kinase inhibitor imatinib. Patients who present with accelerated phase or blast crisis should be treated with combination therapy, including imatinib, interferon alpha or chemotherapy.

The age of this patient makes allogeneic stem cell transplantation from a donor too risky a procedure to be considered.

#### A6: What is the long-term outcome?

Chronic myeloid leukaemia consists of three distinct phases.

- *Chronic phase:* relatively easy to control blood counts with imatinib monotherapy. Patient remains relatively well with few symptoms.
- *Accelerated phase:* the blood counts become more difficult to control, often swinging from too low to too high.

- *Blast crisis:* the clinical picture becomes more akin to acute leukaemia, with increasing constitutional symptoms and marrow failure, i.e. low platelets, anaemia and high WCC. Further chromosomal abnormalities, in addition to the Philadelphia chromosome, often occur at this stage. Patients at this stage become resistant to conventional therapies and the prognosis is very poor.

Overall survival without transplantation has historically been around 5–6 years, but survival is much longer in patients who have a good response to imatinib. If there is a poor initial response to imatinib, the dose can be increased or interferon or cytosine arabinoside can be added; alternatively, one can switch from imatinib to one of the other tyrosine kinase inhibitors – dasatinib or nilotinib. With the exception of allogeneic stem cell transplantation, none of the therapies is thought to be curative, but transplantation is now reserved for patients who fail to respond to tyrosine kinase inhibitors.

## CASE 9.5 – A 63-year-old-man presents with a left-sided TIA.

### A1: What are the likely diagnosis and the possible differential diagnoses?

This patient is suffering from recurrent TIAs and has a high Hb, red cell count (erythrocytosis), WCC (leucocytosis) and platelet count (thrombocythaemia). This combination is highly suggestive of polycythaemia rubra vera (PRV); in this condition TIAs occur because of high whole blood viscosity caused by increased red cells and also increased platelet 'stickiness'. One still needs to consider the common causes of TIAs (systemic emboli resulting from atrial fibrillation, mural thrombus after a myocardial infarction, carotid artery disease).

### A2: What are the relevant points to elicit from the history?

It is important to know whether the patient has any symptoms suggestive of an alternative underlying condition, such as palpitations (atrial fibrillation) or previous chest pain (mural thrombus). Headaches and pruritus are typical of PRV, and one should ask directly if the patient has experienced amarousis fugax.

### A3: What are the possible clinical signs?

One should examine to ascertain if the patient has an irregular tachycardia (atrial fibrillation), carotid bruits or cardiac murmurs. The spleen is typically enlarged in PRV, and there may be plethoric facies and excoriations caused by itching and scratching.

### A4: What additional investigations are indicated?

Polycythaemia is classified as true (real increase in red cell mass) and false (reduction in plasma volume). True polycythaemia is further subclassified as primary (PRV) or secondary to some other pathology within the patient, such as hypoxic lung or cardiac disease or renal cell carcinoma. In patients with suspected polycythaemia, if the haematocrit is below 0.60 in males or below 0.56 in females, the diagnosis of true polycythaemia will need to be confirmed by blood volume studies (directly measuring red cell mass and plasma volume). In equivocal cases, oxygen saturation, a chest radiograph and abdominal ultrasonography should also be performed to rule out pulmonary, cardiac and renal causes of polycythaemia.

In PRV, 95 per cent of patients have a mutation of the *JAK2* gene. It is thought that around 5 per cent of patients with PRV do not have the *JAK2* mutation, but a high uric acid or high vitamin B12 level, along with a low erythropoietin level, with or without splenomegaly, is very suggestive of primary polycythaemia.

This patient also requires an electrocardiogram (ECG), carotid Doppler ultrasonography, an echocardiogram or computed tomography (CT) of the head, depending on his symptoms and clinical signs.

### A5: What is the treatment?

The patient requires urgent hospital intervention to begin red cell venesection. As the platelet count is so high, hydroxycarbamide or the platelet-lowering agent anagrelide should be commenced to reduce the platelet count to normal levels along with antiplatelet therapy (aspirin or clopidogrel).

### A6: What is the long-term outcome?

Long-term management includes regular venesection to keep the haematocrit below 0.45, antiplatelet therapy (aspirin or clopidogrel) and 'mild' chemotherapy (e.g. hydroxycarbamide) to reduce the platelet count to normal levels. Specific inhibitors of *JAK2* are undergoing clinical trials. Overall survival for PRV is typically more than 10 years, but thrombosis, progression to acute myeloid leukaemia (up to 20 per cent of patients) and myelofibrosis (up to 15 per cent of patients) are life-threatening complications.

## CASE 9.6 – A 23-year-old man is brought into A&E having become acutely unwell while shopping.

### A1: What are the likely diagnosis and the possible differential diagnoses?

The clinical history is one of sudden collapse and shock following what appears to be a relatively short period of ill-health. The differential diagnosis includes acute blood loss, sepsis (including meningitis), pancreatitis, hypoglycaemia, cerebral pathology (fits, thrombosis, haemorrhage) and cardiac problems (infarction, arrhythmia). The patient's blood count shows that there is marrow failure, with inability to produce red cells, neutrophils and platelets. This can occur with many conditions, but the high WCC (presumably blasts) indicates that the patient has acute leukaemia. This is completely in keeping with the fairly rapid onset of his symptoms.

### A2: What are the relevant points to elicit from the history?

This would need to be from a third party and would focus on features of anaemia (e.g. lethargy, palpitations, dyspnoea), low neutrophil count (infections) and low platelet count (nose bleeds and bruising). It would also be necessary to exclude other possibilities for his collapse (e.g. type 1 diabetes, heavy drinking, epilepsy).

### A3: What are the possible clinical signs?

Clinically the patient is shocked – low blood pressure, tachycardia, tachypnoea. The high temperature is very suggestive of septic shock precipitated by neutropenia. The most common organisms are Gram-negative bacteria, but Gram-positive sepsis is also possible. There may be ecchymoses related to the low platelet count.

### A4: What additional investigations are indicated?

The patient needs assessment of renal and liver function, calcium, urate, glucose and amylase, arterial blood gases, blood and urine culture, ECG and chest radiograph. Coagulation studies should be done to investigate the possibility of disseminated intravascular coagulopathy (DIC), possibly precipitated by a Gram-negative septicaemia. This diagnosis can be confirmed by measuring fibrinogen degradation products such as D-dimers. Cerebral imaging should be considered urgently to rule out or confirm intracerebral bleeding.

### A5: What is the treatment?

The patient is shocked, and therefore raising the blood pressure to allow adequate organ perfusion is essential. Crystalloids are required, but correction of the abnormal coagulation with fresh frozen plasma or cryoprecipitate (which is a better source of fibrinogen than fresh frozen plasma) will also help.

Placement of a central venous line to measure central venous pressure and aid fluid replacement and a urinary catheter to assess urine output should be considered. If fluids alone do not adequately raise the blood pressure, inotropes should be instituted. If respiratory failure ensues, assisted ventilation will be required.

Platelet transfusions will raise the platelet count and reduce the risk of fatal haemorrhage. The immediate commencement of broad-spectrum antibiotics with activity against both Gram-negative and Gram-positive bacteria is critical if the patient is to survive.

Although the patient is very anaemic, this is not the source of shock. Red blood cell transfusions will raise the Hb and potentially aid oxygen delivery to the tissues, but this is potentially dangerous because the patient has a very, very high WCC, and a sudden increase in intravascular cells via transfusion has a very high risk of precipitating hyperleucostasis, which can be catastrophic. Correction of the anaemia can usually wait until the WCC has been reduced with chemotherapy. If a red cell transfusion is thought to be potentially of benefit, this should be given very slowly.

## A6: What is the long-term outcome?

Septic shock associated with neutropenia has a very high mortality rate, but assuming the patient survives this immediate life-threatening complication, the cure rate for acute leukaemia ranges from 20 per cent to 80 per cent, depending on the particular prognostic type.

**OSCE counselling case**

OSCE COUNSELLING CASE 9.2 – **What advice would you give a GP who writes to you about a 37-year-old African Caribbean woman with mild fluctuating neutropenia (0.8–1.5×10⁹/L; normal range 2.0–8.0×10⁹/L) over the past 4 years?**

This woman has long-standing isolated but fluctuating neutropenia. The normal range quoted for most haemocytometers is usually based on an Anglo-Saxon white population and therefore may not be appropriate for all ethnic groups. African Caribbean individuals are well described as having lower neutrophil counts (as low as $0.5 \times 10^9$/L) but have no increased infective risk. For this patient, the neutrophil count may well be 'normal'. Other causes of isolated neutropenia should be considered, including autoimmune disorders (e.g. systemic lupus erythematosus, rheumatoid arthritis), drugs (angiotensin-converting enzyme [ACE] inhibitors), and familial and chronic benign neutropenia. Systemic problems of the bone marrow are highly unlikely (e.g. cancer – haematopoietic and non-haematopoietic, vitamin B12 and folate deficiency) because this condition has not deteriorated over 4 years. Cyclical neutropenia, a rare cause of neutropenia, is a possible differential diagnosis but, as the patient has no predisposition to infections, no further investigations are required.

Overall, the GP should be reassured, but regular monitoring every 12 months or so would be advisable until the diagnosis is clear.

## HAEMOGLOBINOPATHIES

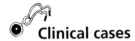

### Clinical cases

### For the case scenarios given, consider the following:

> **Q1**: What are the likely diagnosis and the possible differential diagnoses?
> **Q2**: What are the relevant points to elicit from the history?
> **Q3**: What are the possible clinical signs?
> **Q4**: What additional investigations are indicated?
> **Q5**: What is the treatment?
> **Q6**: What is the long-term outcome?

### CASE 9.7 – A 3-year-old girl is referred with failure to thrive.

The patient is the first child born to Asian parents, who have recently moved to the UK. There was no family history of note. On examination the girl is pale and slightly icteric, with frontal skull bossing. Her pulse is 110/min and regular, with no obvious added heart sounds. On auscultation the chest is clear. Abdominal examination reveals distension with hepatomegaly 3 cm and splenomegaly 5 cm below the costal margins.

Investigations reveal the following:

- Hb 5.1 g/dL (normal range 11.5–16.5 g/dL)
- MCV 58 fL (normal range 80–100 fL)
- MCH 19 pg (normal range 27–33 pg)
- WCC 9.1×10⁹/L (normal range 4–11.0×10⁹/L)
- platelets 317×10⁹/L (normal range 150–400×10⁹/L)
- ferritin 12 ng/mL (normal range 6–81 ng/mL)
- folate 4.1 ng/L (normal range 2.1–20 ng/L)
- vitamin B12 273 ng/L (normal range 130–900 ng/L)
- iron 18 µmol/L (normal range 10–30 µmol/L)
- iron-binding capacity 60 µmol/L (normal range 40–75 µmol/L)
- sodium 142 mmol/L (normal range 135–145 mmol/L)
- potassium 4.8 mmol/L (normal range 3.4–5.0 mmol/L)
- urea 5.0 mmol/L (normal range 2.5–7.0 mmol/L)
- creatinine 79 µmol/L (normal range 50–100 µmol/L)
- total protein 71 g/dL (normal range 60–80 g/dL)
- albumin 33 g/dL (normal range 35–50 g/dL)
- bilirubin 38 µmol/L (normal range 1–22 µmol/L)
- AST 65 IU/L (normal range 19–48 IU/L)
- ALP 71 IU/L (normal range 30–115 IU/L)
- LDH 1584 U/L (normal range 200–500 U/L).

## CASE 9.8 – An 18-year-old African woman awoke with shortness of breath and bilateral chest pain.

The woman is admitted through A&E. She was previously well, apart from a cough the previous day, but she awoke this morning with shortness of breath and bilateral chest pain. She says she had a similar episode 3 years earlier shortly after arriving in the UK from Nigeria. On examination she is very distressed and tachypnoeic. Her temperature is 39.7 °C. General examination is unremarkable, apart from the respiratory system and a chronic skin ulcer above the right medial malleolus. Her respiratory rate is 36/min, with reduced air entry and percussion note at the right midzone. There are widespread bilateral coarse crepitations.

Investigations reveal the following:

- Hb 6.8 g/dL (normal range 11.5–16.5 g/dL)
- MCV 84 fL (normal range 80–100 fL)
- MCH 29 pg (normal range 27–33 pg)
- WCC $17.1 \times 10^9$/L (normal range $4–11.0 \times 10^9$/L)
- platelets $619 \times 10^9$/L (normal range $150–400 \times 10^9$/L)
- ferritin 45 ng/mL (normal range 6–81 ng/mL)
- folate 6.2 ng/L (normal range 2.1–20 ng/L)
- vitamin B12 416 ng/L (normal range 130–900 ng/L)
- sodium 139 mmol/L (normal range 135–145 mmol/L)
- potassium 4.8 mmol/L (normal range 3.4–5.0 mmol/L)
- urea 11.2 mmol/L (normal range 2.5–7.0 mmol/L)
- creatinine 169 µmol/L (normal range 50–100 µmol/L)
- total protein 64 g/dL (normal range 60–80 g/dL)
- albumin 34 g/dL (normal range 35–50 g/dL)
- bilirubin 42 µmol/L (normal range 1–22 µmol/L)
- AST 58 IU/L (normal range 19–48 IU/L)
- ALP 71 IU/L (normal range 30–115 IU/L)
- LDH 1381 U/L (normal range 200–500 U/L)
- arterial blood gases:
  - pH 7.36 (normal range 7.35–7.45)
  - $PO_2$ 6.9 kPa (normal range 11.3–14.0 kPa)
  - $PCO_2$ 5.1 kPa (normal range 4.7–6.0 kPa)
- chest radiograph: widespread shadowing, especially at the right midzone.

## 👥 OSCE counselling case

OSCE COUNSELLING CASE 9.3 – **If two parents who are carriers of sickle-cell disease have three children, what is the chance of no child being a carrier or suffering from full-blown sickle-cell disease?**

## 🔑 Key concepts

To work through the core clinical cases in this section, you will need to understand the following key concepts.

The area of haemoglobinopathies is a test of your knowledge of ethnicity, hereditary diseases, erythropoiesis, paediatrics, and the hazards and benefits of blood transfusions. In keeping with most fatal hereditary conditions, haemoglobinopathies mostly have autosomal recessive inheritance but with variable penetrance. Different types of haemoglobinopathy occur in different areas of the world, but with globalization they are becoming a more common clinical problem in the UK. Management can be split into preventive, prophylactic and therapeutic.

## Answers

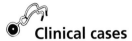

## Clinical cases

### CASE 9.7 – A 3-year-old girl is referred with failure to thrive.

### A1: What are the likely diagnosis and the possible differential diagnoses?

There are only four conditions that give rise to hypochromic (low MCH)/microcytic (low MCV) anaemia: iron deficiency, thalassaemia major, anaemia of chronic disease, and hereditary sideroblastic anaemia (usually X-linked recessive inheritance, i.e. affects boys). The normal ferritin, iron and iron-binding capacity rule out iron deficiency and anaemia of chronic disease. The raised bilirubin, AST and LDH indicate ineffective erythropoiesis or haemolysis, which is characteristic of thalassaemia major. Thalassaemic conditions are found in many different ethnic groups, including Mediterranean, Middle Eastern and Asian.

### A2: What are the relevant points to elicit from the history?

Thalassaemia major is the result of the inability to produce either alpha- or beta-globin chains due to hereditary genetic defects in the respective genes. Thalassaemia major is the result of inheriting two genetic defects – one from each parent, i.e. autosomal recessive inheritance. Over 100 different genetic defects have been described. Very severely affected fetuses may not be viable, leading to stillbirth. You need to ask whether there is any family history of stillbirth or anaemia and whether the two parents are related, i.e. consanguineous.

### A3: What are the possible clinical signs?

Children present with failure to thrive, pallor and shortness of breath (caused by anaemia), mild jaundice (resulting from ineffective erythropoiesis and haemolysis), abdominal distension (hepatomegaly and splenomegaly caused by extramedullary haematopoiesis, haemolysis and later iron overload) and bony enlargement (resulting from marrow hyperplasia – frontal bossing, maxillary and parietal bone enlargement).

### A4: What additional investigations are indicated?

A blood film will reveal a severe hypochromic/microcytic anaemia with erythroblasts present in the peripheral blood, and with target cells and basophilic stippling. If there is inability to produce either alpha- or beta-globin chains, the developing erythroid cell will try to produce other types of Hb to compensate.

Haemoglobin electrophoresis will detect absent or reduced HbA and the presence of abnormal haemoglobins, e.g. HbF, HbH (β4), HbBarts (γ4) and HbA2. In some patients who are carriers of alpha-thalassaemia, Hb electrophoresis may be normal and more sophisticated tests such as globin chain synthesis may be required. As the underlying molecular changes are characterized, molecular genetic studies are being increasingly used for diagnostic purposes.

Having identified that a patient has or is a carrier of thalassaemia, it is necessary to screen family members. Any identified carriers should have genetic counselling to make them aware of the risks for any future children. Advice regarding antenatal screening or possible termination of future pregnancies needs to be given by counsellors experienced in this field.

## A5: What is the treatment?

The mainstay of treatment for affected individuals is a red cell transfusion programme. This not only relieves symptoms but also prevents the bony overgrowths that occur.

If children are treated early, splenomegaly may not occur. If there is a delay in diagnosis or starting a transfusion programme, splenomegaly and hypersplenism may occur, which increases transfusion requirements. In this situation splenectomy may be performed but due to infective problems, this is usually deferred until after the age of 5 years. Immunization with pneumococcal, meningococcal C and *Haemophilus influenzae* vaccines and long-term prophylactic antibiotics is required by all patients after splenectomy.

Among the many risks of blood transfusion is iron overload, which occurs as a result of regular blood transfusions. Each unit of blood contains 250 mg iron, and regular monitoring of ferritin to detect early iron overload is required.

This iron accumulation damages normal tissues, including the liver, pituitary, heart, gonads and pancreas, and therefore treatment with the iron chelator desferrioxamine (subcutaneous) with or without deferiprone is required. Iron excretion by desferrioxamine is increased by vitamin C supplementation. Regular eye and hearing assessments are necessary for all patients on long-term desferrioxamine. Deferasirox is a relatively new drug replacing desferrioxamine as the first-choice iron chelator in many areas of the world. Monitoring of renal and hepatic function is required. If organ damage due to iron overload has occurred, hormone replacements (e.g. insulin) may be required.

As regular blood transfusions are the mainstay of therapy, immunization against hepatitis B is recommended.

The underlying problem is one of failure of the developing red cells to produce adequate Hb. Haematopoietic stem cell transplantation from a suitable allogeneic donor is hazardous, with many possible pitfalls (including death), but is potentially curative.

## A6: What is the long-term outcome?

People who are carriers of thalassaemia have a normal life expectancy. Before iron chelation therapy became widespread, people with thalassaemia used to die by the age of 20–30 years. In theory, well-chelated patients should have a normal life expectancy, but in reality they often die prematurely. Stem cell transplantation is potentially curative, provided that patients do not succumb to transplantation complications.

## CASE 9.8 – **An 18-year-old African woman awoke with shortness of breath and bilateral chest pain.**

### A1: What are the likely diagnosis and the possible differential diagnoses?

This young African woman presents with respiratory failure and chest pain. The differential diagnosis includes pulmonary embolism, chest infection, asthma and sickle-cell crisis (chest syndrome). The clinical picture is not typical of asthma, and the anaemia and biochemical pictures of haemolysis are not explained by pulmonary embolism alone. The clinical examination and chest radiograph are highly suggestive of a chest infection, but this alone does not completely explain the clinical picture and blood results. Intractable skin ulceration over the malleoli is a common feature of sickle-cell disease. The patient's clinical presentation and investigations are highly suggestive of a sickle-cell crisis, probably precipitated by a chest infection.

Haemoglobin S (HbS) is insoluble and forms crystals when deoxygenated. This distorts the red blood cells, giving them their characteristic shape and blockage of the microcirculation, leading to ischaemia and infarction.

## A2:  What are the relevant points to elicit from the history?

Sickle-cell disease has a highly variable clinical course, with some patients having a virtually normal life and others succumbing in infancy to crises or infection. It is important to ascertain whether the patient is known to have sickle-cell disease or has had previous crises or if one of her parents or siblings is known to have sickle-cell disease or to be a sickle carrier. Precipitating factors known to lead to sickle crises, including hypoxia (altitude), surgery, trauma, cold, infections and dehydration, should be sought.

## A3:  What are the possible clinical signs?

Anaemia (pallor, tachycardia, tachypnoea) is universal as a result of chronic intravascular haemolysis. Acute sickle-cell crisis is caused by acute occlusion of the microcirculation, leading to tissue hypoxia and organ infarction on a background of intravascular red cell haemolysis. Clinical signs are highly variable, depending on the predominantly affected organ. Acute pain – bony (e.g. long bones, vertebrae, ribs) or abdominal (e.g. spleen, liver, gut infarction) – is very common. Splenomegaly is common in young children, but ultimately splenic infarction leading to hyposplenism supervenes. Cerebral vessel occlusion can manifest as hemiparesis, paraparesis, fits, loss of or reduced consciousness and blindness. The combination seen in this patient of fever, leucocytosis, dyspnoea, chest pain and pulmonary infiltrate is often referred to as 'acute chest syndrome'. The clinical and chest radiograph findings are non-specific and hence do not distinguish sickling within the chest from a chest infection.

  Chronic sickle-cell disease leads to ischaemic necrosis of joints and secondary arthritic changes. High-output cardiac failure as a result of a combination of chronic anaemia, myocardial and pulmonary microinfarction often leads to premature death. Renal impairment caused by papillary necrosis and proliferative retinopathy is a late manifestation. Hepatomegaly is usually modest, but pigmented gallstones and biliary disease are common. Leg ulcers are a common typical feature.

## A4:  What additional investigations are indicated?

First you need to confirm the diagnosis of sickle-cell disease. This is most easily done by looking at the blood film. Blood film changes of hyposplenism (target cells, Howell–Jolly bodies, thrombocytosis) will also be seen. The presence of HbS can be confirmed with a Sickledex test and Hb electrophoresis.

## A5:  What is the treatment?

General measures to treat any underlying precipitating factor (e.g. analgesia, antibiotics, rehydration, oxygen therapy) are essential. The patient should be anticoagulated with heparin (unless contraindicated) because she has a very high risk of thrombosis.

  Blood transfusion of red cells dilutes HbS, improving microvascular circulation and oxygen delivery; it also temporarily suppresses HbS production. Partial exchange transfusion is usual.

  All patients with sickle-cell disease should take oral folic acid. Regular blood transfusions of red cells to keep the level of HbS below 30 per cent will effectively prevent crises occurring. As long-term blood transfusions are potentially very hazardous, this approach should probably be reserved for high-risk periods, such as before surgery or during pregnancy.

  Hydroxyurea (hydroxycarbamide) increases production of HbF, which has a protective effect on sickling cells and reduces crises.

  Patients with sickle-cell disease are hyposplenic and should therefore receive pneumococcal, meningococcal C and *H. influenzae* immunization and life-long penicillin. Allogeneic haematopoietic stem cell transplantation is potentially curative but carries a high risk. It may have a role in selected patients, such as children with strokes.

## A6:  What is the long-term outcome?

In the developing world many patients with sickle-cell disease die in childhood from crises or infection. With good medical care, many patients survive into middle age.

**OSCE counselling case**

OSCE COUNSELLING CASE 9.3 – **If two parents who are carriers of sickle-cell disease have three children, what is the chance of no child being a carrier or suffering from full-blown sickle-cell disease?**

As sickle-cell disease is an autosomal recessive condition, each parent must have one normal gene and one sickle gene. Thus, each individual child has a one in four chance of not being a carrier and not having sickle-cell disease. Thus, the chance of all three children not being carriers or having full-blown sickle-cell disease is $1/4 \times 1/4 \times 1/4 = 1$ in 64.

## REVISION PANEL

- Iron deficiency occurs when iron intake/absorption does not balance iron loss, i.e. bleeding. A thorough history is essential to establish the aetiology of the iron deficiency and direct investigations.
- Macrocytic anaemia with neurological deficit is pernicious anaemia until proved otherwise.
- A raised globulin should always raise the possibility of underlying myeloma.
- Very high white counts are a medical emergency, and urgent assistance from a haematologist is essential.
- Polycythaemia is very common and needs to be properly investigated and the correct management instituted.
- Shock in the setting of marrow failure (neutropenia) should always be suspected to be due to sepsis and treated immediately with broad-spectrum antibiotics.
- Always remember that normal ranges may differ between different ethnic groups.
- Thalassaemia should be considered in any patient presenting with microcytic anaemia from one of the high thalassaemia prevalence areas of the world.
- Sickle-cell crisis is a medical emergency with a high rate of potential complications. Advice from a clinician experienced in looking after patients with sickle-cell disease should be sought.

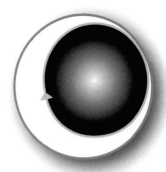

# 10 Oncology emergencies

*Daniel Rea*

## Questions

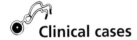

### Clinical cases

## For each of the case scenarios given, consider the following:

> **Q1**: What is the likely diagnosis?
> **Q2**: What aspects of the physical examination are most relevant?
> **Q3**: What investigations would be performed?
> **Q4**: How would the diagnosis be confirmed?
> **Q5**: What would be the initial management?
> **Q6**: What issues need to be addressed following acute management?

### CASE 10.1 – A 66-year-old man complains of recent-onset bilateral leg weakness, polydipsia, constipation and difficulty passing urine.

A 66-year-old man has been sent to the accident and emergency (A&E) department with a 10-day history of progressive lower limb weakness. In addition, he complains of low thoracic back pain. He complains of frequency and difficulty passing urine, constipation and excessive thirst. He was diagnosed with early prostate cancer 2 years ago and is being treated with goserelin, a luteinizing hormone-releasing hormone (LHRH) agonist. In other respects, he is in good health. He lives alone in a second-floor flat.

### CASE 10.2 – A 48-year-old woman develops fever 10 days after adjuvant chemotherapy for early breast cancer.

A 48-year-old woman presents to A&E while visiting a relative. She complains of feeling unwell and has a temperature of 38 °C. She underwent a mastectomy and reconstructive surgery 6 weeks earlier for a node-positive invasive breast cancer. Ten days ago she started her first cycle of a planned programme of chemotherapy at a hospital 200 miles away. She does not know what drugs she was given. She is normally fit and well with no other medical complaints. She has a respiratory rate of 24/min, her pulse is 120 beats/min and her blood pressure is 95/60 mmHg.

### CASE 10.3 – A 59-year-old smoker has dyspnoea and arm and facial swelling.

A 59-year-old man presents to his general practitioner (GP) with a 1-week history of progressive facial swelling, swelling of both arms, and shortness of breath on climbing a flight of stairs. He has smoked 20 cigarettes a day for 40 years and works as a garage foreman. He is sent to A&E following a chest radiograph that shows a widened mediastinum and a right hilar mass. He had a previous chest radiograph 6 months earlier, which was normal apart from some patchy shadowing in the left midzone, which is no longer present.

## OSCE counselling cases

### OSCE COUNSELLING CASE 10.1 – 'How will I cope at home if complete recovery is not achieved?'

The 66-year-old man with prostate cancer and leg weakness, described in Case 10.1, is now clinically stable and awaiting imaging investigations. He is aware of the likely cause of his symptoms and signs.

### OSCE COUNSELLING CASE 10.2 – 'How long have I got to live?'

The patient in Case 10.1 asks how long he has to live.

## 🔑 Key concepts

To work through the core clinical cases in this section, you will need to understand the following key concepts.

- Cytotoxic chemotherapy involves the use of drugs with a narrow therapeutic index, so side effects are common and can be life-threatening.
- Prompt intervention usually results in complete resolution of acute toxicity, but late toxicities may be slow to resolve or irreversible.
- As acute toxicity is reversible, aggressive management of severe complications is appropriate, even in patients with advanced incurable malignancy.
- Short-term neutropenia is very common after cytotoxic chemotherapy of common solid malignancies, but it requires intervention only when accompanied by infection. When the risk of febrile neutropenia is high, primary or secondary prophylaxis with growth factors will reduce the risk of neutropenic complications.
- Acute complications of malignancy require prompt assessment and, where invasive intervention is appropriate, this should be introduced as soon as possible to relieve symptoms and limit the extent of damage and disability. Supportive care and symptom relief should be introduced immediately. Acute complications of malignant disease rarely resolve completely and often mark a transition into a new phase of the patient's illness. Careful assessment of the consequences of a new complication is required and may have implications for future prognosis, physical and psychological health. They usually indicate failure of current therapy and indicate a need to review this.

## Answers

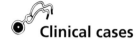
### Clinical cases

### CASE 10.1 – **A 66-year-old man complains of recent-onset bilateral leg weakness, polydipsia, constipation and difficulty passing urine.**

### A1: What is the likely diagnosis?

A1: The likely diagnosis is spinal cord compression secondary to bone metastasis from prostate cancer that has become refractory to first-line endocrine therapy. This is complicated by hypercalcaemia as a result of widespread bone involvement.

### A2: What aspects of the physical examination are most relevant?

- hydration status
- functional status (how well can the patient walk?)
- presence of spinal tenderness
- presence of a sensory level
- degree and extent of lower limb weakness, muscle tone and reflexes
- sacral sensation, anal tone and presence of clinically detectable bladder distension.

### A3: What investigations would be performed?

- whole-spine magnetic resonance imaging (MRI)
- urea and electrolytes (U&Es)
- creatinine, calcium, albumin and prostate-specific antigen (PSA)
- full blood count (FBC) and international normalized ratio (INR).

### A4: How would the diagnosis be confirmed?

Whole-spine MRI will identify the presence and level of spinal cord compression. Imaging of the whole spine will identify additional lesions that will affect decision-making and permit treatment planning. Corrected serum calcium will establish the presence of hypercalcaemia, which may be accompanied by biochemical evidence of dehydration and renal failure.

### A5: What would be the initial management?

- high-dose dexamethasone
- intravenous (IV) rehydration, followed by IV bisphosphonate
- catheterization if in retention
- spinal decompression and stabilization as treatment of choice if technically achievable and multiple levels of compression excluded
- urgent radiotherapy to the sites of compression if surgery is contraindicated.

## A6: What issues need to be addressed following acute management?

The prognosis after spinal cord compression is generally poor, with a median survival of 12 months. Functional status is superior for patients treated surgically, however. Postoperative radiation will be required, and second-line options for treatment for advanced prostate cancer should be considered, such as chemotherapy or second-line hormone therapy. Rehabilitation after treatment will depend on the degree of neurological recovery and may require extensive physiotherapy. Physiotherapy, occupational therapy and nursing assessment of the patient and his home environment will be required to facilitate discharge planning. Home adjustments or relocation may be needed. Ongoing monitoring of hypercalcaemia and maintenance bisphosphonates are needed. Long-term control may be achieved with oral bisphosphonates but, if unsuccessful, regular IV bisphosphonates are required.

## CASE 10.2 – A 48-year-old woman develops fever 10 days after adjuvant chemotherapy for early breast cancer.

### A1: What is the likely diagnosis?

This is very likely to be neutropenic sepsis. Virtually all cytotoxic drugs cause myelosuppression, and infection is a frequent complication of myelosuppression. Infection can progress rapidly and may be fatal if uncontrolled.

### A2: What aspects of the physical examination are most relevant?

Examination should focus on assessment of the severity of presumed infection and the potential source of infection. Vital signs should be confirmed. Surgical wounds should be examined, including donor sites for reconstruction. Respiratory and abdominal examinations are important. Examination of the oral cavity and perineal area should be performed, noting ulceration and the presence of candidiasis. The peripheral circulation should be assessed and any evidence of widespread bleeding noted such as ecchymoses or petechiae.

### A3: What investigations would be performed?

- FBC, including differential white blood cell count (WCC)
- arterial blood gases (performed after platelet count has confirmed this is safe)
- blood cultures, including separate cultures from indwelling lines
- U&Es and creatinine C-reactive protein (CRP)
- urine culture and swabs from any open wounds
- chest radiograph
- sputum culture if produced.

### A4: How would the diagnosis be confirmed?

Neutropenia will be confirmed by blood count. Arbitrarily, neutropenia is defined as an absolute neutrophil count below $1.0 \times 10^9$/L. Associated thrombocytopenia may also be present; if detected, coagulation status should be assessed, including D-dimers, because disseminated intravascular coagulation can complicate severe sepsis.

### A5: What would be the initial management?

Rapid IV fluids should be commenced initially using plasma expanders where hypotension is present. Broad-spectrum IV antibiotics should be administered using the regimen recommended by the local hospital neutropenic sepsis policy. Where a source of infection is suspected, such as a respiratory focus, secondary antibiotics should be added, again following the local protocol. An allergy history should be obtained and a recent antibiotic history noted, which may influence drug choice. Pulse oximetry and blood gas evaluation may indicate the need for oxygen supplementation. The patient should be catheterized if she is not passing urine freely or if hypotension persists after fluid load. If hypotension does not respond adequately to fluid load, the patient should be managed in a high-dependency or intensive care environment. Inotropic support may be required to maintain adequate cardiac output. Severe metabolic acidosis may require correction, and artificial ventilation may be needed. The use of granulocyte colony-stimulating factors (G-CSFs) in established neutropenic sepsis is controversial but is commonly given to patients with severe sepsis and marked neutropenia. The requirement for IV antibiotics and length of inpatient stay is reduced. Patients with low-risk febrile neutropenia without sepsis and moderate neutropenia above $0.5 \times 10^9$/L can be discharged early, provided adequate support is available

## A6: What issues need to be addressed following acute management?

Neutropenic sepsis in solid tumours (non-leukaemic) usually responds promptly to standard treatment, and most patients make a full uncomplicated recovery after the return of normal neutrophil function. Intravenous antibiotics are generally administered for at least 24h after resolution of fever, with appropriate oral antibiotics thereafter until all signs of infection have resolved. If fever does not settle within 48h, full clinical review should take place. Repeat cultures should be taken, microbiological advice sought and a change in antibiotics considered. The possibility of a viral or fungal infection should also be considered and treated if appropriate. The treating oncologist should be notified of the details of the episode and will need to take all the patient's circumstances into account when deciding appropriate modification of the treatment programme. Consideration of dose reduction or prophylaxis against future neutropenic sepsis is an appropriate strategy if further chemotherapy is used.

## CASE 10.3 – A 59-year-old smoker has dyspnoea and arm and facial swelling.

### A1: What is the likely diagnosis?

This is superior vena cava obstruction (SVCO) secondary to malignancy. The patient's smoking history and the rapid appearance of the radiological abnormality make the most likely diagnosis small cell lung cancer, but it is not possible to reliably exclude a non-small cell lung cancer or a high-grade lymphoma. The symptoms could be caused by venous thrombosis, although this does not explain the abnormal radiology. There may be associated thrombus.

### A2: What aspects of the physical examination are most relevant?

Full examination is required but should focus particularly on the respiratory and circulatory systems. The presence of clubbing should be noted, and the chest and upper body should be examined for venous distension and diversion. The neck veins should be examined and the degree of facial swelling noted. Periorbital swelling may be present, and the patient's ability to close his eyes should be assessed. A paradoxical pulse and reduced-output state may indicate coexistent cardiac tamponade. Examination of the entire body for evidence of metastatic deposits is required. Lymph node masses and liver involvement may help with identification of source for histological confirmation and assist staging assessment.

### A3: What investigations would be performed?

Computed tomography (CT) will define the mediastinal abnormality more accurately than chest radiograph and identify areas of external compression and associated thrombus. Computed tomography should include the abdomen to complete staging of the malignancy. Phlebography will establish patency of the superior vena cava and should be performed in conjunction with percutaneous stent insertion. Bronchoscopy should be performed to obtain a tissue diagnosis and indication of the presence of a primary bronchogenic neoplasm. Full blood count, INR, U&Es, creatinine, calcium and liver function tests are useful ancillary investigations; low sodium could indicate syndrome of inappropriate antidiuretic hormone secretion (SIADH), which would favour a diagnosis of small cell lung cancer. High calcium would indicate a possible squamous cell carcinoma or bone involvement. Tumour markers are of modest value, a high carcinoembryonic antigen (CEA) level being indicative of a probable adenocarcinoma, and a high lactate dehydrogenase (LDH) possibly indicating a lymphoid malignancy.

## A4: How would the diagnosis be confirmed?

Phlebography or CT will confirm the clinical diagnosis of SVCO, but both may be needed for complete evaluation. Histological diagnosis of the type of malignancy can usually be obtained at bronchoscopy, but if no malignancy is seen CT-guided biopsy or mediastinoscopy may be required to sample areas of suspected malignancy. An accurate tissue diagnosis is increasingly important, as treatment is increasingly tailored towards tumour type. Molecular markers are used in assessing the potential benefit of targeted therapies. The most important reason for a tissue diagnosis in this case is to identify or rule out a potentially curable condition such as high-grade lymphoma.

## A5: What would be the initial management?

Radiologically guided stent placement provides the optimal means to palliate SVCO, resulting in rapid relief of symptoms. Anticoagulation should commence after stent placement. High-dose corticosteroids may provide temporary relief of symptoms but could make interpretation of lymphoma histology more difficult and should therefore be avoided if possible until a tissue diagnosis has been obtained. The underlying disease should be treated correctly. A bulky high-grade lymphoma causing SVCO should be treated initially with chemotherapy, which may be curative. A small cell lung cancer has a high response rate to chemotherapy, and localized disease will respond well to radiotherapy, but treatment is non-curative. Non-small cell lung cancer presenting with SVCO is very unlikely to be amenable to surgical resection but can be usefully palliated by either chemotherapy or radiotherapy.

## A6: What issues need to be addressed following acute management?

Assuming that this patient does indeed have small cell lung cancer, stenting should successfully relieve the obstruction and he will start to respond to chemotherapy. The long-term outlook is bleak, however, with a median survival of around 12 months. The patient may need psychological support and help adjusting to his fatal prognosis. He may need to retire on ill-health grounds and require help accessing appropriate financial support. Irrespective of his physical requirements, he and his family or close friends should be seen by a lung cancer support nurse or specialist palliative care nurse (Macmillan Nurse), who can help explore all of the above issues and help him access appropriate support as and when required. Close communication between hospital and community-based care is essential for the optimal future management of this patient. If an alternative diagnosis such as adenocarcinoma of the bronchus is reached, then the options for additional palliative treatment with biological agents such as epidermal growth factor receptor (EGFR) antagonists will need to be assessed by mutational analysis of the EGFR gene.

## OSCE counselling cases

### OSCE COUNSELLING CASE 10.1 – 'How will I cope at home if complete recovery is not achieved?'

The reality is that complete recovery after spinal cord compression is unusual unless diagnosed very early, when minimal cord damage has taken place. In the case described, it is very difficult to predict the outcome. The patient is likely to be shocked and frightened by the diagnosis and needs time to adjust to the change in circumstances. It is reasonable to suggest that detailed discussion be deferred until the extent of residual deficit is known, so there can be a realistic assessment of what the patient will be able to do and how independent he will be. In discussing treatment options, the patient can expect to have the best- and worst-case scenarios described and an indication of how likely any of the possible outcomes are. Rather than guess at these, it is entirely appropriate to request specialist assistance at this stage.

### OSCE COUNSELLING CASE 10.2 – 'How long have I got to live?'

All doctors encountering patients with terminal malignant disease will be asked this question. The atmosphere and environment in which this issue is discussed are important. An explanation that the answer is complicated and will take time is acceptable, provided that you return soon; where possible, anticipating the question that is going to be asked will allow you to control the circumstances.

You need to establish that the patient is ready to discuss this question and that you are sure that he wishes to hear an answer to the question. The patient may be expressing a whole series of anxieties about the terminal illness and not really wish to be confronted with a direct answer in weeks or months. Ensure that the patient has the appropriate support from relatives or friends. If this is not possible, an additional member of staff who knows the patient well should be present and willing to stay with him or her after you leave. It is important to find time to talk about the question and the patient's reaction to your answers.

You should explain that estimating prognosis is inaccurate on an individual basis, with wide variations between patients. Ask the patient to tell you what he thinks the prognosis may be; you can then guide him forwards or backwards in his estimate. Avoid being too specific by providing a median survival figure; giving a sensible range is a better way to illustrate the likely prognosis. You will need to gauge how the patient is reacting during the conversation, taking things more slowly when he displays unease. Avoid becoming a source of unrealistic expectations, but always try to conclude the discussion on an optimistic aspect of the consultation.

## REVISION PANEL

- Spinal cord compression from metastases may present with difficulty walking and 'off legs'. If in doubt, an urgent MRI should be performed and treatment commenced with dexamethasone.
- Neutropenic sepsis should be considered in any febrile patient receiving cytotoxic therapy. Virtually all cytotoxic drugs cause myelosuppression, and infection is a frequent complication of myelosuppression. Infection can progress rapidly and may be fatal if uncontrolled.
- Neutropenia will be confirmed by blood count. Arbitrarily, neutropenia is defined as an absolute neutrophil count below $1.0 \times 10^9$/L. Thrombocytopenia and anaemia may also be present and must be treated accordingly.
- Superior vena cava obstruction is an emergency and should be considered in a smoker with progressive facial swelling, swelling of both arms and shortness of breath. A CT scan of the chest will establish the diagnosis.

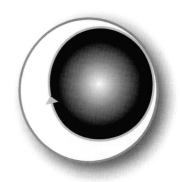

# 11 Neurology

*Stuart Weatherby*

## DISORDERS OF CONSCIOUSNESS

## CEREBROVASCULAR DISEASE

## DISEASES OF PERIPHERAL NERVES

# HEADACHE

| Questions | |
|---|---|
| Clinical cases | 334 |

| Answers | |
|---|---|
| Clinical cases | 336 |

# CENTRAL NERVOUS SYSTEM DEMYELINATION

| Questions | |
|---|---|
| Clinical case | 344 |

| Answers | |
|---|---|
| Clinical case | 345 |

# DISORDERS OF CRANIAL NERVES

| Questions | |
|---|---|
| Clinical cases | 347 |

| Answers | |
|---|---|
| Clinical cases | 348 |

# MOVEMENT DISORDERS

| Questions | |
|---|---|
| Clinical cases | 351 |

| Answers | |
|---|---|
| Clinical cases | 352 |

# MISCELLANEOUS NEUROLOGICAL DISORDERS

| Questions | |
|---|---|
| Clinical cases | 354 |
| OSCE counselling case | 355 |

| Answers | |
|---|---|
| Clinical cases | 356 |
| OSCE counselling case | 361 |
| Revision panel | 362 |

# DISORDERS OF CONSCIOUSNESS

## Questions

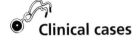

### Clinical cases

## For each of the case scenarios given, consider the following:

> **Q1**: What are the issues that need to be discussed with a patient newly diagnosed with epilepsy?
> **Q2**: What issues in the given history support or refute a particular diagnosis?
> **Q3**: What additional features would you seek to support a particular diagnosis?
> **Q4**: What clinical examination would you perform, and why?
> **Q5**: What investigations would be most helpful, and why?
> **Q6**: What treatment options are appropriate?

### CASE 11.1 – A 58-year-old previously well man suffers an episode of loss of consciousness just after leaving the golf club bar with his friends.

The patient smells of urine, seems a bit dazed, has a mild headache and feels achy but otherwise is normal. He cannot recall anything about the incident. He is a smoker.

### CASE 11.2 – A 24-year-old woman who is known to have epilepsy started fitting after a family argument. An ambulance was called.

The ambulance team tell you that when they arrived at the hospital the patient had been fitting for 30 min. She is still fitting when she arrives in hospital and appears non-responsive. Her body is thrashing violently on the bed. Her eyes are screwed tightly shut. Her oxygen saturation is 99 per cent air. Her pupils react to light and her plantar responses are down-going. The rest of the examination is normal.

### CASE 11.3 – A 21-year-old woman presents with a history of an episode of loss of consciousness 3 months ago.

The patient is otherwise well and plays hockey for the university's first team. Her friends witnessed her loss of consciousness and have come to the clinic with her. The event occurred while she was socializing in a hot and busy pub. After standing for 25 min waiting to be served at the crowded bar, she felt light-headed and became very pale and sweaty, her vision darkened and she crumpled down on to the floor. She was unrousable for a few seconds but then came round quickly, with no confusion. While she was unrousable, her limbs were observed to jerk two or three times. A medical student who was in the pub told her that she had had an epileptic 'fit'. Examination is normal and no postural blood pressure drop is noted.

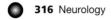 OSCE counselling case

## OSCE COUNSELLING CASE 11.1 – 'Will the epilepsy have any future implications for me?'

A 22-year-old woman is admitted to hospital following a witnessed epileptic seizure. What are the issues that need to be discussed with a patient newly diagnosed with epilepsy?

## Key concepts

To work through the core clinical cases in this section, you will need to understand the following key concepts.

### OVERVIEW OF EPILEPTIC SEIZURE TYPES

The classification of epileptic seizures can seem confusing, because multiple terms are used. Seizure type can be described on the basis of the clinical phenotype or on the basis of the underlying aetiology. The following simplified classification permits an understanding of the relevance of various terminologies. There are two main types: generalized and focal (see www.ilae-epilepsy.org/ctf/over_frame.html for more details).

- *Focal seizures:* only part of the brain (the focus) is affected. Consciousness is not lost, although it may be impaired. Partial seizures are sometimes called 'localization-related seizures', because an underlying structural abnormality is implied.
- *Generalized seizures:* the 'whole brain' is affected, and the key clinical feature is loss of consciousness. A generalized seizure may involve the whole brain at onset (primary generalized seizure – the whole brain has a predisposition to seizure) or may start as a focal seizure that then spreads to involve the whole brain (secondary generalized seizure).

In most adults, epilepsy is of a focal nature, with or without secondary generalization. Structural lesions should be excluded (space-occupying lesions and cerebrovascular disease are more common in elderly people; minor structural lesions, including scarring, focal areas of atrophy and cryptogenic foci, are more common in younger adults).

Initial onset of primary generalized seizures is rare outside of childhood and young adulthood. Although paediatric and rare epilepsy syndromes are outside the scope of this text, it is useful to briefly discuss juvenile myoclonic epilepsy. This is primary generalized epilepsy that usually starts in childhood or adolescence. It is associated with brief episodes of myoclonus (brief generalized single body jerks). Juvenile myoclonic epilepsy requires life-long treatment.

The generalized seizures can be subdivided on phenotypic grounds rather than on the basis of underlying aetiology:

- *convulsive tonic–clonic (generalized convulsions)* – loss of consciousness and tonic and clonic phases of muscular contractions
- *absence type (absence seizures)* with sudden immediate and short-lived loss of consciousness and no loss of postural tone
- *other generalized seizure types* – e.g. myoclonic (this may be brief generalized single body jerks, often throwing the individual to the ground) and atonic (sudden loss of postural tone with collapse to the ground – 'drop attack').

The focal seizures can also be subdivided on phenotypic grounds:

- focal motor seizures
- focal sensory seizures
- secondary generalized seizures.

### MANAGEMENT OF PROLONGED SEIZURES AND STATUS EPILEPTICUS

Secure airway, give oxygen, assess cardiac and respiratory function, and give intravenous (IV) benzodiazepine. Carers in the community may be able to terminate serial seizures by giving rectal diazepam or lorazepam. In the hospital setting, IV lorazepam 4 mg (or diazepam 10 mg) is more appropriate and should be given again after 10 minutes if there is no response. If there is a history of alcohol abuse, IV thiamine should be administered. If there is any suspicion of hypoglycaemia, 50 mL 25% glucose should be given intravenously. (Note that glucose given alone in a patient with alcohol problems can precipitate Wernicke's encephalopathy.)

If fitting persists, the patient should receive phenytoin 18 mg/kg IV at a rate not exceeding 50 mg/min, followed by maintenance doses of about 100 mg every 6–8 h. An alternative is fosphenytoin, a phenytoin pro-drug prescribed in terms of phenytoin equivalent. If fitting persists after 30 min, the patient should be transferred promptly to intensive care for more aggressive treatment to control seizures (e.g. with phenobarbital). It is crucial to diagnose and treat the underlying cause of the seizures and to recognize any associated injuries or complications (e.g. aspiration pneumonia).

## Answers

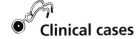

### Clinical cases

#### CASE 11.1 – **A 58-year-old previously well man suffers an episode of loss of consciousness just after leaving the golf club bar with his friends.**

#### A1: What is the likely differential diagnosis?

The likely differential diagnoses are generalized seizure and syncope. In this situation there is very little history on which to base a diagnosis, but it is a commonly occurring scenario. The differential diagnosis essentially breaks down into causes of seizure and causes of syncope. Causes for transient loss of consciousness include the following:

- epilepsy
- cardiac:
  - arrhythmia
  - decreased cardiac output from mechanical causes, e.g. outflow obstruction
- hypovolaemia
- hypotension:
  - vasovagal attack
  - drugs
  - dysautonomia
- vascular:
  - carotid sinus syncope
  - carotid disease
- metabolic:
  - hypoglycaemia
  - anaemia
  - anoxia
- multifactorial:
  - vasovagal
  - cardiac syncope
  - cough syncope
  - micturition syncope.

#### A2: What issues in the given history support or refute a particular diagnosis?

The fact that the patient smells of urine, seems a bit dazed, has a mild headache, feels achy, and cannot recall anything about the incident is most consistent with a generalized convulsive seizure.

Seizures may be classified as generalized (consciousness lost) or partial (consciousness not lost). There is also a variant of partial seizures (complex-partial) in which consciousness is impaired. Epilepsy subtypes are briefly reviewed in 'Key concepts' above.

#### A3: What additional features would you seek to support a particular diagnosis?

The diagnosis of causes of loss of consciousness is fundamentally a clinical issue and based primarily on an accurate history. Insufficient history may be one reason that the misdiagnosis rate for epilepsy is so high (up to 26 per cent in one population-based study, the most common conditions mistaken for epilepsy being syncope and non-epileptic seizures). A corroborative history is essential.

Although the patient says he cannot remember anything about the incident, he should be questioned closely to try to find out how he felt just before he lost consciousness. Did the event truly begin abruptly (consistent with a seizure), or did he feel strange or have *déjà vu* or *jamais vu* symptoms beforehand? (These symptoms are suggestive of a complex-partial seizure that may have then become generalized.) Did he develop a shaking in one side that progressed before he lost consciousness? (These symptoms suggest a partial motor seizure that became generalized.) Alcohol is known to provoke seizures and, as the patient had the event after leaving the golf club bar, he may have been drinking alcohol. Medical problems such as hypoglycaemia in diabetes mellitus can also provoke seizures. A comprehensive past medical and drug history should be obtained. As the patient is a smoker, it is important to question him for constitutional symptoms such as weight loss and cough with haemoptysis.

Witnesses should be interviewed (with the patient's permission) to get a description of the events.

- *What were the circumstances?* In generalized seizures, the event occurs abruptly, frequently without warning, and is not related to posture. The patient often appears normal before the event. In syncope, the patient often feels light-headed beforehand. Some types of syncope are related to circumstances, e.g. standing suddenly (postural hypotension), coughing (cough syncope), urination (micturition syncope – generally in men), in association with palpitations (syncope related to arrhythmia) or anxiety (e.g. in vasovagal syncope).
- *What did the patient look like?* Generalized seizures are usually of a tonic–clonic type and the patient tends to fall stiffly (tonic) and then start a coarse generalized limb shaking (clonic). This tends to go on for around 30 s, during which the patient is unresponsive to all stimuli. If examined during this period, the pupils are unreactive to light and the plantar responses are up-going. The patient may bite his tongue and be incontinent of urine. When the patient regains consciousness, he is often confused (postictal confusion) with aching muscles and a headache. In generalized seizures, the patient may be cyanosed or look normal. It is common for oxygen saturations to be low during a prolonged generalized tonic–clonic epileptic seizure. Often convulsive seizures of this type occur singly or in groups of two or three. Prolonged series of such seizures without regaining consciousness in between is called convulsive status epilepticus and requires urgent treatment. In syncope, the patient often appears pale shortly before and during the event. The period of loss of consciousness tends to be very brief (seconds). There is no confusion afterwards.

## A4:  What clinical examination would you perform, and why?

- Look in the patient's mouth for evidence of tongue biting (this can occur during a generalized seizure).
- A common cause for seizures in this age group is cerebrovascular disease. Evidence of ischaemic heart disease should be sought. Postural hypotension, arrhythmia and cardiac murmurs can also be associated with syncopal events.
- Neurological examination should concentrate on looking for lateralizing signs. These may occur as a result of a focal cerebral lesion, e.g. from a stroke or a space-occupying lesion. Fundoscopy, if it identifies papilloedema, suggests the presence of raised intracranial pressure from a space-occupying lesion.
- The patient smokes, so the possibility of a cerebral metastasis from a bronchogenic carcinoma should be considered.
- If there is a history of alcohol excess, it is important to assess for signs of chronic liver disease.

## A5:  What investigations would be most helpful, and why?

- *BM stick* – allows rapid measurement of glucose

- *electrocardiogram (ECG)* – should be done in all patients because epilepsy and cardiac causes of loss of consciousness can be difficult to distinguish; if arrhythmias are suspected, a 24h ECG is helpful
- *full blood count (FBC)* – anaemia and infection can provoke seizures
- *urea and electrolytes (U&Es) and calcium* – hyponatraemia and hypocalcaemia in particular can provoke seizures
- *blood glucose* – hypoglycaemia can provoke seizures
- *brain imaging* – computed tomography (CT) of the brain will exclude a space-occupying lesion and may identify evidence of cerebrovascular disease, and it is often used for rapid assessment; magnetic resonance imaging (MRI) of the brain is better at identifying small structural lesions and is the brain imaging modality recommended by many authorities.

Electroencephalography (EEG) should be performed in all patients to support the diagnosis of epilepsy in patients with a suitable history and to help with seizure classification and localization. It is important to note that a 'normal' EEG does not exclude epilepsy, and a 'non-specifically abnormal' EEG does not necessarily imply an underlying significant neurological problem. Diagnosis of epilepsy is based primarily on a clear history. One reason for the high rate of misdiagnosis in epilepsy may be inappropriate interpretation of the EEG result. A single resting EEG shows abnormalities in only 50 per cent of patients with epilepsy. Sensitivity increases if the EEG is done within 24h of a seizure, repeated or performed after sleep deprivation. Most useful of all is if the EEG can be performed during a seizure with video monitoring of the patient (video-telemetry). Conversely, normal phenomena, artefacts and non-specific abnormalities, occurring in about 20 per cent of the general population, are open to misinterpretation and may yield false-positive results. Correct analysis of the EEG is dependent on the context in which it is performed. If an EEG is requested as a screening tool for a patient with, for example, 'funny turns', it may yield minor abnormalities and cause more diagnostic uncertainty than it solves.

## A6: What treatment options are appropriate?

This patient is likely to have suffered a secondary generalized seizure, but a diagnosis of epilepsy cannot be made on the basis of a single seizure. Infection, drugs and metabolic problems can provoke seizures. Anti-epileptic drugs (AEDs) are therefore not usually started after a first seizure unless the risk of recurrence is thought to be high. Epilepsy may be viewed as a chronic neurological condition characterized by recurrent unprovoked seizures. The nature of the seizures depends on which brain structures are affected.

Anti-epileptic drugs are usually started after the second seizure. Current indications and side-effect profiles for the various AEDs are readily available in the British National Formulary. The principles of treatment are addressed and commonly used first-line monotherapy agents are discussed in brief.

A treatment should be effective, with minimal side effects for the patient. At present there is no clear consensus as to where the balance between efficacy and side effects lies. In circumstances where there is no urgency to start treatment, the decision should ideally be made jointly by the patient and a neurologist. Potentially acceptable side effects will differ from patient to patient; there are particular issues when prescribing for women, because drug interactions with the oral contraceptive pill, safety in pregnancy and breastfeeding need to be taken into account. The aim of treatment is to control seizures with a single agent (monotherapy), although a small proportion of patients may eventually require more than one AED.

There are now a large number of AEDs (including phenytoin, sodium valproate, carbamazepine, lamotrigine, levetiracetam, topiramate, oxcarbazepine, tiagabine and phenobarbital, to name but a few). Some are licensed for use only as adjuncts (i.e. as an add-on treatment in patients with difficult-to-treat epilepsy) and should not be initially used as monotherapy.

At present, commonly prescribed first-line monotherapy AEDs in patients who do not require urgent treatment include sodium valproate, lamotrigine and carbamazepine. Lamotrigine and sodium valproate are accepted as suitable for primary generalized seizures, partial/secondary generalized seizures, and epileptic seizures of uncertain nature. Carbamazepine is not generally used for primary generalized seizures because it may worsen this seizure type significantly.

## CASE 11.2 – **A 24-year-old woman who is known to have epilepsy started fitting after a family argument. An ambulance was called.**

### A1: What is the likely differential diagnosis?

Non-epileptic seizure disorder is overwhelmingly likely in this scenario. Before making this diagnosis, however, it is important to be confident that the other important diagnosis of prolonged generalized tonic–clonic seizure (status epilepticus) has been excluded. Status epilepticus is defined as continuous epileptic seizures for more than 30 min or recurrent seizures over 30 min with failure to regain consciousness in between events. Untreated, status epilepticus carries a high mortality; it occurs in 3–7 per cent of patients with epilepsy.

### A2: What issues in the given history support or refute a particular diagnosis?

A2: Onset during a stressful event can be suggestive of a psychogenic factor. Epileptic seizures can be triggered by stressful events, however, so this feature is rather non-specific. The fact that the patient is known to have epilepsy does not support either an epileptic or a non-epileptic aetiology. A significant number of patients (about 30 per cent) have mixed epileptic and non-epileptic seizure disorders.

### What additional features would you seek to support a particular diagnosis?

This case demonstrates the importance of making a diagnosis before starting potentially dangerous treatments. Non-epileptic seizure disorder is considered to have a psychogenic basis. Non-epileptic attacks are found to be most common in women aged 20–50 years. Factors that may play a part in their onset often include a personal or family history of psychiatric disorder or depression, previous significant life events such as bereavement, or a history of physical, sexual or emotional abuse.

### A4: What clinical examination would you perform, and why?

The fact that the patient's eyes are tightly shut suggests a volitional component to the muscle activity. This would not be expected to occur in status epilepticus. Wild thrashing, hip thrusting, normal pupillary responses, normal oxygen saturations and normal plantar responses are suggestive of non-epileptic seizures. The patient may respond to deep pain stimuli during the seizure. In status epilepticus, the patient is completely unresponsive.

### A5: What investigations would be most helpful, and why?

An EEG should be done. Although it seems rather self-evident, it is important to emphasize that non-epileptic seizures are *not* epileptic seizures. Correct identification of non-epileptic seizures is particularly important to prevent inappropriate transfer to intensive care for epilepsy management. An EEG performed during the seizure will be normal in a non-epileptic seizure but would be expected to show epileptiform discharges during generalized status epilepticus. Serum prolactin is often elevated during and shortly after a prolonged generalized tonic–clonic seizure. It is not generally significantly elevated by a non-epileptic seizure. It should be remembered, however, that prolactin levels can also be increased by drugs (e.g. phenothiazines). This can occasionally cause diagnostic confusion.

### A6: What treatment options are appropriate?

Patients with non-epileptic seizure disorder require a psychotherapeutic approach to help control their condition. The fits self-terminate. Status epilepticus is a potential differential diagnosis in this situation; the management of status epilepticus is outlined in 'Key concepts' above.

## CASE 11.3 – **A 21-year-old woman presents with a history of an episode of loss of consciousness 3 months ago.**

### A1: What is the likely differential diagnosis?

The likely differential diagnoses are syncope (simple faint – vasovagal syncope), cardiac arrhythmias, hypoglycaemia, hyperventilation, drug-related or -provoked, and epilepsy. This history is highly suggestive of syncope and is most likely to be a vasovagal event.

### A2: What issues in the given history support or refute a particular diagnosis?

The symptoms related to posture, and the fact that the patient became pale and felt light-headed before losing consciousness (i.e. a relatively long premonitory period), suggest impairment of cerebral blood flow. The facts that the patient crumpled to the floor rather than falling stiffly, and that loss of consciousness was very short-lived and with rapid recovery, are also highly suggestive of a syncopal event.

The circumstances of the events (a hot, crowded situation) are highly suggestive of vasovagal syncope. The fact that the patient is otherwise very active would suggest that a primary cardiac arrhythmogenic or structural lesion is less likely (although it does not entirely exclude it).

A few short-lived and transient limb-jerking movements are compatible with a syncopal event (and are *not* diagnostic of epilepsy), although longer-lasting jerking movements of the limbs are more suspicious of epileptic seizures.

### A3: What additional features would you seek to support a particular diagnosis?

Is there is a past or family history of epilepsy or heart problems? Did the patient have palpitations before the event (more suggestive of an arrhythmia)? Was there any incontinence or tongue biting with the episode of loss of consciousness? This is common with epileptic seizures but not in syncope.

Remember that a patient may not volunteer aspects of a history that are potentially embarrassing, and direct questioning may be needed to elicit this information.

### A4: What clinical examination would you perform, and why?

One would not usually expect to find any abnormalities in the general or neurological examination. During examination, however, particular attention should be paid to excluding abnormalities in the cardiac system (e.g. arrhythmias, heart murmurs). A postural blood pressure drop may sometimes be found.

### A5: What investigations would be most helpful, and why?

An ECG would help to further discount the (unlikely) possibility of a primary cardiac/arrhythmogenic cause. Otherwise, no other investigations are necessary at present.

Importantly, an EEG is not indicated; if performed, it may complicate matters – a substantial proportion of 'normal' EEGs may show minor alterations in wave morphology that can confuse the unwary.

If the patient has further events, further investigation with a 24h ECG may identify disorders of heart rhythm. If an arrhythmogenic cause is strongly suspected and the 24h ECG is normal, a cardiac 'memo' can be helpful. If a structural cause is strongly suspected, an echocardiogram can identify evidence of outflow obstruction. Tilt-table testing is sometimes helpful in patients with severe and frequent episodes of syncope if cardiac abnormalities have been excluded.

### A6: What treatment options are appropriate?

This patient requires reassurance that the episode was a faint rather than an epileptic seizure. She should try to avoid precipitating activities.

## ⚥ OSCE counselling case

## OSCE COUNSELLING CASE 11.1 – 'Will the epilepsy have any future implications for me?'

Epilepsy is a long-term diagnosis. Issues surrounding AED choice, seizure triggers (fatigue, alcohol and other drugs, stress, occasionally photosensitivity), specific issues for women, driving regulations, safety in the home, and the cognitive effects of epilepsy and AEDs must be discussed with the patient. It is important to document in the notes that this has been done, for medicolegal reasons. A useful checklist is available from the Scottish Intercollegiate Guidelines (www.sign.ac.uk). Comprehensive guidelines are also available from the National Institute for Health and Clinical Excellence (www.nice.org.uk).

The following issues need to be discussed.

- Explain what epilepsy is.
- Discuss the side effects of the various AED options.
- Discuss triggers to seizures, e.g. lack of sleep, infections, drugs, poor compliance with AED medication.
- Discuss sudden unexplained death in epilepsy (SUDEP). There are around 500 cases of SUDEP in the UK every year, which is more than the annual number of cases of cot deaths. The causes are not clear, but SUDEP appears to be more frequent in people with poor seizure control and who are non-compliant with treatment. All patients with epilepsy should be informed about SUDEP, but it is important to do this at an appropriate time and not necessarily at the time of diagnosis.

The following issues should also be discussed.

### Issues for women

Women taking one of the enzyme-inducing anticonvulsants (including carbamazepine, phenytoin and topiramate) may need to take a high-dose oral contraceptive because the low dose is likely to be less effective.

The risk that children of parents with epilepsy will themselves develop epilepsy is only about 5 per cent, unless the parent has a clearly hereditary form of the disorder. Patients should be managed in an obstetric clinic with access to a physician specializing in epilepsy. Use of the long-established AEDS during pregnancy appears to be associated with an approximate two- or threefold increase in the risk of major congenital malformations in women with epilepsy. The risk of malformation appears to be dose-related, and a higher rate is seen in women receiving two or more drugs. The risks appear to be greatest with sodium valproate. Risks may be minimized by taking folic acid supplements, so it is important for a patient to try to plan pregnancy in advance (or to take 5 mg folic acid per day if there is a possibility of conception). Pre-pregnancy and post-delivery vitamin K is also recommended to prevent haemorrhagic disease of the newborn. No pharmaceutical company guarantees that their product is safe during pregnancy. Patients should generally continue treatment in pregnancy, as the risks of stopping (e.g. injury during a fit, fetal hypoxia in prolonged generalized seizures) are generally greater than the risks of continuing.

### Lifestyle

Consider employment and relationship issues, and inform the patient about driving issues. The doctor has a legal obligation to explain to the patient who has had an epileptic seizure that he or she must inform the Driver and Vehicle Licensing Agency (DVLA) and must not drive until the medical panel of the DVLA has considered the case. The patient is under a legal obligation to inform the DVLA.

The following apply if the patient holds a group 1 licence (normal car licence). After an unprovoked single seizure, the stipulation of the DVLA is that the patient must not drive until he or she has been fit-free for 6 months. If the patient has had more than one seizure, the stipulation is that a period of

12 months of seizure freedom is required before returning to driving. DVLA guidelines on episodes of loss of consciousness are occasionally updated and vary depending on the type of licence, whether a seizure was provoked, and in episodes of 'unexplained' loss of consciousness (e.g. when the patient presents alone with no recall about the event) whether there is a high or low risk of recurrence. The DVLA website shows the current recommendations for driving after many types of illness (www.dft.gov.uk/dvla/medical/ataglance.aspx).

No driving restrictions are currently required for a simple faint for a normal driving licence (group 1). If the faints are recurrent, then the three 'Ps' should apply on each occasion – an identifiable provocation, a prodrome and a postural element.

After syncope with a high risk of recurrence, if the cause is identified and treated, the DVLA usually allows a patient to drive 4 weeks later. If the cause is not identified, the stipulation is usually 6 months off driving (assuming there are no further events).

## Stopping AED after 2 years of seizure freedom

Some 70–80 per cent of fits will stop with a single AED. After a period of seizure freedom, it is appropriate to discuss the pros and cons of stopping treatment because the epilepsy may have remitted. After being fit-free after 2 years of monotherapy, the probability of remaining seizure-free in the following 2 years is approximately 80 per cent if the AED is continued and about 55–60 per cent if the AED is discontinued. It is important to note that some primary epilepsy syndromes such as juvenile myoclonic epilepsy will not remit, and the patient will require life-long treatment.

# CEREBROVASCULAR DISEASE

## Questions

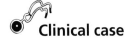

### Clinical case

### For the case scenario given, consider the following:

> **Q1**: What is the likely differential diagnosis?
> **Q2**: What issues in the given history support or refute a particular diagnosis?
> **Q3**: What additional features would you seek to support a particular diagnosis?
> **Q4**: What clinical examination would you perform, and why?
> **Q5**: What investigations would be most helpful, and why?
> **Q6**: What treatment options are appropriate?

CASE 11.4 – **A previously well 39-year-old man attends the accident and emergency (A&E) department with a left-sided headache, neck pain and slight word-finding difficulty after a mild whiplash injury 2 h earlier.**

He says his right arm 'doesn't feel right'. His wife has noticed a slight drooping of his eyelid on the left.

# Answers

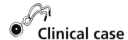
## Clinical case

### CASE 11.4 – A previously well 39-year-old man attends A&E with a left-sided headache, neck pain and slight word-finding difficulty after a mild whiplash injury 2 h earlier.

#### A1: What is the likely differential diagnosis?

The likely differential diagnoses are dissection of the left carotid artery, migraine with aura, left-sided intracerebral haemorrhage, and cerebrovascular disease causing a left-sided stroke in the middle cerebral artery territory. The most likely cause is a dissection of the left carotid artery.

#### A2: What issues in the given history support or refute a particular diagnosis?

Carotid artery dissection is a significant cause of stroke in patients younger than 40 years. Dissections are usually subadventitial (between the media and adventitia or within the media), creating a false lumen that can cause stenosis, occlusion or pseudo-aneurysm of the vessel. Simultaneously, the dissection may cause the formation of a thrombus, from which fragments embolize. Strokes resulting from carotid dissection may thus have a haemodynamic or embolic origin. In this case, a major clue to the cause of this patient's stroke is that he has a painful drooping left eyelid, which suggests the possibility of Horner's syndrome. Horner's syndrome is caused by damage to the sympathetic supply to the eye. The sympathetic fibres travel with the carotid artery, and carotid dissection may damage these fibres. Horner's syndrome consists of ptosis, miosis, enophthalmos and sometimes loss of sweating on one half of the face. It is important to consider a carotid dissection in any case of painful Horner's syndrome.

As in this patient, carotid artery dissections have non-specific presenting symptoms such as neurological deficits and headache. They often occur at a relatively young age and in previously healthy individuals, either spontaneously or after various degrees of trauma.

Neurologists manage stroke in all age groups. This patient is very young to have significant cerebrovascular disease. The other causes mentioned would not generally be expected to cause Horner's syndrome, but they remain possibilities. Each aura symptom in migraine usually lasts only 20 minutes.

#### A3: What additional features would you seek to support a particular diagnosis?

If the patient does not have a previous or family history of migraine, this reduces the possibility of migrainous aetiology. Is there a history suggestive of a connective tissue disorder such as Marfan syndrome (a heritable condition that affects the connective tissue characteristics, including tall stature, lax joints, lens dislocation and cardiovascular abnormalities) or Ehlers–Danlos syndrome (heritable disorders of connective tissue, characterized by skin extensibility, joint hypermobility and tissue fragility caused by a defect in collagen)? These connective tissue disorders can predispose to arterial dissections.

#### A4: What clinical examination would you perform, and why?

Signs of an upper motor neuron pattern sensorimotor deficit in the right arm, and signs of Horner's syndrome should be found. It is important to search for evidence of a head injury and, given the history of neck pain, to exclude evidence of spinal cord damage (bilateral limb weakness and sensory loss).

## A5: What investigations would be most helpful, and why?

Computed tomography of the brain will in most circumstances be adequate to demonstrate ischaemic damage in the middle cerebral artery distribution, although MRI is more sensitive. Ultrasonography of carotid arteries is fast, convenient, non-invasive and highly sensitive, and may identify a dissection. Invasive contrast arteriography is more accurate but carries a greater risk. Non-invasive alternatives include CT and magnetic resonance angiography (MRA). Electrocardiography and echocardiography may also be performed to rule out a cardiac source of cerebral emboli in many cases of 'young stroke'.

## A6: What treatment options are appropriate?

Formal anticoagulation for a period of months is usually favoured, although the evidence base for this is relatively poor. In practice, the choice between anticoagulation agents and aspirin is made depending on various circumstances (e.g. severity of stroke, length of time since dissection).

# DISEASES OF PERIPHERAL NERVES

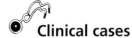

## Clinical cases

### For each of the case scenarios given, consider the following:

> **Q1**: What is the likely differential diagnosis?
> **Q2**: What issues in the given history support or refute a particular diagnosis?
> **Q3**: What additional features would you seek to support a particular diagnosis?
> **Q4**: What clinical examination would you perform, and why?
> **Q5**: What investigations would be most helpful, and why?
> **Q6**: What treatment options are appropriate?

### CASE 11.5 – A 29-year-old man presents with a 10-day history of progressive ascending leg weakness and numbness.

He suffered a 'stomach bug' while on holiday in Spain about 3 weeks ago. He was previously well.

### CASE 11.6 – A 65-year-old man with type 2 diabetes (requiring insulin for the past 5 years) presents with a progressive ascending symmetrical numbness and burning.

The symmetrical numbness and burning discomfort have involved his feet (and more recently his ankles) over the past 8 years.

### CASE 11.7 – A pregnant 35-year-old woman presents with a 4-month history of tingling in her left hand.

This is worse at night and often wakes her. She finds that hanging her left arm down outside the bed or shaking the left hand may help. She was previously well.

# Answers

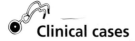

## Clinical cases

### CASE 11.5 – **A 29-year-old man presents with a 10-day history of progressive ascending leg weakness and numbness.**

#### A1: What is the likely differential diagnosis?

The likely differential diagnoses are Guillain–Barré syndrome (acute inflammatory demyelinating polyneuropathy [AIDP]), botulism, diphtheria and acute intermittent porphyria.

#### A2: What issues in the given history support or refute a particular diagnosis?

The story of ascending numbness and weakness about 10 days after an acute infection is typical of Guillain–Barré syndrome, which is an acute peripheral neuropathy causing weakness, paraesthesia and hyporeflexia. Progression generally stops 5 weeks after onset, and maximal weakness typically occurs at 2 weeks. The weakness is almost always symmetrical. Around 60 per cent of patients have a gastrointestinal or respiratory infection 1–3 weeks before onset. Mortality of the disease is in the range 5–10 per cent; the condition does not tend to recur. Cranial nerves may be involved in 45–75 per cent of cases and may be the dominant clinical feature, e.g. the Miller Fisher syndrome (a variant with ophthalmoplegia, ataxia and areflexia). A process similar to Guillain–Barré syndrome (chronic inflammatory demyelinating polyneuropathy [CIDP]) may occur over a period of months.

Botulism is often a food-borne disease, caused by the bacterium *Clostridium botulinum*, but wound botulism is increasingly recognized in people who inject drugs. Although there can be an incubation period, the symptom progression is very rapid. Early oropharyngeal symptoms, ciliary paralysis (fixed pupils) and normal sensation distinguish botulism from Guillain–Barré syndrome.

Diphtheria is an acute infectious disease caused by *Corynebacterium diphtheriae*. There is often a high fever and a tonsillar/pharyngeal membrane. The condition is now rare due to immunization programmes.

Acute intermittent porphyria, an autosomal dominant metabolic problem with increased production and excretion of porphobilinogen, can also cause a rapidly advancing symmetrical peripheral neuropathy. It is rare, however, and there are often accompanying features of abdominal pain.

#### A3: What additional features would you seek to support a particular diagnosis?

The neuropathy may progress to involve the respiratory muscles, and the patient may reach a critical state without any obvious prior clinical deterioration. The patient should be questioned about whether he has shortness of breath, particularly when lying flat (respiratory muscle weakness is more apparent in this position).

#### A4: What clinical examination would you perform, and why?

Guillain–Barré syndrome is an acute peripheral neuropathy. Examination should reveal a symmetrical global weakness of the legs and a reduction in sensation to all modalities in a stocking distribution. Reflexes become diminished and then absent as the disease progresses.

An important part of the clinical examination is to assess respiratory function. Forced vital capacity (FVC) measurements are essential; FVC is the volume of air expelled by a forced maximal expiration from a position of full inspiration. A peak expiratory flow rate, as used in assessing patients with asthma, is *not* appropriate and should not be used.

## A5: What investigations would be most helpful, and why?

- *FVC:* as the natural history of the condition is that it will continue to deteriorate over 5 weeks, regular FVC measurements are essential to detect incipient hypoventilatory respiratory failure.
- *Lumbar puncture:* an elevated cerebrospinal fluid (CSF) protein would be expected but may remain normal in 10 per cent of patients. It may take 1–2 weeks after the onset of weakness for the elevation in CSF protein to become apparent. The CSF white cells should remain normal; if they are significantly elevated (e.g. >50), an associated human immunodeficiency virus (HIV) infection should be considered.
- *Neurophysiology – nerve conduction studies:* these may be normal in the first 2–3 weeks but are then likely to demonstrate evidence of demyelination, with conduction block, slowed distal latencies and decreased motor conduction velocities.
- *Blood tests, U&Es, antibody tests, vitamin B12 and folate, serological studies for infection (e.g. Mycoplasma, Campylobacter):* blood investigations may identify low sodium (e.g. from syndrome of inappropriate antidiuretic hormone secretion [SIADH]). Vitamin B12 deficiency would not really be expected to cause such a rapidly progressive neuropathy, but it is possible and is a treatable cause of neuropathy; if the lumbar puncture was normal, it should be considered further.

## A6: What treatment options are appropriate?

Intravenous immunoglobulin (IVIG) and plasma exchange therapy are comparable in terms of efficacy. Most patients generally receive IVIG because it is easier to administer and may shorten recovery time by 50 per cent. As the patient is likely to be relatively immobile, prophylaxis with low-molecular-weight (LMW) heparin should be considered.

Effective management involves monitoring the patient closely to look for complications, in particular progressive respiratory failure, cardiac arrhythmias and autonomic instability. It is important to note that that a chronic form of Guillain–Barré syndrome (CIDP) exists, characterized by a progressive or relapsing demyelinating polyneuropathy over 3 months. The findings on investigation are generally very similar to those of Guillain–Barré syndrome, although patients with CIPD may also respond to corticosteroids.

## CASE 11.6 – A 65-year-old man with type 2 diabetes (requiring insulin for the past 5 years) presents with a progressive ascending symmetrical numbness and burning.

### A1: What is the likely differential diagnosis?

The likely diagnosis is chronic sensory peripheral neuropathy caused by diabetes mellitus.

### A2: What issues in the given history support or refute a particular diagnosis?

The patient has had diabetes mellitus for long enough to develop complications. The slow progression, in a symmetrical fashion, affecting a stocking distribution, is typical of a peripheral neuropathy. The burning discomfort is consistent with neurogenic pain.

### A3: What additional features would you seek to support a particular diagnosis?

Although the likely cause is a chronic peripheral neuropathy caused by diabetes mellitus, one should take care before making such assumptions. The problem could be multifactorial. Other causes of a peripheral neuropathy should be excluded.

A history of chronic excess alcohol intake, vitamin B12 and folate deficiency, thyroid disease, renal failure, autoimmune diseases (which may cause a vasculitic neuropathy) or paraproteinaemia (e.g. multiple myeloma) should be sought.

## A4: What clinical examination would you perform, and why?

Examination should reveal a stocking sensory loss with loss of ankle jerk reflexes. Often dorsal column sensation (vibration sense, joint position sense, light touch) is preferentially affected. Look for other complications of diabetes mellitus (e.g. retinopathy, cerebrovascular disease, ischaemic heart disease, peripheral vascular disease, renal failure).

## A5: What investigations would be most helpful, and why?

The following blood tests should be done:

- glucose
- glycated haemoglobin (HbA1c)
- urea and electrolytes
- vitamin B12 and folate
- thyroid function tests
- immunoglobulins and electrophoresis.

The blood tests are to identify other causes of a peripheral neuropathy and also to assess longer-term diabetic control (HbA1c).

Neurophysiological studies of nerve conduction are often useful in classifying whether the neuropathy is predominantly demyelinating (loss of the myelin insulation around the nerves, causing slow conduction velocity) or axonal (thinning of the nerve fibres, causing small-amplitude responses). Demyelinating peripheral neuropathies are more frequently the result of acquired causes and may be aggressive, but they are more often treatable. A cause should be identifiable in almost all cases. Axonal neuropathies are generally more indolent and slowly progressive.

In this case, the cause is likely to be a diabetic peripheral neuropathy. In many cases of slowly progressive axonal peripheral neuropathy, however, investigations do not always reveal an identifiable cause. The neuropathy is then termed an idiopathic axonal peripheral neuropathy.

## A6: What treatment options are appropriate?

Treatment is symptomatic treatment of the pain with drugs such as amitriptyline and gabapentin. Treatment of the cause, in this case optimizing diabetic control, will slow progression of the neuropathy.

## CASE 11.7 – A pregnant 35-year-old woman presents with a 4-month history of tingling in her left hand.

### A1: What is the likely differential diagnosis?

The likely differential diagnoses are left carpal tunnel syndrome, left ulnar neuropathy and left cervical root lesions.

The main sensory supply to the hand is from median and ulnar nerves (and a minimal contribution in the anatomical snuffbox from the radial nerve). Carpal tunnel syndrome is a compressive problem affecting the median nerve.

### A2: What issues in the given history support or refute a particular diagnosis?

The most likely diagnosis is carpal tunnel syndrome. Carpal tunnel syndrome is more common in conditions where the carpal tunnel becomes narrowed, such as during pregnancy, trauma, rheumatoid arthritis and hypothyroidism. Worsening of symptoms at night and relief on shaking the affected hand are typical of carpal tunnel syndrome. The sensory disturbance in median/ulnar lesions affects only the hand. The sensory disturbance associated with cervical root lesions is more extensive and extends above the hand. It should be emphasized that cervical root lesions in patients of this age group are very uncommon (although they occur with greater frequency in elderly people).

### A3: What additional features would you seek to support a particular diagnosis?

In carpal tunnel syndrome, although there may be weakness in the median nerve muscles, it is the sensory symptoms that predominate. An ulnar neuropathy typically causes a more pronounced functional deficit than median nerve compression.

### A4: What clinical examination would you perform, and why?

In carpal tunnel syndrome, the sensory symptoms are confined to the anterior aspect of the lateral three and a half fingers. Thenar atrophy may be noted. Weakness of thumb abduction is a useful clinical sign for the motor component of carpal tunnel syndrome. Hyperflexion of the wrist for 60 s may elicit paraesthesia (Phalen's sign). Tapping the volar wrist over the median nerve (Tinel's sign) may produce paraesthesia in the median distribution of the hand.

Complete ulnar nerve paralysis causes a claw hand. Wasting of the small hand muscles results in hyperextension of the fingers at the metacarpophalangeal joints and flexion at the interphalangeal joints. The sensory disturbance of ulnar neuropathy affects the medial one and a half fingers.

Cervical C6, C7 or C8 root damage can cause sensory loss in the hand, although this will extend into the forearm. Muscle weakness will be in the affected myotome and the relevant reflex arcs may be affected.

### A5: What investigations would be most helpful, and why?

Nerve conduction/electromyography (EMG) studies are helpful in confirming the clinical diagnosis.

### A6: What treatment options are appropriate?

For carpal tunnel syndrome, reduction of pressure on the median nerve will provide relief. In this case, fluid retention and oedema are likely to reduce after pregnancy and the symptoms may then remit. Placing the hand in a splint may give symptomatic benefit. Injecting the carpal tunnel with corticosteroid could provide relief. Often surgical release of the carpal tunnel is necessary.

For ulnar nerve palsy, surgical release at the site of compression may be needed.

For cervical root lesions, surgical decompression at the site of the cervical root lesion may be needed. As mentioned earlier, cervical root lesions in this age group are very uncommon.

# HEADACHE

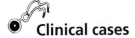

### Clinical cases

## For each of the case scenarios given, consider the following:

> **Q1**: What is the likely differential diagnosis?
> **Q2**: What issues in the given history support or refute a particular diagnosis?
> **Q3**: What additional features would you seek to support a particular diagnosis?
> **Q4**: What clinical examination would you perform, and why?
> **Q5**: What investigations would be most helpful, and why?
> **Q6**: What treatment options are appropriate?

## CASE 11.8 – A 40-year-old woman attends A&E with her worst-ever headache.

The headache started suddenly in the occipital area 5 h ago and was associated with nausea and vomiting and some photophobia. Her neck became stiff after around 2 h.

## CASE 11.9 – A 25-year-old woman presents to A&E with a severe gradual-onset headache.

The headache is right-sided, throbbing and periorbital, and there is associated nausea. The patient has had similar episodic headaches over the past 5 years; they generally last 10 h before settling.

## CASE 11.10 – A 70-year-old woman presents with sharp shooting pains in the region of the left cheek.

The pains last a few seconds and occur several times a day. She finds that yawning or touching the left cheek provokes attacks of the pain.

## CASE 11.11 – A 70-year-old woman presents with a gradual-onset diffuse headache, which is more severe in the left temporal region.

The patient comments that wearing her spectacles has become uncomfortable, and combing her hair exacerbates the pain.

## CASE 11.12 – **A 22-year-old woman presents with a 2-week history of headache of gradual onset.**

The headache is generalized, worse in the morning and exacerbated by coughing and straining. There is associated nausea. She started the combined oral contraceptive pill 6 weeks ago.

## CASE 11.13 – **A 40-year-old man who was previously well presents with a 6-day history of gradual-onset worsening headache, lethargy, myalgia and fever, and by the sixth day altered behaviour.**

The patient is brought to hospital after his wife called an ambulance because he had a generalized seizure.

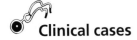

# Answers

## Clinical cases

### CASE 11.8 – **A 40-year-old woman attends A&E with her worst-ever headache.**

#### A1: What is the likely differential diagnosis?

The likely differential diagnoses are subarachnoid haemorrhage, thunderclap headache, bacterial meningitis, viral meningitis, cerebral venous sinus thrombosis and migraine.

#### A2: What issues in the given history support or refute a particular diagnosis?

The history is typical of subarachnoid haemorrhage. This classically presents with sudden-onset, worst-ever headache with nausea, vomiting, photophobia and neck stiffness (although this can take a few hours to develop). The textbook description of subarachnoid haemorrhage is of a sudden-onset, worst-ever headache similar to a blow to the back of the head. If a patient presents in this way, subarachnoid haemorrhage should be at the top of the differential diagnosis. In practice, patients do not always follow the textbook description. A useful operational definition is of sudden-onset, first or worst headache, usually occipital and maximal within moments, which may develop over minutes and lasts at least 1 h. Subarachnoid haemorrhage may occur outside these parameters but is rare.

A thunderclap headache may present in exactly the same manner as a subarachnoid haemorrhage, but does not tend to last longer than an hour.

#### A3: What additional features would you seek to support a particular diagnosis?

The temperature may be mildly elevated by subarachnoid haemorrhage or cerebral venous sinus thrombosis. Bacterial and viral meningitis may cause a high fever. Thunderclap headache is not associated with a fever.

Approximately 1 per cent of all headaches seen in A&E are subarachnoid haemorrhage. The most common differential diagnosis for acute headache admitted to hospital is migraine. The symptoms of migraine tend to evolve, however, and the headache is not usually of sudden onset. The headache is often frontal and may be unilateral. Thunderclap headaches may be recurrent. A history of previous normal investigations for a recurrent headache of this type may preclude the need to exclude subarachnoid haemorrhage on each occasion.

Sudden-onset headache can also occur in other conditions such as cerebral venous sinus thrombosis (although this mode of presentation is rare), which tends to be more common in females. Bacterial meningitis may very rarely present in this fashion, although the patient usually has a more gradual-onset headache and may have a purpuric rash. Viral meningitis is unlikely because the patient often has a prodromal illness and a sudden-onset headache would be exceptional.

#### A4: What clinical examination would you perform, and why?

If the patient has had a subarachnoid haemorrhage, she may have focal neurological signs that give a clue as to the cause of the bleed – e.g. a nerve III palsy suggests a posterior communicating artery aneurysm. If there is elevated intracerebral pressure, fundoscopy may reveal papilloedema. In bacterial meningitis a purpuric rash may be identified and the patient may also have signs of septicaemia.

Patients with subarachnoid haemorrhage, bacterial meningitis, cerebral venous sinus thrombosis or migraine may have focal neurological abnormalities. Viral meningitis and thunderclap headache are not associated with focal neurological deficits.

## A5: What investigations would be most helpful, and why?

Full blood count will show elevated white cells in a bacterial (neutrophilia) or viral (lymphocytosis) meningitis. It will be normal in migraine, thunderclap headache and cerebral venous sinus thrombosis. The FBC would be expected to be normal in subarachnoid haemorrhage.

Uncontrasted CT of the brain will show the presence of blood in about 98 per cent of cases of subarachnoid haemorrhage when done within 12 h.

Lumbar puncture should be carried out after 12 h in patients where the CT brain scan does not show blood. Lumbar puncture is 100 per cent accurate for the presence or absence of subarachnoid haemorrhage if carried out appropriately within 12 h to 2 weeks of symptom onset. It will also identify elevated white cells (as occurs in meningitis). The accurate diagnosis of a subarachnoid haemorrhage is dependent on identifying blood breakdown products in the CSF, rather than the identification of red blood cells (as red cells in the CSF can be due to a subarachnoid haemorrhage or a 'traumatic tap'). Blood within the CSF is broken down into bilirubin and is measurable after 12 h. In a subarachnoid haemorrhage, bilirubin will be identified in the CSF when performed after 12 h, whereas bilirubin breakdown products are not identified in a 'traumatic tap'.

## A6: What treatment options are appropriate?

If investigations reveal subarachnoid haemorrhage, calcium antagonists (e.g. nimodipine) should be given. These reduce the mortality and morbidity from cerebral artery vasospasm provoked by the presence of subarachnoid blood and need to be given to all patients. Non-invasive or invasive angiography should be performed to identify the presence of an aneurysm, which can then be ablated by neuroradiological or neurosurgical techniques.

If investigations reveal an elevated CSF pressure but are otherwise normal, MRI of the brain with venogram sequences will identify or exclude the presence of a cerebral venous sinus thrombosis. The more typical presentation and management of cerebral venous sinus thrombosis are addressed in Case 11.12.

If investigations are normal, the differential diagnosis lies between thunderclap headache and migraine. A thunderclap headache is of sudden onset, whereas migraine headaches are generally of more gradual onset (it is good practice in this situation to retake the initial history). Migraine lasts longer than a thunderclap headache, and features of nausea, vomiting, photophobia and phonophobia are often more pronounced than in thunderclap headache. Furthermore, migraine may be associated with focal neurological symptoms and signs.

Although the history would be unusual for meningitis, it is appropriate to briefly discuss this important condition here. Patients in whom bacterial meningitis is suspected generally have a gradual-onset headache, rash, neck stiffness, nausea, vomiting, photophobia and confusion (although not necessarily all of them). A purpuric rash indicates a more generalized sepsis. In bacterial meningitis, the lumbar puncture results typically show raised protein, low glucose and raised white cells (neutrophils). If the lumbar puncture has been performed after the patient has been on antibiotics (i.e. partly treated bacterial meningitis), the white cells are often lymphocytes. In viral meningitis, the findings are normal (or very slightly raised) protein, normal glucose and raised white cells (lymphocytes). In tuberculous meningitis, the findings are raised protein, low glucose and raised white cells (lymphocytes).

In suspected bacterial meningitis, it is important to start appropriate antibiotics on an empirical basis as soon as possible (i.e. before doing a lumbar puncture). Instituting antibiotic therapy 1–2 h before lumbar puncture will not significantly decrease the diagnostic sensitivity if the culture of the CSF is done together with testing for bacterial antigens and with blood cultures. In most patients, initial empirical therapy with a broad-spectrum cephalosporin (cefotaxime or ceftriaxone), supplemented with ampicillin in young infants and older adults, is appropriate. In patients with suspected bacterial meningitis, it is currently considered appropriate to start corticosteroids at the same time as initiating antibiotics, and to continue steroids for the first 4 days. Most regions have their own local policies, and these should be consulted because the situation regarding antimicrobial treatment may be subject to variation. Bacterial meningitis should be notified to public health physicians, who will contact trace and give prophylactic antibiotics as necessary. In patients who are immunocompromised, patients in whom tuberculous meningitis is suspected, and patients with a recent foreign travel history, other treatment regimens are necessary.

## CASE 11.9 – **A 25-year-old woman presents to A&E with a severe gradual-onset headache.**

### A1: What is the likely differential diagnosis?

The likely diagnosis is migraine.

### A2: What issues in the given history support or refute a particular diagnosis?

Episodic gradual-onset severe headaches in young women are almost always migraine.

### A3: What additional features would you seek to support a particular diagnosis?

The patient should be questioned for other features of migraine. Some patients find that various foodstuffs precipitate their headaches (e.g. cheese, chocolate, red wine, citrus fruit, crisps). There may be a hormonal component to the symptoms, and the headaches may be worse around the time of menstrual periods. Some hours before the onset of headache, patients may suffer premonitory symptoms, such as hunger or anxiety. An aura may precede the headache. Often there is a family history of migraine.

### A4: What clinical examination would you perform, and why?

Examination is normal.

### A5: What investigations would be most helpful, and why?

The diagnosis of migraine is based on history. No investigations are necessary. Migraine is the most common primary headache, affecting 10–20 per cent of the population of the USA. It occurs more commonly in women. The International Headache Society (www.i-h-s.org) has classified all headache types. There are two main types of migraine: migraine with aura and migraine without aura. The cardinal feature of migraine aura is that it evolves slowly; most aura symptoms develop over 5–20 min and usually last less than 60 min. The headache generally follows soon after the aura. Auras vary in type and complexity. Visual auras are the most common and include scotomata (blind spots in the visual field), fortification spectra and geometric visual patterns. Progressive sensory disturbance is the second most common migraine aura. The typical migraine headache is of gradual onset, throbbing and unilateral, although it may be bilateral in a substantial minority of patients. Nausea, vomiting, photophobia and phonophobia are often accompanying features.

### A6: What treatment options are appropriate?

Many patients respond to simple analgesics, especially non-steroidal anti-inflammatory drugs, which are often given with an antiemetic such as metoclopramide. Diclofenac and domperidone suppositories may also be helpful. If these measures do not work, the triptan class of anti-migraine drugs (selective serotonin agonists) may be used. These drugs significantly reduce the severity and duration of the migraine headache, but they are not effective if given during the aura. They should be taken at the onset of the headache. Several guidelines are available for the diagnosis and management of migraine.

The guidelines of the British Association for the Study of Headache are available from www.bash.org. uk. In cases of frequent migraine, prophylactic agents such as beta-blockers or amitriptyline are often considered.

The combined oral contraceptive pill is currently contraindicated in women with migraine with aura, as a result of concerns about increased stroke risk.

Patients with frequent migraines sometimes respond by taking frequent doses of analgesics. This can lead to increased chronicity of the headache and a rebound medication overuse headache. Codeine and other opiates are particularly problematic in this respect.

## CASE 11.10 – **A 70-year-old woman presents with sharp shooting pains in the region of the left cheek.**

### A1: What is the likely differential diagnosis?

The likely differential diagnosis is trigeminal neuralgia.

### A2: What issues in the given history support or refute a particular diagnosis?

Trigeminal neuralgia tends to occur in people aged over 60 years and is more common in women. It is characterized by brief paroxysms of pain localized in the maxillary or mandibular divisions of the trigeminal nerve.

### A3: What additional features would you seek to support a particular diagnosis?

Attacks may be triggered by yawning or touching the area of skin innervated by the mandibular branch of the trigeminal nerve. It is important to note that involvement of the ophthalmic branch is very rare.

### A4: What clinical examination would you perform, and why?

Examination is usually normal but may reveal altered sensation in the area of skin innervated by the mandibular branch of the trigeminal nerve.

### A5: What investigations would be most helpful, and why?

Magnetic resonance imaging is generally used to exclude a vascular or other compressive lesion of the relevant divisions of the trigeminal nerve.

### A6: What treatment options are appropriate?

Medical treatments include carbamazepine, gabapentin and amitriptyline.

If the pain is refractory to medical treatments, neurosurgical procedures including microvascular decompression (to separate the trigeminal nerve from a compressing blood vessel) and percutaneous glycerol rhizolysis (injecting glycerol to damage the trigeminal fibres causing the pain) may be considered.

## CASE 11.11 – **A 70-year-old woman presents with a gradual-onset diffuse headache, which is more severe in the left temporal region.**

### A1: What is the likely differential diagnosis?

The likely differential diagnoses are temporal arteritis and a space-occupying lesion.

## A2: What issues in the given history support or refute a particular diagnosis?

In a patient of this age, it is always worth bearing in mind the possibility of a space-occupying lesion. This history is, however, typical of temporal arteritis.

Temporal arteritis is more common in people aged over 70 years, especially in women. It is a medium-/large-vessel vasculitis. Affected vessels are infiltrated by lymphocytes, plasma cells and multinucleated giant cells, often in a patchy fashion. Temporal arteritis is closely linked to polymyalgia rheumatica (a clinical syndrome characterized by severe aching and stiffness in the neck, shoulder girdle and pelvic girdle). Temporal pain and tenderness are characteristic, and the patient may complain of pain when wearing spectacles and combing her hair.

## A3: What additional features would you seek to support a particular diagnosis?

The patient may have constitutional symptoms such as malaise, lethargy, weight loss and night sweats. She may notice increasing discomfort in the jaw when talking or chewing (jaw claudication).

The inflammatory process in the blood vessels may occur throughout various areas of the body and cause ischaemia. Visual loss, stroke, angina and arterial aneurysms may all be associated.

## A4: What clinical examination would you perform, and why?

There is likely to be tenderness over the temporal arteries, which may have diminished or absent pulses.

## A5: What investigations would be most helpful, and why?

An erythrocyte sedimentation rate (ESR) is usually (but not always) elevated and gives additional support to the clinical diagnosis. Abnormal liver function tests may occur, and the FBC may show an anaemia, leucocytosis or thrombocytosis. If the patient has typical symptoms, brain imaging is not necessary.

As this condition occurs in elderly people, and the headache phenotype can be rather variable, CT of the brain may be helpful to exclude a space-occupying lesion if there is clinical uncertainty over the diagnosis. Furthermore, a raised ESR can be associated with other conditions (e.g. myeloma, infections, cancers). In cases of diagnostic uncertainty, these conditions may need to be excluded.

Definitive diagnosis is achieved by temporal artery biopsy to identify the inflammatory lesions described above. The inflammation tends to be patchy and may not always appear in a single biopsy.

## A6: What treatment options are appropriate?

Corticosteroids should be started immediately after clinical diagnosis. It is not necessary to perform a temporal artery biopsy first, because the inflammatory changes generally persist for 2 weeks. Treatment is usually with high-dose prednisolone orally, although if vision is threatened high-dose IV methylprednisolone infusions may be used initially. The response to treatment is typically rapid, within 48 h. In most cases it is usual to start the patient on 60 mg prednisolone and to slowly wean the dose down over several months once the symptoms are under control. If the ESR was initially raised, it can be used to guide treatment. When a patient gets to a dose of around 10 mg prednisolone, the dose reduction process is much slower (e.g. 1 mg/month). Often a dose threshold is found, below which the symptoms return, and the patient may therefore require long-term corticosteroids. If the patient is placed on long-term steroids, it is necessary to consider monitoring of bone density using a dual-energy X-ray absorptiometry (DEXA) scan and instituting 'bone protection' with drugs such as bisphosphonates to reduce the likelihood of steroid-induced osteoporosis.

## CASE 11.12 – **A 22-year-old woman presents with a 2-week history of headache of gradual onset.**

### A1: What is the likely differential diagnosis?

The likely differential diagnoses are cerebral venous sinus thrombosis, idiopathic intracranial hypertension and brain tumour.

### A2: What issues in the given history support or refute a particular diagnosis?

This history is typical of both cerebral venous sinus thrombosis and idiopathic intracranial hypertension. The phenotype of the headache is of raised pressure (headache worse in the morning and exacerbated by coughing and straining), and other causes of raised pressure (e.g. brain tumour) are possible and need to be excluded. Prothrombotic states (e.g. combined oral contraceptive pill) predispose to cerebral venous sinus thrombosis. Cerebral venous sinus thrombosis and idiopathic intracranial hypertension are more common in women.

### A3: What additional features would you seek to support a particular diagnosis?

Ask for symptoms of lateralizing weakness or sensory disturbance. This suggests underlying structural lesions and would be consistent with a brain tumour or possibly cerebral venous sinus thrombosis. Idiopathic intracranial hypertension does not cause limb weakness. Disturbance of visual function (particularly enlargement of the blind spots) may occur in both idiopathic intracranial hypertension and cerebral venous sinus thrombosis. Impairment of consciousness can occur in brain tumours with oedema, and in cerebral venous sinus thrombosis; it does not occur in idiopathic intracranial hypertension.

### A4: What clinical examination would you perform, and why?

Patients with idiopathic intracranial hypertension are almost always female and overweight. Examination of visual function is important. Visual fields may be affected in both conditions (enlarged blind spots and constricted visual fields). Fundoscopy may reveal papilloedema. General neurological examination may reveal lateralizing signs.

### A5: What investigations would be most helpful, and why?

Although CT of the brain is useful to exclude a tumour, the most appropriate imaging investigation is MRI of the brain with venogram sequences. This is more sensitive in identifying a cerebral venous sinus thrombosis. Recent evidence suggests that D-dimers are often elevated in patients with acute and subacute cerebral venous sinus thrombosis, but their measurement is not sensitive enough to confirm or exclude the condition definitively. It is important to monitor vision carefully, because visual loss can occur rapidly in both cerebral venous sinus thrombosis and idiopathic intracranial hypertension. An early sign is development of enlargement of the blind spots, which can be detected by clinical examination of the visual fields (but much more sensitively by formal charting of the visual fields).

If imaging studies are normal, then the likely diagnosis (if the patient is overweight and has papilloedema) is idiopathic intracranial hypertension. A lumbar puncture with CSF measurement will confirm the diagnosis by identifying raised intracranial pressure (pressure >25 cmH$_2$O).

### A6: What treatment options are appropriate?

If investigations identify a brain tumour, oncological and neurosurgical opinions should be sought.

If investigations identify cerebral venous sinus thrombosis, the generally accepted treatment is formal anticoagulation, initially with heparin and then with warfarin for 3–6 months. Medications associated with hypercoagulable states, such as the combined oral contraceptive pill, should be discontinued.

If investigations identify idiopathic intracranial hypertension, it is important to stop any medication that may precipitate the condition (e.g. combined oral contraceptive pill, tetracycline antibiotics). Idiopathic intracranial hypertension occurs almost exclusively in people who are overweight; weight loss is the mainstay of treatment. Medications such as carbonic anhydrase inhibitors (e.g. acetazolamide) and diuretics (e.g. furosemide) are also used to reduce the CSF pressure.

It is important to realize that progressive visual field loss in idiopathic intracranial hypertension and cerebral venous sinus thrombosis is often asymptomatic. By the time the patient notices an impairment of visual acuity (a late-stage symptom in raised intracranial pressure), a significant degree of permanent visual loss may already have occurred. Regular monitoring of visual fields, both clinically and with formal perimetry, as part of the assessment of optic nerve function, together with visual acuity, colour vision and fundoscopy, is vital. Idiopathic intracranial hypertension is a more chronic condition than cerebral venous sinus thrombosis and requires longer-term monitoring of visual function.

If a patient with either of these two conditions develops progressive visual loss that does not respond to medication, neurosurgical procedures to protect optic nerve function should be considered (CSF diversion such as lumboperitoneal shunt, or optic nerve sheath fenestration). Although lumbar puncture can acutely reduce CSF pressure, the effect is transient. Repeated lumbar punctures do not help with longer-term management.

## CASE 11.13 – A 40-year-old man who was previously well presents with a 6-day history of gradual-onset worsening headache, lethargy, myalgia and fever, and by the sixth day altered behaviour.

### A1: What is the likely differential diagnosis?

The likely differential diagnoses are encephalitis, brain abscess and brain tumour.

### A2: What issues in the given history support or refute a particular diagnosis?

A brain tumour or abscess could present in this fashion. The prodrome of a viral-type illness is suggestive of encephalitis, however, as is the progressive evolution of symptoms. The altered behaviour and subsequent fit suggest involvement of the substance of the brain, as occurs in encephalitis. In meningitis, behaviour change does not occur unless there is more extensive involvement (meningoencephalitis) or the patient has systemic infection.

### A3: What additional features would you seek to support a particular diagnosis?

A history of close contacts with infectious diseases, travel abroad, tick or insect bites, or predisposition would increase the probability of an infectious cause.

### A4: What clinical examination would you perform, and why?

Lateralizing neurological signs suggest a structural lesion within the brain but will not distinguish a cause. Similarly, papilloedema will suggest raised intracranial pressure but may occur in all of the above causes. If the patient has a metastatic brain tumour, general examination may reveal evidence of the primary tumour. Fever, however, is not generally a feature of a brain tumour.

### A5: What investigations would be most helpful, and why?

Computed tomography of the brain will essentially exclude an intracerebral mass lesion and may be done rapidly (it can be useful particularly if the patient is confused), but the imaging modality of choice is MRI. This will better identify the nature of a space-occupying lesion and is much more sensitive at picking up the changes that occur in encephalitis. Herpes simplex virus encephalitis is the most common and treatable encephalitis in the UK, and abnormalities are frequently noted in the temporal lobes on MRI.

An EEG is helpful if further consideration is being given to a potential diagnosis of encephalitis. It will generally be abnormal, showing increased slow-wave activity and possibly epileptiform discharges. In herpes simplex virus encephalitis, characteristic EEG changes of lateralized periodic complexes at regular intervals of 2–3 s are seen.

A lumbar puncture is not generally helpful in investigating brain tumours. It is contraindicated in brain abscesses. If imaging excludes a mass lesion and significant oedema, a lumbar puncture can be helpful to investigate encephalitis. In herpes simplex virus encephalitis, the CSF is often under increased pressure with raised white cells (lymphocytes), elevated protein and modestly reduced glucose (i.e. the lumbar puncture results may be similar to those in tuberculous or fungal meningitis). Polymerase chain reaction of the CSF is likely to detect the presence of herpes simplex virus 1 or 2. General blood investigations (including FBC and U&Es) should be performed in all patients – SIADH occurs reasonably frequently in encephalitis.

## A6: What treatment options are appropriate?

In this patient, the mostly likely diagnosis is encephalitis. The aetiology of encephalitis is usually infectious and is most commonly the result of herpes simplex virus 1 or 2, although varicella zoster virus, Epstein–Barr virus, cytomegalovirus, measles, mumps, rubella, tick-borne disease and rickettsiae may also cause encephalitis. Outside the UK, other infective agents such as West Nile virus and Japanese B virus should be considered. In the immunocompromised patient, fungal and parasitic agents should be considered. With the exception of herpes simplex virus and varicella zoster virus encephalitis, the viral forms of encephalitis are not currently treatable. Symptomatic treatment is necessary in all patients. The antiviral agent aciclovir given IV for 10–14 days reduces both mortality and morbidity in herpes simplex virus and varicella zoster virus encephalitis. Aciclovir is given in all patients because clinically it is not possible to distinguish between the various forms of encephalitis. If there is significant cerebral oedema, treatment with the osmotic diuretic mannitol or corticosteroids needs to be considered (e.g. dexamethasone). If therapy is started early, the survival rate is over 90 per cent, although neuropsychiatric sequelae are common. If seizures are present, anticonvulsants should be started and continued for some months once the condition has resolved.

In practice antibiotics (as used for empirical bacterial meningitis therapy) are often started on admission (because bacterial meningitis is sometimes initially considered). If the investigations suggest a brain tumour, the imaging characteristics may suggest that this is either primary or secondary (i.e. metastatic). Further investigation to identify the site of the primary tumour and liaison with neurosurgeons and oncologists are indicated. If investigations suggest a brain abscess, investigation as to the source and whether there are predisposing factors (e.g. immunodeficiency) must be carried out. Liaison with neurosurgical colleagues is necessary because drainage and excision are often used. Non-surgical management (e.g. with a prolonged course of brain-penetrating antibiotics) is usually reserved for patients with an abscess in a difficult site for surgery.

# CENTRAL NERVOUS SYSTEM DEMYELINATION

## Questions

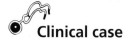

### Clinical case

**For the case scenario given, consider the following:**

> **Q1**: What is the likely differential diagnosis?
> **Q2**: What issues in the given history support or refute a particular diagnosis?
> **Q3**: What additional features would you seek to support a particular diagnosis?
> **Q4**: What clinical examination would you perform, and why?
> **Q5**: What investigations would be most helpful, and why?
> **Q6**: What treatment options are appropriate?

### CASE 11.14 – A 35-year-old white woman presents with a 3-day history of progressive numbness below the umbilicus, with mild weakness of the lower limbs and urinary frequency.

Five years previously the patient had a subacute episode of uncomfortable visual loss in the right eye with full recovery over a week.

## Answers

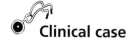

## Clinical case

CASE 11.14 – **A 35-year-old white woman presents with a 3-day history of progressive numbness below the umbilicus, with mild weakness of the lower limbs and urinary frequency.**

### A1: What is the likely differential diagnosis?

The likely differential diagnoses are inflammation of the spinal cord (transverse myelitis) and spinal cord compression.

### A2: What issues in the given history support or refute a particular diagnosis?

The most likely cause is inflammation of the spinal cord (transverse myelitis). The symptoms of lower limb weakness, a sensory level at the umbilicus and urinary dysfunction localize the problem to the thoracic cord. In patients of this age group, the gradual-onset history is suggestive of transverse myelitis, although a gradual onset may also occur in certain causes of spinal cord compression (e.g. tumour, epidural abscess). The previous history of visual disturbance suggests a previous inflammatory lesion in the optic nerve (optic neuritis) and that this event is also the result of central nervous system (CNS) inflammation (transverse myelitis). (A spinal cord infarction would be of sudden onset but would cause the same examination findings.)

### A3: What additional features would you seek to support a particular diagnosis?

A preceding viral illness is suggestive of an inflammatory cause. Back pain is often a feature of spinal cord compression (trauma, tumour, epidural abscess), although mild back discomfort can occur in transverse myelitis. In cases of spinal cord compression caused by epidural abscess, the patient may be systemically unwell with a fever.

### A4: What clinical examination would you perform, and why?

First, it is important to localize the lesion. In a thoracic spinal cord lesion, the patient should have increased tone in the legs, a pyramidal pattern of weakness and a sensory level on the trunk. Lower limb reflexes will be brisk and plantar responses up-going. A fever may occur in an epidural abscess. Mild pyrexia is compatible with a transverse myelitis.

Vertebral tenderness occurs in an epidural abscess and may occur in spinal cord tumour. Although the patient has made a full symptomatic recovery from her previous visual problem, examination may reveal impaired colour vision and a pale optic disc in the affected eye (both signs of optic nerve damage).

### A5: What investigations would be most helpful, and why?

The subacute progressive onset after a viral infection in a previously well young woman is typical of transverse myelitis. Spinal cord compression, e.g. from a tumour, can present in a similar manner but is rare. Compression from an intervertebral disc would be unlikely in patients of this age group, and compression from an epidural abscess or spinal abscess is often (but not exclusively) associated with fever and localized spinal tenderness. Transverse myelitis is inflammation of the spinal cord. It may occur in isolation or in the setting of another illness. It may be associated with infections (viral or bacterial, e.g. *Mycoplasma pneumoniae*, *Borrelia* spp., syphilis, tuberculosis), autoimmune disease (e.g. systemic lupus erythematosus, Sjögren's syndrome, sarcoidosis). Occasionally vitamin B12 deficiency can produce a spinal cord syndrome that may mimic transverse myelitis. In the western world, transverse myelitis in patients of this age group is most frequently associated with multiple sclerosis (MS). It is likely that this patient has MS because she has had a previous event consistent with inflammation in another part of the CNS (the optic nerves).

Magnetic resonance imaging at this level will help to distinguish between an inflammatory and a compressive lesion in the thoracic spinal cord. It is important, however, to image the whole spinal cord because occasionally lesions higher up can produce a similar clinical picture. Imaging of the brain and cervical spine is necessary because MS causes a characteristic pattern of inflammation in the brain, and inflammatory changes may also be identified within the cervical spine.

A lumbar puncture may be helpful to look for further evidence of CNS inflammation. Oligoclonal bands unique to the CSF are consistent with the underlying cause of the symptoms being MS. Visual-evoked potentials examine the integrity of the visual pathways by showing the patient a flashing chessboard pattern on a monitor and attaching electrical 'pick-ups' over the visual cortices. These may also provide paraclinical evidence of more widespread inflammatory problems within the CNS (as found in MS).

Multiple sclerosis is an idiopathic autoimmune inflammatory disease of the CNS characterized by inflammation and demyelination of the white matter in the brain and spinal cord. It is the most common neurological disease to affect young adults. The aetiology is uncertain, although both genetic and environmental factors are known to be important. In common with various autoimmune diseases, the condition occurs more frequently in women. Onset is usually between the ages of 30 and 40 years. Typically, patients initially suffer relapsing episodes of neurological dysfunction, with full or partial remissions (relapsing–remitting MS). The relapses may be provoked by infection.

After about 10 years, patients tend to slowly become more disabled, even between relapses (secondary progressive phase MS).

Common forms of neurological disturbance in MS include transverse myelitis, optic neuritis (a subacute, usually unilateral visual loss, with pain on eye movement and a relative afferent pupillary defect, i.e. the pupil of the affected eye does not respond to light but the consensual reflex is maintained – there is usually a full clinical recovery), and brainstem or cerebellar disturbances.

A definite diagnosis of MS is given when a patient has had at least two attacks of demyelination (hence 'multiple') at two different sites in the CNS at different time points. Visual evoked potentials may provide paraclinical evidence of demyelination within the clinically unaffected visual system and provide some evidence of lesions disseminated in the site. Magnetic resonance imaging provides similar information and is more useful. Multiple sclerosis produces high-signal inflammatory lesions in the brain in a periventricular distribution, and inflammatory changes may also be found in the cervical spinal cord. Other autoimmune or connective tissue disorders may cause changes in the brain and spinal cord that can be identified on MRI, but the periventricular pattern is fairly specific to MS.

If a patient presents with an episode of transverse myelitis without a significant past history, he or she has a 'clinically isolated syndrome'. It is uncertain whether this could be a one-off event, or the first symptom of MS. The presence of periventricular lesions on brain MRI, or oligoclonal bands in the CSF, is highly suggestive that the patient will have further neurological events affecting the CNS and thus be diagnosed with MS.

## A6: What treatment options are appropriate?

Intravenous corticosteroids, usually given as 1 g prednisolone IV every day for 3 days, are the treatment of choice for all relapses in MS. Corticosteroids speed up the rate of recovery but do not modulate the disease process itself. If there are frequent and problematic relapses, disease-modifying therapies (interferon beta or copolymer) can reduce the relapse rate. Emerging data are showing encouraging results for a large number of immunomodulatory treatments (e.g. fingolimod, natalizumab, alemtuzumab), some of which may influence the rate of disability progression.

# DISORDERS OF CRANIAL NERVES

## Questions

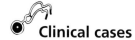

### Clinical cases

**For each of the case scenarios given, consider the following:**

**Q1**: What is the likely differential diagnosis?
**Q2**: What issues in the given history support or refute a particular diagnosis?
**Q3**: What additional features would you seek to support a particular diagnosis?
**Q4**: What clinical examination would you perform, and why?
**Q5**: What investigations would be most helpful, and why?
**Q6**: What treatment options are appropriate?

CASE 11.15 – **A 35-year-old man who has recently had a viral infection presents with a 48-h history of progressive-onset drooping of the left side of his face.**

He has noticed his sense of taste is worse and noises seem louder.

CASE 11.16 – **A 55-year-old man with diabetes presents with a 4-day history of progressive painful right periorbital pain, drooping of the right eyelid and double vision.**

When he lifted his eyelid he noted that his right eye seemed to be deviated 'down and out' and he is unable to move it.

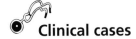

## Answers

### Clinical cases

#### CASE 11.15 – A 35-year-old man who has recently had a viral infection presents with a 48-h history of progressive-onset drooping of the left side of his face.

#### A1: What is the likely differential diagnosis?

The most likely diagnosis is Bell's palsy – an acute inflammatory lower motor neuron lesion of the facial nerve. This may be associated with a viral infection and may occur in all age groups and in both sexes. Maximum facial paralysis generally occurs in 48 h and in almost all cases within 5 days.

The facial nerve runs through the parotid gland, and so parotid tumours may cause a facial nerve palsy. In this situation, the onset may be more insidious.

There are a number of other causes of lower motor neuron facial palsies: Guillain–Barré syndrome, myasthenia gravis, sarcoidosis (a multisystem granulomatous inflammatory disease) and Lyme disease (caused by the tick *Borrelia burgdorferi*) can cause lower motor facial paralysis but are rare and usually bilateral. Moreover, one would expect additional signs and symptoms.

#### A2: What issues in the given history support or refute a particular diagnosis?

Bell's palsy may be associated with a viral infection, particularly herpes simplex virus. It is important to remember that the facial nerve runs through the parotid gland, and parotid tumours may cause facial nerve palsy; in this case, however, the onset would be expected to be insidious.

Hyperacusis (painful sensitivity to noise) occurs because of involvement of a branch of the facial nerve supplying the stapedius muscle, which acts to damp the ossicular chain. Taste sensation to the anterior two-thirds of the tongue is affected because the trigeminal nerve fibres that run in the chorda tympani nerve and supply the tongue join and travel with the facial nerve.

An upper motor neuron facial weakness is unlikely with this history, partly because other associated symptoms of sensory motor disturbance would be expected.

#### A3: What additional features would you seek to support a particular diagnosis?

Bell's palsy affects only the facial nerve, and more extensive symptoms would therefore be unlikely. In cases of parotid tumour, the patient may have noted swelling of the cheek.

#### A4: What clinical examination would you perform, and why?

Examination should confirm features of a left lower motor neuron facial lesion, such as left-sided facial weakness, difficulty in closing the left eye and an inability to furrow the left side of the forehead.

The forehead is bilaterally innervated by the facial nerve. In an upper motor neuron lesion causing unilateral facial paralysis, the forehead is therefore spared.

It is important to examine the patient for signs of a viral herpes zoster skin rash in the external auditory canal and mucous membranes of the oropharynx; this combination of Bell's palsy and herpes zoster is termed Ramsay Hunt syndrome.

## A5: What investigations would be most helpful, and why?

Bell's palsy is a clinical diagnosis. In practice, if examination reveals only a lower motor neuron facial nerve palsy, then no other investigations are needed at this stage.

## A6: What treatment options are appropriate?

If the eyelid does not close properly, the cornea can be damaged. The eye must be protected (e.g. taped shut), particularly during sleep.

Around 80 per cent of patients with Bell's palsy recover within a month. Early recovery of some motor function in the first 5 days is a favourable prognostic sign. A short course of oral corticosteroids combined with an antiviral agent is associated with improved recovery. If the patient does not recover it is worth reconsidering the cause. Ultrasonography of the parotid gland will identify a tumour causing compression of the facial nerve. Brain imaging will help identify tumours that invade the temporal bone and can cause facial palsy. A lumbar puncture will help in identifying evidence of Lyme disease and other infective agents.

## CASE 11.16 – **A 55-year-old man with diabetes presents with a 4-day history of progressive painful right periorbital pain, drooping of the right eyelid and double vision.**

### A1: What is the likely differential diagnosis?

The likely differential diagnoses are compressive right nerve III palsy and infarction of the right nerve III.

### A2: What issues in the given history support or refute a particular diagnosis?

The hallmarks of a nerve III palsy are unilateral ptosis and ophthalmoplegia, the eye being deviated down and out.

### A3: What additional features would you seek to support a particular diagnosis?

If the cause of nerve III palsy is compression, the pupil of the affected eye will be fixed and dilated (pupil-involving nerve III palsy). If the cause of nerve III palsy is infarction of the nerve, the pupil of the affected eye is unaffected (pupil-sparing nerve III palsy). Enlargement of the pupil is a sign of compression because the pupilloconstrictor fibres are located peripherally in the nerve. Infarction of nerve III characteristically involves the central portion of the nerve but spares the peripheral fibres.

Pain may be a feature of both compression and infarction of cranial nerve III. Nerve III infarction is common in people with diabetes and hypertension. It is important, however, not to assume that this patient has a nerve III infarct just because he has a vascular risk factor.

### A4: What clinical examination would you perform, and why?

Pupillary examination is important to help distinguish between a compressive nerve III palsy and a vascular cause, for the reasons outlined above. In a nerve III palsy, the ptosis is often quite profound. The eye should be deviated down and out.

As a rule of thumb, all cases of painful pupil involving nerve III palsies suggest a compressive cause.

### A5: What investigations would be most helpful, and why?

If the patient has a painful pupil-involving nerve III palsy, an urgent CT scan of the brain and a CT angiogram are needed.

The acute onset of a painful pupil-involving nerve III palsy suggests a rapidly expanding lesion such as an aneurysm, most commonly of the posterior communicating artery. It is vital not to miss this. There is a significant risk of the aneurysm bursting and causing a subarachnoid haemorrhage. Computed tomography and CT angiography are likely to identify an aneurysm. If an aneurysm is identified, it is important to liaise with neurosurgical and neuroradiological colleagues to consider clipping the aneurysm or endovascular ablation.

If no aneurysm is identified, other causes of compressive nerve III palsy should be considered, such as tumours, carcinomatous lesions of the skull base or cavernous sinus, inflammatory lesions of the nerve or orbit, and giant cell arteritis. These are often accompanied by other symptoms or signs, however. An ESR and MRI of the brain (with contrast or with venogram sequences) are helpful in identifying these other causes.

In a pupil-sparing nerve III palsy, imaging may show evidence of cardiovascular disease and vascular risk factors should be explored.

# MOVEMENT DISORDERS

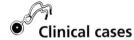

## Clinical cases

## For each of the case scenarios given, consider the following:

**Q1**: What is the likely differential diagnosis?
**Q2**: What issues in the given history support or refute a particular diagnosis?
**Q3**: What additional features would you seek to support a particular diagnosis?
**Q4**: What clinical examination would you perform, and why?
**Q5**: What investigations would be most helpful, and why?
**Q6**: What treatment options are appropriate?

## CASE 11.17 – A 60-year-old woman attends with gradual-onset very slowly progressive tremor in both hands over 10 years.

The tremor is not present at rest. The patient finds it difficult to drink or to use cutlery. She comments that her grandfather, mother and brother had or have similar symptoms. She finds that a small tot of whisky helps ease the tremor.

## CASE 11.18 – A 25-year-old man with 'psychiatric problems' presents with a progressive 2-year history of 'movement problems' (at rest and on intention) and slurring of speech.

The patient's cousin died in his teens of a 'liver problem'.

# Answers

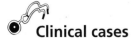

## Clinical cases

### CASE 11.17 – **A 60-year-old woman attends with gradual-onset very slowly progressive tremor in both hands over 10 years.**

**A1:** What is the likely differential diagnosis?

The likely diagnosis is benign essential tremor.

**A2:** What issues in the given history support or refute a particular diagnosis?

Benign essential tremor is familial in 50 per cent of cases (autosomal dominant), and there may be a striking improvement with alcohol. It tends to affect both hands. It is slowly progressive.

**A3:** What additional features would you seek to support a particular diagnosis?

The tremor is characteristically coarse, affects the upper limbs distally, and is exacerbated by sustained postures. Cerebellar tremor is different because it is particularly evoked when attempting fine coordinated movements.

**A4:** What clinical examination would you perform, and why?

Other than the coarse symmetrical tremor, more prominent when the patient holds her hands outstretched, no other abnormalities are identified.

**A5:** What investigations would be most helpful, and why?

Benign essential tremor is a clinical diagnosis, and investigations are not generally necessary. Occasionally, in the early stages, benign essential tremor can be confused with Parkinson's disease.

**A6:** What treatment options are appropriate?

Propranolol or primidone may be appropriate. Not all patients require treatment, however, and often the treatment response is poor.

### CASE 11.18 – **A 25-year-old man with 'psychiatric problems' presents with a progressive 2-year history of 'movement problems' (at rest and on intention) and slurring of speech.**

**A1:** What is the likely differential diagnosis?

The likely differential diagnoses are an organic movement disorder (Wilson's disease), a drug-related movement disorder and a psychogenic movement disorder.

**A2:** What issues in the given history support or refute a particular diagnosis?

Progressive onset tremor in a patient with a psychiatric problem may be a drug-related tremor caused by antipsychotic medication. It is possible that the patient has a dyskinesia from antipsychotic medication (which can also cause parkinsonian-type symptoms). An alternative is that he has a psychogenic movement disorder.

In any young patient with a movement disorder, it is important to consider and exclude the diagnosis of Wilson's disease. Wilson's disease is an autosomal recessive inherited condition caused by mutation in the ATP7B gene on chromosome 13q. The gene is expressed predominantly in liver, kidney and placenta and, to a lesser extent, in heart, brain, lung, muscle and pancreas; the result is an excess of tissue copper deposition. Liver disease is the most common presenting problem in children. Neurological features are a more common mode of presentation in adults. About 35–50 per cent of patients present with neurological or psychiatric symptoms. The condition is important because it is treatable. If left untreated, however, it is fatal. As this young man has a psychiatric history and a family history of liver disease, it is highly likely that the diagnosis is Wilson's disease.

## A3: What additional features would you seek to support a particular diagnosis?

It is important to find out the patient's psychiatric medication and doses. Antipsychotics can cause dyskinesia. Even if the patient is on high doses of antipsychotic medication, Wilson's disease must be excluded.

## A4: What clinical examination would you perform, and why?

Typical findings in Wilson's disease are irregular random brief abrupt movements of the arms (chorea). A brown crescentic deposit in the periphery of the iris, known as the Kayser–Fleischer ring, is often found, particularly in patients with significant neurological involvement; this is a granular deposit of copper. If the patient has brown eyes, the deposit may not be easy to visualize. Signs of liver disease may also be present.

## A5: What investigations would be most helpful, and why?

The following investigations may be helpful:

- slit-lamp microscope examination to identify the Kayser–Fleischer ring
- low serum copper level
- low serum caeruloplasmin level
- increased 24h urinary copper level
- MRI of the brain often shows changes in the basal ganglia.

## A6: What treatment options are appropriate?

Copper-chelating agents such as penicillamine are appropriate, with monitoring of serum copper to guide treatment.

# MISCELLANEOUS NEUROLOGICAL DISORDERS

## Questions

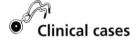

### Clinical cases

## For each of the case scenarios given, consider the following:

> **Q1**: What is the likely differential diagnosis?
> **Q2**: What issues in the given history support or refute a particular diagnosis?
> **Q3**: What additional features would you seek to support a particular diagnosis?
> **Q4**: What clinical examination would you perform, and why?
> **Q5**: What investigations would be most helpful, and why?
> **Q6**: What treatment options are appropriate?

## CASE 11.19 – A 30-year-old woman presents with a 3-month history of feeling generally lethargic, intermittent drooping of her left eye and intermittent double vision.

The patient feels her muscles are generally weaker. These symptoms are worse towards the end of the day. She has also noticed that her voice is weaker, again worse at the end of the day.

## CASE 11.20 – A previously well 50-year-old man presents with a 5-month history of progressive weakness in his upper and lower limbs.

The symptoms initially affected the patient's hands, the right more than the left. He comments that the muscles in his hands have got 'thinner' and he has noticed some 'flickering' of the muscles in his arms. There are no sensory symptoms.

## CASE 11.21 – A 50-year-old man presents with a 12-month history of gradual-onset tremor in his right hand.

The tremor is present at rest, and the patient feels that it is aggravated by stress. His handwriting is deteriorating and getting smaller, and he feels that his movements are generally slower. Otherwise his health is good.

##  OSCE counselling case

### OSCE COUNSELLING CASE 11.2 – 'Will I be able to look after myself in 6 months?'

A 35-year-old woman is told she has multiple sclerosis and is concerned that she will not be able to look after herself.

## Answers

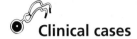
**Clinical cases**

### CASE 11.19 – **A 30-year-old woman presents with a 3-month history of feeling generally lethargic, intermittent drooping of her left eye and intermittent double vision.**

#### A1: What is the likely differential diagnosis?

The likely differential diagnoses are myasthenia gravis and Lambert–Eaton myasthenic syndrome (LEMS).

#### A2: What issues in the given history support or refute a particular diagnosis?

The history is typical of myasthenia gravis, caused by antibodies against acetylcholine (ACh) nicotinic postsynaptic receptors at the neuromuscular junction. Myasthenia gravis has a bimodal age distribution and predominantly affects young adults aged 20–30 years and people over the age of 50 years. Myasthenia gravis is characterized by fluctuating weakness worsened by exertion. Weakness increases during the day and improves with rest. The hallmark of the history and examination is significant fatiguing of the muscles with use.

It can be difficult in practice to distinguish LEMS from myasthenia gravis. Both conditions present with increasing weakness after exertion, and there are also some clinical differences. It is rare for LEMS to present with double vision or dysphagia. In LEMS, the muscles of the trunk, shoulder and pelvic girdle are most frequently involved. It is caused by an autoimmune attack directed against the voltage-gated calcium channels on the presynaptic motor nerve terminal. Fifty per cent of LEMS cases are associated with an underlying neoplasm, particularly small cell carcinoma of the lung.

In this clinical case, the patient is young. LEMS tends to affect people in older age groups, and occurrence at the age of 30 years would be very unusual.

#### A3: What additional features would you seek to support a particular diagnosis?

The patient should be questioned to determine whether she has fatiguing weakness in other muscle groups. In around 25 per cent of patients, myasthenia gravis is confined to the eye muscles, and the clinical features are therefore limited to ptosis and diplopia (ocular myasthenia). The disorder may spread to other areas (generalized myasthenia) over years, however. In generalized myasthenia, the weakness tends to involve predominantly ocular, facial and bulbar muscles (weakness of speech and swallowing) and axial muscles (especially weakness of head flexion).

A history of drug use should be sought. A number of drugs, including aminoglycosides, tetracyclines, penicillamine, beta-blockers, lithium and corticosteroids, can worsen myasthenic symptoms and may therefore provoke symptom onset.

Myasthenia gravis can be associated with autoimmune diseases, and symptoms of thyroid dysfunction should be sought.

#### A4: What clinical examination would you perform, and why?

On examination the patient has a mild ptosis of the left eye. Eye movements appear normal, but after you have finished testing them the patient complains that the double vision seems to be starting again. There is mild proximal muscle weakness. Sensory and reflex examinations are normal.

If the diagnosis of myasthenia gravis is suspected, it is important to actively assess the patient for fatiguability of muscle power. This is an add-on to the general neurological examination and so will be found only if it is specifically considered. One method is to continually or repeatedly test power in a particular muscle group (e.g. up-gaze of the eyes to demonstrate a fatiguable ptosis). Sensory examination and deep tendon reflexes are normal. In LEMS, reflexes are often depressed. It is very important to remember that respiratory muscle weakness may occur, and FVC measurements should be made. Testing for signs of thyroid disease or an enlarged thymus should be carried out.

## A5: What investigations would be most helpful, and why?

Anti-ACh receptor antibodies are present in around 85 per cent of patients with generalized myasthenia gravis and 50 per cent of patients with pure ocular myasthenia gravis. Thyroid abnormalities are associated in about 4 per cent of patients. Computed tomography of the chest is needed because a proportion of patients with myasthenia gravis have a thymoma. Anti-smooth muscle antibodies are present in about 84 per cent of patients with thymoma under 40 years of age.

Edrophonium is a short-acting acetylcholinesterase inhibitor. It potentiates neuromuscular transmission by reducing breakdown of ACh at the neuromuscular junction. A positive edrophonium test shows a significant improvement in muscle power after administration. The test is usually carried out in a double-blind fashion. The test is not used frequently nowadays because of concerns about cardiac side effects. A therapeutic trial of pyridostigmine may provide the same information.

In myasthenia gravis, neurophysiological studies show a decremental response to repetitive stimulation. As fatiguability of respiratory muscles may result in hypoventilatory failure, FVC measurements may be needed to monitor respiratory function.

In LEMS, anti-voltage-gated calcium channel antibodies can be identified with a blood test. Neurophysiological tests often show a marked and progressive increment in the amplitude of response (often termed 'incremental response').

## A6: What treatment options are appropriate?

Pyridostigmine is a longer-acting acetylcholinesterase inhibitor and is helpful for symptomatic control in myasthenia gravis. It may be sufficient in patients with mild ocular symptoms only. Patients with generalized myasthenia gravis also need disease-modifying therapy. Immunosuppression with corticosteroids followed by steroid-sparing agents (e.g. azathioprine) is the standard oral medication of choice. As a short-term dip in myasthenic control may occur when steroids are started, it is common practice to start treatment in hospital and to increase the steroid doses very slowly. Intravenous Ig or plasma exchange can be useful in producing improvement more rapidly. If the patient is found to have a thymoma, it should be surgically removed. In young patients with thymic hyperplasia and high anti-ACh receptor antibodies, thymectomy appears to induce remission in a proportion of patients (although there is no comprehensive evidence base for this).

An underlying malignancy requires treatment. For LEMS, treatment with 3,4-diaminopyridine may be effective. Plasma exchange and IVIG are also helpful.

## CASE 11.20 – A previously well 50-year-old man presents with a 5-month history of progressive weakness in his upper and lower limbs.

### A1: What is the likely differential diagnosis?

The likely differential diagnoses are motor neuron disease (MND), progressive cervical myeloradiculopathy (progressive compression of the cervical cord and cervical nerve roots), multifocal motor neuropathy and myasthenia gravis.

## A2: What issues in the given history support or refute a particular diagnosis?

The most likely diagnosis in this case is MND. Motor neuron disease is a progressive degenerative disorder of motor neurons. As the motor neuron pathway starts within the CNS (in the Betz cells) and travels peripherally, the clinical features of MND may be predominantly upper motor neuron or lower motor neuron, or both. Motor neuron disease usually starts in the fourth to seventh decades of life. It is universally fatal, with a mean disease duration of 3 years. It begins insidiously with weakness (which may be asymmetrical), muscle atrophy or fasciculations in one or more limbs. As the disease progresses, the weakness becomes more symmetrical. It is likely that the 'thinning' of the muscles described by the patient represents atrophy and that the flickering is fasciculations. There are no abnormalities of sensation in MND. No loss of anal sphincter tone occurs, because smooth muscles are not involved.

## A3: What additional features would you seek to support a particular diagnosis?

The most common form of MND involves a combination of upper and lower motor neuron features. Lower motor neuron signs include atrophy and fasciculations, while upper motor neuron (corticospinal tract) signs include up-going plantar response, spasticity and brisk tendon reflexes. More rarely, the disease predominantly affects the motor nuclei of the lower brainstem and causes weakness of the muscles of the jaw, tongue and pharynx (termed 'progressive bulbar palsy'). If lower motor neuron features predominate, the appearances may be similar to myasthenia gravis or LEMS (helpful distinguishing features include the fact that eye signs are common in myasthenia gravis but do not occur in MND, and wasting and fasciculations do not occur in myasthenia gravis or LEMS). If the features are of a dominant lower motor neuron problem of the limbs, a rare form of motor peripheral neuropathy called multifocal motor neuropathy is a possible differential diagnosis (helpful distinguishing features include the fact that in multifocal motor neuropathy there is often little wasting of the muscles). High cervical cord compression (involving exiting nerve roots, i.e. cervical myeloradiculopathy) can mimic the more typical cases of MND where there are mixed upper and lower motor neuron signs. With a spinal cord lesion, however, sphincter function is often affected, whereas sphincter function is preserved in MND.

## A4: What clinical examination would you perform, and why?

Examination normally shows mixed upper and lower motor neuron features.

## A5: What investigations would be most helpful, and why?

Serum creatine phosphokinase is often elevated in MND, but this is non-specific. Magnetic resonance imaging of the cervical spine excludes a cervical cord lesion. In MND, neurophysiological studies show denervation in the muscle groups of at least three different segments of the body (because MND is a diffuse process) and no sensory abnormalities. In multifocal motor neuropathy, neurophysiological studies identify conduction block. The neurophysiological features of myasthenia gravis and LEMS are discussed in Case 11.19.

## A6: What treatment options are appropriate?

Treatment is symptomatic support, although symptomatic treatments for complications (cramps, spasticity, drooling, dysphagia, ventilatory failure) are the mainstay of managing this disease. As the disease progresses, speech and swallowing may become so weak that vocal communication and oral feeding are impossible. A communication board may help the patient with communication, and a percutaneous gastrostomy feeding tube may be necessary to maintain adequate nutrition.

Ventilatory failure as a result of progressive muscle weakness develops in the later stages of the disease. Nocturnal hypoventilation may cause early-morning headache and lethargy. Non-invasive respiratory support (e.g. nocturnal ventilatory support using a tight-fitting mask) can help alleviate these symptoms.

The use of invasive ventilation (e.g. ventilation via tracheostomy) is a complex issue. It will prolong life but may well prolong suffering. It may also result in an altered mode of death (e.g. pneumonia). To try to accommodate the patient's wishes, it is important to discuss these issues at an appropriate, but relatively early, stage in the disease.

Riluzole is a disease-modifying therapy with a modest effect. It results in a modest decrease in risk of tracheostomy or death by about 20 per cent over 12 months of treatment. It does not cause symptomatic improvement, however, and does not prevent death. Side effects such as fatigue, nausea and worsening liver function may necessitate discontinuing treatment.

## CASE 11.21 – **A 50-year-old man presents with a 12-month history of gradual-onset tremor in his right hand.**

### A1: What is the likely differential diagnosis?

The likely differential diagnosis is Parkinson's disease.

### A2: What issues in the given history support or refute a particular diagnosis?

Although other conditions (e.g. benign essential tremor, vascular parkinsonism, 'Parkinson plus' syndromes) can cause diagnostic confusion, this history is particularly suggestive of Parkinson's disease.

### A3: What additional features would you seek to support a particular diagnosis?

The cardinal features of Parkinson's disease are tremor, bradykinesia and rigidity. Patients are often noted to have an 'expressionless' face, and their handwriting becomes smaller (micrographia). They have poor arm swing and may have stooped posture (particularly later in the disease course). Frequent falls, shuffling gait, difficulty in initiating movements and 'freezing up' occur later in the disease course.

Some patients with cerebrovascular disease may have a parkinsonian appearance. This tends to manifest in a slow, stiff, rigid-type gait, and tremor is not a major feature.

### A4: What clinical examination would you perform, and why?

The tremor is 'pill rolling' (imagine rolling a pill between the index finger and thumb), which occurs at rest and *not* by intention. This is an important difference from cerebellar tremor, which is typically brought out by testing limb coordination (e.g. when attempting to touch the tip of the examiner's moving finger).

The tone will appear generally increased (rigidity), and movements (especially rapid alternating movements) will be slower (bradykinesia).

### A5: What investigations would be most helpful, and why?

In typical cases the diagnosis is made on clinical grounds alone.

### A6: What treatment options are appropriate?

Treatment is symptomatic and does not alter the disease course. If the patient does not have functional limitation, treatment can be deferred. In this particular case, the patient appears to be limited and it would be appropriate to begin treatment.

There is an argument for trying to delay drug treatment in Parkinson's disease for as long as possible. The earlier treatment is started, the earlier the patient starts to develop difficult side effects such as unwanted movements (dyskinesias). These issues should be discussed with the patient. The gold standard, most efficacious treatment is L-dopa, which must be combined with a peripheral decarboxylase inhibitor to minimize peripheral side effects such as nausea and vomiting. There is evidence, however, that treatment with L-dopa may be associated with an earlier onset of limiting dyskinesia, relative to the newer, but less efficacious dopamine agonists that boost in vivo dopamine production. Currently it is usual practice to delay the use of L-dopa and to begin treatment with a dopamine agonist. Treatment response in the early years of the disease is very good. L-Dopa is added in when the effects of the dopamine agonists are no longer sufficient.

Dopamine is known to play a part in the reward system of the brain. It is increasingly recognized that dopaminergic drugs, including dopamine agonists, may produce significant behavioural side effects. Patients may become hypomanic or hypersexualized or indulge in compulsive behaviours such as compulsive gambling, eating disorders or punding (repetition of complex behavioural patterns such as collecting). Rasagaline, a relatively new monoamine oxidase inhibitor type B, is increasingly used as early monotherapy in Parkinson's disease, in part because of this syndrome.

In later disease, the disease itself and the effects of treatment become more unpredictable. Higher doses of medication may be required to control symptoms, but these may cause limiting dyskinesias. Catechol-O-methyltransferase inhibitors are used as treatment adjuncts, e.g. to prolong the duration of action or minimize the dose of L-dopa. Apomorphine given subcutaneously is used in the late stage, when patients are poorly responsive to oral treatment; this reduces the duration of the 'off' periods when patients are unable to move. Neurosurgery (deep brain stimulation) may benefit carefully selected patients who have symptoms that cannot be controlled with medication.

**OSCE counselling case**

## OSCE COUNSELLING CASE 11.2 – 'Will I be able to look after myself in 6 months?'

The patient must be informed by a senior doctor and given time to ask any questions that they may have. The patient should have family members with them if they wish. Offering a follow-up consultation soon afterwards is useful to address any issues that the patient later thinks of. Specialist nurses play a particularly valuable role in this follow-up.

It should be explained that patients with MS have a tendency to inflammation within the brain and spinal cord, and that they may therefore experience episodes (termed 'relapses') of weakness, sensory problems or visual disturbance.

Patients are often very frightened that they may quickly become disabled. At diagnosis, it is important to try to help the patient be positive about the condition. It can be helpful to explain that a significant proportion of patients do not suffer significant fixed deficit for many years, and that there is even a category of 'benign' MS. It is also helpful to explain that there are effective symptomatic treatments for MS. In addition, if a relapse causes a significant functional deficit, corticosteroid pulses speed recovery. If there are frequent and problematic relapses, disease-modifying therapies can reduce the relapse rate, and some may influence the progression of disability.

It should be explained that the cause of MS is unknown but that there is a genetic susceptibility and infections can trigger relapses. Pregnancy is not a problem in MS, and in fact there is often a slight improvement during pregnancy. The risk of MS occurring in the children of patients with MS is about 3–5 per cent. The patient should be offered the contact details of the MS Society, which can offer support and advice. As MS is a chronic neurological disease, all patients receive regular follow-up. Many regions also have specialist nurse support for this condition.

## REVISION PANEL

- Seizures may be classified as generalized (consciousness lost) or partial (consciousness not lost).
- Epilepsy is a long-term diagnosis. Issues surrounding AED choice, seizure triggers (fatigue, alcohol and other drugs, stress, occasionally photosensitivity), specific issues for women, driving regulations, safety in the home, and the cognitive effects of epilepsy and AEDs must be discussed with the patient.
- Carotid artery dissection is a significant cause of stroke in patients under the age of 40 years.
- Ascending numbness and weakness about 10 days after an acute infection is typical of Guillain–Barré syndrome, which is an acute peripheral neuropathy causing weakness, paraesthesia and hyporeflexia.
- A chronic peripheral neuropathy may be caused by diabetes mellitus, chronic excess alcohol intake, vitamin B12 and folate deficiency, thyroid disease, renal failure, autoimmune diseases (which may cause a vasculitic neuropathy) and paraproteinaemia (e.g. multiple myeloma).
- Carpal tunnel syndrome is common in conditions where the carpal tunnel becomes narrowed, such as in pregnancy, trauma, rheumatoid arthritis and hypothyroidism. Worsening of symptoms at night, and relief on shaking the affected hand, are typical of carpal tunnel syndrome. It is an example of an isolated mononeuropathy.
- Symptoms of a subarachnoid haemorrhage are a sudden-onset worst-ever headache, similar to a blow to the back of the head. There may be focal neurological signs that give a clue as to the cause of the bleed – e.g. a nerve III palsy suggests a posterior communicating artery aneurysm.
- Other causes of headaches include bacterial meningitis, viral meningitis, cerebral venous sinus thrombosis, benign intracranial hypertension, giant cell arteritis and migraine.
- Trigeminal neuralgia tends to occur in people aged over 60 years and is more common in women. It is characterized by brief paroxysms of pain localized in the maxillary or mandibular divisions of the trigeminal nerve.
- Symptoms of lower limb weakness, a sensory level at the umbilicus and urinary dysfunction of gradual onset are suggestive of a transverse myelitis, although a gradual onset may also occur in certain causes of spinal cord compression (e.g. tumour, epidural abscess).
- Multiple sclerosis is an idiopathic autoimmune inflammatory disease of the CNS characterized by inflammation and demyelination of the white matter in the brain and spinal cord.
- Bell's palsy is an acute inflammatory lower motor neuron lesion of the facial nerve. Other causes of lower motor neuron facial palsies include Guillain–Barré syndrome, myasthenia gravis, sarcoidosis and Lyme disease.
- Wilson's disease may result in irregular random brief abrupt movements of the arms (chorea). A brown crescentic deposit in the periphery of the iris, known as the Kayser–Fleischer ring, is often found, particularly in patients with significant neurological involvement.
- Parkinson's disease is associated with the triad of tremor, bradykinesia and rigidity.

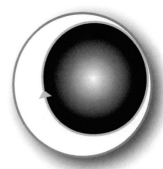

# 12 Infectious diseases

*Chris Ellis*

## Questions

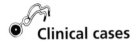

### Clinical cases

## For each of the case scenarios given, consider the following:

> **Q1**: What is the likely diagnosis or differential diagnosis?
> **Q2**: What investigations should be performed?
> **Q3**: What would be the initial management?
> **Q4**: What is the prognosis?

### CASE 12.1 – A 26-year-old man presents with fever, headache and confusion.

A 26-year-old executive presents with a 1-week history of headache and 2 days of confusion. He has a temperature of 39 °C. He returned 3 weeks previously from a 2-week safari in Kenya. Full blood count (FBC) and biochemical profile are normal; computed tomography (CT) shows no abnormality.

### CASE 12.2 – A 30-year-old woman presents with prolonged fever of unknown origin.

A 30-year-old woman is referred with a 6-month history of fever in the evenings, often accompanied by a faint erythematous rash with aches and pain, some of which clearly arise from the joints. She has not lost weight. She has already been investigated extensively, with a normal chest radiograph and abdominal CT. Rheumatoid antibodies and antinuclear antibodies (ANA) are both negative. On examination you find a faint macular rash, a temperature of 39 °C, a 3 cm smooth liver enlargement and 1 cm glands in both axillae. Cardiovascular examination is unremarkable. Blood cultures have yielded no growth.

### CASE 12.3 – A 30-year-old woman has fainted and has fever and a rash.

The patient was well until 48 hours before presentation. Her illness began with nausea and vomiting, and later she felt feverish. On the morning of admission she got up, and then felt faint and briefly lost consciousness. On admission her temperature is 39 °C, her pulse is 110/min, and her blood pressure is 100/60 mmHg supine. There is a diffuse erythematous rash on her face and trunk, which blanches on pressure. She is menstruating.

### CASE 12.4 – A 30-year-old man presents with productive cough, feverishness and weight loss.

A 30-year-old Somali man who has lived in the UK for 2 years presents with 1 month of productive cough, feverishness and weight loss. On examination, he is thin but otherwise no abnormality is detected. A chest radiograph shows patchy consolidation of the right upper zone. There is no significant past medical history.

## CASE 12.5 – **A 36-year-old woman presents with fever, headache and a rash.**

A 36-year-old female university lecturer presents with 3 days of fever, headache and a rash that she describes as 'a return of her suntan'. Four weeks earlier she returned from a 2-week holiday in Kenya. She is on no medication. She has several 1 cm diameter glands in her neck, pharyngitis and a maculopapular rash on her trunk. Her temperature is 38 °C.

## CASE 12.6 – **A 22-year-old man presents with persistent diarrhoea and weight loss.**

A 22-year-old male medical student presents 6 weeks after returning from his elective period in Nepal. While there, he had two episodes of watery diarrhoea and took a single dose of ciprofloxacin on each occasion; his symptoms settled within 48 h. He was well on return but developed watery diarrhoea 1 week later, which has persisted; he now reports five or six motions a day, with some abdominal distension and excessive flatus. He has lost 6 kg in the past 2 weeks.

## 👥 OSCE counselling cases

OSCE COUNSELLING CASE 12.1 – 'I am a 26-year-old builder. Last year I fell off a ladder and had to have my spleen removed. Someone in the pub told me I can die of septicaemia. Was he right, and what can I do about it?'

OSCE COUNSELLING CASE 12.2 – 'I am a gay man who has one regular partner, but occasionally I have sex with new male acquaintances. Although I try to remember to "play safe", I don't think I have always succeeded. I am fully fit and, as far as I know, none of my partners is HIV positive. Would you advise me to be tested?'

OSCE COUNSELLING CASE 12.3 – 'I am a 24-year-old mother of a 6-month-old baby girl. My widowed mother was recently in hospital for a hip replacement, and her wound was infected with methicillin-resistant *Staphylococcus aureus* (MRSA). I love my mother but don't want her in my home as she could infect my baby. In any case, shouldn't she have been kept in hospital?'

## Key concepts

The following are definitions of sepsis, often referred to in the literature as systemic inflammatory response syndrome (SIRS).

- Sepsis: two or more of:
  - temperature >38 °C or <36 °C
  - pulse >90/min
  - respiratory rate >20/min
  - white blood cell count (WBC) >12 000 or <4000.
- Severe sepsis: sepsis with one or more of:
  - hypotension
  - confusion
  - oliguria
  - hypoxia
  - acidosis
  - disseminated intravascular coagulation (DIC).
- Septic shock: severe sepsis with hypotension despite fluid resuscitation.

# Answers

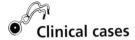

## Clinical cases

### CASE 12.1 – A 26-year-old man presents with fever, headache and confusion.

#### A1: What is the likely diagnosis or differential diagnosis?

Headache, fever and confusion suggest encephalitis, but this man is at risk of falciparum malaria, which can produce a picture identical to encephalitis (so-called cerebral malaria). The differential diagnosis therefore includes two conditions for which early treatment can be literally vital – herpes simplex encephalitis and falciparum malaria.

#### A2: What investigations should be performed?

A haematological sample should be sent immediately to look for malarial parasites, which will usually be seen as rings within erythrocytes. It is crucial that the request be made specifically, because automated cell counters do not detect malarial parasites. The normal CT excludes cerebral swelling, and so it is safe to perform a lumbar puncture; the cerebrospinal fluid (CSF) may contain lymphocytes and erythrocytes in keeping with a primary encephalitis.

#### A3: What would be the initial management?

It would be prudent to cover both of the treatable life-threatening possible diagnoses, unless the blood film conclusively confirms falciparum malaria. Malaria should be covered by intravenous (IV) quinine (consult the current British National Formulary for details, and confer with the regional infectious diseases department), and IV aciclovir will cover herpes encephalitis.

#### A4: What is the prognosis?

The prognosis of severe malaria is good, provided the patient survives the first few days, but during that period the full sepsis syndrome may be encountered, with acute renal failure, disseminated intravascular coagulation (DIC) and adult respiratory distress syndrome (ARDS).

About a third of patients with herpes encephalitis die, a third survive with varying degrees of permanent brain damage, and a third eventually make a virtually complete recovery. Early treatment is crucial to a good outcome, but even patients who are treated very promptly may have permanent brain damage.

### CASE 12.2 – A 30-year-old woman presents with prolonged fever of unknown origin.

#### A1: What is the likely diagnosis or differential diagnosis?

This is adult systemic Still's disease. Patients who have been pyrexial for several weeks usually turn out to have occult infection, occult neoplasm (lymphoma or non-obstructing cancers, e.g. renal) or a connective tissue disorder. This story is typical of systemic Still's disease in young adults.

#### A2: What investigations should be performed?

First-line investigations for pyrexia of unknown origin are FBC and biochemical profile, blood culture, midstream urine, and chest radiograph (with malarial parasites requested specifically and urgently if the patient has been in a malarial area in the preceding 3 months). If these are unhelpful, proceed to ANA and imaging of the abdomen (ultrasonography is usually available first, but CT is necessary if ultrasonography is inconclusive and no other diagnosis has emerged).

Adult Still's disease is underrecognized, partly because there is no specific test. It has some definite features, however:

- daily fever (typically early evening)
- arthralgia/arthritis
- negative rheumatoid factor and negative ANA
- two of: leucocytosis; rash-transient erythema, often with fever; serositis (e.g. pleural effusion); hepatomegaly; splenomegaly; generalized lymphadenopathy.

## A3: What would be the initial management?

A trial of corticosteroids should be the initial management. Clinicians are often reluctant to give steroids to patients for fear of lighting up occult infection. In practice, this is almost never a problem. Prolonged steroid therapy can, indeed, lead to activity of dormant tuberculosis (TB), but it makes little difference to most bacterial infections. Furthermore, the response in conditions such as Still's disease is usually rapid and decisive so that, if the patient is not apyrexial and dramatically improved within 3 days, the therapy should be reconsidered.

## A4: What is the prognosis?

The prognosis is usually good. It may take several months before the patient can be weaned off steroids entirely, and relapses are common for about 5 years after the first episode, after which they usually cease. A minority of patients develop an established connective tissue disorder such as a rheumatoid disorder.

## CASE 12.3 – **A 30-year-old woman has fainted and has fever and a rash.**

### A1: What is the likely diagnosis or differential diagnosis?

There is enough evidence to justify treating this woman for presumed septic shock. A possible focus of infection could be the genital tract; a tampon should be sought and, if present, removed. Toxic shock syndrome (TSS) is a specific form of septic shock caused by toxins liberated by staphylococci, which may colonize the vagina and multiply on tampons or cause soft tissue infection such as cellulitis.

### A2: What investigations should be performed?

Any patient with sepsis should be examined carefully for a focus, including careful inspection for evidence of skin or soft tissue infection, and evidence of focal infection in the thorax, abdomen and pelvis. Blood cultures must be taken. A chest radiograph is mandatory because pneumonia may not be apparent clinically. When appropriate, the vagina should be examined and a tampon or intrauterine contraceptive device (IUCD) removed and cultured.

Sepsis is a clinical diagnosis based on a constellation of abnormalities (see 'Key concepts' above). A positive blood culture (bacteraemia) supports it, and in this case isolation of a toxin-producing *S. aureus* from a tampon would confirm TSS. The critical practical point is, however, that immediate management will not be affected by what the laboratory may report later.

### A3: What would be the initial management?

Initial management includes IV fluids, which should be given as rapidly as possible, and high-dose IV broad-spectrum antibiotics to ensure specific cover for any likely focus. In this case, standard broad-spectrum cover should be augmented by a potent anti-staphylococcal agent such as flucloxacillin. When pneumonia is suggested clinically or radiologically, treatment should be augmented with cover for atypical pathogens (e.g. a macrolide such as clarithromycin or a quinolone). When appropriate, the focus of infection (tampon, IUCD; aspirate or drain fluctuant areas in soft tissue infection) should be removed.

## A4: What is the prognosis?

The prognosis depends very much on the promptness and thoroughness of immediate intervention. Complete recovery is the aim, but the more the initial intervention is delayed, the more likely is progression to a full sepsis syndrome, with circulatory collapse, acute renal failure, ARDS and DIC.

## CASE 12.4 – A 30-year-old man presents with productive cough, feverishness and weight loss.

### A1: What is the likely diagnosis or differential diagnosis?

Pulmonary TB is overwhelmingly the most likely diagnosis. Acute bacterial pneumonias typically progress more rapidly. The absence of a previous history makes bronchiectasis unlikely.

### A2: What investigations should be performed?

Sputum should be sent for TB microscopy and culture. If TB is confirmed, the patient should be tested for human immunodeficiency virus (HIV) after appropriate counselling.

### A3: What would be the initial management?

It is common practice for patients with this presentation to receive an antibacterial appropriate for community-acquired pneumonia (e.g. amoxicillin plus a quinolone or a macrolide such as clarithromycin), pending confirmation of the diagnosis of TB. There is an argument for avoiding quinolones in this context because they have anti-tuberculous activity and it is important to avoid promoting resistance to agents that may be needed in the future to treat TB. Once the diagnosis is confirmed, the patient should be treated with a combination of rifampicin, isoniazid, pyrazinamide and ethambutol for 2 months, reducing to rifampicin and isoniazid for a further 4 months. He will need careful supervision to ensure compliance and recovery. If he is smear-positive (acid-fast bacilli seen on Ziehl–Neelsen staining), he will be highly infectious and will remain so until 2 weeks after the start of treatment. Consider isolating him in hospital for this period.

The patient should be officially notified to the consultant in communicable disease control, who will arrange for screening of household contacts and, if appropriate, of acquaintances and colleagues.

### A4: What is the prognosis?

The prognosis is good. Over 95 per cent of compliant patients with the drug-sensitive strain of TB are cured at the end of the conventional 6-month course of treatment, with a relapse rate of no more than 2 per cent. Most relapses occur within 1 year of stopping treatment. If the patient is HIV-positive, treatment should still cease at 6 months, but the relapse rate will be higher.

## CASE 12.5 – A 36-year-old woman presents with fever, headache and a rash.

### A1: What is the likely diagnosis or differential diagnosis?

Falciparum malaria must be considered in any patient with a fever within 3 months of return from an endemic area. It would not cause lymphadenopathy or a rash. This could be a non-specific viral infection, glandular fever (primary Epstein–Barr virus infection) or a primary HIV illness.

### A2: What investigations should be performed?

A blood sample asking for malaria parasites and a glandular fever screen should be done.

is no reason why colonized patients should not go home, if they are fit enough to manage. If they are admitted to hospital, they may have the depressing experience of being nursed in a side room, because there is some evidence that this reduces the likelihood of transmission to others. Common sites for colonization are the nostrils and wounds. If there is no evidence of an inflammatory response, there is no imperative to treat the patient; if wounds are inflamed, the choice of antibiotic should be guided by sensitivity testing, although there may be no alternative to IV agents such as vancomycin. Colonization can be treated with topical antiseptics in an attempt to eliminate MRSA if readmission to hospital is likely to be necessary within 1 year.

## REVISION PANEL

- Consider sepsis if two or more of the following are present: temperature >38 °C or <36 °C; pulse >90/min; respiratory rate >20/min; white blood cell count >12 000 or <4000.
- Always consider falciparum malaria in a traveller returning from an endemic area. Failure to treat results in acute renal failure, DIC and ARDS.
- Patients who have been pyrexial for several weeks usually turn out to have occult infection, occult neoplasm (lymphoma or non-obstructing cancers, e.g. renal), a connective tissue disorder or rarely Still's disease.
- Toxic shock syndrome is a specific form of septic shock caused by toxins liberated by staphylococci, which may colonize the vagina and multiply on tampons or cause soft tissue infection such as cellulitis.
- Consider pulmonary TB in any person with a chronic productive cough, weight loss and night sweats.
- Primary HIV infection may present as a glandular fever-like illness, often with a rash in patients in whom the underlying diagnosis is not yet established. Other front-door presentations include *P. carinii* pneumonia (typically 3–4 weeks of dry cough, with more recent shortness of breath on effort or fever), oral candidiasis and generalized lymphadenopathy.
- Offer pneumococcal vaccine and life-long prophylactic penicillin to splenectomized patients.

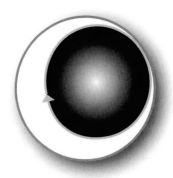

# 13 Dermatology

*Nevianna Tomson*

# MALIGNANT MELANOMA

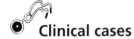

### Clinical cases

## For each of the case scenarios given, consider the following:

> **Q1**: What is the likely differential diagnosis?
> **Q2**: What issues in the given history support the diagnosis?
> **Q3**: What additional features in the history would you seek to support a particular diagnosis?
> **Q4**: What clinical examination would you perform, and why?
> **Q5**: What investigations would be most helpful, and why?
> **Q6**: What treatment options are appropriate?

## CASE 13.1 – A 40-year-old woman presents with a brown mark on her leg.

A 40-year-old woman presents with a 3-month history of a gradually enlarging brown mark over her left shin. It has bled spontaneously on two occasions and appears to have become darker over the past few weeks.

## CASE 13.2 – An 80-year-old woman attends the accident and emergency (A&E) department after a fall at home. She comments that the 'age spot' on her forehead has become 'more noticeable'.

An 80-year-old woman attends A&E after a fall at home. The attending casualty officer incidentally notices a dark brown and black-coloured mark over her forehead. It is entirely asymptomatic and has been present for many years. The patient comments that it has become more noticeable over the past few months.

## CASE 13.3 – A 62-year-old man presents with a brown mark under his thumbnail.

A 62-year-old African Caribbean man presents to his general practitioner (GP) having developed a dark-brown longitudinal streak under his right thumbnail. It has appeared in the past 2 months and is asymptomatic.

## 👥 OSCE counselling cases

### OSCE COUNSELLING CASE 13.1 – 'My mother died of melanoma. Is there anything I should do?'

A 20-year-old woman has come to see you concerned about her risk of developing malignant melanoma. She tells you that her mother died aged 35 years from metastatic malignant melanoma, and her maternal aunt has recently been diagnosed at the age of 50 years with melanoma. Does the woman have an increased risk of developing melanoma? What can she do to minimize her risk of melanoma in the future?

### OSCE COUNSELLING CASE 13.2 – 'What happens now that I have been diagnosed with malignant melanoma?'

A 49-year-old man has recently had a suspicious mole excised from his back. The histology has confirmed this to be a malignant melanoma. He attends the dermatology clinic and is told the diagnosis. What is the next step in his management?

## Key concepts

To work through the core clinical cases in this section, you will need to understand the following key concepts.

Malignant melanoma is an invasive malignant tumour of melanocytes that usually develops in skin that was previously normal, but may arise in a pre-existing mole. The leg is the most common site in women and the back in men, although malignant melanoma can affect any site of the body. Acral lentiginous melanoma is the most common melanoma in oriental and black patients but is rare in white patients. It occurs on palmar and plantar skin and under the nails. Mucosal melanoma may occur in the oral cavity, around the anus or on the genitalia but is rare.

The main diagnostic feature of malignant melanoma is the history of change in a pigmented lesion. The Glasgow Seven-Point Check List and the American ABCDE System have been devised to help with diagnosing malignant melanoma. The Glasgow system lists three major features – change in size, irregularity in colour and irregularity of outline – and four minor features – diameter >6mm, inflammation, bleeding, itching or change in sensation.

Excision biopsy of the mole is suggested in the presence of one major feature. The presence of minor features adds to the suspicion of melanoma. In the UK, the American ABCDE system is mainly used:

- A: asymmetry of the shape of the lesion
- B: irregularity of the border
- C: variation in colour
- D: diameter of the lesion (increase in diameter)
- E: elevation (mole becomes raised or nodular).

A malignant melanoma usually looks different from the patient's other moles.

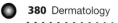

## Answers

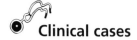

## Clinical cases

### CASE 13.1 – **A 40-year-old woman presents with a brown mark on her leg.**

#### A1: What is the likely differential diagnosis?

The likely differential diagnoses are malignant melanoma, benign mole, seborrhoeic wart, dermatofibroma, freckle, solar lentigo and pigmented basal cell carcinoma (BCC).

#### A2: What issues in the given history support the diagnosis?

The patient gives a clear history of a pigmented lesion that is changing in size and colour. Both of these features suggest malignant melanoma. Melanomas may appear black or have irregular pigmentation with shades of white, red, blue, brown or black. Associated symptoms such as itching or bleeding can also signify that a melanoma is developing but are less important than change in size, shape and colour.

#### A3: What additional features in the history would you seek to support a particular diagnosis?

It is important to establish how the lesion began. Was there a pre-existing mole? If so, when did it start to change? Determine how the lesion has changed. Is it simply a change in diameter, or has its outline become more irregular? Benign moles usually have a symmetrical even outline, whereas malignant melanomas tend to have an irregular edge with one area advancing more than the rest of the lesion. Finally, determine whether there is any family history of skin cancer, in particular malignant melanoma.

#### A4: What clinical examination would you perform, and why?

Examine the lesion in detail. Remember ABCDE. A dermatoscope may be used to examine the lesion more closely and in trained hands improves diagnostic accuracy. If a malignant melanoma is suspected, a general examination to look for secondary metastases is mandatory, paying particular attention to any cervical, axillary or inguinal lymphadenopathy and examining for hepatomegaly.

#### A5: What investigations would be most helpful, and why?

The only way to confirm a melanoma is to excise the lesion and send it for histological analysis. This will determine the Breslow thickness of the melanoma (a measurement, in millimetres, of how deeply tumour cells are invading from the epidermis of the skin into the dermis). The Breslow thickness is related directly to prognosis and will determine whether further tests need to be done. The TNM cancer grading system is used to determine the stage of the melanoma (0–IV) using the Breslow thickness to determine the tumour stage (T), the number of involved lymph nodes to determine the lymph node staging (N), and the presence and number of distant metastases (M). In general, melanomas greater than 2 mm in Breslow thickness are in stage IIB and above; it is recommended that these patients have further investigations, including full blood count (FBC), liver function tests (LFTs), lactate dehydrogenase (LDH), and a computed tomography (CT) scan of the chest, abdomen and pelvis to look for metastases. Patients with tumours that are over 1 mm in Breslow thickness are usually offered a sentinel lymph node biopsy, a new technique that is used to identify the lymph node that drains tissue fluid from the area of the melanoma. The node is then removed to see whether it contains cancer cells.

## A6: What treatment options are appropriate?

Surgical excision is the only definitive treatment for malignant melanoma. Initially the mole is removed with a 2 mm margin of normal skin and analysed for Breslow depth. National Cancer Guidelines recommend a second re-excision of the scar to prevent local recurrence of the melanoma. If the melanoma is of Breslow thickness less than 1 mm, then a 1 cm re-excision is recommended. For lesions of Breslow thickness over 1 mm, a re-excision of 2–3 cm may be recommended. Chemotherapy may be used to palliatively treat metastatic disease, but this is often as part of clinical trials.

## CASE 13.2 – An 80-year-old woman attends A&E after a fall at home. She comments that the 'age spot' on her forehead has become 'more noticeable'.

### A1: What is the likely differential diagnosis?

The likely differential diagnoses are lentigo maligna, lentigo maligna melanoma, solar lentigo, simple or senile lentigo, malignant melanoma, seborrhoeic keratosis and café-au-lait spot.

### A2: What issues in the given history support the diagnosis?

Lentigo maligna is an in situ malignant melanoma. It can closely resemble other pigmented lesions, such as simple or solar lentigos and flat seborrhoeic keratosis. It appears as a flat pigmented lesion with colours that may vary from light tan to dark brown or black. It gradually enlarges but is otherwise asymptomatic. Its margin is usually irregular. It becomes thickened and nodular as it invades through the basement membrane and is then known as lentigo maligna melanoma.

### A3: What additional features in the history would you seek to support a particular diagnosis?

Lentigo maligna typically occurs over sun-exposed areas. Most patients give a history of significant sunlight exposure throughout their lives. Ask the patient whether the lesion is more noticeable because it has enlarged or developed an irregular border or colour.

### A4: What clinical examination would you perform, and why?

Examine the lesion in detail for irregularity in border and colour, and measure its size. In particular, note any nodularity that may suggest progression to lentigo maligna melanoma. Examine the patient for lymphadenopathy.

### A5: What investigations would be most helpful, and why?

Magnification of the lesion by dermoscopy can be useful in trying to distinguish lentigo maligna from simple lentigo and early seborrhoeic keratosis. Incisional or excisional biopsy of the lesion is necessary, however, to confirm the diagnosis of lentigo maligna and distinguish it from lentigo maligna melanoma.

### A6: What treatment options are appropriate?

Ideally, lentigo maligna should be excised surgically. It usually occurs in elderly people, however, and is often quite sizeable at presentation. Dermatologists sometimes prefer to observe these lesions and monitor with serial photographs or perform an incisional biopsy to sample a large part of the lesion.

Excision can be undertaken, especially if the lesion becomes thickened and is suspected to have developed into lentigo maligna melanoma. Early lentigo maligna can also be treated with radiotherapy.

## CASE 13.3 – A 62-year-old man presents with a brown mark under his thumbnail.

### A1: What is the likely differential diagnosis?

The likely differential diagnoses are subungual melanoma, trauma, linear melanonychia (straight, longitudinal, brown/black, evenly pigmented line – common in the nails of black people but very rarely in white people), and fungal nail infection.

### A2: What issues in the given history support the diagnosis?

In the absence of a history of trauma, a subungual melanoma must be considered as the most likely diagnosis.

### A3: What additional features in the history would you seek to support a particular diagnosis?

Ask the patient whether he recalls any trauma to the nail. Are any of the other nails affected in a similar way?

### A4: What clinical examination would you perform, and why?

Examine the nail carefully. In subungual melanoma, the pigment under the nail is deep and often irregular. Deep red/purple colours or pinpoint russet areas suggest haemorrhage from trauma. Look out for Hutchinson's sign – a flat pigmented irregular patch of skin over the nail fold, highly diagnostic of subungual melanoma. The nail may also be deformed and may split as the melanoma underneath thickens. The patient must be examined for metastatic spread.

### A5: What investigations would be most helpful, and why?

A nail biopsy is the only way to confirm or refute the diagnosis.

### A6: What treatment options are appropriate?

The melanoma is surgically excised, which frequently necessitates amputation of the digit.

## 👥 OSCE counselling cases

### OSCE COUNSELLING CASE 13.1 – 'My mother died of melanoma. Is there anything I should do?'

The incidence of melanoma is rapidly increasing. In the UK, it has been estimated that the lifetime risk of developing malignant melanoma is 1 in 91 for men and 1 in 77 for women. Ultraviolet (UV) light is considered to be the most important factor. Intense and infrequent exposure once or twice a year appears to carry a greater risk than chronic continuous sunlight exposure. Fair-skinned people, people with red hair, blue eyes and poor tanning capacity, and people who burn frequently when exposed to sunlight have the greatest risk of developing melanoma.

Most malignant melanomas occur sporadically, but 2–10 per cent of patients diagnosed with malignant melanoma give a positive family history of melanoma in one or more first-degree relatives. This may be a result of inheritance of specific melanoma susceptibility genes or grouping of other known risk factors, such as similar skin type, sun exposure and the number of pigmented naevi in family members.

Prevention of melanoma is extremely important. Patients must be educated on the dangers of UV radiation and sunburn, and the importance of using photoprotection, including clothing, to cover sun-exposed areas and high-factor sunscreens. Patients should also be educated on the features of malignancy to look out for, in order to help with early detection and treatment of malignant melanoma in the future.

### OSCE COUNSELLING CASE 13.2 – 'What happens now that I have been diagnosed with malignant melanoma?'

The patient may need to have the following, depending on the Breslow depth of the melanoma:

- full clinical examination to look for metastases
- investigations to look for metastatic spread of the melanoma – FBC, LFTs, LDH and CT scan of the chest, abdomen and pelvis
- patients with tumours over 1 mm in Breslow thickness are usually offered a sentinel lymph node biopsy
- further excision of the scar with a 1–3 cm margin to minimize the risk of local recurrence in the future
- follow-up for up to 5 years to exclude local recurrence or metastatic spread; at each visit the patient should have the scar examined and a general examination to look for cervical, axillary and inguinal lymphadenopathy and hepatomegaly. The patient should be taught how to self-examine the scar and how to look for lymphadenopathy.

# NON-MELANOMA SKIN CANCER

## Questions

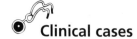

### Clinical cases

**For each of the case scenarios given, consider the following:**

**Q1**: What is the likely differential diagnosis?
**Q2**: What issues in the given history support the diagnosis?
**Q3**: What additional features in the history would you seek to support a particular diagnosis?
**Q4**: What clinical examination would you perform, and why?
**Q5**: What investigations would be most helpful, and why?
**Q6**: What treatment options are appropriate?

### CASE 13.4 – **A 70-year-old man presents with an ulcer on his scalp.**

A 70-year-old man presents with an ulcer over the vertex of his scalp. He has been losing his hair since the age of 30 years and noticed the sore appearing 6 months ago. It has increased in size and bleeds on minimal trauma.

### CASE 13.5 – **A 48-year-old man presents with a lump on his cheek that is getting bigger.**

A 48-year-old man who works as a landscape gardener presents to his GP, having noticed a small lump appearing over his right cheek about a year ago. It has been slowly increasing in size but is otherwise asymptomatic.

### CASE 13.6 – **An 82-year-old woman presents with two red patches on her shin.**

An 82-year-old woman has come to see you with two red scaly patches over her right shin. She is not sure how long they have been present because they are not giving her any symptoms. Two years ago she had some solar keratoses over her forehead that were treated with cryotherapy.

**OSCE counselling case**

## OSCE COUNSELLING CASE 13.3 – 'What can I do to reduce my risk of more skin cancers in the future?'

A 42-year-old woman has recently had two nodular BCCs excised from her face. She attends for a routine follow-up visit.

# Key concepts

To work through the core clinical cases in this section, you will need to understand the following key concepts.

Actinic keratoses (solar keratoses) are areas of chronic sun-induced skin damage occurring on exposed sites (face, balding scalp, ears, dorsum of hands). They are usually multiple and appear as rough red scaly lesions. Small lesions are more easily felt than visualized. They are considered premalignant and have the potential to progress to squamous cell carcinoma (SCC). A variety of treatments are available, the most commonly used being cryotherapy, 5-fluorouracil (5FU) cream, diclofenac gel and curettage.

Bowen's disease is another name for intraepidermal squamous cell carcinoma (in situ SCC). It occurs predominantly in elderly people over sun-exposed sites (usually over the lower legs). Lesions present as a red plaque with a variable amount of scale and enlarge slowly over time. They are typically asymptomatic but may itch, ulcerate or bleed. Often they are misdiagnosed as eczema or psoriasis. In a fifth of patients, multiple lesions occur. Progression to invasive SCC has been reported in about 5 per cent of patients. Treatment of Bowen's disease is with cryotherapy, 5FU cream, diclofenac gel, photodynamic therapy or surgical excision/curettage.

Basal cell carcinoma (rodent ulcer) is the most common skin cancer. It originates from the basal cells of the lower epidermis and is locally destructive but rarely metastasizes. It is common on the head and neck and over the back and chest. It presents as an asymptomatic nodule that slowly enlarges and may occasionally bleed. It is often diagnosed incidentally. Ideally, it should be surgically removed by excision, but a superficial BCC or multiple BCCs may be removed by curettage and cautery. Superficial BCCs may be medically treated with 5FU cream, imiquimod cream, photodynamic therapy or cryotherapy. Occasionally, radiotherapy may be used.

Squamous cell carcinoma is a malignant tumour that arises from keratinocytes and has the potential to metastasize. It presents on sun-exposed sites (face, ears, balding scalp, dorsum of hands, forearms, lower legs) as a tender lump or ulcer that enlarges quite rapidly and fails to heal. Surgical excision is the treatment of choice, but radiotherapy may also be used.

## Answers

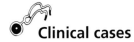

### Clinical cases

---

## CASE 13.4 – A 70-year-old man presents with an ulcer on his scalp.

### A1: What is the likely differential diagnosis?

The likely differential diagnoses are SCC, solar keratosis, Bowen's disease, ulcerated BCC, keratoacanthoma and viral wart.

### A2: What issues in the given history support the diagnosis?

A non-healing ulcer over a sun-exposed area raises the possibility of an SCC. Patients may report that the lesion crusts over or bleeds when traumatized (e.g. on combing hair) or spontaneously.

### A3: What additional features in the history would you seek to support a particular diagnosis?

Ultraviolet irradiation is the most common cause, so it is important to ask about previous sun exposure. Has the patient worked outdoors or lived abroad? Has he received psoralen and ultraviolet A (PUVA) treatment or used sunbeds in the past? Ask about X-ray irradiation, used in the past to treat tinea capitis, eczema and psoriasis, which may have been a predisposing factor. Squamous cell carcinomas are also well known to arise in scars, such as those from previous burns. Immunosuppressants also predispose to non-melanoma skin cancers, and SCCs are common in recipients of organ transplants. Also enquire about any family history of skin cancer.

### A4: What clinical examination would you perform, and why?

Examine the ulcer and measure its size. The rest of the skin must also be examined for other sun-induced cutaneous premalignant and malignant conditions, such as solar keratosis, Bowen's disease and BCC. Look also for any clinical signs of metastasis, paying particular attention to the regional lymph nodes.

### A5: What investigations would be most helpful, and why?

The lesion must be biopsied or excised to confirm the diagnosis histologically.

### A6: What treatment options are appropriate?

The treatment of choice is surgical excision with a 4mm margin of normal skin excised with the tumour. Radiotherapy is also very effective and typically used for patients who refuse surgery, patients with non-resectable tumours, and where tumour margins are ill-defined. Patients are followed up to look for clinical signs of recurrence.

## CASE 9.5 – A 48-year-old man presents with a lump on his cheek that is getting bigger.

### A1: What is the likely differential diagnosis?

The likely differential diagnoses are BCC, epidermoid cyst, sebaceous hyperplasia, intradermal naevus, seborrhoeic keratosis, viral wart, SCC and keratoacanthoma.

## A2:  What issues in the given history support the diagnosis?

A BCC must be considered when there is a history of a slowly enlarging lump over a sun-exposed site. It generally starts as an asymptomatic papule that becomes nodular and ulcerates centrally.

## A3:  What additional features in the history would you seek to support a particular diagnosis?

Ask the patient about exposure to UV light, X-ray irradiation and use of immunosuppressant medication, as you would when an SCC is suspected.

## A4:  What clinical examination would you perform, and why?

Examine the lesion and measure its diameter. The lesion classically appears as a pearly papule or nodule with telangiectasia and a raised rolled edge (nodular BCC). Basal cell carcinomas are usually subdivided into types:

- *superficial BCC* – flat red patches usually over the trunk; a rolled, pearly, telangiectatic border may be visible
- *nodular/cystic BCC* – as described above
- *multifocal BCC* – these start as nodules that expand, with areas of apparent regression between them; there are fine strands of tumour connecting the nodules, however
- *morphoeic BCC* – elevated smooth firm plaque that is often misdiagnosed as a scar; may appear pearly with telangiectasia
- *pigmented BCC* – as for nodular BCC, but with pigmented margins; a pigmented BCC may be mistaken for malignant melanoma.

## A5:  What investigations would be most helpful, and why?

A diagnostic biopsy may be performed for histological confirmation of the type of BCC. Lesions that look classical for BCC, however, are best excised with a 4 mm margin of normal skin.

## A6:  What treatment options are appropriate?

Surgical treatment can be by excision with a 4 mm margin or curettage and cautery for small, multiple and superficial lesions. Cryotherapy is sometimes used for superficial or multiple lesions. Radiotherapy may be more appropriate in elderly people and in people who refuse surgery. Patients do not require follow-up if the BCC has been completely excised, but they are often followed up if the BCC is treated in another way as there is then a higher risk of recurrence.

## CASE 13.6 – **An 82-year-old woman presents with two red patches on her shin.**

## A1:  What is the likely differential diagnosis?

The likely differential diagnoses are Bowen's disease, actinic keratosis, SCC, BCC, eczema, psoriasis and seborrhoeic keratosis.

## A2:  What issues in the given history support the diagnosis?

A red scaly patch on the lower leg of an elderly woman is typical of Bowen's disease. Most lesions are asymptomatic and go unnoticed by the patient.

### A3: What additional features in the history would you seek to support a particular diagnosis?

Lesions of Bowen's disease show gradual radial growth. Ask the patient about symptoms such as bleeding or ulceration, which may occur as the lesion enlarges. Most lesions are caused by chronic UV light irradiation, so ask the patient about sun exposure.

### A4: What clinical examination would you perform, and why?

Examine the lesions and record the diameter of each. Look for induration, erosion or ulceration of the plaques, which may suggest malignant transformation into SCC. Examine the rest of the skin for other premalignant or malignant lesions.

### A5: What investigations would be most helpful, and why?

The diagnosis is usually made on clinical examination and can be confirmed by biopsy of the lesion.

### A6: What treatment options are appropriate?

Cryotherapy with liquid nitrogen, topical 5FU cream or imiquimod cream is usually used and is very effective, although it may lead to ulceration, particularly when treating lesions on the lower limbs of elderly people. Curettage and cautery or occasionally excision can also be used. Photodynamic therapy is usually reserved for large or multiple lesions.

## 👫 OSCE counselling case

### OSCE COUNSELLING CASE 13.3 – 'What can I do to reduce my risk of more skin cancers in the future?'

Prevention of skin cancer involves educating patients about the disease in order to change their behaviour and lifestyle. Advise the patient to limit her exposure to UV light by wearing suitable clothing to cover her trunk and limbs, and a wide-brimmed hat to protect her scalp, face and ears. She should avoid going outdoors during the middle of the day when the sun is at its strongest ('Between eleven and three, hide under a tree'). A sunscreen of sun protection factor 30 or above should be applied to any sun-exposed site. She should also be educated to examine her skin regularly for any new lesions so that any skin cancers can be detected early and treated.

# ECZEMA

## Questions

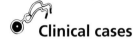

### Clinical cases

**For each of the case scenarios given, consider the following:**

**Q1**: What is the likely differential diagnosis?
**Q2**: What issues in the given history support the diagnosis?
**Q3**: What additional features in the history would you seek to support a particular diagnosis?
**Q4**: What clinical examination would you perform, and why?
**Q5**: What investigations would be most helpful, and why?
**Q6**: What treatment options are appropriate?

### CASE 13.7 – An 18-year-old girl presents with painful weeping lesions over her face.

An 18-year-old girl attends A&E complaining of painful weeping lesions over her face. These started 2 days ago over her chin and have now spread to involve her entire face. She has had eczema since she was a baby, but it has not been active for the past 2 years. Last week she had a cold sore over her upper lip.

### CASE 13.8 – A 24-year-old woman with sore red hands.

A 24-year-old hairdresser has developed painful red scaly lesions over the palmar aspect of both hands. She has noticed small blisters and weeping areas when it is very severe. While she was on maternity leave last year her hands improved, but since she has returned to work the condition has flared up again.

## ㅤ OSCE counselling cases

### OSCE COUNSELLING CASE 13.4 – 'Which creams should I use for my baby's eczema?'

A mother comes to see you with her 6-month-old baby. He developed eczema soon after birth, with red dry areas over his cheeks, limb flexures and abdomen, and dry scale (cradle cap) over his scalp. She has been prescribed lots of different creams by different GPs each time she takes him to the surgery and is not sure where to use each cream. Explain to her what general measures she can take to help improve the child's eczema, and explain where and how to use emollients and topical steroids.

### OSCE COUNSELLING CASE 13.5 – 'I have been referred for patch testing. What does this involve?'

A 42-year-old man has been referred to the contact dermatitis clinic for patch testing. He is a keen gardener and suspects the eczema over his hands results from contact with plants in the summer months. Explain to him what patch testing involves.

## Key concepts

To work through the core clinical cases in this section, you will need to understand the following key concepts.

There are several different types of eczema.

- *Atopic eczema* is a chronic pruritic inflammatory disorder, mainly affecting children but sometimes persisting into adulthood. It is characterized by relapses and remissions. It is frequently associated with other atopic disorders such as asthma and hayfever.
- *Seborrhoeic eczema* is a chronic eczematous disorder with erythema and scaling distributed over the face (glabella, alae of the nose, eyebrows, sideburns, ears), scalp, flexures and upper trunk. It is typically associated with overgrowth of the yeast *Pityrosporum ovale* (also known as *Malassezia furfur*) and may be asymptomatic.
- *Discoid eczema* is characterized by coin-shaped raised erythematous lesions occurring over the trunk and limbs. It usually occurs in older people, but it can also present in young adults. Secondary infection with staphylococci is common.
- *Pompholyx eczema* is characterized by pruritic vesicular eruptions over the palms, soles and sides of the digits. It usually occurs in young people and is associated with excessive sweating and warm weather.
- *Varicose eczema* is characterized by pruritic red eczematous patches over the shins. It commonly occurs secondary to venous hypertension. Varicose veins are often visible. Other changes may include oedema of the lower limbs, induration and hyperpigmentation caused by haemosiderin deposition in the skin. Ulceration may be precipitated by minor injury or infection.
- *Contact dermatitis* is an irritant or allergic eczematous reaction caused by an external substance coming into contact with the skin. Irritant contact dermatitis can affect anyone if they are exposed to a sufficient concentration of the irritant agent and for enough time. Allergic contact dermatitis is a delayed-type hypersensitivity allergic reaction that occurs only in predisposed people on every encounter with the allergen.

# Answers

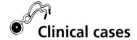
## Clinical cases

### CASE 13.7 – **An 18-year-old girl presents with painful weeping lesions over her face.**

#### A1: What is the likely differential diagnosis?

This is eczema herpeticum. Impetigo caused by staphylococci or streptococci (or a combination of these) is also a possibility, although it is more common in children.

#### A2: What issues in the given history support the diagnosis?

Eczema herpeticum is the most likely diagnosis in the light of the recent cold sore. Contrary to popular belief, this does not occur only when the eczema is in an active phase.

#### A3: What additional features in the history would you seek to support a particular diagnosis?

Start by finding out when, where and how the lesions began, whether the GP gave any treatment, whether the patient used any over-the-counter medication, and whether there was any improvement or deterioration from the medication. Are any other members of the family or friends affected in a similar way? Painful and weeping lesions indicate infection, so it is important to establish whether the patient has been feeling unwell in any way (e.g. fever, rigors). Finally, find out more about her past medical history and how her eczema was managed in the past.

#### A4: What clinical examination would you perform, and why?

Examine the patient's skin and document the extent and morphology of the lesions. Vesicles, yellow crusts or a combination of these is usually present. Look for associated lymphadenopathy. Examine the patient's eyes for any conjunctival involvement, as left untreated this may lead to corneal scarring and blindness.

#### A5: What investigations would be most helpful, and why?

Bacterial and viral swabs of the vesicle fluid or crusts will confirm the organism responsible. If the patient is pyrexial, blood cultures must be taken. An FBC may show a raised white cell count (WCC). C-reactive protein (CRP) will also be elevated in infection.

#### A6: What treatment options are appropriate?

Oral aciclovir 200 mg five times a day for 5 days is the treatment of choice for eczema herpeticum. If the infection is severe, intravenous (IV) aciclovir may be used. If the diagnosis is in doubt or secondary bacterial infection is also suspected, it is best to add in flucloxacillin and penicillin. Topical emollients will provide symptomatic relief and, once the infection has been treated, topical corticosteroids are usually necessary to treat the eczema. If there is eye involvement, an urgent assessment by an ophthalmologist is needed to exclude corneal ulceration, which may lead to blindness if left untreated.

The patient should be nursed in a side room and warned to avoid close physical contact with friends and family, because the herpes virus is contagious. Once the infection has been treated, it is important to educate the patient on management of her eczema with daily use of emollients and topical corticosteroids over areas of active eczema. Bath oils and soap substitute emollients are useful to prevent dryness of the skin. Antihistamines can also be used to control pruritus.

## CASE 13.8 – **A 24-year-old woman with sore red hands.**

### A1: What is the likely differential diagnosis?

The likely differential diagnoses are allergic contact dermatitis, irritant contact dermatitis, pompholyx eczema, tinea and psoriasis.

### A2: What issues in the given history support the diagnosis?

Allergic contact dermatitis is a delayed hypersensitivity reaction. Once the individual has been sensitized to a given allergen, dermatitis recurs on every subsequent exposure. Frequently the allergen responsible is encountered in the workplace and the dermatitis remits at weekends or holidays. Lesions are often pruritic or sore, and blisters are common with severe reactions. The distribution reflects the areas of contact with the allergen. Industrial dermatitis is commonly seen over the palms of the hands; the dorsum of the hands and wrists are typically affected with allergy to rubber gloves; and the earlobes and navel are affected with allergy to nickel in earrings and metal jeans studs.

### A3: What additional features in the history would you seek to support a particular diagnosis?

The history is very important when allergic contact dermatitis is suspected. The distribution of dermatitis may give a clue to the responsible allergen, as indicated above. Common allergens responsible for contact dermatitis include metal (nickel and cobalt in costume jewellery), rubber, perfumes, nail varnish, plants, hair dyes, cosmetics, and colophony in adhesive dressings such as plasters. Ask the patient about any hobbies she has that may bring her into contact with potential allergens. Find out whether she has tried any topical preparations and whether they have improved or exacerbated the problem. Topical anaesthetics, antihistamines and rarely corticosteroids may occasionally be the culprit allergen.

### A4: What clinical examination would you perform, and why?

Determine whether the dermatitis is confined to the palms of the hands or whether other areas are also involved. In palmoplantar psoriasis, the soles of the feet may be similarly involved. There may also be other clues for psoriasis, such as scaly plaques over the extensor surfaces of the limbs, scaling of the scalp, or pitting and onycholysis of the nails. On the other hand, tinea is almost always unilateral, and there may be a history or clinical evidence of athlete's foot as the source of infection.

### A5: What investigations would be most helpful, and why?

The diagnosis of allergic contact dermatitis can be confirmed by patch testing (see OSCE counselling case 13.5). If tinea is suspected, skin scrapings from the lesion can be taken and sent for mycology to look for the presence of fungus. In weeping lesions, superimposed infection can be identified by sending skin swabs for microbiology.

### A6: What treatment options are appropriate?

If possible, the antigen should be completely removed from the patient's environment. This usually leads to complete recovery. This is not always possible, however, so the patient should be advised to avoid contact with the allergen as much as she can, e.g. by wearing rubber gloves when handling the allergen. Topical corticosteroids will provide symptomatic relief, but the dermatitis will recur on exposure to the allergen. In very severe cases, a short course of systemic steroids may be used.

## ♟♟ OSCE counselling cases

### OSCE COUNSELLING CASE 13.4 – 'Which creams should I use for my baby's eczema?'

Simple measures can help with the management of eczema. Skin contact with irritants such as woollen clothing (the clothing layer next to the skin should always be 100 per cent cotton), fragranced soaps and bubble baths should be avoided. Preventing the child from overheating will help reduce pruritus. This includes ensuring that bath water is not too warm and that the room temperature is controlled.

The daily use of emollients to prevent dryness of the skin is vital. These should be used at least first thing in the morning and after a bath at night, and more frequently in the winter months and if the skin is still dry. A soap substitute such as emulsifying ointment is good to help with skin hydration; a bath oil can also be added to the bath water. Some emollients, soap substitutes and bath oils also contain an antibacterial agent that is useful in treating and preventing infection, especially in children who often scratch at their eczema. The child should have a bath each night and then have an emollient applied. Olive oil is an effective emollient for the scalp in babies with cradle cap. A topical corticosteroid should be applied to areas of active eczema. Parents should be advised to use topical steroids sparingly, as liberal and continual use leads to thinning of the skin (skin atrophy). Ointment preparations are generally better than creams at hydration, but creams are used in preference over weeping areas, where ointments tend to slide off. A 20 min gap between emollient and steroid application will prevent dilution of the steroid. Topical steroids should not be used over areas of infected eczema. Occasionally a topical antibiotic and corticosteroid combination is prescribed for areas of mildly infected eczema. In children with severe eczema, a technique known as 'wet wrapping' can be very effective at controlling the disease. This is done by applying emollients or weak topical steroid cream to the skin and wrapping the child in moist gauze bandages.

If there is no evidence of infection and topical steroids have been ineffective, topical tacrolimus cream or topical pimecrolimus cream may be used in children over the age of 2 years. These immunomodulatory creams control the eczema by suppressing the immune system locally in the skin. They have been used widely in the UK only for the past 10 years and their long-term effects are unknown, but they are considered to be safe and, unlike steroid creams, they do not lead to thinning of the skin.

### OSCE COUNSELLING CASE 13.5 – 'I have been referred for patch testing. What does this involve?'

When allergic contact dermatitis is suspected, patch testing is performed, whereby the suspected allergen is placed in direct contact with the skin. About 30 commonly encountered allergens are used in a standard battery, and other potential allergens are added, such as a range of plants in suspected plant-induced contact dermatitis, or the patient's own cosmetics in facial dermatitis. The allergens are placed in individual aluminium wells and applied to the patient's back with adhesive tape. They are left in place for 48 h and then removed. The skin is inspected at 96 h for areas of dermatitis corresponding to the application site of each allergen. Positive readings are interpreted with the clinical context in mind because they may not be relevant to the patient's symptoms.

# PSORIASIS

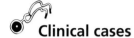

## Clinical cases

### For each of the case scenarios given, consider the following:

> **Q1**: What is the likely differential diagnosis?
> **Q2**: What issues in the given history support the diagnosis?
> **Q3**: What additional features in the history would you seek to support a particular diagnosis?
> **Q4**: What clinical examination would you perform, and why?
> **Q5**: What investigations would be most helpful, and why?
> **Q6**: What treatment options are appropriate?

## CASE 13.9 – A 33-year-old woman presents with dry red patches over her elbows and knees.

A 33-year-old woman presents with dry red scaly patches of skin over the elbows and knees. These have come on gradually over the years and are asymptomatic. She also has dandruff. This has recently become much worse and is causing her great embarrassment.

## CASE 13.10 – A 54-year-old man presents with reddened skin.

A 54-year-old man has developed redness and discomfort of the skin over his trunk and limbs. He was diagnosed with chronic plaque psoriasis in his twenties. On examination, he is pyrexial and has confluent erythema over his chest, back, abdomen, arms and legs.

## ⁂ OSCE counselling cases

### OSCE COUNSELLING CASE 13.6 – 'Can I have some tablets instead of creams for my psoriasis?'

A 40-year-old woman has had chronic plaque psoriasis affecting her trunk, limbs and scalp for 20 years. This has been reasonably well controlled with topical preparations. She has recently read an article in a magazine describing a 'miracle tablet that cures psoriasis'. She tells you that she is fed up with her messy creams and wants to have this tablet. What systemic therapies are commonly used to treat psoriasis? When are they used, and what does a specialist need to take into consideration when initiating treatment? What monitoring is required?

### OSCE COUNSELLING CASE 13.7 – 'Can I use a sunbed to treat my psoriasis?'

A 22-year-old woman has recently been diagnosed with psoriasis. She tells you that her aunt also has the condition, which has almost completely cleared with UV treatment given by her specialist. She wants to know if buying a sunbed to use at home will help her psoriasis. Explain to her why it is not recommended for her to use a sunbed at home. What types of UV treatment are available for the treatment of psoriasis?

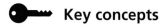 **Key concepts**

To work through the core clinical cases in this section, you will need to understand the following key concepts.

Psoriasis is a common chronic hyperproliferative and immunological condition, characterized by well-demarcated erythematous silvery scaled plaques, typically in a symmetrical distribution over extensor surfaces and in the scalp.

There are several types of psoriasis.

- *Chronic plaque psoriasis/psoriasis vulgaris* is characterized by well-defined, usually symmetrical raised red plaques with thick silvery scale, most commonly over the extensor surfaces of the elbows and knees, although it may occur at any skin site. The scalp is usually affected, and there may be nail involvement.
- *Flexural psoriasis* may occur alongside chronic plaque psoriasis. There are well-defined areas of erythema affecting the flexures (groin, perianally, axillae, umbilicus, inframammary folds).
- *Guttate psoriasis* usually affects adolescents and young adults, occurring days or a few weeks after a severe streptococcal throat infection. A history of this is not always obtained, however. It presents with widespread drop-like ('guttate') red papules with silvery scale over the trunk and limbs. It resolves within a few months but may recur in some patients.
- *Palmoplantar pustular psoriasis* is characterized by pustules occurring over the palms and soles, on the background of well-defined red scaly plaques. It is usually bilateral, and there may be psoriasis elsewhere.
- *Erythrodermic psoriasis:* worsening psoriasis can develop into erythroderma, a term used to describe abnormal reddening of the skin affecting over 90 per cent of the total body surface area. Patients are usually unwell and may be pyrexial. The redness is the result of capillary proliferation. Erythroderma may also be caused by eczema, drugs or cutaneous T-cell lymphoma (also known as mycosis fungoides).
- *Generalized pustular psoriasis* is an extreme form of psoriasis with extensive small sterile pustules and underlying erythema covering the skin. It can be provoked by abrupt cessation of potent steroids or a reduction in immunosuppressive treatment for psoriasis, or may be the result of concurrent infection, pregnancy or alcohol excess. There is a significant associated mortality.
- *Psoriasis of the nails:* about a third of patients with psoriasis and a quarter of patients with psoriatic arthropathy and psoriasis have nail changes. These may occur in isolation, however. Changes include pitting, onycholysis and subungual hyperkeratosis.
- *Psoriatic arthropathy:* arthropathy occurs in 8–10 per cent of patients with psoriasis, but it may also occur in the absence of skin changes. It may present in different forms, most commonly asymmetrical arthritis, symmetrical polyarthritis, ankylosing spondylitis and arthritis mutilans.

# Answers

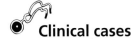

## Clinical cases

### CASE 13.9 – **A 33-year-old woman presents with dry red patches over her elbows and knees.**

**A1:** What is the likely differential diagnosis?

The likely differential diagnoses are psoriasis, eczema and tinea.

**A2:** What issues in the given history support the diagnosis?

The distribution of the lesions is characteristic of psoriasis. Apart from its cosmetic appearance, which causes significant distress to some patients, the condition is usually asymptomatic. Both eczema and tinea are typically pruritic.

**A3:** What additional features in the history would you seek to support a particular diagnosis?

It is important to find out how the condition has progressed up to now. Has it got gradually worse over the years, or does it come and go? Is it worse at any particular time of year? Most patients find that their psoriasis is worse in the winter and improves with sun exposure in the summer months. Find out whether there are any other exacerbating or relieving factors. Alcohol, nicotine, beta-blockers, lithium and antimalarial drugs can all make psoriasis worse. Enquire about nail and scalp involvement and whether the patient has any joint pains. Ask the patient about her family history – a third of patients with psoriasis recall a family member with the condition.

**A4:** What clinical examination would you perform, and why?

Examine the skin, scalp and nails for changes consistent with psoriasis. Plaques vary in size and shape and may coalesce into large areas. Pay particular attention to the elbows, knees and natal cleft as these are typical sites for psoriasis plaques. The Auspitz sign may be elicited by scraping away the surface of a scaly plaque to reveal tiny bleeding points from the dilated superficial capillaries.

**A5:** What investigations would be most helpful, and why?

Psoriasis is a diagnosis made clinically, and usually no investigations are necessary. If tinea is suspected, skin scrapings sent for mycology may differentiate between the diagnoses.

**A6:** What treatment options are appropriate?

There are many treatments for psoriasis. Daily emollients are used alongside other topical preparations such as coal tar, dithranol, corticosteroids and vitamin D analogues, some being available in combined preparations. For scalp psoriasis, tar shampoos and topical corticosteroid scalp applications usually achieve good results. Psoralen and ultraviolet A treatment (PUVA), or short-wave UV (UVB) radiation without psoralen, also known as TL-01, can be used for widespread psoriasis. The number of treatments that can be given to a patient in their lifetime is limited because UV radiation increases the risk of skin malignancies. Cytotoxic drugs such as methotrexate, ciclosporin and oral retinoids can be very effective for severe psoriasis but require careful blood monitoring to avoid complications. Patients with severe psoriasis who have not shown a response to these conventional systemic agents may be offered treatment with a new class of agents known as biologics (etanercept, adalimumab, infliximab, ustekinumab). These are administered by injection or infusion every week or every few weeks and may be highly effective, but they are very expensive and patients need to be selected carefully before treatment.

## CASE 13.10 – **A 54-year-old man presents with reddened skin.**

### A1: What is the likely differential diagnosis?

Causes of erythroderma include psoriasis, eczema, drugs and cutaneous T-cell lymphoma (also known as mycosis fungoides).

### A2: What issues in the given history support the diagnosis?

Erythroderma is a term used to describe abnormal reddening of the skin affecting over 90 per cent of the total body surface area. In this case, the patient's psoriasis is most probably the cause.

### A3: What additional features in the history would you seek to support a particular diagnosis?

Find out when the patient's symptoms began. Was there a preceding illness (e.g. sore throat) or did the patient become unwell once the skin erythema developed? What is the extent of the patient's psoriasis normally, and how is it managed? Determine whether there have been any changes made to his psoriasis treatment recently. Abrupt cessation of topical corticosteroids or oral immunosuppressive medication can precipitate erythroderma. An increase in alcohol consumption can cause an exacerbation of psoriasis.

### A4: What clinical examination would you perform, and why?

Erythrodermic psoriasis is deep red in colour. It may also be exfoliative, with scaling or peeling of the skin. Thick white or silvery scaly plaques may cover the body or be confined to the extensor surfaces of the elbows and knees. In most patients with psoriasis, there is also scalp involvement, which may vary from fine flakes to thick scaly plaques. The nails may also be affected, with pitting, ridging or onycholysis.

### A5: What investigations would be most helpful, and why?

The diagnosis is usually made on history and examination. An FBC may show a leucocytosis, and inflammatory markers such as CRP or erythrocyte sedimentation rate (ESR) may be raised. An infection screen (e.g. blood cultures, chest radiograph) is necessary if there is any history or sign of infection. It is important to monitor renal function because vasodilation leads to increased percutaneous water loss, with consequent decreased urine output, which may lead to renal failure. Liver function must also be measured if the patient admits to excess alcohol consumption.

### A6: What treatment options are appropriate?

Correction of hypovolaemia and hypothermia and treatment of concomitant sepsis are vital in the early stages of erythroderma. Emollients are applied daily. Systemic therapy (e.g. retinoids, methotrexate, ciclosporin) is usually needed to control the underlying psoriasis. Corticosteroids and UV light therapy are usually avoided.

## 👥 OSCE counselling cases

### OSCE COUNSELLING CASE 13.6 – 'Can I have some tablets instead of creams for my psoriasis?'

The decision to start systemic therapy can be difficult and is made by a specialist. It is generally a long-term commitment, using drugs with potential side effects, which require careful monitoring. The patient must be told that the drug is not a cure for psoriasis and that the disease usually returns to its previous state after stopping treatment. Drug interactions may occur, so it is important to take a drug history before initiating treatment. Systemic therapies are used to treat erythrodermic psoriasis, generalized pustular psoriasis, and extensive psoriasis where other therapy has failed, multiple admissions to hospital have been necessary or the disease interferes with function or restricts the patient's quality of life.

The most commonly used systemic therapies are methotrexate, ciclosporin and acitretin.

Methotrexate is given as a once-weekly dose of 0.2–0.4 mg/kg. A test dose of 2.5–5 mg is given before starting therapy to detect idiosyncratic myelosuppression, which may occur within 7–10 days (an FBC is necessary). Bone marrow toxicity may occur, so the FBC must be monitored. Regular LFTs are needed because hepatotoxicity may occur. Occasionally a liver biopsy is necessary if hepatic fibrosis is suspected. Methotrexate is excreted by the kidneys so renal function is also monitored. It is teratogenic in early pregnancy; all women need adequate contraception and must be told to avoid pregnancy for at least 3 months after cessation of treatment.

Ciclosporin is given as either a low-dose regimen (2.5 mg/kg/day, increased slowly) or a high-dose regimen (5 mg/kg/day). These are usually well tolerated. The risk of nephrotoxicity means that careful monitoring of renal function is vital. Treatment is usually limited to a few months at a time, as long-term ciclosporin increases the risk of renal damage. There is also a risk of hypertension, and blood pressure checks are mandatory.

Acitretin is taken as tablets, usually 20–30 mg a day; higher doses lead to side effects. Hyperlipidaemia and hepatotoxicity may occur, so monitoring of cholesterol, triglycerides and liver function is necessary. Acitretin is highly teratogenic and should be avoided in women of childbearing age. Unlike methotrexate and ciclosporin, acitretin is not immunosuppressive.

### OSCE COUNSELLING CASE 13.7 – 'Can I use a sunbed to treat my psoriasis?'

Ultraviolet treatment can be very beneficial for the treatment of psoriasis, but it must be initiated by a specialist and given in a controlled manner. The dose given (in joules per square centimetre, or $J/cm^2$) depends on the patient's skin type. There is a risk of cutaneous malignancy, which is cumulative and becomes highly significant after a total dose of $1200 J/cm^2$. People with psoriasis often require repeated courses of UV treatment to keep the disease under control. A record is kept of the cumulative exposure, which is kept to a minimum where possible. It is not recommended that patients use sunbeds because there is no monitoring of the dose given.

PUVA, or UVB radiation without psoralen, can be used in the treatment of psoriasis. Psoralens may also be applied topically or added to the bath before UVA exposure (bath PUVA). Treatment is usually given two to three times a week for about 20 treatments to obtain clearance of the disease. Multiple courses of treatment are usually necessary in a patient's lifetime. Patients must be warned of the risks of developing cutaneous malignancies.

# PRURITUS

## Questions

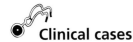

### Clinical cases

## For each of the case scenarios given, consider the following:

> **Q1**: What is the likely differential diagnosis?
> **Q2**: What issues in the given history support the diagnosis?
> **Q3**: What additional features in the history would you seek to support a particular diagnosis?
> **Q4**: What clinical examination would you perform, and why?
> **Q5**: What investigations would be most helpful, and why?
> **Q6**: What treatment options are appropriate?

### CASE 13.11 – A 36-year-old Asian woman presents with a 2-month history of generalized pruritus.

The patient has no associated rash. She has been feeling tired for a few months now but has no other symptoms. On examination, she has pale conjunctivae.

### CASE 13.12 – An 88-year-old man who lives in a residential home has developed a generalized itchy rash.

The rash is particularly bad over the patient's hands, arms, groin and thighs. The itching is worse at night and prevents him from sleeping. Some of the other residents at the home have developed a similar itchy rash.

## ⚇ OSCE counselling case

### OSCE COUNSELLING CASE 13.8 – 'I have been told I have urticaria. What is this?'

A 33-year-old man has had intermittent episodes of a nettle-like rash over his body for the past 6 months. Each episode lasts for a few hours. He has not identified any triggers but has noticed that the rash becomes less itchy and fades slowly after taking antihistamine tablets. He has been told the diagnosis is urticaria. Explain to him what this diagnosis means. Are there any investigations he can have to determine the cause?

##  Key concepts

To work through the core clinical cases in this section, you will need to understand the following key concepts.

The common causes of generalized pruritus include:

- *haematological:*
  - iron deficiency anaemia
  - polycythaemia rubra vera
  - paraproteinaemia
- *hepatic disease:*
  - extrahepatic obstructive jaundice
  - primary biliary cirrhosis
  - cholestasis of pregnancy
- *renal disease:*
  - chronic renal failure
- *endocrine disease:*
  - hyper- or hypothyroidism
  - diabetes mellitus
- *internal malignancy:*
  - lymphoma
  - leukaemia
  - abdominal cancer
  - bronchial carcinoma
- *drugs:*
  - oral contraceptive pill (causes cholestasis)
  - opiates (cause histamine release)
  - alcohol and drug withdrawal
- *psychological.*

The common pruritic skin disorders are eczema, scabies, urticaria, insect bites, lichen planus, drug eruptions, bullous pemphigoid, dermatitis herpetiformis and polymorphic light eruptions.

## Answers

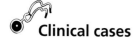

### Clinical cases

---

### CASE 13.11 – **A 36-year-old Asian woman presents with a 2-month history of generalized pruritus.**

#### A1: What is the likely differential diagnosis?

Causes of generalized pruritus must be considered (see 'Key concepts' above).

#### A2: What issues in the given history support the diagnosis?

The most likely diagnosis is pruritus secondary to iron deficiency anaemia. Patients with anaemia often have non-specific symptoms and complain of lethargy. The pale conjunctivae also suggest anaemia.

#### A3: What additional features in the history would you seek to support a particular diagnosis?

Find out whether the patient has any other associated symptoms. The tiredness and pale conjunctivae suggest anaemia, although iron deficiency in the absence of anaemia can also cause pruritus. Is there anything in the history to suggest iron deficiency? Is she vegetarian or vegan, and does she eat a balanced diet? Enquire about any history of blood loss (e.g. bleeding per rectum, heavy menstrual blood loss). Find out whether the pruritus occurs at any specific time (e.g. pruritus after a hot bath is classically associated with polycythaemia). Are there symptoms suggesting internal malignancy such as weight loss, haemoptysis, chronic cough, fevers or night sweats? Drugs such as opiates and their derivatives may also cause pruritus, so ask the patient about any medication she is taking.

#### A4: What clinical examination would you perform, and why?

A full general examination is necessary to look for coexisting skin disease or a cause for the pruritus. Often, the only positive findings are the excoriations caused by the patient scratching. Look for scabies burrows in the finger webs or pruritic papules over the genitals. Examine for evidence of chronic liver disease, hypo- or hyperthyroidism, and renal failure or malignancy, all of which may present with pruritus.

#### A5: What investigations would be most helpful, and why?

An FBC to look for anaemia or polycythaemia rubra vera is necessary. Iron studies (ferritin, total iron-binding capacity) can determine whether iron deficiency is present. It may be necessary to investigate further for a cause with faecal occult blood, e.g. by sigmoidoscopy. Liver function tests may indicate cholestasis. Renal function tests may reveal uraemia secondary to chronic renal failure as the cause of pruritus. Thyroid function tests may show thyrotoxicosis or hypothyroidism. Diabetes can also cause generalized pruritus, so check the patient's fasting glucose.

#### A6: What treatment options are appropriate?

Treatment is that of the underlying cause. Prevent dryness of the skin that can cause or exacerbate pruritus. Menthol in aqueous cream can be very soothing. Bath oils and emollients used as soap substitutes can also provide symptomatic relief. Antihistamines may provide symptomatic relief. A sedating antihistamine may help the patient sleep at night, but a non-sedating antihistamine is better for daytime use so it does not interfere with driving and work.

## CASE 13.12 – **An 88-year-old man who lives in a residential home has developed a generalized itchy rash.**

### A1: What is the likely differential diagnosis?

The likely differential diagnoses are scabies, eczema, tinea corporis and tinea cruris and drug eruption.

### A2: What issues in the given history support the diagnosis?

Itching that is particularly bad over the hands and groin area and is worse at night suggests a diagnosis of scabies, especially if other members of the family or residential home are also complaining of pruritus. The itch intensifies with time and, apart from sparing the face, affects the whole body.

### A3: What additional features in the history would you seek to support a particular diagnosis?

A very observant patient may have noticed the scabies burrows and describe them as very pruritic, but usually they go unnoticed. Ask whether the patient has any small itchy lumps between the fingers, around the nipples, or on the buttocks and genitalia. Pruritic papules on the penis or scrotum are characteristic of scabies. Find out whether the patient has tried any treatments – topical corticosteroids are often wrongly prescribed if the rash is mistaken for eczema, and they often provide temporary symptomatic relief from itching but actually make the condition worse.

### A4: What clinical examination would you perform, and why?

Finding a scabies burrow is diagnostic. Look carefully over the webs of the fingers, dorsum of the hands, around the wrists and on the palms. Multiple serpiginous slightly raised linear tracks of a few millimetres in length are characteristic. The *Sarcoptes scabiei* mite may be just visible as a black dot at one end of the burrow. The pruritus and rash associated with scabies are a result of an allergic reaction to the mite's faeces and present as an extremely itchy erythematous papular eruption. Multiple excoriations are often present, and bruising from vigorous scratching may occur.

### A5: What investigations would be most helpful, and why?

The diagnosis is made on history and examination, although occasionally a mite can be carefully extracted from a burrow using a fine needle and visualized under the microscope.

### A6: What treatment options are appropriate?

Scabies is easily treatable, but the patient must apply the treatment correctly and be warned that the itching (which is caused by an allergic reaction to the mite's faeces) typically persists for a few weeks after the mite has been eradicated. The treatment should be applied to all the skin areas except the face. Most lotions for scabies need to be applied and left on for 12–24h before being washed off. Usually two applications applied 7 days apart are recommended – the treatment kills the mite but not the eggs, and it is possible for new eggs to hatch a week later and lead to reinfestation. Permethrin 5% cream or malathion 0.5% lotion is usually used. Close contacts such as family members and carers may also need treatment. Other measures include washing the patient's bedding, towels and undergarments at a high temperature. As the itch and eczema persist for weeks, application of crotamiton, with or without a topical corticosteroid, and a sedating antihistamine tablet can provide symptomatic relief.

## 👬 OSCE counselling case

### OSCE COUNSELLING CASE 13.8 – 'I have been told I have urticaria. What is this?'

Urticaria is a term used to describe intermittent transient itchy red swellings of the skin that occur secondary to histamine and other vasoactive substances being released from granules within mast cells in blood vessels. Angio-oedema occurs if the mucous membranes are also involved, with swelling around the eyes and of the lips, tongue and larynx. This may be life-threatening because of the possibility of asphyxia. Patients often describe the rash as itchy wheals and blisters, 'nettle rash' or 'hives'. They typically appear as raised annular areas with a red periphery and central pallor. The rash lasts for several hours and the skin appears completely normal afterwards. In most patients, a cause is never identified (idiopathic urticaria), but the following are some common causes of urticaria:

- *drugs* – aspirin and other non-steroidal anti-inflammatory drugs, antibiotics (especially penicillin and cephalosporins), angiotensin-converting enzyme (ACE) inhibitors
- *foods* – e.g. nuts, dairy products, shellfish, dyes, additives
- *infection* – focal sepsis
- *physical* – cold, heat, UV light, pressure
- *blood transfusion reactions*.

Treatment involves avoiding any identified precipitating cause and controlling the symptoms with antihistamines. If there is a history of angio-oedema leading to anaphylaxis, the patient must be provided with an adrenaline injection for self-administration.

The diagnosis is usually made on the history alone. Investigations are rarely helpful. Blood tests are usually normal and therefore not indicated. It can be helpful to ask the patient to make a list of things ingested in the 24 h before each attack to try to identify the trigger. An elimination diet may be worth trying. Skin-prick and radioallergosorbent (RAST) tests are often positive in a non-specific way, but the results must be interpreted in the clinical context.

# ACNE

## Questions

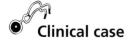
**Clinical case**

### For the case scenario given, consider the following:

**Q1**: What is the likely differential diagnosis?
**Q2**: What issues in the given history support the diagnosis?
**Q3**: What additional features in the history would you seek to support a particular diagnosis?
**Q4**: What clinical examination would you perform, and why?
**Q5**: What investigations would be most helpful, and why?
**Q6**: What treatment options are appropriate?

### CASE 13.13 – A 17-year-old girl presents to her GP complaining of spots over her face for the past 4 years.

The patient has tried multiple over-the-counter acne preparations, with no improvement. She is very concerned about the scarring left behind.

## 👥 OSCE counselling case

### OSCE COUNSELLING CASE 13.9 – 'Can I have isotretinoin for my acne?'

A 23-year-old woman has been treated for acne with various topical preparations and different courses of antibiotics for the past 2 years, with little success. Her friend was recently given isotretinoin tablets, which have cured her acne. The patient wishes to have the same treatment. What are the indications for prescribing isotretinoin? What are the side effects that she needs to know about before starting treatment?

## 🔑 Key concepts

To work through the core clinical cases in this section, you will need to understand the following key concepts.

Acne is a chronic disorder of the pilosebaceous apparatus of the skin. It results from overactivity of the sebaceous glands and blockage of its ducts, leading to the formation of open (blackheads) and closed (whiteheads) comedones. The sebaceous glands are under the control of androgens and produce sebum, which may be converted into comedogenic and irritant free fatty acids by the anaerobic bacterium *Propionibacterium acnes* within the pilosebaceous duct.

There are various treatments for acne. The choice of treatment depends on the disease severity and the individual patient.

- *Topical therapy* is used for mild acne and as an adjunct to other acne treatments. Examples include benzoyl peroxide, retinoic acid, antibiotics and salicylic acid.
- *Systemic antibiotics* such as tetracyclines and erythromycin are used to treat acne that does not respond to topical treatment alone.
- *Hormone therapy:* a combined preparation of cyproterone acetate and ethinylestradiol (co-cyprindiol) reduces sebum production and is helpful in some patients.
- *Systemic retinoid therapy:* 13-cis-retinoic acid (isotretinoin) is a synthetic derivative of vitamin A. It acts by reducing sebum secretion by 90 per cent, microorganisms (especially *P. acnes*), plugging of the pilosebaceous ducts and inflammation. It also influences epithelial proliferation and differentiation so that the sebaceous glands return to their prepubertal state.

# Answers

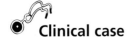

## Clinical case

### CASE 13.13 – A 17-year-old girl presents to her GP complaining of spots over her face for the past 4 years.

**A1: What is the likely differential diagnosis?**

The likely differential diagnoses are acne vulgaris, rosacea (usually occurs from the fourth decade onwards) and perioral dermatitis (may be secondary to misuse of topical corticosteroids).

**A2: What issues in the given history support the diagnosis?**

Acne is a very common problem in adolescents. The hallmark of acne is the comedone, which may be open (blackhead) or closed (whitehead). The characteristic lesions and their distribution give the diagnosis away.

**A3: What additional features in the history would you seek to support a particular diagnosis?**

Find out when the lesions started and their distribution. Do they affect only the face, or are the patient's back, chest or upper arms also involved? Ask the patient to describe the lesions – are they small papules or large cysts? What type of scars do the lesions leave when they resolve? Post-inflammatory hyperpigmentation is common and appears as a brown mark when the lesion resolves. It is not a permanent scar but can take many months to fade away. The colour tends to be more intense in patients with darker skin. Pitted atrophic scars ('ice-pick scars') may occur after severe nodulocystic acne and are permanent. Rarely, patients may have hypertrophic or keloid scarring, which is disfiguring.

**A4: What clinical examination would you perform, and why?**

The skin may appear greasy with red papules, pustules, comedones, and sometimes nodules, cysts, post-inflammatory hyperpigmentation and pitted or hypertrophic scars. Determine the distribution of the acne.

**A5: What investigations would be most helpful, and why?**

The diagnosis is made on history and clinical examination. If the lesions look infected, a swab may be sent for microbiology. Bear in mind that pustules are typically sterile.

**A6: What treatment options are appropriate?**

Topical benzoyl peroxide is antibacterial and comedolytic. Combined preparations with an antibiotic are also available. It can be very drying and cause irritation, so the treatment is started at the weakest concentration. Topical antibiotics alone are also used. Topical retinoic acid is a keratolytic agent and useful for comedonal acne and post-inflammatory hyperpigmentation. Salicylic acid can also be used as a keratolytic agent. Systemic antibiotics are the mainstay of acne treatment. Tetracyclines (oxytetracycline, doxycycline, minocycline, lymecycline), erythromycin or trimethoprim can be very effective but need to be taken for at least 3–6 months before a benefit is seen. As a rule, acne over the trunk responds slower than facial acne, and antibiotics may need to be continued for longer. For antibiotic-resistant acne or severe acne leading to scarring, systemic retinoid therapy is the treatment of choice.

**OSCE counselling case**

## OSCE COUNSELLING CASE 13.9 – 'Can I have isotretinoin for my acne?'

Isotretinoin is used in the treatment of the following:

- nodulocystic acne – severe chronic acne that is usually resistant to standard therapy; it is most frequent in males and presents with deep painful papules and nodules that lead to scars, occasionally with keloid formation
- acne leading to scarring
- antibiotic-resistant acne
- acne causing significant psychological distress to the patient.

Isotretinoin is given as 1 mg/kg/day in tablet form for 16 weeks. The effect is usually evident within 6 weeks. One course is usually sufficient to clear most patients' acne.

The main side effect noticed by patients is dryness of the skin and mucous membranes; patients must be advised to use an emollient and lip balm to alleviate this. Patients who usually wear contact lenses are advised to wear spectacles instead during the treatment period. Nosebleeds may occur in patients with a predisposition. Isotretinoin is metabolized through the liver and may cause hyperlipidaemia; liver function tests and cholesterol and triglyceride levels are taken before starting and during treatment. Patients should be warned of the risk of depression – there have been cases of suicide reported in patients receiving treatment with isotretinoin, and therefore depression is a relative contraindication to starting treatment.

It is vital that patients are informed that the drug is highly teratogenic, especially as most female patients on treatment are of childbearing age. A pregnancy test is mandatory before starting therapy. Patients are entered into a pregnancy prevention programme whereby they are prescribed treatment each month only if they have a negative pregnancy test. Patients are counselled to use two forms of contraception (oral contraception and a barrier method) during treatment and for at least 3 months after cessation of treatment.

## REVISION PANEL

- A malignant melanoma may arise de novo or present as a pre-existing mole that is enlarging and changing in colour. It usually looks different from the patient's other moles.
- A suspected melanoma must be excised urgently so that it can be analysed for Breslow depth. The Breslow depth is a good prognostic indicator and determines whether further investigations are needed.
- Melanoma may present as an enlarging freckle in elderly people (lentigo maligna).
- Subungual melanoma presents with discoloration under a nail, which may mimic haemorrhage from trauma.
- Actinic keratoses result from chronic sun damage and usually occur as rough red asymptomatic lesions that are often multiple and on sun-exposed sites.
- Actinic keratosis and Bowen's disease (in situ SCC of the skin) can progress to SCC and must be treated.
- Treatment for actinic keratosis, Bowen's disease and superficial BCC can be with cryotherapy, 5FU, imiquimod cream, photodynamic therapy or surgery (curettage and cautery or excision).
- SCCs must be excised urgently, as they have the potential to metastasize. Patients need follow-up after excision for early detection of recurrence.
- A BCC is best excised, but it does not need follow-up if removed completely as they very rarely metastasize.

- Atopic eczema is the most common type of eczema and is typically associated with hayfever and asthma.
- Infected eczema can be a dermatological emergency. Eczema herpeticum can also affect the eye and lead to corneal scarring and blindness.
- Patients with suspected contact dermatitis must be patch-tested to identify the allergen(s) responsible.
- The treatment of eczema includes patient education, emollients, soap substitutes and topical steroids for exacerbations.
- Patients with eczema should be advised to limit the use of topical steroids and use them sparingly, as continual use leads to skin atrophy.
- Psoriasis can affect the skin, scalp, nails and joints
- Erythrodermic psoriasis can be a life-threatening emergency, and the patient may be systemically unwell.
- Topical treatments for psoriasis include emollients and preparations containing coal tar, dithranol, corticosteroids and vitamin D analogues.
- PUVA or UVB radiation without psoralen (TL-01) can be used for widespread psoriasis, but patients should be warned that phototherapy increases the risk of skin cancer.
- Severe psoriasis can be treated with systemic agents such as methotrexate, ciclosporin and acitretin, or with biologic injections or infusions, which can be prescribed only by a dermatologist.
- Patients presenting with pruritus can be subdivided into those with pruritus and a rash where the itch is secondary to the skin condition, and those presenting without a rash, in which case an internal or medical cause is usually responsible for the itching.
- Blood investigations are necessary for patients presenting with pruritus in the absence of a skin rash.
- If scabies is suspected, look for burrows in the finger webs and on the hands.
- Scabies is highly infectious, and all contacts need to be treated at the same time as the patient.
- If urticaria is accompanied by angio-oedema, the patient must be given an adrenaline injection for self-administration to use in case of anaphylaxis.
- The hallmark of acne is the comedone, which may be open (blackhead) or closed (whitehead).
- Acne can lead to scarring, which may be permanent and disfiguring.
- If topical acne treatments have been ineffective, systemic antibiotics should be prescribed for at least 3–6 months.
- In women with acne, the oral contraceptive pill containing cyproterone acetate can be effective in treating acne.
- If systemic antibiotics have been ineffective, or the acne is severe, oral isotretinoin can be given. This needs careful monitoring, especially in female patients.

# Index

# Contents

# Acknowledgements

I would like to thank everyone who has worked so hard to complete this book – Cathy Dickens and the PasTest team. Thanks especially to my fellow editor, Cathy, whose excellent teaching eased my early passage through basic surgical training and whose subsequent advice, friendship and *joie de vivre* is invaluable.

I have been fortunate enough to be surrounded by fantastic friends and colleagues. There are too many to list everyone by name (but you know who you are) and I appreciate all your support.

Thanks to my family and last, but certainly not least, thanks to my husband Roy, for backing me up, making me laugh and who is a constant and irreplaceable source of patience and good cheer.

# Preface

This book is an attempt to help surgical trainees pass the MRCS exam by putting together the revision notes they need. It was written (in the main) and edited by trainees for trainees and while we do not claim to be authorities on the subjects by any means, we hope to save you some work by expanding our own revision notes and putting them in a readable format. Originally written when we were SHOs, as time has passed and we have ourselves climbed the surgical ladder, we have updated the text but have tried to keep the style of the books as accessible and informal as possible. Medical students interested in surgery may also find it a good general introduction to the surgical specialties.

Now in its third incarnation we have refined this edition further to cover the evolving MRCS syllabus in two volumes. These two books have been designed to be used together and in conjunction with the existing PasTest MRCS Part B OSCE's volume. Although the format of surgical examinations in the UK has changed to include OSCE assessment, the principles of core surgical knowledge remain the same, and often a good exam answer starts with a structured summary followed by expansion of individual points. We have, therefore, arranged each topic in this format, and we have used boxes, bullet points and diagrams to highlight important points. There is additional space around the text for you to annotate and personalise these notes from your own experience.

My dad is fond of saying that the harder you work, the luckier you get, and I have always found this to be true – so GOOD LUCK!

Ritchie Chalmers

# Picture Permissions

# Contributors

**Editors**

**Claire Ritchie Chalmers BA PhD FRCS**
*Breast Surgery*

**Catherine Parchment Smith BSc(Hons) MBChB(Hons) FRCS(Eng)**
*Abdominal Surgery*

**Contributors**

**Sam Andrews MA MS FRCS (Gen)**
Consultant General and Vascular Surgeon, Maidstone Hospital and Medway Foundation NHS Trust
*Vascular Surgery*

**Paul M Brennan BSc (Hons) MB BChir MRCS**
ECAT Clinical Lecturer, Honorary Specialist Registrar Neurosurgery, Edinburgh Cancer Research Centre, University of Edinburgh Department of Clinical Neurosciences, NHS Lothian
*Neurosurgery (elective)*

**Mary M Brown MBChB FRCS(UROL)**
Consultant Urological Surgeon, Department of Urology, Gartnavel General Hospital, Glasgow
*Urological Surgery*

**Sylvia Brown MD MRCS MBChB**
ST7 in General Surgery, Southern General Hospital, Glasgow
*Endocrine Surgery*

**Nicholas E Gibbins MD, FRCS (ORL-HNS)**
ENT Specialist Registrar, Department of Otolaryngology, Guy's Hospital, London.
*Endocrine Surgery / Head and Neck Surgery*

**Jennifer McIlhenny MBChB MSc MRCS**
ST3 in General Surgery, Department of General Surgery, Western Infirmary, Glasgow.
*Breast Surgery*

**Mr Sai Prasad, M.D, FRCS**
Consultant Cardiothoracic Surgeon, Department of Cardiothoracic Surgery, Royal Infirmary of Edinburgh, Edinburgh
*Cardiothoracic Surgery*

**Arin K Saha BA (Hons) MBBChir MA (Cantab) MRCS (Eng) MD**
Registrar in General Surgery, Pinderfields Hospital, Yorkshire and the Humber Deanery.
*Abdominal Surgery*

**Karen S Stevenson PhD, MRCS, MBChB, BSc(Med Sci)**
Specialty Registrar in General Surgery, Dept of Renal Transplant Surgery, Western Infirmary, Glasgow
*Transplant Surgery*

**George Tse MSc, MRCSEd, MBChB, BSc (Hons)**
Kidney Research UK, Clinical Training Fellow, Centre For Inflammation Research, University of Edinburgh
*Cardiothoracic Surgery*

**Ravinder S Vohra PhD, MRCS**
Lecturer in General Surgery, Queen Elizabeth Hospital Birmingham, Birmingham
*Abdominal Surgery*

# Contributors to Previous Editions

**Sudipta Banerjee MBChB DLO FRCS (ORL-HNS)**
Specialist Registrar, North Western Deanery
*Ear, Nose, Head and Neck*

**Juliette Murray FRCS**
Consultant In Breast Surgery, Wishaw General
Hospital, Lanarkshire, Scotland
*Paediatric surgery*

**Robert S. Boome MBChB(CT) FRCS(Ed) FCS (Orth) SA**
Consultant Orthopaedic Surgeon,
Department of Orthopaedics and Trauma,
Bradford
Royal Infirmary, Bradford
*Orthopaedics*

**Luke Devey MA BM BCh MRCSEd**
MRC Clinical Research Training Fellow, Tissue
Injury and Repair Group, MRC Centre for
Inflammation Research, Edinburgh
*Cardiothoracic Surgery*

**Nigel Gummerson MA(Oxon) MRCS**
Specialist Registrar in Orthopaedics/Trauma
Surgery, Yorkshire Deanery
*Orthopaedics*

**Christopher J. Hammond BM BCh MA MRCS**
Specialist Registrar in Radiology, Leeds
General Infirmary, Leeds
*Elective Neurosurgery and Spinal Surgery*

**Jonathan D.M. Harrison MBChB Dm FRCS**
Consultant General and Colorectal Surgeon,
Department of General Surgery, Harrogate
District Hospital, Harrogate
*Abdomen*

**Sarah Heap MBChB MRCS**
Senior House Officer in Vascular Surgery,
Manchester Royal Infirmary, Manchester
*Orthopaedics*

**Catherine Hernon BSc MBChB AFRCS(Ed)**
Specialist Registrar Plastic Surgery, Yorkshire
Rotation *Orthopaedics*

**Mark Lansdown BSc MB BCh MCh FRCS**
Consultant Surgeon, Leeds Teaching Hospitals
NHS Trust, Leeds
*Endocrine Surgery*

**James McK. Manson BSc FRCS ChM**
Consultant Upper-Gastrointestinal Surgeon,
Department of Gastro-Intestinal Surgery,
Singleton Hospital, Swansea
*Abdomen*

**Catherine R. Tait MBChB(Hons), MRCS(Eng), MD**
Surgical Fellow, Department of Breast Surgery,
Leeds General Infirmary, Leeds
*Breast, Endocrine Surgery*

**Jake Timothy FRCS(Eng) FRCS(SN)**
Consultant Neurosurgeon and Spinal Surgeon,
Department of Neurosurgery, Leeds General
Infirmary, Leeds
*Elective Neurosurgery and Spinal Surgery*

**Philip Turton MBChB FRCS(Gen Surg) MD(Hons)**
Consultant Breast and Oncoplastic Breast
Surgeon, Honorary Senior Lecturer in
Breast Surgery, The Breast Unit, St James's
University Hospital, The Leeds Teaching
Hospitals Trust, Leeds
*Breast*

**Sunjay Jain MD FRCS (Urol)**
Clinical Lecturer in Urology, University of
Leicester, Leicester

**Professor Kilian Mellon MD FRCS (Urol)**
Professor of Urology, University of Leicester,
Leicester

# Introduction

## A    The Intercollegiate MRCS Examination

The Intercollegiate MRCS examination comprises two parts: Part A (MCQ) and Part B (OSCE)

### Part A (written) : Multiple Choice Questions (MCQ)

Part A is a four hour MCQ examination consisting of two 2hr papers taken on the same day.  The papers cover generic surgical sciences and applied knowledge, including the core knowledge required in all nine specialties.  The marks for both papers are combined to give a total mark for Part A although there is also a minimum pass mark for each paper. There are no limits as to the number of times that you can attempt this part of the exam.

Paper 1 - Applied Basic Sciences MCQ paper

Paper 2 - Principles of Surgery-in-General MCQ paper

There are 135 questions per paper and two styles of question. The first type of question requires the single best answer. Each question contains five possible answers of which there is only one single best answer. An example of this type of question from the college website is:

A 67-year-old woman is brought to the emergency department having fallen on her left arm.

There is an obvious clinical deformity and X-ray demonstrates a mid-shaft fracture of the humerus. She has lost the ability to extend the left wrist joint. Which nerve has most likely been damaged with the fracture?

A   The axillary nerve
B   The median nerve
C   The musculocutaneous nerve
D   The radial nerve
E   The ulnar nerve

The second type of question is an extended matching question. Each theme contains a variable number of options and clinical situations. Only one option will be the most appropriate response to each clinical situation. You should select the most appropriate option. It is possible for one option to be the answer to more than one of the clinical situations. An example of this type of question from the college website is:

Theme: Chest injuries

Options

A Tension pneumothorax
B Aortic rupture
C Haemothorax
D Aortic dissection
E Ruptured spleen
F Cardiac tamponade

For each of the situations below, select the single most likely diagnosis from the options listed above. Each option may be used once, more than once or not at all.

1. A 24-year-old man is brought into the emergency department having been stabbed with a screwdriver. He is conscious. On examination he is tachypnoeic and has a tachycardia of 120 beats/minute. His blood pressure is 90/50 mmHg. He has a small puncture wound below his right costal margin. A central venous line is inserted with ease, and his central venous pressure is 17 cm. A chest Xray shows a small pleural effusion with a small pneumothorax. He has received two units of plasma expander, which has failed to improve his blood pressure.
2. A 42-year-old man is admitted following a road traffic accident complaining of pains throughout his chest. He was fit and well prior to the incident. He is tachypnoeic and in considerable pain. His brachial blood pressure is 110/70 mmHg and his pulse rate is 90 beats/minute. Both femoral pulses are present though greatly diminished. A chest Xray shows multiple rib fractures and an appreciably widened upper mediastinum. Lateral views confirm a fractured sternum. An eCG shows ischaemic changes in the V-leads.

Further examples of the two types of question are available on the college website and in the PasTest MRCS Practice Question Books.

The questions cover the entire syllabus and are broken down into:

### Paper 1

**Applied Surgical Anatomy** - 45 questions. This includes gross anatomy as well as questions on developmental and imaging anatomy:-

| Topic | Number of questions |
|---|---|
| Thorax | 6 |
| Abdomen, pelvis, perineum | 12 |
| Upper limb, breast | 8 |
| Lower limb | 6 |

| | |
|---|---|
| Head, neck and spine | 9 |
| Central, peripheral and autonomic nervous systems | 4 |

**Physiology -** 45 questions. This includes 12 questions on general physiological principles covering thermoregulation, metabolic pathways, sepsis and septic shock, fluid balance, metabolic acidosis/alkalosis, and colloid and crystalloid solutions

**System specific physiology :-**

| Topic | Number of questions |
|---|---|
| Respiratory system | 6 |
| Cardiovascular system | 6 |
| Gastrointestinal system | 4 |
| Renal system | 6 |
| Endocrine system (including glucose homeostasis) | 4 |
| Nervous system | 3 |
| Thyroid and parathyroid | 4 |

## **Pathology** - 45 questions.

This includes 20–22 questions on general principles of pathology:-

| Topic | Number of questions |
|---|---|
| Inflammation | 3 |
| Wound healing and cellular healing | 1-2 |
| Vascular disorders | 3 |
| Disorders of growth | 3 |
| Tumours | 6 |
| Surgical immunology | 3 |
| Surgical haematology | 1-2 |

**System specific pathology** (22–26 questions):-

| Topic | Number of questions |
|---|---|
| Nervous system | 1-2 |
| Musculoskeletal system | 3 |
| Respiratory system | 1-2 |
| Breast disorders | 4 |
| Endocrine systems | 1-2 |
| Genitourinary system | 3 |
| Gastrointestinal system | 5 |
| Lymphoreticular system | 1-2 |
| Cardiovascular system | 3 |

## Paper 2

**Clinical Problem Solving -** 135 questions. This includes 45 questions on **Principles of Surgery in General** and 90 questions on **Surgical Specialties:-**

**Principles of Surgery in General**

| Topic | Number of questions |
|---|---|
| Perioperative care | 8 |
| Post-operative care | 4 |
| Surgical techniques | 6 |
| Management/legal topics | 4 |
| Microbiology | 6 |
| Emergency medicine | 9 |
| Oncology | 8 |

| Surgical Specialties Topic | Number of questions |
|---|---|
| Cardiothoracic | 6 |
| Abdominal | 9 |

| | |
|---|---|
| Upper gastrointestinal | 4-5 |
| Hepatobilary and pancreatic | 5 |
| Colorectal | 6 |
| Breast | 4-5 |
| Endocrine | 6 |
| Vascular | 7 |
| Transplant | 3 |
| ENT | 6 |
| Oro-maxillo-facial | 2 |
| Paediatrics | 6 |
| Neurosurgery | 6 |
| Trauma/orthopaedics | 7-8 |
| Plastics | 6 |
| Urology | 7 |

It is therefore important that you cover the entire syllabus in order to pick up the greatest number of marks.

**Part B:  Objective Structured Clinical Examination (OSCE)**

To be eligible for Part B you must have passed Part A. The OSCE will normally consist of 18 examined stations each of 9 minutes' duration and one or more rest/preparation station. Although the MRCS remains an exam for the core part of Surgical Training, six of the stations will be examined in a specialty context and the other 12 reflect generic surgical skills. You must specify your choice of specialty context stations at the time of your application to sit the exam. This structure may change in the future, check the website for the most up to date information.

These speciality stations will examine the following broad content areas:

1. Anatomy and surgical pathology
2.  Applied surgical science and critical care
3. Communication skills in giving and receiving information and history taking.
4. Clinical and procedural skills

Speciality areas are:
* Head and Neck
* Trunk and Thorax

- Limbs (including spine)
- Neurosciences

Each station is manned by one or two examiners and is marked out of 20 with a separate 'overall global rating' of:
- Pass
- Borderline Pass
- Borderline Fail
- Fail

There are 4 domains assessed throughout the exam which are areas of knowledge, skill, competencies and professional characteristics that a candidate should demonstrate. These are:
- Clinical Knowledge
- Clinical and Technical skill
- Communication
- Professionalism

The overall mark is calculated from both the mark out of 20 and the overall global rating. In order to pass the exam you need to achieve the minimum pass mark and also a minimum competence level in each of the four content areas and in each four domains.

The OSCE and preparation for it are covered in depth in the PasTest MRCS Part B (OSCE) handbook.

# B  Candidate Instructions for Part A (MCQ)

Candidates who are late by no more than 30 minutes for the exam may be allowed entry at the discretion of the senior invigilator but will not be given extra time. You may not leave in the first 60 minutes or the last 15 minutes of the examination and then you must wait until answer sheets and question booklets have been collected from your desk.

Each desk in the examination hall will be numbered and candidates must sit at the desk that corresponds to their examination/candidate number.

Candidates must bring proof of identity to each examination, such as a current passport or driving licence that includes your name, signature and a photograph. Once seated this should be placed on the desk ready for inspection.

Pencils and all stationery will be provided. Mobile phones and electronic devices (including pagers and calculators) must be switched off and are not permitted to be on the desk or on your person during the exam. Failure to comply with this will lead to suspension from the exam.

Dress comfortably. You are allowed to take a small bottle of water or a drink in to the exam hall with you.

There are equal marks for each question. Marks will not be deducted for a wrong answer. However, you will not gain a mark if you mark more than one box for the same item or question. The answer sheets are scanned by machine. If you do not enter your answer to each question correctly and clearly on the answer sheet the machine which scores your paper may reject it. Mark each answer clearly as faint marking may be misread by the machine. If you need to change an answer, you should make sure that you rub it out completely so that the computer can accept your final answer.

Many candidates find it easier to mark their answers on the question booklet first and transfer them to the answer sheet later. If you do this, you should allow time to transfer your answers to the answer sheet before the end of the examination. No extra time will be given for the transfer of answers.

## C    Preparing for the MCQ exam

The MRCS` exam and syllabus is being constantly updated and the best way to keep up to date with its requirements is via the website 'http://www.intercollegiatemrcs.org.uk' which contains information on :

- Examination dates
- Regulations
- Guidance notes
- Domain descriptors
- Application Forms
- Syllabus
- Candidate Feedback
- Annual reports

Different people prepare for MCQ examinations in different ways. The key to success is to do as many practice questions as possible. You may prefer to revise a topic before undertaking practice questions or use practice questions to highlight areas of lack of knowledge and direct your learning.

The PasTest book series also includes practice SBAs and EMQs for Part A of the MRCS. In addition over 4000 practice questions are available from PasTest Online Revision including apps for android and i-phones.

## D    The Syllabus

The syllabus essentially remains the same although it is structured differently every few years. The most up to date version can be found on the intercollegiate website. The syllabus from 2012 has been structured in 10 modules:

**Module 1:  Basic Sciences** (to include applied surgical anatomy, applied surgical physiology, applied pharmacology (centred around the safe prescribing of common drugs), surgical pathology (principles underlying system-specific pathology), surgical microbiology,  imaging (principles, advantages and disadvantages of various diagnostic and interventional imaging methods)

**Module 2: Common surgical conditions** (under the topics of gastrointestinal disease; breast disease; vascular disease; cardiovascular and pulmonary disease; genitourinary disease; trauma and orthopaedics; diseases of the skin, head and neck; neurology and neurosurgery; and endocrine disease).

**Module 3: Basic Surgical skills** (including the principles and practice of surgery and technique)

**Module 4: The Assessment and Management of the Surgical Patient** (decision making, team working and communication skills)

**Module 5: Peri-operative care** (pre-operative, intra-operative and post-operative care including the management of complications)

**Module 6 Assessment and management of patients with trauma** (including the multiply injured patient)

**Module 7: Surgical care of the paediatric patient**

**Module 8: Management of the dying patient**

**Module 9: Organ and tissue transplantation**

**Module 10: Professional behaviour and leadership skills** (including communication, teaching and Training, keeping up to date, managing people and resources within healthcare, promoting good health and the ethical and legal obligations of a surgeon)

# CHAPTER 1

# Abdominal Surgery

## Catherine Parchment Smith, Arin K. Saha and Ravinder S. Vohra

## 1.1 Anterior abdominal wall

### Layers of the abdominal wall

 **In a nutshell ...**

When you make an incision in the anterior abdominal wall you will go through several layers:
- Skin
- Subcutaneous fat
- Superficial fascia
- Deep fascia (vestigial)
- Muscles (depending on incision)
- Transversalis fascia
- Extraperitoneal fat
- Peritoneum

### Skin

The skin has horizontal Langer's lines over the abdomen. Dermatomes are also arranged in transverse bands.

### Deep fascia

This is a vestigial thin layer of areolar tissue over muscles.

### Superficial fascia (Scarpa's fascia)

- Absent above and laterally
- Fuses with deep fascia of leg inferior to inguinal ligament
- Very prominent in children (can even be mistaken for external oblique!)
- Continuous with Colles' fascia over perineum (forms tubular sheath for penis/clitoris and sac-like covering for scrotum/labia)

### Muscles

 **In a nutshell ...**

The muscles you'll pass through depend on the incision site:
- External oblique
- Internal oblique
- Rectus abdominis
- Transversus abdominis
- Pyramidalis
- Rectus sheath

- **External oblique** is a large sheet of muscle fibres running downwards from lateral to medial like a 'hand in your pocket'. Medially, the external oblique becomes a fibrous aponeurosis which lies over the rectus abdominis muscle (see below), forming part of the anterior rectus sheath
- **Internal oblique** is a second large sheet of muscle fibres lying deep to the external oblique and at right angles to it. Medially, it forms a fibrous aponeurosis which splits to enclose the middle portion of rectus abdominis as part of the anterior and posterior rectus sheath
- **Transversus abdominis** is the third large sheet of muscle lying deep to the internal oblique and running transversely. Medially, it forms a fibrous aponeurosis which contributes to the posterior rectus sheath lying behind rectus abdominis
- **Rectus abdominis** and its pair join at the linea alba in the midline to form a wide strap that runs longitudinally down the anterior abdominal wall. It lies within the rectus sheath formed by the aponeuroses of the three muscles described above. It is attached to the anterior rectus sheath, but not to the posterior rectus sheath, by three tendinous insertions. These insertions are at the level of the xiphisternum, umbilicus and halfway between (giving the 'six-pack' appearance in well-developed individuals!). The blood supply of rectus abdominis is through the superior epigastric artery (a terminal branch of the internal thoracic artery) and the inferior epigastric artery (a branch of the external iliac artery) which anastomose to form a connection between the subclavian and external iliac systems (Fig. 1.1). The superior epigastric artery is the pedicle on which a TRAM flap is raised for breast reconstruction. The nerve supply to the recti is segmental from T6 to T12 and

the nerves enter the sheath laterally and run towards the midline (so are disrupted in Battle's incision – see Figure 1.3)
- **Linea alba** is a fibrotendinous raphe running vertically in the midline between the left and right rectus abdominis muscles. It is formed by the fusion of the external oblique, internal oblique and transversus abdominis aponeuroses. They fuse in an interlocking/ interdigitating structure through which epigastric hernias may protrude. The linea alba provides an avascular and relatively bloodless plane through which midline laparotomy incisions are made. It is easier to begin a laparotomy incision above the umbilicus, where the linea alba is wider, thicker and better defined than below the umbilicus
- **Pyramidalis** is a small (4 cm long) unimportant muscle arising from the pubic crest and inserting into the linea alba. It lies behind the anterior rectus sheath in front of rectus abdominis. This is the only muscle you go through in your lower midline laparotomy incision and it is not as bloodless as the linea alba which it underlies

## Rectus sheath

 **In a nutshell ...**

Any incision over rectus abdominis will go through the anterior rectus sheath. Arrangement of the rectus sheath is best considered in three sections:
- Above the level of the costal margin
- From the costal margin to just below the umbilicus
- Below the line of Douglas

- **Above the level of the costal margin:** the anterior rectus sheath is formed by the external oblique aponeurosis only. There is no internal oblique or transversus abdominis aponeurosis at this level. Therefore there is no posterior rectus sheath and rectus abdominis lies directly on the fifth to seventh costal cartilages
- **From the costal margin to just below the umbilicus:** the anterior rectus sheath is formed by the external oblique aponeurosis and the anterior leaf of the split internal oblique aponeurosis. It is attached to rectus abdominis by tendinous intersections. The posterior rectus sheath is formed by the posterior leaf of the internal oblique aponeurosis and the transversus abdominis aponeurosis

- **Below the line of Douglas:** about 2.5 cm below the umbilicus lies a line called the 'arcuate line of Douglas' (Fig. 1.1). At this level, the posterior rectus sheath (ie the posterior leaf of the internal oblique aponeurosis along with the transversus abdominis aponeuroses) passes anterior to rectus abdominis. Therefore, below the arcuate line of Douglas there is no posterior rectus sheath. Rectus abdominis lies directly on transversalis fascia, which is thickened here, and called the 'iliopubic tract'. The anterior rectus sheath is now formed by all the combined aponeuroses of the external oblique, internal oblique and transversus abdominis muscles

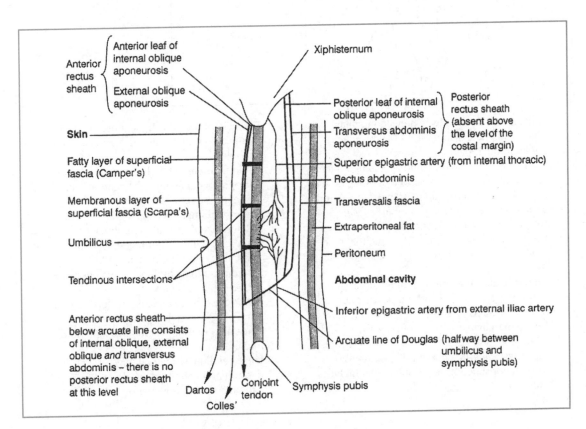

**Figure 1.1 Sagittal section of the abdominal wall**

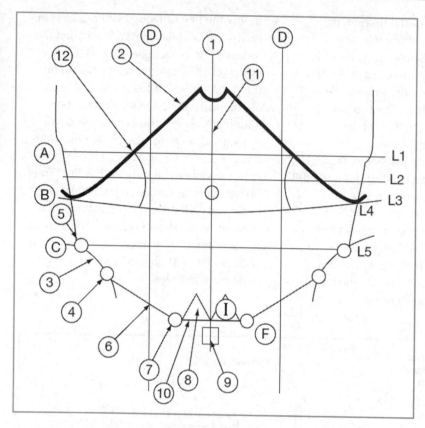

**Figure 1.2 Surface landmarks of the anterior abdominal wall**

(A) **Transpyloric line:** halfway between jugular notch and pubic symphysis at L1; this plane passes through pylorus, pancreatic neck, duodenojejunal flexure, fundus of gallbladder, tip of ninth costal cartilage, hila of kidneys; also it is the level of termination of the spinal cord.

(B) **Subcostal line:** under lowest rib (rib 10 at L3).

(C) **Intertubercular/transtubercular line:** between two tubercles of iliac crest (L5); note that plane of iliac crests (supracristal plane) is higher (at L4).

(D) **Midclavicular line:** through midinguinal point, halfway between ASIS and symphysis pubis.

(1) **Xiphoid process:** xiphisternal junction is at T9.

(2) **Costal margins:** ribs 7–10 in front; ribs 11 and 12 behind; tenth costal cartilage is lowest at L3.

(3) **Iliac crest:** anterior superior iliac spine (ASIS) to posterior superior iliac spine (PSIS); highest point L4.

(4) **ASIS**.

(5) **Tubercle of iliac crest:** 5 cm behind ASIS at L5.

(6) **Inguinal ligament:** running from ASIS to pubic tubercle.

(7) **Pubic tubercle:** tubercle on superior surface of pubis; inguinal ligament attaches to it, as lateral end of the superficial inguinal ring.

(8) **Superficial inguinal ring:** inguinal hernia comes out above and medial to pubic tubercle at point marked (I); femoral hernia below and lateral to pubic tubercle at point marked (F).

(9) **Symphysis pubis:** midline cartilaginous joint between pubic bones.

(10) **Pubic crest:** ridge on superior surface of pubic bone medial to pubic tubercle.

(11) **Linea alba:** symphysis pubis to xiphoid process midline.

(12) **Linea semilunaris:** lateral edge of rectus crosses costal margin at ninth costal cartilage (tip of gall bladder palpable here).

**Contents of the rectus sheath**

- Rectus abdominis
- Pyramidalis
- Segmental nerves
- Segmental vessels from T7 to T12
- Superior and inferior epigastric vessels (see Figure 1.1)

Layers of the abdominal wall divided in three common incisions

| Midline laparotomy | Kocher's incision | Gridiron appendicectomy incision |
|---|---|---|
| Skin | Skin | Skin |
| Subcutaneous fat | Subcutaneous fat | Subcutaneous fat |
| Scarpa's fascia | Scarpa's fascia | Scarpa's fascia |
| Linea alba | Medially:<br>Anterior rectus sheath<br>Rectus abdominis<br>Posterior rectus sheath | |
| | Laterally:<br>External oblique<br>Internal oblique<br>Transversus abdominis | External oblique<br>Internal oblique<br>Transversus abdominis |
| Fascia transversalis | Fascia transversalis | Fascia transversalis |
| Preperitoneal fat | Preperitoneal fat | Preperitoneal fat |
| Parietal peritoneum | Parietal peritoneum | Parietal peritoneum |

**Diseases of the umbilicus**

**Congenital**

- Cord hernias
- Gastroschisis
- Exomphalos

**Tumours**

- Primary
  - Benign (papilloma, lipoma)
  - Malignant (squamous cell carcinoma [SCC], melanoma)
- Secondary
  - Breast
  - Ovarian
  - Colon (via lymphatic, transcoloemic and direct spread along falciform ligament)

Endometriosis

**Hernias**

- Childhood (umbilical)
- Adult (paraumbilical)

**Fistula**

- Urinary tract (via urachal remnant)
- Gastrointestinal tract (via vitelloin-testinal duct)

**Suppurations**

- Primary
  - Obesity
  - Pilonidal
  - Fungal infections
- Secondary
  - From intra-abdominal abscess

## Surface markings of abdominal organs and vessels

- **Gallbladder:** tip of right ninth costal cartilage where linea semilunaris intersects the costal margin (Figure 1.2)
- **Spleen:** under ribs 9, 10 and 11 on the left; long axis lies along rib 10; palpable in infants
- **Pancreas:** lies along the transpyloric plane (L1)
- **Kidney:** from the level of T12 to L3; the hilum lies on the transpyloric plane (L1); right kidney is lower; kidneys move 2–5 cm in respiration
- **Appendix:** McBurney's point is the surface marking of the base of the appendix one third of the way up the line joining the anterior superior iliac spine to the umbilicus
- **Aortic bifurcation:** at the level of L4 vertebra to left of midline

- **External iliac artery:** palpable at midinguinal point halfway between ASIS and symphysis pubis

## Abdominal incisions

**The ideal abdominal incision**
- Allows easy and rapid access to relevant structures
- Allows easy extension (if necessary)
- Favours secure healing in the short term (no dehiscence) and in the long term (no herniation)
- Leaves patients relatively pain-free postoperatively
- Gives a satisfactory cosmetic appearance

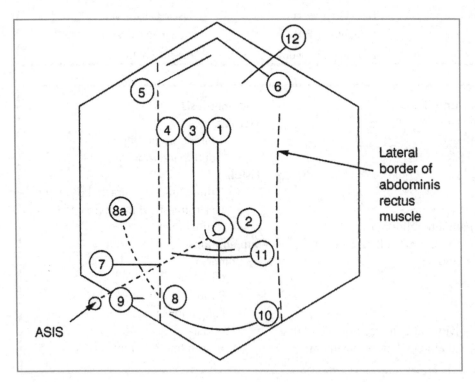

Figure 1.3 Abdominal incisions

## Figure 1.3 Abdominal incisions

(1) **Midline incision through linea alba:** provides good access. Can be extended easily. Quick to make and close. Relatively avascular. More painful than transverse incisions. Incision crosses Langer's lines so it has poor cosmetic appearance. Narrow linea alba below umbilicus. Some vessels cross the midline. May cause bladder damage.

(2) **Subumbilical incision:** used for repair of paraumbilical hernias and laparoscopic port.

(3) **Paramedian incision:** 1.5 cm from midline through rectus abdominis sheath. This was the only effective vertical incision in the days when catgut was the only available suture material. Takes longer to make than midline incision. Does not lend itself to closure by 'Jenkins rule' (length of suture is 4 × length of wound). Poor cosmetic result. Can lead to infection in rectus sheath. Other hazards: tendinous intersections must be dissected off; need to divide falciform ligament above umbilicus on the right; if rectus is split more than 1 cm from medial border, intercostal nerves are disrupted leading to denervation of medial rectus (avoid by retracting rectus without splitting).

(4) **Pararectal 'Battle's' incision:** now not used because of damage to nerves entering rectus sheath and poor healing leading to postoperative incisional hernias.

(5) **Kocher's incision:** 3 cm below and parallel to costal margin from midline to rectus border. Good incision for cholecystectomy on the right and splenectomy on the left – but beware superior epigastric vessels. If wound is extended laterally too many intercostal nerves are severed. Cannot be extended caudally.

(6) **Double Kocher's (rooftop) incision:** good access to liver and spleen. Useful for intrahepatic surgery. Used for radical pancreatic and gastric surgery and bilateral adrenalectomy.

(7) **Transverse muscle-cutting incision:** can be across all muscles. Beware of intercostal nerves.

(8) **McBurney's/gridiron incision:** classic approach to appendix through junction of the outer and middle third of a line from the anterior superior iliac spine (ASIS) to the umbilicus at right angles to that line. May be modified into a skin-crease horizontal cut. External oblique aponeurosis is cut in the line of the fibres. Internal oblique and transversus abdominis are split transversely in the line of the fibres. Beware: scarring if not horizontal; iliohypogastric and ilioinguinal nerves; deep circumflex artery.

(8a) **Rutherford–Morrison incision:** gridiron can be extended cephalad and laterally, obliquely splitting the external oblique to afford good access to caecum, appendix and right colon.

(9) **Lanz incision:** lower incision than McBurney's and closer to the ASIS. Better cosmetic result (concealed by bikini). Tends to divide iliohypogastric and ilioinguinal nerves, leading to denervation of inguinal canal mechanism (can increase risk of inguinal hernia).

(10) **Pfannenstiel's incision:** most frequently used transverse incision in adults. Excellent access to female genitalia for caesarean section and for bladder and prostate operations. Also used for bilateral hernia repair. Skin incised in a downward convex arc into suprapubic skin crease 2 cm above the pubis. Upper flap is raised and rectus sheath incised 1 cm cephalic to the skin incision (not extending lateral to the rectus). Rectus is then divided longitudinally in the midline.

(11) **Transverse incision:** particularly useful in neonates and children (who do not have the subdiaphragmatic and pelvic recesses of adults). Heals securely and cosmetically. Less pain and fewer respiratory problems than with longitudinal midline incision but division of red muscle involves more blood loss than longitudinal incision. Not extended easily. Takes longer to make and close. Limited access in adults to pelvic or subdiaphragmatic structures.

(12) **Thoracoabdominal incision:** access to lower thorax and upper abdomen. Used (rarely) for liver and biliary surgery on the right. Used (rarely) for oesophageal, gastric and aortic surgery on the left.

## 1.2 Hernias

### In a nutshell ...

A hernia is a protrusion of all or part of a viscus through the wall of the cavity in which it is normally contained.

Types of abdominal hernias:

Groin:
- Inguinal
- Femoral

Umbilical

Paraumbilical

Incisional

Epigastric

Spigelian

Lumbar

Gluteal

Sciatic

### Groin hernias

Inguinal and femoral hernias are two of the most common types of hernia. Their repairs make up a large proportion of elective surgery.

### All groin hernias

All hernias are more common on the right than on the left (may be due to later descent of right testis or previous appendicectomy)

### Incidence of groin hernias

**Male children**
- 4% of male infants have indirect inguinal hernia
- Risk of incarceration is high in babies
- Presents as lump in the groin when child cries
- Indirect inguinal > direct inguinal > femoral (very rare)

**Female children**
- All groin hernias rare in female children
- Presence of bilateral hernias should alert clinicians to possible testicular feminisation syndrome
- Hernias in female children may contain an ovary in the hernia sac which must be reduced at surgery
- Indirect inguinal > direct inguinal > femoral (very rare)

**Male adults**
- Direct inguinal > indirect inguinal > femoral

**Female adults**
- Indirect inguinal > femoral > direct (rare)

# Inguinal hernias

## Anatomy of the inguinal region

### Inguinal canal

This is an oblique intermuscular slit, 6 cm long, above the medial half of the inguinal ligament between the deep and superficial rings. It transmits the spermatic cord in the male and the round ligament of the uterus in the female.

### Deep inguinal ring

This is an oval opening in the transversalis fascia, 1.3 cm above the inguinal ligament, midway between the ASIS and the pubic tubercle. This is the midpoint of the inguinal ligament – just lateral to the midinguinal point. The deep ring is bounded laterally by the angle between the transversus abdominis and the inguinal ligament. It is bounded medially by the transversalis fascia and the inferior epigastric vessels behind this.

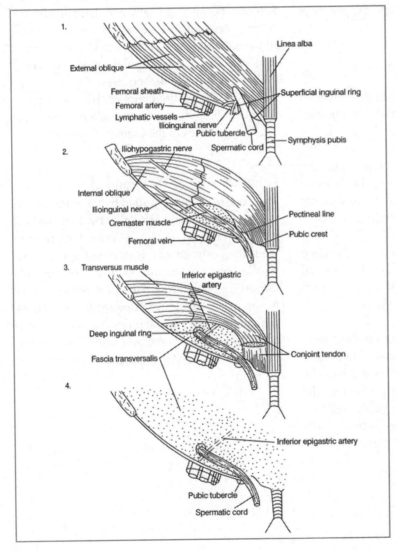

**Figure 1.4 Anatomy of the inguinal region:**

1. With skin and cutaneous fat removed
2. With external oblique removed
3. With internal oblique removed
4. With transversus muscle removed

### Superficial inguinal ring

This is a triangular opening in the external oblique aponeurosis. The lateral crus attaches to the pubic tubercle. The medial crus attaches to the pubic crest near the symphysis. The base of the superficial ring is the pubic crest.

### Floor of the inguinal canal

The inguinal ligament forms most of the floor of the inguinal canal. The lacunar ligament forms the medial part of the floor, filling in the angle between the inguinal ligament and the pectineal line.

### Ceiling of the inguinal canal

Lateral to medial, this is formed by transversus abdominis, internal oblique and the conjoint tendon.

**Transversus abdominis** arises lateral to the deep ring from the lateral half of the inguinal ligament. It arches over the roof of the inguinal canal to become the conjoint tendon.

The **internal oblique** arises in front of the deep ring from the lateral two-thirds of the inguinal ligament and, lying superficial to transversus abdominis, behaves in the same way.

The **conjoint tendon** is formed by the fusion of the aponeurosis of the internal oblique and transversus abdominis. It arches over the canal, forming the medial roof, strengthening the posterior wall. It inserts into the pubic crest and the pectineal line at right angles to the lacunar ligament, which forms the floor here.

Transversus abdominis, the internal oblique and conjoint tendon can contract and lower the roof of the inguinal canal, thereby strengthening it. They are supplied by L1 from the iliohypogastric and ilioinguinal nerves. These nerves are at risk in the muscle-splitting incision for appendicectomy, which leads to increased risk of direct hernia.

### Anterior wall of the inguinal canal

The anterior wall is formed mostly by the external oblique strengthened laterally by the internal oblique. The superficial ring is a defect in the anterior wall. The anterior wall is strongest opposite the weakest point of the posterior wall – the laterally placed deep ring. Here, the anterior wall is strengthened by the internal oblique fibres that originate anterior from the lateral two-thirds of the inguinal ligament.

### Posterior wall of the inguinal canal

The posterior wall is formed by the transversalis fascia, strengthened medially by the conjoint tendon. The deep ring is a defect in the posterior wall. The posterior wall is strongest opposite the weakest point of the anterior wall – the medially placed superficial ring. Here, the posterior wall is strengthened by the conjoint tendon fibres, formed from the internal oblique and transversus abdominis as they curve over to insert posteriorly into the pubic crest and the pectineal line.

**Contents of the inguinal canal in the male**

**Vas**

**Arteries:**
- Testicular
- Artery to vas
- Cremasteric

**Veins:** pampiniform plexus

**Lymphatic vessels:** the testis drains to the para-aortic lymph nodes; the coverings of the testis drain to the external iliac nodes

**Nerves:**
- Genital branch of genitofemoral (supplies cremaster muscle)
- Sympathetic nerves accompanying arteries
- Ilioinguinal nerve (enters via anterior wall of canal, not via internal ring, and runs in front of spermatic cord) supplies skin of inguinal region, upper part of thigh and anterior third of scrotum or labia

**Processus vaginalis:** obliterated remains of peritoneal connection to tunica vaginalis

All of these are in the spermatic cord except the ilioinguinal nerve

**Coverings of the spermatic cord**
- Internal spermatic fascia (from transversalis fascia)
- Cremasteric fascia (from internal oblique and transversus abdominis)
- External spermatic fascia (from external oblique)

The inguinal canal is a natural point of weakness in the abdominal wall. There are several features that normally reduce this weakness:
- The rings lie some distance apart (except in infants)
- The anterior wall is reinforced by the internal oblique in front of the deep ring
- The posterior wall is reinforced by the conjoint tendon opposite the superficial ring
- When abdominal pressure increases, the internal oblique and transversus abdominis contract, lowering the roof
- When abdominal pressure increases, we automatically squat so the anterior thigh presses against the inguinal canal and reinforces it

## Indirect inguinal hernias

 **In a nutshell ...**

- 60% of adult male inguinal hernias are indirect
- 4% of male infants have indirect inguinal hernias

Indirect inguinal hernias are the most common type of groin hernia in children. They are thought to be caused by the congenital failure of the processus vaginalis to close (saccular theory of Russell).

**Predisposing factors for indirect hernia**

- **Males:** bigger processus vaginalis than in women
- **Premature twins or low birthweight:** processus vaginalis not closed
- **Africans:** the lower arch in the more oblique African pelvis means the internal oblique origin does not protect the deep ring
- **On the right side:** right testis descends later than the left
- **Testicular feminisation syndrome:** genotypic male but androgen-insensitive so phenotypically female
- **Young men:** direct hernias become more common with age
- **Increased intraperitoneal fluid:** from whatever cause, eg cardiac, cirrhotic, carcinomatosis, dialysis; tends to open up the processus vaginalis

The indirect inguinal hernia sac is the remains of the processus vaginalis. The sac extends through the deep ring, inguinal canal and superficial ring. The inferior epigastric artery lies medial to the neck. In a complete sac the testis is found in the fundus. In an incomplete sac, the sac is limited to the canal or is inguinoscrotal or inguinolabial. The indirect hernia commonly descends into the scrotum.

## Direct inguinal hernias

 **In a nutshell ...**

- 35% of adult male inguinal hernias are direct
- 5% of adult male inguinal hernias are a combination of direct and indirect

The direct inguinal hernia is an acquired weakness in the abdominal wall which tends to develop in adulthood (unlike indirect hernias which are common in children) and are therefore the most common groin hernias in old men.

The direct inguinal hernia sac lies behind the cord. The inferior epigastric artery lies lateral to the neck. The hernia passes directly forwards through the defect in the posterior wall (fascia transversalis) of the inguinal canal. This hernia does not typically run down alongside the cord to the scrotum, but may do so.

## Femoral hernias

### Anatomy of the femoral region

#### Femoral sheath

The femoral sheath is a downward protrusion into the thigh of the fascial envelope lining the abdominal walls. It surrounds the femoral vessels and lymphatics for about 2.5 cm below the inguinal ligament. The sheath ends by fusing with the tunica adventitia of the femoral vessels. This occurs close to the saphenous opening in the deep fascia of thigh.

The anterior wall is continuous above with fascia transversalis and the posterior wall is continuous above with fascia iliacus/psoas fascia. It does not protrude below the inguinal ligament in the fetal position.

The femoral sheath exists to provide freedom for vessel movement beneath the inguinal ligament during movement of the hip.

> **Contents of the femoral sheath**
> - **Femoral artery:** in lateral compartment
> - **Femoral veins:** in intermediate compartment
> - **Lymphatics:** in medial compartment or femoral canal
> - **Femoral branch (L1) of genitofemoral nerve:** pierces the anterior wall of the femoral sheath running on the anterior surface of the external iliac artery
>
> Note that the femoral nerve lies in the iliac fossa between the psoas and the iliacus behind the fascia, so it enters the thigh outside the femoral sheath.

## Femoral canal

The femoral canal is the medial compartment of the femoral sheath containing lymphatics. It is about 1.3 cm long with an upper opening called the 'femoral ring'.

The femoral canal allows lymph vessels to be transmitted from the lower limbs to the abdomen and is also a dead space into which the femoral vein can expand when venous return increases. The femoral canal is the path taken by femoral hernias.

> **Contents of the femoral canal**
> - Fatty connective tissue
> - Efferent lymph vessels from deep inguinal nodes
> - Deep inguinal node of Cloquet (drains penis/clitoris)

## Femoral ring

The top of the femoral canal is called the femoral ring. It is covered by the femoral septum – a condensation of extraperitoneal tissue. This is pushed downwards into the canal in a hernia.

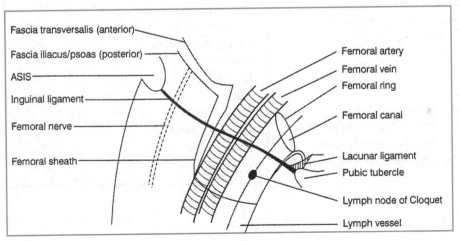

**Figure 1.5 The femoral region**

## Boundaries of the femoral ring

- **Anteriorly:** inguinal ligament
- **Posteriorly:** superior ramus of pubis and pectineal ligament
- **Medially:** lacunar ligament or iliopubic tract
- **Laterally:** femoral vein

These are also the margins of the neck of a femoral hernia. Note that three of the four boundaries are rigid, so a femoral hernia is prone to strangulation.

The lacunar ligament may have to be incised to release a strangulated hernia, risking bleeding from the accessory (abnormal) obturator artery.

## Epidemiology of femoral hernia

In females, indirect inguinal hernias are still more common than femoral hernias. However, they are found 2.5 times more commonly in females because:

- The inguinal ligament makes a wider angle with the pubis in the female
- Enlargement of the fat in the femoral canal of fat middle-aged women stretches the femoral canal; this fat disappears in old age, leaving a bigger canal
- Pregnancy increases intra-abdominal pressure and stretches the fascia transversalis

## Mechanics of femoral hernia

The femoral hernia enters the femoral canal through the femoral ring. The hernia arrives in the thigh next to the saphenous opening of the femoral sheath. The cribriform fascia over the saphenous opening becomes stretched over the hernia. The hernia enlarges upwards and medially into the superficial fascia of the inguinal ligament. Typically it lies between the superficial external pudendal and superficial epigastric veins, compressing the saphenous vein as it emerges through the saphenous opening.

## Characteristics of a typical femoral hernia

- Small (hard to find in an obese patient)
- Not reducible
- No cough impulse
- Often contains only omentum
- May contain a knuckle of bowel (most common site for Richter's hernia)
- More common on the right
- 35–50% of all strangulated groin hernias in adults are femoral hernias

## Differential diagnosis of femoral hernia

Inguinal hernia:

- Femoral hernia emerges below and lateral to pubic tubercle
- Inguinal hernia emerges above and medial to pubic tubercle

Saphena varix
Enlarged lymph node
Lipoma
Femoral artery aneurysm
Sarcoma
Ectopic testis
Obturator hernia
Psoas bursa
Psoas abscess

# Management of groin hernias

Diagnosis of a groin hernia is usually clinical. However, various imaging methods are available to confirm the diagnosis and assess anatomy in cases that are not straightforward (ultrasonography, contrast herniogram, computed tomography [CT] / magnetic resonance imaging [MRI]). In a contrast herniogram, water-soluble contrast media is injected into the peritoneal cavity through the anterior abdominal wall. The patient is positioned prone and pooling of contrast into the hernia sac is looked for on a radiograph. This is now rarely performed.

**European Hernia Society Guidelines for the Treatment of Inguinal Hernia in Adult Patients (2009)**

**Primary unilateral:** mesh repair (Lichtenstein's or endoscopic repair if expertise is available)

**Primary bilateral:** mesh repair (Lichtenstein's or endoscopic)

**Recurrent inguinal hernia:** modify technique in relation:

- If previously anterior – open preperitoneal mesh or endoscopic approach
- If previously posterior – Lichtenstein's totally extraperitoneal (TEP) is preferred to transabdominal preperitoneal (TAPP) repair in the case of endoscopic surgery

**Prophylactic antibiotics** are not recommended in low-risk patients or in endoscopic surgery

**Anaesthesia:**

ASA 1/2: always consider day surgery

ASA 3/4: consider local anaesthesia or day surgery

## Indications for groin hernia repair

| Elective (to be prioritised by job) | Indirect Symptomatic direct | Rate of strangulation of inguinal hernia is 0.3–2.9% per year; increased risk if irreducible or indirect |
|---|---|---|
| Prompt | Irreducible inguinal hernia History of less than 4 weeks | Greater risk of strangulation in first 3 months after appearance |
| Urgent | All femoral hernias | 50% strangulate within 1 month |
| Emergency | Painful irreducible hernias | |

# Repair of inguinal hernia

 **In a nutshell ...**

Main aims of inguinal hernia repair:
- Reduce hernia contents
- Remove hernia sac
- Repair defect

**Main approaches**

For primary uncomplicated inguinal hernias:
- Lichtenstein's mesh repair
- Laparoscopic repair

Other recognised techniques:
- Shouldice technique
- McVay–Cooper ligament operation

Herniotomy for children is a different operation from herniorraphy for adults as there is no need to repair the posterior wall of the inguinal canal in children because there is no defect there.

**CHAPTER 1**

 **Op Box: Open repair of inguinal hernia (mesh or Shouldice)**

### Mesh repair

This is the method of choice for nearly all elective open inguinal hernia repairs in the UK and is also used in incarcerated or even strangulated emergency hernia repairs where there is no gross contamination by pus or bowel contents.

- Reinforce posterior wall of inguinal canal with Prolene mesh
- Apply mesh on transversalis fascia and internal oblique muscle
- Slit lateral end to accommodate spermatic cord
- Suture inferior margin of mesh to inner surface of inguinal ligament using continuous Prolene or nylon suture
- Fix medial and superior margins to internal oblique muscle using interrupted sutures
- Medial end should reach pubic tubercle
- Suture lateral tail ends to one another around the cord, ensuring that the gap left in the mesh for the cord is enough to admit the little fingertip (therefore no cord damage) but will not admit a whole finger (therefore no hernia recurrence)

### Shouldice repair

This is a recognised method for open inguinal hernia repair and is useful when a mesh is contraindicated (eg in a strangulated hernia with pus or bowel contents contaminating the inguinal canal).

- Cremaster muscle should always be divided to give good access to the deep ring
- Margins of the deep ring are dissected from the cord
- Fascia transversalis is opened from the deep ring medially down to the pubic tubercle
- Fascia transversalis is cleaned of extraperitoneal fat to expose: the deep surface of the conjoint tendon above and medially; and the fascia transversalis as it plunges into the thigh below and laterally to become the anterior layer of femoral sheath
- Lower lateral fascia transversalis flap is sutured to the undersurface of the conjoint tendon
- Upper flap is overlapped and sutured to anterior surface of lower lateral flap of the fascia transversalis (this reconstructs the posterior wall of the inguinal canal)
- Suturing is taken laterally to make a new deep ring flush with the emergent cord
- Repair is reinforced medially by suturing the conjoint tendon to the aponeurosis of external oblique

### Closure of Shouldice and mesh repairs

- Same for both methods
- Inspect for potential femoral hernia before closure
- Close external oblique aponeurosis with continuous absorbable suture (eg PDS) over the cord
- Close Scarpa's fascia with interrupted Vicryl
- Close skin with undyed subcuticular Monocryl
- Draw down ipsilateral testicle to the bottom of the scrotum

## Postoperative advice after open repair of inguinal hernia

- Often home the same day
- Eat, drink and mobilise on waking
- Back to sedentary job within 2 weeks
- Back to heavy lifting, strenuous sports and manual labour in 6 weeks
- Safe to drive when performing an emergency stop does not cause any discomfort (advise them to check with their insurance company if they are in doubt)
- Oral analgesia may be needed for a few days
- Follow-up is usually by GP only unless there is an ongoing audit

## Complications of open repair of inguinal hernia

- Haematoma
- Wound infection and mesh infection
- Recurrence
- Testicular atrophy or ischaemic orchitis due to cord damage in males
- Temporary postoperative urinary retention due to pain in elderly people or men with pre-existing prostatic symptoms

---

### Intraoperative hazards of open repair of inguinal hernia

**Damage to the ilioinguinal nerve**
This may be cut when the canal is entered (causing sensory loss in the lower groin or scrotum) or sutured into the mesh, causing chronic pain if care is not taken.
In large or emergency hernias where damage or entrapment of the nerve is unavoidable, the nerve should be cut as proximally as possible because numbness is preferable to pain.

**Damage to the cord structures in the male**
- Vas
- Testicular artery
- Pampiniform plexus of veins
This may lead to reduced fertility, ischaemic orchitis or varicocele respectively.

**Orchidectomy**
Very occasionally in an emergency situation with a large incarcerated or strangulated inguinoscrotal hernia, or in the elective patient with enormous chronic inguinoscrotal hernias or recurrent open hernias, it may impossible to preserve the cord and it might be necessary to remove the cord and testicle to achieve safe closure of the posterior wall. These patients should have the risk explained in the consent.

## Advantages and disadvantages of mesh repair

| Advantages | Disadvantages |
|---|---|
| Easier to learn and perform for trainees | Risk of infection (avoid haematomas and use prophylactic antibiotics) |
| Lower recurrence rate (1 in 1000) | |
| Tension-free repair | |
| Reduced analgesic requirement | |

## Advantages and disadvantages of Shouldice repair

| Advantages | Disadvantages |
|---|---|
| Low risk of infection Indicated in presence of strangulated bowel where mesh is not recommended | Technically more difficult than mesh repair |
| | High standard of training needed |
| Low recurrence rate in the right hands | Surgical time longer than with mesh repair |
| | Tension-free repair difficult to perform |
| | Postop analgesic requirement higher than with mesh repair |

This technique was perfected by the Shouldice Clinic. Recurrence rate is <1% there, but approaches 3.5% elsewhere. Trainee surgeons at the Shouldice Clinic must assist in 50 hernia repairs then perform 100 hernia repairs under supervision before being allowed to repair inguinal hernias independently.

## Other types of inguinal hernia repair

**Laparoscopic repair** is a popular and recognised form of hernia repair. There are two types: transabdominal preperitoneal (TAPP) or totally extraperitoneal (TEP) repair. Laparoscopic inguinal hernia surgery should be performed only by appropriately trained surgeons. Laparoscopic repair is associated with an increase in operation time; however, there is a shorter recovery time when compared with open hernia repair. Both TAPP and TEP procedures are associated with a reduction in wound-related infections, haematoma, persistent numbness and pain compared with open repair. The rates of recurrence is similar for laparoscopic and open repair.

In the **McVay–Cooper ligament operation** the fascia transversalis is opened and the upper medial flap is sutured to the iliopectineal ligament (Cooper's ligament).

The Bassini (darn) repair is no longer recommended due to high recurrence rates.

## Inguinal hernia repair in children

In the repair of inguinal hernias in children:
* Herniotomy alone is sufficient
* The hernia is reduced, the sac divided and ligated but there is no need to repair the posterior wall of the canal as there is no weakness there

- Mesh or darn herniorrhaphy is not indicated

Ovaries should be looked for in females and reduced at the time of surgery. The possibility of testicular feminisation syndrome should be considered in female children with bilateral hernias.

## Repair of femoral hernias

### In a nutshell ...

**Main aims**
- Reduce hernia contents
- Remove peritoneal sac
- Repair defect

**Three main approaches**
- Low crural (Lockwood)
- High inguinal (Lotheissen)
- High extraperitoneal (McEvedy)

Laparoscopic repair can also be performed.

## RCS guidelines on repair of femoral hernias

- Recommends high inguinal approach except in thin females, where a low crural approach is acceptable
- Advises high extraperitoneal approach in complex, recurrent or obstructed hernias

## Groin hernia repair under local anaesthetic

The advantages of any surgery under local anaesthetic (LA) are discussed fully in Book 1. They include removing the risk of general anaesthesia, as well as decreased cost and shorter patient stay. Groin hernia repair is an ideal operation to be performed under local or regional anaesthesia, especially when combined with day-case surgery. This is likely to become more popular with the increasing use of preoperative ultrasound-guided transversus abdominis plane (TAP) block. The anaesthetic agents, precautions and complications are discussed in Book 1. LA is not suitable for obese, anxious or uncooperative patients, or in complex or recurrent hernias.

### Method of administering LA in groin hernia repair
- Subcutaneous weal in line of incision
- Deep injection at ilioinguinal and iliohypogastric nerves (one finger-breadth medial to ASIS)
- Further injection deep to proposed incision
- Deep infiltration as needed
- Bupivacaine block before closure in both GA and LA

## Op box: Femoral hernia repair 1: crural (low) approach (Lockwood's approach)

### Indications

All femoral hernias should be repaired within a month of diagnosis if the patient is fit, due to the high risk of strangulation.

The low approach is the simplest approach and the most often used for elective repair. It is a controversial approach for an incarcerated or strangulated hernia because it is difficult to resect compromised bowel through this incision (if compromised bowel slips through the canal back into the abdomen, laparotomy is needed to retrieve it).

**Preop preparation:** similar to inguinal hernias.

- Suitable for day case?
- Local, spinal or general anaesthetic? Urgent or emergency repair?
- Open or laparoscopic? Crural, inguinal or extraperitoneal approach?
- Social circumstances for discharge?
- Patient must be consented (mention relevant hazards and complications; see below)
- The correct side should be marked and shaved
- GA cases with comorbidity may need appropriate work-up and anaesthetic review

**Position:** supine.

**Incision:** oblique incision 1 cm below and parallel to the medial inguinal ligament.

### Procedure

- Expose and open the femoral sac in the subcutaneous tissue
- Examine contents and reduce into the abdomen
- In an elective repair usually only omentum is present
- Compromised bowel should never be returned to the abdomen
- Once contents are reduced into the abdomen, transfix the sac neck using Vicryl and excise it 1 cm distal to the ligation
- Suture the inguinal to the pectineal ligaments for 1 cm laterally with interrupted nylon sutures on a J-shaped needle, tying the sutures only once they have all been placed
- Take care to protect the laterally located femoral vein and avoid constricting it

### Intraoperative hazards

- Damage to the femoral vein, bladder or hernial sac contents
- Failure to identify Richter's hernia
- Bleeding from an abnormal obturator artery

**Closure:** close subcutaneous tissue using Vicryl; close skin with subcuticular Monocryl

**Postop:** as for inguinal hernia repair although recovery from this approach is usually faster.

### Complications

- Wound infection
- Haematoma
- Missed Richter's hernia
- Recurrence is rare

## Op box: Femoral hernia repair 2: high inguinal approach (Lotheissen's approach)

- Can be done for elective femoral hernias or emergency irreducible femoral hernias where a bowel resection is considered unlikely
- Approaches femoral canal through inguinal canal
- Dissection is the same as for inguinal hernia repair but the transversalis fascia is opened to expose femoral vessels and the canal beneath it
- The disadvantage is that it disrupts the normal inguinal canal but it is ideal, therefore to repair a coexisting inguinal hernia
- Provides better access to the contents of the peritoneal sac than the low approach, but it is not ideal for access to strangulated contents or in patients with bowel obstruction (which may need a bowel resection); the high extraperitoneal approach is better for these strangulated hernias (see the next op box)

**Preop preparation**
- As for crural approach (see previous op box)
- Also consent for additional hazards and complications listed below

**Position**: supine.

**Incision**: 2.5 cm above medial two-thirds of inguinal ligament along a skin crease, as for inguinal hernia repair.

**Procedure**
- Deepen incision to external oblique aponeurosis
- Ligate and divide superficial veins
- With scissors slit along fibres of external oblique as far as the superficial inguinal ring
- Identify the ilioinguinal nerve (preserve if possible)
- Protect the cord with a sling
- Once in the inguinal canal, divide the posterior fascia transversalis to access the femoral canal
- Open the femoral hernia sac
- Examine the contents and reduce if safe to do so (ie no bowel with compromised viability)
- Transfix the neck of the sac and ligate and divide it 1 cm distal to the ligature
- Repair the femoral canal defect by suturing the pectineal ligament to the medial inguinal ligament
- Reconstitute the transversalis fascia (otherwise recurrence rate is high)
- Examine inguinal hernia orifices

**Intraoperative hazards**
- As for inguinal and low crural femoral hernia repair
- Damage to the ilioinguinal nerve
- Damage to the cord structures in the male
- Damage to contents of the hernia sac

## Op box: Femoral hernia repair 2: high inguinal approach (Lotheissen's approach)

- Damage to the femoral vein
- Failure to identify Richter's hernia
- Bleeding from an abnormal obturator artery

**Closure:** as for inguinal hernia repair.

- Close external oblique aponeurosis with a continuous absorbable suture (eg PDS) over the cord
- Close Scarpa's fascia with interrupted Vicryl
- Close skin with undyed subcuticular Monocryl
- Draw down ipsilateral testicle to the bottom of the scrotum

**Postop:** as for inguinal hernia repair.

- Often home the same day
- Eat, drink and mobilise on waking
- Back to sedentary job within 2 weeks
- Back to heavy lifting, strenuous sports and manual labour in 6 weeks
- Safe to drive when performing an emergency stop does not cause any discomfort (advise them to check with their insurance company if they are in doubt)
- Oral analgesia may be needed for a few days

Follow-up is usually by GP only unless there is an ongoing audit.

### Complications

- Haematoma
- Wound infection
- Recurrence of femoral or inguinal hernia
- Testicular atrophy or ischaemic orchitis due to cord damage in males
- Temporary postoperative urinary retention due to pain in elderly people or men with pre-existing prostatic symptoms

**Op box: Femoral hernia repair 3: high extraperitoneal approach (McEvedy's approach)**

### Indications
- Most useful approach for strangulated hernia because it facilitates bowel resection if necessary
- Safest approach for an emergency femoral hernia with either a red, hot, tender, irreducible hernia or evidence of bowel obstruction or both
- Also used for bilateral hernias through Pfannenstiel's incision

### Preop prep
- As for femoral hernia repair 1 (crural approach) plus: catheterise to minimise risk to bladder

#### *For strangulated femoral hernias:*
- Include consent for laparotomy and bowel resection
- Give intravenous (IV) antibiotics preoperatively
- Group and save

#### *For femoral hernias with bowel obstruction:*
- Give IV fluid
- Check potassium
- Pass a nasogastric (NG) tube and urethral catheter preoperatively
- Consent for laparotomy and bowel resection
- Group and save

**Position:** supine.

### Incision
- Make transverse incision 6 cm above and parallel to inguinal ligament over lateral border of rectus sheath
- Divide rectus sheath vertically at the lateral border to expose peritoneum

### Procedure
- Move peritoneum and bladder away from the back of the anterior abdominal wall exposing the femoral canal and the neck of the sac
- Reduce sac into the wound (divide lacunar ligament to facilitate this)
- Open sac and examine contents
- If bowel looks doubtful, wrap it in a warm pack for 10 minutes and re-inspect
- If bowel is non-viable, resect it and do an end-to-end anastomosis
- Reduce contents of sac
- Transfix neck of sac with a Vicryl suture and excise it 1 cm distal to ligature
- Close defect by medial apposition of inguinal and pectineal ligaments, protecting and avoiding compression of femoral vein laterally
- Use strong, non-absorbable suture and a J-shaped needle
- After repair, the femoral canal should just admit the tip of the little finger

## Op box: Femoral hernia repair 3: high extraperitoneal approach (McEvedy's approach)

**Intraoperative hazards**
- Damage to bladder
- Damage to femoral vein, bleeding
- Damage to adjacent small bowel or mesentery during mobilisation and resection

**Closure**
- Repair rectus with continuous, non-absorbable sutures
- Close subcutaneous tissue with Vicryl
- Subcuticular Monocryl or clips to skin

**Postop**
- Without bowel resection, as for high inguinal approach (see previous op box)
- With small-bowel resection may need a couple of days longer in hospital with gradual introduction of diet

**Complications**
- Infection
- Haematoma
- Incisional hernia
- Plus, if small bowel was resected:
  - Postoperative ileus
  - Adhesions
  - Anastomotic stricture

## Summary of postoperative complications of inguinal or femoral groin hernia repair

**Wound complications**
- Bleeding
- Haematoma
- Sepsis
- Sinus

**Scrotal complications**
- Ischaemic orchitis
- Testicular atrophy
- Hydrocele
- Genital oedema
- Damage to vas and vessels

**Special complications**
- Nerve injuries
- Persistent postop pain
- Compression of femoral vessels
- Urinary retention
- Impotence

**General complications**
- Chest infection
- DVT
- PE
- Cardiovascular problems
- Visceral injury

**Operation failure**
- Recurrence
- Missed hernia
- Dehiscence
- Mortality

## Other abdominal hernias

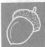 **In a nutshell ...**

- Paraumbilical
- Spigelian
- Umbilical (see 'Paediatric surgery')
- Lumbar
- Incisional
- Gluteal
- Epigastric
- Sciatic

## Paraumbilical hernia

**In a nutshell ...**

Paraumbilical hernia is a protrusion of the peritoneal sac and contents (often omentum) through a defect in the linea alba adjacent to the umbilicus, rather than through the cicatrix itself (as in true paediatric umbilical hernias). They are common in obese adults and are at high risk of strangulation due to the small neck.

More common within increasing age; M = F
- **Causes:** increased intra-abdominal pressure, eg ascites, multiple pregnancy, malignancy, chronic obstructive pulmonary disease (COPD) or obesity

- **Anatomy:** the sac protrudes through a defect in the linea alba near the umbilical cicatrix but, unlike the true umbilical hernia, not through the cicatrix itself. Progressively increases in size. Usually contains extraperitoneal fat or omentum and very occasionally transverse colon or small bowel. The neck of the sac is often very narrow compared with the sac contents, and very fibrous. Contents adhere to each other, to coverings and to the omentum
- **Coverings:** skin, superficial fascia, rectus sheath, transversalis fascia and sac. These stretch and fuse into a thin membrane through which peristalsis may be seen
- **Complications:** redness, excoriation, ulceration, gangrene, pendulousness, infection, faecal fistula, strangulation, incarceration and obstruction
- **Clinical features:** usually irreducible. May present with pain due to incarceration and subacute obstruction. Strangulation is common due to narrow neck

### Surgical repair of paraumbilical hernia

This may have significant mortality in old patients with large hernias. Problems include:
- Patients tend to be old or obese with comorbidity
- High risk of strangulation
- Difficult anatomy and reduction
- May have increased intra-abdominal pressure after reduction, which exacerbates respiratory problems; preoperative weight loss and chest physiotherapy may help

## Op box: Mayo's operation for paraumbilical hernia ('vest over pants')

### Indications
- Elective (reducible or asymptomatic incarcerated)
- Prompt (symptomatic, non-tender, incarcerated)
- Emergency (strangulated, incarcerated and tender or obstructed)

Many of these patients are obese, and a non-symptomatic incarcerated hernia is a management problem in a patient with significant comorbidity who is at risk from a GA. The patient and surgeon must weigh up the risks of elective surgery with the benefits of preventing possible future emergency surgery.

### Preop preparation
In an elective patient with significant comorbidity liaison with anaesthetist and preop work-up may be needed.

*For strangulated (red, hot, tender, irreducible) emergency hernias:*
- Include consent for laparotomy and bowel resection
- Give IV antibiotics preoperatively
- Group and save

*For paraumbilical hernias with bowel obstruction:*
- Give IV fluid
- Check potassium
- Pass an NG tube and urethral catheter preoperatively
- Consent for laparotomy and bowel resection
- Group and save

**Position**: supine.

**Incision**: excise stretched skin as a horizontal ellipse.

### Procedure
1. Deepen incision to rectus sheath to expose neck of sac
2. Enlarge incision laterally to give a long transverse exposure
3. Open sac near neck where adhesions are least likely
4. Examine and return protruding bowel
5. Excise protruding omentum to lessen volume of contents
6. Remove sac and overlying skin
7. Ensure any adherent bowel or omentum is mobilised away from the peritoneal surface of the rectus
8. Bring up lower edge of rectus and fix with non-absorbable mattress sutures to behind the upper flap (the 'pants')
9. Pull down upper flap to overlap the lower flap (the 'vest')

## Op box: Mayo's operation for paraumbilical hernia ('vest over pants')

**Mesh repair:** for defects >3 cm.
- Follow steps 1–7
- Close the defect with interrupted non-absorbable sutures
- Suture a polypropylene mesh onto the anterior rectus sheath over the defect with non-absorbable interrupted sutures

**Intraoperative hazards**
- Unable to reduce contents – enlarge defect by incising linea alba and trim redundant omentum
- Devascularisation of umbilical skin – it is better to excise skin of doubtful viability and refashion the cicatrix
- Suturing of omentum or bowel into wound – enlarge the defect so you have a good view and be sure that the internal edges are clear of adherent bowel and omentum; each stitch should be placed under direct vision
- Bleeding – ensure haemostasis of omentum before returning it to the abdomen
- Bowel resection – this is less common than in incarcerated groin hernias, but necessitates an enlarged midline laparotomy incision
- Multiple smaller defects nearby (epigastric hernias) – join them together and close as one larger incision; mesh is usually advisable in these cases

**Closure**
- Subcutaneous fine suction drain to prevent seroma
- Vicryl to Scarpa's fascia ('fat stitch' to close dead space)
- Anchor skin to the linea alba with a subcutaneous Vicryl stitch to refashion an umbilical depression – do not let the stitch come through the skin as it will be a conduit for infection
- Clips or subcuticular Monocryl to skin

**Postop**
- Drain out and home within 24 hours if drainage minimal and no bowel resection needed
- Eat, drink and mobilise early
- Oral analgesia may be needed for a few days
- No follow-up needed except for audit
- Back to sedentary work within 2 weeks; heavy lifting, strenuous sport and manual labour in 6 weeks

**Complications**
- Infection
- Haematoma; seroma
- Loss of umbilicus (no matter how unsightly their infected, discoloured, bulging, chronic paraumbilical hernia was preoperatively, patients are often very put out by the loss of their umbilicus so must be consented for this)
- Recurrence

## Incisional hernia

 **In a nutshell ...**

A diffuse extension of peritoneum and abdominal contents though a weak scar.

### Incidence of incisional hernia
- 6% of abdominal wounds at 5 years
- 12% at 10 years
- M = F

### Clinical features of incisional hernia

Can present as a lump increasing in size, subacute intestinal obstruction, incarceration, pain, strangulation, skin excoriation and, rarely, spontaneous rupture (more common in caesarean section and gynaecological wounds). Smaller incisional hernias can cause persistent discomfort in abdominal wound caused by impalpable extraperitoneal protrusion.

### Surgical repair of incisional hernia
- **Layer-to-layer anatomical repair:** if there is no tissue loss
- **Mesh repair:** usually the preferred type of repair. The mesh can be inserted in the space between the abdominal muscles and the peritoneum (sublay); across defect (inlay) or over any of a wide variety of simple repairs (onlay).
- **Keel repair:** sac is invaginated by successive lines of non-absorbable sutures

### Recurrence rates
- Vary from 1% to 46%
- Low (10%) with mesh

---

**Causes of incisional hernia**

**Technical failure by surgeon**
- Postop haematoma, necrosis, sepsis
- Inept closure
- Drains or stomas
- Inappropriate incision

**Tissue factors**
- Age
- Immunosuppression
- Diabetes
- Jaundice
- Renal failure
- Malignant disease
- Infection

**High-risk incisions**
- Lower midline
- Upper midline
- Lateral muscle splitting
- Subcostal
- Parastomal
- Transverse

**Preop conditions**
- Cardiopulmonary disease
- Obesity
- Local skin/tissue sepsis

---

## Epigastric hernia

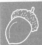

**In a nutshell ...**

Protrusion of extraperitoneal fat or peritoneum through one of the lozenge-shaped fissures commonly found between latticed fibres of the linea alba.

Epigastric hernias can occur in children or adults and may cause disproportionate epigastric pain and upper gastrointestinal (GI) symptoms. They are cured by excision of the sac and repair of the linea alba. Thirty per cent have coexisting intra-abdominal disease causing upper GI symptoms and so should be fully investigated.

## Spigelian hernia

**In a nutshell ...**

Protrusion of peritoneum through bands of the internal oblique muscle as the muscle enters the semilunar line.

These are also known as **semilunar line hernias** and account for 1% of abdominal hernias. Most occur below the umbilicus adjacent to the line of Douglas. It is usually deflected laterally by the external oblique and can be found near the iliac crest. The sac may enter the rectus sheath and be confused with rectus muscle haematoma. They are more common in women than men. They present as an aching lump, and are diagnosed by ultrasound scan. They can strangulate. Repair is by excision of the peritoneal sac and closure of the aponeurotic defect.

## Lumbar hernia

**In a nutshell ...**

Occur spontaneously, or after:
- Renal operations
- Lumbar abscesses
- Paralysis of lateral lumbar muscles by poliomyelitis or spina bifida

## Other types of hernia

Other rarer types of hernia include gluteal (through greater sciatic notch) and sciatic (through lesser sciatic notch).

## 1.3 Complications of hernias

**In a nutshell ...**

- Incarceration
- Obstruction
- Strangulation
- Reduction en masse
- Richter's hernia
- Maydl's hernia
- Pantaloon hernia
- Afferent loop strangulation
- Littre's hernia
- Spontaneous rupture of hernia sac
- Traumatic rupture of hernia
- Involvement in peritoneal disease process
- Sliding hernia
- Herniation of female genitalia

## Incarceration

The contents are fixed in the sac because of their size or adhesions. The hernia is irreducible but the contents are not necessarily strangulated or obstructed.

## Obstruction

The lumen of the bowel is obstructed by the neck of the hernia itself or the fibrosis or swelling of the peritoneum or bowel. The afferent loop will be distended, but the efferent will be empty.

## Strangulation

In strangulation, the blood supply to the contents of the hernia is cut off, leading to ischaemia. When a loop of gut is strangulated, there will also be intestinal obstruction. The swelling and oedema increase the strangulation, which normally starts with venous obstruction, leading to oedema, arterial obstruction and finally ischaemia.

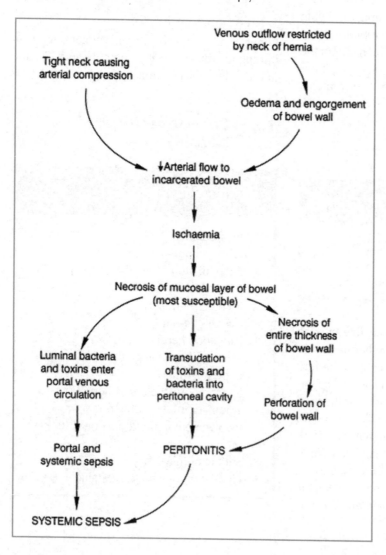

**Figure 1.6 Pathophysiology of bowel strangulation**

The longer the strangulated length of bowel, the more the consequent systemic morbidity.

The more distal the bowel is strangulated, the more toxicity and morbidity.

The constricting agent is usually the neck of the peritoneal sac, which is often fibrosed and rigid where it crosses the parietal defect.

In **indirect hernias**, the constriction is caused by the deep ring or the superficial ring. In **direct hernias**, the constriction is caused by the defect in the fascia transversalis.

The **femoral hernia** is more constricting due to the inflexible neck (three of its four margins are rigid). The constriction is due to the fibrosis of the peritoneum of the neck of the sac rather than the femoral ring itself, which is why the femoral vein is rarely obstructed. The saphenous vein may be occluded by the fundus as it exits from the femoral sheath.

In an **umbilical hernia** the rigid aponeurotic margins around the peritoneal sac are the constricting agents.

The clinical features of strangulation include pain and tenderness in an irreducible hernia. Strangulated hernias containing small bowel are more frequently on the right due to the anatomy of the mesentery.

### Reduction en masse

This is a complication that can occur when an apparently incarcerated hernia is reduced manually without surgery by pressure on the groin. In reduction en masse the entire hernia sac (Figure 1.7) complete with strangulating neck is reduced out of sight through the abdominal wall. If this happens in an inguinal hernia the cord is foreshortened and the testicle is drawn up. Traction on the testicle causes pain and a tender mass is felt in the abdomen (Smiddy's sign).

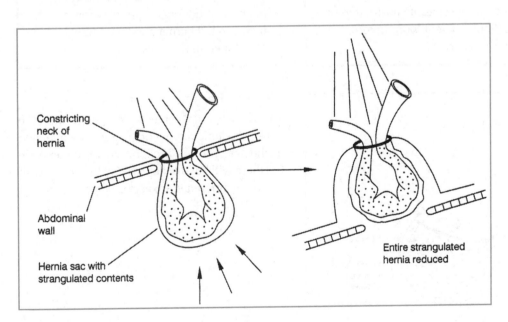

Constricting neck of hernia

Abdominal wall

Hernia sac with strangulated contents

Entire strangulated hernia reduced

Figure 1.7 Reduction en masse of a hernia

Pushing a hernia back into the abdomen without surgery may relieve obstruction or strangulation, and is occasionally acceptable in a patient with a very short history of non-tender incarceration who is unfit for or unwilling to have surgery. It does, however, risk a number of serious complications (see box on 'Complications of reducing an incarcerated hernia'), so if the hernia does not reduce fairly easily, it is best not to persist in fit adults. Manual reduction is, however, the initial treatment of choice of an incarcerated groin hernia in children (see box 'Incarcerated hernia in infants').

---

### Complications of reducing an incarcerated hernia

- Rupture of the bowel at the neck of the sac
- Return of devitalised bowel to the abdomen
- Reduction en masse
- Even after successful reduction, returned bowel can develop a stricture at either of two sites of constriction of efferent and afferent loops (internal stenosis of Garr)

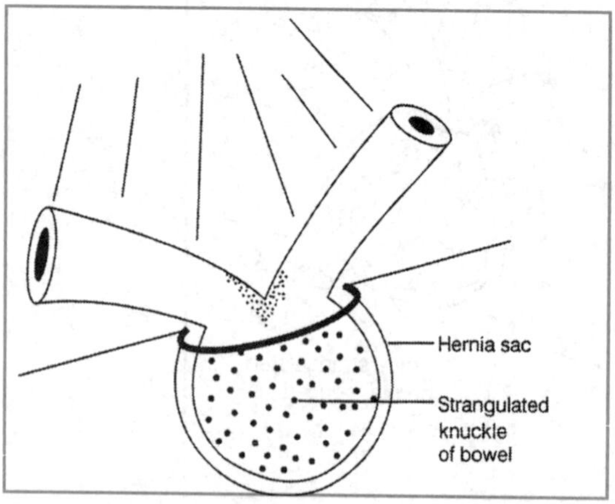

---

### Incarcerated hernia in infants

Presents as a painful irreducible lump in the groin.

Bile-stained vomiting indicates obstruction.

Treatment

- Resuscitation
- IV fluids
- NG tube ('drip and suck')

Hernia must be reduced promptly.

Reduction by taxis is safe in children.

May need opiate analgesia and sedation for reduction.

It is never appropriate to leave a painful irreducible lump in the groin of a child with bile-stained vomiting overnight without either reduction or surgery.

Reduction en masse is very rare but it is wise to continue 'drip and suck' overnight after successful reduction.

Definitive surgery on the hernia should be carried out after 48–72 hours when oedema has settled.

There is a 30% risk of testicular atrophy in children undergoing surgery for incarcerated hernia and this should be mentioned in the consent.

---

### Richter's hernia

This is a partial enterocele when only the anti-mesenteric margin of the gut is strangulated in the sac. The obstruction may be incomplete but there will be a tender, irreducible hernia with a varying amount of toxaemia and gangrene.

Hernia sac

Strangulated knuckle of bowel

**Figure 1.8 Richter's hernia.**

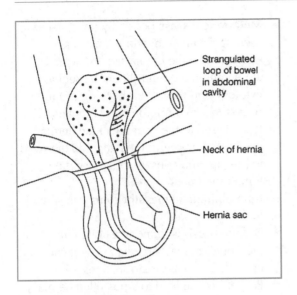

**Figure 1.9 Maydl's hernia**

### Maydl's hernia

This occurs when a W-shaped loop of small gut lies in the hernia sac and the intervening loop is strangulated within the main abdominal cavity. This is seen in very large hernial sacs, especially in developing countries.

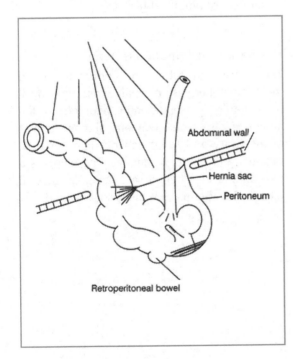

**Figure 1.10 Sliding hernia**

### Sliding hernia (hernia en glissade)

The bowel can be opened in error in these cases if the surgeon mistakes it for the sac.

This occurs when the sac wall is composed in part by retroperitoneal viscus, such as caecum or colon. The bowel forms part of the hernia but anatomically lies outside the cavity of the sac. In children, sliding hernias of the bladder (in boys) or ovary and tubes (in girls) can occur. Large hernias in old people may contain huge loops of sigmoid or caecum with only a small sac in the upper part. Surgical treatment should be carried out with care because there is a danger of opening the bowel instead of the sac. The patulous redundant sac is removed, hernia contents are mobilised and reduced.

## Pantaloon hernia

This occurs when direct and indirect sacs straddle the inferior epigastric artery.

## Afferent loop strangulation

Another rare problem, seen in large hernias when gut of the afferent loop becomes entwined about the afferent and efferent loops.

## Littre's hernia

This is a hernia sac containing a strangulated Meckel's diverticulum. It can progress to gangrene, suppuration, and formation of a local fistula.

## Spontaneous rupture of a hernia sac

This can occur in incisional hernia. It is surprisingly benign and peritonitis is rare. It needs an urgent laparotomy. The adhesions and oedema at the neck of the sac probably prevent the main peritoneal cavity from immediate contamination.

## Traumatic rupture of hernia

This is usually due to blunt trauma to the abdomen or a hernia when it is 'down'. It can occur during overenthusiastic attempts at reduction. Rupture usually occurs at the neck of the sac. Urgent laparotomy is needed.

## Involvement in the peritoneal disease process

- **Mesothelial hyperplasia:** repeated incarcerations of the gut in the hernial sac during infancy can lead to local peritoneal hyperplasia. This is an exuberant reactive phenomenon, not a malignant condition such as adult peritoneal mesothelioma, from which it must be distinguished

- **Metastatic disease** occurs by transcoelomic seeding or direct invasion. If ascites or thickening in the hernia sac is detected at operation, the fluid should be sent for cytology and the sac for histology. Only occurs in 1 in 3 million hernia repairs. It is advised to then complete the hernia operation and return the patient to the ward to prepare and consent for appropriate further treatment
- **Intra-abdominal mesothelioma** can spread to the hernia sac
- **Endometriosis** is found most often in incisional hernias after gynaecological operations or caesarean sections
- **Peritonitis** can lead to a pus-filled hernia sac
- **Appendicitis** can be found in inguinal, femoral or umbilical hernias

## Herniation of female genitalia

The ovary and tubes are commonly found in inguinal hernias in small girls. They must be carefully preserved and returned to the abdomen. In older women, sliding hernias of the ovary and tubes can occur in femoral, inguinal and obturator hernias. The uterus is a rare finding in a hernia sac, but pregnancy in incarcerated hernias has been documented.

# SECTION 2
# Oesophagus

## 2.1　Anatomy and physiology of the oesophagus

**In a nutshell ...**

The oesophagus is a muscular tube extending from the cricoid cartilage (C6) to the cardiac orifice of the stomach (T10 and left seventh costal cartilage):

- Length is 25 cm
- Divided into upper third, middle third and lower third
- Each third has a different relation, blood supply, venous drainage, lymph drainage and muscle structure
- Each third is approached differently for surgery

## Anatomy of the oesophagus

### Histology

- Running the whole length there is an inner circular and outer longitudinal muscle and a submucosal layer with sparse mucous glands (fewer in the middle)
- The mucosa is thickened and muscularised
- The epithelium is stratified, squamous, non-keratinised up to the gastro-oesophageal junction

## Gross anatomy and surgical approach

|  | Upper (cervical) | Middle (thoracic) | Lower (thoracic and abdomen) |
|---|---|---|---|
| **Relations** | C6, C7<br>Trachea<br>Thyroid<br>Recurrent laryngeal nerve<br>Thoracic duct | Ti body<br>Descending aorta<br>Thoracic duct<br>Trachea and left main bronchus<br>Right pulmonary artery<br>Pericardium<br>Arch of the aorta<br>Azygos vein | Pierces diaphragm 2.5 cm left of midline at TlO<br>1–2 cm in abdomen<br>Through left crus fibres of diaphragm<br>Right crus fibres form sling<br>Left lobe of liver and left triangular ligament<br>Left gastric artery<br>Left inferior phrenic artery |
| **Blood supply** | Inferior thyroid artery | Oesophageal branches from aorta and bronchial arteries | Branches from left gastric and left inferior phrenic arteries |
| **Venous drainage** | Inferior thyroid vein<br>Vertebral vein<br>Brachiocephalic | Azygos and hemi-azygos veins | Left gastric vein draining to the portal system (porto-systemic anastomosis at T8) |
| **Lymph** | To deep cervical nodes | Posterior mediastinal and tracheobronchial nodes | Left gastric and celiac nodes |
| **Muscles** | Skeletal | Mixed | Smooth |
| **Nerves** | Recurrent laryngeal<br>Sympathetic from middle cervical ganglion | Vagus (left vagus eventually runs anteriorly on abdominal oesophagus, lying closer to it than the right vagus, which eventually runs posteriorly)<br>Sympathetic trunk<br>Greater splanchnic nerve | Vagus forms anterior and posterior vagal plexuses |
| **Surgical approach** | Between trachea and carotid sheath | From the right<br>In front of the vertebral canal, transecting azygos arch<br>Beware posterior vessels and thoracic duct | From the left<br>Above the diaphragm<br><br>Beware heart and inferior pulmonary vein |

# Physiology of swallowing

## In a nutshell ...

**Swallowing is initiated voluntarily – thereafter it is entirely a reflex.**
Touch receptors in the pharynx are set off. These impulses are sent to the medulla and lower pons (swallowing centre). Impulses from the swallowing centre are transmitted to the:
- Pharynx and oesophagus via cranial nerves
- Oesophagus via the vagus

The three phases of swallowing are:
- Oral
- Pharyngeal
- Oesophageal

### Oral phase
- Tongue sends bolus of food to pharynx and initiates reflexes by touch receptors
- Nerves involved are V (sensory) and XII (voluntary motor)

### Pharyngeal phase
- Takes less than 1 second (during which time respiration is inhibited):
  - Soft palate is pulled up
  - Vocal cords are pulled together
  - Upper oesophageal sphincters relax
  - Superior constrictor muscle contracts
- Peristaltic wave is initiated
- Nerves involved are IX (sensory) and V, IX and X (autonomic)

### Oesophageal phase
- Upper oesophageal sphincter reflexly constricts

- Peristaltic wave (primary peristalsis) continues at 5 cm/second
- Receptive relaxation ahead of the food bolus relaxes the lower oesophageal sphincter (LOS), permitting entry to the stomach; this is mediated by inhibitory neurones in the myenteric plexus
- If food remains in the oesophagus, distension initiates secondary peristalsis which starts above the site of distension and moves down
- Nerves involved are X (sensory) and V, IX and X (autonomic)

## Lower oesophageal sphincter

The lower oesophageal sphincter is a term that encompasses a combination of anatomical and physiological factors that permit the gastro-oesophageal junction (GOJ) to allow food boluses from the oesophagus into the stomach while preventing the gastric juices of the stomach running up into the oesophagus.

The normal resting tone of the LOS is >5 mmHg (varying from 0 to 30) over a distance of >1 cm.

This complex mechanism can become dysfunctional, causing pain or difficulty swallowing (eg in achalasia where the LOS resting pressure is high) or conversely allowing backflow of gastric contents (eg in scleroderma reflux oesophagitis where the LOS resting pressure is low).

### Anatomical factors accounting for the lower oesophageal sphincter
- **A zone of circular smooth muscle in the distal oesophagus:** under control of the intramural plexus, this region has a sustained resting tone which relaxes only when swallowing occurs (similar to an internal sphincter)

- **The right crus of the diaphragm forms a sling around the oesophagus** as it passes into the abdomen and contracts when intra-abdominal pressure increases ('pinchcock' action), thus preventing the stomach contents from being 'squeezed' into the oesophagus; it acts as an external sphincter
- **The angle of His:** the oesophagus does not pass into the abdomen in a straight line; this angle of entry acts as a valve to help stop reflux
- The lower portion of the oesophagus lies not in the chest but in the abdomen
- **There is an intraluminal mucosal flap** at the level of the GOJ which acts like a valve
- **Efficient gastric emptying:** if there is a physical distal obstruction or physiological slowing of the passage of gastric contents, the LOS will be overcome and there will be reflux and vomiting

---

**Endocrine and neural control of the lower oesophageal sphincter**

| | |
|---|---|
| Gastrin | Contracts |
| Cholecystokinin (CCK) | Relaxes |
| Secretin | Relaxes |
| Acetylcholine | Contracts |
| Vasoactive intestinal peptide (VIP) | Relaxes |
| Noradrenaline | Relaxes |
| Nitric oxide (NO) | Relaxes |

---

## 2.2 Pain and difficulty swallowing

 **In a nutshell ...**

Dysphagia and odynophagia are often symptoms of oesophageal disease and usually need urgent investigation by upper GI endoscopy to exclude carcinoma of the oesophagus. If nothing is found, barium swallow, manometry and pH studies may be helpful.

### Dysphagia

- Difficulty – not pain – on swallowing; it may be associated with an uncomfortable sensation of bolus arrested during progression at the level of the pharynx, oesophagus or gastro-oesophageal region
- Progressive dysphagia over several weeks, starting with solids and leading to liquids, is typical of oesophageal cancer

### Odynophagia

- This is the correct term for pain on swallowing and is usually felt within 10–15 seconds of swallowing

The causes of dysphagia and odynophagia usually overlap.

# Causes of painful/difficult swallowing

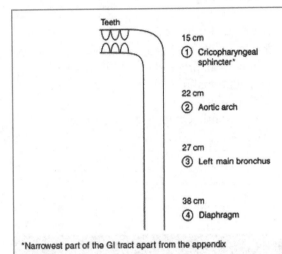

Teeth

15 cm
① Cricopharyngeal sphincter*

22 cm
② Aortic arch

27 cm
③ Left main bronchus

38 cm
④ Diaphragm

There are several areas of narrowing of the oesophagus which are important because:

- Swallowed foreign bodies can lodge
- There is a slight delay in the passage of food or fluids
- Strictures develop following the drinking of caustic fluids
- Common sites of carcinoma
- Difficulty passing a gastroscope may occur

*Narrowest part of the GI tract apart from the appendix

**Figure 1.11 Areas of narrowing of the oesophagus**

## Anatomical causes

### Intrinsic lesions (in the oesophageal wall or lumen)

- Malignancy
- Cricoid web
- Inflammatory/peptic stricture

### Extrinsic lesions

- Lymphadenopathy
- Bronchial carcinoma
- Left atrial enlargement in mitral stenosis

## Functional causes

### Difficulties in initiating swallowing

Neurological causes include:

- Motor neurone disease
- Post-stroke
- Globus hystericus

### Oesophageal dysmotility

- Diffuse oesophageal spasm
- Scleroderma

Dysphagia is part of the syndrome of gastro-oesophageal reflux disease (GORD) and may be an indication of severe disease.

> **Conditions in which odynophagia (pain on swallowing) is a feature**
> **Inflammation**
> - Reflux oesophagitis
> - Peptic oesophageal ulceration
>
> **Infection**
> - Thrush
> - Herpes
> - Viral and bacterial pharyngitis
>
> **Spasm**
> - Diffuse oesophageal spasm

## Assessment of painful/difficult swallowing

### History

Ask about heartburn, weight loss, timescale, progression (eg solids to liquids), previous surgery, previous endoscopy findings and risk factors (see individual pathologies described below).

### Examination

Look for anaemia, cachexia, neck lymphadenopathy and abdominal masses.

## Investigating painful/difficult swallowing

### Upper GI endoscopy

This is usually the first investigation:
- If normal, proceed to barium swallow
- If abnormal result:
  - Lesion – biopsy
  - Extrinsic compression – CT scan

---

 **Procedure box: Upper gastrointestinal endoscopy**

Endoscopy is invaluable for the evaluation of the oesophagus, stomach and duodenum by allowing imaging and biopsy.

**The endoscope**

This is a flexible tube containing a fibreoptic viewing lens (fibreoptic endoscope) or video camera (video endoscope), light source, irrigation/suction/biopsy channels and directional control wires.

**The patient**
**Consent**

Empty stomach: fasted overnight (if elective) or have the stomach drained or washed out by a nasogastric (NG) tube if there is obstruction; intubation should be considered in emergency cases such as haematemesis where there is a risk of aspiration.

Assess risks: such as previous surgery, bleeding disorders, mechanical heart valves, comorbidity and anticoagulants/antiplatelets.

**Prepare for procedure:**
- Lidocaine throat spray ± sedation (usually midazolam)
- Regular obs and sats monitored by a dedicated team member
- Patient lies on left side, neck flexed and tooth-guard inserted

**The examination**

Your aim is to intubate the duodenum initially, then carry out a full examination on withdrawal of the scope.

*Intubate duodenum*
- Direct visualisation during intubation is safer than blind intubation

- Warn the patient about gagging and get him or her to swallow as you intubate the oesophagus
- Entry into the stomach via the oesophagus; follow the rugae
- Identify the pylorus and intubate the duodenum
- Turn right (posteriorly) into D2 and advance as far into the duodenum as practicable
- Take biopsies for coeliac disease here if indicated

### Examine duodenum

- Withdraw the endoscope, examining on your way out
- Pay particular attention to the proximal duodenum (the duodenal bulb), which is the hardest to visualise and is at the site of most of the duodenal pathology

### Examine oesophagus

Note and measure the distance from the incisors of:

- The LOS (a narrowed area closing the GOJ lumen)
- The Z-line (where white oesophageal squamous mucosa meets pink gastric columnar mucosa)
- The diaphragmatic hiatus (a brief narrowing seen when the patient sniffs)

Examine the rest of the oesophageal mucosa on withdrawing the scope slowly.

### The procedures

If pathology is encountered at diagnostic endoscopy, several procedures can be performed:

- Biopsy (for histology or CLO test)
- Snare (of polyps)
- Sclerotherapy (of bleeding varices or ulcers)
- Banding (of varices)
- Haemostasis (diathermy, argon, laser, etc)
- Balloon or bougie dilation (of oesophageal strictures)
- Stenting (often done radiologically, depending on local expertise)
- Percutaneous endoscopic gastrostomy (for feeding tube)

These procedures are described in detail in relevant sections in this and other chapters.

### The risks

- Reaction to sedation
- Aspiration
- Perforation (<1 in 3000 for elective diagnostic upper endoscopy)
- Bleeding

The last three are more common with blind intubations, emergency endoscopies and therapeutic procedures.

In the UK, the Joint Advisory Group (JAG) of GI endoscopy was formed to maintain high standards of training and quality assurance in GI endoscopy.

### Barium swallow

These radiological contrast studies target the oesophagus and stomach, and are useful if endoscopy is not possible due to patient condition, lack of cooperation or obstructing pathology. They can also provide useful information on dysmotility conditions.

### Manometry

An NG tube containing a pressure transducer is passed into the oesophagus. Squeeze and resting pressures are measured at various levels of the oesophagus. It detects peristaltic waves, which normally travel down the oesophagus at 5 cm/s (not in achalasia). The normal resting pressure of the LOS is 10–15 mmHg over at least 2 cm in the closed state. Squeeze pressures of up to 100 mmHg should be generated in response to wet and dry swallows during the test. The test usually takes 20–30 minutes to perform.

### pH studies

A naso-oesophageal wire containing a pH probe is placed in the lower oesophagus for 24 hours. This is attached to a mobile transducer which the patient carries around while recording in a diary when he or she is eating, lying down, sleeping or feeling pain. The patient must stop any antireflux treatment a week before.

On average, during the 24-hour test oesophageal pH is <4 for:
- 1.5% of the total time
- 2.3% of the upright time
- 0.6% of the supine time

Significantly longer times than this (eg >4% of total time) indicate reflux. This test does not account for duodenal (biliary) reflux which is alkaline.

The DeMeester score is a composite measure of reflux episodes and length of time that the pH is measured at <4.

### Computed tomography

This may be indicated if a suspicious lesion is identified (for confirmation and staging) or extrinsic compression is seen (for diagnosis).

Functional diagnoses (such as globus hystericus) can be made only in patients with normal results on endoscopy, barium swallow, pH and manometry.

## 2.3 Gastro-oesophageal reflux disease

 **In a nutshell ...**

The term 'reflux' refers to symptoms caused by the presence of gastric contents within the oesophagus. The clinical definition is an oesophageal pH of <4 for >4% of a 24-hour period on pH monitoring.

### Epidemiology of gastro-oesophageal reflux disease

GORD is the most common upper GI diagnosis made. Most people have some degree of reflux, especially after meals; 7% of healthy people have heartburn; 5% will eventually need an operation.

Reflux is usually (but not always) associated with hiatus hernia. Of people aged >50 years, 50% have a hiatus hernia. A third of these patients have reflux.

## Aetiology of gastro-oesophageal reflux

 **In a nutshell ...**

**Three factors normally keep gastric juices out of the oesophagus:**
- Oesophageal clearance
- LOS competence
- Gastric clearance

If any of these is affected, the risk of reflux increases.

### Oesophageal clearance

Efficient clearance normally relies on:
- Gravity
- Saliva flow
- Normal motility (lost in motility disorders such as scleroderma)
- Fixation for efficient peristalsis (lost in hiatus hernia)

### Lower oesophageal sphincter competence

Resting LOS pressure should be >5 mmHg over a distance of >1 cm. LOS pressure is reduced in certain groups:
- Smokers
- Women on the oral contraceptive pill (OCP)
- People on atropine
- Pregnant women

### Gastric clearance

This relies on:
- Normal secretion
- Rapid clearance
- Normal nerve supply

Thus, gastric outlet obstruction can lead to reflux. Duodenogastric reflux (eg after gastric resection) worsens symptoms. Obese and pregnant people have reduced gastric clearance due to increased intra-abdominal pressure.

Smoking and alcohol are also risk factors.

## Clinical features of gastro-oesophageal reflux

- Epigastric/retrosternal/interscapular pain ('heartburn' is pathognomonic)
- Angina-type pain (reflux may be exercise-related)
- Odynophagia (especially when swallowing hot drinks)
- Reflux of food (this is not vomiting; it is effortless, especially on bending)
- Globus (lump in throat); the cricopharyngeal 'bar' may be seen on barium swallow
- Pulmonary aspiration (nocturnal coughing; hoarse voice); this is known as 'gastric asthma'

## Diagnosis of gastro-oesophageal reflux

- **History:** effect of posture and antacids. Patients aged <55 with no worrying symptoms or risk factors require a urease breath test or a stool antigen test to rule out *Helicobacter pylori*. If positive this should be eradicated and, if negative, a trial of medical therapy (proton pump inhibitor or PPI) for 1 month should be given. Investigate further if there is a history of weight loss, anaemia, anorexia, family history or Barrett's oesophagus. All patients aged >55 with new symptoms of GORD should be investigated. If symptoms in young patients do not resolve after medical treatment, further investigations should be performed

- **Endoscopy** is the first investigation of choice for reflux (see section 2.2). It makes the diagnosis in 70% of cases and can confirm it by biopsy. Importantly, endoscopy can also diagnose other pathologies (eg Barrett's oesophagus). It can also show changes proximal to the squamocolumnar junction
- **Biopsy** is diagnostic in 80%. Tissue from 5 cm above the GOJ shows increased eosinophils and hypoplasia
- **pH monitoring** is the gold standard for diagnosing reflux because it is 90% sensitive (see Section 2.2). Most upper GI specialists insist on pH monitoring and oesophageal manometry before a surgical antireflux procedure as objective evidence of the indications for surgery and the results of surgery
- **Oesophageal manometry** is used preoperatively (see Section 2.2)
- **Barium swallow** is useful for diagnosing hiatus hernia, but is not a definitive investigation for reflux
- **Bernstein acid perfusion test** reproduces reflux symptoms in 70% of cases. HCl 0.1 mmol/l is introduced into the oesophagus at a rate of 6 ml/min, 5 cm above the GOJ. This is rarely done now

---

**Stages of endoscopically detected oesophagitis**

| | |
|---|---|
| Stage I | Discrete linear ulceration |
| Stage II | Areas of more confluent oesophagitis |
| Stage III | Circumferential oesophagitis |
| Stage IV | Stricture formation |

Note that 30% of patients with significant reflux will have a normal endoscopy.

---

# Complications of gastro-oesophageal reflux disease

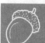 **In a nutshell ...**

- Oesophageal strictures
- Barrett's oesophagus (see Section 2.8)
- Bleeding

## Oesophageal stricture

The most common cause of benign oesophageal strictures is GOR. Endoscopy and biopsy diagnose 95% of cases.

---

**Non-reflux causes of benign oesophageal strictures**

| Drugs | Disease |
|---|---|
| Slow K | TB |
| Tetracycline | Crohn's disease |
| NSAIDs | |
| Lye | |

---

Benign strictures are treated by dilation, using either balloon dilators or tapered bougies (which may be silicone, mercury-filled or Celestin). These are usually 44–45 French (about 15 mm in diameter). The dilation is carried out under endoscopic or radiological control, although frequent attenders can be taught how to self-dilate at home using soft silicone dilators.

Surgery involves an antireflux procedure such as a laparoscopic Nissen fundoplication in the first instance. Oesophageal replacement is rarely needed and is indicated by certain criteria, eg young people, recurrent stricture, undilatable stricture (rare) or a shortened oesophagus.

## Barrett's oesophagus

Barrett's oesophagus is defined as an acquired condition in which any portion of the normal squamous lining has been replaced by a metaplastic columnar epithelium which is visible macroscopically. This should be confirmed histologically. It represents the extreme end of the pathophysiological spectrum of GORD (see Section 2.8). Patients with Barrett's oesophagus exhibit an increased risk of malignant transformation when compared with the general population.

## Bleeding

Bleeding is rare in reflux disease unless there is severe erosive oesophagitis. In such situations anaemia may occur, but usually reflux does not explain anaemia or bleeding so another cause should be sought.

## Treatment of gastro-oesophageal reflux

### Medical treatment of gastro-oesophageal reflux

This works for 90% of patients:

- Conservative treatment: lose weight, raise bed-head, decrease size of evening meal, reduce alcohol intake
- Antacids (helps 36% of patients)
- Metoclopramide: increases LOS pressure and increases gastric emptying; it helps about half the patients
- $H_2$-receptor blockers (eg cimetidine 800 mg twice daily and ranitidine 150 mg twice daily)
- PPIs, eg omeprazole and lansoprazole: 90% short-term healing

## Surgical treatment of gastro-oesophageal reflux

Most antireflux surgery involves some form of stomach wrap around the lower oesophagus. This limits reflux by decreasing hiatus hernia and increasing LOS tone. It may also have the effect of a flap valve:

- **Nissen 360° fundoplication:** the fundus is mobilised (usually by dividing the short gastric arteries). It is wrapped around the oesophagus and then sutured to itself on the other side. This can be done laparoscopically. It is called 'floppy' because you should be able to pass your finger within the wrap. The success rate is high (up to 90%). Complications include gas bloat (5%), dysphagia (5%) and recurrent reflux (5%)
- **Toupe:** a posterior (270°) partial fundoplication
- **Dor:** an anterior partial (180°) fundoplication
- **Belsey mark IV:** a transthoracic fundoplication. It is less satisfactory than Nissen fundoplication
- **Hill repair:** in this repair, the fundoplicated GOJ is fixed to the median arcuate ligament of the diaphragm
- **Angelchik prosthesis:** this is a silicone collar with two tapes, anchored below the diaphragm. It can increase dysphagia. The prosthesis can migrate or cause erosion. It costs more than Nissen fundoplication. It is now rarely performed
- **Roux-en-Y procedure:** this is indicated if reflux is recurrent. There is high morbidity and mortality (see Section 3, Stomach and duodenum)

## 2.4 Hiatus hernia

### In a nutshell ...

**Sliding hiatus hernia (type 1):** this is a cephalad displacement of the GOJ and proximal stomach through the diaphragmatic hiatus into the posterior mediastinum. The stomach is covered anteriorly by a sac of peritoneum but is bare posteriorly.

**Paraoesophageal hernia (type 2):** this is when the GOJ remains in its normal position below the hiatus and the stomach herniates into the chest next to the oesophagus. The stomach is completely covered in peritoneum. Initially only the fundus herniates, but eventually the entire stomach can enter the chest.

**Type 3 hiatus hernia:** this has elements of both sliding and paraoesophageal hiatus hernias.

**Gastric volvulus:** this may occur when a type 2 or 3 hiatus hernia enlarges so much that the entire stomach is herniated anterior to the oesophagus upside down in the chest with the pylorus located at the diaphragm (organoaxial rotation). Typically the sliding hiatus hernia is discovered incidentally while investigating coexisting symptoms such as reflux and, although it rarely needs treatment, it is corrected by reflux surgery. On the other hand, paraoesophageal hiatus hernias commonly present with symptoms and surgical repair is indicated.

### Epidemiology of hiatus hernia

Hiatus hernia can be demonstrated radiologically in 50% of the population, and in 80% of GORD patients; 95% are sliding hernias. Other types of hiatus hernia (described above) are relatively rare. Paraoesophageal hernias are more common in elderly people (aged >70).

### Investigating a hiatus hernia

**Chest radiograph** can be diagnostic. Lateral chest radiograph (rarely performed) shows an air–fluid level in the posterior mediastinum.

**Barium swallow** confirms the diagnosis and may define the extent of a large intrathoracic hiatus hernia.

**Endoscopy** rules out oesophagitis and checks the position of the GOJ (may be high in a shortened oesophagus).

### Presentation and management of hiatus hernia

**Sliding hiatus hernias** are associated with, but not known to be the cause of, GORD. There is no indication for surgical repair of an asymptomatic sliding oesophageal hiatus hernia, but surgical antireflux procedures for persistent reflux resistant to medical treatment involve reducing any coexisting hiatus hernia.

**Paraoesophageal hernias** may present with:
- postprandial breathlessness (due to lung compression)
- early satiety
- dysphagia
- history of reflux that has spontaneously improved over time
- respiratory distress
- bleeding gastric ulcer/gastritis
- rupture or gangrene of the intrathoracic stomach

Patients with a large paraoesophageal hiatus hernia may develop complications, so even asymptomatic paraoesophageal hiatus hernias should be repaired if the patient is fit.

Surgery involves reduction of the hernia, excision of the sac, narrowing of the hiatus plus a fundoplication to prevent future reflux. The elective procedure is now usually done laparoscopically. A transthoracic approach is preferred in a strangulated or ruptured gastric volvulus.

## 2.5 Motility disorders

 **In a nutshell ...**

**Causes of oesophageal dysmotility**
*Primary*
- Achalasia
- Diffuse oesophageal spasm

*Secondary*
- Autoimmune rheumatic disorders (eg scleroderma)
- Chagas' disease
- Diabetes mellitus
- Amyloid
- Intestinal pseudo-obstruction
- Myasthenia gravis

## Achalasia

 **In a nutshell ...**

Achalasia usually presents as difficulty swallowing and retrosternal chest pain. It is characterised by a high LOS pressure and failure of the relaxation of the sphincter. There is also poor peristalsis throughout the oesophagus.

### Epidemiology of achalasia
- Absence of relaxation of the LOS affects 1 in 100 000 people
- Usually affects people aged 30–60
- 5% of cases occur in childhood

### Pathogenesis of achalasia
Pathogenesis is unknown. There a number of theories, including inheritance, and a neurotropic virus affecting the vagal nucleus may be responsible. There is degeneration of the nitric oxide-secreting inhibitory neurones, and loss of the receptive relaxation reflex. There is also generalised degeneration of the myenteric plexus and vagal efferents, with loss of ganglionic cells.

### Early phase
- Vigorous achalasia and chest pain
- Simultaneous peristaltic contractions

### Later phase
- Dilatation of the oesophagus with retention of solids and liquids
- Dysphagia and regurgitation
- Liquids and solids equally difficult to swallow (unlike mechanical obstruction)

## Investigating achalasia

- **Endoscopy:** essential to rule out fixed mechanical obstruction (long-standing achalasia is a risk factor for squamous cell cancer of the oesophagus due to chronic stasis and retention)
- **Barium swallow:** shows a 'bird's beak' abnormality of the LOS with a dilated oesophagus; typically there is no gastric air bubble; there may be food residue in the oesophagus or no emptying of contrast into the stomach
- **Manometry:** manometry is the key diagnostic test. Characteristic manometric features of achalasia include absence of peristalsis and incomplete relaxation of the LOS with a normal or high LOS pressure (normal resting pressure is 0–30 mmHg)

**Complications of achalasia** include nocturnal aspiration, bronchiectasis, and lung abscess. Carcinoma develops in 3% of cases, usually a squamous cell carcinoma (SCC) in the midoesophagus, which is bulky with poor prognosis.

## Treatment of achalasia

- **Conservative management:** medical management offers virtually no benefit
- **Balloon dilation:** to a pressure of 300 mmHg for 3 minutes. This works in approximately 70% of patients but there is a 3% perforation rate
- **Heller's cardiomyotomy:** a 7-cm single myotomy at the GOJ (recognised by small transverse extramucosal veins). Reflux after myotomy is common and many recommend combining myotomy with an antireflux procedure
- **Injection of botulinum toxin:** injection into the LOS under endoluminal ultrasound control is a new treatment with limited long-term success

## Pseudo-achalasia

This typically occurs in those aged >50. It is caused by carcinoma of the LOS, cardia or extrinsic tumour (eg pancreas, lymphoma). There is increased resistance on passing the endoscope (unlike true achalasia).

## Diffuse oesophageal spasm

Of patients admitted with 'anginal' chest pain 30% have normal angiograms. Some of these have diffuse oesophageal spasm (DOS). Retrosternal pain radiating to the jaw and interscapular region is described and the patient is clammy and pale. The symptoms are intermittent and hard to diagnose but manometry may reveal a 'nutcracker oesophagus' with high-amplitude peristalsis of long duration. Nifedipine and reassurance are the mainstay of treatment.

## Chagas' disease

Chronic infection with *Trypanosoma cruzi*, a parasite native to Brazil, causes destruction of intermuscular ganglion cells. This leads to a clinical picture very similar to achalasia. It is also associated with cardiomyopathy, megacolon, megaduodenum and megaureter.

## Scleroderma (systemic sclerosis)

Of scleroderma patients, 80% have oesophageal involvement. Oesophagitis is also seen in CREST (**c**alcinosis, **R**aynaud's phenomenon, **o**esophagitis, **s**cleroderma and **t**elangiectasia) syndrome. An adynamic oesophagus and GOR lead to the formation of a stricture. The LOS is found to be hypotensive on manometry, unlike in achalasia. Medical treatment or a partial fundoplication (avoiding chronic dysphagia) is the treatment option.

Other autoimmune rheumatic disorders associated with oesophageal dysmotility include the following:

- Rheumatoid arthritis
- Dermatomyositis
- Polymyositis
- Systemic lupus erythematosus (SLE)

## 2.6 Oesophageal perforation

### Causes of oesophageal perforation

#### Spontaneous rupture

Spontaneous rupture usually results in a torn left posterior aspect of the oesophagus, just above the cardia. Classically, patients present with severe chest pain/upper abdominal pain after an episode of vomiting (Boerhaave syndrome). This may lead to cardiovascular collapse. Clinically, there may be subcutaneous emphysema. Chest radiography typically shows a pneumothorax, mediastinal gas and pleural effusion. A water-soluble contrast swallow is helpful. Early diagnosis is the key to a successful outcome.

#### Penetrating injury

This is rare because the oesophagus is smaller than other vital intrathoracic organs. Resection may be needed.

#### Instrumental perforation

There are five typical sites of perforation during endoscopy (Figure 1.12).

The clinical picture may be less acute and dramatic than with spontaneous rupture; however, mediastinitis usually develops.

Mediastinitis is a dangerous condition that can lead to severe systemic disturbance and cardiovascular collapse. Cardiac dysrhythmias are common (tachycardia, atrial fibrillation). Classically, mediastinal 'crunch' (like footsteps on soft snow) may be heard with the heart sounds.

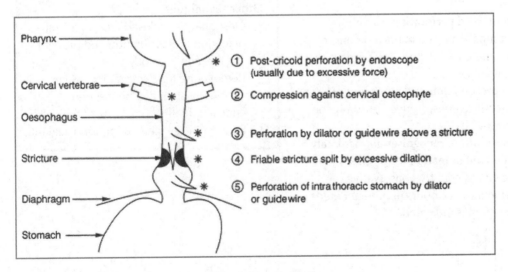

**Figure 1.12 Typical sites of perforation during endoscopy**

## Diagnosis of oesophageal perforation

Early diagnosis of oesophageal perforation reduces the risks of complications and mortality.

A plain chest radiograph can show pleural effusions, pneumomediastinum and subcutaneous emphysema in up to 90% of patients, but can also be normal if taken early. A contrast study remains the gold standard in diagnosis of oesophageal perforation. CT is useful when perforations are difficult to locate or diagnose.

## Treatment of oesophageal perforation

There is some controversy about non-surgical vs surgical management depending on the type of perforation. The following are the principles of initial management:

- Resuscitation
- Nil by mouth
- Broad-spectrum antibiotics
- Parenteral nutrition
- PPIs and analgesia

Principles for the different types of presentation are as follows:

- **Small contained perforation** (intramural or mediastinal): may be managed conservatively, with contrast study after 5 days to confirm healing
- **Delayed presentation** (2 days or longer after injury): manage conservatively; usually too friable to suture
- **Large perforation, recognised immediately with little contamination** (eg at endoscopy in a starved patient): try conservative management for 12 hours; if patient deteriorates, surgery is indicated

- **Boerhaave syndrome** (rupture induced by vomiting): early surgery is recommended because there is usually massive contamination

In any of these cases, signs of peritonitis almost always indicate surgery.

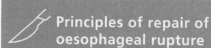

### Principles of repair of oesophageal rupture

This is usually performed through a thoracotomy:

- Incise muscle layer of oesophagus to see mucosal defect (always larger than the muscle defect)
- Strengthen repair by intercostal flap or fundus of stomach
- Excise any abnormal strictures
- May proceed to excision of oesophagus with delayed or immediate reconstruction (if so, a gastrostomy for feeding should be considered)

**Other techniques**

- Oesophagus is closed around a T-tube placed in the perforation and brought out through the body wall
- Remove the tube several weeks later
- A covered stent can be inserted endoscopically
- Endoscopic placement of fibrin sealant

> **Complications of oesophageal perforation**
>
> | | |
> |---|---|
> | Mediastinitis | Pneumothorax |
> | Pyothorax | Haemomediastinum |
> | Subcutaneous | Chest infection |
> | emphysema | Peritonitis |
> | Chylothorax | Pleural effusion |
> | | Pneumoperitoneum |

## 2.7 Other benign oesophageal disorders

> **In a nutshell ...**
>
> - Pharyngeal pouch (see Chapter 5, Head and Neck Surgery)
> - Infective oesophagitis
> - Oesophageal atresia (see Paediatric Surgery)
> - Oesophageal web (see Chapter 5, Head and Neck Surgery)
> - Oesophageal ring (Schatzki's ring)

### Infective oesophagitis

The oesophagus is particularly susceptible to infection in some patients:

- Immunocompromised patients (viral oesophagitis)
- Patients on broad-spectrum antibiotics (fungal oesophagitis)

The most common infections include the following:

- Herpes simplex
- Cytomegalovirus (CMV)
- Candidiasis (thrush)

## Oesophageal ring (Schatzki's ring)

This is a band of connective tissue at the squamocolumnar junction of the lower oesophagus. It may be covered in squamous or columnar epithelium. These rings cause dysphagia because they constrict the lumen. It is not known what causes them. Balloon or bougie dilation and antireflux medication control the symptoms.

## 2.8 Barrett's oesophagus

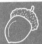

> **In a nutshell ...**
>
> - In 1950 Barrett described a gastric-lined oesophagus
> - It is a latent, irreversible, metaplastic response to reflux
> - The current definition is endoscopically visible columnar metaplasia within the oesophagus, irrespective of length, with intestinal metaplasia on histological examination
> - The previous definition of 3 cm of columnar metaplasia is out of date (because of what is known as 'short segment' Barrett's oesophagus)
> - The British Society of Gastroenterologists currently recommend surveillance endoscopy every 2 years in patients with biopsy-proven non-dysplastic changes. Practice still varies between institutions
> - High-grade dysplasia is associated with a focus of invasive adenocarcinoma in 30–40% of patients
> - If the changes persist after intensive acid suppression and are confirmed by two expert pathologists, oesophagectomy is recommended
> - If unfit for surgery, endoscopic ablation or mucosal resection can be considered

## Aetiology of Barrett's oesophagus

Barrett's oesophagus is the consequence of prolonged severe reflux. It is thought to be due to the combined effect of gastric acid, bile and pancreatic juice. The normal squamous epithelium becomes repeatedly damaged and there is clonal selection of a metaplastic epithelial type of cell, which is more resistant or suited to the reflux environment. Not all patients with severe reflux develop Barrett's oesophagus.

## Epidemiology of Barrett's oesophagus

Most cases go undiagnosed during the patient's lifetime, but it is estimated that 1% of the UK population has a Barrett's oesophagus.

## Barrett's oesophagus and cancer

Once established, there is a small but significant risk of progression to cancer:

Barrett's oesophagus
↓
Dysplasia
↓
Adenocarcinoma

The incidence of adenocarcinoma of the oesophagus in patients with Barrett's oesophagus is increased to 1% per year. Although this represents a 40- to 80-fold increase in risk (a 50-year-old has a 1 in 4 chance of adeno-carcinoma developing during the next 25 years) no more than 5% of patients with Barrett's oesophagus will actually die of oesophageal cancer.

## Follow-up of Barrett's oesophagus

This is a controversial area. However, the British Society of Gastroenterologists have formulated some recent guidelines:

- Two-yearly endoscopic surveillance with systematic biopsy (four-quadrant every 2 cm) is currently recommended for patients with Barrett's oesophagus with no dysplastic cells on biopsy (despite low death rate and limitations of treatment). High-quality evidence for this intervention is still lacking
- If low-grade dysplasia is present on biopsy, further biopsies should be performed after intensive acid suppression for 8–12 weeks followed by 6-monthly surveillance
- High-grade dysplasia is associated with a focus of invasive adenocarcinoma in 30–40% of patients. If the changes persist after intensive acid suppression and are confirmed by two expert pathologists, oesophagectomy is recommended. However, surveillance-detected tumours are at an earlier stage and have a 5-year survival rate after resection of >85%
- If unfit for surgery, endoscopic ablation or mucosal resection can be considered

## Treatment of Barrett's oesophagus

### Metaplasia and dysplasia

Medical or surgical treatment of reflux does not usually lead to regression of metaplasia. Evidence suggests that successful antireflux surgery normalises cancer risk (but may take up to 20 years). Ablation of abnormal mucosa (with laser, argon-beam diathermy or photodynamic therapy associated with medical/surgical antireflux therapy) results in squamous regeneration. However, it is not clear whether this decreases or removes the malignant risk.

### High-grade dysplasia and cancer

Most experts agree that high-grade dysplasia (confirmed by a second pathologist) should be treated by resection in patients fit for oesophagectomy. Invasive adenocarcinoma detected on surveillance biopsies should also be treated by resection. Of patients with high-grade dysplasia 50% will have invasive adenocarcinoma.

## 2.9 Oesophageal carcinoma

### In a nutshell ...

- The incidence of adenocarcinoma of the oesophagus in the western world is now higher than SCC of the oesophagus
- Adenocarcinomas mainly arise in the lower third of the oesophagus, often in a region of Barrett's oesophagus, whereas SCCs arise throughout the oesophagus
- The type of surgery depends on the position of the cancer, but after resection a neo-oesophagus is commonly formed from the stomach
- Overall 5-year survival rate is 25% despite careful patient selection

### Epidemiology of oesophageal carcinoma

- More males than females (3M:1F)
- Rare in people aged <40
- Increased incidence in 'Asian oesophageal cancer belt' (stretches from eastern Turkey, Iran, northern Afghanistan, to northern China and India). High incidences are also found in South Africa and Kenya

- Greater geographical variation in incidence than any other tumour. In high-incidence areas, the occurrence of oesophageal cancer is 50- to 100-fold higher than in the rest of the world

### Site of oesophageal carcinoma

Thought to be most common at points of physiological narrowing of oesophagus (see Figure 1.11). In the western world, the lower oesophagus and GOJ are by far the most common sites of oesophageal tumours.

### Pathology of oesophageal carcinoma

- **Adenocarcinomas** account for 65% of oesophageal cancers in the UK and their incidence is increasing in the USA at a rate of 5–10% per year. Adenocarcinomas mainly arise in the lower third of the oesophagus and at the GOJ. A predisposing factor is Barrett's oesophagus
- **Squamous cell carcinomas** can arise at any level within the oesophagus and the current incidence appears static
- **Oat cell carcinoma** is rare, with a poor prognosis
- **Other rare tumours** are adenoid cystic carcinoma, melanoma and carcinoid

## Aetiology of oesophageal carcinoma

| Risk factors associated with oesophageal cancer | |
| --- | --- |
| **Adenocarcinoma** | **Squamous cell carcinoma (SCC)** |
| Barrett's oesophagus | High alcohol intake |
| GORD | Tobacco use |
| Obesity | Nitrosamines in diet |
| High fat intake | Vitamin C deficiency |
| Cigarette smoking | Vitamin A deficiency |
| High alcohol intake | Coeliac disease |
| | Strictures |
| | Lye |
| | Webs |
| | Achalasia |
| | Peptic ulcer disease |

## Presentation of oesophageal carcinoma

Oesophageal carcinoma may present with the following features:
- Dysphagia and/or odynophagia
- Retrosternal discomfort
- Atypical chest pain
- Pseudo-achalasia
- Fluid regurgitation leading to bouts of coughing, aspiration, and even chest infection
- Hoarseness (right recurrent laryngeal nerve palsy)
- Anaemia (rare)
- Massive haematemesis
- Lymphadenopathy

## Diagnosis and staging of oesophageal carcinoma

Upper GI endoscopy is the mainstay of diagnosis. CT, endoscopic ultrasonography (EUS), positron emission tomography (PET)/CT, laparoscopy/thoracoscopy are all used in staging patients with disease.

Staging is based on the TNM classification:
- **Stage 1:** T1 N0 M0
- **Stage 2a:** T2 or T3 + N0 M0
- **Stage 2b:** T1 or T2 + N1 M0
- **Stage 3:** T3 or T4 + N1 M0
- **Stage 4:** any T or N + M1

T1, tumour invading the lamina propria but not reaching the submucosa; T2, tumour invading into but not beyond the muscularis propria; T3, tumour invading the adventitia but not the adjacent structures; T4, tumour invading the adjacent structures; N1, regional lymph node involved; M1, metastasis present.

## Management of oesophageal carcinoma

### Preoperative preparation
- Correct urea and electrolytes (U&Es)
- Correct anaemia
- Optimise nutrition:
  - Withdraw solid food
  - Start high-protein liquid diet
  - Enteral feed via an NG tube (if necessary)
- Optimise respiratory function:
  - Encourage patient to give up smoking
  - Intensive physiotherapy
  - Treat any chest infection

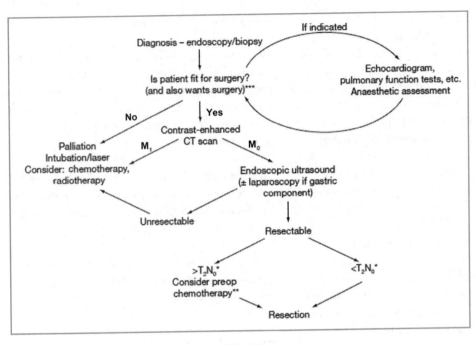

Figure 1.13
Algorithm for
management
of oesophageal
carcinoma

\* $T_2$ means that the tumour has not breached the muscularis propria.

\*\* If preoperative chemotherapy is given, it is important to carry out a CT scan before surgery to ensure that no metastases have developed.

\*\*\* In upper-third cricopharyngeal tumours many would consider radiotherapy to be the primary treatment of choice.

## Surgical approaches to the oesophagus

### In a nutshell ...

The oesophagus can be approached via the:
- Neck
- Right or left chest
- Abdomen

Almost any combination of these approaches has been described. The most common approaches are:
- Ivor Lewis procedure
- McKeown three-phase oesophagectomy
- Trans-hiatal resection

- **Ivor Lewis procedure:** this is an initial laparotomy and mobilisation of the stomach, preserving the right gastroepiploic arcade, followed by a right thoracotomy during which the tumour is resected and the mobilised stomach brought up to anastomose to the oesophagus
- **McKeown three-stage oesophagectomy:** this is an Ivor Lewis procedure plus a neck incision. The stomach is brought all the way up to the neck and an anastomosis is made between the stomach and the cervical oesophagus
- **Trans-hiatal resection:** this is a laparotomy and a neck incision. The oesophagus is mobilised by blunt dissection from above or below. The stomach is used as a conduit and brought up to the neck and a cervical anastomosis carried out as in the three-phase procedure
- **Laparoscopic-assisted approaches:** various combinations of minimally invasive approaches including thoracoscopy- and laparoscopy-assisted have been attempted. Serious complications can occur, such as bleeding from the azygos vein, intercostal vessels and the aorta, and injury to the tracheobronchial tree and recurrent laryngeal nerve. Some studies have reported shortened intensive care unit (ICU) and hospital stay, with similar anastomotic leak and respiratory complication rates when compared with open surgery. However, clear advantages of the minimally invasive methods have not yet been demonstrated

There is no convincing evidence that any particular approach to the oesophagus is significantly better than any other in terms of surgical morbidity, mortality or long-term survival. The location and stage of the primary tumour should dictate the surgical approach used. Trans-hiatal resection is probably not suitable for patients with middle- or upper-third tumours.

The only surgical factor that affects long-term survival is negative resection margins (both longitudinal and circumferential). There is no convincing evidence that radical lymphadenectomy for adenocarcinoma significantly influences long-term survival.

The stomach is the most commonly used conduit after resection for oesophageal cancer, but if the stomach is not available for any reason, then the colon or small bowel can be used.

The overall operative mortality rate for oesophagectomy remains around 10% but in the best units in the UK it is now well under 5%.

## The role of chemotherapy and radiotherapy

Oesophageal cancer is associated with poor outcomes. It is therefore unsurprising that multiple neoadjuvant and adjuvant regimens have been studied. The results of the major trials are summarised below:

- Neoadjuvant radiotherapy – failed to show any benefit when compared with surgery alone
- Adjuvant radiotherapy – improves local disease control and may have a benefit in those who have had a pallative resection
- Neoadjuvant chemotherapy – did not alter the rate of resection, rate of complete resection or postoperative complications, but was associated with a significant survival advantage
- Adjuvant chemotherapy – appears to improve survival at 5 years
- Neoadjuvant chemoradiotherapy – compared with surgery alone, neoadjuvant chemoradiation and surgery improve survival and reduced locoregional cancer

recurrence. It also produces a higher rate of complete resection

- Chemoradiotherapy as a *definitive* therapy – provides a reduction in mortality at 1–2 years and reduction of local recurrence rate when compared with radiotherapy alone

## Outlook of oesophageal carcinoma

 **In a nutshell ...**

Only about 30% of patients with oesophageal carcinoma are appropriate for resection. Despite such selection the overall 5-year survival rate in most UK series is about 25%. In the last 30 years what has improved in the management of oesophageal carcinoma is staging/assessment and the short-term results after surgery due to improvements in surgery, anaesthesia and perioperative care. Unfortunately, what has not improved is the natural history of the disease.

## Postoperative treatment of oesophageal cancer

- Minimise pain, preferably using a thoracic epidural
- Minimise respiratory failure by:
  - Careful patient selection
  - Preoperative physiotherapy
  - Postoperative intensive care
  - Good pain control
- Minimise postoperative nutritional deficiency (eg site a feeding jejunostomy during the operation)

## Palliative management of advanced oesophageal cancer

- **Stenting:** a self-expanding metal stent via fibreoptic endoscopy, with or without radiological control can be deployed. It can keep the oesophagus patent; however, a special diet needs to be followed or the stent can become blocked. Problems include migration of the stent or tumour growing over or through it
- **Argon plasma coagulation (APC):** again, effective in relieving dysphagia and bleeding

Tracheo-oesophageal fistula is an incurable, dangerous complication of oesophageal carcinoma. Insertion of a covered endo-oesophageal stent is the usual treatment:

- **Chemotherapy:** good for adenocarcinomas but patients need to be fairly fit to tolerate it
- **Radiotherapy:** better for SCC. It may produce strictures or fistulation subsequently
- **Laser treatment:** good for short, intrinsic tumours to restore swallowing. It may need repeating. There is a danger of perforation
- **Surgery:** no longer indicated in incurable cases

# SECTION 3

# Stomach and duodenum

## 3.1 Anatomy of the stomach

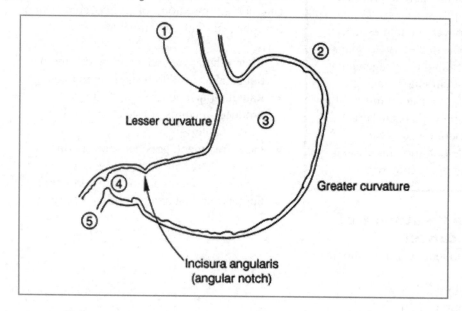

Figure 1.14
**Structure of the stomach**

(1) **Cardia:** most fixed part of the stomach – left of midline at T10 – cardiac orifice (gastro-oesophageal junction) has four factors guarding it against reflux: 1, lower oesophageal muscle fibres; 2, fibres of right crus; 3, mucosal flaps of muscularis mucosa; 4, difference between intrathoracic and intra-abdominal pressure.

(2) **Fundus:** projects above cardia. Usually touches diaphragm. Full of swallowed air.

(3) **Body:** largest part of stomach, from fundus to incisura angularis, which is a prominent feature that does not change with peristalsis.

(4) **Pylorus:** from incisura angularis to gastro-duodenal junction: pyloric antrum – proximal dilated portion; pyloric canal; pyloric sphincter – thickened circular muscle; pylorus – narrow lumen of pyloric sphincter.

(5) **Pyloric opening:** in recumbent position with stomach empty lies right of midline at L1.

## Muscle layers of the stomach

- Outer longitudinal
- Inner circular
- Incomplete innermost oblique

The innermost layer loops over the fundus. It is thickest at the notch between the oesophagus and the stomach. It is oblique when the stomach is empty. It is vertical when the stomach is full and the trunk is erect (supporting the weight of the gastric contents).

## Relations of the stomach

Three double layers of peritoneum form important connections between the stomach and other organs:

1. The **lesser omentum** is a double layer from the liver to the lesser curvature of the stomach
2. The **gastrocolic ligament** is the peritoneum running from the greater curvature of the stomach to the transverse colon (it is continuous with the **greater omentum** which is the large apron of fat lying inferior to the transverse colon)
3. The **gastrosplenic omentum** runs from the stomach to the spleen

The posterior relations of the stomach are referred to as the **stomach bed** and include many clinically important structures:

- Peritoneum (anterior and posterior wall of the lesser sac)
- Left crus and dome of the diaphragm
- Upper left kidney and adrenal
- Pancreas, spleen and splenic artery
- Transverse mesocolon
- Aorta and coeliac trunk
- Coeliac ganglia and lymph nodes

## Blood supply of the stomach

The blood supply of the stomach is summarised in Figure 1.15:

- The lesser curvature is supplied by branches from the left and right gastric arteries (may be double) running between layers of lesser omentum; these branches meet in an end-to-end anastomosis
- The fundus and the upper left side of the greater curvature are supplied by the short gastric arteries from the splenic artery running in the gastrosplenic ligament
- The lower greater curvature is supplied by the left and right gastroepiploic arteries (rarely double) from the splenic and gastro-duodenal artery running between two layers of greater omentum; they may or may not anastomose

---

### Surgical implications of gastric blood supply

The rich blood supply of the stomach has implications in gastric surgery, where much of the arterial supply may be disrupted. For example:

- In an oesophagectomy, the stomach is made into a tube which is mobilised into the chest to replace the resected oesophagus. Under these conditions the right gastric artery (which is also sometimes divided) and the right gastroepiploic are the only blood supply to the entire stomach tube
- In a Polya gastrectomy, where the left gastric artery has been divided, the gastric stump is supplied only by the short gastrics

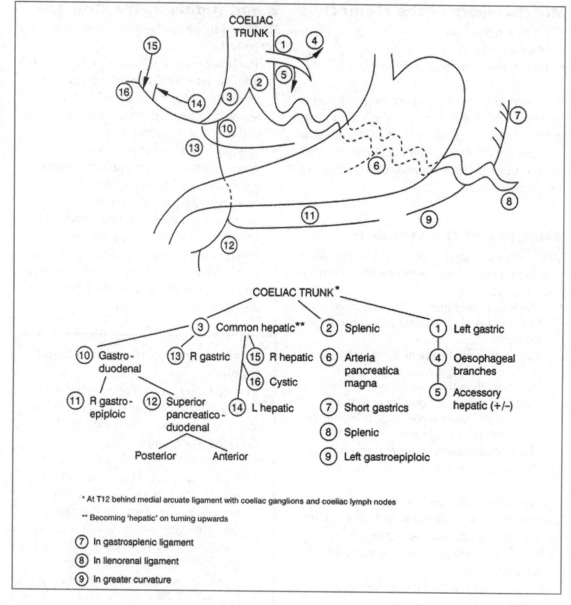

Figure 1.15 Blood supply of the stomach

## Venous drainage of the stomach

Veins follow arteries and drain into portal veins but there are two exceptions. Firstly, there is no gastroduodenal vein. Secondly, the prepyloric vein of Mayo overlies the pylorus and drains into the portal or right gastric vein.

Oesophageal branches are one of the five portosystemic anastomoses.

## Lymphatic drainage of the stomach

- Lymphatic drainage is to the coeliac nodes via a network of freely anastomosing vessels (Figure 1.16)
- Valves direct lymph in the direction shown in Figure 1.16

## Nerve supply to the stomach

- The sympathetic nerve supply to the stomach is from the coeliac plexus and runs with the vessels
- The parasympathetic nerve supply to the stomach is via the vagus nerves, which are shown in Figure 1.17

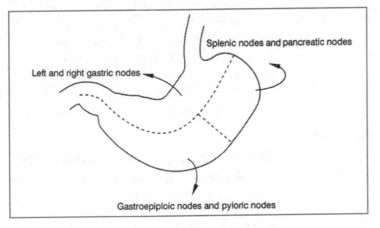

**Figure 1.16 Lymphatic drainage of the stomach**

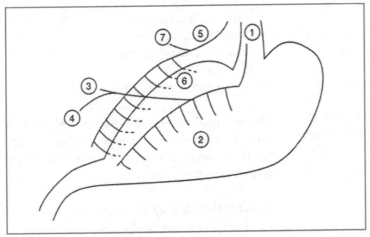

**Figure 1.17 Nerve supply to the stomach**

(1) Anterior vagal trunk: mostly left vagus. At the gastro-oesophageal junction, it lies in contact with the anterior oesophagus. Runs down lesser omentum with the left gastric artery. Double in 20% of people.
(2) Gastric branches.
(3) Large hepatic branches.

(4) Branches to pyloric antrum.
(5) Posterior vagal trunk: mostly right vagus. Lies in loose tissue behind and to the right of the right oesophageal margin. Runs in lesser omentum behind anterior trunk. Rarely double.
(6) Numerous branches to posterior of stomach.
(7) Large coeliac branch: coeliac ganglia.

## Histology of the stomach

At the cardio-oesophageal junction, the stratified squamous epithelium changes to single-layered columnar epithelium. This epithelium has specific characteristics in different areas of the stomach.

### Cardia

- Short glands
- Mucus-secreting cells only

### Body

- Mucus-secreting cells
- Peptic cells that secrete pepsin
- Parietal cells that secrete acid and intrinsic factor
- Gastric pits with test tube-like glands

### Pylorus

- Mucus-secreting cells
- Gastrin-producing (G) cells
- Somatostatin-secreting D cells
- Enterochromaffin (EC) cells
- Serotonin- and endorphin-secreting cells

There is no external landmark between the acid-secreting body cells and the pyloric G cells.

## 3.2 Anatomy of the duodenum

 **In a nutshell ...**

The duodenum is the first part of the small bowel.
- It runs from the pylorus of the stomach to the jejunum
- It curves over the convexity of the aorta and the inferior vena cava
- Its structure is described and relations listed in Figure 1.18

## Blood supply of the duodenum

The **duodenal cap** (the most common site of bleeding duodenal ulcers) is supplied by branches of many arteries, including the:
- Hepatic artery
- Common hepatic artery
- Gastroduodenal artery
- Superior pancreaticoduodenal artery
- Right gastric artery
- Right gastroepiploic artery

The **proximal duodenum** (proximal to the bile duct) is supplied by the superior pancreatico-duodenal artery (a branch of the hepatic artery from the coeliac trunk).

**Distal to the bile duct** the duodenum is supplied by the inferior pancreaticoduodenal artery (a branch of the superior mesenteric artery).

The veins correspond with the arteries, with some blood also entering the small prepyloric vein.

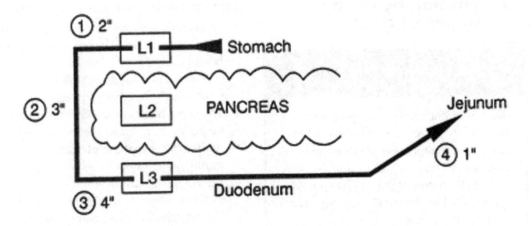

**Figure 1.18 Structure and relations of the duodenum:**

(1) **First part:** 2 inches long. Runs right, upwards and backwards. The first inch is intraperitoneal and the rest is retroperitoneal. Forms the lower border of the epiploic foramen. Lies behind the right lobe of the liver. Posterior relations include the interior vena cava, right kidney, liver pedicle (superiorly) and gastroduodenal artery (this is the one that bleeds in a posterior penetrating duodenal ulcer).

(2) **Second part:** 3 inches long, running inferiorly to the right of the head of the pancreas. The bile duct and main pancreatic duct open at the major duodenal papilla (ampulla of Vater) on the posteromedial wall, 4 cm from the pylorus. (The accessory pancreatic duct opens 2 cm proximal to this at the minor duodenal papilla.) The second part of the duodenum is retroperitoneal and is crossed by the transverse mesocolon attachments. It lies in front of the hilum of the right kidney.

(3) **Third part:** the longest part, it is retroperitoneal, 4 inches long, and running transversely inferior to the pancreas and behind the transverse mesocolon and curls of jejunum. The superior mesenteric artery and vein travel in front of the third part of the duodenum. This is a crucial surgical relationship, particularly when performing a pancreaticoduodenectomy.

(4) **Fourth part:** the last inch of retroperitoneal small intestine before the duodenojejunal flexure (D-J flexure). The duodenum is retroperitoneal, whereas the jejunum hangs from a mesentery. The ligament of Treitz fixes the duodenojejunal flexure to the left psoas fascia. There are four paraduodenal recesses around the D-J flexure which can cause internal hernias (rare).

## Lymphatic drainage

Lymph from the duodenum drains to the coeliac and superior mesenteric nodes.

## Nerve supply of the duodenum

- Parasympathetic supply of the duodenum is from the vagus nerve
- Sympathetic supply of the duodenum is from the coeliac and mesenteric plexus
- Nerves run with the blood vessels

## 3.3 Physiology of the upper GI tract

### In a nutshell ...

The movement of food through the GI tract and its digestion are controlled by a complex combination of neural and hormonal feedback mechanisms:

- **Neural control** of the GI system is mediated by the enteric and extrinsic nervous systems
- **Hormonal control** of the GI system is mediated by blood-borne, paracrine and neurocrine hormones

**Physiology of the upper GI tract**

**Neural control**

- Enteric nervous system
  - Meissner's plexus
  - Auerbach's plexus
- Extrinsic nervous system
  - Sympathetic from coeliac plexus
  - Parasympathetic from vagus

**Hormonal control**

- Blood-borne hormones (eg gastrin, secretin, CCK)
- Paracrine hormones (eg histamine, somatostatin)
- Neurocrine hormones (eg VIP, GRP)

**Movement of food through the GI tract**

- Inner circular, outer longitudinal layer
- Peristalsis
- Migrating myoelectric complex
- Different muscular activity in each section of GI tract

CCK, cholecystokinin; GRP, gastrin-releasing hormone; VIP, vasoactive intestinal hormone.

## The enteric nervous system

- The enteric nervous system consists of two interlinking nerve plexuses running in the bowel wall (Figure 1.19):
  - Submucosal Meissner's plexus
  - Myenteric Auerbach's plexus
- The nerve plexus of the GI tract contain 108 neurones (as many as the spinal cord)
- **Auerbach's myenteric plexus:** consists mostly of motor neurones to smooth muscle cells of muscularis externa:
  - These motor neurones usually produce acetylcholine as a neurotransmitter for muscarinic receptors
  - The inner circular muscle is more richly innervated than the longitudinal muscle
- **Meissner's submucosal plexus:**
  - Consists mostly of **secretomotor neurones** to the glandular, endocrine and epithelial cells
  - These secretomotor neurones usually produce acetylcholine and VIP neurotransmitters to stimulate effector cells, but >25 other neuromodulatory substances have been identified
- Auerbach's and Meissner's plexuses both have:
  - Sensory neurones and interneurones which form intrinsic reflex arcs that respond to intestinal pH, luminal pressure and pain
  - Connections with the sympathetic and parasympathetic nervous systems, which modulate their motor and secretory activity

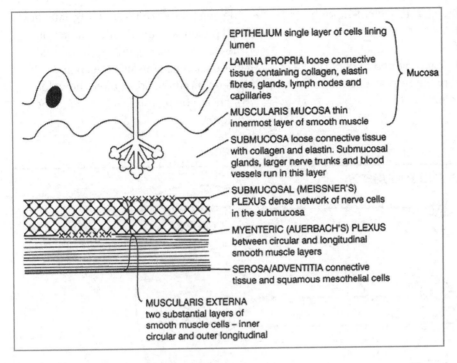

EPITHELIUM single layer of cells lining lumen

LAMINA PROPRIA loose connective tissue containing collagen, elastin fibres, glands, lymph nodes and capillaries

MUSCULARIS MUCOSA thin innermost layer of smooth muscle

Mucosa

SUBMUCOSA loose connective tissue with collagen and elastin. Submucosal glands, larger nerve trunks and blood vessels run in this layer

SUBMUCOSAL (MEISSNER'S) PLEXUS dense network of nerve cells in the submucosa

MYENTERIC (AUERBACH'S) PLEXUS between circular and longitudinal smooth muscle layers

SEROSA/ADVENTITIA connective tissue and squamous mesothelial cells

MUSCULARIS EXTERNA two substantial layers of smooth muscle cells – inner circular and outer longitudinal

**Figure 1.19 The nerve plexuses within the bowel wall**

## The extrinsic nervous system

### In a nutshell ...

The GI system is supplied with sympathetic nerves from the coeliac plexus and parasympathetic nerves from the vagus.

- Functions of extrinsic nerves:
  - Act on and modulate the enteric nervous system
  - Influence secretory and motor activities
  - Regulate blood supply
- Sympathetic nerves convey afferent pain impulses and efferent vasomotor impulses (run with blood vessels)
- Parasympathetic innervation is via the vagus nerve

- 90% of the parasympathetic nerves carry sensory afferent impulses which form extrinsic reflex arcs
- The vagus also increases motility and secretion of the stomach and innervates the pyloric sphincter (so transection of the vagus trunks reduces gastric acid secretion and causes gastric stasis)

## Neural control of the stomach

Neural control of the stomach occurs in three stages:

1. **Cephalic stage** (Figure 1.20):
   - An excitatory stage responsible for saliva production
   - Some pancreatic juice production
   - 10% of gastric secretion
2. **Gastric stage:**
   - Responsible for 80% of gastric secretion
   - Mediated by a short gastric reflex and a long vagus reflex

- There is also an inhibitory element to the gastric stage

3. **Intestinal stage:**
   - The final stage of gastric neural control
   - Mostly inhibitory but responsible for 10% of gastric secretion

- The acid, increased osmolarity, fatty acids and peptides in the duodenum act on the stomach via neural and hormonal feedback mechanisms to decrease gastric motility and regulate the volume of chyme being propelled through the pylorus

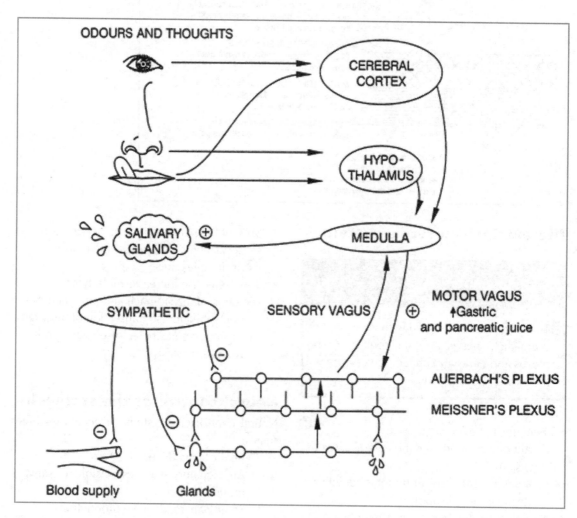

Figure 1.20 Cephalic stage of neural control of the stomach

# Hormonal control of the GI tract

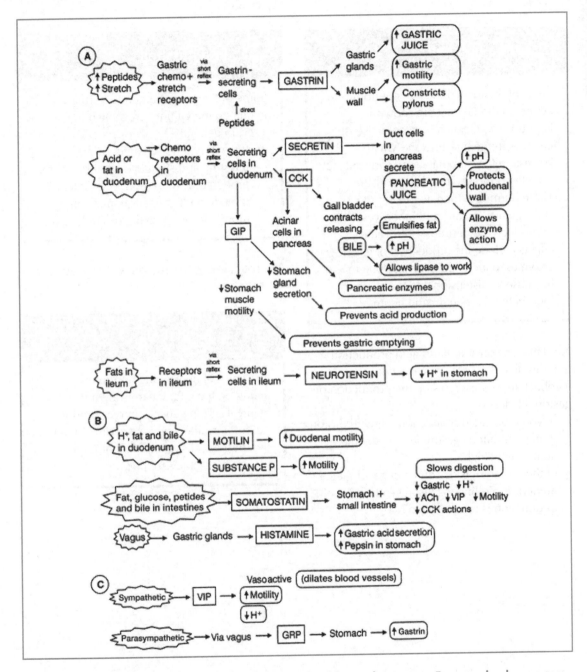

Figure 1.21 Hormonal control of the GI tract: A, blood-borne hormones; B, paracrine hormones; C, neurocrine hormones

## Blood-borne hormones acting on the GI tract

### In a nutshell ...

Some of the many blood-borne hormones acting on the GI tract are shown in Figure 1.21. In general, receptors sense changes in the intestine and via an intrinsic reflex stimulate secretory cells to secrete hormones into the bloodstream. These hormones then act on remote cells, glands, organs and blood vessels to produce the desired result. The effects include the production of gastric enzymes, pancreatic juice and bile in response to distension and undigested food in the duodenum and ileum.

Note that gastrin stimulates acid production and this acid then operates as a negative feedback mechanism to stop the production of gastrin. Hence:
- If you block acid production (eg with proton pump inhibitors) gastrin levels become abnormally high
- If there is an outside source of gastrin (eg a tumour in Zollinger–Ellison syndrome) acid production is uncontrolled

## Paracrine hormones acting on the GI tract

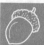

### In a nutshell ...

Some of the many paracrine hormones acting on the GI tract are shown in Figure 1.21. In general:
- Receptors sense changes in the intestine and stimulate local hormone production. These hormones interact directly on local cells, glands and muscle to produce the desired result

## Neurocrine hormones acting on the GI tract

### In a nutshell ...

Examples of neurocrine hormones acting on the GI tract are shown in Figure 1.21. In general, nerves produce neurotransmitters which act directly on the muscle cells, glandular cells and blood vessels they supply.

# Movement of food through the GI tract

## In a nutshell ...

Food is moved through the GI tract by peristalsis, a coordinated muscular movement made possible by the electrophysiology of the smooth-muscle bowel walls. These movements are reinforced by the intermittent migrating myoelectric complex (MMC).

Each part of the GI tract has characteristic motility:

- Swallowing and oesophageal motility were described in Section 2
- Gastric motility is described below
- Motility of the small bowel is described in Section 7
- Motility of the large bowel is described in Section 8
- The physiology of defecation is described in Section 9

## Electrophysiology of GI tract motility

There are two layers of smooth muscle, an inner circular and an outer longitudinal layer, which run along the entire length of the GI tract.

- GI smooth muscle cells are electrically coupled so that they tend to work as a functional unit
- A resting membrane potential oscillates with a characteristic rhythm, controlling the rate of regular contractions

## Peristalsis

- Contractions of the smooth muscles of the GI tract wall mix and propel the contents of the lumen
- Waves of contractions vary in frequency:
  - 13/min in the duodenum on average
  - 8/min in the ileum on average
- Hormones and neurotransmitters affect the force and strength
- The vagus increases the rate of peristalsis

## Migrating myoelectric complex

- MMC is characterised by 70- to 90-minute periods of quiescence, interrupted by periods of vigorous and intensely propulsive contractions lasting 3–6 minutes
- These contractions sweep the stomach and small bowel clear of debris from the previous meal (the housekeeper of the bowel)

## Gastric motility

The proximal stomach (fundus and body):

- Stores ingested food
- Is responsible for secretion of acid, pepsin and intrinsic factor

The distal stomach (antrum and pylorus):

- Grinds the food into fine particles (chyme)
- Empties the stomach in little spurts into the duodenum and small bowel

Relaxation of LOS is caused by the oesophageal peristaltic wave. This initiates receptive relaxation of the stomach, triggered by the movement of the pharynx:

- Distension of the stomach by food leads to increased secretion and motility mediated by local and vasovagal reflexes
- Contractions of the body of the stomach mix food with gastric juice
- More forceful contractions in the antrum cause a churning action

- The pyloric sphincter closes as waves arrive, allowing only small volumes (about 3 ml/min) into the duodenum
- Feedback by hormones and neurones ensures that gastric emptying is not faster than neutralisation of gastric acid and processing of the chyme by the duodenum and jejunum
- Gastric emptying takes 3–4 hours:
  - Liquids first
  - Fats last
- The 'gastric slow wave' is a basic electrical rhythm every 20 seconds when feeding
- There are 10 minutes of activity every 100 minutes when fasting – hunger pangs!

## Vomiting

- A protective, involuntary mechanism for clearing the stomach of noxious substances
- Action is controlled by a vomiting trigger zone in the medulla, which receives afferent nerve impulses from the intestinal viscera, kidneys, bladder, uterus, cerebral cortex and semicircular canals of the ear
- The receptors for these impulses lie on the floor of the fourth ventricle (and are directly stimulated by opiates, digoxin and anaesthetic agents)
- Efferent nerves stimulated by the vomiting trigger zone are the cranial nerves V, VII, IX, X and XII
- The process of vomiting is associated with several autonomic responses:
  - Salivation
  - Vasoconstriction (and therefore pallor)
  - Sweating
  - Dizziness
  - Tachycardia
  - Sequence of events:

Anorexia and nausea
↓
Retching
↓
Airway protected by closure of larynx and nasopharynx
↓
Pylorus and oesophageal sphincters relax
↓
Duodenum contracts
↓
Diaphragm and abdominal wall contract and stomach contents are expelled

- In persistent vomiting (eg due to gastric outlet obstruction) certain biochemical changes occur:
  - Metabolic alkalosis
  - Hypokalaemia
  - Hypochloraemia
  - Paradoxical aciduria
- In addition, in infants you see:
  - Hypoglycaemia
  - Jaundice
- During vomiting there is loss of sodium and water, potassium, acid and chloride which are expelled in the gastric juices; the body's main priority is to restore volume (salt and water) to avoid shock
- The kidney reacts by increasing the absorption of sodium (and therefore retains fluid) in exchange for potassium, which is lost in the urine

As potassium stores are low due to the vomiting, the potassium runs out and the kidney has to look for another cation to exchange for sodium.

The kidney then uses hydrogen ions in exchange for sodium and excretes them in the urine, causing an aciduria. This is paradoxical because, due to the acid lost in the vomit, there is already a serum metabolic alkalosis. The kidney would normally respond to a metabolic alkalosis by absorbing hydrogen ions but, because reabsorbing sodium and water is the main priority here, the kidney is found to be secreting hydrogen ions into the urine in the presence of a metabolic alkalosis, thereby worsening the alkalosis.

The reason for all this is that the kidney is trying to replace lost salt and water. We can replace this saline intravenously and therefore prevent all these sequelae. If the saline has potassium in it as well, the metabolic disturbances can be minimised.

Infants become quickly hypoglycaemic due to lack of food and there is an idiopathic glucuronyl transferase activity impairment causing mild jaundice.

## Gastric physiology

### Functions of the stomach

**In a nutshell ...**

**Functions of the stomach**
**Reservoir**
**Mixer**
- Mechanised food breakdown and mixing with secretions

**Secretor**
- Water and electrolytes
- Acid
- Mucus
- Bicarbonate ($HCO_3^-$)
- Proteases
- Intrinsic factor
- Gastrin

**Digester** (aids in digestion)
- Iron
- Calcium
- Vitamin B12
- Proteins

**Gatekeeper**
- Regulates passage of food into duodenum
- Prevents bacterial contamination

### The stomach as reservoir

The fasting stomach has a volume of 50 ml and a pressure of <1 kPa. Pressure remains low until more than a litre has entered the stomach. Thus the stomach can act as a reservoir, tolerating large volumes without its pressure receptors causing the food to be forced onwards as they do in the rest of the GI tract.

How does the stomach maintain this low pressure?

Laplace's law states that in a sphere:

$$P = 2T/r$$

where $P$ is the pressure, $T$ the tension in the wall and $r$ the radius of the sphere.

Therefore as the radius of the stomach increases, pressure will increase **only** if the tension in the wall increases too.

The stomach maintains a low pressure by maintaining a low wall tension. It does this in two ways:
1. Plasticity: the gastric smooth muscle has a low resting tone even when it is stretched
2. Receptive relaxation: distension of the stomach wall causes vasovagal feedback, which reduces the tone of the stomach muscle

Thus (up to a point!) the stomach muscle wall tension and therefore the intragastric pressure stay low as the radius of the stomach increases.

## The stomach as mixer

- The stomach mixes food with digestive juices, churning it around and only allowing small amounts of fully mixed food (chyme) out of the pylorus at a time; this is done using peristaltic waves travelling towards the pylorus, gaining intensity as they travel (the pyloric pump)
- The pylorus contracts as the wave reaches it, allowing only a small amount of gastric juice through into the duodenum, and forcing the rest to splash back into the stomach (retropropulsion)
- Thus the boluses of food churn around, getting mixed with digestive juices and ground into chyme (trituration)
- The waves of peristalsis originate from pacemaker interstitial cells of Cajal on the proximal greater curve

## The stomach as secretor

- The stomach is a secretory organ (Figure 1.22)
- From its gastric glands which empty into the lumen it produces 2–3 l/day of gastric juice
- Gastric juice consists of water, electrolytes, mucus, acid and enzymes
- The stomach also produces hormones from the APUD (amine precursor uptake and decarboxylation) cells in the mucosa and releases them into the bloodstream

The stomach also secretes the following:
- **Histamine** from the enterochromaffin-like (EC) cells in the gastric mucosa, stimulated by the vagus nerve
- **Intrinsic factor** from the parietal cells, stimulated by the same things that stimulate gastric acid release, ie vagus, gastrin and histamine (remember that in pernicious anaemia, anti-parietal cell antibodies cause deficiency of intrinsic factor and vitamin B12)
- **Gastrin** from the G cells in the antral mucosa and upper small bowel (this hormone is not secreted into the gastric lumen but into the bloodstream; its regulation and actions are summarised in the box below)

---

**Gastrin**
**Stimulated by:**
- Products of digestion, caffeine, alcohol, via direct stimulation of G-cell receptors
- Vagus via acetylcholine receptors
- Distension via intrinsic nerve reflexes

**Inhibited by:**
- Increased acidity, secretin, somatostatin

**Stimulates:**
- Gastric secretion by parietal cells
- Pepsinogen secretion
- Intrinsic factor secretion
- Enhances gastric motility
- Increases LOS tone to prevent reflux

---

**Composition of gastric fluid**
- 70 mmol/l $Na^+$
- 10 mmol/l $K^+$
- 10 mmol/l $Cl^-$

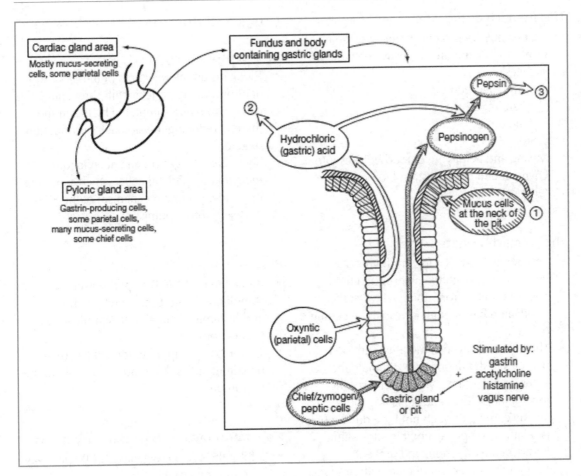

**Figure 1.22 Gastric gland secretions**

(1)  **Mucus:** a thick sticky glycoprotein that adheres to the gastric mucosa. Also secreted by cells of the gastric mucosa. It:
- Lubricates passage of food
- Protects underlying mucosa from digestion by acid and pepsin
- Stores hydrogen carbonate, which acts as a buffer, allowing a pH gradient of 2 in the lumen and 7 at the cell surface

(2)  **Hydrochloric acid:** produced by oxyntic (parietal) cells deep in the pit using ATP-driven proton pumps (exchanging $H^+$ for $K^+$) and chloride pumps (exchanging $Cl^-$ for $HCO_3^-$). It:
- Activates pepsinogens into active pepsins
- Allows the pepsins to function at their optimal pH
- Reduces ferric iron in the diet to ferrous iron, which can be absorbed by the gut
- Enhances solubility of iron and calcium in the duodenum (hence iron deficiency anaemia post-gastrectomy)
- Inhibits bacterial colonisation

In addition, acid in the duodenum stimulates secretin, which reduces gastric acid secretion (negative feedback).

(3)  **Pepsin:** produced by chief/zymogen/peptic cells deep in the gastric pit as a precursor pepsinogen, which is converted to its active form by reaction with hydrochloric acid. It:
- Breaks down food proteins into smaller proteins and polypeptides
- Digests 20% of the proteins in the average meal
- Is inactivated when the duodenal contents are neutralised by bowel

## The stomach as digester

- Digests 20% of proteins in the average meal, using pepsin (the only digestive enzyme it secretes)
- Aids the digestion of:
  - Vitamin B12
  - Calcium
  - Iron
- Mixing and acidifying of food boluses into chyme facilitates digestion later on in the GI tract

## The stomach as gatekeeper

- The stomach sends a few millilitres of chyme out through the pylorus at a time, and is inhibited from doing so when the duodenum has enough chyme to be getting on with
- The acid, fats, hyperosmolality and food particles in the duodenum stimulate the enterogastric reflex, which increases the tone of the pylorus and stops any more chyme coming through until the duodenum is relatively empty again; this allows time for adequate digestion, and prevents overloading of the circulation with products of digestion
- After a gastrectomy this reflex is lost, so uncontrolled volumes of food arrive in the duodenum, causing 'dumping' syndromes (covered later in this section)

## Drugs and the stomach

### H$_2$-receptor antagonists

- Block histamine receptors of the acid-producing parietal cells, preventing the cells from being stimulated by histamine, thereby reducing the stomach's production of acid
- There are also gastrin and acetylcholine receptors on parietal cells, which stimulate the acid-secreting mechanism of the H$^+$/K$^+$ ATPase 'proton' pump

### Proton pump inhibitors

- Block the H$^+$/K$^+$ ATPase pump itself (so stimulation by gastrin, acetylcholine, and histamine is unable to stimulate acid production)
- The proton pump inhibitors (PPIs) are benzimidazoles that bind irreversibly to the proton pump

### Non-steroidal anti-inflammatory drugs

- Inhibit the cyclo-oxygenase (COX) pathway in gastric mucosal cells
- This decreases prostaglandin (PG) synthesis, which is needed for the integrity of these cells (causing ulceration of the stomach lining)

### Cigarettes

- Smokers have accelerated gastric emptying, increased acid production and decreased pancreatic bicarbonate secretion (all making a more acidic duodenum)
- They also cause impaired healing

# 3.4 Peptic ulceration

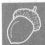 **In a nutshell ...**

**Peptic ulcers are chronic, usually solitary lesions. They occur in:**
- Duodenum (80%)
- Stomach (19%)
- Duodenum and stomach (4%)
- Other sites (1%) where gastric acid can damage the mucosa (eg oesophagus, gastroenterostomy, stoma, jejunum, Meckel's diverticulum)

**Predisposing factors for peptic ulceration include:**
- *Helicobacter pylori*
- **Smoking and alcohol:** decrease pyloric competence, leading to more acid in the duodenum
- **Drugs:** non-steroidal anti-inflammatory drugs (NSAIDs) and corticosteroids both affect mucosal defences
- **Stress:** burns, major surgery, 'type A' personalities
- **Associated diseases:** alcoholic cirrhosis, chronic renal failure (CRF), chronic obstructive pulmonary disease (COPD), hyperparathyroidism; these all increase serum calcium, which increases gastrin production
- **Familial:** there is a threefold increase in the incidence of duodenal ulcers in relatives; duodenal ulcers are also most common in HLA-B5 and blood group O people
- **Gastrin secretion:** see box on Zollinger–Ellison syndrome below. Gastric hypersecretion can also result from hyperplasia of the antral G cells of the stomach

Endoscopy is the gold standard investigation. Medical management has replaced surgery as the mainstay of treatment, but complications of peptic ulceration may still need surgical management.

# Epidemiology of peptic ulceration

- The **incidence** is increasing worldwide but decreasing dramatically in developed countries; this may be because of increased medical anti-ulcer and *H. pylori* treatment or a decrease in smoking, or because of both:
  - Duodenal ulcers develop in 0.8% of the population per year
  - Gastric ulcers develop in 0.2% of the population per year
- The **peak age** for duodenal ulcer is increasing (25–50 years worldwide but higher in developed countries); gastric ulcers occur in older age groups (>50)
- There is a 3:1 male:female ratio for gastric ulcers, and 4:1 for duodenal ulcers
- Mortality is higher in poor people

# Aetiology of peptic ulceration

- *H. pylori* infection (see below)
- Peptic ulcers are caused by the action of gastric acid and pepsin on the mucosa of the GI tract
- There is some controversy about whether it is increased acid secretion or a decrease in mucosal defences that is more important
- Duodenal ulceration is thought to be mostly due to increased acid production
- Gastric ulceration, on the other hand, is thought to be mostly due to the breakdown in mucosal defence against acid and pepsin

---

**Mucosal defences against peptic ulceration**

**Extramucosal**

- 'Mucous cap': a hydrophobic gel layer secreted by mucus cells
- Buffer layer: hydrogen carbonate is trapped in the mucous cap, buffering the acid
- Bicarbonate secretion: leads to a pH gradient from 2 in the lumen to 7 on the epithelial surface

**Mucosal**

- Luminal cell resistance to acid
- Mucosal integrity (prostaglandin helps to maintain this so is reduced when taking NSAIDs; other growth factors also help and are inhibited by alcohol)
- Tight cell–cell junctions

**Microvascular**

- The microcirculation neutralises acid and removes toxic substances; smoking-related microvascular disease reduces this blood flow

---

# *Helicobacter pylori* infection

- *H. pylori* is a Gram-negative flagellated spiral microaerophilic bacillus specific for human gastric mucosa that exists deep in the mucous layer
- About 50% of the world population is colonised with *H. pylori*
- It produces the enzyme urease, creating an alkaline microenvironment
- *H. pylori* is probably causative in duodenal ulcer and may be associated with gastric ulceration

## Association of *H. pylori* and peptic ulcer

| Clinical features | Cases with *H. pylori* infection (%) |
|---|---|
| Duodenal ulcer | 90–100 |
| Gastric ulcer | 70–75 |
| Dyspeptic symptoms (but no visible ulcer) | 50 |
| No symptoms (normal volunteers) | 20 |

### Conditions associated with *H. pylori* infection
- Duodenal ulceration
- Gastric ulceration
- Atrophic gastritis
- Gastric MALT (mucosa-associated lymphoid tissue) lymphoma
- Ischaemic heart disease
- Gastric cancer

Researchers have found that *H. pylori* leads to gastric mucosal injury in several ways:
- It produces a toxin which induces **vacuole formation** in cells
- It produces **ammonia** which is toxic to gastric epithelial cells
- It adheres to the epithelial cells (necessary for colonisation) and **disrupts the cell surface** using proteases and lipases, thus allowing acid to diffuse into the cell
- *H. pylori* infection **increases gastric acid secretion** (it returns to normal when *H. pylori* is eradicated)
- *H. pylori* infection at the antrum **increases gastrin production** via ammonia and cytokines
- *H. pylori* infection stimulates an **immune response** which damages epithelial cells

### Detecting *H. pylori*
#### Culture
- The best way (but never used because it is so slow and technically difficult)
#### Serology
- Fast and easy (but detects antibodies in serum which can persist for 6–12 months after eradication)
#### Quick urease, eg CLO (*Campylobacter*-like organism) test
- Antral biopsy is placed in a culture medium containing urea and a pH-sensitive indicator. If *H. pylori* is present, ammonia is produced and the pH indicator changes colour (eg turns from yellow to red [positive] in the CLO test)
- Problems are the following:
  - Test best read after 24 hours
  - Can be false-negative in people on PPIs
  - Requires endoscopy (so not suitable for routinely confirming eradication)
#### Carbon-13 urea breath test
- Non-invasive, sensitive and specific test
- Ingested urea is labelled with non-radioactive carbon-13; it is split into ammonia ($NH_3$) and $^{13}C$-labelled $CO_2$ by *H. pylori*
- Labelled $CO_2$ can be detected in patients' breath samples using mass spectrometry
- Test is best done near the laboratory as the equipment is very specialised and transport of specimens difficult
#### Histology
- Modified Giemsa stain detects *H. pylori* in endoscopic biopsy samples if the sample comes from an infected area
- Other stains can be used
- Needs an endoscopic biopsy (more invasive than other tests)

---

### Zollinger–Ellison syndrome

This is an association between a gastrin-secreting tumour of the pancreatic islet cells and gastric hypersecretion, which leads to single or multiple gastroduodenal and jejunal ulceration.

High levels of acidity produce a typical clinical picture:

- Epigastric pain
- Nausea
- Vomiting
- Severe diarrhoea (the only symptom in 10% of patients)
- The tumours themselves (gastrinomas) are typically in the pancreas but can occur anywhere within a triangular area around the head of the pancreas
- Sixty per cent of gastrinomas are malignant and half of these have metastasised at presentation

Zollinger–Ellison syndrome is part of the multiple endocrine neoplasia (MEN) type I syndrome (see Chapter 4, Endocrine Surgery) in 25% of cases, and these gastrin-secreting pancreatic tumours are often associated with parathyroid tumours.

Zollinger–Ellison syndrome is diagnosed by the following:

- Fasting serum gastrin (unreliable) elevated on at least three occasions
- Demonstrated raised basal and pentagastrin-stimulated acid secretion
- Secretin stimulation test showing 100% increase in serum gastrin in response to infusion of secretin

---

## Pathology and histology of peptic ulceration

### Site of peptic ulceration

- 80% are solitary
- 80% occur in the duodenum, of which 90% are in the first part of the duodenum (on the anterior wall, within a few centimetres of the pyloric ring)
- 19% occur in the stomach (usually the lesser curvature at the border of the body/antrum)

### Gross pathology of peptic ulceration

Chronic peptic ulcers have standard (virtually diagnostic) gross and microscopic appearances:

- 50% are <2 cm in diameter
- 10% are >4 cm in diameter (usually in stomach)
- Usually round or oval
- Sharply punched-out defect with straight walls and level margins (margin heaping is a sign of malignancy)
- Depth varies from superficial to deep; deep ulcers penetrate the muscularis mucosa and may perforate completely
- Base is usually smooth and clean with no exudate due to peptic digestion; vessels may project into base and lead to haemorrhage
- Underlying scarring causes spokes or spicules
- Surrounding mucosa usually oedematous and reddened

## Histology of peptic ulceration

**Zone 1**  Superficial thin layer of necrotic fibrinoid debris

**Zone 2**  Active cellular neutrophil infiltrate

**Zone 3**  Active granulation tissue with mononuclear leucocytes

**Zone 4**  Solid fibrous or collagenous scar; local arteries thick and thrombosed

## Clinical presentation of peptic ulceration

### Duodenal ulcer

- Epigastric pain during fasting
- Pain at night (2–4am typically)
- Relieved by food and antacids
- Relapsing and remitting (2 weeks of symptoms every few months)
- Penetrating posterior ulcers cause severe constant pain that radiates to the back
- 10% of duodenal ulcers are painless

### Gastric ulcer

- Epigastric pain induced by eating
- Patient loses weight
- Nausea and vomiting more common than with a duodenal ulcer
- Iron deficiency anaemia is common

## Investigating peptic ulcers

### Endoscopy

This is the gold standard as it diagnoses inflammation and gastric ulcers can be biopsied:

- 10% of all gastric ulcers are malignant
- At least six biopsies should be taken from the edge of any gastric ulcer seen (not the necrotic centre)
- CLO test can be used to test for *H. pylori*

## Double-contrast barium meal

This is rarely done:

- Barium meal will identify hiatus hernia and most ulcers (but will miss inflammation)
- Biopsies are not possible

## Tests for *H. pylori*

*H. pylori* infection can be tested for in a number of ways (see box on page 82).

## Gastric acid secretion test

If there are multiple ulcers and Zollinger–Ellison syndrome is suspected, gastrin, pentagastrin and secretin stimulation tests are useful (see Section 5, Biliary tree and pancreas).

## Treatment of peptic ulcers

 **In a nutshell ...**

**Medical (common)**
Acid suppression
- H$_2$-receptor blockers
- PPIs

*H. pylori* treatment
- Triple therapy (including antibiotics and acid suppression)
- Followed by long-term acid suppression

**Surgical (very rare)**
Gastric ulcer:
- Billroth I and II
- Vagotomy, pyloroplasty and excision of ulcer
- Vagotomy, antrectomy and Roux-en-Y

Duodenal ulcer:
- Truncal vagotomy
- Selective vagotomy
- Highly selective vagotomy

**CHAPTER 1**

## Medical treatment of peptic ulcers

 **In a nutshell ...**

**Test for *H. pylori***

If the result is negative, treat with a full-dose PPI for 1 or 2 months.

If the result is positive, treat with eradication therapy:

- Amoxicillin 1 g plus clarithromycin 500 mg plus either lansoprazole 30 mg or omeprazole 20 mg (twice daily)

Or

- Clarithromycin 250 mg plus metronidazole 400 mg plus either lansoprazole 30 mg or omeprazole 20 mg (twice daily)

Prescribe a PPI or $H_2$-receptor antagonist long-term.

Advise avoidance of known precipitants for the person, such as smoking.

For people taking NSAIDs or low-dose aspirin (antiplatelet therapy):

- Stop NSAIDs whenever possible and offer alternative analgesia
- For people on low-dose aspirin: while the ulcer is healing, stop aspirin, continue aspirin (at a dose of 75 mg daily) or switch to clopidogrel

After healing of the ulcer, if a person requires continued use of an antiplatelet drug, the options are low-dose aspirin with a PPI (at a dose licensed for gastroprotection) or clopidogrel alone.

These recommendations are based on those made by the National Institute for Health and Clinical Excellence (NICE) and Cochrane reviews:

- There is evidence from a Cochrane review that PPIs are effective in healing peptic ulcers and prevent the risk of rebleeding
- Although NICE guidance offers the choice of full-dose PPI or an $H_2$-receptor antagonist, evidence suggests that PPIs are more effective in reducing rebleeding in those with acute peptic ulcer bleeding
- Evidence from a Cochrane review indicates that, in people with duodenal ulcers and *H. pylori* infection, eradication therapy is the most effective treatment to heal the ulcer and prevent recurrence
- Evidence from a systematic review indicates that, in people with peptic ulcers and *H. pylori* infection, 7-day PPI-based triple therapy was sufficient for ulcer healing

## Surgical treatment of peptic ulcers

This is now very rarely done and is included here for completeness. It is still brought up in exams because it can test the candidate's understanding of anatomy and physiology.

### Indications for elective surgery

- Failure of medical treatment (eg non-healing or frequently relapsing ulcer)
- Complications, or the reasonable expectation of complications (haemorrhage, perforation, obstruction)
- Any non-healed gastric ulcer (biopsies are not always reliable)

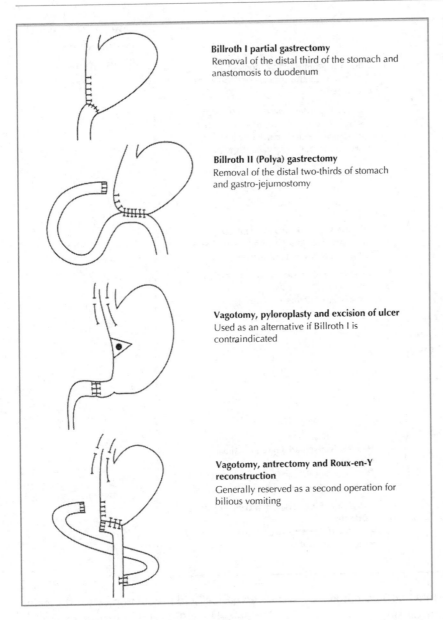

**Figure 1.23 Surgical treatment of a gastric ulcer**

**Billroth I partial gastrectomy**
Removal of the distal third of the stomach and anastomosis to duodenum

**Billroth II (Polya) gastrectomy**
Removal of the distal two-thirds of stomach and gastro-jejumostomy

**Vagotomy, pyloroplasty and excision of ulcer**
Used as an alternative if Billroth I is contraindicated

**Vagotomy, antrectomy and Roux-en-Y reconstruction**
Generally reserved as a second operation for bilious vomiting

- A giant gastric ulcer (>3 cm diameter) is not an indication for surgery, but must be removed if it has not healed after 6–8 weeks of medication

## Surgical treatment of gastric ulcer

- Principles of surgery for gastric ulcer are removal of the ulcer along with the gastrin-secreting zone of the antrum
- Most authorities recommend a formal gastrectomy involving at least the distal third of the stomach
- The two classic operations are Billroth I and Billroth II or Polya, shown in Figure 1.23 (Polya is the name of a Hungarian surgeon)

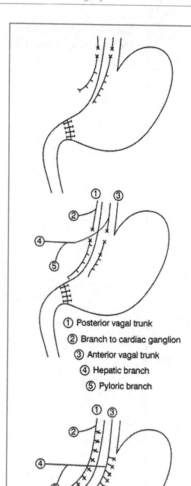

**Truncal vagotomy and pyloroplasty**
Cuts both vagal trunks at level of abdominal oesophgus:

- If stomach is denervated, this causes gastric stasis so a drainage procedure is needed (gastrojejunostomy or pyloroplasty)
- Similar complications to gastrectomy

**Selective vagotomy and pyloroplasty**
Denervation of stomach with preservation of nerve supply to the intact pylorus:

- Generally preserves coeliac and hepatic branches of the vagus
- Still needs a drainage procedure

① Posterior vagal trunk
② Branch to cardiac ganglion
③ Anterior vagal trunk
④ Hepatic branch
⑤ Pyloric branch

**Highly selective/parietal cell/proximal vagotomy**
Only branches to fundus and body are cut, leaving antral nerves intact:

- Does not disrupt coeliac, hepatic or pyloric branches
- No diversion procedure needed
- High recurrence rate

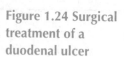

Figure 1.24 Surgical treatment of a duodenal ulcer

- These operations are much less common now that PPIs are so successful
- Complications of gastric surgery are discussed below

## Surgical treatment of duodenal ulceration

- Surgery for duodenal ulcer aims to reduce the acid secretions of the stomach by dividing the vagus nerve

- Decreasing acid production was historically achieved by a Billroth I or II gastrectomy, but this was superseded by vagotomy, which was in turn superseded by successful medical treatment
- Nowadays very few trainee upper-GI surgeons get to do an elective anti-peptic ulcer vagotomy for duodenal ulceration. As many patients who have had their operations still attend surgical clinics

or may come to further surgery, a good understanding of the procedures and complications is useful (Figure 1.24)

- If the vagus nerve is divided proximally gastric stasis results, so a drainage procedure (eg pyloroplasty) is needed
- Elective surgery for duodenal ulcer is seldom performed nowadays because medical treatment is so successful

## Postoperative complications

 **In a nutshell ...**

The postoperative problems of gastric and duodenal surgery depend on the precise operation carried out. They fall into several categories:

**Problems around the anastomoses**

- Obstruction
- Leaks
- Oesophagitis
- Bleeding
- Alkaline reflux gastritis and vomiting

**Problems due to vagus nerve transection**

- Diarrhoea
- Gastric atony
- Gastric outlet obstruction
- Gallstones

**Problems due to loss of stomach capacity and function**

- Dumping
- Vitamin B12 deficiency and iron deficiency anaemia
- Malnutrition

**Gastric remnant cancer**

**Pancreatitis**

## Problems around the anastomoses

### Obstruction

- Afferent loop obstruction
- Efferent loop obstruction
- Gastric outlet obstruction

These tend to occur in the early postoperative period. Small-bowel obstruction due to stricturing or adhesions can occur later.

### Leaks

- Anastomotic leak
- Duodenal stump leak

### Oesophagitis

This can be worsened by alkaline reflux into the stomach or by gastric outlet obstruction.

### Bleeding

This can be:

- Immediately postoperative
- Delayed due to leak or sepsis
- Long-term due to gastritis or oesophagitis

### Alkaline reflux gastritis

- Involves reflux of duodenal contents into the stomach due to the gastroenteric anastomosis in a Billroth I or II
- Leads to epigastric pain, bilious vomiting and weight loss; alkaline contents can also cause a nasty oesophagitis that is not detected by normal pH monitoring
- Treatment is with colestyramine, antacids and occasionally Roux-en-Y gastrojejunostomy, which avoids the problem by allowing drainage of the alkaline duodenal contents into the jejunum distal to the gastroenteric anastomosis (see Figure 1.23)

- The number of patients who get symptomatic alkaline reflux gastritis is small, and there are other long-term problems with a Roux-en-Y (such as a paretic, non-functioning Roux loop – 'Roux loop syndrome', which is a serious complication); for this reason Billroth II is still a useful option in the first instance

## Problems due to vagus nerve transection

### Effects of a truncal vagotomy

 **In a nutshell ...**

- Decreased acid secretion
- Faster gastric emptying
- Gastric outlet obstruction (unless pyloroplasty performed)
- Gallbladder denervation (leading to steatorrhoea and gallstones)
- Diarrhoea
- Dumping syndrome

Truncal vagotomy (see Figure 1.24) denervates the GI tract from the stomach to the mid-transverse colon, including the gallbladder and pancreas, with the effects described below:

- **Decreased acid secretion** due to loss of cholinergic stimulation of the parietal cell:
  - Responsiveness to gastrin and histamine is decreased
  - Basal acid secretion is reduced by 80%
  - Stimulated acid secretion is reduced by 50% (of course this is not a complication but the aim of the operation)

- **Faster gastric emptying** due to loss of vagally mediated receptive relaxation:
  - Causing higher intragastric pressure
  - This contributes to post-vagotomy diarrhoea and dumping syndromes (see below)
- **Gastric outlet obstruction** due to loss of vagal relaxation of the pylorus:
  - This is more likely if there is pyloric scarring or oedema caused by the ulceration
  - This is the reason why a pyloroplasty is always done with a truncal vagotomy (but opening up the pylorus surgically contributes to post-vagotomy diarrhoea)
- **Gallbladder denervation** increases stasis (and therefore the risk of gallstones) and reduces bile and pancreatic secretion:
  - An increase in undigested fat in the faeces contributes to post-vagotomy diarrhoea (although frank steatorrhoea is rare)
- **Severe diarrhoea** occurs in 10% of patients post-truncal vagotomy because of:
  - Dumping syndrome
  - Faster gastric emptying
  - Pyloroplasty
  - Steatorrhoea

Post-vagotomy diarrhoea is treated with small, low-residue meals, codeine and loperamide

### Effects of a highly selective vagotomy

This restricts vagal denervation to the proximal stomach, preserving antral, pyloric and pancreaticobiliary function (see Figure 1.24). A pyloroplasty is not required and the above side effects are far less common.

# Problems due to removal of the stomach (worse in total gastrectomies)

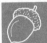

## In a nutshell ...

- Dumping syndrome
- Anaemia and malnutrition
- Carcinoma of gastric remnant
- Pancreatitis

## Dumping syndrome

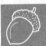

## In a nutshell ...

Dumping syndrome is a group of cardiovascular and GI symptoms resulting from rapid gastric emptying after truncal vagotomy and pyloroplasty or gastric resection. It arises because of destruction of the pylorus which normally controls gastric emptying. Early dumping is essentially due to hypovolaemia and late dumping is essentially due to hypoglycaemia.

After eating the stomach normally regulates the slow and carefully timed release over several hours of small amounts of well-digested and mixed chyme to the duodenum in response to a sensitive feedback mechanism. Without the pylorus to control the flow, or the stomach to act as a reservoir, the entire contents of the meal in a patient after pyloroplasty or gastric resection lands in the duodenum.

Early and late dumping have two very different physiological explanations and clinical effects. They occur in about 10% of patients immediately after gastric resection but remain a long-term problem for only 1–2%.

### Early dumping

Features (within 5–45 minutes of eating):
- Sweating
- Palpitations
- Dizziness
- Flushing
- Tachycardia
- Abdominal pain
- Nausea
- Diarrhoea

Early dumping is due to hypovolaemia. The proximal small bowel is flooded or 'dumped' with gastric contents, rather than the contents being squirted through the pylorus over a period of 1–2 hours, so there is a huge flux of bile, pancreatic juice and succus entericus into the upper GI tract, which causes a large fluid shift.
- It tends to improve with time and small dry meals
- Subcutaneous somatostatin injections can limit symptoms

### Late dumping

- Less common
- Tends not to feature GI symptoms
- Features (within 2–4 hours of eating)
- Sweating
- Palpitations
- Dizziness
- Tachycardia

Late dumping is due to rebound hypoglycaemia (in response to an abnormally high level of carbohydrate in the small bowel). This stimulates release of enteroglucagon, which sensitises islet cells to stimuli, resulting in overproduction of insulin and the symptoms of hypoglycaemia.

Small dry meals and glucose sweets help symptoms.

### Anaemia and malnutrition

*Iron*
- Absorption depends on the reaction of dietary iron ($Fe^{2+}$) with gastric acid to become the easily absorbed $Fe^{3+}$
- Without this, iron deficiency anaemia may result
- It is worsened by the vitamin B12 deficiency (see below)

*Vitamin B12*
- This enters the stomach bound to salivary R protein
- Intrinsic factor is secreted in the stomach and travels down the GI tract with vitamin B12
- In the duodenum pancreatic trypsin hydrolyses the R protein from vitamin B12 to make it available for binding to intrinsic factor (only when bound to intrinsic factor can vitamin B12 be absorbed in the terminal ileum, where it enters the circulation and becomes an essential element in red blood cell synthesis)
- Vitamin B12 deficiency leads to macrocytic anaemia
- It is clear that losing the stomach (no intrinsic factor), transecting the vagus (reduced pancreatic secretions), bypassing the duodenum (no opportunity to hydrolyse R protein) or removing the terminal ileum (only site of vitamin B12 absorption) can all lead to a megaloblastic anaemia (treat with vitamin B12 injections)

*Calcium*
- Also rendered more absorbable by the acidic environment of the stomach
- Therefore calcium deficiency may occur post-gastrectomy

*Malnutrition*
- Malabsorption may occur due to the fast transit of undigested food through the GI tract and dumping syndrome
- Reduced appetite
- Early satiety (due to loss of reservoir in gastrectomies or increased gastric pressure in vagotomy), unpleasant dumping syndrome and reflux symptoms may lead to reduced appetite

These factors in an already debilitated postoperative patient may result in malnutrition.

### Carcinoma of the gastric remnant

Gastrectomy for benign disease predisposes to development of adenocarcinoma of the stomach (threefold over 20 years). The cause is unknown, but it is thought to be related to metaplasia. Prognosis is usually poor.

### Pancreatitis

Increased gallstone formation due to gallbladder denervation and altered pancreatic anatomy and drainage pattern may cause recurrent pancreatitis.

## 3.5 Complications of peptic ulceration

### In a nutshell ...

Complications of peptic ulceration are the fourth most common cause of perioperative death.
The main complications of peptic ulceration are:
- Haemorrhage
- Perforation
- Gastric outlet obstruction
- Recurrent ulceration

## Haemorrhage

Peptic ulceration is responsible for 44% of all upper GI haemorrhages; oesophagitis and gastritis/erosions account for a further 44%. In 2007, the overall mortality rate of patients admitted with acute GI bleeding was 7%, because:
- A third of patients with peptic ulcer haemorrhage have no previous history or diagnosis of peptic ulcer disease
- There is an increasing elderly population

### Clinical assessment of a suspected bleeding peptic ulcer

Presentation is haematemesis, melaena or, rarely (in a torrential bleed), blood per rectum. History and examination should concentrate on calculating a pre-endoscopic Rockall score (see table below).

### Investigating a bleeding peptic ulcer

The 2008 Scottish Intercollegiate Guidelines Network (SIGN) guidelines suggest the following:
- Patients with an initial **Rockall score of 0** should be considered for early discharge with outpatient investigations
- Patients with an initial **Rockall score >0** should have an endoscopy

| | Score | | | | |
|---|---|---|---|---|---|
| **Variable** | **0** | **1** | **2** | **3** | |
| **Age (years)** | <60 | 60–79 | >80 | | |
| **Shock** | Systolic blood pressure (SBP) >100 mmHg and heart rate (HR) <100 beats/min | SBP >100 mmHg and HR >100 beats/min | SBP <100 mmHg | | **Initial score** |
| **Comorbidity** | Nil | | Cardiac failure, Ischaemic heart disease, major morbidity | Renal failure, liver failure, metastatic cancer | |
| **Diagnosis** | Nil or Mallory–Weiss tear | All other diagnoses | GI malignancy | | **Additional criteria for full score** |
| **Stigmata of recent haemorrhage** | Nil | | Blood, adherent clot, spurting vessel | | |

If the initial (pre-endoscopic) score is >0 there is a significant mortality (score 1, predicted mortality rate 2.4%; score 2, predicted mortality rate 5.6%), suggesting that only those scoring 0 can be safely discharged.

### Major endoscopic stigmata of recent haemorrhage

| Stigmata | Risk of ongoing bleed or rebleed |
|---|---|
| Pulsatile or oozing haemorrhage | > 85% |
| Fresh clot on ulcer | 85% |
| Adherent clot on ulcer | 50% |
| Visible vessel in base of ulcer | 40% (eg dark spot, red spot, elevated tubular structure, defect in base of ulcer) |

### Management of a bleeding peptic ulcer

The management of a bleeding gastric or duodenal ulcer is summarised in Figure 1.25. The principles are as follows:

- Assessment and resuscitation:
  - Shocked patients should receive prompt volume replacement
  - Red cell transfusion should be considered after loss of 30% of the circulating volume
- Endoscopy is the first-line investigation and can identify and often treat the bleeding point and should be performed within 24 hours of the initial presentation.

## Endoscopic control of haemorrhage

In the presence of major signs of recent haemorrhage, endoscopic therapy significantly reduces the risk of rebleeding. Methods include the following:

- Injections:
  - Adrenaline: typically a 0.5–1 ml aliquot of 1 in 100 000 adrenaline into **each** of the four quadrants of the ulcer base
  - Ethanol
  - Variceal sclerosants
- Heater probe
- Clips
- Bipolar electrocoagulator
- Nd:YAG (neodymium:yttrium–aluminium–garnet) laser

Once haemostasis has been achieved by endoscopic therapy, **pharmacological therapy** is usually started:

- **Acid suppression** (the aim of acid suppression is to maintain intragastric pH >6 to stabilise clots and prevent rebleeding). A meta-analysis of 24 randomised controlled trials (RCTs) involving 4373 patients confirmed that PPIs significantly reduce the rate of rebleeding and the need for surgery. Subsequent analyses have also shown that when high-dose PPI treatment (omeprazole 80 mg bolus injection followed by 8 mg/h intravenous infusion for 72 h) is used, there is a significant reduction in mortality)
- **Tranexamic acid** (the role of fibrinolytic inhibitors in GI bleeding is unclear)
- *H. pylori* **eradication:** the *H. pylori* infection rate in patients with bleeding peptic ulcers is 79.8% (95% CI 78–81%). Delayed tests suggest that it may be even higher, so patients should have eradication therapy

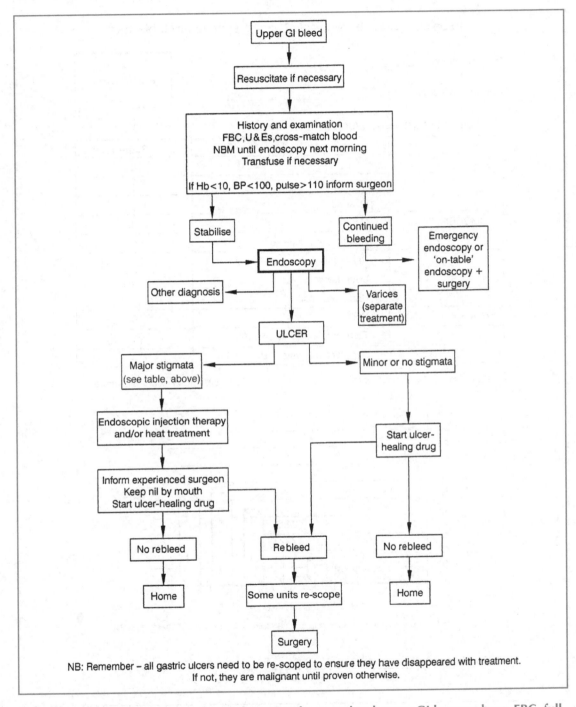

**Figure 1.25 Summary of management of suspected non-variceal upper-GI haemorrhage. FBC, full blood count; NBM, nil by mouth; U&Es, urea and electrolytes**

CHAPTER 1

To be completed by Medical / Nursing staff for all GI bleeds

Date of admission: _____

Admitting consultant: _____

PATIENT LABEL

## Rockall score (pre-endoscopic)

| | | Score |
|---|---|---|
| AGE | Under 60 | 0 |
| | 60–80 | 1 |
| | Over 80 | 2 |
| COMORBIDITY | None | 0 |
| | Heart / Lung disease | 2 |
| | Renal failure Liver failure Carcinomatosis | 3 |
| SHOCK | None | 0 |
| | Tachycardia only, pulse >100 | 1 |
| | Hypotension, systolic BP <100 | 2 |

Low risk – total score 2 or less          High risk – total score 3 or more

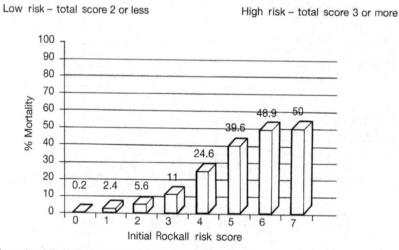

Observed mortality: National audit 3981 cases of acute upper GI bleeding (Rockall et al GUT 1996 38:316-321)

Patient's score: _____

Figure 1.26 Rockall classification of upper GI bleed

## Rebleeding after endoscopy

Early endoscopy should be repeated if:
- The initial endoscopy was suboptimal due to difficult access or poor visualisation
- Rebleeding is life-threatening

### Digital subtraction angiography
- Assists the localisation of bleeding points and simultaneous selective coil transcatheter embolisation using coils and polyvinyl alcohol and gelatin sponge
- Currently only small cohort studies have demonstrated high rates of success in stopping bleeding (98%), a reduction in rebleeding within 30 days (68–76%) and low complication rates (5%)
- In addition, a single retrospective study showed no difference in rebleeding or mortality when embolisation was compared with surgery despite the more advanced age and greater prevalence of heart disease in the embolisation group

## Indications for emergency surgical treatment of a bleeding peptic ulcer

### Absolute indications for surgery
- Continued bleeding (particularly in the presence of a spurting vessel at endoscopy that does not stop with adrenaline)
- Lesions that invariably rebleed (aortoenteric fistula)

### Relative indications
- One rebleed in hospital (two rebleeds in patients aged <60 years)
- Transfusion requirements of:
  - 4 units in 24 hours (patients aged >50)
  - 6 units in 24 hours (patients aged <50)

- Shortage of whole blood

Scores (eg Rockall classification) done by staff on admission can give an early indication of the mortality risk of a patient with an upper GI bleed (Figure 1.26).

## Principles of emergency surgical treatment of bleeding peptic ulcer
- Stop bleeding by under-running bleeding vessel with a suture (usually all that is required)
- Conservative or definitive surgery depends on:
  - Condition of patient
  - Experience of surgeon
  - Cause of ulcer
  - Previous medical treatment
- Definitive treatment for bleeding duodenal ulcer:
  - Vagotomy and pyloroplasty or proximal gastric vagotomy (not done now)
- Definitive treatment for bleeding gastric ulcer:
  - Resection of ulcer to prevent rebleeding and exclude malignancy (vagotomy is not needed)
- In some very large or persistently rebleeding ulcers a distal gastrectomy with Billroth II/Polya reconstruction may be indicated

# Perforation

Perforation from peptic ulcer is more common and more serious in elderly age groups (mortality rate of 20% in those aged >70) but can occur in younger people.

## Clinical features of a perforated peptic ulcer

- The classic presentation is sudden severe epigastric pain with developing peritonitis
- 50% have no history of peptic ulcer disease
- 80% have a pneumoperitoneum on an erect chest radiograph
- After 12 hours bacterial peritonitis develops and the mortality rate increases with time

## Principles of management of a perforated peptic ulcer

- Prompt diagnosis
- Vigorous resuscitation
- Early laparotomy
- In some cases conservative treatment is advised (see below)

### Preoperative care

- Fluid resuscitation
- Monitor urine output
- Correct electrolyte imbalance
- Nasogastric (NG) tube
- Antibiotics (eg cefuroxime and metronidazole)
- Analgesia (usually opioids)
- Central venous pressure (CVP) measurement if in doubt about fluid replacement

## Non-surgical management of a perforated peptic ulcer

This is controversial.

### Advantages of non-surgical management

- Reported mortality rate of <5% in selected patients
- May be the only course of action in unfit patients
- More popular now that PPIs encourage rapid healing

### Disadvantages of non-surgical management

- Up to 28% eventually need surgery
- May miss gastric cancer or perforation from another viscus (eg colon)
- Regular assessment needed
- Surgeon must be ready to operate at any time if patient deteriorates
- Older patients do less well

### Mainstays of non-surgical management

- Nil by mouth
- NG tube
- Intravenous (IV) fluid
- Broad-spectrum antibiotics
- Continued reassessment (any sign of sepsis, hypotension or hypoxia should prompt the team to consider urgent surgery)

Note that the results of conservative treatment of a perforated gastric ulcer are very poor, so a contrast study to ensure that the ulcer is duodenal is wise before embarking on a trial of conservative treatment.

## Surgical management of perforated duodenal ulcer

- Simple closure by approximation of ulcer edges or use of omental patch is the most common procedure
- Vigorous peritoneal lavage is essential
- More extensive surgery is rarely necessary and is contraindicated unless the following three criteria are satisfied:
  - The patient is cardiovascularly stable
  - No established peritonitis is present
  - A surgeon with sufficient experience is available
- In some centres, this will be done laparoscopically
- Studies suggest that laparoscopic repair is associated with less analgesic use, shorter hospital stay, less wound infection and lower mortality rate; however, associated with longer operating times and more suture-site leakage when compared with open repair

## Surgical management of perforated gastric ulcer

This is much less common than perforated duodenal ulcer, and there are a number of treatment options:

- Simple closure
- Billroth II/Polya resection
- Billroth I resection
- Truncal vagotomy with excision of ulcer and pyloroplasty
- Over-sewing of ulcer

# Gastric outlet obstruction

Duodenal ulceration can cause stricturing and narrowing of the first part of the duodenum, leading to gastric outlet obstruction, also called **pyloric stenosis**, but an obstructing tumour is a much more common cause nowadays.

## Clinical presentation of gastric outlet obstruction

- Projectile vomiting of undigested food but no bile
- Epigastric pain
- Weight loss
- Dehydration
- Electrolyte imbalance (hypochloraemic, hypokalaemic, metabolic alkalosis)

Findings may include the following:
- Palpable distended stomach
- Visible peristalsis
- Succussion splash
- Mild cases: inflammation and obstruction may resolve with gastric lavage, acid suppression therapy and bedrest
- More severe cases: may be hard fibrotic strictures with a dilated, atonic stomach

## Management of gastric outlet obstruction

One of the problems in this situation is the uncertainty as to whether the cause of the stenosis is definitely benign. Biopsies can often be equivocal. In straightforward cases endoscopy may be diagnostic and balloon dilatation may be therapeutic. Surgery should be deferred until fluid and electrolyte abnormalities have been corrected.

Traditionally, surgical options for benign pyloric stenosis have been:
- Gastroenterostomy
- Rarely, truncal vagotomy + gastroenterostomy/antrectomy

However, as benign pyloric strictures are rarer nowadays, and undiagnosed malignancy is a risk, it is often safer to do a resection and reconstruction such as a Billroth II.

Scarred gastric ulcers are rare nowadays but give rise to an 'hour-glass' deformity and are treated by surgery.

## Recurrent ulceration

Common reasons for recurrence include:

- Incomplete vagotomy
- Inadequate gastric resection
- Zollinger–Ellison syndrome
- Carcinoma
- Smoking
- *H. pylori*
- Hypercalcaemia
- Ulcerogenic drugs

Recurrence can occur months after the original operation and present with bizarre pain. Treatment is with PPIs and eradication therapy if necessary.

## 3.6   Gastric carcinoma

### In a nutshell ...

Gastric cancer is a common and important tumour. It is often diagnosed too late for curative procedures in the UK, although it is detected earlier in countries such as Japan, where it is more common. The main surgical treatment modalities are partial and total gastrectomies.

## Incidence of gastric carcinoma

- Third most common cause of cancer death in men in the UK
- In the UK, 10 000 new cases per annum
- Very common in Japan
- Incidence falling in Europe and USA
- 80% are aged >65 years
- Distal carcinomas are more common in lower social classes
- Proximal (cardia) tumours are more common in higher social classes
- More common in men than women (2M:1F)

## Aetiology of gastric carcinoma

### Chronic gastritis

- There is a known association between chronic gastritis and gastric cancer
- Of superficial cancers, 94% are found in areas of gastritis

### Pernicious anaemia

- The incidence of gastric cancer is raised in patients with chronic atrophic gastritis
- One type (autoimmune type A) is associated with pernicious anaemia caused by anti-parietal cell antibodies
- There is a fivefold increased risk of gastric cancer in young patients with pernicious anaemia
- Another type of chronic atrophic gastritis is environmental type B, related to:
  - *H. pylori*
  - Toxic and dietary agents
  - Previous surgery leading to bile reflux
- Of all patients with pernicious anaemia 10% develop gastric cancer in 10–20 years

### Family history

- Genetic factors are implicated by variations in races, which persist despite emigration
- Risk of stomach cancer in relatives of an affected patient is four times greater than that in those with no affected relative
- Gastric cancer is most common in people with blood group A
- Napoleon and his father and grandfather all died of gastric cancer

### Environmental factors

Diet, alcohol and tobacco are implicated in the development of gastric cancer but links have not been proved.

## *H. pylori* infection

There is undoubtedly a higher prevalence of *H. pylori* in patients with gastric cancer when compared with the normal population, but a causative link has not been proved.

## Previous gastric surgery

Studies show an increased risk of gastric cancer after surgery for benign disease. The risk seems to be related to intestinal metaplasia at the anastomosis spreading into the gastric remnant.

## Premalignant conditions

### Gastric polyps

- Adenomatous gastric polyps (25%) have a chance of malignant change, unlike hyperplastic polyps (75%), which rarely become malignant

### Gastric ulcers

- The appearance of a gastric cancer in a chronic gastric ulcer has been recorded, but it is thought that this is usually due to an error in diagnosis

### Hypertrophic gastropathy (Ménétrier's disease)

- This is a rare disorder involving rugal-fold hypertrophy, hyperplasia of mucus-producing cells, parietal cell atrophy producing hypochlorhydria and protein-losing enteropathy
- Of reported cases, 15% developed gastric cancer

## Site of gastric cancers

There has been a change in the anatomical subsite distribution of gastric cancer:

- Increased incidence in the proximal stomach, particularly around the cardia
- Decreased incidence in the distal stomach
- This leads to an increasing incidence of cancers around the GOJ, and it can be difficult to tell which are oesophageal and which are gastric
- Siewert classified tumours of the GOJ:
  - Type I is true lower oesophageal adenocarcinoma, usually arising from Barrett's oesophagus
  - Type II is true junctional tumour
  - Type III is an upper gastric tumour

## Pathology of gastric cancers

Gastric cancers have four macroscopic appearances:

1. **Malignant ulcer:** with raised, everted edges
2. **Polypoid tumour:** proliferating into the stomach lumen
3. **Colloid tumour:** massive gelatinous growth
4. **Linitis plastica** (leather-bottle stomach): caused by submucosal infiltration of tumour with marked fibrous reactions producing a small, thickened, contracted stomach

## Microscopic pathology

Tumours are all adenocarcinomas with varying degrees of differentiation. One method of classification (Lauren classification) divides these adenocarcinomas into two types.

### Intestinal type

- Poor prognosis
- Composed of malignant glands

### Diffuse type

- Better prognosis
- Composed of single or small groups of malignant cells

## Spread of gastric cancers

### Local spread

- Often well beyond the visible tumour
- Oesophagus may be infiltrated (spread to duodenum is rare)
- Adjacent organs may be directly invaded

### Lymphatic spread

- Commonly along the nodes of the lesser and greater curves
- Lymph drainage from the cardiac end of the stomach may invade the mediastinal nodes and thence the supraclavicular nodes of Virchow on the left (Troisier's sign)
- At the pyloric end, involvement of the subpyloric and hepatic nodes may occur
- The Japanese Research Society for Gastric Cancer has designated four tiers of nodes likely to be involved according to the location of the main tumour
- These are groups of nodes, the involvement of which indicates increasingly advanced disease (which correlates with survival)

### Bloodstream dissemination

- Occurs via the portal system to the liver and thence occasionally to the lungs and the skeletal system

### Transcoelomic spread

- May produce peritoneal seedlings and bilateral Krukenburg's tumours due to implantation in both ovaries

## Clinical features of gastric cancer

The diagnosis is commonly made only when the disease is advanced. Symptoms are effects of the tumour, of metastases or general features of malignant disease.

### Local symptoms and signs

- Epigastric pain: may radiate into the back, suggesting pancreatic involvement
- Vomiting: especially with pyloric obstruction
- Dysphagia: especially with tumours of the cardia
- Perforation or haemorrhage
- Mass in the upper abdomen on examination

### Symptoms and signs of metastases

- Jaundice
- Abdominal distension due to ascites
- More rarely, chest infections or bone pain suggesting metastases in the lungs or skeleton
- Enlarged liver or nodes, jaundice or ascites on examination

### General features of gastric cancer

- Anorexia
- Weight loss
- Anaemia

## Differential diagnosis of gastric cancer

There are five common diseases that give a similar clinical picture of a slight lemon-yellow tinge, anaemia and weight loss. These are:

- Carcinoma of the stomach
- Carcinoma of the caecum
- Carcinoma of the pancreas
- Pernicious anaemia
- Uraemia

The principal differential diagnosis of gastric carcinoma is a benign gastric ulcer.

## Investigating gastric cancer

### Gastroscopy
This is the investigation of choice and the first investigation that should be carried out in any patient suspected of gastric malignancy:

- The advantage of fibreoptic endoscopy is that a suspicious lesion can be biopsied. Biopsies from large malignant ulcers are notoriously difficult to take, because there are large areas of benign inflamed and necrotic material within the tumour. At least six to eight biopsy specimens should be taken from the edge of the tumour

A gastric ulcer should not be considered benign just because it has responded to medical treatment; it should be re-endoscoped and rebiopsied until it has completely disappeared.

### Computed tomography
- Tumours at the cardia are best demonstrated following gastric distension with 600–800 ml water
- Distal body and antral tumours are best evaluated in the prone position

### Endoscopic ultrasonography
- Superior to CT for the local staging of gastric carcinoma
- Higher-frequency transducers can evaluate the subgroups suitable for endoscopic mucosal resection
- The presence of direct invasion into adjacent structures can be assessed
- Lymph nodes can be easily assessed

## Management of gastric cancer

### Preoperative optimisation
Optimising lung function and nutritional status are important in the preoperative period:

- Patients should give up smoking
- High-risk patients should undergo preoperative physiotherapy
- Consider placement of a nasojejunal or percutaneous jejunostomy feeding tube if there is obstruction or malnourishment
- A critical care bed may need to be arranged
- The anaesthetist should be warned of any major problems and may require further tests of pulmonary or cardiac function

### Staging of gastric cancer
Full staging of the tumour is usually impossible until laparotomy (as shown in the table).

**TNM staging system for gastric carcinoma**

| Stage | Clinical pathology | 5-year survival rate |
|-------|-------------------|----------------------|
| I | Radical resection T1, N0, M0 | 80% |
| II | Radical resection T2–4, N0, M0 | 40% |
| III | Radical resection Tx–4, N0, M0 | 20% |
| IVA | Palliative resection Tx–4, N1–3, M0–1 | <5% |
| IVB | No resection T4, N0–3, M0–1 | <5% |

T1, tumour invading the lamina propria but not reaching the submucosa; T2, tumour invading into but not beyond the muscularis propria; T3, tumour invading the adventitia but not the adjacent structures; T4, tumour invading the adjacent structures. N1, 1–2 lymph nodes involved; N2, 3–6 nodes involved; N3, >7 nodes involved. M1, metastasis present.

## Curative surgery for gastric cancer

This is only applicable to people without widespread metastases. Many patients in this country present with advanced disease with little prospect of surgical cure, but some have early T1 or T2 N0 lesions which may have been found by chance. These patients have a good chance of survival postoperatively (see table above).

### Principles of curative surgery

- Removal of the lesion by partial, subtotal or total gastrectomy
- Removal of lymph nodes to a level determined by the site and extent of the tumour
- Restoration of the continuity of the GI tract
- Creation of a reservoir in the case of total gastrectomy

### Partial/subtotal gastrectomy

- Possible methods of reconstruction include Billroth I, Polya and Roux-en-Y (see Figure 1.23)
- Subtotal gastrectomy removes four-fifths of the stomach
- As it is commonly for distal tumours, the entire pylorus is usually removed as well

### Extended gastrectomy

- For GOJ tumours
- Includes resection of the distal oesophagus

### Total gastrectomy

- Performed for middle-third tumours
- Methods of reconstruction after a total gastrectomy include Roux-en-Y, oesoph-agojejunostomy with or without a jejunal pouch, and variations of these
- The 5-year survival rates for radical gastrectomy vary according to stage (see table above)

## Dissection 1 (D1) and dissection 2 (D2) gastrectomies

This has been one of the most controversial topics in the whole of surgery:

- Studies demonstrate that nodal involvement indicates a poor prognosis and more aggressive surgical approaches to remove involved lymph nodes are gaining popularity
- The Italian Gastric Cancer Study Group compared D1 (perigastric lymph nodes) with D2 (hepatic, left gastric, coeliac and splenic arteries, as well as those in the splenic hilum) in 2010. This RCT found that the postoperative morbidity rate (18% versus 12%) and mortality rate (2.2% versus 3%) were no different between the groups
- D2 dissections are now generally recommended over D1 dissections. A pancreas- and spleen-preserving D2 lymphadenectomy is suggested because it provides more staging information and may provide a survival benefit

## Palliative surgery for gastric cancer

Many patients with gastric cancer can only be offered palliation. Symptoms most commonly requiring palliative surgery are:

- Obstruction
- Haemorrhage
- Pain

### Principles of palliative surgery

- Perform surgery only if it will significantly extend or improve quality of life
- The procedure should be tailored to each patient's symptoms and wishes
- Theoretically the optimal operation is palliative resection if this is practicable, because it is the treatment of choice for obstruction and haemorrhage, and it is also

effective for ulcer-type pain (but not for pain related to extragastric extension and metastatic disease)
- However, this is rarely possible without considerable morbidity, so the modern options of stents and palliative chemotherapy are often preferable to surgical resection
- Discussion with the oncologist beforehand at the multidisciplinary team (MDT) meeting may identify other procedures that can be performed while the patient is on the table, such as inserting a Hickman line for palliative chemotherapy or a jejunostomy feeding tube
- Apart from resection, other procedures available are bypass, intubation and exclusion

## Adjuvant therapy for gastric cancer

- **Adjuvant radiotherapy:**
  - The British Stomach Cancer Group reported lower rates of local recurrence in patients who received postoperative radiotherapy than in those who underwent surgery alone
  - The Gastrointestinal Tumor Study Group revealed higher 4-year survival rates in patients with unresectable gastric cancer who received radiotherapy and chemotherapy than in those who received chemotherapy alone (18% vs 6%)
- **Intraoperative radiotherapy:**
  - Method of delivering radiotherapy allows for a high dose to be given while in the operating room so that other critical structures can be avoided
  - A National Cancer Institute study showed that, although the median survival duration was higher (21 months vs 10 months) in the IORT group, this was not statistically significant

- **Adjuvant chemotherapy:**
  - Recent meta-analyses compared 13 randomised trials and showed that adjuvant systemic chemotherapy was associated with a significant survival benefit (odds ratio for death 0.80; 95% CI 0.66–0.97)
  - Subgroup analysis suggests that this effect is exaggerated in node-positive patients
- **Adjuvant chemoradiotherapy:**
  - The Intergroup 0116 study patients who received the adjuvant chemoradiotherapy demonstrated improved disease-free survival rates (from 32% to 49%) and improved overall survival rates (from 41% to 52%) compared with those who were observed
- **Neoadjuvant chemotherapy:**
  - Attempts to downstage disease to increase resectability, determine chemotherapy sensitivity, reduce the rate of local and distant recurrences and improve survival
  - Both a European and a US RCT have demonstrated a survival benefit when patients were treated with three cycles of preoperative chemotherapy followed by surgery and then three cycles of postoperative chemotherapy, compared with surgery alone

## Postoperative management of gastric cancer

This older group of patients, often with comorbidity, undergo a laparotomy and major surgery. They need careful postoperative care. Intensive care overnight is often indicated because postoperative ventilation and sedation have benefits for more frail patients. An epidural is invaluable for controlling pain and improving outcome.

Look out for important immediate postoperative complications:

- Chest infection
- Pulmonary embolus
- Anastomotic leak

Total gastrectomies are associated with adverse long-term nutritional effects:

- Weight loss can be corrected by dietary supplementation
- After total gastrectomy all patients become vitamin $B_{12}$-deficient and need 3-monthly injections within 6–12 months
- Many patients develop iron deficiency anaemia after a total gastrectomy and this will also have to be looked for
- Malabsorption of fat and protein is common
- Absorption of glucose usually increases, producing early hyperglycaemia and late hypoglycaemia

## Other stomach tumours

### Lymphoma

- The stomach is the most common extranodal primary site for non-Hodgkin's lymphoma, and primary gastric lymphoma accounts for 5% of all gastric neoplasms
- In addition, secondary lymphoma is commonly seen in the stomach (secondary to either a lymphoma arising elsewhere in the GI tract or to primary nodal disease)

---

**Kiel classification of primary gastric lymphomas**

**B-cell lymphomas (98%)**

- Mucosa-associated lymphoid tissue (MALT)
  Low grade
  High grade (with or without low grade component)
- Low with mixed high grade
- Mantel cell
- Burkitt-type
- Others

**T-cell lymphoma (rare)**

- Enteropathy-associated
- Non-enteropathy-associated

---

Clinical features of gastric lymphomas

- Gastric lymphomas may look like diffuse gastritis, localised ulcers or polypoid tumours, and mainly occur in the distal stomach
- The mean age of presentation is 60 years
- Symptoms are similar to those of gastric cancer (rather than those of lymphoma)
- Anaemia and epigastric mass are common presentations; obstruction and perforation are rare

## Diagnosis of gastric lymphomas

- This is difficult, with appearances of gastritis and benign ulcer leading to poor diagnostic accuracy on endoscopy
- Biopsy provides a positive tissue diagnosis in only 60–80% of cases, with difficulty in getting deep enough biopsies to pick up the submucosal infiltration
- Endoscopic ultrasonography is the best preoperative diagnostic and staging investigation

## Treatment of gastric lymphomas

- 66% of lesions are resectable and the overall 5-year survival rate is 24%
- Prognosis depends on the stage of disease and resectability
- There is some controversy among surgeons and oncologists over treatment of both primary and secondary lymphoma in the stomach, and the role of primary chemotherapy alone, surgery with adjuvant chemotherapy or surgery alone
- Patients should be discussed in an MDT meeting
- A full-thickness, high-grade, solitary primary gastric lesion may result in perforation when the tumour melts away on chemotherapy; a patient on chemotherapy is not in a good condition for emergency surgery for this condition, with a high mortality
- On the other hand, a patient with diffuse, low-grade disease may be completely cured by chemotherapy or *H. pylori* eradication and never come to surgery
- Patients with extragastric nodal disease are also more likely to be best treated by chemotherapy
- In general these patients do better than those with gastric adenocarcinoma

---

**MALT lymphoma**

MALT lymphoma is thought to be a type of primary gastric lymphoma distinct from other extranodal lymphomas.

- 'Peyer's patches' of organised lymphoid tissue occur through many parts of the GI tract, but not in the stomach (which does not normally contain lymphoid tissue)
- Organised MALT follicles in the stomach are associated with *H. pylori* infection
- *H. pylori* is found in 92% of patients who have gastric MALT lymphoma, but a causal link has yet to be proved
- *H. pylori* eradication can lead to complete cure or regression of MALT lymphoma, and chemotherapy may be indicated, but there is usually no role for surgery

---

## GI stromal tumours (GISTs)

This includes the group of tumours previously classified as leiomyosarcomas, leiomyomas and sarcomatous lesions of the stomach.

- There are four groups:
  - Tumours showing differentiation towards muscle cells (the largest category)
  - Tumours showing differentiation towards neural elements
  - Tumours showing dual differentiation
  - Tumours lacking any differentiation
- The last two groups are regarded as malignant and account for about 1% of primary stomach cancers
- GISTs are often not identified until they are quite large
- They originate from smooth muscle and are often slow-growing
- It is difficult to distinguish benign from malignant tumours in this group

### Presentation of GISTs

- 75% of patients present with either haematemesis or melaena
- Patients may have a palpable abdominal mass

### Diagnosis of GISTs

- Endoscopy
- Endoscopic ultrasound-guided biopsy

### Management of GISTs

- Surgery involves local excision without lymphadenectomy. Lateral submucosal spread is unusual, so removal of the tumour with a cuff of normal stomach is adequate. For large tumours a formal gastric resection may be necessary
- Prognosis and follow-up depend on whether the tumour is benign or malignant, its size, and whether it is high grade or low grade. In one small series, no patient with a benign tumour had a recurrence or metastasis, but all those with a high-grade malignancy had died within 3 years
- Adjuvant therapy may be indicated in some high-grade tumours
- In general, these tumours do much better than gastric adenocarcinomas
- A tyrosine kinase inhibitor, imatinib (Glivec), has recently been shown to show significant survival benefit in patients following surgical excision of certain subtypes of GISTs (KIT positive)

## Neuroendocrine tumours of the stomach

This group includes tumours also known as carcinoids, endocrine and neuroendocrine tumours. These tumours have the following features:

- Arise from the endocrine cells of the stomach, such as G cells or EC cells (carcinoids)
- Account for fewer than 1% of all gastric tumours
- May be benignly behaving, well-differentiated tumours or high-grade, malignantly behaving tumours
- May be non-functioning or functioning (eg resulting in hypergastrinaemia)
- There is an association with:
  - Chronic atrophic gastritis
  - Hypertrophic gastropathy
  - Zollinger–Ellison syndrome
  - MEN type I syndrome

### Diagnosis of neuroendocrine tumours of the stomach

- Endoscopy and biopsy
- Gastrin stimulation tests
- CT to exclude hepatic metastases (common in carcinoid-type tumours) should be performed if indicated
- Associated MEN I tumours should be looked for

### Management of neuroendocrine tumours of the stomach

- Surveillance (for small sporadic benign tumours)
- Endoscopic ablation, resection or transmural excision
- Laparoscopic wedge resection
- Malignant neuroendocrine tumours and sporadic cases that are 1–2 cm in diameter should be treated by formal resection as for adenocarcinomas of the stomach
- Patients with symptoms of carcinoid syndrome may be treated with somatostain analogues. The addition of α-inteferon may be of benefit in patients resistant to somatostain analogues alone
- Prognosis depends on grade; sporadic tumours do less well than those associated with hyperplasia, but in general these tumours do better than gastric carcinoma

## Squamous cell carcinoma of the stomach

- Extremely rare
- Presentation and treatment is similar to adenocarcinoma

## 3.7 Gastritis

### Acute gastritis and stress ulcers

- Acute gastritis is a transient inflammatory response that is not associated with permanent gastric mucosal abnormality
- It tends to occur in response to specific insults such as alcohol, drugs or dietary indiscretion
- Endoscopy shows inflamed mucosa which may bleed on contact
- Acute stress erosions are associated with:
  - Severe burns (Curling's ulcers)
  - Brain damage (Cushing's ulcers)
  - Alcohol
  - NSAIDs
  - Major surgery
  - Trauma
  - Stay on an ICU
- They are 1–2 cm in size and are found in the stomach and the first part of the duodenum
- Acute stress erosions differ from peptic ulcers:
  - They are multiple not single
  - They have no predilection for the antrum and lesser curve
  - They do not reach the musculararis propria
- The main surgical significance of acute gastritis is that it presents as acute abdominal pain and should be differentiated from peptic ulcer disease

## Chronic gastritis

Chronic gastritis is very common. There are two main types.

### Type A gastritis

- Associated with parietal cell antibodies
- Tends to be associated with reduced acid secretion
- May lead to vitamin B12 malabsorption
- May present as pernicious anaemia
- Has a familial or genetic predisposition

### Type B gastritis

- Involves the pyloric region, extending up along the lesser curve
- Causes:
  - Duodenogastric reflux
  - Post-gastric surgery
  - Pernicious anaemia
  - Chronic alcohol ingestion
  - NSAIDs
  - Cigarette smoking

The surgical significance of chronic gastritis is the increased risk of gastric carcinoma in patients with gastritis and its presentation with abdominal pain. In 90% of patients with a gastric cancer, atrophic gastritis with intestinal metaplasia can be demonstrated. Patients with known chronic gastritis may be at higher risk of developing cancer.

## 3.8 Congenital abnormalities of the stomach

Congenital hypertrophic pyloric stenosis is covered in Paediatric Surgery, Book 1.

## Gastric diverticula

- True gastric diverticula are rare, usually asymptomatic, incidental findings on endoscopy or barium meal
- Surgical treatment is not usually needed, but the existence of these diverticula should be recognised so that they are not confused with more serious pathology

## Gastric duplication and cysts

- This is a tubular structure lined by gastric epithelium intimately applied to the wall of the stomach
- 15% communicate with the stomach but most have no outlet
- Do not usually present until the early teens, although they are present at birth
- Must be distinguished from hydatid cysts, dermoid cysts and enterogenous cysts
- Surgical treatment is not usually required, but a gastric duplication cyst can be opened and drained

## Gastric mucosal diaphragm

- A rare defect that does not usually present until adulthood
- There is a mucosal diaphragm close to the pylorus with a small hole in it that can be enlarged endoscopically

## Ectopic gastric mucosa

- This is most commonly found in Meckel's diverticulum where it may cause ileal ulceration and can be complicated by bleeding
- Ectopic gastric mucosa has also been reported in the tongue, duodenum and biliary tract
- Conversely, ectopic pancreatic tissue can be present in the stomach wall

## 3.9 Congenital abnormalities of the duodenum

Duodenal atresia is covered in Paediatric Surgery, Book 1.

## Ectopic and annular pancreas

- Annular pancreas results in a ring of pancreatic tissue around the second portion of the duodenum, which may cause obstruction
- Ectopic pancreatic tissue can exist in the wall of the duodenum and may be seen on a barium meal
- Surgical treatment is not usually needed for ectopic pancreas unless it causes obstruction

## Megaduodenum

- Enlargement of the first, second and proximal ends of the third part of the duodenum is a rare condition
- Whether this is an acquired or congenital disease is controversial, but it has been reported that Auerbach's plexus was absent from this section of the duodenum in one case
- This pattern of dilatation has also been seen after major surgery or after application of plaster cast to the trunk
- Megaduodenum has also been termed 'superior mesenteric artery syndrome' because the level of obstruction is the site where the duodenum is crossed by the superior mesenteric artery
- The symptoms are bilious vomiting and a barium meal confirms the diagnosis
- Treatment is initially conservative with NG intubation and IV fluids, but occasionally bypass gastro- or duodenojejunostomy is necessary

## Duodenal diverticula

- These are more common than gastric diverticula and arise close to the ampulla of Vater
- Intraluminal diverticulum is a failure of recanalisation, leaving a sac in the lumen of the duodenum, also arising from the region of the ampulla of Vater
- These do not usually require surgical intervention but may cause confusion on diagnostic investigation, and can make ERCP (endoscopic retrograde cholangiopan-creatography) very difficult or impossible

## 3.10 Other conditions of the stomach and duodenum

### Gastric volvulus

The stomach can rotate in an organoaxial axis (60%) or mesenterioaxial axis (30%). It can occur at any age but is typically found in elderly people. It may present in two ways:

1. If uncomplicated there may be surprisingly mild symptoms of epigastric abdominal distension, retching and an inability to pass an NG tube
2. If the stomach becomes gangrenous it will present as an emergency with a shocked patient

Gastritis or bleeding gastric ulceration may also occur. A paraoesophageal hiatus hernia is often associated with the organoaxial type of volvulus (see Section 2.4, Oesophagus). Surgery involves repair of the paraoesophageal defect.

## Ingested foreign bodies

- Ingested foreign bodies that have successfully passed through the pharynx and the cardia will usually pass through the rest of the GI tract and will not need surgery
- Psychiatrically disturbed patients who ingest large numbers of unusual items should also be treated expectantly unless they develop evidence of perforation
- A **trichobezoar** is a hairball caused by habitual chewing of hair, which can be large enough to fill the entire stomach (usually removable endoscopically)
- Collections of vegetable elements such as leaves and seeds (a **phytobezoar**) may occur in post-gastrectomy patients where there is some obstruction to the efferent loop; endoscopic removal is the first line of treatment of these also

## Duodenal tumours

### Benign duodenal tumours

- Seen at 1% of endoscopies
- Include adenomas, GISTs, lipomas and carcinoid tumours
- Presentation is usually GI haemorrhage

### Malignant duodenal lesions

- Rare, but account for a third of small-bowel cancers
- Most common types are adenocarcinomas, lymphomas and carcinoids
- Presentation is usually obstruction, jaundice due to obstruction of the ampulla of Vater or a palpable mass
- The 5-year survival rate for all duodenal cancers is about 25%

The duodenum is the most common extracolonic site of tumours in patients with **familial adenomatous polyposis** and these patients should therefore be screened endoscopically.

# Morbid obesity

- A third of the western population are classified as 'obese', ie have a body mass index (BMI) $\geq 30\,kg/m^2$
- Projected figures suggest that this will rise to affect 60% of men and 50% of women by 2050
- Increased risk for many serious health conditions such as ischaemic heart disease, stroke, type 2 diabetes mellitus, certain types of cancers and premature death

## Surgery for obesity

- Severe obesity is defined as a BMI of >40 or >35 in the presence of related comorbid conditions
- Prevention is still the best cure; this makes up the cornerstone of the 2011 NICE guidelines
- Once obesity is present, non-surgical options have so far proved to be largely ineffective, but include behavioural therapy; various medical therapies have been tested
- There are two types of surgical procedures: restrictive and restrictive with malabsorption

## Gastric restriction

- Many techniques create a mechanical barrier to the ingestion of food:
  - Vertical banded gastroplasty
  - Silastic ring gastroplasty
  - Gastric banding

## Gastric bypass (restrictive and malabsorptive)

- This procedure results in weight loss by shortening the length of intestine available for digestion and absorption
- Creation of a small pouch with a volume of about 20 ml, and the distal stomach and the proximal small bowel are bypassed by anastomosing the gastric pouch to the divided jejunum. The biliary pancreatic limb is anastomosed to the small bowel between 100 and 150 cm from the point of division of the jejunum

## Success of surgical procedures

The Swedish Obesity Study reported a 10-year follow-up in 4000 operated patients in 2007:

- Weight loss from baseline was stabilised at 25% in the gastric bypass group, 16% in the sleeve gastrectomy group and 14% in the banding group when compared with controls

In a recent meta-analysis involving over 20 000 operated patients:

- The 30-day mortality rate was 0.1% for the purely restrictive procedures and 0.5% for gastric bypass
- Diabetes was completely resolved in 76.8% of patients and resolved or improved in 86.0%
- Hyperlipidaemia improved in 70%
- Hypertension was resolved in 61.7% of patients and resolved or improved in 78.5%
- Obstructive sleep apnoea was resolved in 85.7% of patients

## Complications

- Anastomotic leaks
- Anaemia
- Stomal ulcer
- Incisional hernia
- Intestinal obstruction
- Protein malnutrition

## Trauma to the stomach and duodenum

### Blunt external trauma

- Deceleration injuries, typically in road traffic accidents (RTAs), can lead to rupture of the stomach or duodenum
- Rupture of the stomach is more likely when it is full and may occur as an isolated injury
- Rupture of the duodenum against the spine is more likely to be associated with injuries to the pancreas

These injuries have a high mortality if untreated, and good management depends on prompt resuscitation, diagnosis and laparotomy, as covered in Trauma in Book 1.

## Penetrating injuries of the abdomen

- Usually caused by stab wounds
- Affect the stomach far more often than the duodenum
- Recent management strategies involve a more expectant policy in patients without evidence of hypovolaemia or peritonitis

## Iatrogenic perforation of the stomach and duodenum

Endoscopy and endoscopic procedures can result in perforation of the stomach and duodenum, in the following ways:

- Over-inflation of a stomach with a necrotic lesion
- Use of Nd:YAG laser for endoscopic tumour ablation
- ERCP sphincterotomy
- Forcing the endoscope past (or dilating) a friable constricting tumour

Iatrogenic perforation may need surgical repair but can often be treated conservatively with:

- Nil by mouth
- NG suction
- IV fluids
- IV antibiotics

# SECTION 4

# Liver and spleen

## 4.1 Anatomy of the liver

### Gross anatomy of the liver

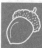

**In a nutshell ...**

- At 1.5 kg the liver is the largest gland in the body
- It is wedge-shaped and has an upper diaphragmatic surface and a postero-inferior visceral surface
- It consists of four lobes – **right, left, quadrate** and **caudate**
- The right lobe may have an additional caudal projection called Riedel's lobe

**The diaphragmatic or upper surface** of the liver is:

- Convex and lies under the diaphragm, predominantly under cover of the ribs
- Made up of anterior, superior, posterior and right surfaces
- Mostly covered by peritoneum, by which it is attached to the diaphragm

Viewed from the diaphragmatic surface, the left and right lobes of the liver are divided by the falciform ligament (Figure 1.27).

**The posteroinferior or visceral surface** is moulded to adjacent viscera and irregular in shape, and lies in contact with the abdominal oesophagus, stomach, duodenum, right colic flexure, right kidney, right adrenal gland and gallbladder.

Viewed from the visceral surface, the left and right lobes of the liver are divided by an H-shaped arrangement of structures formed by the following:

- Porta hepatis (the crossbar of the 'H')
- Ligamentum teres
- Inferior vena cava (IVC)
- Gallbladder

The caudate and quadrate lobes of the liver lie within the limbs of this 'H' (Figure 1.29).

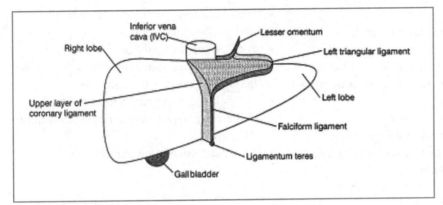

Figure 1.27 Anterior view (front) of the liver – this shows the right, anterior and superior parts of the diaphragmatic surface of the liver

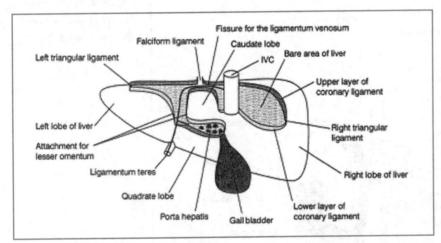

Figure 1.28 Posterior (back) view of the liver – this shows the posterior part of the diaphragmatic surface and the visceral surface of the liver

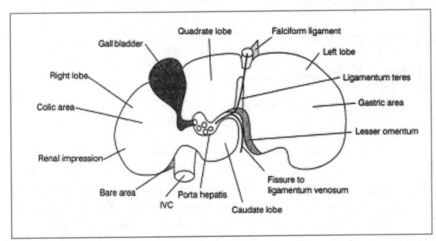

Figure 1.29 Inferior (undersurface) view of the liver – this shows the visceral surface of the liver as seen at laparotomy when looking into the abdomen with the lower border of the liver retracted up towards the costal margin

## Porta hepatis

The porta hepatis is the hilum of the liver.

It lies in the free edge of the lesser omentum, anterior to the epiploic foramen, and is approximately 5 cm long.

The porta hepatis consists of the following:

- Common hepatic duct – divides to become right and left hepatic ducts

- Hepatic artery – divides to become the right and left hepatic arteries
- Portal vein – formed from the superior mesenteric vein (SMV) and the splenic vein behind the neck of the pancreas
- Sympathetic nerve fibres from the coeliac axis and parasympathetic nerve fibres from the vagus
- Lymphatic vessels and lymph nodes

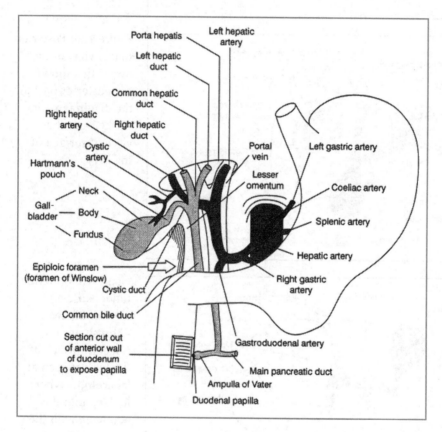

Figure 1.30 Structures entering and leaving the porta hepatis

## Peritoneal attachments

The liver is enclosed in peritoneum except for a small posterior bare area. The peritoneum is reflected from the liver onto the diaphragm and stomach in a double layer, forming various ligamentous attachments (see Figure 1.28).

- **The falciform ligament** is a two-layered fold of peritoneum ascending from the umbilicus to the anterior and superior surface of the liver. It has a free sickle-shaped lower border containing the ligamentum teres. The upper layer of the coronary ligament is formed from the right leaf of the falciform ligament and extends around the bare area of the liver, meeting the lower layer of the coronary ligament to form the right triangular ligament (see Figure 1.28)

- **The ligamentum teres** is the obliterated remains of the left umbilical vein which, in utero, brings blood from the placenta back to the fetus. It runs from the umbilicus in the free edge of the falciform ligament and passes into a fissure on the visceral surface of the liver to the porta hepatis
- **The ligamentum venosum** is the fibrous remnant of the fetal ductus venosus that shunts blood from this left umbilical vein into the IVC, short-circuiting the liver. It runs in a fissure on the visceral surface
- **The left triangular ligament** is formed from the left leaf of the falciform ligament and is continuous with the lesser omentum (see Figure 1.28)
- **The lesser omentum** arises from the edges of the fissure for the ligamentum venosum and the porta hepatis and passes down to the lesser curvature of the stomach. The porta hepatis (see Figure 1.30) runs in the free edge of the lesser omentum where it forms the anterior wall of the epiploic foramen (the entrance to the lesser sac)

## Blood supply of the liver

The liver receives 1500 ml blood/minute:

- 30% of this is from the coeliac artery via the hepatic artery carrying oxygenated blood
- 70% of this is from the portal vein which brings venous deoxygenated blood rich in the products of digestion that have been absorbed from the GI tract

### Arteries

The normal blood supply consists of right and left branches of the common hepatic artery. Anatomical variation is common:

- In 30% of the population there are one or two accessory arteries
- The right accessory artery usually arises from the superior mesenteric artery (SMA) and travels to the left of the common bile duct in the porta hepatis
- The left accessory artery arises from the left gastric artery and runs to the left lobe of the liver via the gastrohepatic ligament

### Portal system

- The portal vein is formed by the splenic vein and the SMV posterior to the pancreatic neck
- It receives tributaries from:
  - Right and left gastric veins
  - Pancreaticoduodenal veins
  - Cystic veins
  - Paraumbilical veins

### Blood flow in the liver

- Branches of the hepatic artery and portal vein run along with the bile ductules, forming portal triads at the corners of each liver lobule (Figure 1.31)
- Arterial and venous blood is conducted to the central vein of each liver lobule by liver sinusoids
- The central veins drain into the right, middle and left hepatic veins, which open directly into the IVC
- A number of small short veins also drain directly from the posterior surface of the liver to the IVC
- The falciform ligament anatomically divides the liver into right and left lobes, but the watershed of blood supply between the right and left hepatic arteries occurs to the right

of the falciform ligament (corresponding to a plane running from the gallbladder bed to the IVC)

- The caudate and quadrate lobes (segments I and IV) are anatomically part of the right lobe of the liver but are supplied by the left hepatic artery and portal vein, ie functionally part of the left lobe

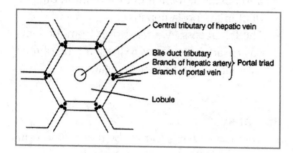

Figure 1.31 Arrangement of lobules in the liver

## Liver segments

The liver is divided into eight segments, each of which is independent and has its own triad of vessels (an artery, vein and bile duct). Segments are arranged according to the position of the right, middle and left hepatic veins. Sizes of segments are variable but their position is constant.

Surgically this is very useful, allowing resection of individual or groups of segments:

- Caudate lobe – segment I
- Left lobe – segments II and III
- Quadrate lobe – segment IV
- Right lobe – segments V to VIII

**Riedel's lobe** is a projection of normally functioning liver tissue downwards from the right lobe of the liver. It may cause diagnostic difficulties by giving a false impression of hepatomegaly.

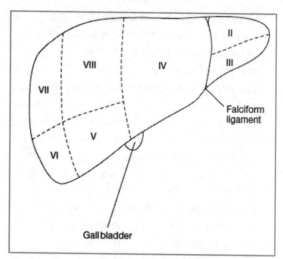

Figure 1.32 The functional segments of the liver as seen from an anterior view of the 'ex vivo' liver (you cannot see segments VI or VII from the front when the liver is in the patient but you can in the flattened-out dissection specimen that you might get in your viva)

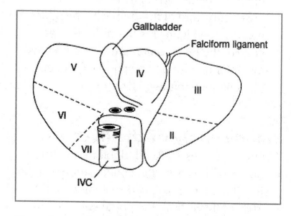

Figure 1.33 The functional segments of the liver as seen from an inferior view

## Lymphatics of the liver

The liver produces more than a third of all body lymph. The lymph vessels leave the liver via the porta hepatis. The draining lymph nodes are the coeliac nodes and the posterior mediastinal nodes.

## Nerve supply of the liver

The nerve supply of the liver is derived from the sympathetic and parasympathetic nerves by way of the coeliac plexus. The anterior vagal trunk gives rise to a large hepatic branch which passes directly to the liver.

## Histology of the liver

- The segments are divided into acinar units which are centred on the portal triad
- Sheets of hepatocytes run through the acini separated by sinusoidal spaces
- Blood flows into the sinusoidal spaces (space of Disse) which are lined with endothelial cells and contain a large number of macrophages (Kupffer cells) for ingestion of bacteria
- Within each acinar unit there are therefore zones of tissue radiating away from the central arteriole which are subject to decreasing levels of oxygenation:
  - Zone 1 – closest to the arteriole
  - Zone 2 – middle zone
  - Zone 3 – closest to the venule
- Hepatocytes in zone 3 are most susceptible to disease processes by effects of toxins whereas those in zone 1 are most likely to be capable of regeneration
- Regeneration occurs remarkably quickly
- This is due to cellular hyperplasia which quickly alters the architecture of the liver
- It is stimulated by either removal of liver tissue or fibrosis in surrounding tissue
- This initiates production of hepatocyte growth factors and stimulates a cytokine cascade

## 4.2  Physiology of the liver

### In a nutshell ...

**The functions of the liver are:**
- Metabolism and heat production
- Bile production
- Excretion
- Storage
- Detoxification
- Other (endocrine, reticuloendothelial, fetal haematopoiesis, vitamin D activation)

## Metabolism of the liver

### In a nutshell ...

The portal venous system delivers the products of digestion (fats, proteins and carbohydrates) to the liver where they are metabolised into a form that can be utilised by the body. As a metabolic centre the liver produces heat, contributing to core body temperature.

### Fat metabolism

Thirty per cent of chylomicrons from intestinal lacteals are transported to the liver to be made into triglycerides, phospholipids and cholesterol. The liver synthesises and secretes very-low-density lipoproteins (VLDLs). It provides cholesterol for use by the body and excretes the excess in bile (see page 148). The liver can also facilitate β-oxidation of fatty acids if energy is needed from fats (eg in starvation or diabetic ketoacidosis).

- **Starvation:** in starvation, ketone bodies produced in the liver from the oxidation of fatty acids are circulated to the cells of the body for use as a metabolite in the place of glucose. Gluconeogenesis also occurs from the liver and the cells use glucose in preference to ketones. The level of ketone bodies in the circulation is controlled by insulin, which inhibits further lipolysis if serum ketone levels rise. Excess ketones are excreted in the urine (hence ketones in the urinalysis of patients starved for surgery is a normal finding)
- **Diabetic ketoacidosis:** in diabetic ketoacidosis, however, there is a severe insulin deficiency and excessive glucagon production; thus the liver is stimulated to carry out lipolysis, gluconeogenesis and glycogenolysis, resulting in an over-production of glucose. This glucose cannot be utilised by the cells of the body in the absence of insulin and, although some of the excess is excreted in the urine, blood glucose levels rise. Furthermore, in the absence of insulin the level of ketone bodies in the serum is not controlled, so, although ketones are excreted in the urine, serum ketone levels also rise

Fat-soluble vitamins (DEKAs) are also delivered to the liver and stored there.

### Protein metabolism

Absorbed peptides are broken down by the liver into their constituent amino acids, producing ammonia as a byproduct. The liver also synthesises all non-essential amino acids. From these amino acids, the liver manufactures 25 g/day of plasma proteins and enzymes, including serum albumin, prothrombin 2, fibrinogen and blood-clotting factors. All the plasma proteins are produced by the liver except the γ-globulins, which are produced by plasma cells.

### Carbohydrate metabolism

Under the control of insulin, glucagon and other hormones, the liver is responsible for the storage and release of glucose in the form of glycogen, thereby keeping the serum glucose level constant:

- **Glycogenesis** is the conversion of glucose into glycogen for storage when the blood glucose level is high
- **Glycogenolysis** releases glucose into the blood by breaking down these stores of glycogen when the blood glucose level is low
- **Gluconeogenesis** converts amino acids, lipids and carbohydrates into glucose if needed (eg in starvation)

Glycogen is also stored in skeletal muscle.

### Excretion

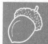 In a nutshell ...

The liver breaks down and solubilises many of the waste products of the body and then excretes them, either into the bloodstream, for excretion in the urine, or into the bile, for excretion into the faeces. These waste products include:
- Ammonia
- Lipid-soluble substances
- Hormones
- Bacteria and foreign particles
- Cholesterol
- Bile pigments
- Toxins and drugs

## Ammonia

Ammonia is formed by the breakdown of proteins and is converted into urea in the liver. The basic reaction in the liver needs a lot of energy in the form of ATP. In severe liver disease the blood urea ($NH_4^+$) level falls and the ammonia levels ($NH_3$) rises. Urea is excreted by the kidney via the urea cycle.

## Lipid-soluble substances

This includes drugs, hormones, bilirubin, steroids and phenols. These substances are made soluble and then conjugated with glucuronic acid, glycine or glutathione. They can then be excreted into the bile (see Section 5.2).

## Hormones

These also get inactivated in the liver, and include the following:
- Protein hormones (insulin, antidiuretic hormone [ADH])
- Steroid hormones (oestrogen)
- Catecholamines

Signs of increasing blood levels of oestrogen in liver failure include gynaecomastia, microgonadism and palmar erythema.

## Bacteria and foreign particles

These are removed from the bloodstream by filtration. Kupffer cells are part of the reticuloendothelial system and line the hepatic sinusoids. They remove bacteria, toxins and damaged or abnormal red blood cells from the circulation.

## Cholesterol

Cholesterol (see Section 5.2) is produced by the liver as a side effect of fat metabolism and is excreted in the bile.

---

**The cytochrome P450 system**

Drugs and toxins are metabolised by the liver in two stages:
- **Phase 1** (involving the cytochrome P450 system) increases solubility but does not necessarily detoxify the drug. Phenytoin, warfarin, halothane, indometacin and ciclosporin are prepared for excretion by this system.
- **Phase 2** reduces toxicity and further increases solubility.

**Clinical implications**
- Some drugs increase the activity of the cytochrome P450 system (eg barbiturates, phenytoin, rifampicin, lidocaine). This leads to an increased excretion and therefore reduced effectiveness of the drugs listed above that are solubilised by the cytochrome P450 system (eg a patient may have reduced effect of ciclosporin if started on rifampicin)
- Some drugs inhibit the cytochrome P450 system (eg erythromycin, ketoconazole, cimetidine). This leads to a reduced clearance of the drugs listed above that are solubilised by the system (eg a patient on warfarin may become over-anticoagulated if started on cimetidine)
- Paracetamol produces toxic metabolites after it has been through the cytochrome P450 system. Therefore liver toxicity is a delayed side effect of paracetamol overdose.

**CHAPTER 1**

### Bile pigments

Bilirubin (see Section 5.2) is produced as a side effect of red blood cell degradation and is excreted in the bile and urine.

### Toxins and drugs

The liver is important to doctors because it metabolises the drugs and toxins that we give to patients. The mechanism by which this is achieved has implications for drug interactions (see box below).

## Bile production

This is covered in detail in Section 5.2. Bile is produced continuously by the liver and is stored in the gallbladder. Between 500 ml and 1500 ml of bile is produced each day.

## Storage by the liver

- **Glycogen:** the liver stores energy in the form of glycogen that can be converted into glucose if needed by the cells of the body (see above)
- **Vitamins:** fat-soluble (DEKA) vitamins; vitamin B12 (> 3 years' supply!)
- **Minerals:** iron, copper, ferritin

## Vitamin D activation

Vitamin D is converted to 25-hydroxycalciferol in the liver. This step is essential for calcium absorption and metabolism (see Chapter 4, Endocrine Surgery).

---

 **In a nutshell ...**

Bile consists of:

**Substances being excreted**
- Bile pigments (from red blood cells)
- Cholesterol (from fat metabolism)
- Fat-soluble drugs and toxins

**Substances being secreted to aid digestion**
- Bile salts (to emulsify fats)
- Inorganic salts including bicarbonate ions (to neutralise duodenal contents)
- Lecithin (to aid solubility of cholesterol)
- Water

## Liver function tests

### Markers of synthetic function
Prothrombin time (PT):
- Liver is major synthetic site for all clotting factors except von Willebrand factor (vWF)
- Factors II, VII, VIII and X are vitamin K-dependent

Albumin:
- Plasma protein synthesised by the liver
- Half-life is 20 days so can be used as an indicator of chronic liver synthesis
- Functions:
  - Osmotic
  - Binds and transports, eg bilirubin, calcium and drugs
- Low measured values due to decreased production (poor hepatic synthesis, small-bowel malabsorption, malnutrition) or increased protein loss (ascites, increased breakdown in catabolic states, eg severe illness and infection, nephrotic syndrome, enteropathies and inflammatory gut conditions, burns)

### Markers of excretory function
- Bilirubin: conjugated/unconjugated fraction (see Section 4.3)

### Markers of bile duct or hepatocyte damage
Alkaline phosphatase (ALP):
- Different isoenzymes present in liver, bone, intestine, placenta and kidney
- Located in walls of bile duct cannuliculi
- Increased synthesis occurs in presence of increasing concentrations of bile acids associated with biliary stasis

Alanine and aspartate transaminases or aminotransferases (ALT and AST):
- AST also found in cardiac and skeletal muscle; ALT is liver-specific
- Intracellular enzymes leak from damaged hepatocytes

$\alpha$-Glutamyl transpeptidase ($\alpha$-GT):
- Enzyme located in the biliary tree
- Production induced by certain drugs and alcohol

# CHAPTER 1

## 4.3 Jaundice

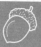

### In a nutshell ...

Jaundice is defined as an elevation of the serum bilirubin (normal 9 µmmol/l) and is clinically detectable at 35 µmmol/l. Bilirubin metabolism is outlined in Figure 1.37 (in Section 5). Jaundice is usually classified as pre-hepatic, hepatic or post-hepatic.

Bilirubin is conjugated in the liver, so high levels of unconjugated bilirubin indicate a pre-hepatic cause (eg haemolysis), whereas high levels of conjugated bilirubin indicate a post-hepatic cause (eg gallstones). In clinical practice, the hepatic and post-hepatic forms often coexist, eg cholestasis may produce secondary damage to the liver (biliary cirrhosis). Conversely, liver cirrhosis or metastatic disease may cause bile duct compression.

## Classification of jaundice

Classically, deranged liver function tests (LFTs) are described as having either a 'hepatocellular' (inflammatory) or a 'cholestatic' (obstructive) picture. As an inflammatory pathology progresses, hepatocyte oedema and swelling cause partial intrahepatic cholestasis due to obstruction of canaliculi. Equally, as biliary obstruction progresses, backwash of bile towards the hepatocytes causes inflammation and hepatocyte damage. As either pathology progresses, this can cause the picture to become slightly mixed.

### Common drugs that may cause these pictures

| Hepatic jaundice | Obstructive 'cholestatic' jaundice |
|---|---|
| Paracetamol | Co-amoxiclav |
| Amiodarone | Flucloxacillin |
| Diclofenac | Erythromycin |
| Fluconazole | Co-trimoxazole |
| Heparin | Captopril |
| Labetolol | Phenothiazides |
| Diltiazem | |

### History of a jaundiced patient

| Important aspects | Suggests |
|---|---|
| Recent travel | Hepatitis |
| Drug addiction | |
| Joint pains | |
| Anorexia | |
| Malaise | |
| Alcohol addiction | Cirrhosis |
| Fat intolerance | Gallstones |
| Recurrent right upper quadrant pain | |
| Weight loss | Malignancy |
| Constant epigastric boring pain | |
| Family history of blood disorders | |
| Bruising tendency | Hepatocellular damage |
| Pale stool, dark urine | Obstructive jaundice |
| Pruritus | |

## CLASSIFICATION OF JAUNDICE

| | Pre-hepatic | Hepatic jaundice | Post-hepatic (obstructive) jaundice* |
|---|---|---|---|
| Causes | **Increased breakdown of red blood cells**<br>Spherocytosis<br>Haemolytic anaemia<br>Incompatible blood transfusion<br>Resorption of haematoma | **Decreased conjugation**<br>Cirrhosis<br>Hepatitis<br>Prematurity<br>Crigler–Najjar syndrome (congenital inability to conjugate bilirubin due to enzyme inhibition)<br>Gilbert syndrome (7% population, exacerbated by intercurrent illness),<br>Dubin–Johnson syndrome<br>**Decreased hepatocyte uptake**<br>Sepsis<br>Drug and toxin reactions<br>**Liver tumours (primary or secondary)** | **Common or segmental bile duct obstructions**<br>Gallstones<br>Biliary stricture (intra-/extrahepatic eg primary sclerosing cholangitis, primary biliary cirrhosis, chronic cholangitis, traumatic or iatrogenic stricture)<br>Tumour (intra-/extrahepatic eg cholangiocarcinoma, ampullary carcinoma, pancreatic cancer)<br>**Canaliculi obstruction**<br>Inflammatory swelling of hepatocytes due to hepatitis or cirrhosis; cholestasis due to drug reaction |
| Jaundice | **Mild jaundice**<br>Bilirubin rarely >100 μmol/litre unconjugated | **Variable jaundice**<br>May be conjugated or unconjugated | **Variable jaundice**<br>Bilirubin may exceed 1000 μmol/litre conjugated |
| Urine | **Normal colour**<br>Bilirubin not present<br>Urobilinogen raised | **Dark**<br>Bilirubin may be present | **Dark**<br>Bilirubin present<br>Urobilinogen absent (no enterohepatic circulation) |
| Stool | **Normal colour**<br>Increased urobilinogen | **Normal colour** | **Pale stools**<br>Stercobilinogen down |
| Alkaline phosphatase | Normal | **Mildly raised due to swollen hepatocytes blocking ducts**<br>**Very high in primary biliary cirrhosis** | **Very high**<br>Massively upregulated by increasing bile concentrations in the ducts |
| Aminotransferase | Normal | **Typically very high, especially in acute viral hepatitis or cirrhosis**<br>Severe damage to hepatocytes can elevate levels to thousands | **Normal or moderately raised due to bile backwash** |
| Prothrombin time (PT) | Normal | **Prolonged and not correctable with vitamin K**<br>Most sensitive sign of liver damage | **Prolonged but correctable with vitamin K** |

*May result in secondary liver damage causing misleading results, so can be difficult to distinguish from hepatic jaundice.

### Examining a jaundiced patient

| Important aspects | Suggests |
|---|---|
| Spider naevi | Stigmata of chronic liver disease |
| Palmar erythema | |
| Finger clubbing | |
| Ascites | |
| Splenomegaly | Portal hypertension and cirrhosis |
| Prominent abdominal wall veins | |
| Xanthomas | Biliary cirrhosis |
| Kayser–Fleischer rings in iris | Wilson's disease |
| Large knobbly liver | Malignant disease |

## Investigating jaundice

A simplified scheme for investigating jaundice is shown in Figure 1.34. Many tools can aid in the diagnosis of the cause of the jaundice. These are described in the following pages.

### Blood tests

- **Serum bilirubin** is raised by definition. The presence of raised conjugated bilirubin suggests that the jaundice is either hepatic or post-hepatic
- **LFTs** may be useful in determining the degree of hepatic damage. The results of serum biochemistry in jaundiced patients are shown in the table 'Classification of jaundice'
- **Haematological investigations** (red blood cell fragility, Coombs' test, reticulocyte count) can confirm a haemolytic cause

- **PT** and **APTT** (activated partial thromboplastin time) should be checked before any invasive investigations are performed
- **Hepatitis screen** should be performed before invasive procedures if possible

### Urinalysis

- Bilirubin in the urine indicates obstructive jaundice
- Excess urobilinogen suggests pre-hepatic or hepatic jaundice
- Absence of urobilinogen in the urine suggests obstructive jaundice

### Analysis of faeces

- This is the basis of occasional biochemistry vivas and MCQs but in reality is rarely done
- Absence of bile pigments indicates a hepatic or post-hepatic cause
- Raised faecal urobilinogen suggests pre-hepatic jaundice
- Faecal occult blood tests may be positive in the presence of bleeding oesophageal varices or an ampullary carcinoma bleeding into the duodenum

### Plain radiographs

Ten per cent of gallstones are radio-opaque and may be seen on a plain abdominal radiograph. Plain radiographs may also show:

- Calcification in chronic pancreatitis
- Lung metastases in malignant disease
- An air cholangiogram if there is a fistula between the intestine and biliary tree, or if gas-forming organisms are present in severe cholangitis
- An enlarged gallbladder as a soft-tissue mass in the right upper quadrant

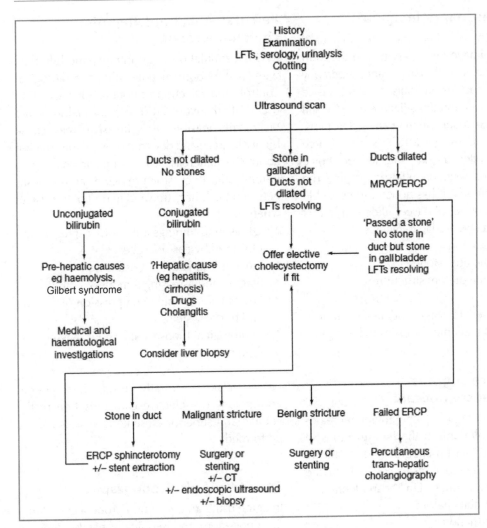

Figure 1.34
Investigating
jaundice

## Ultrasonography

This is an essential baseline investigation in a jaundiced patient. It can show the following:

- Gallstones in the gallbladder (but may miss stones in the duct)
- Dilated bile ducts (a common hepatic duct of >8 mm diameter at the porta hepatis is abnormal)
- The level of obstruction (in 90% of cases)
- The cause of obstruction (may be diagnosed but the degree of accuracy varies)
- Intrahepatic tumour deposits, abscesses, cysts or cirrhosis (can be diagnosed and biopsied under ultrasound control)
- A mass in the pancreas (can be assessed and measured but may be difficult to diagnose)
- Splenomegaly
- Upper abdominal varices
- Alteration in portal flow dynamics associated with hypertension, compression or invasion
- Lymph node enlargement
- Ascites

## Magnetic resonance imaging

Magnetic resonance imaging (MRI) is used increasingly to image the biliary tree in the form of magnetic resonance cholangiopancreatography (MRCP). This has revolutionised non-invasive imaging of the liver and the biliary tree. ERCP still has a role in intervention (stenting, sphincterotomy, removing duct stones) but MRCP is now, where it is available, often the investigation of choice for dilated ducts seen on ultrasonography. The main benefits are that it has none of the possible complications of ERCP (see Procedure box overleaf) and can be used to diagnose:

- Biliary obstruction
- Common bile duct stones
- Malignant bile duct obstruction

MRI is also used to stage and assess tumour operability and it enables biopsies to be taken.

## Endoscopic retrograde cholangiopancreatography

Endoscopic retrograde cholangiopancreatography has revolutionised the investigations of the biliary tree (see Procedure box). It allows diagnostic and therapeutic access to both the bile and pancreatic ducts. ERCP can identify:

- Details of ductal anatomy
- Level of obstruction
- Nature of obstruction
- Stones and stricturing tumours
- Congenital ductal abnormalities
- Acquired abnormalities, such as early chronic pancreatitis

Biopsies may be taken and therapeutic measures, such as sphincterotomy, stone extraction, dilatation and stenting of strictures, can be performed.

## Percutaneous trans-hepatic cholangiography

PTC is cannulation of an intrahepatic bile duct with a fine-bore needle under radiological control, and injection of contrast. It provides a useful alternative if ERCP is unavailable or not technically feasible. It is invasive, may cause biliary leakage and does not provide information about the pancreas. It is useful for delineating intrahepatic duct strictures and anastomoses between the biliary tree and jejunum. It is useful when:

- Ultrasound findings are equivocal (eg view obscured by gas or ascites)
- ERCP is equivocal or unsuccessful
- Staging and assessing tumour operability
- Looking for invasion/compression of arterial and portal systems
- Radiological biopsies of tumour masses are required

IV contrast is usually used, but arterial portography by selective catheterisation of the coeliac and superior mesenteric vessels can be performed.

## Endoscopic ultrasonography

Imaging using an ultrasound probe inserted into the duodenum endoscopically has become an indispensable tool in the assessment of biliary and pancreatic pathology in recent years. It is particularly useful in imaging the area of the pancreatic head and the bile duct. It can pick up microlithiasis (very small stones) that are missed by any other modality. Perhaps the most useful function is the ability to do an endoscopic ultrasonography (EUS)-guided biopsy of a periampullary mass. This is done with a needle that comes out of the side of the endoscope. It has the great advantage that there is no danger of seeding cells into the peritoneum, as can happen with a percutaneous CT-guided biopsy.

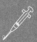

# Procedure box: Endoscopic retrograde cholangiopancreatography (ERCP)

## Indications
- Diagnostic indications:
  - Dilated ducts on ultrasonography with rising LFTs
  - Pre-cholecystectomy to confirm clear ducts
  - Assessing suspected benign or malignant pancreatic pathology
  - Assessing suspected benign or malignant duct pathology
- Therapeutic indications:
  - Removing stones in the ducts before or after surgery
  - Stenting or dilating strictures
  - Sphincterotomy

## Pre-procedure
- Check clotting
- Patient starved for 6 hours
- Trained endoscopic team essential
- Consent for complications (see below)
- Oxygen, suction and ERCP equipment in fluoroscopic room

## Contrast medium
- Non-ionic to reduce pancreatitis (usually iodine)
- Low concentration to visualise stones in bile duct
- Higher concentration to visualise pancreatic ducts

## Procedure
- Left lateral position
- Local anaesthetic throat spray
- IV sedation
- IV broad-spectrum antibiotics
- Hyoscine butyl bromide given to reduce duodenal peristalsis
- Side-viewing duodenoscope introduced by mouth
- Ampulla identified
- Selective cannulation of both bile and pancreatic ducts
- Visualisation by radiography
- Overfilling of pancreatic duct avoided

## Therapeutic modalities available
- Sphincterotomy
- Stone extraction
- Balloon dilation of strictures
- Stenting of tumours

## Causes of failure to cannulate bile duct
- Duodenal diverticulum
- Previous surgery
- Impacted stone
- Ampullary stenosis
- Subampullary tumour
- Technical difficulty

## Complications of ERCP
- Mild self-limiting pancreatitis (3%)
- Severe life-threatening pancreatitis (0.1%)
- Contrast reactions
- Bacteraemia
- Septicaemia
- Perforation and haemorrhage in therapeutic cases

## Radionuclide scanning

A gamma-emitting isotope, which is taken up by the liver, is injected into the patient. Depending on the choice of isotope, different areas are imaged and captured by a gamma camera, eg:

- Technetium-99m-labelled sulphur colloid is taken up by Kupffer cells of the reticuloendothelial system of the liver and spleen
- Gallium-67 citrate is useful to detect hepatomas
- Technetium-labelled white blood cells (WBCs) can demonstrate liver abscesses
- Technetium-99m-labelled iminodiacetic acid compounds ([$^{99m}$Tc]HIDA) are secreted in the bile and so outline the biliary tree

Most radionuclide scanning has been supplanted by ultrasonography, CT, MRCP and ERCP in recent years. The exception to this is HIDA scanning, which is still very useful as a functional scan of the biliary tree, especially the gallbladder. If a patient has an HIDA scan and is given an IV injection of cholecystokinin (CCK) or an oral fatty meal, the gallbladder will contract. The ejection fraction of the gallbladder should be at least 50%. If it is in the region of 20% or 30% it suggests an abnormal gallbladder, which can be a source of pain even in the absence of stones.

## Arteriography

Although not used to investigate the biliary system directly, selective arteriography of the hepatic and coeliac arteries and SMAs can give valuable information before hepatic or pancreatic surgery. Once more widely used, it has now been largely supplanted by EUS, laparoscopic ultrasonography and spiral CT. Arteriography provides information about anatomical variants, and therapeutic embolisation can also be employed for vascular, non-operable tumours.

## Barium studies

These are not routine investigations in jaundiced patients but can give information about:

- Duodenal distortion due to adjacent tumours
- Gastric carcinoma
- Oesophageal varices

## Oral cholecystogram

Not generally helpful in jaundiced patients because the uptake and excretion of the dye are impaired in the damaged liver.

## Management of jaundice

This depends on the underlying cause. In general, while investigations are being carried out, it is essential to preserve renal function with adequate hydration and monitoring of urinary output, and then proceed to definitive treatment.

## 4.4 Portal hypertension

The surgeon's input into this area is now very small. Portal hypertension and oesophageal varices are now managed largely by gastroenterologists and radiologists.

 **In a nutshell ...**

The normal portal pressure is between 8 and 10 mmHg. Portal hypertension is an acute or chronic increase in this pressure (>12 mmHg). Increased portal pressure results from either increased portal blood flow (arteriovenous [AV] fistula, increased splenic blood flow) or obstruction to portal venous flow. The causes of obstruction are shown in the box below and are classified according to the site of the block.

The four important effects of portal hypertension are:

- Splenomegaly (see Section 4.10)
- Ascites
- Development of a collateral portosystemic circulation (which leads to oesophageal varices)
- Hepatic failure and its sequelae

**Causes of portal hypertension**

Worldwide, post-viral hepatitis is the most common cause.
In developed countries, alcoholic cirrhosis is the principal cause.

**Pre-hepatic causes**
Portal venous thrombosis
Compression of portal vein by lymph nodes, tumour or pancreatitis

**Hepatic causes**
Cirrhosis of the liver
Multiple hepatic metastases

**Post-hepatic causes**
Budd–Chiari syndrome (thrombosis of hepatic vein)

**Cardiac causes**
Constrictive pericarditis
Right heart failure
Pulmonary causes
Pulmonary hypertension

**Other rare causes**
Splenic vein thrombosis
AV fistula
Tropical splenomegaly
Immunological (lupoid)
Schistosomiasis
Chronic active hepatitis
Early primary biliary cirrhosis (PBC)
Congenital hepatic fibrosis
Sarcoidosis
Toxins
Metabolic (eg Wilson's disease)
Drugs (eg methotrexate, vitamin A)
Caval abnormality
Constrictive pericarditis
Tumour invasion of hepatic vein

## Splenomegaly

Splenomegaly occurs because of:

- Portal hypertension
- Leucopenia and thrombocytopenia causing hypertrophy of the splenic substance itself

See Section 4.10.

## Ascites

Ascites is due to a combination of:

- Raised portal pressure (not enough to cause ascites on its own)
- Low serum albumin (decreased intravascular osmotic pressure)
- Increased aldosterone activity with sodium and water retention
- Increased lymphatic pressure in the cirrhotic liver, resulting in lymph transudation from both the liver and the intestine

In metastatic disease it may also be a feature of widespread peritoneal malignancy.

### Causes of ascites

- **Portal hypertension (see also box 'Causes of portal hypertension')**
- **Hypoproteinaemia:**
  - Kidney disease associated with albuminuria
  - Cirrhosis of the liver
  - Cachexia of wasting diseases, malignancy and starvation
  - Protein-losing enteropathies
- **Chronic peritonitis:**
  - Physical
    - Post-irradiation
    - Talc granuloma
  - Infection
    - Tuberculous peritonitis
  - Neoplasms
    - Peritoneal metastases
    - Mucus-forming tumours (pseudo-myxoma peritonei)
- **Chylous ascites:**
  - Congenital abnormalities
  - Trauma
  - Primary or secondary lymph gland disease

## Management of ascites

### Diagnostic ascitic tap

- Total protein, amylase, albumin
- Exclude malignancy: cytology
- Infection screen: white cell count (WCC), microscopy and culture

### General measures

- Low-salt diet
- Fluid restriction
- Potassium-sparing diuretics, eg spirono-lactone (if renal function normal)

### Paracentesis

- Indicated for diuretic-resistant ascites, tense ascites (impairs respiration) and infected ascites
- Performed by introducing a peritoneal catheter (eg Bonanno) under aseptic conditions and under antibiotic cover
- It is important to replace fluid drained with IV albumin solution (eg 100 ml of 20% human albumin solution per 3 litres drained). Close monitoring of renal function is also important. Aim for a daily fluid weight loss of not more than 0.5–1.0 kg/day

## Peritoneal venous shunting

- A surgical measure for resistant ascites
- A tube is channelled subcutaneously between the peritoneal cavity and the internal jugular vein
- A chamber with a one-way valve is inserted under the skin and patients compress the chamber to pump ascitic fluid out from the abdomen

## The collateral portosystemic circulation

There are five main areas of portosystemic anastomosis that decompress the obstructed portal system by diverting blood flow:

1. **Between the left gastric vein and the oesophageal veins** (oesophageal varices)
2. **Between the superior and inferior rectal veins** (rectal varices in the same position as haemorrhoids – these are NOT the same as haemorrhoids, which are vascular cushions full of arterial blood)
3. **Along the obliterated umbilical vein to the superior and inferior epigastric veins** (caput medusae on the anterior abdominal wall)
4. **Retroperitoneal anastomoses** (veins of Retzius)
5. **Diaphragmatic anastomoses** (can cause intraoperative bleeding)

As a result of its catastrophic effect, haemorrhage from bleeding oesophageal varices is the most significant surgical presentation of portal hypertension.

Oesophageal varices account for 10% of cases of upper GI bleeding but cause 50% of deaths.

## Management of oesophageal variceal haemorrhage

Eleven per cent of patients undergoing endoscopy for upper GI bleeding have variceal bleeding. The large majority have bleeding oesophageal varices (90%). Variceal haemorrhage has a poor prognosis and prompt recognition and treatment are required.

The outcome for patients with variceal haemorrhage is closely related to the severity of the underlying liver disease. The severity of liver disease is stratified by the Child–Pugh grade (see page 132); the 3-year mortality rate after endoscopic treatment for bleeding varices is reported as 32% for Child's A, 46% for Child's B and 79% for Child's C.

Patients presenting with variceal bleeding should be assessed and resuscitated as for any other patient with an upper GI bleed. There should be a high index of suspicion when there is a history of previous variceal bleeding, known liver disease, or clinical assessment identifies stigmata of chronic liver disease or portal hypertension, such as jaundice, ascites, splenomegaly, encephalopathy, caput medusae or spider naevi.

### Immediate resuscitation takes priority

- In patients with suspected variceal bleeding, endoscopy should be performed once appropriate resuscitation has been undertaken

## Control the acute bleeding

### Variceal banding

RCTs and meta-analyses have clearly demonstrated that banding and ligation are superior to sclerotherapy in producing control of bleeding, reducing all-cause mortality and death caused by it. Banding may be technically difficult in cases of continued bleeding, and sclerotherapy may then be necessary (see below).

### Drug treatment of oesophageal varices

- Somatostatin, octreotide and lanreotide: reduce splanchnic and hepatic flow
- Vasopressin: causes generalised vasoconstriction but its use is controversial
- Terlipressin (Glypressin): an analogue of vasopressin that has a longer action and fewer systemic effects
- Recent evidence from the SIGN guidelines supports the use of terlipressin for 48 hours and octreotide or high-dose somatostatin each for up to 5 days after a variceal bleed

### Balloon tamponade

Insertion of a double-ballooned Sengstaken–Blakemore or Minnesota tube into the oesophagus controls variceal bleeding **temporarily** by direct compression at the bleeding site.

### Sclerotherapy of varices

Injecting sclerosant, such as ethanolamine, into bleeding varices is usually undertaken at the initial emergency endoscopy to control acute bleeding. It is successful in about 70% of cases, and may be repeated to prevent rebleeding. If two attempts of sclerotherapy fail, a more major intervention is indicated.

## Prevent recurrent bleeding

### Intrahepatic shunt

Transjugular intrahepatic portosystemic shunt (TIPSS) is a radiological technique for creating a portosystemic shunt and diverting blood directly to the systemic venous circulation. The principle is to reduce the portal pressure gradient by short-circuiting the liver. It is indicated in uncontrolled or recurrent bleeding or in end-stage patients awaiting transplantation. In the short term the intervention might be effective but in the long term the stents tend to block.

### Extrahepatic shunt

In long-term elective treatment, extrahepatic shunt or oesophageal transection is the alternative to repeated sclerotherapy. These shunts require a surgical procedure and may be indicated in patients with failed endoscopic treatment. They are rarely performed. The following are the three main extrahepatic shunts:

1. **Total shunt** (portacaval)
2. **Partial shunt** (narrow-diameter portacaval graft)
3. **Selective shunt** (distal splenorenal)

### Oesophageal transection (rare)

The aim of oesophageal transection is to interrupt the gastric oesophageal portosystemic anastomosis. Early oesophageal transection has compared favourably with injection sclerotherapy, but it requires a laparotomy and dissection in the presence of established portal hypertension and opening of the stomach, all of which are hazardous in the acutely bleeding patient. It is rarely performed now, with the usual procedure for uncontrollable variceal bleeding being banding, terlipressin ± tamponade and TIPSS while being considered for transplantation.

## Liver transplantation

The underlying liver disease causing oesophageal varices is often not reversible, and liver transplantation may offer the only definitive treatment. Liver transplantation is used for end-stage liver disease with intractable portal hypertension. It is not suitable for cases of pre-hepatic obstruction with good liver function, and is used with caution for cases with a persisting underlying cause.

# 4.5 Clinical evaluation of liver disease

## History of liver disease

Taking a history for liver disease

| Symptoms | Suggests |
|---|---|
| Anorexia | Malignancy |
| General malaise | |
| Joint pains | |
| Fever | |
| Weight loss | |
| Constant epigastric boring pain | |
| Fat intolerance | Gallstones |
| Recurrent right upper quadrant pain | |
| Pale stool, dark urine | Obstructive jaundice |
| Pruritus | |
| Previous/current haematemesis | Varices |

**Complications of variceal haemorrhage**

- Aspiration
- Hepatic decompensation (encephalopathy, ascites, liver failure)
- Malnutrition
- Infections from enteric organisms
- Pneumonia
- Hypoxia
- Renal failure
- Alcohol withdrawal

## Aetiology of liver disease

- Recent travel abroad
- Tattoos, drug abuse (particularly intravenous), blood transfusions
- Alcohol addiction (CAGE questions)
- Sexual history
- Occupational history:
  - Solvent exposure
  - Dirty water – Weil's disease
- Family history (eg malignancy, blood disorders, Wilson's disease, $\alpha_1$-antitrypsin)
- Medications:
  - Antibiotics (eg rifampicin)
  - Alternative herbal medications
  - Overdose and psychiatric history
  - Diet history (eg non-alcoholic steatohepatitis [NASH] in obesity)

## Examination in liver disease

- Signs of malignancy (hard, knobbly liver; Courvoisier's sign; look for primary)
- Stigmata of chronic liver disease:
  - ± Hepatomegaly (liver may enlarge or shrink and fibrose)
  - Jaundice
  - Spider naevi (seen in distribution of superior vena cava [SVC])
  - Palmar erythema and Dupuytren's contracture

- Finger clubbing and leukonychia
- Gynaecomastia, testicular atrophy and loss of body hair
- Encephalopathy (confusion, eg serial 7s; liver flap)
- Purpura and bruising
- Portal hypertension:
  - Ascites
  - Splenomegaly
  - Prominent abdominal wall veins
  - Signs of right heart failure
- Other signs:
  - Excoriation marks (pruritis)
  - Needle marks (drug use)
  - Xanthomas (commonly primary or secondary biliary cirrhosis)
  - Kayser–Fleischer rings in iris (Wilson's disease)

---

**Causes of hepatomegaly**

**Cirrhosis**
- Alcoholic
- Primary biliary cirrhosis (PBC)

**Neoplastic**
- Metastases
- Primary hepatocellular carcinoma (HCC)
- Haematological malignancy (eg lymphoma)

**Infection**
- Schistosomiasis
- Multiple liver abscesses

**Vascular**
- Budd–Chiari syndrome
- Congestion from right heart failure

**Other**
- Metabolic (haemochromatosis and Wilson's disease)
- Polycystic liver disease

---

# Scoring systems in liver disease

Child's scoring is used to stage liver disease of any aetiology and gives prognostic information as to disease progression. Some versions substitute nutritional status for the ascites category.

### Child–Pugh classification of liver disease

|  | Child's A | Child's B | Child's C |
|---|---|---|---|
| Albumin (g/l) | >35 | 28–35 | <28 |
| Bilirubin (µmol/l) Prothrombin time (s) | Normal <17 | 20–50 18–20 | >50 >20 |
| Ascites | None | Slight | Moderate |
| Encephalopathy | None | Grade 1–2 | Grade 3–4 |

### Hepatic encephalopathy grading

| Grade 1 | Mild confusion |
|---|---|
| Grade 2 | Drowsiness; inappropriate behaviour |
| Grade 3 | Somnolent (but rousable); confusion |
| Grade 4 | Coma |

# Investigating liver disease

Should be guided by the results of a thorough history and examination, and initially followed by simple investigations:

- **Blood:**
  - Plasma biochemistry (renal and liver function tests)
  - Full blood count (clotting, haemoglobin and mean corpuscular volume [MCV])
  - Random alcohol if suspected
  - Tumour markers: $\alpha$-fetoprotein (AFP), carcinoembryonic antigen (CEA)
  - Hepatitis B surface and core antigens, hepatitis C
  - Ferritin (haemochromatosis – iron)

- Caeruloplasmin (Wilson's disease – copper)
- Serum liver autoantibodies and immunoglobulins
- Cholesterol and triglycerides
- **Urine**
- **Ultrasonography:**
  - Bile duct sizes and gallstones
  - Tumour (intrahepatic/extrahepatic)
  - Liver size
  - Splenomegaly
  - Patency of portal vessels
- **Liver biopsy:**
  - For non-malignant parenchymal disease
  - May be performed percutaneously under local anaesthetic, radiologically via transjugular approach, laparoscopically or at open laparotomy
  - Complications include bleeding (haemoperitoneum or haemobilia), fistula formation, pneumothorax and damage to other organs
- **Other investigations:**
  - ERCP
  - MRCP
  - Percutaneous hepatic cholangiography
  - HIDA scanning
  - Hepatic angiography

## 4.6    Cirrhosis

 **In a nutshell ...**

Cirrhosis is a group of conditions in which there is chronic hepatic injury with healing occurring by regeneration and fibrosis. This fibrosis leads to further cell damage and destruction of hepatic architecture, progressing to liver failure and portal hypertension. There is an increased risk of HCC, particularly on a background of viral hepatitis.

The causes are many and some are listed in the box 'Causes of cirrhosis'. The most common are alcohol, viral hepatitis, primary biliary cirrhosis and, in the tropics, schistosomiasis and secondary biliary cirrhosis:

- **Primary biliary cirrhosis** is a distinct clinical entity thought to have an autoimmune pathogenesis. It occurs mainly in middle-aged women
- **Secondary biliary cirrhosis** is caused by damage or compression of the bile duct, leading to recurrent cholangitis
- **Schistosomiasis** is very common in South America, Africa, the Middle East and East Asia. It is caused by *Schistosoma* species, a parasite carried in freshwater snails, and infestation causes fibrosis, leading to portal hypertension but not a true cirrhosis

### Causes of cirrhosis (common causes*)
**Infection**
- Hepatitis B and C*
- Schistosomiasis

**Toxins**
- Alcoholic liver disease*
- Drug induced

**Autoimmune/primary**
- Primary biliary cirrhosis*
- Primary sclerosing cholangitis
- Chronic active hepatitis

**Metabolic**
- Haemochromatosis
- Wilson's disease
- $\alpha_1$-Antitrypsin deficiency
- Galactosaemia
- Type IV glycogen storage disease
- NASH (eg obesity, total parenteral nutrition [TPN])

**Other**
- Sarcoidosis

Cirrhosis can be suggested by ultrasonography and CT but the diagnosis can be confirmed only on histology.

The main complications of cirrhosis are liver failure, ascites and portal hypertension. Abdominal surgery is very hazardous in a patient with cirrhosis as surgery leads to an increased risk of hepatic decompensation with ascites, haemorrhage and renal failure.

## 4.7 Liver masses

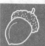

### In a nutshell ...

**Differential diagnosis of a liver mass**
**Benign** (common – 1% of all postmortem examinations)
Adenoma
Focal nodular hyperplasia
Haemangioma
Cyst (simple/parasitic) – see Section 4.10
Abscess (pyogenic/amoebic) – see Section 4.9
**Malignant**
Primary HCC
Intrahepatic cholangiocarcinoma
Sarcomas
Secondary metastatic disease (most common malignancy)

## Benign liver tumours

### Adenoma
- Seen in young women; associated with use of the oral contraceptive pill
- Presents incidentally or with bleeding after rupture (30%)

- May be single or multiple, of variable size (1–30 cm)
- Treatment is removal if it is expanding or there is doubt about the diagnosis

### Focal nodular hyperplasia
- Also seen in young women
- Discrete subcapsular lesions that have an obscure aetiology and are usually symptomless
- Growth can cause pain

### Haemangioma
- Benign mesenchymal tumours
- Can cause bleeding or be mistaken for metastatic tumours

## Primary malignant liver tumours

### Hepatocellular carcinoma
- Also known as hepatoma, HCC is rare in the UK and the USA but common worldwide
- May arise spontaneously or more frequently in cirrhotic livers, usually due to viral hepatitis or alcohol
- The tumour forms a large solitary mass or multiple foci throughout the liver
- The clinical picture occurs late: hepatomegaly, bloodstained ascites, rapid progression and distant metastasis
- Prognosis and treatment options depend on the number and distribution of tumours and whether spontaneous or on a cirrhotic background. People with cirrhosis are not usually resected due to risks of decompensation of the residual liver tissue. Spontaneous (non-cirrhotic) HCC can be surgically resected

- Large tumours from either background can undergo chemoembolisation of their arterial supply before resection or liver transplantation. Primary hepatomas have been treated with 5-fluorouracil and doxorubicin with some success
- Prognosis is poor in spontaneous cases but better in those tumours that arise on a background of cirrhosis

## Cholangiocarcinoma

- Much less common than HCC
- Cholangiocarcinoma is an adenocarcinoma arising from the biliary tree
- May be intrahepatic or extrahepatic
- Predisposing factors include the following:
  - Primary sclerosing cholangitis (PSC)
  - Anabolic steroids
  - Liver fluke infestation
  - Thorotrast radiological contrast administration
- Usually presents with jaundice
- Very poor prognosis; minimal response to chemotherapy; can occasionally be resected
- Very occasionally may be a candidate for liver transplantation (if entirely intrahepatic in nature with no evidence of extrahepatic disease, eg on a background of PSC)

## Angiosarcoma

- A rare, malignant vascular tumour
- Can be either primary or secondary spread from the spleen
- Predisposing factors include: cirrhosis, arsenic, vinyl chloride and anabolic steroids

## Metastatic disease of the liver

Metastases are by far the most common liver neoplasm. The metastatic deposits can arise by portal or systemic blood, or direct spread.

---

**Cancers that commonly metastasise to liver**
- Colorectal
- Pancreatic
- Cholangiocarcinoma
- Bronchus
- Breast
- Melanoma
- Renal
- Neuroendocrine, including carcinoid

---

### Clinical presentation of liver metastases
- **Early** (often asymptomatic):
  - Found on staging an identified primary
  - Incidental finding on imaging for another pathology
- **Late:**
  - Hepatomegaly (large, hard, irregular liver)
  - Jaundice (must have significant volume of liver replaced by tumour or an element of intrahepatic duct compression to develop jaundice)
  - Hepatorenal syndrome and renal failure
  - Portal vein obstruction producing oesophageal varices and ascites
  - IVC obstruction producing leg oedema

### Synchronous/metachronous metastases
- Synchronous metastases are found at the same time as the primary tumour
- Metachronous metastases develop at a later stage after resection of the primary (may be years later)
- In general, multiple and synchronous metastases have a worse prognosis than solitary and metachronous metastases

CHAPTER 1

Many are now found early due to investigations at the time of presentation and radiological surveillance after resection of the primary tumour

### Poor prognostic factors for liver metastases

- Bilobar disease
- Large numbers of metastases
- Venous invasion (portal or hepatic)
- Absence of a pseudocapsule
- Extrahepatic disease
- Recurrence and re-resection

The management of colorectal metastases is covered in Section 8, Large bowel.

## Management of liver neoplasms

### In a nutshell ...

Each case should be assessed individually for type of tumour, distribution of disease, total tumour burden, presence of extrahepatic disease and ability to withstand major surgery. Many will require a combination of techniques. Options for the management of neoplastic liver disease include the following:

- Surgical resection
- Radiofrequency- or cryoablation
- Chemoembolisation
- Chemotherapy
- Transplantation

## Surgical resection

- Surgery may be considered in primary HCC and cholangiocarcinoma, and in metastases from colorectal, renal and neuroendocrine primaries
- Resection may be combined with another modality (eg preoperative chemotherapy for multiple small lesions; right-sided resection plus radiofrequency ablation of solitary tumour in the remaining lobe)
- Distribution of the lesions is more important than the total number. Resection is based on the pattern of liver segmentation
- Adequate margins are approximately 1 cm of surrounding liver tissue but increasingly surgeons are attempting more radical resection and this may not be adequate for tumour clearance
- Staged resection can be performed to avoid liver insufficiency in large resections
- Intraoperative vascular occlusion techniques allow excision of lesions lying near the vena cava

## Ablation techniques

- These involve inserting an ultrasound-guided needle into the centre of the tumour and ablating it with alcohol, freezing or heating by radiofrequency
- They can be performed percutaneously, laparoscopically or at open surgery
- Ablation is indicated for small lesions, as an adjunct to surgery and in frail patients who will not tolerate major resection

## Hepatic artery chemoembolisation

- Infusion of chemotherapeutic agents through the hepatic artery is a technique predominantly used for HCC and malignant neuroendocrine tumours
- Portal vein embolisation can decrease the likelihood of liver insufficiency occurring after extensive liver resection by inducing hypertrophy in the future remnant liver. This may be used in hilar cholangiocarcinoma
- Other therapies are experimental or used as part of a multimodality treatment
- Brachytherapy, in which radioactive implants are placed at laparotomy, has been used to decrease recurrence in selected patients after surgical resection. Tumour-specific immunotherapy regimens have been attempted in advanced disease that is resistant to conventional therapy, especially renal carcinoma

## 4.8   Liver infections

### In a nutshell ...

**Liver abscesses**
- Portal
- Biliary
- Trauma
- Direct extension
- Viral hepatitis
- Hepatitis A
- Hepatitis B
- Hepatitis C

## Liver abscesses

### Sources of infection

- Arterial: as part of a general septicaemia (unusual)

- Portal: from an area of suppuration drained by the portal vein, eg appendicitis can result in portal pyaemia
- Biliary: resulting from an ascending cholangitis
- Spread: from adjacent infection such as subphrenic abscess or acute cholecystitis
- Trauma: followed by secondary haemorrhage and added infection

### Clinical features of liver abscesses

- High swinging temperature and rigors
- Abdominal pain and a tender palpable liver
- Jaundice

### Investigating liver abscesses

- Chest radiograph shows:
  - Elevation of the right diaphragm
  - Right pleural effusion
  - Basal pulmonary collapse
  - Fluid level below the diaphragm
- Ultrasonography is usually diagnostic
- CT scans and isotope liver scans may also be helpful
- Blood cultures should be taken before antibiotics are commenced

### Management of liver abscesses

- **Antibiotic treatment** should be targeted to the causative organism
- If a localised abscess is identified on ultrasonography, **percutaneous aspiration under ultrasound control** is often successful
- **Surgery** is indicated if the abscess ruptures, causing peritonitis, or if percutaneous aspiration fails
- **Laparoscopy** can be useful both diagnostically and therapeutically
- Liver abscesses secondary to severe cholangitis require urgent bile duct

drainage, usually by **endoscopic sphincterotomy**

- Abscesses due to *Entamoeba histolytica* are a special type of portal infection. An enzyme produced by the protozon destroys the liver tissue. Metronidazole is the antibiotic of choice

## Viral hepatitis

### In a nutshell ...

This is essentially a medical condition, but its surgical implications include the following:

- Sequelae such as HCC, cirrhosis, portal hypertension
- Risks of transmission to the surgeon
- Differential diagnosis of jaundice

### Causative agents

There are several separate viral agents (hepatitis viruses A–G):

- **Hepatitis A** spreads by the faecal–oral route and by nasal droplets. Children and young adults are usually affected
- **Hepatitis B** is transmitted by inoculation with contaminated syringes or by transfusion of blood or plasma from an infected patient. The blood in these individuals contains the Australia antigen and is highly infective. Any age may be infected
- **Hepatitis C** – similar transmission to type B, but risks of infection are much higher

### Clinical features of viral hepatitis

Both hepatitis B and C can lead to chronic infection, cirrhosis and tumour formation. There is a prodromal period of a few days with anorexia, fever, malaise and vomiting. The patient becomes jaundiced, with dark urine. The liver is palpable and tender.

### Treatment of viral hepatitis

Supportive, with rest and avoidance of alcohol.

### Complications of viral hepatitis

- Hepatic failure
- Massive liver necrosis (rare)
- Relapse
- Post-hepatic cirrhosis

Hepatitis viruses are a risk for hospital workers, who should all be immunised against hepatitis B.

## 4.9   Liver cysts

### Simple cysts

- Simple cysts are solitary or multiple
- They are usually asymptomatic and rarely need intervention. They are commonly found incidentally or (rarely) cause hepatomegaly
- Their main clinical implication is differentiation from more significant liver pathology. Occasionally they may require de-roofing surgically if very large or recurrent

### Polycystic liver disease

- Polycystic liver disease is often associated with adult polycystic disease of the kidneys and pancreas
- Liver function is compromised in only a few cases, and the renal disease complicating the associated polycystic kidney disease is more often the clinical problem

- Most patients are asymptomatic, but hepatomegaly, bleeding into the cysts or obstruction of the biliary or venous outflow may cause problems
- Surgical treatment is less successful than in solitary cysts and is reserved for symptomatic patients

## Hydatid cysts

These occur as a result of liver infestation with *Echinococcus granulosus*, a parasite of dogs, sheep and humans that is endemic in China and the Mediterranean.

### Clinical features of hydatid cysts

Symptoms are often non-specific and include pain, incidental findings or jaundice.

The active cyst may:
- Rupture into the peritoneal cavity, alimentary canal or biliary tree, which can result in an anaphylactic reaction
- Undergo supra-added infection with bacteria
- Press on intrahepatic bile ducts and produce obstructive jaundice

### Investigating hydatid cysts

- Ultrasonography or CT scan
- Serological tests specific for hydatid antibodies
- Eosinophilia and plain abdominal radiographs are not diagnostic but may arouse suspicion

### Management of hydatid cysts

- Treatment with albendazole may shrink or cure the cysts
- Calcified asymptomatic cysts are usually dead and should be left alone

- Enlarging subcapsular cysts are likely to cause complications and may need surgery
- At laparotomy, aspiration with or without cyst excision is recommended but recurrence is likely. Care should be taken not to spill the contents into the abdomen

## 4.10 The spleen

 **In a nutshell ...**

The spleen is the largest lymphoid organ and was previously considered dispensable, with splenectomy being the only procedure for management of its disorders until the 1970s. As awareness of its functions and of the side effects of removal have become known, the management of splenic disease/trauma has become more conservative.

## Functions of the spleen

- **Immune functions:** antigen processing, IgM and opsonin production
- **Filtering:** macrophages are important in removing cellular and non-cellular material, including bacteria such as pneumococci and defective or old red cells and platelets
- **Haematopoiesis:** in the fetus, and later if demand exceeds marrow capacity
- **Iron re-utilisation**
- **Platelet pooling**

## Anatomy of the spleen

- The numbers 1, 3, 5, 7, 9, and 11 summarise the anatomy of the spleen – it measures 1 × 3 × 5 inches, weighs 7 oz and lies between ribs 9 and 11 in the left hypochondrium
- Its long axis lies along the tenth rib

- On its medial aspect the kidney leaves an impression posterior to the hilum with the posterior leaf of the greater omentum (the lienorenal ligament) passing from the hilum to the kidney. The tail of the pancreas lies within the lienorenal ligament. The anterior leaf (gastrosplenic ligament) joins the hilum to the greater curve of the stomach, the area between the leaves forming part of the boundary of the lesser sac
- There is a notch in the anterior surface of the spleen, left over from its embryonic development
- As a pathological spleen enlarges, it grows towards the umbilicus, and needs to double in size before it extends beyond the costal margin and becomes palpable
- The blood supply is from the splenic artery (from the coeliac axis) which enters the hilum via the lienorenal ligament and divides into smaller segmental branches (up to four). Venous drainage is via the splenic vein to the portal system
- 'Accessory spleens' (splenunculi) occur in 1 in 10 people and result from the failure of fusion of embryonic segments. They are usually found along the splenic vessels or peritoneal attachments and may be multiple

## Trauma to the spleen

This is usually due to blunt trauma to the abdomen or lower ribs. Injury may occur due to more minor trauma in children (caused by the proportionally larger spleen and less robust rib cage) or in adults with splenomegaly. The main signs are those of haemorrhage and may follow four presentations.

### Injury involving the capsule with continuing bleeding

Usually presents with evidence of haemorrhage that continues to be unstable despite resuscitation.

### Extracapsular rupture

A small tear may initially be closed by adherent omentum or clot. Patients initially have evidence of haemorrhage and often left shoulder-tip referred pain (Kehr's sign). A period of recovery follows, lasting hours to days. There may then be a second more profound bleed, with collapse, shock and generalised abdominal pain.

### Intracapsular rupture leading to haematoma formation

This is initially contained due to the shock, but as blood pressure is elevated further bleeding occurs, leading to intraperitoneal rupture.

### Intracapsular rupture

With haematoma formation only, presents with pain and minimal evidence of blood loss.

### Investigating splenic trauma

If the patient is haemodynamically stable the possibility of splenic injury can be assessed with ultrasonography or CT scanning (both have diagnostic accuracy of >90%) although most trauma protocols recommend CT to exclude intra-abdominal injuries.

If the patient is unstable with obvious abdominal injuries, laparotomy is indicated after initial attempts at resuscitation.

Diagnostic peritoneal lavage is indicated only if there is doubt as to the cause of hypovolaemia (eg in unconscious, multiply injured patients). Some argue that it has no role, because less invasive investigations can be carried out if the patient is stable and immediate laparotomy is indicated if the patient is unstable.

## Management of splenic trauma

### Conservative management

- Non-surgical management can be cautiously undertaken if there is absence of progressive haemorrhage (<4-unit transfusion in 48 hours) and no other intra-abdominal injuries
- Non-surgical treatment is recommended in children and, where possible, bleeding will usually stop within 12 hours
- Patients should be closely observed for at least 7–10 days due to the risk of secondary rupture

### Surgical management

- Where laparotomy is required every effort should be made to conserve the spleen, with experience showing that it is possible to conserve enough to be of value in 30–50% of cases
- Small tears may be managed by pressure and haemostatic agents, and fractures can be sutured with large liver needles
- Arterial branch ligation may be of benefit and may aid partial splenectomy
- Multiple fractures may be treated by omental wrapping or enclosing the spleen within a mesh bag
- Occasionally total splenectomy is required, sometimes combined with implantation of splenic fragments within the omentum. There is evidence that these fragments function, though their efficacy is unknown

## Splenomegaly

The normal spleen weighs 200 g, but this can be massively increased by various pathological processes. Gradual splenomegaly may develop with minimal symptoms, but sudden enlargement usually causes upper abdominal discomfort. Massive enlargement may compress the stomach, leading to early satiety/weight loss.

## Causes of splenomegaly

**Infection**
*Bacterial*
- Typhoid
- Typhus
- TB
- Septicaemia
*Spirochaetal*
- Syphilis
- Leptospirosis
*Viral*
- Glandular fever
*Protozoal*
- Malaria
- Kala-azar

**Cellular infiltration**
- Amyloidosis
- Gaucher's disease

**Collagen diseases**
- Felty syndrome
- Still's disease

**Autoimmune disorders**
- Rheumatoid arthritis
- Systemic lupus erythematosus

**Haemolytic anaemias**

**Cellular proliferation**
- Myeloid and lymphatic leukaemia*
- Pernicious anaemia
- Polycythaemia rubra vera
- Spherocytosis
- Thrombocytopenic purpura
- Myelosclerosis

**Congestion**
- Portal hypertension usually due to cirrhosis*
- Hepatic vein obstruction
- Chronic congestive heart failure

**Infarction**
*Emboli from*
- Bacterial endocarditis
- Left atrium in atrial fibrillation
- Left ventricle after myocardial infarction
*Splenic artery or vein thrombosis*
- Polycythaemia
- Retroperitoneal malignancy

**Space-occupying lesions**
- Cysts
- True solitary cysts
- Polycystic disease
- Hydatid cysts
*Angioma*
*Lymphosarcoma*
*Lymphoma*

*Most common causes.

**Hypersplenism** is defined as splenomegaly with associated anaemia, leucopenia or thrombocytopenia. There is compensatory bone marrow hyperplasia.

# Splenectomy

## Indications for splenectomy

### Trauma
- Immediate
- Iatrogenic
- Delayed
- Spontaneous rupture

### Neoplastic/staging
- Lymphomas including Hodgkin's
- Chronic leukaemias
- Massive haemangiomas (rare)
- Secondary carcinomas (rare)
- With gastrectomy for cancer
- With distal pancreatectomy
- Unexplained splenomegaly

### Hypersplenism
- Haemolytic anaemias
- Immune thrombocytopenic purpura
- Neutropenia
- Tropical splenomegaly
- Myelosclerosis

### Portal decompression
- Bleeding varices with splenic vein thrombosis
- Conventional splenorenal shunt

### Infections
- TB
- Hydatid cyst
- Splenic abscess

### Other
- Splenic artery aneurysm
- Non-parasitic splenic cyst
- Torsion of wandering spleen

 Principles of splenectomy

### Indications
As described in the box 'Indications for splenectomy' above.

### Preop preparation
- Correct anaemia and clotting. Platelet count can be improved with preoperative steroids or immunoglobulin therapy
- Treat any infection
- Immunise patient against encapsulated bacteria (pneumococci, meningococci and *Haemophilus influenzae* b 2–4 weeks preoperatively
- Cross-match 4 units. Early discussion with transfusion department is useful if there is a history of repeated transfusions as they may have autoantibodies
- For emergency splenectomy the preoperative preparation is resuscitation as outlined above

## Principles of technique
### For elective open splenectomy
**Incision:**
- Upper midline or subcostal or thoracoabdominal
- Early ligation of splenic artery alongside body of pancreas
- Mobilisation of spleen by division of short gastrics
- Splenic artery divided at hilum
- Splenic vein divided next
- Beware of greater curve of stomach, pancreatic tail and left colic flexure
- Search for splenunculi that could cause recurrence

### For laparoscopic splenectomy
**Indications:**
- Small or moderate non-malignant spleens (eg ITP)
- Spleen is morcellated and sucked out via port so is not suitable for histological assessment of cancer

### For emergency splenectomy
- Pack all quadrants to control bleeding
- If bleeding is controlled, inspect spleen to see if it is salvageable
- If bleeding is profuse, deliver spleen immediately to wound by digitally dissecting the lienorenal ligament
- The vessels may be ligated individually or en masse and the spleen removed

### Postop
- Normal changes seen in the blood after splenectomy include:
  - A transient neutrophilia
  - Increased size and number of platelets
  - Presence of nucleated red cells and target cells

### Complications of splenectomy
- Intraoperative haemorrhage
- Gastric/colonic perforation
- Pancreatic trauma leading to wound dehiscence/pancreatic fistula
- Postoperative haematoma that can become infected, leading to abscess formation
- Increased risk of sepsis, including overwhelming post-splenectomy infection

### Overwhelming post-splenectomy infection
Caused by infection by one of the encapsulated organisms normally destroyed by the spleen – *Streptococcus pneumoniae*, *Neisseria meningitidis* or *Haemophilus influenzae*.
- Infection with these pathogens can lead to overwhelming sepsis with mortality rate of 50–90%
- Incidence is approximately 2% in children and 0.5% in adults; highest incidence is in those undergoing splenectomy for lymphoreticular malignancy
- All patients should have prophylaxis following splenectomy

### Current guidelines for post-splenectomy prophylaxis
- Risk explained to patient, with card to carry
- Immunisation with Pneumovax, Hib and meningococcal vaccines; remember boosters at 5–10 years
- Antibiotic prophylaxis with amoxicillin (erythromycin if allergic) until age 15 only – NOT lifelong
- Patients should commence amoxicillin at first sign of febrile illness
- Malaria prophylaxis if required

# SECTION 5

# Biliary tree and pancreas

## 5.1 Anatomy of the biliary system

### In a nutshell ...

The biliary system is concerned with collecting bile from the liver (where it is manufactured), storing it and transporting it to the duodenum, where it enters the GI tract. The anatomy reflects this function.

Bile capillaries lying in the portal triads at the corners of the liver lobules collect bile and drain it into branches of the hepatic duct.

The right and left hepatic ducts fuse in the porta hepatis to form the 4-cm-long **common hepatic duct**.

This joins with the cystic duct (also 4 cm long, but does vary hugely), draining the gallbladder, to form the common bile duct (10 cm long).

The **common bile duct** (CBD) commences about 4 cm above the duodenum then passes behind it to open at a papilla on the medial aspect of the second part of the duodenum. The CBD usually joins the main pancreatic duct in a dilated common vestibule (the ampulla of Vater).

Occasionally, the bile and the pancreatic ducts open separately into the duodenum.

The opening of the ampulla is guarded by the muscular sphincter of Oddi. The structures entering and leaving the hilum of the liver are arranged in the free edge of the lesser omentum, forming the anterior boundary of the foramen of Winslow (see Figure 1.30 in Section 4, Liver and spleen).

### The gallbladder

The gallbladder normally holds 50 ml bile. It functions as a bile reservoir and concentrator. It lies in a fossa separating the right and quadrate lobes of the liver. The duodenum and transverse colon lie inferior to it and an inflamed gallbladder can ulcerate or fistulate into either of these structures.

The muscular sac is divided into a fundus, a body and a neck that opens into the cystic duct via a dilated Hartmann's pouch (Figure 1.35). Gallstones commonly lodge in Hartmann's pouch, which may not be present in a non-pathological gallbladder.

The mucosa of the biliary tree is lined by columnar cells and bears mucus-secreting glands. The gallbladder is supplied by the cystic artery, which is usually a branch of the right hepatic artery. The cystic artery lies in a triangle (**Calot's triangle**) formed by the inferior border of the liver, the cystic duct and the common hepatic duct. Gangrene of the gallbladder is rare because, even if the cystic artery becomes thrombosed in acute cholecystitis, there is a rich secondary blood supply coming in from the liver bed. Gangrene may occur in the unusual event of a gallbladder on an abnormally long mesentery undergoing torsion, which will destroy both its sources of blood supply.

There is no vein accompanying the cystic artery. Small veins pass from the gallbladder through its bed directly into the liver.

Errors in gallbladder surgery are frequently the result of failure to appreciate the variations in the anatomy of the biliary system (Figure 1.35). This is why it is so important to identify the structures of Calot's triangle before dividing any structure. The gallbladder and ducts are subject to numerous anatomical variations that are best understood by considering their embryological development. During development of the biliary tree, the ducts and gallbladder are temporarily solid due to proliferation of the epithelial lining.

If recanalisation fails to occur, this can lead to atresia of the gallbladder, bile duct or hepatic duct. Most commonly, biliary atresia occurs at the level of the porta hepatis.

## Embryological development of the liver, pancreas and biliary tree

In week 3 of gestation the liver bud appears as an outgrowth of endodermal epithelium at the distal end of the foregut (Figure 1.36). The hepatic cell strands of the liver bud penetrate the mesodermal septum transversum that lies between the pericardial cavity and the stalk of the yolk sac.

The connection between the liver bud and the foregut (the bile duct) gives rise to a ventral outgrowth which will form the gallbladder and cystic duct.

The epithelial liver cords mingle with the vitelline and umbilical veins, forming the hepatic sinusoids. They also form the parenchyma and lining of the biliary duct.

The mesoderm of the septum transversum forms the haematopoietic cells, Kupffer cells and connective tissue cells.

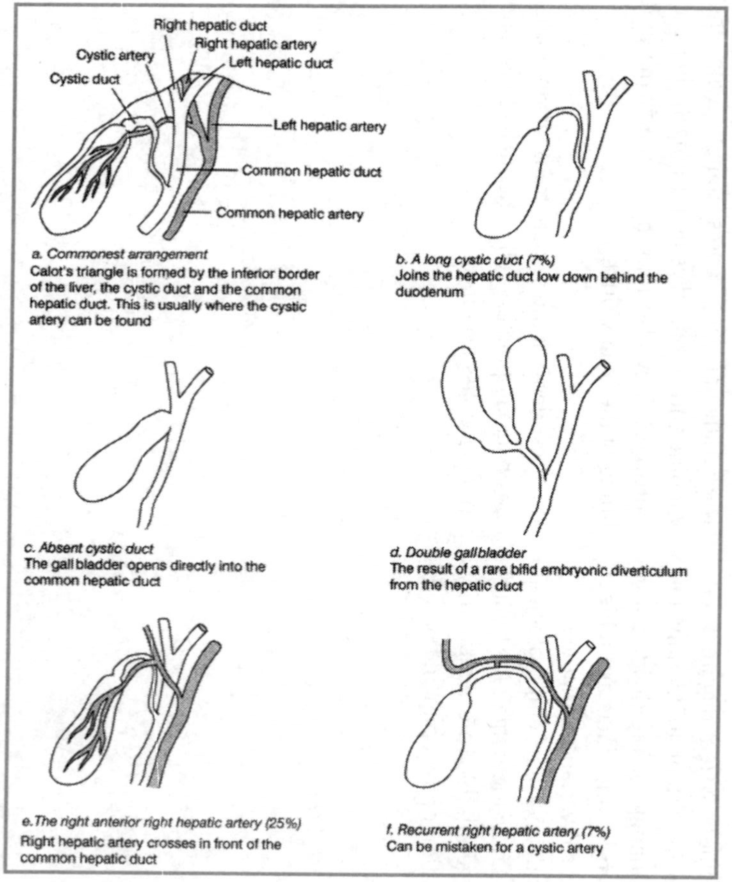

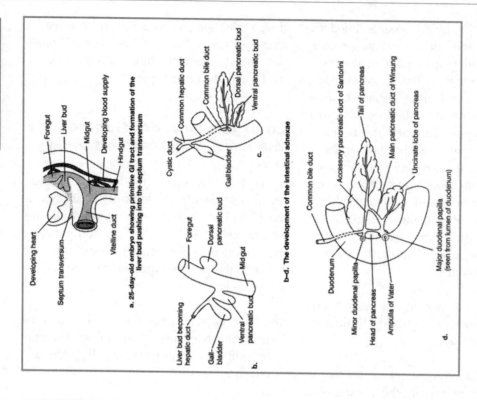

Figure 1.36 Embryology of the pancreas and biliary tree

**a. 25-day-old embryo showing primitive GI tract and formation of the liver bud pushing into the septum transversum**

- Developing heart
- Septum transversum
- Foregut
- Liver bud
- Midgut
- Developing blood supply
- Hindgut
- Vitelline duct

**b.**
- Liver bud becoming hepatic duct
- Foregut
- Dorsal pancreatic bud
- Gall-bladder
- Ventral pancreatic bud
- Mid gut

**c.**
- Cystic duct
- Common hepatic duct
- Common bile duct
- Dorsal pancreatic bud
- Gall bladder
- Ventral pancreatic bud

**d.**
- Common bile duct
- Accessory pancreatic duct of Santorini
- Tail of pancreas
- Main pancreatic duct of Wirsung
- Uncinate lobe of pancreas
- Major duodenal papilla (seen from lumen of duodenum)
- Ampulla of Vater
- Head of pancreas
- Minor duodenal papilla
- Duodenum

**b–d. The development of the intestinal adnexae**

Figure 1.35 Variations in biliary anatomy

**a. Commonest arrangement**
Calot's triangle is formed by the inferior border of the liver, the cystic duct and the common hepatic duct. This is usually where the cystic artery can be found
- Right hepatic duct
- Right hepatic artery
- Left hepatic artery
- Left hepatic duct
- Common hepatic duct
- Common hepatic artery
- Cystic artery
- Cystic duct

**b. A long cystic duct (7%)**
Joins the hepatic duct low down behind the duodenum

**c. Absent cystic duct**
The gall bladder opens directly into the common hepatic duct

**d. Double gall bladder**
The result of a rare bifid embryonic diverticulum from the hepatic duct

**e.The right anterior right hepatic artery (25%)**
Right hepatic artery crosses in front of the common hepatic duct

**f. Recurrent right hepatic artery (7%)**
Can be mistaken for a cystic artery

# 5.2 Physiology of the biliary tree

**In a nutshell ...**

Bile consists of:

**Substances being excreted:**
- Bile pigments (from red blood cells)
- Cholesterol (from fat metabolism)
- Fat-soluble drugs and toxins

**Substances being secreted to aid digestion:**
- Bile salts (to emulsify fats)
- Inorganic salts including bicarbonate ions (to neutralise duodenal contents)
- Lecithin (to aid solubility of cholesterol)
- Water

Bile is produced in the liver under the control of a negative feedback mechanism. It is stored in the gallbladder and secreted under the control of hormones (CCK, secretin) and nerves (vagus, cephalic reflex).

## Composition and function of bile

### Bilirubin

Bilirubin is a bile pigment that is a byproduct of the degradation of the haem groups of haemoglobin. Bilirubin is conjugated by the liver so that it can be excreted in the faeces as stercobilinogen and in the urine as urobilin. Bilirubin blood levels may rise if the breakdown of red blood cells increases (haemolysis), there is liver failure or the flow of bile is interrupted (in obstructive jaundice from gallstones or ampullary tumours). Bile pigments that are not excreted are recirculated to the liver (Figure 1.37).

### Cholesterol

Cholesterol is excreted in the bile and needs both lecithin and bile salts to solubilise it enough to be transported. Failure to solubilise all the cholesterol predisposes to gallstone formation. The bile is the only route of excretion of cholesterol so the liver is responsible for the regulation of serum cholesterol.

### Bile salts (or acids)

Bile salts are mostly cholic acid and chenode-oxycholic acid. These are steroid molecules which act as detergents and emulsify fats in the duodenum so that they can be absorbed. They make up 50% of the dry weight of bile. They are synthesised from cholesterol by hepatocytes by conjugating it with glycine and taurine; 4 g/day are secreted, mostly to be reabsorbed in the ileum (for a summary see box 'The enterohepatic circulation of bile salts' and Figure 1.38).

Bile salts consist of a fat-soluble hydrocarbon ring with several charged groups around it so that it can mix with fat and water. In clusters called micelles they increase fat solubility by emulsifying the fat, leading to its easier digestion by water-soluble lipases to glycerol, glycerides and fatty acids. Micelles also help to transport

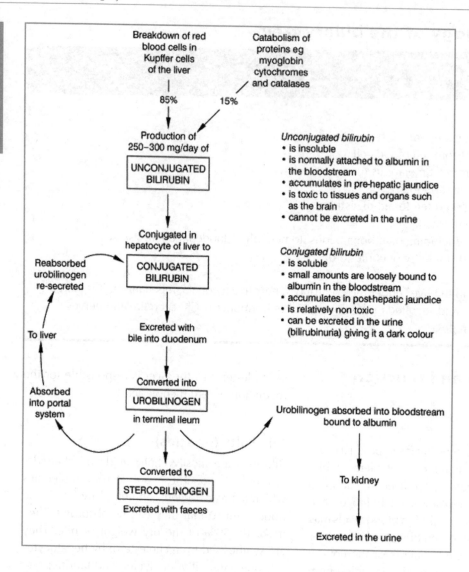

Figure 1.37
Bilirubin
metabolism

*Unconjugated bilirubin*
• is insoluble
• is normally attached to albumin in the bloodstream
• accumulates in pre-hepatic jaundice
• is toxic to tissues and organs such as the brain
• cannot be excreted in the urine

*Conjugated bilirubin*
• is soluble
• small amounts are loosely bound to albumin in the bloodstream
• accumulates in post-hepatic jaundice
• is relatively non toxic
• can be excreted in the urine (bilirubinuria) giving it a dark colour

cholesterol out of the liver so that it can be excreted into the gut.

### Inorganic salts

These are mostly sodium chloride and sodium bicarbonate. The concentration of bicarbonate ions is high (alkaline) and allows for the neutralisation of gastric acid in the duodenum. This enables the appropriate digestive enzymes to function.

### Lecithin

This increases the solubility of cholesterol, allowing more to be excreted with the help of the bile salts.

### Water

Ninety-seven per cent of bile is water. Some is reabsorbed in the gallbladder, which concentrates bile.

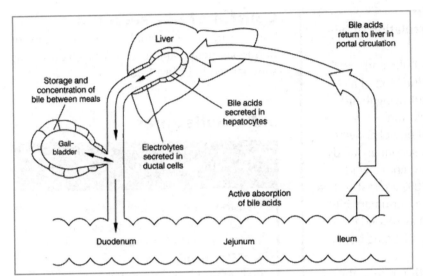

Figure 1.38
Enterohepatic
circulation of bile

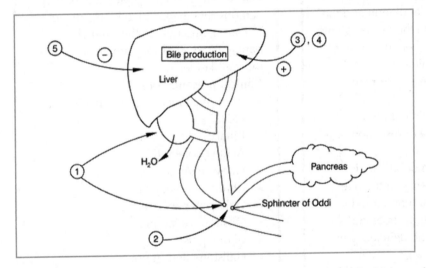

Figure 1.39 Control of
gallbladder secretion

(1) **CCK:**
- Contracts the gallbladder
- Opens the sphincter of Oddi
- Is secreted in response to acid, calcium, fatty acids and amino acids in the duodenum
- Injection can be given during an HIDA scan to assess gallbladder function

(2) **Cephalic reflex:** opens sphincter of Oddi in response to food in mouth

(3) **Secretin:** increases hepatic bile production; increases water and bicarbonate content

(4) **Vagus:** acts as secretin; stimulated in the cephalic and gastric stages of digestion

(5) **Level of bile salts:** high level of recirculated bile salts decreases new production in the liver (feedback mechanism)

### The enterohepatic circulation of bile salts

- Primary bile acids (cholic and chenodeoxycholic) function to aid solubility of lipids, allowing their absorption in the jejunum
- Bacteria in the small bowel convert the primary acids to secondary acids (lithocholic and deoxycholic acid)
- Of these acids 80–90% are reabsorbed in the terminal ileum as primary bile salts, or in the colon as secondary bile salts, with 10–20% being newly synthesised daily
- Reabsorbed bile acids return to the liver via the portal circulation and the remainder are lost in the faeces, giving them a dark colour (hence pale stools in obstructive jaundice)
- Recirculation of these acids may occur twice per meal
- The enterohepatic circulation is disrupted by disease or resection of the terminal ileum
- Failure of resorption of bile acids leads to their deficiency in the bile, causing steatorrhoea (undigested fat in the stool – so that stools float and are looser than usual) and deficiency in fat-soluble vitamins
- High concentrations of excreted bile acids in the colon cause diarrhoea

## Control of bile secretion

This involves a complex combination of hormonal, neural and feedback mechanisms, as summarised in Figure 1.39.

## 5.3 Gallstones

 **In a nutshell ...**

Gallstones are common:
- 20% of gallstones are cholesterol
- 5% are bile pigment stones
- 75% are mixed

Gallstones can be asymptomatic or they can obstruct the gallbladder by impacting in Hartmann's pouch, the CBD or pancreatic duct as they are passed out of the gallbladder.

**Clinical presentations**
- Asymptomatic/incidental finding (20%)
- Biliary colic
- Acute cholecystitis
- Empyema/mucocele
- Chronic cholecystitis
- Gallstone pancreatitis
- Obstructive jaundice
- Cholangitis
- Gallstone ileus (rare)

**Investigations**
- LFTs, ultrasonography and MRCP ± ERCP

**Treatments**
- Preop ERCP ± sphincterotomy ± stone extraction
- Cholecystectomy (open or laparoscopic) ± bile duct exploration and clearance

# Epidemiology of gallstones

- 10% of British women in their 40s have gallstones
- Affects more women than men (2F:1M)
- Incidence increases with age and certain nationalities (eg Mediterranean)
- There is a genetic predisposition, so ask about family history

The saying that gallstones occur in fair, fat, fertile females of 40 is slightly inaccurate, but can be a useful reminder of the typical patient.

# Pathogenesis of gallstones

There are three common varieties of gallstones:

- **Cholesterol stones (20%):**
  - Occur as solitary stones, in pairs or as multiple mulberry stones
  - May be associated with high cholesterol, pregnancy, diabetes and the oral contraceptive pill (OCP)
  - The 'strawberry gallbladder' is cholesterosis of the gallbladder with a mucosa studded with submucous collections of cholesterol
  - Bile salts and phospholipids hold insoluble cholesterol in suspension so a decrease of either increases gallstones
- **Bile pigment stones (5%):**
  - Small, black, irregular, multiple, gritty and fragile stones
  - Occur in excess of circulating bile pigment (eg haemolytic anaemia)
- **Mixed stones (75%):**
  - Multiple and faceted, and may collect in similarly sized groups (generations of stones)
  - They originate because of precipitation of cholesterol

# Other predisposing factors

- Excess mucus production by the gallbladder
- Infection of the biliary tract
- Metabolic factors
- Stasis (eg in pregnancy)
- Ileal dysfunction (prevents reabsorption of bile)
- Obesity, hypertriglyceridaemia
- Chronic liver disease

# Pathological effects of gallstones

## Silent gallstones

Twenty per cent of patients with gallstones are asymptomatic.

## Obstruction of the gallbladder

A gallstone may become impacted in Hartmann's pouch, causing an obstruction to the exit of the gallbladder. This causes a chemical cholecystitis because water is absorbed from the bile in the gallbladder and it becomes concentrated. This is usually sterile at first but then it may become secondarily infected from organisms secreted from the liver into the bile stream. Occasionally, if the gallbladder is empty of bile when outlet obstruction occurs, mucus secretion continues and distends the gallbladder, forming a **mucocele**.

## Movement of a stone into the CBD

This may be asymptomatic. The stone may distend the cystic duct, causing colicky pain (biliary colic). It may obstruct the CBD, causing jaundice and proximal duct dilatation. As it progresses to the sphincter of Oddi into the duodenum the obstruction can affect the pancreatic duct, causing acute pancreatitis.

Stones in the CBD can be asymptomatic or can present with any combination of:

- Biliary colic
- Obstructive jaundice
- Secondary biliary cirrhosis
- Cholangitis
- Pancreatitis

**Differential diagnoses of stones in the CBD** include the following:

- With jaundice (75%):
  - Malignant obstruction (eg cancer of the pancreas – often painless jaundice)
  - Acute hepatitis
  - Other causes of jaundice (see table 'Classification of jaundice' in Section 4.3)
- Without jaundice (25%):
  - Renal colic
  - Intestinal obstruction
  - Angina

### Ulceration of a stone through the wall of the gallbladder

Gallstones may erode into the duodenum or colon. Impaction of a stone in the distal ileum results in intestinal obstruction (gallstone ileus).

## Clinical presentation of gallstones

### Biliary colic

This is pain probably resulting from distension of the gallbladder outlet or duct system when a stone becomes impacted.

**Typical clinical features** include the following:

- Colicky right hypochondrial or epigastric pain
- Pain radiating to the lower pole of the right scapula
- Restless patient rolling in agony

- Sweaty, nauseous, vomiting patient

The episode may resolve when the stone is passed along the duct or falls back into the gallbladder. Differential diagnosis includes renal colic, intestinal obstruction and angina.

### Acute cholecystitis

In 95% of cases inflammation of the gallbladder due to chemical or bacterial cholecystitis is a sequela of obstruction of the cystic duct by gallstones.

### Typical clinical features of acute cholecystitis

- History of previous dyspepsia, fat intolerance or biliary colic
- Right upper quadrant (RUQ) pain becoming more severe, constant and localised after a day or two
- Fever, toxaemia, leucocytosis, rigors

On examination there is rebound tenderness and guarding in the RUQ, Murphy's sign (see table 'Specific signs on examination of the abdomen' in Section 6.1). A mass may be palpable if the gallbladder is distended.

### Complications of acute cholecystitis

- Empyema of gallbladder
- Perforation of the gallbladder, causing peritonitis
- Obstructive jaundice, even if ductal stones have passed, due to local oedema
- Acalculous acute cholecystitis can occur in 5% of cases: if a single causative stone has been passed; in typhoid fever; in critically ill individuals

## Differential diagnoses of acute cholecystitis

- Perforated duodenal ulcer
- Acute pancreatitis
- Right-sided basal pneumonia
- Acute appendicitis

## Chronic cholecystitis (gallbladder dyspepsia)

This is almost always associated with gallstones that repeatedly inflame the gallbladder, resulting in fibrosis and thickening of the entire gallbladder wall. Long-standing dyspeptic symptoms punctuated by episodes of cholecystitis are typical. Differential diagnoses include peptic ulceration, hiatus hernia and angina.

## Gallstone pancreatitis

Transient blocking of the ampulla of Vater by passing stones can trigger acute pancreatitis, especially if the stones are numerous and small. Pancreatitis is dealt with in Section 5.7.

## Obstructive jaundice

Patients with a CBD stone may present with acute-onset obstructive jaundice. It may be distinguished clinically from a malignant cause of jaundice because the onset is acute, there is usually a history of pain and the gallbladder is not usually palpable (Courvoisier's law). Ultrasonography and MRCP can confirm the diagnosis, and ERCP is therapeutic.

## Acute cholangitis

This is due to infection of the bile in the biliary tree. It develops in the presence of bile duct obstruction and biliary infection. Charcot's triad of pain, fever and jaundice alerts the surgeon to the diagnosis, but it should be suspected in anyone with a biliary obstruction who develops septicaemia. These patients can get very sick very fast. Antibiotics and resuscitation are the mainstays of the initial emergency treatment. Decompression of the biliary tree by endoscopic, radiological or surgical means, depending on the patient and the pathology, should be planned as the definitive management.

---

**Factors predisposing to acute cholangitis**

- Stones in the CBD
- Biliary stricture
- Post-biliary reconstructive procedures
- Post-bile duct instrumentation (eg ERCP)

---

## Gallstone ileus

Chronic perforation of an inflamed gallbladder forming a cholecystoenteric fistula can lead to a gallstone becoming lodged in the GI tract, usually at the level of the ileocaecal valve or at the site of Meckel's diverticulum 2 feet (60 cm) proximal to the ileocaecal valve. The patient, usually elderly, presents with a history of RUQ pain and an acute small-bowel obstruction. The radiograph (if you are lucky!) may show an opacity in the right iliac fossa and air in the biliary tree. A CT scan is usually diagnostic.

After resuscitation and nasogastric decompression, an urgent laparotomy is indicated. The gallstone should be milked back up the terminal ileum to a healthy bit of bowel and removed through a small enterotomy. Definitive treatment of the fistula is best left until the acute episode has settled. If the removed stone is faceted, look for another stone.

## Empyema and emphysema of the gallbladder

This is a severe form of acute cholecystitis that occurs mainly in elderly people. Unlike uncomplicated acute cholecystitis, there is pus in the gallbladder (which may be palpable as a tender mass) and the patients are very septic. Early surgery prevents perforation, which has a high mortality. Emphysematous cholecystitis presents similarly in elderly or immunocompromised people as a result of a gangrenous gallbladder infected with the gas-forming *Clostridium perfringens*. Urgent surgery is equally vital for these two groups of patients. Percutaneous radiologically guided decompression is useful as a temporising measure to improve the fitness of an unfit septic patient for a more definitive procedure.

## Investigating gallbladder disease

This is described in detail in the section on jaundice in Section 4.3. Ultrasonography, liver function tests (LFTs) and MRCP/ERCP are the mainstays of diagnosis of gallbladder disease. A CT scan may be useful in obstructive jaundice where malignancy is suspected.

## Management of gallstone disease

### Acute cholecystitis

The principles of treatment of an acute cholecystitis attack include:

- Admission to hospital
- Pain relief with opiates
- Intravenous fluids
- Broad-spectrum antibiotics
- Elective cholecystectomy, either during that admission or 6 weeks after discharge

**Cholecystectomy** is recommended after an attack of cholecystitis because:

- There is a high risk of recurrent attacks
- There is a risk of life-threatening complications, such as perforation of the gallbladder, pancreatitis or obstructive jaundice, in future attacks
- There has been controversy about whether to perform a cholecystectomy early during the admission for cholecystitis or 6 weeks later, after the attack has settled

---

### When to perform a cholecystectomy

There has been controversy about whether to perform a cholecystectomy early during the admission for cholecystitis or 6 weeks later, after the attack has settled.

There have been three recent systematic reviews to investigate just this issue. These have found that there is no significant difference in operative morbidity or mortality between the two groups.

Importantly, there is no significant difference in the risk of conversion to open surgery between the two groups. However, in those patients who were randomised to delayed surgery, 18% required emergency laparoscopic cholecystectomy due to non-resolution of symptoms or symptom recurrence before the planned elective procedure.

Early cholecystectomy does have advantages and should be the treatment of choice in people with acute cholecystitis. Patients with multiple comorbidites and relative contraindications for cholecystectomy may be treated conservatively.

## Chronic cholecystitis

If a patient is diagnosed as having chronic cholecystitis, an elective cholecystectomy is indicated.

## Stones in the CBD

This is a controversial topic with many factors to consider. There are several ways to approach a stone in the CBD. It may pass on conservative treatment (thankfully the most common outcome). If there is a history of jaundice ± dilated ducts on ultrasonography, many surgeons would request a preoperative MRCP to confirm that the ducts are clear before surgery. This is preferable (if available) to a diagnostic ERCP, which has higher morbidity. If the ducts are clear, cholecystectomy can be performed safely. If there is a stone in the CBD it can be removed either via ERCP preoperatively or at the time of surgery. The latter option necessitates an intraoperative exploration of the CBD. A problem arises if the cholecystectomy is laparoscopic, which most are. A laparoscopic exploration of the bile duct is a skilled procedure and, unless the operator is suitably experienced, there may be long operating time, significant morbidity and significant conversion to open surgery.

## Asymptomatic stones

There is controversy over the management of asymptomatic gallstones. If left alone, only 7% of asymptomatic gallstones needed surgery for gallstone-related disease within 5 years, so prophylactic surgery is not indicated. However, 44% of patients with symptomatic gallstones eventually require surgery, thus justifying a cholecystectomy.

## Medical treatment of gallstones

- All patients with gallstones are advised to keep to a low-fat diet. Oral bile salts (eg chenodeoxycholic acid) are used to dissolve small, non-calcified stones in a functioning gallbladder in patients not suitable for surgery. These criteria only account for about 15–25% of patients with gallstones. The disadvantages include the following:
- Prolonged treatment for months (necessary)
- Attacks of biliary colic as fragments of stone are passed
- Recurrence (common)

Lithotripsy (ultrasonic destruction of small stones) is possible and can be combined with percutaneous aspiration of debris under ultrasound control. These methods have limited applications.

## Cholecystectomy

Open cholecystectomy is being replaced by the laparoscopic operation except when contraindicated. A recent Cochrane review has concluded that there are no significant differences in mortality and complications between the laparoscopic and the open techniques. The laparoscopic operation has advantages over the open operation with regard to duration of hospital stay and convalescence.

**Op box: Open cholecystectomy**

**Preop**
- Ultrasonography, LFTs and clotting screen
- Exclude peptic ulcer disease and hiatus hernia if diagnosis in doubt
- Encourage weight loss and smoking cessation
- Decide if intraoperative cholangiogram is likely

**Incision**
- Traditionally right subcostal (Kocher's)
- Right paramedian is often used as it is less painful and provides good access

**Procedure**
- Thorough laparotomy, especially duodenum, caecum and oesophageal hiatus
- Free duodenum and hepatic flexure of colon from gallbladder
- Clamp on fundus and clamp on Hartmann's pouch
- Most surgeons do a fundus-first open cholecystectomy (alternatively, the peritoneum over the cystic duct may be divided as in a laparoscopic procedure)
- Identify Calot's triangle
- Divide cystic artery between ligatures
- Perform cholangiogram if indicated
- Divide the cystic duct between ligatures
- Dissect the gallbladder from the liver bed (anterograde removal)
- In difficult cases (eg fibrotic or acutely inflamed gallbladder) the dissection can be fundus-first (retrograde removal)
- Ensure haemostasis
- A drain may be placed next to the liver bed

**Closure**
- In layers or mass closure with non-absorbable sutures; clips or subarticular suture to skin

**Postop**
- Analgesia, early chest physiotherapy, oral fluid day 1
- Drain out at 24 h if <100 ml drainage
- Home day 5 if all well

**Surgical hazards**
- Damage to hepatic duct or CBD
- Damage to hepatic artery

**Complications**
- Haemorrhage from slipped tie or from gallbladder bed
- Biliary leak
- Missed stone in bile duct or cystic duct stump
- Biliary stricture from damage to biliary tree
- Wound complications

## Op box: Laparoscopic cholecystectomy

**Preop**

As with open cholecystectomy, plus:
- Ensure that there are no contraindications to laparoscopic cholecystectomy
- Consent patient for conversion to an open operation, preferably stating the operating surgeon's conversion rate

**Procedure**
- Induce a pneumoperitoneum through a 10-mm subumbilical incision. Three further incisions are made under laparoscopic vision:
  - 10-mm incision in the midline just below the xiphisternum
  - 5-mm incision in the midaxillary line on the transpyloric plane
  - 5-mm incision in the anterior axillary line 5 cm below the costal margin
- Perform a laparoscopic survey of the entire abdomen
- Identify the structures of Calot's triangle as in the open operation
- Divide the cystic artery between LigaClips and then widely open Calot's triangle to ensure that the structure at the inferior margin of the triangle is the cystic duct
- Perform cholangiogram if indicated
- Divide cystic duct between LigaClips
- Dissect gallbladder from the liver by a combination of blunt dissection and cautery
- Check the liver bed for haemostasis
- Remove the gallbladder through the subumbilical or subxiphisternal port
- A drain can be brought out through one of the right-sided ports
- The abdomen is exsufflated and the instruments withdrawn

**Closure**
- Close linea alba 10-mm incisions with non-absorbable sutures or PDS Staples or Monocryl to skin. Some surgeons use glue

**Postop**
- Fully mobilised and eating by the next day
- Home after 24 hours if all well

**Surgical hazards**
- Requiring conversion to an open operation
- Injury to the bowel or great vessels during insufflation
- Damage to CBD, portal vein or right hepatic artery
- Failure to complete procedure
- Common duct stones
- $CO_2$ retention due to absorption of intraperitoneal $CO_2$
- Accidental perforation of the gallbladder and scattering of calculi

**Complications**
- As for open operation but fewer wound and general complications
- Post-site hernia

> **Relative contraindications to laparoscopic cholecystectomy**
> - Jaundice
> - Cirrhosis
> - Previous upper abdominal surgery
> - Surgeon not familiar with equipment or technique
> - Acute cholecystitis (empyema/gangrene)
> - Morbid obesity
> - Pregnancy

### Intraoperative cholangiography

Intraoperative cholangiography has two main functions:

1. Image common duct stones
2. Decrease risk of biliary injury

There has been a great deal of debate about whether cannulation of the biliary tree and contrast radiography during cholecystectomy are necessary. The argument for intraoperative cholangiography is that it:

- Defines anatomical variations
- Confirms that the duct about to be divided is the cystic duct
- Visualises stones in the CBD (occur in 10% of cholecystectomies) which, if overlooked, would lead to persistent obstructive jaundice and risk of postoperative cholangitis and bile leak

Some surgeons suggest that an intraoperative cholangiography should be performed only on selected patients, including those with:

- Abnormal CBD seen on ultrasonography
- Wide cystic duct seen on operation
- An elevated alkaline phosphatase or bilirubin within the 6 months preceding the operation

- difficulty in identifying anatomy or suspicion of intraductal stones during the operation

Opponents of intraoperative cholangiography claim that there is no convincing evidence that the procedure decreases the incidence, rate or risk of CBD injury. Preoperative MRCP is a safe, non-invasive way of checking that the ducts are clear.

The options available to the surgeon who finds a stone in a bile duct during a laparoscopic cholecystectomy are:

- Leave the stone and do a postoperative ERCP
- Convert to an open procedure
- Attempt laparoscopic retrieval using balloon, basket, cholendoscope or by performing a laparoscopic choledochotomy

### Endoscopic retrograde cholangiopancreatography

ERCP is described in detail in Section 4.3. Diagnostic ERCP is being replaced by MRCP but therapeutic ERCP is invaluable to the upper GI surgeon. This technique has revolutionised the treatment of choledocholithiasis (stones in the CBD). The CBD is successfully cleared in 94% of cases, usually using a balloon, basket or sphincterotomy.

ERCP is less likely to be successful in difficult cases, such as those with:

- Aberrant anatomy
- Periampullary diverticulum
- Prior upper GI surgery
- Difficult stones, eg those that are >15 mm, intrahepatic, impacted, multiple
- Stricture associated with the stone

## 5.4 Other disorders of the biliary tree

### In a nutshell ...

- Carcinoma of the gallbladder
- Gallbladder disease in children
- Primary sclerosing cholangitis
- Benign bile duct stricture
- Bile duct carcinoma

## Carcinoma of the gallbladder

### Pathology of gallbladder carcinoma

- Carcinoma of the gallbladder is rare
- It affects more females than males (4F:1M)
- 90% are adenocarcincomas and 10% squamous cell carcinomas (SCCs)
- It is associated with gallstones in 95% of cases
- It spreads to the liver, either directly or via the portal vein and via lymphatics to the porta hepatis

### Clinical features of gallbladder carcinoma

This carcinoma is often discovered incidentally during cholecystectomy. Gallbladder cancer is the fifth most common GI cancer in the USA and the most common hepatobiliary cancer. Gallbladder cancer arises in the setting of chronic inflammation; the presence of gallstones increases the risk of gallbladder cancer four- to fivefold. In addition, abnormal anatomy, eg congenital defects with anomalous duct junctions and choledochal cysts, increases the risk of gallbladder cancer.

### Treatment of gallbladder carcinoma

Survival is correlated with the tumour, node, metastasis (TNM) staging system. Most patients unfortunately have regional disease or distant metastases at presentation. Thus, the prognosis is generally poor (current 5-year survival rate of about 15–20%):

- Stage IA disease (T1, N0, M0) – simple cholecystectomy (should be curative)
- Stage IB disease (T2, N0, M0) – extended cholecystectomy (5-year survival rate of 70–90%)
- Stage IIB disease (T1–3, N1, M0) – extended cholecystectomy (5-year survival rate of 45–60%)
- Stage III disease (T4, any N, M0) – is generally not surgically curable (1-year survival rate for advanced gallbladder cancer is less than 5%, with a median survival of 2–4 months)

## Gallbladder disease in children

The development of the gallbladder and biliary tree is discussed in Section 5.1. The following are the main childhood disorders:

- Extrahepatic biliary atresia
- Choledochal cysts
- Inspissated bile syndrome (can occur secondary to haemolysis)
- Spontaneous perforation of the CBD (rare)
- Acute gallbladder distension (often after respiratory tract infections)
- Benign inflammatory tumours of the bile ducts

## Primary sclerosing cholangitis

This is a chronic fibrosing inflammatory condition of the biliary tree that affects young adults – in the intrahepatic and extrahepatic ducts. The gallbladder and the pancreas may also be affected.

It is of unknown aetiology but it is associated with ulcerative colitis in 50–70% of cases. Patients may be at increased risk of developing bile duct carcinoma.

Presentation is usually progressive jaundice and RUQ pain. Cholangiography shows strictures. LFTs show a high alkaline phosphatase. Immunological studies are also useful.

Treatment is symptomatic with steroids with an average survival of 5–7 years. Liver transplantation is the only definitive treatment. For details about liver transplantation, see Transplant Surgery.

## Benign bile duct stricture

These are most often postoperative or associated with gallstones. Other causes include parasitic infestations, acute cholecystitis, chronic pancreatitis and sclerosing cholangitis.

Investigations are aimed at identifying the level of the stricture and excluding a malignant cause. Percutaneous trans-hepatic cholangiography is useful because ERCP cannot image the biliary tree proximal to the stricture. Ultrasonography is less invasive.

Treatment is ballooning, stenting, or excision and reconstruction (hepaticojejunostomy).

## Bile duct carcinoma

This is very uncommon and accounts for only 0.2% of GI malignancies. Unlike carcinoma of the gallbladder, it affects men and women equally.

Predisposing factors include the following:
- Bile duct stones (in 20–30%)
- Sclerosing cholangitis

- Ulcerative colitis
- Cysts of the bile duct
- Parasitic infestation

Bile duct carcinoma is an adenocarcinoma that appears macroscopically as a small nodule, a papillary lesion or a diffuse stricture; 50% occur in the hepatic duct and 50% in the cystic duct and CBD.

## Clinical features of bile duct carcinoma

Jaundice (90%), pain (30%), ascites (40%), anorexia, weight loss and anaemia.

## Investigating bile duct carcinoma

This depends on the presentation, site of tumour and planned management and includes:
- Ultrasonography
- CT
- ERCP
- Positron-emission tomography (PET)-CT

## Management of bile duct carcinoma

### Curative surgery
- Potentially curable lesions are surgically resected
- This operation traditionally has high morbidity and mortality (approximately 20%); however, dedicated specialist centres have reported mortality rates of only 5%
- Distal tumours have a higher resectability rate

## Palliation

Of all patients, 80–90% have incurable lesions. The aim is to relieve obstruction. Techniques include:

- Bypass procedures, such as hepaticojejunostomy or Roux-en-Y
- Intraoperative insertion of internal or intero-external stents
- Percutaneous biliary stenting
- Percutaneous biliary drainage
- Endoscopic transpapillary stenting
- Radiotherapy
- Photodynamic therapy

In frail, older patients with concurrent disease, non-surgical measures are preferred.

## 5.5 Anatomy of the pancreas

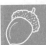 **In a nutshell ...**

The pancreas lies retroperitoneally in the transpyloric plane. It is divided into a head, neck, body and tail:
- **The head** lies in the C-shaped curve of the duodenum. It has an uncinate process that hooks behind the superior mesenteric vessels
- **The neck** lies in front of the superior mesenteric and portal veins
- **The body** passes to the left and upwards behind the lesser sac, forming part of the stomach bed. The lesser sac can become distended with fluid from acute pancreatitis, forming a pseudocyst
- **The tail** lies within the splenorenal ligament, touching the hilum of the spleen

## Gross anatomy of the pancreas

The pancreatic duct of Wirsung drains most of the pancreas into the major duodenal papilla. It is joined by the CBD at or before the ampulla of Vater. The uncinate process is drained by the accessory duct of Santorini, which opens into the duodenum at the minor duodenal papilla. Although the uncinate lobe is an inferior part of the pancreas, it drains into the minor duodenal papilla, which is 2 cm above or proximal to the major ampulla for developmental reasons (see Figure 1.36).

The important posterior relations of the pancreas are the following:
- Inferior vena cava (IVC)
- Superior mesenteric vessels
- Crura of the diaphragm
- Coeliac plexus
- Left kidney and adrenal gland
- Splenic artery (along the upper border of the pancreas)
- Splenic vein, inferior and superior mesenteric veins draining into the portal vein behind the neck of the pancreas
- CBD (lies within the pancreas itself)

A neoplasm at the head of the pancreas can therefore cause obstructive jaundice, portal vein obstruction or IVC obstruction.

## Blood supply of the pancreas

Blood supply is from the splenic and pancreaticoduodenal arteries. The corresponding veins drain into the portal system; the lymphatics drain largely to superior mesenteric nodes.

## Embryology of the pancreas

The embryology of the pancreas is shown in Figure 1.36. It develops from a large dorsal bud from the duodenum and a smaller ventral bud from the CBD. The ventral bud swings round posteriorly to fuse with the dorsal bud, trapping the superior mesenteric vessels between the two parts. The ducts of these two buds of the pancreas then communicate, and that of the smaller takes over the main pancreatic flow to form the main duct, leaving the original duct of the larger portion of the gland as the accessory duct.

Rarely, the two developing segments of the pancreas completely surround the second part of the duodenum (annular pancreas) and may produce duodenal obstruction. Ectopic pancreas nodules can be found in the stomach or small bowel.

## Structure of the pancreas

### In a nutshell ...

The pancreas is lobulated and encapsulated. The lobules are made up of serous secretory cells draining via their ductules into the main ducts (exocrine glands). Between these alveoli lie the islets of Langerhans which secrete insulin, not into the ducts but directly into the circulation (endocrine glands).

### Exocrine pancreas

The structure of the exocrine pancreas resembles that of the salivary glands and accounts for 98% of the volume of the pancreas:

- Acinar cells form acini, which each drain into an intercalated duct forming the functional unit of the exocrine pancreas
- Acini are organised into lobules which drain via intralobular and extralobular ducts into the pancreatic duct
- The pancreas is innervated by branches of the vagus nerve, which stimulate secretion of both acinar and islet cells
- Postganglionic sympathetic nerves from the coeliac and superior mesenteric plexus tend to be inhibitory to secretion

### Endocrine pancreas

- The endocrine cells of the pancreas reside in the islets of Langerhans
- These tiny (100-nm diameter) clusters of specialised cells account for less than 2% of the volume of the pancreas
- They have a good blood supply and are innervated by the vagus and sympathetic nerves
- The islets consist of separate types of cells secreting hormones:
  - Insulin from $\beta$ cells
  - Glucagon from $\alpha$ cells
  - Somatostatin from $\delta$ cells
  - Pancreatic polypeptide from F cells

## 5.6 Physiology of the pancreas

### In a nutshell ...

**Exocrine pancreas**
- Acinar secretion (enzymes)
- Duct secretion (water, bicarbonate, sodium)

**Endocrine pancreas**
- Insulin
- Glucagon
- Somatostatin
- Pancreatic polypeptide

## Exocrine pancreas

### Composition of pancreatic juice

- **Acinar secretion** (digests duodenal contents): trypsinogen, chymotrypsinogen, procarboxylase, procarboxypeptidases, phospholipase, amylase, lecithin, sodium chloride, water
- **Duct secretion** (increases pH of duodenal contents): bicarbonate, sodium ions, water

### Secretion of pancreatic juice

Digestive enzymes are stored in an inactive form to prevent autodigestion. Granules containing inactive pro-enzymes fuse with cell membrane and exocytose. Trypsinogen is converted to trypsin by enterokinase in the duodenum. Trypsin then converts the other inactive enzymes into their active forms. The duct cells secrete bicarbonate in exchange for chloride ions. The bicarbonate concentration increases as the secretion rate increases.

### Stimulation of pancreatic secretion

- **Parasympathetic vagal stimulation:** in response to cephalic and gastric phase
- **Secretin:** in response to acid in the duodenum
- **CCK:** in response to peptides, amino acids, fatty acids in the duodenum

## Endocrine pancreas

As well as acting as an exocrine gland, the pancreas also acts as an endocrine gland, secreting several hormones directly into the bloodstream from the islets of Langerhans.

### Insulin from β cells

The main effects of insulin are to promote fuel storage. It consists of two straight-chain peptides held together by disulphide bands. Secretion is stimulated by:

- Glucose
- Protein
- Gastrointestinal peptides
- Cholinergic and β-adrenergic stimuli

Its release is inhibited by circumstances requiring fuel mobilisation, such as fasting or exercise.

---

**Insulin stimulates:**
- Muscle glucose uptake
- Storage of glucose as glycogen
- Protein synthesis

**Insulin inhibits:**
- Adipose tissue lipolysis
- Ketogenesis
- Hepatic glycogenolysis
- Gluconeogenesis
- Glucose release
- Muscle proteolysis

---

Insulin acts through a plasma membrane receptor with tyrosine kinase activity. This leads to modulation of the activities of enzymes involved in glucose and fatty acid metabolism. Insulin also affects the gene expression of numerous enzymes and proteins.

Insulin decreases plasma levels of:

- Glucose
- Free fatty acids
- Ketoacids
- Branched-chain amino acids

Insulin deficiency (diabetes mellitus) leads to:
- Hyperglycaemia
- Loss of lean body mass
- Loss of adipose tissue mass
- Growth retardation
- Metabolic ketoacidosis

## Glucagon from α cells

Glucagon is a single-chain polypeptide released in response to hypoglycaemia and amino acids. Glucagon promotes mobilisation of glucose by stimulating hepatic glycogenolysis and gluconeogenesis. It also increases fatty acid oxidation and ketogenesis. The mechanism of action is modification of enzyme activities by phosphorylation. Cyclic AMP is its second messenger.

Glucagon increases plasma levels of:
- Glucose
- Free fatty acids
- Ketoacids

The insulin:glucagon ratio controls the relative rates of glycolysis and gluconeogenesis. The two hormones have antagonistic effects at numerous steps in hepatic metabolism.

## Somatostatin from δ cells

Somatostatin is a neuropeptide produced by the δ cells. It reduces the rate of digestion by decreasing:
- Motility of the GI tract
- GI secretions
- Digestion and absorption of nutrients
- Secretion of insulin and glucagon

It is secreted in response to meals and avoids overload of the portal venous system with the products of digestion.

## Pancreatic polypeptide from F cells

This is the least clearly understood of the pancreatic hormones. It is a small polypeptide, secreted from the F cells of the islets of Langerhans. Its production is stimulated by a drop in blood sugar or protein and fasting. It slows food absorption and helps regulate variations in the rate of digestion.

## 5.7 Pancreatitis

### In a nutshell ...

**Acute pancreatitis** is an acute inflammation of the pancreas typically presenting with abdominal pain and raised pancreatic enzymes in the blood and urine.
**Chronic pancreatitis** is a continuing inflammatory disease, characterised by irreversible morphological change and typically causing pain ± permanent loss of function.

## Aetiology and predisposing factors

This has long been remembered by the medical student mnemonic **GET SMASH'D** (see overleaf). Gallstones and alcohol account for over 80% of cases in the UK.

---

**Aetiology and predisposing factors of pancreatitis**

**G**allstones and biliary tract disease (40% of cases)

**E**thanol- (alcohol-) related (40%)

**T**oxins and drugs (eg steroids, thiazides, diuretics, oestrogens, azathioprine)

**S**urgery or trauma, including ERCP

**M**etabolic (eg primary hyperparathyroidism, uraemia, diabetic coma, hyperlipidaemia, pregnancy)

**A**utoimmune and inherited

**S**nake bite and infections (eg mumps)

**H**ypothermia

**D**uodenal obstruction

---

## Pathology of pancreatitis

### Initiation of condition

Acinar damage is caused by activated pro-enzymes due to either hypersecretion and ductal obstruction or reflux of duodenal content back into pancreatic ducts.

### Pancreatic necrosis

Once the initial insult has occurred, proteolytic enzymes damage blood vessels, leading to ischaemia and haemorrhage. Further enzymes from the ischaemic pancreas leak into the bloodstream causing systemic effects. The main enzymes liberated in pancreatitis are **trypsin**, **lipase** and **amylase**.

### Types of pancreatitis

- **Acute mild/oedematous pancreatitis:** there is usually complete resolution
- **Acute severe/necrotising/haemorrhagic pancreatitis:** there is a variable degree

of tissue destruction in and around the pancreas; there is a risk of a protracted and complicated clinical course

- **Pancreatic phlegmon:** an inflammatory mass involving the pancreas and retroperitoneal tissues that can be identified by CT scan or seen at laparotomy
- **Sterile pancreatic necrosis:** necrotising pancreatitis without infection; outcomes include gradual resolution, pseudocyst formation or infected necrosis

### Complications of pancreatitis

- **Infected pancreatic necrosis:** necrotising pancreatitis complicated by bacterial infection, frequently leading to generalised sepsis, multiorgan failure and death
- **Pseudocyst:** fluid collections are frequently seen around the pancreas on early scans, but most resolve spontaneously; a pseudocyst is a persistent loculated collection of fluid rich in amylase and usually within the lesser sac
- **Infected pseudocyst:** late infection of an established pseudocyst that can be distinguished from the more serious condition of infected pancreatic necrosis
- **Pancreatic abscess:** a circumscribed collection of pus that can develop from the third week onwards; it does not contain necrotic tissue and may be suitable for percutaneous drainage
- **Other local complications:** include phlegmon, ascites, pseudo-aneurysm
- **Systemic complications:** often life-threatening in severe pancreatitis and may need support on the high dependency unit (HDU) or intensive care unit (ICU). They include respiratory, cardiac and/or renal insufficiency, malnutrition, systemic inflammatory response syndrome, coagulopathies and multiorgan dysfunction

## Clinical features of pancreatitis

In the UK, the incidence of acute pancreatitis is rising and currently the range is 150–400 cases per million of the population. The median age at onset depends on the aetiology. Alcoholic pancreatitis is more common in men, whereas gallstone pancreatitis is more common in women. Clinical features are systemic and local (see box below) but the typical presentation is an acute abdomen in a systemically unwell patient. Differential diagnoses include the following:

- Acute cholecystitis
- Peritonitis
- Peptic ulcer disease
- High intestinal obstruction
- Myocardial infarction

---

### Symptoms and signs of pancreatitis

**Local**

- Epigastric pain radiating to the back
- Acute abdomen – tender, rigid, silent abdomen with distension
- Jaundice due to pancreatic oedema/ gallstone
- Ascites
- Abscess formation
- Grey Turner's and Cullen's signs (bruising in the flanks and umbilicus respectively)

**Systemic**

- Shock due to retroperitoneal fluid loss and vasoactive substances from the pancreas
- Respiratory failure due to acute respiratory distress syndrome (ARDS) and effusions
- Renal failure due to hypovolaemia and direct effects of enzymes

**Metabolic changes**

- Hypocalcaemia
- Hypoglycaemia
- Hypomagnesaemia

---

## Investigating pancreatitis

- **Serum amylase/lipase:** over 200 Somogyi units is abnormal and over three times above the reference range is diagnostic; this varies with the situation. The actual value has no correlation with the severity of the attack
- **Other blood tests:** full blood count or FBC (increased WCC); U&Es; LFTs; albumin; magnesium; glucose; calcium; triglycerides; C-reactive protein (CRP)
- **Blood gases:** hypoxia and acidosis occurs in severe cases
- **Urinary amylase** (rarely done)
- **Erect chest and abdominal radiographs**
- **Ultrasonography:** to rule out gallstones
- **Contrast-enhanced CT scan:** shows pancreas more clearly than ultrasonography and can determine what percentage of the gland is enhancing and what percentage is necrotic
- **MRCP/ERCP:** to assess the presence of a CBD stone

## Scoring systems for pancreatitis

Severity scales of pancreatitis are used as research tools and correlate well with prognosis and chance of admission to an ICU. They are also used clinically to indicate the severity of the attack.

**Ranson's criteria**

**On initial assessment**
- Age >55 years
- WCC >16 × 10⁹/l
- Blood glucose >11 mmol/l
- Lactate dehydrogenase (LDH) >350 IU/l
- AST >250 IU/l

**Within 48 hours**
- Haematocrit decrease >10%
- BUN (blood urea nitrogen) increase >1.8 mmol/l
- Calcium <2 mmol/l
- $PaO_2$ <60 mmHg (8 kPa)
- Base deficit >4 mmol/l
- Fluid sequestration >6 l

The higher the score, the worse the prognosis.

**Glasgow scoring system**
- WCC >15 × 10⁹/l
- Blood glucose >10 mmol/l
- LDH >600 IU/l
- AST/ALT >100 IU/l
- Serum urea >16 mmol/l (no response to IV fluids)
- $PaO_2$ <60 mmHg (8 kPa)
- Calcium <2 mmol/l
- Albumin <32 g/l

More than three positive criteria on either scoring system constitute a severe attack.

# Predictors of a severe attack of pancreatitis

## Initial assessment (clinical)
- Clinical impression (a very subjective marker, but surprisingly accurate)
- BMI >30 kg/m²
- APACHE score* >8

- Older age
- Male
- Alcoholic pancreatitis
- Short time to onset of symptoms
- Evidence of organ failure

## Biochemical and radiologic predictors
- Haem
- CRP >150mg/l
- Serum creatinine
- Pleural effusion on chest X-ray
- CT showing necrosis

*APACHE (Acute Physiology and Chronic Health Evaluation) score is a severity-of-disease classification system. It is calculated from 12 physiological measurements such as blood pressure, body temperature, heart rate, etc.

# Management of pancreatitis

## Immediate resuscitation and assessment
- Analgesia
- Oral or, if not tolerated, nasogastric or nasojejunal feeding
- NG tube (controversial)
- IV fluids
- Oxygen
- Catheterisation
- Sliding-scale insulin regimen if necessary

Later management includes systemic management, detection treatment of necrosis and prevention of recurrence.

## Systemic management

All patients with severe pancreatitis should be managed on an HDU or ICU to support and monitor the various systems:

- The cardiovascular system may need CVP monitoring, and inotropes in severe cases
- Renal failure may necessitate dialysis
- Respiratory failure may lead to the need for ventilation
- Metabolic problems may indicate intravenous calcium gluconate or intramuscular magnesium
- Enteral or total parenteral nutrition (TPN) may be needed

## Prevention of complications

- No consensus on the use of prophylactic antibiotics, but there is some evidence that they improve survival in severe attacks

## Local management

- Urgent ERCP should be performed in patients with proven gallstone acute pancreatitis with a CBD stone or cholangitis. This should be performed within the first 72 hours. All patients undergoing early ERCP require endoscopic sphincterotomy regardless of the presence of a stone
- All patients with gallstone pancreatitis should undergo a cholecystectomy during the same admission or within the next 2 weeks

---

### Pancreatic necrosis

A contrast-enhanced CT scan will show:

- How much of the pancreas has necrosed
- If there is any peripancreatic fluid

In a patient with pancreatic necrosis the peripancreatic fluid may be aspirated and sent for culture. There are stronger indications for pancreatic necrosectomy in patients with an infected necrosis than in those with sterile necrosis.

A **necrosectomy** involves removing the dead pancreatic tissue (described by one upper GI surgeon as being like purple bubble gum!) and introducing a lavage system that can be used postoperatively. There is increased use of minimally invasive techniques involving retroperitoneal endoscopy.

---

## 5.8  Pancreatic carcinoma

 **In a nutshell ...**

Pancreatitic cancer is the eighth most common cancer in the UK and the third most common GI cancer. Over 50% of patients have distant metastases at the time of diagnosis and 5-year survival is extremely poor.

# Incidence of pancreatic carcinoma

Peak incidence is at 60–80 years.

# Predisposing factors for pancreatic carcinoma

- Age (median age is 69 years and the incidence increases linearly after 50 years)
- Smokers (30% arise in smokers)
- Patients with diabetes (associated with a twofold increase)
- Chronic pancreatitis (associated with a 26-fold increase)

# Pathology of pancreatic carcinoma

Most commonly these are ductal adenocarcinomas: 75% occur in the head, 15–20% in the body and 5–10% in the tail. Macroscopically this is a big, grey–white diffuse tumour with ill-defined borders. The tumour tends to spread into and along the main pancreatic duct (of Wirsung) and the bile duct. It is aggressively invasive locally, spreading to the duodenum, local lymph nodes, portal vein and nerve sheaths. It metastasises to the liver.

Rarer types of tumour include:
- Carcinoma in situ (CIS)
- Intraductal carcinoma
- Papillary carcinoma
- Adenosquamous carcinoma
- Osteoclast (giant cell) carcinoma
- Cystadenocarcinoma
- Lymphoma

Carcinoma of the pancreas is one of the periampullary tumours but it should be differentiated from the other malignancies in that area:
- Ampullary carcinoma
- Duodenal carcinoma
- Lower bile duct carcinoma

These other periampullary tumours present similarly but have much better resection and survival rates compared with pancreatic carcinoma.

# Presentation of pancreatic carcinoma

Typical clinical features of pancreatic cancer include:
- Weight loss, malaise, nausea, fatigue
- Jaundice (71%)
- Pain
- Pancreatitis (5% – usually in a young age group)

Tumours of the head of the pancreas tend to present with obstructive jaundice, nausea, weight loss and weakness. A palpable mass may be felt in the RUQ because, unlike in gallstone disease, the gallbladder tends to be normal, thin-walled and distensible (see Courvoisier's law under Section 5.3). In tumours of the body and tail, only 20% present with jaundice. Pain, diabetes and hepatomegaly can indicate a tumour in this site. They tend to present late. Trousseau's sign is a migratory superficial thrombophlebitis associated with pancreatic cancer.

# Diagnosis of pancreatic carcinoma

This relies on clinical suspicion of vague symptoms such as:
- Upper abdominal pain and backache with a negative ultrasound scan and endoscopy
- Unexplained weight loss with no other signs
- Pancreatitis in the absence of gallstones
- Newly diagnosed diabetes, especially if patients are aged >70 years at presentation

## Investigating pancreatic carcinoma

- **Ultrasonography** may show a 'double-duct' sign (both the CBD and the pancreatic duct are dilated)
- **Contrast-enhanced CT** ± **PET** gives information about the spread and resectability
- **Endoscopic ultrasound** ± **FNA** is highly sensitive and specific in diagnosis; in appropriate hands a negative EUS is almost 100% specific

- **ERCP and biopsy** are again very accurate in diagnosis and a stent can be inserted if patients are jaundiced, but this is controversial
- **MRI** can be useful but endoscopic or ERCP biopsies are better because the tract will be removed with the specimen

An example of an algorithm used in a British hospital for investigating suspected pancreatic carcinoma is shown in Figure 1.40.

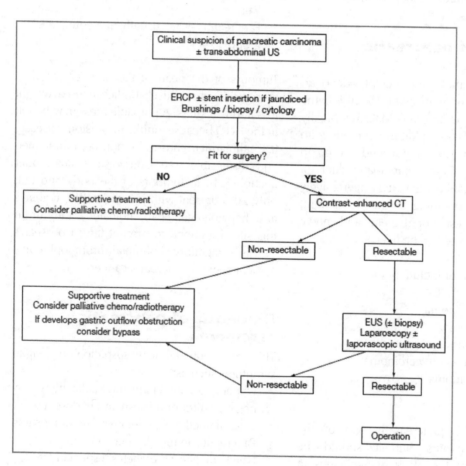

**Figure 1.40 Investigation of pancreatic cancer**

## Surgical management of pancreatic carcinoma

The principles of surgery are different for cancers of the head (**periampullary cancers**) and cancers of the **body** and **tail** of the pancreas. Both need meticulous preoperative preparation, as described in the box below.

---

**Preop preparation for pancreatic cancer**

- **Clotting:** deranged clotting can be corrected with vitamin K
- **Thrombosis:** subcutaneous heparin may be required when clotting is corrected
- **Sepsis:** intraoperative IV antibiotics
- **Drainage:** biliary obstruction can be relieved by ERCP stent or external drainage. Surgery is more hazardous if the bilirubin is >150 units; it causes bleeding, depresses immune function and slows healing; however, some surgeons believe that stenting allows the bile to become infected and increases infective complications (especially external drainage). A large randomised controlled trial is needed

---

## Periampullary cancers

This term encompasses true cancers of the head of the pancreas, duodenal cancers, ampullary cancers and lower bile duct cancers.

Overall, periampullary cancers have a resection rate of 40% although only about 20% of true carcinomas of the head of the pancreas are operable. Whipple's resection is the preferred technique (Figure 1.41). Ampullary carcinomas can be locally resected if the patient cannot withstand major surgery, or if there is convincing evidence that the lesion is benign, but, if the postoperative specimen shows malignancy, recurrence is common and outlook is dire. No benefit has been shown by performing a total pancreatectomy.

## Carcinoma of the body and tail of the pancreas

- Late presentation leads to an overall resection rate of <7%
- Prognosis is poor – most patients have died within 5 months
- Cystadenocarcinomas are rare but have a 5-year survival rate of 50% if resected
- Adjuvant therapy has no proven role
- Histological confirmation of these tumours is crucial because neuroendocrine tumours and lymphomas in the pancreas have different prognoses and require different treatment

### Prognosis

- Overall 1-year survival rate is 24%; 5-year survival rate is 3%
- In those who undergo resection, median survival is only between 12 and 19 months
- The 5-year survival rate is 15–20% (the best predictors of postoperative survival are tumour size <3 cm, no nodal involvement and negative resection margins)

Despite this some patients are still offered surgery because:
- It is the only intervention that carries any chance of cure, however slim
- It has a palliative role in avoiding recurrent jaundice
- An apparent tumour of the body may have originated at the head of the pancreas and have a better prognosis

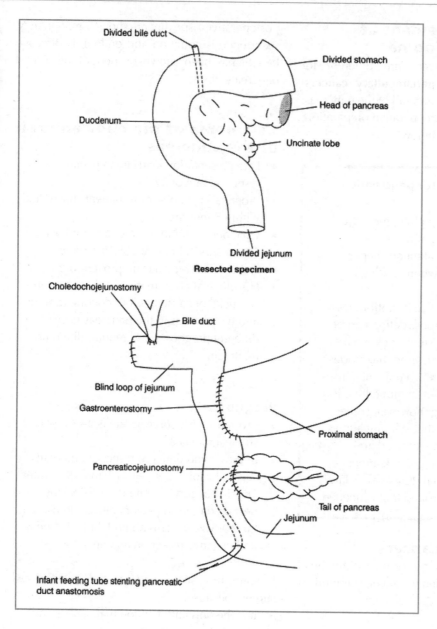

Figure 1.41 Whipple's operation

## Palliative management of pancreatic carcinoma

Symptomatic treatment aims to alleviate problems such as:

- Obstructive jaundice
- Pain
- Duodenal obstruction

Modalities of treatment include:

- Endoscopic or percutaneus trans-hepatic stenting
- Bypass procedures
- Chemical splanchnectomy
- Coeliac block
- Radiation/chemotherapy (there is still ongoing controversy regarding adjuvant and/or neoadjuvant therapy)

## 5.9 Other pancreatic tumours

### In a nutshell ...

**Benign**
- Adenoma
- Cystadenoma
- Islet cell tumours
- Zollinger–Ellison tumour (non-β-cell gastrinoma)
- Insulinoma (β-cell tumour)
- Glucagonoma
- VIPoma

**Malignant**

*Primary*
- Carcinoma (see Section 5.8)
- Cystadenocarcinoma
- Malignant islet cell tumour

*Secondary*
- Invasion from carcinoma of stomach or bile duct

## Adenoma and cystadenoma

These are rare and present in an identical way to malignant pancreatic tumours. The diagnosis is almost always postoperative because it is virtually impossible to differentiate malignant and benign lesions preoperatively. Resection is, nevertheless, the procedure of choice due to the risks of misdiagnosing a malignant lesion or the benign lesions that progress to cancer.

## Gastrinoma

This is a rare tumour of the non-β-cells of the pancreatic islets of Langerhans that can lead to overproduction of gastrin. Only 17% of cases have a single pancreatic tumour. They tend to have multiple metastases and can also occur in the duodenum:

- 30% of gastrinomas are associated with other endocrine tumours (MEN I) especially parathyroid adenomas
- 60% of gastrinomas are malignant at diagnosis

Clinical presentation is peptic ulceration in 90% of cases. These can be single, multiple or treatment-resistant ulcers and may occur outside the stomach or duodenal bulb. Diarrhoea, GI bleeding and perforation are other presentations.

Diagnosis is by a pentagastrin secretion study and fasting serum gastrin levels. Treatment is initial stabilisation of the patient, proton pump inhibitors (PPIs), and resection only if a defined tumour is localised by ultrasonography or CT. In those with diffuse, metastatic or poorly localised tumours, vagotomy and pyloroplasty or total gastrectomy may be the only options.

## Insulinoma

This is twice as common as a gastrinoma but still rare (annual incidence of 1 per million of the population). Unlike gastrinomas, most insulinomas are solitary tumours of the β cells of the pancreas. Clinical presentation is due to hypoglycaemia, including:

- Episodes of disturbed consciousness
- Episodes of odd behaviour
- Patient feels well between attacks

Diagnosis is by:
- Blood glucose
- Plasma insulin
- Glucagon test
- Ultrasonography
- CT

Treatment is excision due to the malignant potential of the tumours. Finding the tumour, even if localised by imaging techniques, can be difficult because it may be as small as 5 mm in size. If the tumour cannot be found, a distal pancreatectomy may be indicated.

## Glucagonoma

Tumours of the pancreatic α cells of the pancreas are extremely rare. They present with a bullous rash and diabetes. Treatment is as for insulinoma.

## Vasoactive intestinal peptide-secreting tumour (VIPoma)

Vasoactive intestinal peptide (VIP)-secreting tumours are very rare and present with:
- Watery diarrhoea
- Hypokalaemia
- Achlorhydria

Plasma VIP levels are raised and resection of the tumour is curative.

## Cystadenocarcinoma

This is a rare, slow-growing tumour; 90% occur in middle-aged women. Tumours may present as an abdominal mass or obstructive jaundice. If technically feasible, resection should be undertaken. If not, prolonged survival may occur even in untreated malignant cases because the tumour is not very aggressive.

## 5.10 Other disorders of the pancreas

### Pancreatic cysts

The classification of pancreatic cysts is shown in the box. They present as firm, large, rounded, upper abdominal swellings. Initially, the cyst is apparently resonant because of the loops of gas-filled bowel in front of it, but as it increases in size it becomes dull to percussion. True cysts require surgical excision. False cysts are drained. This may be performed at laparotomy, laparoscopically, radiologically or endoscopically by drainage or anastomosis into the stomach or the small bowel.

---

**Classification of pancreatic cysts**

**True cysts (20%)**
- Congenital polycystic disease of the pancreas
- Retention
- Hydatid
- Neoplastic (cystadenoma/cystadenocarcinoma)

**False cysts (80%)** (usually a collection of fluid in the lesser sac)
- After acute pancreatitis
- After trauma to the pancreas
- After perforation of a posterior gastric ulcer (rare)

---

## Pancreatic trauma

This can result from blunt or penetrating trauma and is associated with other injuries in 90% of cases. Pancreatic trauma is classified into the following:

- **Minor:** injury does not involve main ducts
- **Intermediate:** distal injury ± duct disruption
- **Major:** injury to the head of the pancreas or pancreaticoduodenal injury

Retroperitoneal injury is notoriously difficult to diagnose clinically, with minimal clinical findings.

Some of the following non-specific investigations may suggest pancreatic injury:

- Raised serum amylase
- Plain abdominal film: air bubbles – along the right psoas margin, along the upper pole of the right kidney, along the lower mediastinum; obliteration of the psoas shadow; scoliosis; ground-glass appearance due to filling of the lesser sac with fluid
- Gastrografin swallow may show duodenal rupture

During laparotomy, the lesser sac should be explored.

Minor and intermediate pancreatic injury may be treated by simple haemostasis and drainage. Major injury may need distal pancreatectomy and splenectomy or, very rarely, as a last resort, pancreaticoduodenectomy. Postoperative care is important, because more deaths are due to late complications such as sepsis and secondary haemorrhage.

## The pancreas in cystic fibrosis

Cystic fibrosis is the most common inherited disorder in white people. It affects many organ systems, especially the lungs. The abnormally viscous mucus secretion causes progressive exocrine pancreatic insufficiency. Pancreatic enzymes may be taken orally to supplement the failing pancreas. Surgery is rarely needed unless stenosis develops in the lower bile and pancreatic ducts.

# SECTION 6

# Acute abdomen

## 6.1 Acute abdominal pain

**In a nutshell ...**

The acute abdomen is the most frequent referral to the general surgeon on call. This chapter is concerned with the understanding, diagnosis and management of the common causes of acute abdominal pain.

## Physiology of abdominal pain

### Visceral pain

This is pain arising from the abdominal, pelvic and thoracic viscera.

The visceral peritoneum (including the mesentery) is sensitive to stretch and is innervated by autonomic nerves. Afferent fibres from these sensory receptors travel with sympathetic and parasympathetic fibres to reach the central nervous system (CNS).

Visceral pain is generally vague and poorly localised and is generated by stretching of the viscera. Due to activation of the autonomic nervous system, visceral pain may be associated with warmth, flushing, pallor and dizziness.

Visceral pain is poorly localised:
- Foregut pain (stomach and duodenum) is felt in the epigastrium
- Midgut pain (jejunum to transverse colon) is felt in the periumbilical region
- Hindgut pain (transverse colon to anal canal) is felt in the lower abdomen

### Somatic pain

This is pain arising from the surface structures. The neuroreceptors in skin and skeletal muscles detect the type and location of the pain very accurately. Abdominal pain arising from the parietal peritoneum is of the somatic type and can be precisely located to the site of the origin.

### Peritonism

This is pain arising from peritonitis (inflammation of the peritoneum). It can be detected by clinical signs of tenderness, rebound and guarding. It can be localised or generalised. It is eased by lying still and exacerbated by movement.

## Causes of acute abdominal pain

### Inflammation and infection

- Appendicitis
- Cholecystitis
- Diverticulitis
- Pancreatitis
- Salpingitis
- Mesenteric adenitis
- Primary peritonitis
- Crohn's disease
- Ulcerative colitis
- Pyelonephritis
- Terminal ileitis
- *Yersinia* infection
- Meckel's diverticulitis

### Obstruction

- Renal colic
- Biliary colic
- Small-bowel obstruction
- Congenital (bands, atresia)
- Meconium ileus
- Malrotation of gut
- Adhesions
- Hernia
- Intussusception
- Gallstone
- Tumours
- Crohn's disease
- Large-bowel obstruction
- Tumour
- Volvulus
- Inflammatory stricture

### Perforation

- Gastric ulcer
- Duodenal ulcer
- Diverticular disease
- Colon cancer
- Ulcerative colitis
- Lymphoma
- Foreign body perforation
- Perforated cholecystitis
- Perforated appendicitis
- Perforated oesophagus
- Perforated strangulated bowel
- Abdominal trauma

### Infarction

- Torsion of a viscus
- Ischaemic bowel (arterial thrombosis/embolus)
- Venous thrombosis
- Aortic dissection

### Haemorrhage

- Rupture of aortic aneurysm
- Mesenteric artery aneurysm
- Aortic dissection
- Ruptured ovarian cyst
- Ruptured ectopic pregnancy
- Ovarian bleed
- Endometriosis
- Rupture of liver tumour
- Rectus sheath haematoma
- Abdominal trauma

**Non-surgical causes of acute abdominal pain**

**Intra-abdominal**

- Diseases of the liver
- Tumours
- Abscesses
- Primary peritonitis
- Bacteria/TB
- *Candida* spp.
- Glove lubricants
- Infections
- Viral gastroenteritis
- Food poisoning
- Typhoid
- Mesenteric adenitis
- *Yersinia*
- Curtis–Fitz-Hugh syndrome (*Chlamydia* spp. causing right upper quadrant pain)

**Neurological**

- Spinal disorders
- Tabes dorsalis

**Abdominal wall pain**

- Rectus sheath haematoma
- Neurovascular entrapment

**Retroperitoneal**

- Pyelonephritis
- Acute hydronephrosis

**Infections**

- Infectious mononucleosis (Epstein–Barr virus or EBV)
- Herpes zoster

**Metabolic disorders**

- Diabetes
- Addison's disease
- Uraemia
- Porphyria
- Haemochromatosis
- Hypercalcaemia
- Heavy metal poisoning

**Immunological**

- Polyarteritis nodosa
- Systemic lupus

**Haematological**

- Sickle cell disease
- Haemolytic anaemia
- Henoch–Schönlein purpura
- Leukaemia
- Lymphomas
- Polycythaemia
- Anticoagulant therapy

**Intrathoracic**

- Myocardial infarction
- Pericarditis
- Pneumothorax, pleurisy
- Coxsackie B virus
- Strangulation of diaphragmatic hernia
- Aortic dissection
- Boerhaave syndrome
- Right heart failure

## Referred pain

In this phenomenon visceral pain is not perceived in the affected viscus but at a somatic site some distance from the viscus (eg testicular pain is felt in the periumbilical area rather than in the scrotum).

## Radiation of pain

In this phenomenon pain is felt diffusely in and around the region of the affected viscus, in addition to being perceived remotely (eg ureteric colic radiating to the ipsilateral testicle).

Figure 1.42
Sites of acute
abdominal pain

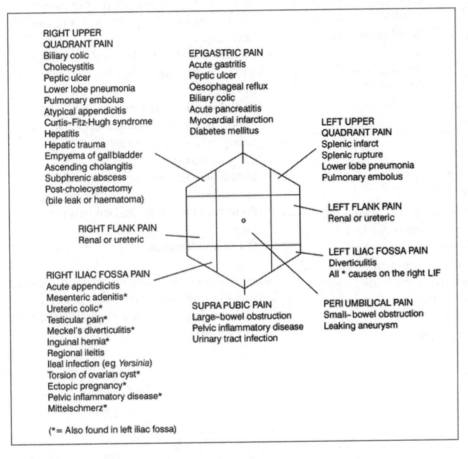

RIGHT UPPER
QUADRANT PAIN
Biliary colic
Cholecystitis
Peptic ulcer
Lower lobe pneumonia
Pulmonary embolus
Atypical appendicitis
Curtis-Fitz-Hugh syndrome
Hepatitis
Hepatic trauma
Empyema of gallbladder
Ascending cholangitis
Subphrenic abscess
Post-cholecystectomy
(bile leak or haematoma)

EPIGASTRIC PAIN
Acute gastritis
Peptic ulcer
Oesophageal reflux
Biliary colic
Acute pancreatitis
Myocardial infarction
Diabetes mellitus

LEFT UPPER
QUADRANT PAIN
Splenic infarct
Splenic rupture
Lower lobe pneumonia
Pulmonary embolus

LEFT FLANK PAIN
Renal or ureteric

RIGHT FLANK PAIN
Renal or ureteric

LEFT ILIAC FOSSA PAIN
Diverticulitis
All * causes on the right LIF

RIGHT ILIAC FOSSA PAIN
Acute appendicitis
Mesenteric adenitis*
Ureteric colic*
Testicular pain*
Meckel's diverticulitis*
Inguinal hernia*
Regional ileitis
Ileal infection (eg Yersinia)
Torsion of ovarian cyst*
Ectopic pregnancy*
Pelvic inflammatory disease*
Mittelschmerz*

SUPRA PUBIC PAIN
Large-bowel obstruction
Pelvic inflammatory disease
Urinary tract infection

PERI UMBILICAL PAIN
Small-bowel obstruction
Leaking aneurysm

(*= Also found in left iliac fossa)

## Sites of acute abdominal pain

Figure 1.42 shows the common sites of abdominal pain and their causes.

## History of acute abdominal pain

A full history from a patient with abdominal pain should include the following:

- **Patient history**

- **Details of the pain:** site, onset, character, radiation, alleviating factors, timing, exacerbating factors and associating features (easily remembered as 'SOCRATES')
- **Review of the relevant systems**
- **Other relevant history:** regular medications and allergies, smoking and drinking, social and family history, review of other systems, anaesthetic problems

Well-recognised sites of radiation of abdominal pain

| Perceived site of pain | Cause of pain |
|---|---|
| Right shoulder tip | Collection under the right diaphragm |
| Left shoulder tip | Collection under the left diaphragm |
| Between scapulae | Gallbladder/thoracic aorta |
| To centre of back | Pancreatitis/aortic aneurysm |
| To ipsilateral testicle | Ureteric colic |
| To ipsilateral flank | Testicular pain |

## Examination of acute abdominal pain

- General overview (does the patient look well/unwell from the end of the bed?)
- Abdominal examination: inspection, palpation, percussion, auscultation; external genitalia (for details see the book *Surgical Short Cases for the MRCS*)
- Rectal examination
- Review of general fitness

## Investigation of acute abdominal pain

- **Bedside tests:** pulse, BP, temperature, urinalysis. Bedside pregnancy tests of urine are mandatory in women of reproductive age with lower abdominal pain to exclude potentially disastrous ectopic pregnancy and to check on pregnancy status in case of later surgery
- **Blood tests:** FBC, U&Es, amylase, group and save, clotting, LFTs, CRP, ABGs (arterial blood gases)
- **Radiological investigations:** erect chest radiograph, plain, supine abdominal radiograph, ultrasonography, CT/MRI, contrast studies
- **Endoscopy:** gastroscopy, colonoscopy, laparoscopy
- **Peritoneal lavage:** limited role except in trauma
- **Other investigations**

Note that, in the acute scenario, urgent laparotomy should not be delayed for time-consuming tests if the clinical indications for surgery are clear.

**SPECIFIC SIGNS ON EXAMINATION OF THE ABDOMEN**

| Sign | Indicates | Definition |
| --- | --- | --- |
| Psoas stretch sign | Appendicitis | Passive extension or hyperextension of the hip increases abdominal pain due to psoas muscle being in contact with the inflamed appendix |
| Rovsing's sign | Appendicitis | Palpation in the left iliac fossa may produce pain at the site of tenderness in the right iliac fossa due to movement of the inflamed parietal peritoneum |
| Grey–Turner's sign | Acute pancreatitis (usually severe haemorrhagic pancreatitis) | Bruising in the flanks due to extravasated blood |
| Cullen's sign | Acute pancreatitis (usually severe haemorrhagic pancreatitis) | Bruising in the area of the umbilicus |
| Murphy's sign | Acute cholecystitis | Patient catches breath due to pain on inspiration while the right hypochondrium is deeply palpated, but not when the left hypochondrium is deeply palpated, due to downward movement of the inflamed gallbladder onto the examining hand during inspiration |
| Boas' sign | Acute cholecystitis | Pain radiating from an inflamed gallbladder to the tip of the right scapula renders an area of skin below the scapula hyperaesthetic |

CHAPTER 1

CHAPTER 1

## 6.2 Common acute abdominal emergencies

### Appendicitis

#### Anatomy of the appendix
- The appendix is a blind-ending tube, usually about 6–9 cm long
- It opens into the posterior medial wall of the caecum, 2 cm below the ileocaecal valve at the point of convergence of the three taenia coli
- It has its own short mesentery (the mesoappendix)
- The appendicular artery is normally a branch of a posterior caecal artery and is an end-artery (thus rendering the appendix susceptible to infarction)

#### Variable sites of the appendix
- **62% are retrocaecal:**
  - Usually free in the retrocaecal fossa
  - May be bound to the caecum leading to poorly localised signs
  - May lie retroperitoneally between the caecum and psoas, leading to the psoas stretch sign (increased pain on passive extension of the right hip)
  - May lie next to the ureter (leading to WBCs in urine)

- **34% are pelvic:**
- Appendix hangs down into the pelvic brim
- Cause more nausea and vomiting
- Easily felt on examination per rectum
- Internal rotation of hip increases pain (obturator sign)
- May have positive psoas stretch sign
- In children pelvic appendicitis may present late because few abdominal symptoms or signs are displayed. Children may have fever and diarrhoea
- Ultrasonography can also help with diagnosis
- **2.5% are paracolic or paracecal**
- **1% are pre-ileal:** with obvious abdominal signs
- **Only 0.5% are post-ileal:** these are harder to diagnose due to poorly localised pain

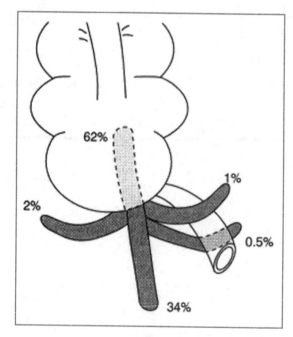

**Figure 1.43 Variable sites of the appendix**

**Rarely:**

- Maldescended caecum leads to right upper quadrant appendicitis
- Long appendix with an inflamed tip can be anywhere (appendix may be up to 25 cm long)
- Transposition of viscera leads to left iliac fossa (LIF) pain (feel for the apex of the heart; if the patient has dextrocardia it is conceivable that the patient has an appendicitis presenting as LIF pain)

## Incidence of appendicitis

This is the most common emergency surgical operation and 80 000 people a year are admitted with this diagnosis in the UK. The incidence has been declining in recent years, which has been hypothesised to be due to changes in diet.

## Pathology of appendicitis

The aetiology is unknown. It may be linked to a lack of fibre, familial tendency or viral infections that increase lymphoid tissue.

The original insult may be due to (or precipitated by) faecoliths, lymphoid tissue hyperplasia, foreign bodies, congenital/inflammatory strictures, tumours or congenital band adhesions.

The appendix wall becomes inflamed and lumen fills with pus

↓

Oedema decreases blood supply leading to infarction

↓

Organisms from the lumen enter devitalised wall

↓

Liquefaction and perforation of appendix occurs

↓

Results in either localised peritonism (if gradual with adhesions) or generalised peritonitis (if frank perforation)

## Clinical features of appendicitis

- **Abdominal pain:** central colicky and vague, localising to right iliac fossa (RIF) after 24 hours and becoming constant
- **Nausea:** ± vomiting and anorexia
- **Pyrexia:** may be present ± high WCC
- **Dry tongue:** coated, with foetor
- **RIF pain:** sharp and localised, worse on movement and found at McBurney's point (a third of the way from the anterior superior iliac spine to the umbilicus). Tenderness, guarding and rebound are features. Rovsing's sign is present (see table in Section 6.1 'Specific signs on examination of the abdomen')

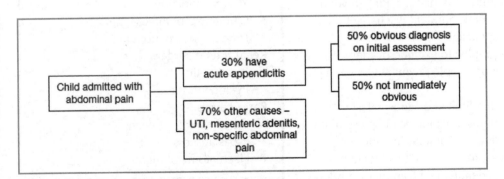

**Figure 1.44 Abdominal pain in children admitted to hospital**

## 'Special' patients

- **Babies:** appendicitis is rare under 3 years of age but has increased mortality. Diarrhoea and vomiting are common
- **Children <5 years:** account for only 7% of cases but 37% of deaths
- **Pregnant women:** appendicitis is less common after 7 months' gestation:
  - 1 in 10 die
  - 3 in 10 have fetal loss
  - 6 in 10 perforate

Problems include nausea mistaken for symptoms of pregnancy, upward displacement of the appendix and guarding masked by the uterus.

## Investigating appendicitis

- **WCC/CRP:** C-reactive protein (CRP) is elevated in >95% of patients with histologically proven appendicitis. A normal WCC/CRP has a >90% negative predictive value for the presence of appendicitis
- **Urinalysis:** pelvic or retrocaecal appendicitis may lead to haematuria or WBC in urine; 30% of children with acute appendicitis have abnormal urinalysis (pyuria or bacteriuria). Urinary or serum hCG (human chorionic gonadotropin) is mandatory in females of reproductive age
- **Cusco's speculum examination:** to exclude pelvic inflammatory disease (PID) in young women (obvious purulent discharge from os, cervical excitation)
- **Ultrasonography:** to exclude ovarian cyst, pyosalpinx or ectopic pregnancy in young women:
  - Although a limited diagnostic test in adults, ultrasonography can be useful for diagnosing appendicitis in children
  - Graded-compression ultrasonography involves identifying the appendix under ultrasound control and pushing on it with the probe to see if there is tenderness
  - In children the inflamed appendix is usually >10 mm diameter
- **Laparoscopy:** especially useful in young women; it may proceed to laparoscopic or open appendicectomy. The popularity of laparoscopic appendicectomy is growing and in many centres has replaced the open operation. Some studies suggest that the laparoscopic approach increases cosmetic satisfaction, decreases surgical site infections and shortens hospital stay. However, there is a significant cost associated with it and a longer operative time
- **Abdominal radiograph:** rarely needed but can be useful if obstruction, perforation or ureteric colic is suspected

---

**Differential diagnosis of appendicitis**
**Mesenteric appendicitis**
**Gastroenteritis**
**Pelvis disorders in females**
- Mittelschmerz
- PID
- Ectopic pregnancy
- Ovarian rupture, bleeding, torsion

**Ileocaecal disorders**
- Meckel's diverticulitis
- Crohn's regional ileitis
- *Yersinia* infection
- Carcinoma of the caecum
- Foreign body perforation

**Renal tract disorders**
- Renal colic
- Pyelonephritis

**Rarer causes**
- Osteomyelitis of pelvis
- Psoas abscess
- Haematoma of rectus

**Op box: Appendicectomy (open and laparoscopic)**

**Preop care**
- Rehydration may be needed
- Antibiotics: one dose preoperatively (usually cefuroxime and metronidazole)
- Consent: must include removal of normal appendix and any other procedure thought necessary at operation (eg removal of Meckel's diverticulum, bowel resection in older patients with atypical symptoms/mass)

**Incisions (see Fig. 1.3) for open appendicectomy**
- McBurney's or gridiron incision
- Lanz incision
- Right paramedian or lower midline (only if carcinoma of caecum is suspected)

**Procedure for open appendicectomy (using McBurney's incision)**
- Incise external oblique in line of fibres
- Split internal oblique and transversus abdominis in the line of their fibres to expose peritoneum
- Incise peritoneum ensuring no bowel in peritoneal fold
- If free pus, send microbiology swab
- Locate caecum and deliver it into the wound using fingers or Babcock's forceps
- Turn caecum to deliver appendix
- Extend incision if necessary or mobilise caecum if difficult
- Divide and ligate mesenteric vessels between clamps
- Base of appendix is crushed, ligated and appendix excised
- Invert stump using purse string
- If appendix is normal, look for Meckel's diverticulum and feel pelvic organs
- If free pus or perforated, wash out with warm saline
- Close in layers

**Procedure for laparoscopic appendicectomy**
(Positioning of ports may vary depending on surgeon preference and position of the appendix base.)

*Perform a diagnostic laparoscopy*
- Place a 10-mm subumbilical port using the open Hassan technique
- Insufflate the abdomen to 12 mmHg and insert the laparoscope (a 30° scope may be used)
- Under direct vision place a 5-mm port in the left iliac fossa (avoid the inferior epigastric vessels)
- Thoroughly visually inspect the abdominal cavity – gentle manipulation of the small bowel and colon may be required and ask the anaesthetist to reposition the patient in a reverse Trendelenburg position (head down) and inspect the pelvis for alternative pathology
- Tilt the patient into a left lateral position, elevating the right side and visualise the appendix

**CHAPTER 1**

*Laparoscopic appendicectomy*
- Place a third (10-mm) port in either the suprapubic region (avoid the bladder) or the right iliac fossa so the instruments easily triangulate around the position of the appendix base
- If the base of the appendix is healthy divide the mesoappendix with careful diathermy and/or clips and use an Endoloop to ligate the base of the appendix. Place a second Endoloop around the base for security and a further Endoloop 1 cm along the appendix body. If the base of the appendix is necrotic then a stapler may be used to remove part of the caecal pole along with the residual appendix
- The appendix can be retrieved by placing it in a collection bag or, if small, through one of the 10-mm ports (the port protects the wound from contamination)
- Suction any free fluid or pus from the pelvis, paracolic gutters and around the liver
- Remove the ports under direct vision
- Close all 10-mm port sites using a J-needle and 1.0 Vicryl

**Postop care**
- Five days of antibiotics if perforated with peritonitis
- Fluids on day 1 (eat when tolerating fluids)

## Complications of appendicitis and appendicectomy
- **Preop complications**
  - Perforation
  - Peritonitis
  - Abscess
- **Early postop complications**
  - Residual abscess
  - Pelvic collection
  - Faecal fistula
  - Ileus
  - Urinary retention
  - Chest problems
  - Thromboembolism
  - Sepsis
- **Late postop complications**
  - Incisional hernia
  - Adhesions
  - Inguinal hernia

### Pelvic collection and appendicectomy
Systematic review of randomised controlled trials (RCTs) has shown a fourfold increase in the incidence of postoperative pelvic collection in patients who have a laparoscopic rather than an open appendicectomy. When performing laparoscopic appendicectomy, it is vital that all pus is aspirated and that, should you decide to wash out the pelvis, all wash is also removed. It is unclear why pelvic collection is more common after the laparoscopic approach but pus and wash fluid may sluice down the right paracolic gutter and lie around the liver while the patient is tilted head down, trickling back into the pelvis when the patient wakes and sits or stands up.

### Effect of perforated appendicitis on subsequent fertility
Decreased fertility is suggested but not proven.

## Conservative treatment of appendicitis

This is advocated if:

- No surgical treatment is available
- Surgery is contraindicated due to poor patient condition
- There is an appendix mass with no peritonitis
- There is late presentation (3–5 days after onset of pain); this is controversial

This non-surgical approach involves a course of antibiotics and observation.

## Interval appendicectomy

This is where appendicectomy is carried out electively some time after successful conservative management. The benefits are not proven and in some studies a third of appendices are normal and a quarter have recurrence.

## Other conditions of the appendix

### 'Grumbling' appendicitis

This is a controversial entity that may be linked to helminth infestation. It may be mimicked by a number of conditions including Crohn's disease, adhesions, salpingitis, recurrent urinary tract infection (UTI) or psychological problems.

### Crohn's disease of the appendix

This is usually associated with Crohn's disease of the ileocaecal region (so local resection of the terminal ileum and caecum may be better than appendicectomy alone).

# Diverticular disease

 In a nutshell ...

**Diverticulum** is an outpouching of the wall of a luminal organ. In diverticular disease, this refers to the colon, but diverticula occur in the rest of the gut and other organs (eg the bladder)

- **Congenital diverticula** involve all layers of the colonic wall (rare)
- **Acquired diverticula** involve areas of colonic mucosa that herniate through the muscular wall of the colon (common)
- **Diverticulosis** means that diverticula are present
- **Diverticular disease** means that diverticula are symptomatic
- **Diverticulitis** refers to acute inflammation of diverticula
- Complicated diverticulitis includes the sequelae of diverticulitis (eg abscesses, fistulas, bowel obstruction, haemorrhage and perforation)

## Epidemiology of diverticular disease

- It is common in developed countries (with low-fibre diets)
- Incidence is increasing
- Incidence increases with age
- 10% of all people aged 40 are affected
- 60% of people aged 80 have diverticulosis

## Aetiology of diverticular disease

Lack of dietary fibre leads to high intraluminal pressures, increased segmentation and muscular hypertrophy in the colonic wall.

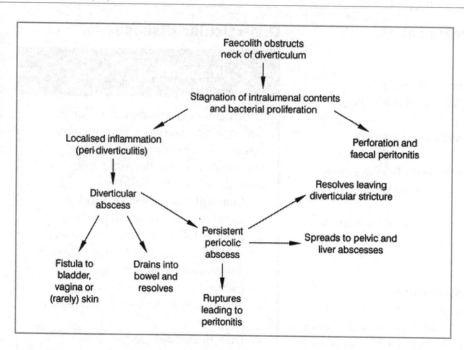

**Figure 1.45 Pathology of diverticulosis**

Acquired diverticula occur at the site of weakness in the now non-compliant colonic wall. The main sites of weakness are where the mesenteric blood vessels penetrate the bowel wall.

## Distribution of diverticulosis
- 45% in sigmoid colon only
- 35% in sigmoid colon and descending colon
- 10% in sigmoid colon, descending colon and transverse colon
- 5% pancolonic
- 5% caecal

## Clinical presentations of diverticulosis

### Diverticular disease
In the absence of inflammation, this may cause a change in bowel habit, pellet-like stools, abdominal discomfort and bloating.

### Uncomplicated diverticulitis
Usually this causes low abdominal pain (often LIF), change in bowel habit ± passage of mucus per rectum. Urinary symptoms, anorexia and nausea can occur. In more severe cases, patients have pyrexia, tachycardia, peritonism, mass, distension and diminished bowel sounds.

### Per rectum bleeding
See also Section 8, Large bowel. This usually occurs in the absence of acute diverticulitis; it is caused by erosion of mural vessels by a diverticulum.

### Pericolic abscesses
These are the result of partial localisation of a diverticular perforation. They can develop in the mesentery, pelvis or retroperitoneum. They can track and 'point' as a perineal, scrotal, psoas or flank abscess. Typical presentation includes tachycardia, spiking temperature and a palpable mass.

## Peritonitis

This is a result of a ruptured pericolic abscess (purulent) or free perforation of a diverticulum (faecal). The patient is acutely unwell with tachycardia, a rigid, silent abdomen, possibly shocked and tachypnoeic.

## Fistulas

These are a result of diverticulitis. Colonic diverticulitis may fistulate into the vagina or uterus (causing faecal vaginal discharge). Colovesical fistulas produce pneumaturia, recurrent UTI and faecaluria. Direct colocu-taneous fistulas may occur but are less common.

## Colonic stricture

Fibrotic healing of recurrent diverticulitis leads to stenosis. These strictures may cause large bowel obstruction or can present on barium or endoscopic investigations for bowel symptoms or abdominal pain.

**Barium enema appearance** of a benign diverticular structure differs from malignant stricture in the following ways:
- Smooth-walled
- No mucosal disruption
- No 'apple-core' appearances
- Diverticular ones tend to be longer strictures

**Endoscopic appearance** differs from malignant stricture as follows:
- Overlying mucosal integrity
- Area of diverticular disease
- Benign biopsies

If doubt persists, a resection should be considered.

## Differential diagnosis of diverticular disease

If patient presents electively:
- Colon carcinoma
- Crohn's colitis
- Irritable bowel syndrome
- Ulcerative colitis (UC)
- Subacute small-bowel obstruction secondary to adhesions

If patient presents as an emergency:
- PID
- Appendicitis
- Complications of ovarian cyst
- Exacerbation of Crohn's disease
- Ischaemic colitis
- Perforated carcinoma of the colon

## Investigating diverticular disease

### Routine tests

**FBC, urine microscopy** (if enterovesical fistula suspected) and **erect chest radiograph** (if perforation suspected), abdominal radiograph (if bowel obstruction or ileus secondary to abscess suspected).

### Imaging studies

**CT** is regarded the best imaging test. It allows diagnosis of diverticular disease, assessment of the extent of the disease, demonstration of stenoses, fistulas and pericolic abscesses.

**Double-contrast barium enema** has largely been replaced in many centres but is useful for measuring the extent of disease. There are problems – it's possible to miss small polyps or carcinoma. **Single-contrast water-soluble enema** is safer if mechanical obstruction or colonic perforation is suspected. **Sinography** can be used to outline the track of an enterocu-taneous fistula. **Cystography** may also be useful.

## Other investigations

**Colonoscopy** is often used as the primary diagnostic tool in elective cases because up to 20% of patients with sigmoid diverticular disease harbour small polyps which can be seen, biopsied or removed. This is contraindicated during an attack of diverticulitis.

## Non-surgical treatment of diverticular disease

### Conservative treatment

In uncomplicated diverticular disease:
* Increased dietary fibre
* Antimuscarinics (eg propantheline bromide)
* Antispasmodics (eg mebeverine hydrochloride)

### Medical treatment

In uncomplicated acute diverticulitis:
* Bowel rest is traditional, but early enteral feeding is gaining in popularity
* IV fluids
* Parenteral antibiotics (eg metronidazole)
* Nasogastric suction if ileus is a feature
* Repeated clinical observation, to detect treatment failure or development of complications
* Outpatient large-bowel investigations after the attack has settled, to exclude other pathology mimicking an attack of diverticulitis

### Radiological guidance

In diverticulitis complicated by abscess formation, percutaneous drainage under radiological guidance is useful. This technique is successful in 75% of patients with a localised collection and avoids emergency laparotomy and temporary colostomy. In addition, laparoscopy and washout have also been shown to be useful. Thus delayed resection with primary anastomosis may then be undertaken when nutritional markers are restored and physical signs of inflammation have resolved.

## Elective surgery

### Indications for elective surgery

* Patients who have recovered from acute diverticulitis but are considered to be at high risk of future attacks (eg one episode in a patient aged <50, or two episodes in patients aged >50, chronically immuno-suppressed patients, proven abscess or perforation treated conservatively)
* Patients with chronic complications of diverticulitis (eg colovaginal and colovesical fistulas, symptomatic large-bowel strictures)
* Patients in whom large-bowel carcinoma cannot be excluded

### Results of elective surgery

* Risk of recurrent diverticulitis after limited colonic resection is similar to that after medically treated diverticular disease (7–15%)
* Main benefit of elective surgery is avoidance of future emergency surgery

## Emergency surgery

Mortality rate increases fivefold when emergency surgery is undertaken. In 30–50% of patients emergency surgery results in a colostomy that is never reversed.

## Indications for emergency surgery

Of patients with acute diverticulitis, 20% undergo a laparotomy, usually for one of the following reasons:

- Faecal peritonitis
- Purulent peritonitis
- Pelvic or intra-abdominal abscess (if not amenable to radiological percutaneous drainage)
- Bleeding that is unresponsive to supportive care
- Bowel obstruction

## Meckel's diverticulum

- Meckel's ileal diverticulum:
  - is in **2%** of people
  - is **2 feet** (60 cm) from the caecum
  - is **2 inches** (5 cm) long
  - (and all of this is true **two**-thirds of the time!)
- It is a true diverticulum, containing all the layers of the intestinal wall
- It is the most common congenital anomaly of the small bowel
- It is a remnant of the omphalomesenteric (vitelline) duct
- The apex is adherent to the umbilicus, or attached to it by a fibrous cord
- It may contain ectopic tissue, most frequently gastric or pancreatic mucosa

## Abdominal pain caused by Meckel's diverticulum

- **Volvulus** or kinking of a loop of small bowel around the fibrous band from the diverticulum to the umbilicus leading to obstruction (in children may present as rectal bleeding and abdominal pain)
- **Haemorrhage or perforation** that may be due to ectopic gastric mucosa being present within it

- **Intussusception** with the diverticulum as the apex of the intussusception
- **Meckel's diverticulitis** clinically identical to appendicitis (50% incidence of perforation)

## Management of Meckel's diverticulum

Meckel's diverticulum may be identified by small-bowel meal or radionuclide scan if gastric mucosa is present, but it is commonly discovered at operation.

## Simple excision of Meckel's diverticulum

This is more difficult if it is broad-based. Many surgeons suggest that incidentally found Meckel's diverticula that are normal should not be resected in patients aged >40.

### Suggested methods of excision

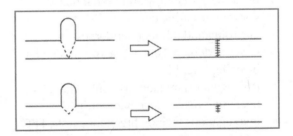

**Figure 1.46 Methods of excision of Meckel's diverticulum**

There is an increased risk of complications if:
- Ectopic mucosa is present
- The diverticulum is >4 cm long
- The base of the diverticulum is <2 cm wide

# Gynaecological causes of acute abdominal pain

Several gynaecological disorders present as an acute abdomen:

- Ruptured ectopic pregnancy
- Endometriosis
- Torsion or rupture of ovarian cyst
- Mittelschmerz (ruptured ovarian follicle)
- PID

## Ectopic pregnancy

- Occurs when a fertilised ovum is deposited outside the uterine cavity
- Affects less than 1% of pregnancies
- Incidence increases with previous salpingitis, intrauterine contraceptive device (IUCD) or previous ectopic pregnancy
- Can occur in sterilised women
- Usually occurs in the fallopian tube; a fertilised ovum lodges in the tube causing vascular engorgement, followed by rupture
- Typical history is a missed period (breast tenderness ± crampy abdominal pain ± systemic disturbance)
- Guarding and rebound tenderness in lower abdomen. Patient may be shocked if bleeding is rapid
- Per vagina examination is contraindicated because it may induce haemorrhage
- Investigations include pregnancy tests, FBC and cross-matching blood
- Early referral to gynaecologist is vital because laparoscopy is the most useful diagnostic test
- Urgent salpingectomy or salpingo-oophorectomy is usually indicated

## Endometriosis

Functioning endometrial tissue is found as deposits outside the uterine cavity:

- Commonly affects the ovaries, fallopian tubes, peritoneum, serosal surface and ligaments of the uterus, sigmoid colon and small bowel
- Affects women aged 30–50
- Symptoms are dysmenorrhoea and low abdominal pain starting 1 week before the period
- Other presentations include low back pain, painful defecation, dysuria, haematuria and partial intestinal obstruction
- Large ovarian endometrial cysts may rupture leading to acute lower abdominal pain, tenderness, guarding and rebound

**Diagnosis** is by laparoscopy or at laparotomy for acute abdomen. **Treatment** is with hormonal manipulation; progesterones or synthetic androgens (eg danazol) are often successful. Complicated endometrial cysts require elective surgery.

## Torsion or ruptured ovarian cyst

- Ovarian cysts are either functional or proliferative
- They can cause acute abdominal pain when they rupture, twist or infarct
- Rupture or torsion produces severe, acute lower abdominal pain with guarding and rebound
- Cysts may be palpable on bimanual examination

**Diagnosis** may be confirmed by ultrasonography or laparoscopy. **Treatment** is surgical excision or aspiration.

## Mittelschmerz (ruptured ovarian follicle)

- Extensive bleeding from a graafian follicle at the time of ovulation can produce severe lower abdominal pain with tenderness and guarding
- Typically occurs midcycle and may have occurred before

**Diagnosis** is confirmed by laparoscopy or at laparotomy when blood is seen in the pelvis.

## Pelvic inflammatory disease

- Syndrome due to ascending infection of the vagina, cervix, endometrium, fallopian tubes ± contiguous structures
- Commonly caused by *Chlamydia trachomatis* or *Neisseria gonorrhoeae*
- Occasionally secondary to GI infection (eg appendicitis) or systemic infection (eg TB)
- Patients present with acute lower abdominal pain and high fever associated with tenderness in the lower abdomen
- On vaginal inspection and examination discharge may be seen, and there is cervical excitation on palpation

**Diagnosis** can be confirmed by laparoscopy.

**Treatment** is by antibiotics (metronidazole and erythromycin) after vaginal and cervical swabs have been taken. An IUCD should be removed if present.

**Complications** include tubo-ovarian abscess, infertility and recurrent infections if partner is not treated.

# Perforation of abdominal viscus

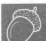 **In a nutshell ...**

Perforation of an abdominal viscus causes sudden onset of acute abdominal pain and peritonitis. Prompt resuscitation is key, and urgent surgery is often indicated.

**Causes of perforation of the abdominal viscus**

**Oesophagus**
- Cancer
- Instrumentation
- Trauma, vomiting

**Duodenum**
- Peptic ulcer

**Colon**
- Diverticular disease
- Carcinoma
- Radiation damage
- Crohn's disease
- Ischaemia
- Tropical infections (typhoid, amoebic infections, TB)

**Stomach**
- Cancer
- Peptic ulcer

**Small bowel**
- Trauma
- Foreign bodies
- Crohn's disease
- Leukaemia, lymphoma
- Peptic ulcer (from ectopic gastric mucosa, eg in Meckel's diverticulum)
- Meckel's diverticulitis
- Potassium chloride tablets (terminal ileum ulceration)

## Clinical presentation of perforation of an abdominal viscus

- Abdominal pain (may be localised to site of perforation initially but becomes generalised)
- Rigid, tender, silent abdomen
- Patient may be systemically unwell, tachycardic, tachypnoeic, febrile, hypotensive
- Shoulder-tip pain and loss of liver dullness on percussion may be elicited
- Symptoms and signs may be minimal in sick elderly patients

## Investigating perforation of an abdominal viscus

- Erect chest radiograph shows free air in 80–90% of visceral perforations
- CT

## Management of perforation of an abdominal viscus

This is described in detail in sections covering each of the underlying conditions. As a general rule, once perforation is confirmed, immediate resuscitation is mandatory and early laparotomy is usually required.

## Inflammatory bowel disease

Ulcerative colitis and Crohn's disease may present as an acute abdomen. Crohn's disease may be mistaken for acute appendicitis or an appendix abscess. It may also present with chronic subacute or even acute small-bowel obstruction, and occasionally causes perforation and presents with severe peritonitis. UC may progress to toxic megacolon which can also perforate. Treatment of these conditions is discussed in Section 8, Large bowel.

## Abdominal wall pain

Pain arising in the abdominal wall rather than the abdominal cavity may occasionally be mistaken for an acute abdomen.

**Neurovascular bundle entrapment** presents as recurrent abdominal pain with one or two trigger points that can be accurately localised using one finger. Injection of local anaesthetic and steroid is diagnostic and may be curative.

**Rectus sheath haematoma** is an uncommon condition that may arise spontaneously after minor trauma or bouts of coughing or sneezing. It may be associated with an underlying disorder of coagulation, degenerative vascular disease, infectious disease or haematological condition (eg leukaemia). The patient presents with acute onset of localised (usually lower) abdominal pain, which is worse when the abdominal muscles are tense. Ultrasonography or CT may reveal the haematoma, and the treatment is conservative.

Note that acute abdominal pain in children is dealt with in the Paediatric Surgery chapter of Book 1.

## 6.3　Intestinal obstruction

### In a nutshell ...

Intestinal obstruction is a term that encompasses impedance to the normal passage of bowel contents through the small or large bowel:

- **Mechanical obstruction** is caused by a physical blockage (complete or incomplete)
- **Functional obstruction** is caused by paralysis of intestinal transit
- **Strangulated obstruction** is the absence of adequate blood supply
- **Simple obstruction** is obstruction with adequate blood supply
- **Closed-loop obstruction** is colonic obstruction with a competent ileocaecal valve that prevents air escaping proximally into the small bowel and thus accelerates large-bowel distension

## Functional obstruction

This is impedance of the normal passage of bowel contents in the absence of a mechanical obstruction. It may affect the small or large bowel. It is usually related to overactivity of the sympathetic nervous system. The two most common clinical presentations are **paralytic ileus** and **pseudo-obstruction**.

### Causes of functional obstruction
**Reflex inhibition of motor activity**
- Postop paralytic ileus
- Spinal injury
- Retroperitoneal haemorrhage
- Head injury
- Chest infection

**Drug-induced**
- Tricyclic antidepressants
- General anaesthetic agents

**Mesenteric vascular diseases**
- Mesenteric arterial embolus
- Mesenteric venous infarction

**Metabolic**
- Hypokalaemia
- Hypothermia
- Diabetic ketoacidosis
- Uraemia

**Peritoneal sepsis**
- Peritonitis
- Pelvic and interloop abscesses

### Paralytic ileus

This is most common after abdominal surgery when the normal short period of postoperative bowel inactivity is prolonged. It is caused or exacerbated by any of the factors listed in the box above. The small bowel undergoes massive distension along its length and, as absorption of fluid from the lumen is impaired, salt and water are lost from the extracellular compartments.

### Clinical features of paralytic ileus

- Recent history of operation or another recognised risk factor
- Typically effortless vomiting and abdominal distension on postoperative day 2 or 3
- No faeces or flatus is passed
- Colicky pain is not usually a feature
- Silence on auscultation

- Plain abdominal radiograph shows gas-distended loops of small bowel and relatively empty colon
- May be gas in the caecum and pelvic colon

It is important to differentiate a paralytic ileus from a mechanical obstruction. Mechanical obstruction tends to occur later in a postoperative phase and is usually associated with colicky abdominal pain and obstructive bowel sounds.

### Prevention of paralytic ileus

To prevent postoperative ileus, avoid unnecessary exposure and handling of the intestine during surgery. It is also important to treat any infections and electrolyte imbalances promptly as they exacerbate the problem.

### Treatment of paralytic ileus

- NG suction
- IV fluid replacement (requirement can be up to 7 l/day)
- Replacement of lost electrolytes (potassium and sodium levels tend to drop and so perpetuate ileus)
- Drug treatments that stimulate peristalsis (eg cisapride) are controversial because they can be dangerous in mechanical obstruction which is often difficult to differentiate

## Pseudo-obstruction

### Clinical features of pseudo-obstruction

This presents as colonic obstruction but a mechanical cause cannot be found:

- Patients are often elderly and bedridden
- Gradual distension of the abdomen and bowel actions cease; bowel sounds may remain and even sound obstructive
- There is little or no abdominal pain and no tenderness

- Abdominal radiographs show a similar picture to mechanical obstruction but gas may be seen in the rectum

### Management of pseudo-obstruction

Once mechanical obstruction is excluded (eg by water-soluble enema or sigmoidoscopy) management is conservative, including the following:

- Correction of fluid and electrolyte imbalances
- Adequate oxygenation and nutritional support
- NG tube not necessary
- Passage of sigmoidoscope and flatus tube usually allows early decompression
- Colonoscopy is useful for investigating and decompressing the bowel
- Prokinetics such as erythromycin or neostigmine can be effective in these patients

### Complications of pseudo-obstruction

- In a grossly distended colon (especially in the presence of a competent ileocaecal valve) caecal rupture may occur
- Regular examination for caecal tenderness is recommended
- Laparotomy may be indicated if the caecum becomes grossly dilated
- Caecal exteriorisation may be required for decompression
- Caecal resection may be required if the caecum is gangrenous
- Tube caecostomy is rarely useful

# Mechanical obstruction

## In a nutshell ...

This common surgical emergency carries a reasonable prognosis if recognised and treated promptly. However, in cases that present late, go undiagnosed or are resuscitated inadequately before surgery, there can be high mortality and morbidity.

- **Small-bowel obstruction** occurs in 80% of cases (usually due to adhesions, hernias or intra-abdominal neoplasia)
- **Large-bowel obstruction** is less common (usually due to tumour, diverticular stricture or sigmoid or caecal volvulus)

## Causes of mechanical obstruction

**Extrinsic**
- Adhesions
- Hernia
- Volvulus
- Intussusception
- Inflammatory masses
- Neoplastic masses
- Congenital bands

**Intrinsic**
- Crohn's disease
- Carcinoma
- TB
- Congenital atresia

**Luminal**
- Gallstones
- Foreign bodies
- Polypoid tumours
- Bezoars
- Parasites

# Physiology of bowel obstruction

## Sequence of events

Fluid and gas accumulate behind the obstruction
↓
Proximal bowel dilates
↓
Peristaltic activity increases (colicky pain)
↓
Eventual inhibition of motor activity (protective mechanism)
↓
Strangulation caused by increased intraluminal pressure or direct vascular occlusion by the obstructing lesion
↓
Venous compromise leads to oedema, which in turn results in arterial compression, ischaemia and intestinal necrosis (this may result in perforation)

## Fluid sequestration

Even in simple (non-strangulated) bowel obstruction, large volumes of fluid can be sequestered in the dilated proximal bowel. Normally:
- 6–9 l/day enters the small bowel
- 1–1.5 l/day enters the large bowel

The shifts of fluid from the intracellular to the extracellular space in obstruction lead to massive fluid and electrolyte imbalances, and may lead to circulatory collapse, shock and death.

Most GI secretions have a similar osmolarity and $Na^+/K^+$ concentration as plasma, thus:
- 140 mmol/l $Na^+$
- 5 mmol/l $K^+$

However, saliva and gastric juice are hypo-osmolar with:

- Low Na$^+$ concentrations (40 and 80 mmol/l, respectively)
- Very high K$^+$ concentrations (15 mmol/l)

As about 1–1.5 litres of saliva and 2 litres of gastric secretions are produced per day, one can see that, in a high small-bowel obstruction with vomiting, dehydration and hypokalaemia are likely. In a more distal small-bowel obstruction, the distended proximal bowel is stimulated to secrete more and is able to absorb less, so fluid becomes sequestered or trapped in the lumen of the small bowel. Usually a 'net absorber', the small bowel now becomes a 'net secretor', with shifts of fluid and electrolytes from the plasma and into the bowel lumen.

Gas also accumulates in the lumen due to:

- Aerophagia (mostly nitrogen)
- Bacterial fermentation
- Diffusion of gases from the plasma as a result of abnormal partial pressures

In strangulated bowel, the bowel wall oedema, intestinal ischaemia, and migration of aerobic and anaerobic bacteria across the intestinal wall lead to further hypovolaemia, generalised sepsis and circulatory collapse.

## Clinical signs and symptoms of mechanical obstruction

These vary depending on the level of the obstruction. The main aims of history, examination and investigation are to:

- Differentiate functional and mechanical obstruction
- Identify any strangulation or bowel ischaemia
- Assess fitness for surgery and resuscitation requirements

A careful history and examination should concentrate on the following findings.

### Pain

- Typically colicky and referred to the central abdomen in simple small-bowel and proximal colon obstruction (embryological midgut)
- In jejunal obstruction the pain comes every few minutes; in ileal and colonic obstruction it comes every half an hour
- It is referred to the central and lower abdomen in distal colon obstruction (embryological hindgut)
- Change from colicky pain to constant abdominal pain may indicate strangulation, ischaemic bowel and a more urgent need for surgery

### Distension

- More pronounced with large-bowel obstruction than with proximal obstruction

### Vomiting

- Occurs early in patients with more proximal intestinal obstruction
- Initially composed of gastric or upper intestinal contents
- Later, intestinal stagnation and bacterial overgrowth occur, leading to effortless faeculent vomiting

### Constipation

- May be complete (no faeces or flatus) or incomplete (some faeces or flatus passed)
- Constipation occurs early in colonic obstruction, but later in small-bowel obstruction

## Tachycardia and hypotension

- May be due to hypovolaemia in simple obstruction (usually responds to fluid resuscitation)
- May be due to ischaemia and sepsis in strangulated obstruction (may be resistant to fluid resuscitation)
- Management of septic shock preoperatively is vital to good outcome

## Temperature

A rise in temperature with tachycardia and peritoneal irritation suggests intestinal ischaemia ± perforation.

## Dehydration

This is seen as decreased tissue turgor and dry mucous membranes.

## Abdominal tenderness

- Simple obstruction leads to poorly localised tenderness that is usually not severe
- Bowel ischaemia causes focal peritonism with guarding over the affected bowel
- RIF tenderness in large-bowel obstruction may indicate closed-loop obstruction with imminent caecal perforation

## Hernial orifices

As one of the most common causes of small-bowel obstruction, it is essential to examine for an incarcerated or strangulated hernia at **all** the hernial orifices.

## Bowel sounds

**Obstructed** bowel sounds are high-pitched with rushes. **Reduced** bowel sounds suggest bowel ischaemia.

## Rectal examination

This is essential because it helps differentiate between functional and mechanical obstruction. In mechanical obstruction, the rectum is often empty and collapsed, but rectal tumours, diverticular masses (felt through the rectal wall), or pelvic malignancy or metastases may be felt. In pseudo-obstruction, a cavernous, ballooned, gas-filled rectum may be detected, with a gush of air or liquid faeces.

Despite all the investigations that are done by the time the consultant comes around in the morning, it may be the SHO who did the per rectum exam who can suggest whether this is likely to be a true mechanical obstruction (needing surgery) or a pseudo-obstruction (needing decompression only).

---

### Why the caecum?

No matter what level of large bowel the obstruction occurs at, chances are that the caecum will be the first place to feel tender, show signs of peritonism and eventually rupture. Even in rectosigmoid obstruction, the caecum may be so gangrenous at operation that a subtotal colectomy rather than a left-sided colectomy will be necessary. The reason for this is Laplace's law.

- **Laplace's law:** as pressure rises, tension in the wall is maximal at the point where the diameter of a tube is greatest

The caecum has the largest radius of any part of the large bowel. Therefore the wall of a dilated colon is most likely to rupture here, no matter where the obstruction is.

---

## Investigating mechanical obstruction

### Blood tests

- FBC
- U&Es
- Amylase
- Cross-match blood

### Radiographs

**Plain abdominal radiographs** are confirmatory in 60% of intestinal obstruction. Abnormally dilated gas-filled bowel loops are seen.

- **In small-bowel obstruction** the following features are seen:
  - Bowel loops with bands (valvulae conniventes) that traverse the diameter of the gut
  - Central bowel loops
  - Pathological dilatation is present if bowel diameter is >5 cm
- **In large-bowel obstruction** the abdominal films show the following:
  - Bowel with bands (haustrae) that incompletely traverse the gut
  - Dilated bowel tends to be peripheral not central
  - Pathological dilatation is present if bowel diameter >8 cm
  - Caecal dilatation is significant if >10 cm

Specific causes of bowel obstruction may be seen in a plain abdominal film:

- **Gallstone ileus:** air in the biliary tree and a radio-opaque calculus in the RIF
- **Sigmoid volvulus:** gross dilatation of the large bowel with the apex of the dilated loop arising from the LIF
- **Caecal volvulus:** gross dilatation of the large bowel in the right lower quadrant (coffee-bean-shaped on plain films)

- **Hernia-induced obstruction:** distended bowel leading to either groin with a localised knuckle of gas-filled bowel in the region of the hernia sac
- **Foreign body-induced bowel obstruction:** radio-opaque foreign bodies may be seen

### Computed tomography

Double-contrast CT identifies 95% of cases of obstruction. CT may show:

- The level of intestinal obstruction
- The cause of obstruction
- The viability of involved bowel, as indicated by circumferentially thickened, high attenuated bowel; congestive changes; haemorrhage in the local mesentery; size of closed-loop obstruction (U-shaped configuration of dilated bowel and associated mesenteric vessels converging towards an apex)
- Liver and lung metastases in the case of malignant obstruction

Adhesions are normally a diagnosis of exclusion if no alternative cause is seen.

### Contrast studies

These have largely been replaced by CT. However, a single-contrast, water-soluble, contrast study (eg with Gastrografin) may be useful and therapeutic in conditions such as intussusceptions.

## Conservative management of mechanical obstruction

### Simple obstruction vs strangulated obstruction

Simple obstruction can initially be managed conservatively with fluid replacement and full investigations before planned definitive surgery if needed. Obstruction complicated by strangulation or ischaemia is a surgical emergency that should be operated on as soon as the patient is resuscitated. For this reason, it is important to assess those features that indicate the risk of strangulation, eg:

- Tachycardia
- Fever
- Tenderness and peritonism
- Leucocytosis
- Nature of obstruction (higher risk of strangulation in incarcerated hernias and an unscarred abdomen)

It is also important to reassess the patient with simple obstruction regularly to ensure that any signs of strangulation are picked up early.

### Non-surgical treatment and resuscitation

Management of obstruction involves the following:

- **Nil by mouth:** intestinal rest; ensures that the patient is ready for theatre at short notice
- **NG decompression:** decompresses the stomach (but not the intestine), reducing the risk of aspiration of gastric contents
- **Analgesia:** more important in strangulated cases
- **Oxygen:** with care in patients with chronic obstructive pulmonary disease (COPD), monitoring saturation and ABGs
- **IV fluid resuscitation:** vital whether or not early surgical intervention is planned, to prevent cardiac and renal complications

In more unwell patients, or those with comorbidity:

- Central venous monitoring
- ABGs

### Management of bowel obstruction

The general rule is 'drip and suck' for up to 48 hours, then surgery if it doesn't settle. Colonic endoscopic stenting means surgery can now be avoided or safely delayed in some cases.

**You must consider surgery if there is:**

- Mechanical obstruction with no previous surgery (virgin abdomen)
- Any sign of strangulation (peritonism, tachycardia, fever, high WCC) or high risk of strangulation (incarcerated hernia)
- Complete obstruction on a Urografin follow-through or enema and no possibility of colonic stenting

**Conservative treatment of mechanical bowel obstruction is only acceptable if:**

- Obstruction has been present for less than 24 hours
- Patient is not fit for surgery or refuses surgery
- Cause of the obstruction is known and surgery is unlikely to be helpful or is very high risk, eg:
  - Patients with multiple admissions for recurrent adhesions that always settle, and with an inoperable battle-scarred abdomen
  - Moribund patients with terminal disseminated malignancy
  - Early postop obstruction thought to be likely to settle (a small-bowel follow-through can determine whether this is a prolonged ileus or a mechanical obstruction)

**Remember:** the threshold for early surgery is lower in children with obstruction because the consequences of missing a mechanical obstruction are dire.

## Surgical management of mechanical obstruction

### In a nutshell ...

Operating on patients with intestinal obstruction aims to:
- Decompress the obstructed bowel
- Correct the cause
- Maintain intestinal continuity
- Avoid iatrogenic injury

### Decompress obstructed bowel

This can be done in the following ways:
- Milking intestinal contents back up to the NG tube which the anaesthetist attaches to the suction
- Using needle decompression
- Decompression via small enterotomy with 'Savage' sucker
- Milking bowel contents through the proximal resection margin
- On-table lavage

### Correct the cause

This cannot always be done at the first operation and depends on the specific cause. If the obstruction cannot be removed, a defunctioning ileostomy or colostomy is an alternative at the first procedure.

### Maintain intestinal continuity

In some cases the bowel is not strangulated, or, if it is, the ischaemia is reversible, in which case no resection is necessary. It is often difficult to determine bowel viability intraoperatively. The following are the most useful criteria:
- Intestinal colour
- Bowel motility
- Presence of mesenteric arterial pulsation

Bowel of dubious viability is wrapped in warm, wet swabs and oxygen delivery is increased. If the bowel is deemed viable it is returned to the abdominal cavity, but if not it may need to be resected.

In the case of bowel resection, if an anastomosis is possible it can be performed at the initial operation. Primary anastomosis should not be carried out if there is:
- Ischaemia of either of the bowel ends
- Tension on the anastomosis
- Peritoneal soiling with faeces or pus
- Gross inflammatory disease, eg Crohn's disease

If primary anastomosis is not possible, one or both bowel ends should be brought out as a stoma rather than risk anastomotic leak.

### Avoid iatrogenic injury

Distended bowel is friable and easily damaged.

### Recurrent (postop) obstruction

In the early postoperative period, functional obstruction (an ileus) is more common than mechanical obstruction (adhesions, undetected distal obstruction, perianastomotic abscess or internal hernia). It is important to distinguish between them and CT may be useful in this setting.

Of patients who have a laparotomy 5–10% may require subsequent treatment for intestinal obstruction. Adhesions may arise around areas of relative ischaemia. Various techniques have been suggested to prevent adhesions:
- Good surgical technique
- No talc or starch on gloves
- Minimise foreign contaminants (suture material) and intestinal content spillage

- Peritoneal irrigation
- Avoid excessive packing with gauze
- Cover anastomosis with omentum
- Use anti-adhesion pharmacological substances (eg bioabsorbable membrane, such as sodium hyaluronidate-impregnated methylcellulose)
- Mechanical prevention (intestinal plication or small intestinal intubation)
- Intestinal stenting in large-bowel obstruction

The placement of an intraluminal stent is a relatively new technique that may become more common, especially in lesions of the descending colon and rectosigmoid junction. It may be used in palliation of malignant colorectal obstruction or to enable patients to avoid emergency surgery if they are temporarily medically unfit.

## Other specific causes of mechanical obstruction

## Volvulus

### In a nutshell ...

A volvulus occurs when a segment of bowel twists through 360°. This often compromises the circulation of the affected segment. It always causes a closed loop obstruction.
'Volvulus' usually applies to the large bowel (eg the sigmoid, the caecum and rarely the transverse colon) but volvulus can occur in segments of the small bowel, especially in the presence of tumour or adhesions

## Sigmoid volvulus

Sigmoid volvulus is responsible for 4% of intestinal obstruction cases in the UK; it is more common in Africa and Asia.

### Predisposing factors for sigmoid volvulus

- Patients are usually elderly, often senile or from a nursing home
- There may be a history of constipation ± laxative abuse for many years
- Redundant sigmoid colon

### Pathogenesis of sigmoid volvulus

The bowel twists in an anticlockwise direction. Circulation is impaired after one and a half twists. It can lead to gangrene, perforation, peritonitis and death.

### Clinical presentation of sigmoid volvulus

Acute abdominal pain, nausea and vomiting are followed by a distended abdomen and absolute constipation. Peritonitis, toxaemia and tachycardia may develop if bowel becomes gangrenous.

### Investigating sigmoid volvulus

Plain abdominal radiograph shows typical distended loop of large bowel full of air. The convexity lies away from the site of obstruction and a bird's-beak narrowing of the colon points towards the site of obstruction.

Barium enema may be helpful in doubtful cases, showing a typical 'ace of spades' deformity. It is contraindicated if gangrene is suspected.

*Treatment of sigmoid volvulus*

Endoscopic decompression should be attempted as soon as possible with insertion of a flatus tube past the twist (if possible) to be left in situ for 24 hours; this may obviate the need for an urgent operation.

Urgent surgery is indicated if the volvulus cannot be untwisted or if signs of gangrene develop. Reduction of the volvulus is followed by sigmoid resection, usually performed with primary anastomosis or exteriorisation of the bowel ends.

Planned surgery after endoscopic decompression may be indicated in recurrent cases if barium studies confirm a grossly redundant sigmoid colon.

### Caecal volvulus

This is less common than volvulus of the sigmoid colon (<1% of all cases of intestinal obstruction in the UK) and is usually due to a lax mesocolon with a mobile caecum. The clinical picture is that of a low small-bowel obstruction. The caecum is visible and distended, lying in the midline or to the left of the abdomen.

Treatment is surgery with reduction of the volvulus. Right hemicolectomy, caecopexy and caecostomy have been advocated.

## Intussusception

This is described in Paediatric Surgery. It can also present in adults with a tumour or lipoma usually acting as the lead point.

## Gallstone ileus

This is responsible for less than 1% of all cases of small bowel obstruction (see Section 5).

## Radiation enteritis

External-beam radiation can result in small-bowel injury. Radiation-induced strictures often present at a delayed interval after radiotherapy. If obstruction results, it is often subacute, allowing time for careful assessment to estimate the length of bowel affected and confirm the diagnosis.

## Mechanical obstruction in children

- Intussusception
- Meconium ileus
- Malrotation and volvulus neonatum

These are discussed in Paediatric Surgery.

## 6.4 Peritonitis

## The peritoneum

### Anatomy of the peritoneum

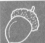 **In a nutshell ...**

The peritoneum is a thin serous membrane. It consists of a single layer of flattened cells (mesothelium).

- The **parietal peritoneum** lines the walls of the abdominal and pelvic cavities
- The **visceral peritoneum** covers the organs
- **Peritoneal fluid** lubricates surfaces and facilitates free movement
- **Extraperitoneal tissue** lies between fascia of abdominal/pelvic wall and the parietal peritoneum; it varies in different regions, forming loose areolar tissue over the lower abdominal wall, a thick fascial layer over iliacus, psoas and in the pelvis, and is fatty over the kidney
- The **peritoneal cavity** is closed in males but has tiny communications with the exterior in females through the uterine tubes
- The **greater sac** is the main component of the peritoneal cavity (Figures 1.48, 1.49)
- The **lesser sac** is a small diverticulum from the greater sac with which it communicates via the epiploic foramen of Winslow (it lies behind the stomach and is also known as the omental bursa)

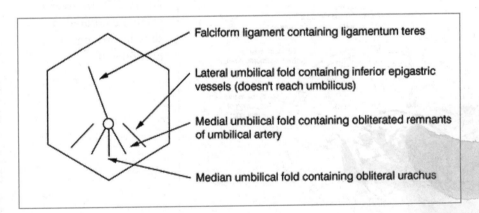

Falciform ligament containing ligamentum teres

Lateral umbilical fold containing inferior epigastric vessels (doesn't reach umbilicus)

Medial umbilical fold containing obliterated remnants of umbilical artery

Median umbilical fold containing obliteral urachus

Figure 1.47 Peritoneal folds of the anterior abdominal wall

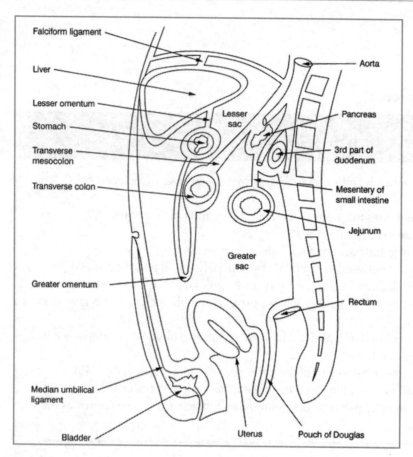

**Figure 1.48 Sagittal section of abdomen showing arrangement of peritoneum**

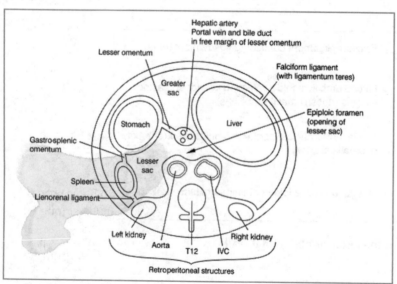

**Figure 1.49 Transverse section of abdomen showing arrangement of peritoneum**

## Borders of the lesser sac

- **Anterior wall:** lesser omentum and stomach
- **Right side:** epiploic foramen and right free border of greater omentum
- **Left side:** hilum of spleen, lienorenal and gastrosplenic ligaments
- **Roof:** peritoneum over caudate lobe of liver
- **Posterior wall:** diaphragm, pancreas, left kidney and adrenal gland and transverse mesocolon

## Functions of the peritoneum

- Movement of viscera
- Absorption of contaminants (contains leucocytes in fluid)
- Seals off infected/ulcerated surfaces
- Suspends viscera in cavity
- Conveys blood vessels, lymphatics and nerves to viscera
- Stores fat (especially greater omentum)

## Terms relating to the peritoneum

### Mesentery

These are two-layered folds of peritoneum attaching the intestines to the posterior abdominal wall, eg to the mesentery of:

- Small bowel
- Transverse mesocolon
- Sigmoid mesocolon

The viscus is suspended by and enclosed in the peritoneum, and the mesentery contains fat, blood vessels and lymphatics, sandwiched between the two layers of the peritoneum.

### Omentum

This is a two-layered fold of peritoneum attaching the stomach to another viscus:

- **Greater omentum:** from the greater curve of the stomach hangs down like an apron in front of the small bowel; it folds back on itself and attaches to the inferior border of the transverse colon
- **Lesser omentum:** runs from the stomach to the liver
- **Gastrosplenic omentum/ligament:** runs from the stomach to the spleen

### Peritoneal ligament

For example, falciform ligament – a double layer of peritoneum attaching the liver to the anterior abdominal wall and diaphragm.

## Boundaries and spaces of the peritoneum

## Boundaries of the epiploic foramen

- **Anterior:** free border of lesser omentum with bile duct, hepatic artery and portal vein
- **Posterior:** IVC
- **Superior:** caudate process of caudate lobe of liver
- **Inferior:** first part of duodenum

The epiploic foramen is the entrance to the lesser sac.

### Subphrenic spaces

- Right and left anterior subphrenic spaces lie between the diaphragm and liver (one on each side of falciform ligament)
- The right posterior subphrenic space lies between the right lobe of liver, right kidney and right colic flexure

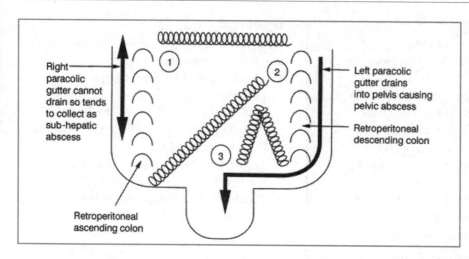

**Figure 1.50 Roots of the mesenteries: (1) transverse mesocolon, (2) mesentery of the small bowel, (3) sigmoid mesocolon**

- The right extraperitoneal space lies between the two layers of the coronary ligament between the liver and diaphragm

For more details on subphrenic abscesses see later in this section.

### Paracolic gutters

These lie on the lateral and medial side of ascending and descending colon (Figure 1.50):

- The right lateral paracolic gutter is in communication with the right posterior subphrenic space
- The left lateral paracolic gutter is separated from the area around the spleen by the phrenocolic ligament but is in communication with the pelvic cavity

### Roots of the mesenteries

The **transverse mesocolon** attaches along the posterior abdominal wall and pancreas (transverse colon is suspended from it).

The origin of the **mesentery of the small bowel** begins on the left posterior abdominal wall near the root of the transverse mesocolon and runs to the right iliac fossa (it is attached to the jejunum and ileum).

The root of the **sigmoid mesocolon** is an inverted V in the left corner of the infracolic compartment (it overlies the bifurcation of the left common iliac vessels and left ureter).

## Peritonitis

### In a nutshell ...

Peritonitis is inflammation of the peritoneum that may be localised (peritonism) or generalised. Peritonitis may be classified according to the causative agent:

- Bacterial peritonitis
- Chemical peritonitis
- Biliary peritonitis
- Pancreatitis
- Blood in the peritoneal cavity
- Meconium peritonitis
- Tuberculous peritonitis
- Drug-induced peritonitis

## Causes of peritonitis

> **Most common causes of peritonitis**
> * Postop complications (30%)
> * Acute appendicitis (20%)
> * Perforated peptic ulcer (20%)

### Bacterial peritonitis

Bacteria enter the peritoneal cavity via four portals:

1. **From the exterior:** penetrating wound or infection at laparotomy
2. **From intra-abdominal viscera:** gangrene of a viscus (eg appendicitis, diverticulitis or intestinal strangulation); perforation of a viscus (eg perforated duodenal ulcer, perforated appendix, rupture of intestine); from trauma (postoperative anastomotic leak)
3. **Via the bloodstream:** as part of a septicaemia ('primary' peritonitis occurs when no obvious infection is demonstrated but is usually secondary to some initial infection)
4. **Via the female genital tract:** acute salpingitis or puerperal infection may lead to peritonitis

### Causative organisms in bacterial peritonitis

| Type of peritonitis | Causative organisms |
|---|---|
| From bowel | Mixed flora (*Escherichia coli, Streptococcus faecalis, Pseudomonas, Proteus, Clostridium, Bacteroides* species) |
| From genital tract | Gonococcus, streptococci |
| Blood-borne | Streptococci, pneumococci, staphylococci, TB |

### Aseptic (chemical) peritonitis

This refers to a perforated duodenal or gastric ulcer. It usually progresses to bacterial peritonitis after several hours. This is one of the most common causes of peritonitis.

### Biliary peritonitis

This may occur as a result of the following:

* **Iatrogenic damage:** leakage from the liver, gallbladder or its ducts after a biliary tract operation. Dislodging a T-tube can also cause leakage. Percutaneous liver biopsy or percutaneous cholangiography can also cause damage to the gallbladder
* **Trauma:** gunshot wounds, stabbing or blunt trauma can rupture the gallbladder
* **Acute cholecystitis:** this rarely leads to biliary peritonitis because, unlike the appendix, the inflamed gallbladder rarely becomes gangrenous or perforates; it tends to become thickened and walled off by adhesions. It also has good blood supply from the liver bed, so is not dependent on one end-artery as the appendix is, which quickly becomes ischaemic. However, perforation of the acutely inflamed gallbladder or transudation of bile through a gangrenous but non-perforated gallbladder may occur
* **Idiopathic:** this is a rare but well-recognised condition in which bile peritonitis occurs without obvious cause, possibly because of a small perforation due to a calculus, which then becomes sealed off

Laparotomy is usually required to deal with any of the above problems.

### Pancreatitis

Acute uncomplicated pancreatitis causes peritonitis but does not require laparotomy.

## Blood in the peritoneal cavity

Blunt abdominal trauma can release blood, pancreatic enzymes and urine into the peritoneal cavity. Blood in the peritoneal cavity causes pain and peritonitis. Sources of bleeding include ovarian cyst, endometriosis, trauma, leaking aortic aneurysm, ruptured ectopic pregnancy, acute haemorrhagic pancreatitis, bleeding disorder, ruptured splenic or hepatic artery aneurysm, intra-abdominal tumour (such as a hepatoma) and torsion of the omentum or bowel.

## Meconium peritonitis

This is intestinal rupture that usually occurs in utero and is therefore sterile. The bowel perforation has usually closed before birth. The most common cause is meconium ileus secondary to cystic fibrosis. Atresia, volvulus or hernia can also be responsible. Plain abdominal radiographs may show intraperitoneal calcification. Treatment involves relief of obstruction and closure of any perforations.

## Tuberculous peritonitis

This is always secondary to TB elsewhere. It spreads from mesenteric lymph nodes, via the female genital tract or from miliary TB. It is rare in the UK but still seen in immigrants and immunocompromised patients. The peritoneum is studded with tubercles in the initial phase, with an accompanying serous effusion. Local abscesses may develop; abdominal viscera become matted together with dense adhesions. Clinically there are three forms:

1. Acute (mimics bacterial peritonitis)
2. Ascitic (serous effusion predominates)
3. Plastic (adhesions, abscesses and obstruction are features)

Treatment is anti-TB chemotherapy and laparotomy for relief of adhesions (if indicated).

## Drugs and foreign bodies

Clinical symptoms similar to acute peritonitis have been described during treatment with **isoniazid** and a β blocker **practolol** (now withdrawn). Intraperitoneal chemotherapy for malignant disease may also cause a peritoneal reaction. **Talc** and **starch** may stimulate foreign body granulomas if introduced into the peritoneal cavity on surgical gloves.

## Pathology of peritonitis

The following are the pathological effects of peritonitis:

- Widespread absorption of toxins from the large inflamed surface
- Associated paralytic ileus leading to loss of fluids, electrolytes and proteins
- Gross abdominal distension with elevation of the diaphragm (can lead to lung collapse and pneumonia)

## Clinical features of peritonitis

- **Signs of underlying condition:** eg appendicitis and peptic ulcer disease
- **Pain:** this is characteristically constant, worse on movement and severe. It may be localised but often becomes generalised. Pain may be referred to the shoulder tip because of diaphragmatic irritation. The abdomen is held rigidly and rebound tenderness is present
- **Signs of ileus:** the abdomen may become distended and tympanitic. Bowel sounds are reduced on auscultation. Vomiting is frequent and may become faeculent
- **Signs of systemic shock:** eg tachycardia, tachypnoea, decreased BP, decreased urine output

## Investigating peritonitis

The diagnosis is usually a clinical one and in many cases an urgent laparotomy is indicated. Investigations are, therefore, of limited value and should not delay prompt treatment unless the diagnosis is in doubt.

Four simple tests are generally needed:

1. **FBC:** usually shows marked leucocytosis and underlying anaemia
2. **U&Es:** can guide fluid resuscitation and enable correction of electrolyte imbalances
3. **Serum amylase:** may help differentiate acute pancreatitis, but may also be elevated in a patient with perforated viscus or other cause of peritonitis
4. **Erect chest radiograph:** will reveal free gas in 80% of cases of a perforated viscus

Other investigations will depend on the underlying pathology.

## Differential diagnosis of peritonitis

Other causes of severe abdominal pain, such as intestinal obstruction, ureteric or biliary colic, tend to lead to restlessness in the patient. Basal pneumonia, myocardial infarction, intraperitoneal haemorrhage or leakage of an aortic aneurysm can lead to misdiagnosis.

## Treatment of peritonitis

- **Analgesia:** usually with IV opiates and an appropriate antiemetic
- **Fluid resuscitation:** with IV crystalloids or colloids depending on degree of dehydration or shock. Hourly urine output measurement is useful so the patient should be catheterised. Electrolyte replacement (especially potassium) is also important.

CVP monitoring indicated in severe cases, or those complicated by comorbidity. Blood cross-matched for surgery

- **NG tube and aspiration:** reduces risk of aspiration pneumonia and alleviates vomiting
- **Antibiotics:** initially broad-spectrum (eg cephalosporin and metronidazole) to cover anaerobic bacteria
- **Oxygen:** essential if the patient is shocked. Hypoxia can be monitored by pulse oximetry or ABG measurements
- **Surgery:** indicated if the source of peritonitis can be removed or closed (eg perforated viscus or gangrenous appendix)
- **Conservative treatment** may be indicated if:
  - The infection has been localised (eg an appendix mass)
  - The cause of the peritonitis is inoperable (eg acute pancreatitis)
  - The patient is not fit for a general anaesthetic

---

**Retroperitoneal tumours**

**Of the kidneys and adrenals**
- Adrenal tumours
- Renal tumours
- Neuroblastomas in children
- Phaeochromocytomas in adults

**Of the pancreas**

**Lots of '-omas'**
- Sarcoma
- Lymphoma
- Haemangioma
- Lipoma
- Teratoma

---

# Subphrenic abscesses

## In a nutshell ...

Two main sequelae of peritonitis:
- Adhesive obstruction (see Section 6.3)
- Intraperitoneal abscesses

Intraperitoneal abscesses occur when peritonitis remains localised or when generalised peritonitis fails to resolve completely; rarely, infection occurs as a result of haematogenous spread.

Localised abscesses are most commonly found in the subphrenic spaces or the pelvis.

## Anatomy of subphrenic abscesses

There are seven anatomical spaces in relation to the abdominal surface of the diaphragm where pus can collect. Four are intraperitoneal (right and left subphrenic and right and left subhepatic), two are perinephric (and, therefore, retroperitoneal), and one is contained above the bare area of the liver so it is also extraperitoneal (Figure 1.51).

## Clinical features of subphrenic abscesses

### General features

Usually, subphrenic infection follows generalised peritonitis after 10–21 days, but it may manifest weeks or months after the original episode. Malaise, nausea, weight loss, anaemia and pyrexia are typical. Many people have a characteristic 'swinging' pyrexia.

### Local features

There may be localising features such as upper abdominal pain, lower chest pain, abdominal or chest wall tenderness. There may be signs of fluid or collapse at the lung base. The abscess may point superficially as described in Figure 1.51. Pain may be referred to the chest wall, loin, upper abdomen, back or shoulder. Hiccoughing may be a feature.

## Diagnosis of subphrenic abscesses

A **WCC** usually shows polymorph leucocytosis.

An **erect chest radiograph** may show any of the following signs:
- Elevation of diaphragm on the affected side
- Diminished or absent mobility of the diaphragm on screening, pleural effusion ± collapse of the lung base
- Gas and a fluid level below the diaphragm

**CT** or rarely **ultrasonography** can accurately localise the collection and drainage under radiological control may be undertaken at the same session.

## Treatment of subphrenic abscesses

### Conservative treatment

In early cases, where there is an absence of gas and free fluid on radiography, broad-spectrum antibiotic therapy may be sufficient. In cases of spreading cellulitis of the subphrenic space, a rapid response to antibiotics may occur, preventing progression to an abscess. Clinical or radiological evidence of a localised abscess collection or failure to respond to antibiotics is an indication for drainage.

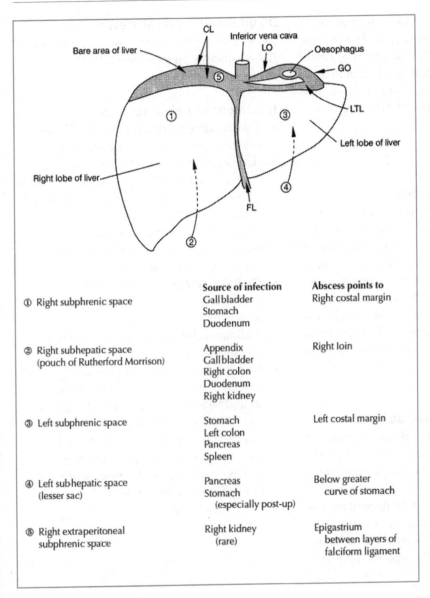

**Figure 1.51 Subphrenic spaces.** CL, coronary ligament; FL, falciform ligament; LTL, left triangular ligament; LO, lesser omentum; GO, gastro-oesophageal ligament

| | Source of infection | Abscess points to |
|---|---|---|
| ① Right subphrenic space | Gallbladder<br>Stomach<br>Duodenum | Right costal margin |
| ② Right subhepatic space (pouch of Rutherford Morrison) | Appendix<br>Gallbladder<br>Right colon<br>Duodenum<br>Right kidney | Right loin |
| ③ Left subphrenic space | Stomach<br>Left colon<br>Pancreas<br>Spleen | Left costal margin |
| ④ Left subhepatic space (lesser sac) | Pancreas<br>Stomach<br>(especially post-up) | Below greater curve of stomach |
| ⑤ Right extraperitoneal subphrenic space | Right kidney<br>(rare) | Epigastrium between layers of falciform ligament |

## Percutaneous drainage under radiological control

Placement of a drainage tube under local anaesthetic by the radiologist avoids both a general anaesthetic and a laparotomy. The drain can be left in place for repeated aspirations or for instilling antibiotics or contrast for subsequent sinograms. Progress can be monitored clinically and radiologically. Deterioration is an indication for surgical drainage.

## Surgical drainage

Depending on the location of the subphrenic abscess (indicated by CT or a superficial swelling), there are two main approaches. The posterior extraperitoneal approach is through the bed of, or below, the twelfth rib. The anterior approach is via a subcostal incision. The cavity should be opened widely and explored to prevent loculi developing, and a large-bore drain inserted as for radiological drainage.

## Pelvic abscesses

### Anatomy of pelvic abscesses

A pelvic abscess is the most common type of intraperitoneal abscess. It may follow any generalised peritonitis but is common after acute appendicitis, gynaecological infections or other pelvic inflammatory disease, including diverticulitis. In the male, the abscess lies between the bladder and the rectum. In the female, the abscess lies behind the uterus and the posterior fornix of the vagina and in front of the rectum (in the pouch of Douglas).

### Clinical features of pelvic abscesses

The general features are similar to those of a subphrenic abscess, ie swinging pyrexia, toxaemia, weight loss and leucocytosis some days after a predisposing condition or operation. The local features which may be present include diarrhoea, mucus discharge per rectum, a tender, boggy mass palpable on rectal or vaginal examination. Occasionally, urinary frequency may occur.

### Diagnosis of pelvic abscesses

Ultrasound and CT scans confirm the diagnosis. There is usually an increase in WCC/CRP.

### Treatment of pelvic abscesses

- **Conservative treatment:** may be all that is necessary because many pelvic abscesses drain spontaneously into the rectum. An early pelvic cellulitis may respond rapidly to a short course of antibiotics, but prolonged antibiotic treatment of an unresolved infection may produce a chronic inflammatory mass, studded with small abscess cavities in the pelvis
- **Digital drainage:** gentle finger pressure at the site of maximal swelling can encourage drainage into the rectum
- **Radiological drainage:** as for subphrenic abscesses (see above)
- **Surgical drainage:** if spontaneous drainage does not occur, the abscess should be formally drained under general anaesthetic with the patient in the lithotomy position. The procedure is performed via a proctoscope or sigmoidoscope. Occasionally, pelvic abscesses drain through the vagina but rectal drainage is usually preferable

# 6.5 Stomas

## In a nutshell ...

There are 100 000 colostomies and 10 000 ileostomies in the UK at present. Incidence is declining due to improved medical treatment of inflammatory bowel disease (IBD) and new stapling techniques enabling low resections to be anastomosed.

**Indications for stomas:**

- **Feeding**, eg gastrostomy after GI surgery, in CNS disease, in coma
- **Decompression**, eg gastrostomy (usually temporary), caecostomy (on-table only)
- **Lavage**, eg caecostomy on-table before resecting distal colonic disease with primary anastomosis
- **Diversion**, eg ileostomy to protect at-risk distal anastomosis, colostomy to achieve bowel rest for Crohn's disease. Loop colostomies and double-barrelled colostomies facilitate closure later but are more difficult to manage
- **Exteriorisation**, eg double-barrelled colostomy (not used for malignancy), resection with end-colostomy and rectal stump (Hartmann's procedure) when primary anastomosis is impossible (eg perforation, ischaemia, obstruction); resection with end-colostomy and mucous fistula (similar to Hartmann's procedure but easier to rejoin); permanent colostomy (eg after abdominoperineal resections in low rectal tumours); permanent ileostomy (eg after panproctocolectomy for ulcerative colitis or familial polyposis coli)

## Selecting a stoma site

| Assess | Avoid | Problem patients |
|---|---|---|
| Before operation | Wound site | Wheelchair-bound |
| With clothes | Bony prominences | Amputees |
| Lying and standing | Existing scars | Obese |
| Good visibility | Umbilicus | Allergies |
| Groin crease/skinfold | | Psychological problems |

## Preoperative preparations

For elective colonic procedures, the following should be considered:

- Laxatives
- Enemas
- Antibiotic prophylaxis
- Deep vein thrombosis (DVT) prophylaxis
- Marking stoma site
- Counselling

# Types of stoma

## Gastrostomy

- **Main indications:** feeding
- **Preop:** empty stomach then fill with air
- **Methods:** commonly endoscopic (percutaneous endoscopic gastrostomy, PEG) under sedation or general anaesthesia (Figure 1.52). May be done as an open procedure or under radiological control

## Jejunostomy

- **Main indications:** feeding
- **Methods:** there are many techniques, the most common being the Witzel jejunostomy. In this (open) method, the jejunostomy is sited 30 cm distal to the ligament of Treitz (duodenojejunal flexure) on the anti-mesenteric border; 10–15 cm of catheter is fed into the distal jejunum lumen, the catheter is fastened to the jejunum at the point of entry through the serosa and then interrupted sutures are used to bring a seromuscular tunnel over the proximal 5–6 cm of the catheter. The jejunostomy tube is brought out through a stab incision in the abdominal wall and the jejunum is sutured to the peritoneal (inner) surface of the anterior abdominal wall

## Ileostomy

### Indications for a temporary ileostomy (usually a loop ileostomy)

- To protect ileorectal anastomosis
- Persistent low intestinal fistula
- Right colonic trauma
- Preliminary to construction of ileoanal reservoir

### Indications for a permanent ileostomy (usually an end-ileostomy)

- Panproctocolectomy for ulcerative colitis, severe Crohn's disease, familial polyposis coli or multiple colonic cancer

Note that 500 ml/day of high-enzyme content fluid is lost from a low-output ileostomy, and 1 l/day in a high-output ileostomy.

## Caecostomy

- **Indications:** a formal caecostomy is seldom performed nowadays but tube caecostomies are still used for on-table lavage, to protect awkward lower anastomoses, and as a decompressing 'blow-hole' for distal colonic obstruction
- **Method:** usually performed with a large-bore catheter through a stab incision in the caecum, protected by a purse string

## Colostomy

### Indications for temporary colostomy

- To protect distal anastomosis
- To defunction a diseased segment (eg for Crohn's disease perineum or severe proctitis)
- If primary anastomosis is not possible after resection (eg in the presence of perforation, sepsis, ischaemia or obstruction)

### Indication for permanent colostomy

- After abdominoperineal resection of low rectal tumours

## Procedure box: Forming an ileostomy

**Preop preparation**
- Counselling and marking preferably by colorectal nurse specialist
- Usually positioned in the right iliac fossa

**Procedure**
- A circular skin defect 2–3 cm in diameter is excised
- A cruciate incision is made in the underlying rectus sheath
- The peritoneum is incised
- The stapled or clamped ileum is passed through the incision in the peritoneum and left to rest outside the abdominal wall with a tissue-holding clamp such as Babcock's, affixed to ensure that it does not fall back into the abdomen
- It is important that the mesentery is not damaged when pulling the bowel through the abdominal wall and that the proximal end is marked in some way
- It is important that the mesentery is not under tension
- The main abdominal wound is closed and dressed
- The intestinal clamp is then removed (or the staple-line excised) to open the bowel
- A 4- to 5-cm spout is formed by everting the stump and suturing the mucosa to the skin with interrupted undyed Vicryl sutures
- A bite of the serosa is taken a few centimetres proximal to the stump with each stitch to evert the stoma
- A drainable transparent stoma bag is fixed over the ileostomy

**Postop**
- The stoma should be observed for ischaemia, retraction and function

**Complications**
- See page 221 for complications of stomas

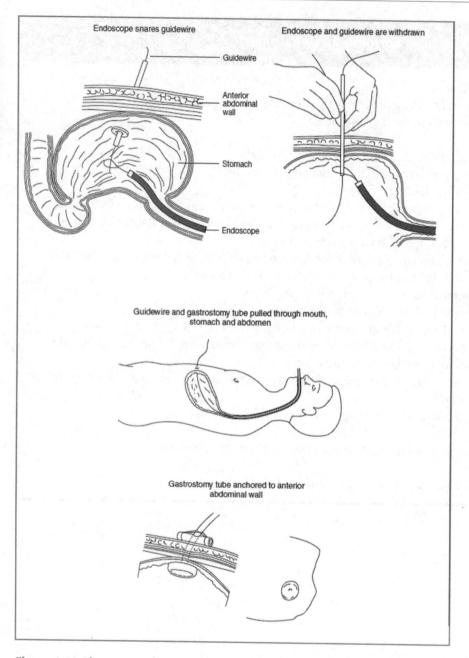

**Figure 1.52 Placement of percutaneous endoscopic gastrostomy tube**

## Loop colostomy (Figure 1.53)

- Used for diversion not resection
- Usually in right transverse colon, proximal to the middle colic artery
- Colostomy bridge is passed around loop of colon through a small avascular window in the mesocolon
- Loop is brought out through the abdominal wall incision
- Bridge is secured, laparotomy wound (if present) is closed, then the stoma is opened and formed

## End-colostomy and rectal stump (Hartmann's procedure)

- Used if a primary anastomosis is contraindicated
- After resection the colostomy is brought out using the proximal end of colon
- Distal (usually rectal stump) is over-sewn and left in the abdomen
- Another laparotomy is required to rejoin the bowel later (unlike in a loop colostomy)

## End-colostomy and mucous fistula

This is used in similar circumstances to Hartmann's procedure but, instead of dropping the rectal stump back into the abdomen, it is brought out as a separate stoma, which – being an efferent limb – produces only mucus. This makes the distal limb more accessible when the bowel is rejoined later. It is also essential if there is a distal stricture forming a 'blow-hole' and preventing a closed-loop obstruction.

## Double-barrelled colostomy

This is used after resection when both limbs of the stoma can be brought to the skin surface adjacent to each other (eg midsigmoid perforation or volvulus). After resection, the proximal and distal limbs of the colon are sutured together along the anti-mesenteric border. This is as easy to close as a loop colostomy and can be closed using a side-to-side stapler at a later date without a laparotomy.

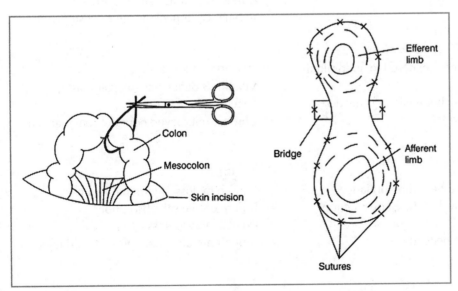

Colon
Mesocolon
Skin incision

Efferent limb
Bridge
Afferent limb
Sutures

**Figure 1.53 Loop colostomy**

### Closure of colostomies

This is best left for 6 weeks until inflammation and oedema have settled, so minimising the risk of a leak. After 10–12 weeks, mobilisation of the bowel may become more difficult because of fibrous adhesion formation.

### Output of colostomies

- **Mid-transverse colon:** 200–300 ml/day; significant enzyme content
- **Low colostomy:** 100 ml/day; virtually no enzyme content

## Complications of stomas

These complications are technical, general and practical.

## Technical problems of stomas

### Ischaemia/gangrene

- Abdominal wall defect too tight
- Injury to mesenteric vessels
- Re-siting is necessary

### Prolapse or intussusception

- When bowel is not anchored to abdominal wall internally
- Reduction is easy but re-siting is needed if prolapse is recurrent

### Parastomal hernia

- May cause difficulties with appliances
- May contain bowel at risk of obstruction/ strangulation
- Re-siting may be needed

### Stenosis

- Poor initial siting
- Ischaemia
- Underlying disease process (carcinoma, IBD)
- Re-siting may be necessary if there is obstruction

### Bowel contents spill over into efferent loop

- Especially in loop colostomy
- Distal bowel is not adequately defunctioned if this occurs
- Split or double-barrelled stomas solve this
- The efferent loop should be sited cephalic to (above) the afferent loop if practicable

## General problems of stomas

### Stoma diarrhoea

- Due to underlying disease
- Due to shortened bowel proximal to stoma
- Due to inappropriate diet
- Can lead to water and electrolyte imbalance, especially after ileostomy

### Nutritional disorders

- Vitamin B deficiency (megaloblastic anaemia)
- Chronic microcytic normochromic anaemia

### Gallstones

- Caused by loss of terminal ileum
- Failure of bile salt absorption
- Excessive water loss
- Patients are also more prone to kidney stones

## Short gut syndrome

- Profuse fluid and electrolyte loss

## Underlying disease

- May cause recurrent symptoms
- Crohn's disease may cause peristomal fistulas or proximal obstruction

## Psychological and sexual problems

- May need counselling and support

## Practical problems of stomas

- **Odour:** advice can be given on hygiene, diet and deodorant sprays
- **Flatus:** this can be improved by diet and special filters
- **Skin problems:** these are usually due to an ill-fitting device. Problems are worsened as the stoma shrinks postoperatively, and can be counteracted by use of a barrier cream or a two-piece appliance. Ileostomies – with their irritant, copious output – can be particularly troublesome. The patient may need a supporting belt if the spout is not big enough
- **Leakage:** transverse loop colostomies are especially prone to leakage. A poor site may be responsible. Methylcellulose paste around the appliance can help
- **Parastomal hernia:** a flexible pouch, supporting belt and filler paste can all help with this problem. Re-siting may be necessary
- **Stoma prolapse:** this requires surgical correction

## Postoperative practicalities and stomas

Stoma appliances must be secure, comfortable, skin friendly, adhesive and odour proof.

Two types of appliance:
1. **One-piece:** adhesive; surrounding pouch adheres to skin; whole appliance is changed
2. **Two-piece:** baseplate with flange; only pouch is changed regularly

Two types of pouch:
1. **Drainable:** used in the immediate postoperative period when output is large and fluid
2. **Closed:** has charcoal filter to release flatus without odour

## Postoperative care

- **Warn/advise patient of problems:** oedematous stoma; copious offensive early output; transparent pouch to monitor stoma
- **Self-care programme:** patients observe how to self-care, then help and finally manage their own stoma
- **Counselling and support:** from stoma-care nurse

## Alternative methods of colostomy management

- **Irrigation:** flushing fluid into the colon via the stoma (no appliance needed); patient needs suitable bathroom facilities; this is not satisfactory for Crohn's disease patients
- **Colostomy plug:** a foam plug that clips to a flange; the plug fills the lumen and blocks the bowel for 8–12 hours

# SECTION 7
# Small bowel

## 7.1 Anatomy and physiology of the small bowel

### In a nutshell ...

- The small bowel consists of the duodenum, the jejunum and the ileum
- Apart from the duodenum, it is an intraperitoneal structure hanging from a mesentery supplied by the superior mesenteric artery and draining into the splenic vein
- The wall is made up of four layers: mucosa, submucosa, muscularis propria and stroma
- Its functions are digestion and absorption of food

### Gross anatomy of the small bowel

- The small bowel is a muscular tube that is about 6 metres long, running from the pylorus of the stomach to the ileocaecal valve

- The anatomy of the duodenum has been covered in Section 3.
- Of the remaining small bowel, the proximal 40% is called the jejunum and the distal 60% the ileum. The transition between the two is not always clear-cut
- The small bowel is intraperitoneal, unlike the duodenum before it and the ascending colon after it (which are retroperitoneal)
- A double layer of peritoneum encloses the small bowel and forms the mesentery from which it is suspended (see Figure 1.48)
- This small-bowel mesentery contains blood vessels, lymphatics and nerves as well as some fat, and is about 15 cm long; it is attached to the posterior abdominal wall by what is known as the 'root of the small bowel'
- The root of the small bowel runs from the duodenojejunal flexure (to the left of the L2 vertebra) diagonally across to the right sacroiliac joint
- The blood supply of the small bowel is from the jejunal, ileal and ileocolic branches of the superior mesenteric artery (see Figure 1.56 in Section 8)
- The veins follow the arteries and drain into the superior mesenteric vein, which joins the splenic vein behind the neck of the pancreas to form the portal vein

- The motor and parasympathetic nerve supply of the small bowel is from the tenth cranial nerve (vagus); preganglionic fibres synapse with the intrinsic neural plexus in the bowel wall
- Sympathetic innervation is from fibres that arise in T9 and T10 and synapse in the superior mesenteric ganglion; pain is carried in sympathetic afferents

> **Relations of the root of the small bowel mesentery (top to bottom)**
> - Third part of the duodenum
> - Aorta
> - Inferior vena cava
> - Right psoas major muscle
> - Right ureter
> - Right gonadal vessels
> - Right iliacus muscle

**Differences between the ileum and jejunum**

|  | Jejunum | Ileum |
| --- | --- | --- |
| Wall | Thick | Thin |
| Valvulae conniventes | Large | Small |
| Diameter | Large | Small |
| Position relative to umbilicus | Around and above | Below |
| Mesentery | Thin | Thick with more fat |
| Arterial arcades | Simple with long terminal vessels | Multiple with short terminal vessels |

The way to remember this is that the long terminal arteries (vasa recta) to the jejunum look more like the letter J than the short stumpy terminal arteries to the ileum, which look like the letter I. And the jejunum is the bigger tube (thicker wall, larger diameter) because it is a bigger word than ileum!

## Histology of the small bowel

The small bowel wall consists of four layers:
- **Mucosa:** the innermost (luminal) surface which in turn consists of three layers:
- **Epithelium** – this layer is made up of:
  - Columnar absorptive cells arranged in finger-like villi
  - Mucus-secreting goblet cells
  - Endocrine enterochromaffin cells
  - Paneth cells
  - Other undifferentiated cells
- **Lamina propria:** this connective tissue layer contains blood vessels, lymphatics and the immunoglobulin-producing plasma cells
- **Muscularis mucosa:** a thin slip of muscle separating the mucosa from the submucosa
- **Submucosa:** this strong connective tissue layer contains:
  - Meissner's nerve plexus (see Figure 1.19 in Section 3)
  - Blood vessels

- Peyer's patches (aggregates of lymphoid tissue especially prominent in the terminal ileum)

**Muscularis propria:** this layer consists of:

- An outer longitudinal layer of muscle
- The myenteric plexus sandwiched between the two muscle layers (see Figure 1.19)
- An inner circular layer of muscle

**Serosa:** this peritoneal outermost layer covers the entire length and circumference of the small bowel

---

**Features of the small bowel that increase absorptive surface area**

**Length**

- 3–10 m (average 6 m)

**Transverse folds**

- Also known as valvulae conniventes/ plica semilunaris/valves of Kecking
- Can be seen at surgery as circular 'wrinkly' ridges in the mucosa

**Villi**

- Finger-like projections of epithelial surface with crypts of Lieberkühn in-between
- Make surface of the small bowel look like a carpet at endoscopy

**Microvilli**

- Hair-like projections on the epithelial cell membrane rich in digestive enzymes
- Can be seen under the microscope as a 'brush border' on luminal surface of the cell membrane

---

# Functions of the small bowel

## Digestion

- **Carbohydrates:** usually make up 30–40% of the western diet. Salivary and pancreatic amylase digest starch into oligosaccharides. Surface enzymes in the brush border of the mucosa of the small bowel break the oligosaccharides into monosaccharides (mostly glucose)
- **Proteins:** activated pepsins in the stomach begin digestion. The majority is by pancreatic proteases: endopeptidases (trypsin, chymotrypsin, elastase) and exopeptidases (carboxypeptidase A and B). Pancreatic secretions are covered in Section 5.6. Digestion is completed by the time proteins reach the midjejunum
- **Fats:** fats are digested by pancreatic enzymes after emulsification by bile salts. Micelles are formed during emulsification, enclosing fats in a bilayer bile-salt disc. Fats are then broken down into components – palmitic, stearic, oleic and linoleic fatty acids – which are absorbed by the intestinal epithelial cells

## Absorption

- **Water:** 10 l/day in, 500 ml/day out. So, **small bowel absorbs about 9.5 l/day**, mostly in the jejunum
- **Potassium:** absorbed at the expense of sodium, using a $K^+/Na^+$ ATPase pump
- **Glucose:** along with other monosaccharides (too big for passive diffusion), glucose is taken up by an active transport system mediated by the $K^+/Na^+$ ATPase pump

- **Amino acids and oligopeptides:** also facilitated by the $K^+/Na^+$ ATPase pump. The small bowel is very efficient at absorbing protein and there is rarely protein malabsorption even after radical small-bowel resection
- **Calcium:** in proximal small bowel by active transport, dependent on the presence of parathyroid hormone and vitamin D (see Chapter 4, Endocrine Surgery)
- **Iron:** if it has been reduced in the stomach to the ferrous ($Fe^{2+}$) form (see Section 3)
- **Fatty acids:** once digested, triglycerides diffuse into the epithelial cells easily with no need for active transport. Within the cytoplasm of the intestinal epithelial cell, they are formed into chylomicrons in order to facilitate absorption into the bloodstream
- **Vitamin B12:** absorbed in the terminal ileum as a vitamin B12–intrinsic factor complex which has been formed in the stomach (see Section 3)
- **Folic acid:** absorbed in the jejunum. Malabsorption may occur if the jejunum is diseased (eg in coeliac disease) or resected. Epanutin, an antiepileptic, inhibits a mucosal enzyme system and results in folic acid being unable to leave the mucosal cells

## What happens after small-bowel resection?

Patients are able to survive without parenteral nutrition with only 80 cm of small bowel, such is its adaptive nature. You should be aware that resecting some sections of the small bowel has specific consequences, however.

### Jejunum

- Reduced absorption of water and electrolytes, fat, protein and carbohydrates results in temporary diarrhoea after total jejunal resection, which settles when the ileum adapts and increases its absorptive capacity
- Folic acid absorption may never recover to previous levels and may have to be supplemented

### Terminal ileum

- Resection of more than 1 metre of terminal ileum reduces the absorption of vitamin B12. This leads to megaloblastic anaemia when the body's stores are depleted (which may take several years) unless vitamin B12 injections are prescribed
- The absorption of bile salts (see Figure 1.38 in Section 5) is reduced, leading to increased risk of gallstones, malabsorption of fats and fat-soluble vitamins (or, as I call them, 'DEKA' vitamins – D, E, K and A)
- Increased amounts of fats and bile salts passing into the colon result in diarrhoea

## 7.2 Imaging and investigating the small bowel

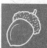

### In a nutshell ...

- Contrast studies
- Endoscopy/capsule endoscopy
- CT
- Angiography
- Isotope studies
- Laparoscopy
- Laparotomy

## Contrast studies

### Small-bowel series (barium follow-through)

- Mainstay of small-bowel investigation for many years
- Relies on passage of orally administered barium into the long, redundant, overlapping small bowel
- Single-contrast
- Adequate to diagnose obstructing lesions or Crohn's disease
- May miss non-obstructing lesions

### Enteroclysis (small-bowel enema)

- Tube passed into proximal jejunum
- Dilute barium and air or methylcellulose insufflation provide double contrast and improved fine detail

## Endoscopy

- **Standard upper endoscopy** visualises the duodenum and proximal jejunum
- **Colonoscopy** can visualise terminal ileum if ileocaecal valve is intubated.
- **Enteroscopy** uses a long, fine, fibreoptic endoscope that is passed transorally into the small bowel. It can be useful for detecting arteriovenous (AV) malformations in patients with GI bleeds of unknown cause

## CT

CT is the most useful image modality for most small-bowel pathology. Spiral CT using oral and IV contrast improves the diagnostic accuracy.

CT allows examination of the following:
- Small-bowel mucosa (eg looking for neoplasms)
- Mesenteric vasculature (eg in mesenteric vein thrombosis)
- Tumour extension or inflammation outside the lumen
- Adjacent organs

MRI is not used as often as CT in small-bowel disease although **MR enterography** has an increasing role in imaging of the small bowel, particularly in the investigation of Crohn's disease.

Ultrasonography is of limited use due to air-filled loops of small bowel.

## Angiography

Most useful in identifying a small-bowel source of GI haemorrhage if the rate of bleeding is >0.5 ml/min.

This can be therapeutic: vasopressin infusion or embolisation can be employed via the angiography catheter to stop the bleeding.

## Isotope studies

Radiolabelled red blood cell scans can identify bleeds of 0.1 ml/min or more; however, localisation is not very precise and the technique is not therapeutic.

## Laparoscopy and laparotomy

Laparoscopy enables direct visualisation of the entire length of the small bowel, biopsy and small-bowel resection.

Laparotomy remains the 'gold standard' for definitively ruling out small-intestinal disease; on-table enteroscopy can also be used.

## 7.3  Intestinal fistulas

### In a nutshell ...

A **fistula** is an abnormal communication between two epithelialised surfaces.
An **intestinal fistula** is an abnormal communication between the intestinal tract and another epithelial surface.
An **internal fistula** is an abnormal communication between two internal epithelialised surfaces, such as the colon and the bladder or the duodenum and the gallbladder.
In an **external fistula** one of the epithelial surfaces is skin.
The table below lists some different types of intestinal fistulas and their clinical presentation.

### Different types of intestinal fistula

| Name | Between | Typical clinical presentation* |
|------|---------|-------------------------------|
| Enterocutaneous | Small bowel and skin | Discharging lesion (usually high output) |
| Enterovesical | Small bowel or colon and bladder | Recurrent urinary tract infection |
| Colovesical | | Pneumaturia, faecaluria |
| Enterocolic | Small bowel or stomach and colon | Diarrhoea, dehydration |
| Gastrocolic | | |
| Rectovaginal | Rectum or colon and vagina | Offensive vaginal discharge |
| Colovaginal | | |
| Cholecystoduodenal | Gallbladder or bile duct and duodenum | Often postoperative or after severe cholocystitis |
| Choledochoduodenal | Gallstone ileus | |
| Colocolic | Two areas of the colon | Diarrhoea |
| Colocutaneous | Colon and skin | Skin lesion discharging faeculent matter |
| | | Skin lesion dischargin faeculent matter (usually low output) |

*All may present with evidence of the underlying disease (such as weight loss, anaemia) or evidence of intra-abdominal sepsis (such as fever, tachycardia, abdominal masses or tenderness).

## Aetiology of fistulas

The box 'Causes of intestinal fistulas' shows the more common causes. A fistula will tend to heal spontaneously in normal circumstances, but certain factors will inhibit spontaneous healing:

- Distal obstruction
- Persistence of underlying disease (eg abscess, carcinoma, inflammatory bowel disease [IBD])
- Epithelialisation of the fistulous tract
- Presence of foreign bodies (such as suture in the fistulous tract)
- Loss of bowel continuity (as occurs after anastomotic breakdown)
- Malnutrition

---

**Causes of intestinal fistulas**

**Iatrogenic**
- Anastomotic leakage
- Percutaneous abscess drainage
- Radiotherapy

**Crohn's disease**
- Spontaneous
- Postoperative

**Carcinoma**
- Direct invasion
- Abscess formation

**Diverticular disease**

**Embryological**

**Traumatic**

---

## Management of fistulas

Management of a patient with an intestinal fistula depends on a number of factors, including the type of fistula, its underlying cause and the condition of the patient. They often present a complex surgical problem, and require a methodical approach and a multidisciplinary team (MDT). The aim of management is to obtain closure of the fistula while keeping the patient in good health.

## SNAP

After initial resuscitation and stabilisation of the patient, the important aspects of management can be remembered with the aid of the mnemonic SNAP:

**S**epsis
**N**utrition
**A**natomy
**P**lan (conservative treatment or surgery)

Special problems include skin care and haemorrhage.

## Sepsis

A fistula is commonly associated with an abscess cavity that may lead to sepsis and death. Evidence of sepsis should be sought and treated as a matter of priority. The presence of an abscess is suggested by the following:

- Persisting pain
- Pyrexia
- Tachycardia
- Leucocytosis/raised inflammatory markers
- Falling serum albumin
- High urinary nitrogen

An abscess can be diagnosed by ultrasonography, CT or fistulography by use of a contrast medium. **Abscesses must be drained surgically or radiologically to control sepsis.** The aim is to convert a complex cavity into a simple fistulous tract which may close spontaneously. No attempt to close the fistula surgically should be made at this stage. Antibiotics should be avoided unless there is evidence of cellulitis or septicaemia.

## Nutrition

The nutritional support and monitoring of fluid and electrolytes should be addressed promptly in the management of patients with fistulas. Large amounts of fluid and electrolytes can be lost in a high-output fistula, and sepsis will increase metabolic requirements.

---

**Multidisciplinary team involved in management of intestinal fistula**

- Surgeons
- Nutritional nurse
- Stoma nurse
- Pharmacist
- Dietitian
- Physiotherapist
- Laboratory staff
- Medical staff
- Radiologists
- Relatives

---

The following are recommended measures to optimise nutrition:

- Documentation and analysis of fistula output and fluid balance
- Regular haematological and biochemical measurements
- Oral intake of food and fluids should be stopped to reduce both fistula output and intestinal secretions
- IV feeding allows intestinal rest and provides adequate nutrition
- Total parenteral nutrition (TPN) is best given through a tunnelled dedicated central venous feeding line

TPN should supply energy, nitrogen, minerals, trace elements and vitamins. Many of these nutrients can be measured in the serum. In the later stages of the high and small-bowel fistulas, jejunal enteral feeding may be considered.

## Anatomy

Diagnosing the cause and extent of the fistula is important, but this should be addressed only once the patient is stable, any sources of sepsis are treated and the nutritional needs are met.

The diagnostic methods used in determining the anatomy of the fistula include the following:

- Fistulography using contrast
- Barium studies of the large and small bowel
- Ultrasound scan
- CT scan
- Injection of diluted methylene blue
- Biochemistry of fistulous output (differentiates between pancreatic, biliary, small-bowel or urinary tract origin)

## Plan

Once information is gained about the anatomy and cause of the fistula, the decision can be made about whether to treat the fistula conservatively or to proceed to surgery. Conservative management is indicated in fistulas that are likely to heal spontaneously.

### Conservative management of intestinal fistulas

Approximately 60% of enterocutaneous fistulas will close within a month of conservative treatment after sepsis has been controlled if the patient is not malnourished. The following are the principles of conservative management:

- Drainage
- Skin protection
- Reduction of fistula output
- Fluid and electrolyte support
- Nutritional support

Drainage is usually achieved by a drainage bag or, rarely, a sump suction system. Skin protection from the proteolytic enzymes in enterocutaneous fistulas is achieved with a number of adhesive devices and pastes under the guidance of an experienced stoma nurse. Fistula output is reduced by ensuring that the patient remains nil by mouth.

Drugs used to reduce secretions include:
- $H_2$-receptor antagonists
- Proton pump inhibitors (PPIs)
- Somatostatin

Throughout a course of conservative treatment, fluid and electrolyte balance must be carefully monitored and maintained, and nutritional support must be continued. If, after 6 weeks, a fistula that should have closed spontaneously has not closed, then the underlying reason for this must be sought and surgical treatment undertaken.

## Surgical treatment of intestinal fistulas

The principles of surgical management of intestinal fistulas are as follows:
- Drain away any septic foci, relieve any distal obstruction, and repair or resect the fistula
- Careful dissection of the adhesions and inflammatory masses is needed
- Temporary exteriorisation of bowel may be necessary because primary anastomosis is not recommended in unfavourable conditions

Another indication for surgery is haemorrhage. Sudden and potentially fatal haemorrhage may occur from eroded vessels within the fistulous tract or associated abscess cavities. Urgent resection is sometimes required, although arterial embolisation may be considered.

# 7.4 Tumours of the small bowel

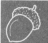

### In a nutshell ...

Although the small bowel makes up most of the length of the GI tract, malignant GI tumours are rarely found there. Below is a brief outline of the benign and malignant tumours found in the small bowel – you need to know them, but not too much detail about them.

**Benign tumours of the small bowel**
- Peutz–Jeghers hamartomas
- Adenoma
- GI stromal tumour (GIST) these do have malignant potential
- Lipoma
- Others (fibromas, schwannomas, neurilemmomas, lymphangiomas and haemangiomas), all of which are generally only removed if symptomatic

**Primary malignant tumours of the small bowel**

These are rare – only 1–2% of all malignant GI tumours are found in the small bowel.

**Including duodenum**
- Adenocarcinoma 40%
- Carcinoid 25%
- Lymphoma 25%
- Sarcoma 10%

**Excluding duodenum**
- Carcinoid 31%
- Adenocarcinoma 29%
- Lymphoma 29%
- Sarcoma 11%

# Peutz–Jeghers hamartomas

Peutz–Jeghers polyps are found in patients with the rare familial Peutz–Jeghers syndrome. The syndrome consists of pigmentation around the lips associated with characteristic intestinal polyps.

- Clinical features of the syndrome:
  - Melanin spots around the lips, buccal mucosa, anal mucosa, and sometimes the face and extremities
  - Numerous hamartomatous polyps throughout the bowel, characteristically in the jejunum and the rest of the small bowel, but less commonly seen in the stomach and large bowel
- Polyps are up to 3 cm in diameter and may be pedunculated; they can be seen on contrast studies
- Complications include intussusception and bleeding
- Treatment is reserved for these complications or for very large or symptomatic individual polyps
- Malignant change in a hamartoma is not significantly higher than in normal tissue (lipomas are also hamartomas). However, people with Peutz–Jeghers syndrome have an increased risk for large-bowel and duodenal carcinoma and other malignancies such as breast and genital tumours

# Adenomas of the small bowel

Adenomatous polyps are common in the large bowel (see Section 8, Large bowel) but are less commonly seen in the small bowel:

- They are often noted in the most commonly visualised area of the small bowel – the duodenum
- They are histologically similar to those found in the large bowel, and can be sporadic or associated with a syndrome such as familial adenomatous polyposis (FAP)
- The polyps are usually asymptomatic, but complications include bleeding, intussusception and malignant change (more of a risk in villous than in tubular adenomas)
- Treatment is controversial: high-risk villous adenomas must be excised; if this cannot be performed endoscopically it may necessitate surgery. If the adenoma is near the ampulla and a focus of malignancy cannot be excluded, Whipple's pancreaticoduodenectomy may have to be performed for a benign lesion – a difficult clinical decision
- Multiple duodenal adenomas in FAP are another clinical dilemma for similar reasons

# Leiomyomas of the small bowel

Leiomyomas are common benign neoplasms that arise from the smooth muscle of the stomach and intestinal wall; they appear on contrast studies as smooth-walled filling defects with intact mucosa. Complications include central necrosis, haemorrhage and obstruction either by the lesion itself or by intussusception.

# Lipomas of the small bowel

Commonly noted in the ileum, lipomas are benign and unimportant unless they cause obstruction or intussusception.

# Gastrointestinal stromal tumours

These spindle-cell neoplasms of varying malignant potential are described in detail in Section 3.6 of Section 3, Stomach and duodenum. They are defined histologically as KIT- (CD117-) positive tumours.

- Common presentations when found in the small bowel are:
  - Asymptomatic, found on CT or contrast studies (as they grow extraluminally they tend not to cause obstruction and may be 10 cm or more before detection)
  - Invasion into adjacent organs
  - Bleeding caused by mucosal ulceration
  - Perforation into the peritoneal cavity causing an acute abdomen
- Treatment is by resection with a cuff of normal tissue although, in recent years, there have been significant successes with the tyrosine kinase inhibitor, imatinib mesylate. The current NICE guidelines suggest that imatinib treatment is recommended as first-line management for unresectable or metastatic tumours. Continuation of treatment is recommended if there is a response.
- Prognosis depends on the size and type of tumour

## Gastrinomas

These most commonly occur in the duodenum and are discussed in Section 3.

## Carcinoids

- Typically found in the terminal ileum
- Also found outside the small bowel, especially in the appendix and rectum
- Carcinoid tumours are neuroendocrine tumours capable of secreting neuroen-docrine substances
- Unlike appendiceal carcinoid tumours, small-bowel carcinoid tumours are frequently symptomatic and commonly cause carcinoid syndrome
- Tumours are usually small but serotonin secretion causes an intense desmoplastic reaction

- Lymph node metastasis is common
- Liver metastases are also common and cause carcinoid syndrome

## Clinical presentation of carcinoids

- Incidental finding
- Obstruction, intussusception or ischaemia (usually due to the inflammation around the tumour, not the small tumour itself)
- Carcinoid syndrome

### Carcinoid syndrome

- Occurs only *if* the carcinoid tumour is secreting vasoactive substances *and* the tumour has metastasised to the liver
- Caused by vasoactive secretions of the carcinoid tumour such as serotonin (5-hydroxytryptamine or 5-HT)
- If produced at the tumour site these peptides enter the portal system and are metabolised by the liver to inactive metabolites such as 5-HIAA (5-hydroxyindoleacetic acid)
- These inactive metabolites then enter the systemic circulation to be excreted through the kidneys
- If there are actively secreting metastases in the liver, the peptides enter the systemic circulation directly and have an effect on the organs to which they are circulated
- **Symptoms** of carcinoid syndrome:
  - Flushing
  - Intractable diarrhoea
  - Bronchospasm
- **Diagnosis** of carcinoid tumour of the small bowel
  - CT
  - Small-bowel follow-through or enema
  - Urinary 5-HIAA levels may be raised if the tumour is secretory

## Management of carcinoid tumour of the small bowel

- Smaller than 1 cm and asymptomatic – local excision
- Bigger than 2 cm – small-bowel resection and lymphatic clearance
- Carcinoid syndrome (by definition metastatic) and other advanced disease – palliative bowel resection, palliative liver resection, chemotherapy (limited) or subcutaneous octreotide

## Prognosis of carcinoid tumour of the small bowel

- Excellent prognosis if incidental, early and no metastases
- 5-year survival rate for metastatic disease (includes most carcinoid syndrome patients) is 30%
- Palliative procedures may improve this

## Adenocarcinoma of the small bowel

- Most common in duodenum; least common in ileum
- Similar aetiology and histology to large-bowel adenoma (see Section 8)
- FAP, Crohn's disease and coeliac disease are risk factors
- **Clinical features** are typically vague and non-specific (thus making these cancers difficult to diagnose) but may include:
  - Abdominal pain
  - Weight loss
  - Obstructive symptoms
  - Anaemia
- They may present as an emergency with:
  - Obstructive jaundice (if periampullary)
  - Haemorrhage
  - Perforation
  - Small bowel obstruction

- **Diagnosis** is aided by:
  - Small-bowel follow-through or small-bowel enema
  - Endoscopy (if duodenal) or colonoscopy (if terminal ileal)
  - CT
  - Enteroscopy
- Management is wide surgical resection with lymphadenectomy, taking involved adjacent bowel loops and organs en bloc:
  - Duodenal tumours require pancreaticoduodenectomy
  - Palliative resection or bypass may be required in advanced cases
  - Outcome reflects late detection of this insidious disease, with 5-year survival rates of 10–20%
  - If caught early, things look brighter, with up to 50% of node-negative patients cured by surgery

## Lymphoma

- Lymphoma is the third most frequent primary malignant tumour of the small bowel after adenocarcinoma and carcinoic
- Lymphoma of the small bowel might be secondary to peripheral lymphoma (see Haematology and Neoplasia in Book 1) or gastric lymphoma (see Section 3) or – in the absence of disease at these sites – may be the primary site for lymphoma
- It arises from the lymphatic tissue of the submucosa which is particularly rich in the ileum; the ileum is therefore the most common site for small-bowel lymphoma
- Sporadic lymphoma of the small bowel occurs in elderly people and presents similarly to small-bowel adenocarcinoma (see above) but may become large enough to present as an abdominal mass
- There is a predisposition to lymphoma in patients with coeliac disease or

immunocompromised patients (such as those with AIDS)

- Diagnosis is by small-bowel enema or follow-through or by CT
- Peripheral lymphadenopathy, haematological abnormality and hepato-splenomegaly are NOT typical of primary small-bowel lymphoma; rather they indicate that the disease in the small bowel is secondary (and therefore not curable by surgical resection)
- Secondary lymphoma is treated by chemotherapy in the traditional way, with surgery reserved for relief of obstruction or debulking
- Primary small-bowel lymphoma is treated by wide surgical resection and lymphadenectomy of the draining nodes, as for adenocarcinoma; any abnormalities of the liver or lymph nodes seen at laparotomy should be biopsied
- Adjuvant chemotherapy and radiotherapy are used if there is residual disease but are controversial in completely resected disease

## 7.5 Bleeding from the small bowel

### In a nutshell ...

There is a proportion of significant or recurrent GI bleeding where the patient has had a normal oesophagogastroduodenoscopy (OGD) and a normal colonoscopy. This is a difficult clinical problem. Some of these patients will have bleeding from the small bowel, and this is difficult to identify due to the limitations of the imaging techniques available.

## Aetiology of small-bowel bleeding

### In a nutshell ...

**Causes of small-bowel bleeds**

Small-bowel neoplasms (see Section 7.4)
Meckel's diverticulum (see Section 6.2)
Angiodysplasia (see Section 8)
Intestinal ulceration
Infection:
- Bacterial
- Viral (eg cytomegalovirus)
Crohn's disease
Coeliac disease
Drug-induced ulcers:
- Potassium tablets
- Enteric or parenteral NSAIDs
Non-specific ulcers

Diagnosis, especially of intermittent small-bowel bleeds, is difficult because:
- OGD and colonoscopy are the first-line investigations of GI bleeding and will not image most of the small bowel
- Capsule endoscopy has an increasing role to play
- Incidental pathology (such as diverticulitis or adenomatous colonic polyps) may be wrongly blamed for the bleed
- Traditional methods of imaging the small bowel (ie contrast studies) are not good at picking up small ulcers or polyps

# Investigating small-bowel bleeding

> **Helpful investigations of a small-bowel bleed**
>
> **Small bowel enteroscopy:** useful but not widely available. May be done on-table through an enterotomy with a colonoscope.
>
> **Mesenteric angiography:** in brisk, active bleeding only. Diagnostic if bleed >1 ml/min and highly specific for anatomical localisation. Can be therapeutic if combined with embolisation or injecting vasoconstrictors.
>
> **Contrast studies:** will only spot obstruction, stricture, diverticulum or large lesions associated with the bleed.
>
> **CT:** may spot obstruction, stricture, diverticulum or a large lesion associated with the bleed. CT angiography may also be used to look for extravasation of contrast but requires rapid bleeding (not suitable if patient haemodynamically unstable).
>
> **Isotope-labelled red blood cell scans:** poor at anatomical localisation but more sensitive than angiography. Will detect bleeding at rates as low as 0.04 ml/min and can re-image over a period of time to allow accumulation of radionuclide.
>
> **Laparotomy:** often unsuccessful and always highly invasive so every attempt should be made to diagnose bleeding source preoperatively. On-table colonoscopy, OGD or enteroscopy via enterotomy can be carried out.

# Management of small-bowel bleeding

Treatments depend on the cause and severity of the bleeding:

- If the lesion is well localised by investigations and bleeding is significant, **surgical excision** is indicated
- Minor self-limiting bleed associated with use of drugs may be managed by simply **avoiding the drug responsible**
- **Mesenteric angiography** can be combined with **embolisation or injection of vasoconstrictor** to stop the bleeding or reduce the rate of a life-threatening bleed; there is a risk of transmural ischaemia and perforation and these need to be explained during the consent procedure

## 7.6    Intestinal ischaemia

 **In a nutshell ...**

The small bowel has a rich arterial supply (25% of the cardiac output) from the superior mesenteric artery (SMA). There is collateral contribution from the coeliac artery and the inferior mesenteric artery (IMA).

**Acute ischaemia of the small bowel can occur due to:**

- Acute embolic or thrombotic occlusion of the SMA (most common cause)
- Non-occlusive mesenteric ischaemia (due to low cardiac output, eg in hypovolaemia or cardiac failure)
- Mesenteric vein thrombosis

Chronic ischaemia of the small bowel is usually secondary to atherosclerosis.

# Acute occlusion of the superior mesenteric artery

Acute occlusion of the SMA is the most common cause of small-bowel ischaemia.

## Aetiology of SMA occlusion

- **Embolic** (usually from the heart after myocardial infarction [MI] or atrial fibrillation [AF]):
  - The emboli typically lodge at the branch of the middle colic artery (the first large branch of the SMA)
  - This spares the first part of the jejunum, supplied by the small jejunal arteries which come off the SMA proximal to the middle colic artery
  - Smaller emboli may lodge more distally causing segmental obstruction
- **Thrombotic** (usually atherosclerotic, perhaps complicated by a low-flow state):
  - This occlusion usually occurs at the origin of the SMA where it comes off the aorta
  - Thrombotic ischaemia therefore does not typically spare the proximal jejunum

## Clinical presentation of SMA occlusion

- Severe non-specific abdominal pain out of proportion to the findings on physical examination
- Vomiting
- Sweating
- High WCC
- Metabolic acidosis

These non-specific findings make intestinal ischaemia difficult to diagnose.

A high index of suspicion is required when a patient presents with the above clinical picture, especially if they have a history of MI, cardiac arrhythmia or peripheral vascular disease (PVD).

## Investigating SMA occlusion

- Mesenteric angiography will distinguish embolic, thrombotic and non-occlusive ischaemia, and diagnose mesenteric vein thrombosis; vasodilators may be selectively infused through the angiography catheter
- CT scan is helpful to exclude some differential diagnoses

## Management of SMA occlusion

### Resuscitate but do not delay

- There is a vicious cycle of bowel ischaemia causing shock and sepsis, which reduces blood flow to the bowel even further
- Preoperative and intraoperative management should be directed towards correcting hypovolaemia, shock and sepsis, but should not delay the definitive procedure

### Restore blood flow

- With an SMA embolus this is done by arteriotomy and embolectomy
- With thrombosis the treatment is an aortomesenteric bypass
- These operations may not be feasible, depending on the patient's state and comorbidity

### Resect necrotic bowel

- Once blood flow is restored as far as possible, any irreversibly necrotic bowel should be resected
- This may involve resecting a large proportion of the small bowel

### Assess viability of dubious bowel

- Sometimes it's difficult to know whether ischaemic bowel will (so does not need to be resected) or will not (leading to necrosis and perforation postoperatively) recover – the latter outcome has a high mortality
- At operation, the potential viability is assessed by:
  - Mesenteric artery pulsations (palpable between surgeon's fingers)
  - Observing bowel peristalsis (stimulated by touch)
  - Colour (black/blue/dusky/pale/pink) of the serosa and the mucosa
  - Sheen (dead bowel is dull not shiny)
- Bowel that is not clearly necrotic but of dubious viability is difficult to manage; a second-look laparotomy at 24–48 hours can be useful

## Non-occlusive mesenteric ischaemia

This usually occurs due to a low-flow state, where there is prolonged mesenteric vasoconstriction.

---

**Causes of low-flow states**
- Congestive cardiac failure
- MI
- Cardiac arrhythmia
- Hypovolaemia
- Sepsis
- Post-cardiac surgery (see Chapter 3)

---

Clinical presentation is similar to occlusive mesenteric ischaemia (see above)

- Angiography will exclude an embolus or thrombus. Vasodilators may be selectively infused through the angiography catheter
- Management consists of correcting the low-flow state and surgery is reserved for cases of peritonitis if the bowel necroses. These patients are often very sick with significant comorbidity so major surgery is fraught with problems

## Mesenteric vein thrombosis

Mesenteric vein thrombosis involves small veins and leads to patchy necrosis. With increasing oedema the arterial supply is compromised and ischaemia develops.

---

**Causes of mesenteric vein thrombosis**
- Idiopathic (the majority)
- Hypercoagulable state:
  - Antithrombin III deficiency
  - Protein C deficiency
  - Protein S deficiency
- Use of the oral contraceptive pill (OCP)
- Portal hypertension
- Sepsis

---

### Clinical presentation of mesenteric vein thrombosis

- Clinical presentation is non-specific with vague abdominal pain, nausea and abdominal distension
- The onset is more insidious than with arterial compromise, and may take weeks
- Eventually ischaemic bowel and even perforation occur with more obvious systemic and abdominal symptoms of shock and peritonitis

## Investigating mesenteric vein thrombosis

- Plain abdominal radiographs show thickened bowel wall
- The WCC is raised
- CT scans can show the actual clot in the superior mesenteric vein
- Mesenteric angiography may be diagnostic
- If the patient presents with peritonitis, the diagnosis is often made at laparotomy
- Hypercoagulable states should be excluded

## Management of mesenteric vein thrombosis

- If caught early enough, anticoagulation may prevent ischaemia and bowel necrosis
- If ischaemia has occurred surgery is usually indicated, and resection of the ischaemic segment with immediate anticoagulation is the treatment of choice
- Lifelong anticoagulation may be indicated if a hypercoagulable state is diagnosed

## Chronic intestinal ischaemia

Known as 'intestinal angina', this occurs in arteriopaths and is usually due to atherosclerotic disease.

- Typical findings are:
  - Postprandial (after meals) abdominal pain
  - Fear of eating
  - Characteristic weight loss
- Diagnosis is by mesenteric angiography
- Treatment is reserved for severe cases and options are:
  - Bypass
  - Endarterectomy
  - Angioplasty

# 7.7 Diverticula of the small bowel

**In a nutshell ...**

The most clinically significant small-bowel diverticula are:
- Duodenal diverticula, which can cause problems with ERCP (see Section 5)
- Meckel's diverticulum, which can contain ectopic gastric mucosa, and develop ulceration, haemorrhage or acute diverticulitis (see Section 8)
- Diverticulosis of the small bowel, usually in the jejunum and ileum

## Jejunoileal diverticulosis

- Occurs in 1% of the population, usually those aged >50
- More common in the proximal jejunum
- Occurs on the mesenteric border; these are false diverticula, ie acquired herniations of the mucosa and the submucosa through the muscular wall of the small bowel
- Thought to occur secondary to pulsion of the intestinal lining through weaknesses of the small bowel where blood vessels penetrate the abdominal wall
- The chronic abdominal pain associated with this condition is thought to be due to this motility disorder rather than to the diverticula themselves
- As in large-bowel diverticula, jejunoileal diverticula may become infected, perforate or bleed
- Treatment in severe cases is resection of the diseased segment

## 7.8    Infectious enteritis

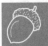

### In a nutshell ...

The pathology and management of bacterial and viral gastroenteritis are beyond the scope of this book. Suffice to say that many patients, especially children, admitted under the surgeons with abdominal pain, change in bowel habit or vomiting, may have an infectious enteritis that is usually self-limiting. There are some infections of the bowel that have particular surgical relevance, and you should know a bit about these. They include *Yersinia enterocolitica*, typhoid and TB.

### Yersinia enterocolitica

- This organism can cause mild gastroenteritis or an invasive ileocolitis
- It usually presents as non-specific, colicky abdominal pain, fever and diarrhoea, but it can masquerade as appendicitis with right iliac fossa tenderness
- Other microorganisms can cause this ileocolitis, which can look just like Crohn's disease clinically, on CT, at laparoscopy or at surgery
- Appendicectomy is wise, but further ileal resection is not indicated
- Diagnosis is made by stool culture or culture of a biopsied lymph node, and treatment is with the appropriate antibiotics

### Typhoid fever

- This is usually caused by *Salmonella typhi* or another of the *Salmonella* species
- Clinical features include:
  - Fevers

- Delirium
- Splenomegaly
- Abdominal pain
- Can cause bowel perforation or haemorrhage due to invasion of the small-bowel mucosa by the bacteria. The terminal ileum is the most common site of perforation
- Diagnosis is by blood and stool cultures
- The infection is treated with the appropriate antibiotics and perforation or haemorrhage is treated surgically

### Tuberculosis

- *Mycobacterium tuberculosis* is common in developing companies and is on the increase in developed countries due to AIDS
- The ileocaecal area is the most common site of intestinal involvement, with:
  - Ulceration
  - Fibrosis
  - Strictures and stenosed bowel segments
  - Fistula formation
  - Matted mesenteric lymph nodes
- Can mimic Crohn's disease but the histological findings of caseating granulomas and the positive ZN test confirm the diagnosis of TB
- Clinical findings may include:
  - Vague chronic abdominal pain
  - Abdominal mass
  - Weight loss
- Pulmonary disease may not be present
- Complications include:
  - Haemorrhage
  - Perforation
  - Obstruction
  - Fistulas
  - Malabsorption
- Treatment is anti-TB therapy for the underlying disease and surgery as indicated for the complications

## 7.9 Radiation small-bowel injury

The way in which radiotherapy works, its indications and the explanation for its effects are detailed in the Oncology chapter of Book 1:

- The small bowel is susceptible to the effects of radiotherapy because it has rapidly dividing cells in its epithelium
- Radiotherapy for pelvic tumours often affects adjacent small bowel
- In addition, postoperative radiotherapy to the pelvis often involves small bowel which has fallen into the pelvis after removal of the affected organ (be it rectum or uterus)

There are two phases of radiation injury affecting the small bowel:

- **Acute radiation enteritis** is due to the sloughing of dead epithelial cells from the bowel:
  - Damage and symptoms are dose-related
  - Crampy abdominal pain, nausea, anorexia and watery diarrhoea are common symptoms
  - Often occurs during the course of radiotherapy so diagnosis is clear
  - Acute radiation enteritis is usually self-limiting
- **Chronic radiation enteropathy** is due to radiation-induced damage to the small blood vessels causing chronic ischaemic changes:
  - Features may include chronic malabsorption, strictures, fistulas or necrosis
  - Symptoms start insidiously and progress slowly; they may be vague and may present a long time after the initial radiotherapy
  - Symptoms vary depending on which of the complications is causing them, and the treatment is likewise targeted to the specific probe

## 7.10 Short-bowel syndrome

 **In a nutshell ...**

This is the result of extensive (>80%) small-bowel resection. Small bowel is a non-renewable resource and only non-viable small bowel or clearly involved small bowel should be resected. One definition of short-bowel syndrome is any patient who needs parenteral nutrition for more than 3 months postoperatively.

Within a couple of days of intestinal resection the bowel dilates, lengthens and thickens and the intestinal villi hypertrophy.

This is **compensatory hyperplasia**, and is the reason why up to 80% of the intestine can often be removed without the need for parenteral nutrition. This occurs in the presence of normal bowel function, but does not occur as efficiently if the bowel is defunctioned or bypassed, or if the patient is not eating (eg on TPN).

The implication of this phenomenon is that early enteral nutrition and prompt restoration of continuity of the bowel allow maximal compensatory hyperplasia, optimising long-term bowel function.

> **Reasons for resecting over 80% of the small bowel**
>
> - Mesenteric ischaemia
> - Crohn's disease
> - Radiation enteritis
> - Necrotising enterocolitis
> - Intestinal atresia
> - Midgut volvulus

> **How to avoid resecting over 80% of the small bowel**
>
> - Early diagnosis and treatment of the above conditions
> - Conservative surgery (and avoidance of surgery) in Crohn's disease
> - Leaving ischaemic bowel of questionable viability until a second-look laparotomy rather than immediately resecting it

## Management of short bowel syndrome

Initial management is with the following:

- Fluid and electrolyte management
- TPN
- Reduction of diarrhoea with opiates and PPIs
- Encourage oral intake until compensatory hyperplasia decreases the need for parenteral feeding
- Aim to wean off TPN if possible

In the long term there are medical and surgical strategies for optimising the absorptive capacity of the small bowel, encouraging compensatory hyperplasia and delaying intestinal transit, including the following:

- Growth hormone (GH)

- Glutamine supplementation (this amino acid is the chief energy source for enterocytes)
- Low-fat, high-carbohydrate, high-fibre diet
- Surgically reversing small-bowel segments
- Colonic interposition
- Recirculating loops
- Retrograde electrical pacing
- Tapering dilated bowel

In extreme cases, intestinal transplantation techniques are being developed. Crucial to these management decisions is the utilisation of a multidisciplinary team, proper nutritional support and referral to tertiary centres for intestinal failure where necessary.

## 7.11 Small-bowel bypass surgery

- Jejunoileal bypass is used in conjunction with stomach volume reduction as part of gastric obesity surgery (see Section 3)
- Bypassing the small bowel is no longer used on its own for obesity surgery, because:
  - Intestinal adaptation restricts its long-term efficiency
  - The electrolyte abnormalities can be fatal
  - Long-term complications include gallstones, kidney stones and cirrhosis of the liver
- There has been some interest in methods to reduce hyperlipidaemia (a risk factor in atherosclerosis and heart disease) by ileal bypass
- If the ileum cannot absorb bile salts, they pass in the stools and new bile salts have to be made from cholesterol stores, thus lowering cholesterol levels

For details of small-bowel obstruction and appendicitis see Section 3 and for Crohn's disease see Section 8.

# SECTION 8
# Large bowel

## 8.1 Symptoms of non-acute abdominal disorders

### In a nutshell ...

Non-acute abdominal disorders commonly present as:
* An abdominal mass
* Indigestion
* A change in bowel habit

### Clinical assessment of an abdominal mass

#### History
* Nature and rate of growth of the mass
* Presence of associated features (weight loss, jaundice, lymphadenopathy, upper GI or bowel symptoms)

## Abdominal mass

### In a nutshell ...

Patients may present having noticed an abdominal mass, or a mass can be noted on examination of a patient with related or unrelated symptoms.
* Causes are many and varied
* Clinical objectives should be to identify the anatomical source of the mass and its pathology
* A mass is usually:
  * A non-pathological abdominal mass
  * A pathologically enlarged organ
  * A solid or cystic tumour (benign or malignant)
* Imaging is usually required to identify the mass

## Examination

- Position
- Shape
- Size
- Surface
- Edge

## Composition

- Consistency
- Fluctuation
- Fluid thrill
- Resonance
- Pulsatility
- Tenderness
- Association with enlargement of palpable organs

## Investigation of an abdominal mass

### Ultrasonography

- Cheap and non-invasive
- Useful for imaging cystic masses and abscesses
- Also visualises many organs well, including liver, gallbladder, spleen, kidneys, bladder, aorta, ovaries and uterine masses

### CT and MRI

Invaluable, especially for retroperitoneal masses. They also give additional information about the relations and operability of the mass, as well as associated lymphadenopathy and distant metastases.

### Other specific investigations

These depend on the nature of the mass:

- Contrast studies
- Endoscopy
- Radioisotope scans

## Non-pathological abdominal masses

An abdominal mass may not always be pathological; other causes may include the following:

- Distended urinary bladder
- Pregnant uterus
- Faeces-filled colon
- Abdominal aorta in a thin individual
- Riedel's lobe of the liver
- Ectopic kidney

## Pathological abdominal masses

Pathological masses are probably most usefully considered according to location, because this is usually the first reliable information that can be determined on examination alone.

### Generalised distension

**The 6 Fs:** this is a useful list of the common causes of generalised distension:

**F**etus

**F**aeces

**F**luid: free (ascites); encysted – see Section 4.4, 'Causes of ascites' and box 'Cystic swellings that can cause abdominal distension'

**F**latus

**F**at

**F**ibroids and other solid tumours – see box 'Solid tumours that can cause abdominal distension'

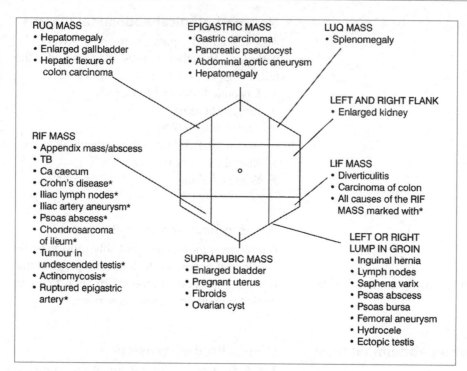

**RUQ MASS**
- Hepatomegaly
- Enlarged gallbladder
- Hepatic flexure of colon carcinoma

**EPIGASTRIC MASS**
- Gastric carcinoma
- Pancreatic pseudocyst
- Abdominal aortic aneurysm
- Hepatomegaly

**LUQ MASS**
- Splenomegaly

**LEFT AND RIGHT FLANK**
- Enlarged kidney

**RIF MASS**
- Appendix mass/abscess
- TB
- Ca caecum
- Crohn's disease*
- Iliac lymph nodes*
- Iliac artery aneurysm*
- Psoas abscess*
- Chondrosarcoma of ileum*
- Tumour in undescended testis*
- Actinomycosis*
- Ruptured epigastric artery*

**LIF MASS**
- Diverticulitis
- Carcinoma of colon
- All causes of the RIF MASS marked with*

**SUPRAPUBIC MASS**
- Enlarged bladder
- Pregnant uterus
- Fibroids
- Ovarian cyst

**LEFT OR RIGHT LUMP IN GROIN**
- Inguinal hernia
- Lymph nodes
- Saphena varix
- Psoas abscess
- Psoas bursa
- Femoral aneurysm
- Hydrocele
- Ectopic testis

Figure 1.54 Sites of abdominal masses. LIF, left iliac fossa; LUQ, left upper quadrant; RIF, right iliac fossa; RUQ, right upper quadrant

## Cystic swellings that can cause abdominal distension

- Ovarian cysts
- Polycystic kidney
- Pancreatic cysts
- Hydatid cysts
- Hydronephrosis
- Urinary bladder
- Mesenteric cysts

## Solid tumours that can cause abdominal distension

- Hepatomegaly
- Splenomegaly
- Pancreatic carcinoma
- Retroperitoneal lymphadenopathy
- Carcinoma of liver
- Retroperitoneal sarcoma
- Nephroblastoma (in children)
- Fibroids
- Large colon cancers
- Polycystic kidneys
- Carcinoma of kidney
- Perinephric abscess
- Ganglioneuroma (in children)

There are certain organs that are specifically felt for on routine abdominal examination in case they are enlarged:

- Liver (hepatomegaly)
- Gallbladder
- Spleen (splenomegaly)
- Aorta
- Kidney

## Hepatomegaly

Physical signs of an enlarged liver

- Descends from the right costal margin
- You cannot get above it
- Moves with respiration
- Dull to percussion up to the level of the eighth rib in the midaxillary line
- Edge can be sharp or rounded
- Surface can be smooth or irregular

Localised enlargement of the liver

- Riedel's lobe
- Secondary carcinoma
- Hydatid cysts
- Liver abscess
- Primary liver carcinoma

**Causes of hepatomegaly**

| With jaundice | Without jaundice |
|---|---|
| **Smooth generalised enlargement** | |
| Infective hepatitis | Heart failure |
| Biliary tract obstruction (gallstones; carcinoma of pancreas) | Cirrhosis |
| Cholangitis | Reticulosis |
| Portal pyaemia | Budd–Chiari syndrome |
| | Amyloid |
| **Knobbly generalised enlargement** | |
| Extensive secondary carcinoma | Secondary carcinoma |
| Cirrhosis | Cirrhosis |
| | Polycystic disease |
| | Primary liver cancer |

### Riedel's lobe

This is an extension of the right lobe of the liver down below the costal margin along the anterior axillary line. It is a normal anatomical variation that is often mistaken for a pathological enlargement of the liver or gallbladder.

### Splenomegaly

The spleen is almost always uniformly enlarged.

Physical signs of an enlarged spleen

- Appears from below the tip of the left tenth rib and enlarges along the line of the rib towards the umbilicus
- Is firm, smooth, and usually spleen-shaped
- Often has a definite notch on its upper edge
- You cannot get above it
- Moves with respiration
- Dull to percussion
- Cannot be balloted

## Causes of splenomegaly

These are listed in Section 4.10.

## Enlarged kidney

### Physical signs of an enlarged kidney

- Smooth and hemi-ovoid
- Moves with respiration
- Not dull to percussion because of overlying colon
- Can be felt bimanually
- Can be balloted or 'bounced' between two palpating hands (depends on the mass reducing into the loin)

### Causes of kidney enlargement

- Hydronephrosis (can be bilateral in distal obstruction)
- Perinephric abscess
- Solitary cysts
- Polycystic disease (usually bilateral)
- Pyonephrosis
- Carcinoma of the kidney
- Nephroblastoma (occasionally bilateral)
- Hypertrophy

Note that a mobile or low-lying kidney can be easily palpable and so seem to be enlarged.

## Enlarged gallbladder

An enlarged gallbladder is usually due to obstruction of the cystic duct or common bile duct:

- Obstruction of the cystic duct is usually by a gallstone and rarely by an intrinsic or extrinsic carcinoma; the patient is not jaundiced and the gallbladder will contain bile, mucus (a mucocele) or pus (an empyema)

- Obstruction of the common bile duct is usually by a stone or a carcinoma of the head of the pancreas; the patient is jaundiced

> **Courvoisier's law**
> In the presence of jaundice, the palpable gallbladder is unlikely to be due to stones.

This is because previous inflammation will have made the gallbladder thick and non-distensible. There are exceptions:

- Stones that form in the bile duct
- Stones in the cystic duct as well as a stone or carcinoma in the bile duct

### Physical signs of an enlarged gallbladder

- Appears from beneath the tip of the right ninth rib
- Smooth and hemi-ovoid
- Moves with respiration
- Cannot feel a space between the lump and the edge of the liver
- Dull to percussion

A gallbladder mass is formed when omentum and bowel adhere to an acutely inflamed gallbladder. It is diffuse and tender and does not move much with respiration.

## Abdominal aortic aneurysm

A normal aorta can be palpated in a thin individual. The size of the aneurysm can be estimated but should be confirmed by ultrasonography. CT is also used after diagnosis to aid in planning treatment decisions. It is diagnosed by its expansile pulsation. Other enlarged organs or masses overlying the aorta may transmit pulsations, giving the false impression of an enlarged aorta, but these pulsations will not be expansile.

## Characteristics of an abdominal aortic aneurysm

- Smooth epigastric mass with distinct lateral margins
- Expansile pulsation
- May extend into the left or (less commonly) the right iliac arteries

Note that the aorta bifurcates at the level of the umbilicus.

## What do you mean by indigestion?

# Indigestion

 **In a nutshell ...**

'Indigestion' is an imprecise term used by patients to describe a number of symptoms. The term may mean epigastric pain, reflux, general abdominal discomfort, abdominal distension or nausea. A careful history can determine the exact nature of the symptoms and suggest a condition that may be responsible.

| Symptoms | Suggests | Investigations |
|---|---|---|
| Burning retrosternal pain<br>Worse on lying down or stooping<br>Can be referred to jaw or arms<br>Associated with acid brash<br>Worse with certain foods (eg citrus fruits) | Reflux oesophagitis | Oesophagoscopy pH studies, manometry |
| Epigastric boring pain during fasting<br>Pain at night relieved by food and antacids<br>Relapsing every few months<br>May radiate to back<br>History of NSAID use | Duodenal ulcer | Endoscopy or barium meal<br>*Helicobacter pylori* serology or breath test |
| Epigastric boring pain, worse after eating<br>Weight loss, nausea<br>Associated with anaemia or melaena<br>History of NSAID use | Gastric ulcer | Endoscopy or barium meal<br>*H. pylori* serology or breath test |
| Right hypochondrial severe colic<br>Radiating to right scapula<br>Vomiting and sweating<br>Worse after fatty food<br>Patient fat, fair, female, fertile in her 40s with a family history of gallstones<br>Jaundice, pale stools, dark urine | Biliary colic | Ultrasound scan of gallbladder<br>LFTs |
| Persistent severe pain in right hypochondrium<br>Fever, malaise<br>Rebound tenderness<br>Jaundice, pale stools, dark urine | Acute cholecystitis | Ultrasound scan of gallbladder<br>FBC<br>LFTs<br>Amylase |

**continued overleaf**

| | | |
|---|---|---|
| Jaundice, fever, malaise, nausea, vomiting<br>Vague upper abdominal pain<br>Tender palpable liver | Hepatitis | Ultrasound scan of liver<br>Serology<br>LFTs |
| Severe constant epigastric pain radiating to back<br>Vomiting, malaise, tachycardia<br>Generalised tenderness and guarding of abdomen<br>History of gallstones or alcohol abuse | Pancreatitis | Ultrasound scan of biliary tree<br>Amylase<br>FBC, U&Es, blood gases, CA (calcium), glucose<br>CT (pancreatitis protocol) |
| Epigastric pain radiating to back<br>Vomiting, dysphagia, haematemesis, melaena, anaemia, jaundice, ascites, weight loss<br>Upper abdominal mass<br>Supraclavicular nodes | Gastric or oesophageal cancer | Endoscopy and biopsy<br>CT of abdomen and chest, EUS<br>FBC |
| Central crushing chest pain radiating to neck and arm associated with exercise<br>History of smoking or familial heart attack | Angina | ECG<br>Cardiac enzymes<br>Exercise stress test |
| Long-standing ache in abdomen<br>Flatulence and intolerance to fatty foods, bloating, loose stools, various non-colonic features (back pain, headache, poor sleep) | Irritable bowel syndrome | Large-bowel investigations are usually normal<br>Air insufflation at sigmoidoscopy reproduces pain |
| LIF pain, change in bowel habit, bloating, mucus or bleeding per rectum | Diverticular disease | Colonoscopy or barium enema |
| Change in bowel habit, blood or mucus per rectum, weight loss, anaemia, malaise | Colonic carcinoma | Colonoscopy or barium enema<br>FBC, CT of chest, abdomen and pelvis |
| LIF pain radiating to epigastrium, worse after meals<br>Diarrhoea, melaena, altered blood<br>History of cardiovascular disease | Vascular insufficiency of the gut | Colonoscopy and biopsy<br>Barium enema shows 'thumbprinting' |

# Change in bowel habit

## In a nutshell ...

A change in bowel habit is an important and common manifestation of bowel disease. This symptom may result from a variety of causes, some of which are self-limiting and relatively innocuous, and some of which are sinister.

A change in bowel habit can be defined as a sustained alteration in:

- Defecation (frequency, periodicity, ease)
- Stool (consistency, appearance, presence of blood or mucus)
- Symptoms (pain on defecation, tenesmus, feeling of incomplete evacuation)

The features characteristic of various important disorders are covered in the relevant sections in this chapter on, for example, colorectal carcinoma (Section 8.6), diverticulitis (Section 6.2) and inflammatory bowel disease (Section 8.4) Three symptoms, however, deserve separate consideration:

- Constipation
- Diarrhoea
- Bleeding per rectum

Change in bowel habit can be a symptom of irritable bowel syndrome.

**Department of Health criteria for defining a group of patients more likely to have bowel cancer for urgent investigation**

- Persistent change in bowel habit (>6 weeks) towards looser stools **with** rectal bleeding
- Persistent change in bowel habit towards looser stools **without** rectal bleeding (aged >60 years)
- Rectal bleeding with a change in bowel habit towards looser stool or increasing stool frequency for 6 weeks or more (aged >40 years)
- Iron deficiency anaemia (<10 g/dl) in all men and postmenopausal women (all ages)
- Right-sided abdominal mass (all ages)
- Palpable intraluminal rectal mass (all ages)
- Rectal bleeding for >6weeks without anal symptoms or change in bowel habit (aged >60 years)

**CHAPTER 1**

## Constipation

### In a nutshell ...

Constipation is a symptom and cannot be considered as a diagnosis until all underlying causes have been excluded. It is defined as infrequent or irregular defecation that may or may not be painful.

The principle of management is to exclude each of the causes described.

### Investigating constipation

*Minimum investigations of constipation*
- Take a careful history, including drug history, gynaecological and psychological history, details of diet, mechanisms of defecation (eg manual assistance in obstructive defecation), obstetric history
- Examination looks for abdominal distension, tenderness and masses
- Rectal examination for fissures, painful piles or perianal sepsis is essential
- Barium studies or colonoscopy must be undertaken to exclude organic obstruction

*Further special tests may be indicated*
- Bowel transit studies can identify an adynamic bowel
- Defecating proctogram (excludes prolapse and looks at perineal muscle function) – see Section 8.3
- Anorectal physiology including electromyography (excludes pudendal neuropathy) – see Section 8.3
- Thyroid function tests
- Pelvic ultrasonography

## Conservative treatment of constipation

### In a nutshell ...

- Advice
- Laxatives
- Behavioural therapy

### Advice

Once the important causes of constipation have been excluded, the first line of management is lifestyle advice that may improve symptoms, including the following:
- Increasing fibre content of the diet
- Increasing exercise
- Never ignoring the need to pass stools
- Eating regular healthy meals

If conservative treatment does not help, laxatives may be needed.

*Laxatives*

Laxatives should be prescribed with caution. Bowel habit can be infrequent without doing any harm and not everyone needs to have a bowel movement every day. Prolonged use of some laxatives can lead to hypokalaemia and atonic non-functioning colon.

| Causes of constipation | Treatment |
|---|---|
| **Organic obstruction** | **Surgery if indicated – other sections in this chapter and Section 6 (Acute abdomen) deal with each condition** |
| • Carcinoma of the colon | |
| • Diverticular disease | |
| • Volvulus, hernias, intussusception | |
| • Crohn's disease strictures | |
| **Adynamic bowel** | **Laxatives, enemas, ACE procedure, colectomy** |
| • Hirschsprung's disease | |
| • Parkinson's disease | |
| • Stroke | |
| • Spinal cord injuries and disease | |
| • Myxoedema | |
| • Pseudo-obstruction | |
| **Diet** | **Dietary advice** |
| • Dehydration | |
| • Starvation | |
| • Lack of dietary fibre | |
| **Painful anal conditions** | **See treatment of individual conditions in Section 9, Perianal conditions** |
| • Fissure in ano | |
| • Prolapsed piles | |
| • Perianal abscess | |
| **Drugs** | **Replace with alternative** |
| • Aspirin | |
| • Opiate analgesics | |
| • Anticholinergics | |
| • Ganglion blockers | |
| • Anticonvulsants | |
| **Habit/psychological** | **Biofeedback/psychology** |
| • Dyschezia (rectal stasis due to faulty bowel habit) | |
| • Depression | |
| • Anorexia nervosa | |
| **Pelvic causes** | **Treat cause as indicated** |
| • Pregnancy and puerperium | |
| • Ovarian and uterine tumours | |
| • Endometriosis | |
| **Defecatory abnormalities** | **See Section 9, Perianal conditions** |
| • Prolapse (obstructive defecation) | **Biofeedback for functional syndromes, surgery for anatomical problems such as prolapse and rectocele** |
| • Reduced anorectal angle | |
| • Functional rectal stenosis (anorectal spasm) | |
| • Outlet syndrome (anismus) | |
| • Pudendal neuropathy | |

| Types of laxative | Indications for use |
|---|---|
| **Bulk-forming drugs**<br>Wheat fibre (Trifyba™)<br>Isphaghula husk (eg Fybogel™)<br>Methylcellulose (Celevac™)<br>Sterculia (Normacol™) | Haemorrhoids<br>Anal fissures<br>Stomas<br>Diverticular disease<br>Irritable bowel |
| **Stimulant laxatives**<br>Bisacodyl<br>Dantron (eg co-danthramer)<br>Docusate sodium (eg Dioctyl™)<br>Senna<br>Sodium picosulfate | Elderly patients<br>Terminally ill patients only<br>Avoiding straining<br>Bowel preparation for surgery or X-ray<br>Chronic slow-transit constipation |
| **Osmotic laxatives**<br>Lactulose<br>Macrogols (eg Movicol™) | Occasional use (eg postop)<br>Chronic slow-transit constipation<br>Hepatic encephalopathy |
| **Bowel-cleaning solutions**<br>Citramag™<br>Fleet™ phospho-soda<br>Klean-Prep™<br>Picolax™ | Bowel preparation before surgery,<br>radiological investigation or endoscopy |
| **Rectal laxatives**<br>Stimulant<br>  • Bisacodyl suppositories<br>  • Glycerol suppositories<br>Faecal softeners<br>  • Arachis oil enema | Postop<br>Can be used as part of biofeedback<br>Postop |
| Osmotic<br>  • Phosphate enema (eg Fleet™)<br>  • Sodium citrate enema<br>  • (eg Fleet™ micro-enema, Micralax™) | Bowel preparation before surgery,<br>radiological investigation or endoscopy<br>Impacted faeces in prolonged constipation |

## Main indications for using laxatives

- Where straining will exacerbate a condition (eg angina or haemorrhoidal bleeding)
- In drug-induced or slow-transit constipation
- Before surgery and radiological procedures
- For expulsion of parasites after anti-helmintic treatment
- In elderly patients or others with an adynamic bowel (eg those with spinal injuries)

### *Behavioural therapy*

Behavioural therapy, biofeedback training or physiotherapy and psychotherapy can be useful in patients with severe idiopathic constipation or faecal soiling in children and adolescents. Patients learn how to control sphincter activity and establish a regular bowel habit.

### *Surgical treatment of constipation*

- A last resort in patients with severe intractable primary constipation (usually restricted to specialist centres)
- Anorectal myectomy has been used in the outlet syndrome but is contraindicated if colonic transit is slow
- Colectomy and ileorectal anastomosis can benefit patients with severe idiopathic slow-transit constipation but can result in diarrhoea
- A proximal colonic stoma through which regular antegrade colonic enemas (ACE procedures) can be performed in selected patients

## Diarrhoea

 **In a nutshell ...**

Diarrhoea can be defined as the passage of more than three loose stools a day. It is due to an increase in the stool water content. The causes of diarrhoea are listed in the box 'Causes of diarrhoea'. A careful history should determine if there is true diarrhoea (as opposed to faecal incontinence, irritable bowel or passage of blood or mucus) and if it is acute or chronic.

### *Causes of diarrhoea*

In **acute diarrhoea**, infective causes are likely. Questions should cover:

- Travel abroad
- Unusual food (eg seafood)
- Diarrhoea among friends or family members

In **chronic diarrhoea**, irritable bowel syndrome is more likely, and colon cancer should be excluded, especially in patients aged >40 years.

## Causes of diarrhoea
### Specific infections
- Food poisoning
  - *Salmonella* spp.
  - *Campylobacter* spp.
  - *Clostridium* spp.
  - Staphylococci
  - *Shigella* spp.
  - *Bacillus* spp.
  - *Giardia* spp.
- Dysentery (amoebic, bacillary)
- Cholera
- Viral enterocolitis

### Loss of absorptive surface
- Bowel resections and short circuits
- Sprue and coeliac disease
- Idiopathic steatorrhoea

### Others
- Pancreatic dysfunction leading to lipase deficiency
- Post-gastrectomy and vagotomy
- Anxiety states
- Lactose intolerance

### Inflammation of the intestine
- Ulcerative colitis
- Tumours of the large bowel
- Diverticular disease
- Crohn's disease

### Drugs
- Antibiotics
- Purgatives
- Digoxin

### Systemic diseases
- Thyrotoxicosis
- Uraemia
- Carcinoid syndrome
- Zollinger–Ellison syndrome

## Investigating diarrhoea

In a short history of acute diarrhoea, suspect infection:

- Take stool and blood cultures
- Check inflammatory markers (WCC, CRP, ESR [erythrocyte sedimentation rate])
- Exclude anaemia (a sign of more severe disease)
- Check urea and creatinine to exclude dehydration, especially in elderly people
- In older people, exclude *Clostridium*, especially if they have been on antibiotics

If the diarrhoea does not settle, the patient is elderly or the history is weeks rather than days, suspect inflammatory bowel disease (IBD) or carcinoma of the colon.

Guidelines recommend bowel investigations in all patients with a significant change in bowel habit (see earlier box 'Department of Health criteria for defining a group of patients more likely to have bowel cancer for urgent investigation').

- Minimum investigation for patients with a sustained change in bowel habit is flexible sigmoidoscopy (in a young person with no risk factors) ± barium enema
- In older (>40 in some units) patients or those with risk factors such as a family history or previous pathology, a full bowel investigation is indicated – this involves colonoscopy, barium enema plus rigid sigmoidoscopy or CT colonography

Further investigations may be targeted towards excluding other suspected causes (see table 'Causes of diarrhoea') such as hyperthyroidism, coeliac disease or lactulose intolerance.

## Treatment of diarrhoea

Treatment of diarrhoea depends on presentation:

- **In acute diarrhoea** it is mainly supportive with oral or IV rehydration and replacement of electrolytes; antibiotics are rarely indicated
- **In chronic diarrhoea** it depends on the aetiology

**Anti-motility agents** include:

- Loperamide (Imodium)
- Diphenoxylate (Lomotil)
- Codeine

These are indicated for short-term control or in intractable conditions such as short-bowel syndrome. They may be contraindicated in some forms of acute infective diarrhoea because they slow the clearance of infective agents.

> **Indications for antibiotic treatment in diarrhoea**
>
> - Severe cases of *Shigella* spp. or *Campylobacter jejuni*
> - Severe cases of *Clostridium difficile*
> - Giardiasis
> - Immunosuppressed patients, babies and the very old infected with *Salmonella* spp.

## Bleeding per rectum

 **In a nutshell ...**

### Major per rectum bleed

A major per rectum bleed can be from the upper or lower GI tract. After appropriate resuscitation it is **investigated first by upper GI endoscopy** and then by large-bowel investigations.

These large upper GI bleeds are most commonly due to:

- Peptic ulcer disease
- Oesophageal varices
- Gastric carcinoma

These conditions are discussed further in Sections 3 and 4.

### Moderate per rectum bleed

Most moderate lower GI bleeds are investigated by one of the following three large-bowel investigations:

- Barium enema (must be combined with rigid or flexible sigmoidoscopy)
- Colonoscopy
- CT pneumocolon

**continued overleaf**

Lower GI bleeds are most commonly due to:

- Diverticular disease
- Angiodysplasia
- Neoplasia
- IBD

### Anal canal-type bleeding

Minor anal canal-type bleeding in young people can be satisfactorily investigated by anal inspection, proctoscopy and flexible sigmoidoscopy alone if there are no worrying features. Anal canal-type bleeding is most commonly due to:

- Haemorrhoids
- Fissures

However, anal cancers, rectal cancers and rectal polyps may also present with anal canal-type bleeding, especially in an older age group, and will be excluded by the above investigations.

---

### When investigating a large per rectum bleed remember – oesophagogastroduodenoscopy (OGD) first!

- There must be heavy bleeding for an upper GI bleed to present with fresh red blood per rectum
- Upper GI causes of a large per rectum bleed are common, often benign and usually treatable
- If an upper GI bleed presenting with fresh red per rectum blood is missed, this is more likely to be imminently fatal than most lower GI causes of a per rectum bleed
- All patients who present with a major per rectum bleed should have an OGD to exclude an upper GI cause before the large bowel is investigated

---

### Causes of lower GI haemorrhage

**Children**

- Meckel's diverticulum
- Juvenile polyps
- IBD
- Intussusception

**Elderly people**

- Diverticular disease
- Angiodysplasia
- Adenomatous polyps
- Carcinoma
- Ischaemic colitis
- IBD
- Radiation proctitis

**Adults**

- IBD
- Adenomatous polyps
- Carcinoma
- AV malformation
- Hereditary telangiectasia
- Haemorrhoids
- Solitary rectal ulcer
- Anal fissure

It is important to differentiate between anal canal-type bleeding and bleeding from the colon.

**Anal canal-type bleeding**

- Usually caused by fissures or haemorrhoids
- Bright-red blood on the paper when wiping after passing a motion
- Not mixed in with the motion
- Anal irritation or pain is a feature

**Bleeding from the colon**

- Dark red blood
- Mixed with faeces
- Associated with slime or mucus
- No anal irritation or pain
- May report abdominal ache, bloating or colic
- Systemic features such as weight loss or malaise may be present

It is often difficult to differentiate between anal canal-type bleeding and bleeding from rectal pathology, which is why sigmoidoscopy is important.

## Patterns of rectal bleeding

The typical pattern of rectal bleeding in common cases is described below.

### Haemorrhoids

See Section 9, Perianal conditions:

- Bright-red blood on the faeces and toilet paper
- Blood may drip into the toilet bowl
- Always exclude other rectal conditions before bleeding is assumed to be from haemorrhoids

### Inflammatory bowel disease

See Section 8.4:

- Small amount of blood mixed with mucus and faeces

- Associated with increased bowel frequency and systemic symptoms such as weight loss and malaise

### Distal colorectal polyps and cancers

See Sections 8.5 and 8.6:

- Bright-red blood or slightly altered streaks of blood
- Can be associated with tenesmus, urgency or a feeling of incomplete defecation

### Proximal colon or caecal tumours

See Section 8.6:

- Can be occult bleeding only
- Commonly presents with iron deficiency anaemia

### Diverticular disease

See Section 6, Acute Abdomen:

- One of the most common causes of major lower GI haemorrhage
- Often brisk and unheralded, and can cause hypovolaemia and shock
- Typically there is a sudden urge to defecate followed by the passage of a dark-red stool. Fresh red blood may be passed in a brisk bleed
- The bleed can be repeated but usually stops spontaneously

### Angiodysplasia

See Section 8.7:

- Presents in a very similar manner to diverticular bleed
- May occur in the presence of diverticulosis, leading to a misdiagnosis
- Predominantly affects older people
- Can be difficult to identify by colonoscopy and arteriography

## Management of lower GI haemorrhage

### Moderate bleeding

This can usually be investigated and treated as an outpatient. An important principle is not to assume the bleed is due to (almost ubiquitous) haemorrhoids until more serious conditions (eg neoplasia, IBD) have been excluded. Different units will have different protocols.

A sensible approach to management involves the following:
- History and general examination
- Anorectal examination
- Proctosigmoidoscopy
- Flexible sigmoidoscopy is adequate for younger patients with anal canal-type, bright-red rectal bleeding and perianal symptoms – this may be done in a 'one-stop' rectal bleeding clinic as an outpatient
- Colonoscopy or double-contrast barium enema is often needed in older patients or those with altered blood and/or worrying symptoms such as weight loss or anaemia
- Treatment of the cause

### Major haemorrhage

This is usually best investigated and treated as an inpatient, at least initially. The following are the important principles:
- Resuscitation takes priority
- Upper GI haemorrhage should be excluded
- Most bleeds stop spontaneously, enabling investigations to be performed as an outpatient
- In the face of continued bleeding, endoscopy is not usually productive and efforts should be made to localise the bleeding point by isotope scanning selective arteriography

- In life-threatening haemorrhage, a laparotomy + on-table enteroscopy is indicated

## Irritable bowel syndrome

In some patients who present with changed bowel habits, no organic disease is discovered on investigation. Some of these will be found to have 'irritable bowel syndrome' (IBS). These patients present with a variety of symptoms.

---

**Symptoms of irritable bowel syndrome**
- Recurrent nausea
- Heartburn
- Epigastric fullness
- Distension and abdominal bloating
- Excessive flatus and per rectum mucus
- Abnormal bowel habit
- Loose or constipated stool (often of small volume)
- Abdominal pain relieved by bowel movements

---

Patients can be subdivided into two types:
1. Spastic constipation (abdominal pain related to disturbed bowel action)
2. Painless diarrhoea (although diarrhoea can be associated with abdominal pain)

There is an association (not invariably) with several psychological or psychiatric disorders:
- Anxiety
- Depression
- Neurosis
- Anorexia nervosa
- Münchausen syndrome

Principles of management of IBS

- Careful assessment including large-bowel investigations – the diagnosis can be made only when other causes of symptoms are excluded
- Offer reassurance and sympathy
- Offer support (eg information groups, dietitians, alternative therapy)

Occasionally, patients may need additional therapies:
- Antispasmodics
- Laxatives
- Constipating agents
- Alternative therapies (eg aromatherapy, acupuncture)
- Joint care with psychologist or psychiatrist
- Anxiolytics (short term)
- Tricyclic antidepressants (low dose)

## 8.2 Anatomy and physiology of the colon

### Anatomy of the colon

 **In a nutshell ...**

The colon consists of the:
- Caecum
- Ascending colon
- Transverse colon
- Descending colon
- Sigmoid colon

It is supplied by the superior and inferior mesenteric arteries and drains into the hepatic portal vein via the superior and inferior mesenteric veins. Sympathetic innervation is from T10 to L2 and parasympathetic innervation is from the vagus and sacral outflow.

### The mesenteries

- Transverse colon always has a mesentery (the transverse mesocolon)
- Sigmoid colon also has a mesentery (the sigmoid mesocolon)
- In most people the ascending and descending colon are plastered onto the posterior abdominal wall so that they have posterior 'bare areas' devoid of peritoneum
- Transverse mesocolon and sigmoid mesocolon carry blood vessels

### The caecum

The caecum is the blind pouch of the large bowel projecting downwards from the start of the ascending colon below the ileocaecal junction. It lies on the peritoneal floor of the right iliac fossa, over the iliacus and psoas fascia, and the femoral nerve.

- The peritoneum covers the front and both sides of the caecum and continues up behind it, forming a variable retrocaecal space
- The taenia coli converge on the base of the appendix, which opens into the postero-medial wall of the caecum
- The terminal ileum is commonly adherent to the left convexity of the caecum for about 2 cm below the ileocaecal junction
- Internally the ileocaecal junction is guarded by the ileocaecal valve, which is not always competent, but which may prevent reflux into the ileum

### The ascending colon

This is the first part of the colon, 15 cm long, running from the ileocaecal junction to the hepatic flexure. It is usually retroperitoneal.

- The ascending colon lies on the iliac and lumbar fascia between the lateral paracolic gutter and medial right infracolic compartment

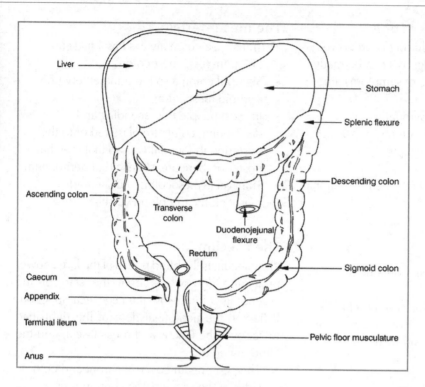

**Figure 1.55 Gross anatomy of the large bowel**

Labels in figure: Liver, Stomach, Splenic flexure, Descending colon, Ascending colon, Transverse colon, Duodenojejunal flexure, Rectum, Sigmoid colon, Caecum, Appendix, Terminal ileum, Pelvic floor musculature, Anus

- The longitudinal muscle of the colon is concentrated into three flat bands, the taenia coli, which sacculate or 'bunch up' the wall of the colon between them
- Appendices epiploicae are bulbous pouches of peritoneum distended with fat; blood vessels supplying them from the mucosa perforate the muscle walls, causing areas of weakness through which mucous membranes can herniate, causing diverticula

### The transverse colon

The second part of the colon is about 45 cm long and extends from the hepatic to the splenic flexure in a loop suspended by its mesentery. It is intraperitoneal.

- The greater omentum, the transverse mesocolon and the transverse colon are fused, so the greater omentum appears to hang from the transverse colon in an apron
- The appendices epiploicae are larger and more numerous than on the ascending colon
- The splenic flexure is much higher than the hepatic flexure

### The descending colon

The third part of the colon is 30 cm long and extends from the splenic flexure to the pelvic brim. It is usually retroperitoneal.

- It lies on the lumbar and iliac fascia, similar to the ascending colon
- Appendices epiploicae are numerous and diverticulosis is common

### Sigmoid colon

The fourth part of the colon is about 45 cm long (but its length varies), and it extends from the descending colon at the pelvic brim to the upper end of the rectum in front of the third piece of the sacrum. It is intraperitoneal.

- The start of the rectum is defined by the end of the sigmoid mesentery, which is the only distinction
- The taenia coli are wider in the sigmoid and fuse distally to form a complete longitudinal coat
- Appendices epiploicae are most common here, as is the incidence of diverticulosis
- The sigmoid mesentery hangs from an upside-down V-shaped base which lies over the bifurcation of the common iliac artery; each limb is about 5 cm long (see Figure 1.50 in Section 6)

# Blood and lymphatic supply of the large bowel

## Arteries

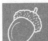 **In a nutshell ...**

The blood supply of the large bowel is shown in Figure 1.56.

- The **superior mesenteric artery** (SMA) supplies the appendix, caecum, ascending and proximal transverse colon
- The **inferior mesenteric artery** (IMA) supplies the rest of the transverse colon, the descending and sigmoid colon, and the upper rectum; it anastomoses with the pudendal vessels in the anal canal

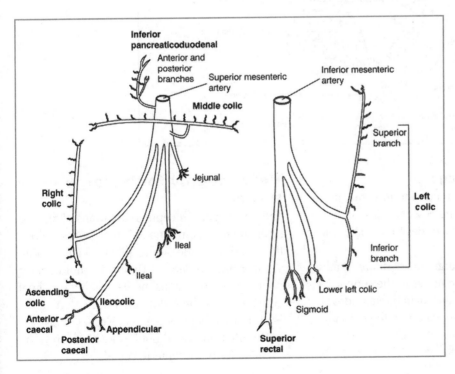

**Figure 1.56 The superior mesenteric artery (left) and the inferior mesenteric artery (right)**

- Arterial disease of the aorta or complications after aortic surgery may occlude these arteries
- The IMA and the small arteries of the transverse colon are especially liable to atherosclerosis
- The marginal artery (of Drummond) is an artery near the gut wall which acts as an anastomosis between the IMA and the SMA; it has clinical relevance because the survival of an anastomosis after division of either of these major arteries may depend on it (it can be absent or poorly developed)

## Veins

- The portal vein drains the blood from the large bowel (Figure 1.57)
- Blood from the right side of the large bowel drains via the **superior mesenteric vein** and ends up in the right hepatic lobe due to the 'streaming' of blood in the portal vein
- Blood from the left side of the large bowel drains via the **inferior mesenteric vein** into the splenic vein and ends up in the left hepatic lobe

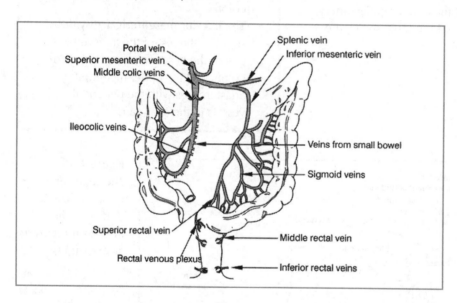

**Figure 1.57 Venous drainage of the large bowel**

## Lymphatic drainage

- Lymphatic vessels tend to follow the arteries
- Left side of the large bowel drains via the superior mesenteric nodes to the para-aortic nodes
- Right side of the large bowel drains via the inferior mesenteric nodes to the superior mesenteric nodes and pancreatic nodes
- Smaller nodes are located on the colonic wall and in the mesentery between the colon and the aorta

## Nerve supply to the large bowel

The main pain receptors are transmitted via sympathetic components that pass along the arteries to the aortic plexus T10–L2 with vasoconstrictor nerves. The main motor fibres come from the vagus nerve to the proximal colon as far as the distal transverse colon.

- The distal large bowel receives a motor supply from sacral outflows which run with the inferior mesenteric vessels

- In the bowel wall is an intramural plexus with connections from the extrinsic nerves
- The smooth muscle fibres are themselves in direct communication with each other by gap junctions

## Physiology of the colon

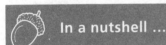

### In a nutshell ...

The main functions of the colon are dehydration and storage of ileal effluent to form faeces.

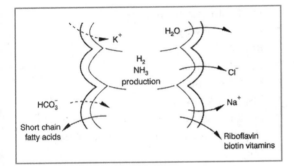

**Figure 1.58 Movement of electrolytes and metabolites across the wall of the colon**

There are three main types of contraction involved in mixing, absorption and transport of colon contents (shown in Figure 1.59). An intrinsic nerve plexus is responsible for contraction; if it is damaged (eg by trypanosomes in Chagas' disease or by drugs such as chlorpromazine or senna) or absent (eg in Hirschsprung's disease), severe constipation or obstruction results.

Various hormones and neurotransmitters can affect the intrinsic plexus (and therefore colon motility):

- Cholecystokinin levels increase after meals and stimulate increased colonic activity
- Colonic activity is reduced by sleep
- Colonic activity is increased by stress
- Many drugs have a potent effect on the colon (eg calcium channel blockers)
- Electrolyte imbalances such as low serum potassium can have a profound effect on smooth muscle function

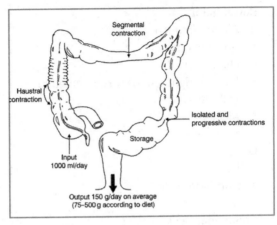

**Figure 1.59 Activity of the large bowel**

## 8.3 Diagnosis of colorectal disease

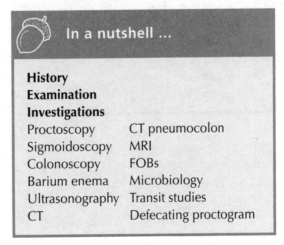

### In a nutshell ...

**History**
**Examination**
**Investigations**

| | |
|---|---|
| Proctoscopy | CT pneumocolon |
| Sigmoidoscopy | MRI |
| Colonoscopy | FOBs |
| Barium enema | Microbiology |
| Ultrasonography | Transit studies |
| CT | Defecating proctogram |

# History of colorectal disease

## History of colorectal disease

**General**
- Weight loss
- Jaundice
- Malaise
- Vomiting
- Anaemia

**Bowel habit**
- Altered frequency
- Constipation
- Diarrhoea
- Blood (bright red, dark red, mixed in with motion)
- Melaena
- Slime

**Drugs**
- Laxatives
- Antidiarrhoeals
- Iron

**Abdominal signs**
- Pain (constant or colicky)
- Distension
- Borborygmi

**Anal and perianal symptoms**
- Pruritus
- Pain on defecation
- Prolapse
- Incontinence
- Discharge
- Tenesmus
- Swelling

# Examination of colorectal disease

## Abdominal examination
- Distension
- Visible peristalsis
- Palpable mass
- Hepatomegaly
- Tenderness

## Anorectal examination
- Inspection
- Pruritus ani
- Perianal warts, abscess, haematoma
- Prolapsing or thrombosed haemorrhoids
- Skin tags
- Anal fistulas and fissures
- Anal/rectal cancer
- Rectocele
- Rectal prolapse
- Faecal soiling
- Inspect on straining
- Digital examination (Figure 1.60)
- Inspect glove for blood, mucus, melaena or pus

There are only three good reasons **not** to do a rectal examination on someone presenting with bowel symptoms or any acute surgical admission:
1. Patient is under 16 years of age
2. Patient has no anus
3. Doctor has no fingers

If you don't put your finger in it, you will put your foot in it and miss an important diagnosis. It is an essential part of a full surgical assessment.

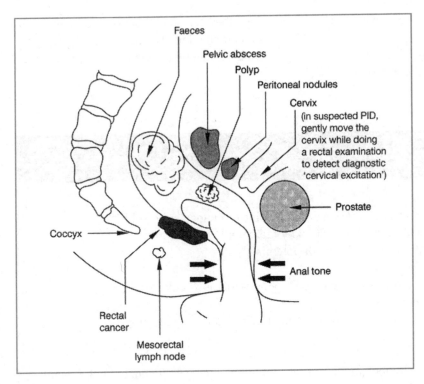

**Figure 1.60 Findings on rectal examination**

Faeces

Pelvic abscess

Polyp

Peritoneal nodules

Cervix
(in suspected PID,
gently move the
cervix while doing
a rectal examination
to detect diagnostic
'cervical excitation')

Prostate

Coccyx

Anal tone

Rectal
cancer

Mesorectal
lymph node

## Investigating colorectal disease

### Proctoscopy

- Enables inspection of the anal canal
- Reveals haemorrhoids, anal and lower rectal polyps, and tumours
- Banding or injection of haemorrhoids and biopsy of mucosa or tumours can be carried out via a proctoscope

### Sigmoidoscopy

#### Rigid sigmoidoscopy

- Can be performed without bowel preparation or sedation in the outpatient clinic
- The rigid sigmoidoscope is 20 cm long and allows visualisation of the rectum (it should be called rectoscopy because the sigmoid

colon is never fully visualised and often not seen at all!)
- The tip of the sigmoidoscope should be advanced only when the lumen is visible
- Sigmoidoscopy reveals abnormalities of mucosa (eg proctitis, IBD) as well as mass lesions (polyps, tumours)
- Biopsies of mucosal lesions should be taken only below 10 cm for fear of bowel perforation
- Biopsies of any protuberant lesions that can be reached should be taken

#### Flexible sigmoidoscopy

- Uses fibreoptic technology or charge-coupled device (CCD)/video technology and a 60- to 100-cm-long endoscope
- Of colorectal carcinomas, 70% are within reach of the flexible sigmoidoscope – this is true sigmoidoscopy because the colon

can be visualised up to and proximal to the splenic flexure

- Specially trained staff maintain the equipment but, with dedicated suites and

staff, they can still be performed in an outpatient clinic. Sedation is rarely needed

- Biopsies can be taken of lesions or mucosa

## Colonoscopy

### Procedure box: Colonoscopy

**Indications**
- Signs and symptoms of mucosal disease (eg bleeding or change in bowel habit)
- Evaluation of mucosal abnormalities found by radiographic techniques
- Surveillance of conditions with malignant potential
- Therapeutic interventions
- Screening of high-risk individuals (eg hereditary non-polyposis colorectal cancer or HNPCC, previous polyps or cancer)
- Colonoscopy is sensitive for mucosal abnormalities and can facilitate biopsies, polypectomy and diathermy of lesions

**The endoscope**
The colonoscope is an instrument about 2 m long (although they vary in length) with several components:
- A viewing system (either a video or fibreoptic) and a light source
- Suction, irrigation and instrumentation channels
- Directional control wires

**Patient preparation**
- **1 week before:** stop iron, bismuth, warfarin, anti-platelets
- **48 hours before:** clear liquid diet
- **12 hours before:** start taking bowel prep, usually Klean-Prep or similar (never osmotic purgatives such as mannitol because they cause hydrogen gas accumulation, which is potentially explosive)
- **Review risk factors:** coagulopathies, cardiopulmonary comorbidity, prosthetic heart valves, drug allergies
- **Consent:** indicating risk of complications
- **Sedation:** as for upper endoscopy, but opiate analgesics are also used because the procedure can be painful due to distension of the colon with air
- **Monitoring:** obs and sats should be regularly monitored by a dedicated team member. Oxygen should be supplied by face mask or nasal cannulae
- **Position:** left lateral (but may be placed supine or prone during the procedure)

continued opposite

## Procedure
- Digital examination first: to exclude stricture or anal canal pathology and confirm there is safe passage for the scope
- Examine rectum, sigmoid colon, transverse colon and descending colon
- Confirm that the caecum has been reached by identifying the ileocaecal valve, triradiate fold and appendiceal orifice, and/or transilluminating the RIF
- Intubation of the terminal ileum is done by experienced endoscopists and is useful (eg in assessing Crohn's disease)
- Biopsy any abnormal mucosa or lesions
- Withdraw the scope, pausing in the rectum to retrovert it and examine the upper anal canal, which is poorly seen on intubation

## Complications
- **Perforation** (<0.5% of diagnostic colonoscopies, <1% of polypectomies) more likely if:
  - The instrument is looped
  - There is pathology damaging the bowel wall such as acute diverticulitis, ischaemia, psuedo-obstruction
  - Therapeutic diathermy is used
- Colonic perforation is a surgical emergency
- **Bleeding** (<1% of all polypectomies): may be immediate (when it can be injected with adrenaline or diathermised) or delayed by several weeks
- **Reaction to drugs used**

---

### JAG Guidelines for Full Certification in Colonoscopy
- Caecal intubation rate >90%
- Polyp detection and removal >10%
- Serious complications <0.5%
- Sedation rates = mean below recommended

### Cleaning of endoscopes
- To prevent exposure of all individuals to potential pathogens
- Cleaning process includes manual cleaning, disinfectant, peracetic acid, isopropyl alcohol and an automatic washer disinfector

---

## Contrast studies

### Single-contrast water-soluble enema
- Urografin, not Gastrografin, is generally used for this study, so it is inaccurate to ask for a 'Gastrografin enema'
- Shows only gross abnormalities (eg mechanical obstruction); does not exclude malignancy in the whole large bowel
- Is typically indicated in an emergency case when the plain abdominal radiograph shows large-bowel obstruction. The differential diagnosis is a pathological obstruction such as cancer (needing surgery) or a pseudo-obstruction needing decompression but very rarely surgery. These two can be differentiated quite well by a water-soluble enema

**Advantages of single-contrast water-soluble enema in the patient with dilated large-bowel loops on plain abdominal radiograph**

- Quick and easy to perform
- Does not need lengthy (and in the truly obstructed patient, dangerous) bowel preparation
- Harmless if it leaks into the peritoneal cavity (in the case of perforation or immediate surgery), unlike barium which is a peritoneal irritant
- In the case of impacted constipation or pseudo-obstruction, has a laxative effect that is often therapeutic
- It gives the radiologist the information that he or she needs about the length and site of the stricture if colorectal stenting is being considered

## Double-contrast barium enema

- Performed by insufflating air after evacuation of barium (and is thus double contrast)
- Reveals fine mucosal detail
- Better diagnostic accuracy than single contrast water-soluble enema
- Extracolonic abnormalities (eg fistulas) are seen more clearly than at endoscopy
- The right colon is revealed in patients in whom colonoscopists could not reach the caecum; however, biopsies and therapeutic snaring of lesions cannot be performed
- The distal 10 cm of the alimentary tract should be visualised by rigid sigmoidoscopy because lesions in this area may not be visualised by barium enema
- It is an acceptable alternative to colonoscopy or CT colonography. The choice of investigation depends on the local resources and expertise

## Ultrasonography

- Useful for identifying liver metastases in patients with colorectal cancer
- Rectal intraluminal ultrasonography can be useful in staging rectal tumours (although MRI is the staging investigation of choice to assess local invasion)
- Intraoperative ultrasonography is the most sensitive technique for identifying hepatic metastases

## Computed tomography

- CT of the chest, abdomen and pelvis is used routinely to stage colorectal cancers preoperatively by detecting distant spread
- Contrast CT may identify gross lesions in patients in whom endoscopy or barium enema is not successful but only CT colonography can exclude a cancer as confidently as a barium enema
- CT is extremely useful in diagnosing a host of non-cancer colon pathology, including inflammation, abscesses or strictures caused by diverticulitis, IBD or ischaemic bowel. It has become an invaluable part of the preoperative work-up of the patient with the acute abdomen

## CT colonography

- In CT colonography, air is insufflated into the colon before a spiral CT. It gives as good a picture as a barium enema, although it is more expensive and less widely available. It can be combined with a staging CT for preoperative cancer work-up
- Remember that a normal CT of the abdomen, even if it is a spiral CT with oral and IV contrast, will not give a good enough resolution of the gut to exclude colonic pathology – CT colonography, however, can

## MRI

- MRI is used to stage rectal cancers preoperatively because it gives good information about the extent of the tumour, invasion of adjacent structures, tissue planes and local lymphadenopathy. Treatment decisions such as whether or not to use preoperative radiotherapy for rectal cancer are based on appearances on MRI. It is also useful in determining the operability of liver metastases
- It is invaluable in assessing anorectal fistulas (see Section 9, Perianal conditions)

## Faecal occult blood test

This test for haemolysed blood can be used to screen patients for colorectal cancer. The faeces are smeared on a filter impregnated with guaiac acid. Hydrogen peroxide is added. The guaiac acid goes blue in the presence of haematin from haemoglobin. The test is not very specific because bleeding from other colonic causes, or even high meat content in the diet, can give false positives.

Although limited as a diagnostic tool, faecal occult blood tests (FOBTs) are non-invasive and useful as a screening tool (see Section 8.6). Some trials have suggested that FOBTs can reduce the mortality from colorectal cancer.

## Microbiological tests

- If infection is suspected, microscopy will show mobile *Amoeba* spp. and parasitic cysts in a fresh stool
- Stool culture will grow bacterial pathogens
- Toxins produced by *Clostridium difficile* can be identified in patients with pseudomembranous colitis

## Transit studies

- Intestinal transit is estimated by following the passage of a known number of ingested radio-opaque markers by plain radiography
- Delay in transit is considered to be present if >80% of markers are still present after 5 days
- This test can be used to investigate constipation

## 8.4 Inflammatory bowel disease

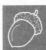 **In a nutshell ...**

IBD is a chronic GI inflammation without identifiable cause. Several inflammatory bowel conditions also exist with a known cause, and these should be excluded:
- Infection
- Antibiotics (pseudomembranous colitis)
- Parasites
- Ischaemic colitis
- Radiation colitis

IBD can be:
- Crohn's disease
- Ulcerative colitis
- Indeterminate colitis (where pathological differentiation between Crohn's disease and ulcerative colitis is impossible)

The pathological findings, clinical presentation, management, complications and prognosis of Crohn's disease and ulcerative colitis are very different.

# Pathology of Crohn's disease and ulcerative colitis

 **In a nutshell ...**

**Crohn's disease**
- Most commonly found in the terminal ileum, but can occur anywhere in the alimentary canal, from mouth to anus
- Involvement is typically transmural with granuloma formation (in 40%), mesenteric fatty encroachment, and risk of fistulation, perforation and obstruction
- Perianal involvement is seen in 75% of patients

**Ulcerative colitis (UC)**
- A mucosal disease that almost invariably involves the rectum and then spreads more proximally in a continuous manner
- Only 15% of cases extend more proximally than the splenic flexure (this group has a greater risk of complications, including cancer)
- In a few cases, the ileum is also affected (backwash ileitis)

## Pathological features of Crohn's disease and ulcerative colitis

| | Crohn's disease | Ulcerative colitis |
|---|---|---|
| Gross pathology | 30% of cases only ileum is affected<br>50% of cases both ileum and colon are affected<br>20% of cases only colon is affected<br>'Skip lesions' of abnormal areas intervening between normal mucosa<br>Any part of alimentary canal affected from mouth to anus | 60% confined to rectum and sigmoid<br>25% extends to splenic flexure<br>15% more proximal than splenic flexure<br>Continuous proximal spread from rectum (no 'skip lesions')<br>Only large bowel affected with occasional 'backwash ileitis' in extensive cases |
| Histology | Whole thickness of bowel wall affected<br>Acute phase: swollen, red, ulcerated bowel<br>Chronic phase: hosepipe thickening with fibrosis, luminal narrowing and obstruction<br>Mucosa: cobblestone appearance<br>Serosa: fatty encroachment<br>Ulcers: can be very deep; fissuring causes adhesion and fistulas between bowel and adjacent structures | Usually limited to mucosa, not affecting muscularis propria<br>Acute phase: swollen, red, ulcerated bowel<br>Chronic phase: regeneration of epithelium; inflammatory pseudopolyps<br>Mucosa: atrophic apart from inflammatory pseudopolyps<br>Serosa: not affected except in toxic megacolon, when all bowel layers are involved<br>Ulcers: small and shallow |
| Microscopic features | Non-caseating epithelioid granulomas in 60–70% of patients<br>Transmural inflammation<br>Fissuring ulcers<br>Lymphoid follicles<br>Mucosal crypt distortion | Granulomas not typical<br>Inflammatory infiltrate confined to lamina propria<br>Crypt abscesses<br>Crypt distortion<br>Metaplasia and dysplasia (can be severe and predisposes to carcinoma) |

## Epidemiology of IBD

Both Crohn's disease and UC are more common in developing countries and in younger adults:

- Crohn's disease affects more females than males
- UC affects both sexes equally
- Incidence of UC is 26 per 100 000 of the population and is static
- Incidence of Crohn's disease is 6 per 100 000 of the population and is rising

## Aetiology of IBD

Of patients with Crohn's disease or UC, 20–30% have a family history of IBD. Aetiology is not clear in either disease but:

- A post-infective theory has been postulated for Crohn's disease
- Autoimmune, environmental and dietary factors have been considered for UC

## Clinical features of IBD

 **In a nutshell …**

- Most common presenting symptom of UC is bloody diarrhoea in an otherwise fit patient
- Presentation of Crohn's disease depends upon the area affected. Anal disease is a useful feature indicating Crohn's disease (affects up to 75% of patients with Crohn's disease)
- Rectal Crohn's disease and UC can be difficult to differentiate

## Typical features of Crohn's disease

- Terminal ileal involvement
- Colitis leading to diarrhoea, mucus and bleeding
- Anal fissure, ulcers, infections and skin tags
- Stricture formation leading to chronic intestinal obstruction
- Local perforation
- Abscess formation
- Fistula to exterior or other organs
- Extraintestinal manifestations
- Anorexia, weight loss, malnutrition, anaemia, nausea

## Typical features of ulcerative colitis

- Bloody diarrhoea with mucus, urgency and incontinence
- Constipation in cases of limited proctitis
- Cramping abdominal pain
- Anorexia, weight loss, malnutrition, anaemia and nausea
- Extraintestinal manifestations

**Symptoms and signs of severe acute colitis**

It is important to recognise patients with severe acute colitis with severe local symptoms as these patients may progress to acute toxic dilatation of the colon and perforation. Symptoms and signs include:

- Frequency of more than 10 stools in 24 hours with blood
- Wasting, pallor, tachycardia, pyrexia
- Tender, distended abdomen

CHAPTER 1

### Clinical features in ulcerative colitis and Crohn's disease

| Symptom | Crohn's disease | Ulcerative colitis |
|---|---|---|
| **Bleeding** | Sometimes | Common |
| **Urgent defecation** | Sometimes | Common |
| **Abdomen** Mass Spontaneous fistulas | Sometimes Sometimes | Rare Never |
| **Anal region** Fissure Ulceration Infection Lesions preceding bowel symptoms | Common Common Common Sometimes | Rare Rare Rare Never |

### Extraintestinal manifestations of inflammatory bowel disease

#### Related to disease activity

- **Skin:** pyoderma gangrenosum, erythema nodosum
- **Mucous membranes:** aphthous ulcers of mouth and vagina
- **Eyes:** iritis
- **Joints:** activity-related arthritis of large joints

#### Unrelated to disease activity

- **Joints:** sacroiliitis, ankylosing spondylitis
- **Biliary tree:** chronic active hepatitis, cirrhosis, primary sclerosing cholangitis
- **Renal:** bile duct carcinoma
- **Integument:** amyloidosis in Crohn's disease, fingernail clubbing

# Investigating inflammatory bowel disease

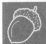 **In a nutshell ...**

Aims of investigations are:
- To make the diagnosis
- To assess the severity of disease

## Sigmoidoscopy

Findings are similar in both Crohn's disease and UC apart from distribution of disease:
- Oedema of mucosa
- Contact bleeding
- Granularity of mucosa
- Ulceration with pus and blood

Biopsies help to distinguish between Crohn's disease and UC. **Sigmoidoscopy should not be performed in acute colitis** (there is a risk of perforation)

## Colonoscopy

- Findings similar to sigmoidoscopy
- Useful for assessing strictures and disease distribution
- Biopsies should be taken
- Useful in surveillance for dysplasia and carcinoma
- **Avoid in acute colitis**

## Barium enema

- Demonstrates extent of macroscopic disease
- Useful for assessing strictures and disease distribution
- Serial biopsies cannot be taken
- **Not appropriate in acute colitis** due to the risk of perforation which would be complicated by barium peritonitis

- Good for distinguishing Crohn's disease from UC
- Identifies fistulas not seen on endoscopy

**Barium enema findings**
**Crohn's disease**
- Discontinuous distribution ('skip lesion')
- Rectal sparing common
- Cobblestone appearance of mucosa
- 'Rose-thorn' ulcers
- Fistulas
- Strictures

**Ulcerative colitis**
- Featureless 'hosepipe' colon
- Decreased haustrae
- Affects rectum and spreads proximally
- Mucosal distortion
- Small ulcers and pseudopolyps
- Shortened colon

### Small-bowel enema/barium meal

- Useful in small-bowel or ileocaecal Crohn's disease
- Mucosal features are similar to those seen in the barium enema
- Long narrowed areas (Kantor's 'string sign') can be seen with proximal dilatation

## Blood tests

The blood tests help to assess the severity of inflammation and also the response to treatment.

**FBC:** anaemia, leucocytosis in sepsis, and platelets raised in acute Crohn's disease.

**ESR, CRP, plasma viscosity (PV):** markers of inflammation, raised in active disease.

**Serum albumin:** tends to be low in patients with active disease.

CHAPTER 1

**IBD inflammatory index:** combined score based on WCC, platelet count, PV and CRP.

**TPMT (thiopurine methyltransferase):** used to detect whether a patient is at risk of developing severe side effects from taking thiopurine medications such as azathioprine.

### Stool microscopy and culture

Done to differentiate between infective colitis and IBD.

## Medical management of inflammatory bowel disease

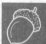

### In a nutshell ...

**Mainstays of medical management:**
* Multidisciplinary approach
* Anti-inflammatory medication
* Immunosuppressants
* Replacement of nutrients, water and electrolytes

### Multidisciplinary approach to IBD

Physicians, surgeons, clinical nurse specialists, stoma therapists, dietitians and patient support groups may all be involved in the management of IBD. More complex cases should be seen in a specialist colitis clinic run jointly by physicians and surgeons with a special interest.

## Anti-inflammatory medication for IBD

### Oral 5-aminosalicylic acid (ASA) preparations (eg mesalazine [Asacol], olsalazine)

* Slow release
* Few side effects
* Often first line of treatment
* Patients are on these drugs long-term as 'preventers' of recurrent flare-ups and complications

### Sulfasalazine (5-ASA and sulfapyridine)

* Suppresses disease activity and maintains remission
* Nausea, vomiting and skin rashes are side effects

## Immunosuppressants for IBD

### Steroids

* Examples are IV hydrocortisone or oral prednisolone
* Used to control exacerbations of colitis. Steroids are very effective but should not be used repeatedly or for long-term management
* Well-known side effects include peptic ulceration, osteoporosis, Cushing syndrome and psychiatric effects
* Withdrawal may lead to recurrent attacks
* Modified-release budesonide causes fewer side effects
* Prolonged high-dose steroids are undesirable and can be an indication for surgery

## Ciclosporin

- Used for acute UC as a second-line drug. It acts by interfering with lymphocyte activation and is a strong immunosuppressant
- It can be given intravenously or as an enema
- Side effects include bone marrow suppression and nephrotoxicity

## Azathioprine

- Immunosuppressive agent used to avoid steroids in resistant Crohn's disease and also in UC in patients who cannot tolerate ciclosporin
- Delayed onset of action and patients are variably responsive, so their TPMT levels need to be checked before deciding on treatment dose

## Topical agents

- Particularly useful in acute attacks of UC because the disease is often restricted to the rectum
- 5-ASA preparations and steroids are available in suppositories, enemas and foam enemas

## Replacement of nutrients, water and electrolytes in IBD

- **Iron** may be needed in chronic cases
- **Oral nutritional supplements** may be needed if markers (eg albumin) are low
- **IV fluids** in acutely unwell, dehydrated patients
- **Potassium supplementation** in acutely unwell patients with severe diarrhoea
- **Parenteral nutrition** in severely malnourished patients

## Other therapies for IBD

- **Infliximab** (anti-tumour necrosis factor or TNF): used by specialists in the management of complex or refractory IBD, especially for the treatment of inflammatory and fistulating perianal Crohn's disease. Recommended groups for treatment include patients who have not responded to conventional therapy and have fistulating disease. It also has a role in UC in patients who have not responded to conventional therapy.
- **Antibiotics:** metronidazole is sometimes prescribed, but in general antibiotics should be given only if specifically indicated for managing bacterial overgrowth in the small bowel or for treating the infective complications of Crohn's disease and perianal Crohn's disease. Metronidazole also has a role after resection of a Crohn's disease segment where there is a primary anastomosis – treatment for 3 months postoperatively is suggested.

## Surgical management of IBD

 **In a nutshell ...**

Surgery is indicated for specific complications or failure of medical management. In Crohn's disease surgery should be limited, whereas in UC it is usually radical.

## Indications for surgery for IBD

- To restore health in patients with chronic disease who have failed medical treatment (eg in nutritional failure)
- To eliminate the risks of side effects of

steroids in patients requiring long-term high-dose steroids
- Premalignant or malignant change on colonoscopic surveillance
- Patients at high risk of developing cancer: usually UC with early onset, extensive colonic involvement and continuous symptoms
- Treatment of complications (usually emergency surgery):
  - Perforation
  - Severe haemorrhage
  - Toxic dilatation (>6 cm megacolon)
  - Stricture causing obstruction
  - Fistulation or abscess formation
  - Sepsis
  - Acute severe attack
- Need to defunction diseased bowel with an ileostomy

## Principles of surgery for IBD

As a result of the differences between Crohn's disease and UC the principles of surgery are not the same.

In **Crohn's disease,** surgery should be as limited as possible and should be reserved for patients with a specific operable problem. This is because:
- Crohn's disease is relapsing and recurrent and can affect the entire length of the GI tract; it cannot be 'cured' by surgery
- Patients may have the disease for a lifetime so it is important to leave as much functioning bowel as possible (40% of patients operated on for Crohn's disease of the small bowel need further surgery within 10 years)
- Complications such as postoperative sepsis and fistulation are common

For these reasons, conservative treatment, limited bowel resection or bowel-preserving procedures (eg stricturoplasty or balloon dilatation) are commonly employed in Crohn's disease.

By contrast, in **ulcerative colitis** radical surgery is often performed. This is because:
- UC is restricted to the large bowel and is always continuous with the diseased rectum; removal of the diseased segment should cure the patient
- patients are at risk of death from perforation or toxic megacolon, so prompt radical surgery is indicated
- patients with long-standing active UC have an increased risk of developing carcinoma of the colon (which panproctocolectomy prevents); this complication is relatively rare in Crohn's disease

### Proctocolectomy with ileostomy

This has been a traditional operation for UC. It eliminates all disease and risk of malignancy. It leaves the patient with a permanent ileostomy. It is still the procedure of choice in many middle-aged and elderly patients. An intersphincteric approach is used when removing the rectum to avoid damage to the pelvic autonomic nerves.

### Sphincter-preserving proctocolectomy with ileal pouch

This is generally regarded as the best operation for patients with UC:
- The rectum is excised leaving the anal canal with an intact sphincter mechanism
- A pouch is constructed from a duplicated or triplicated loop of ileum (J- or W-pouch)
- The pouch is anastomosed to the dentate line

- The desired result is complete continence; results are often good but there is usually frequency of stools (at least four to six a day)

Patients with Crohn's disease are not usually suitable for a pouch because recurrence may affect the ileum used to form it.

### Colectomy with ileorectal anastomosis

This is occasionally used in both UC and Crohn's disease to avoid an ileostomy. The best results are in disease where the rectum is not affected or is only mildly affected. It has fallen from favour due to problems with recurrent disease in the rectum, risk of cancer in the residual rectum and the improved results with pouch surgery. Crohn's disease patients have problems with fistulation and perianal sepsis. In failed cases, a proctectomy is usually indicated.

### Subtotal colectomy with ileostomy ± mucous fistula

This is the operation most indicated in emergency surgery for the following conditions:

- Acute severe attack of colitis resistant to medical therapy
- Perforations
- Toxic megacolon
- Obstruction due to stricture
- Severe haemorrhage
- Fistulation leading to sepsis

Advantages include the following:

- Restoration of health of patient with minimum surgical trauma
- Spares a sick patient the morbidity of a pelvic dissection
- Leaves an intact rectum and anal sphincter for future restorative surgery
- Makes available a specimen for firm histopathological diagnosis

### Surgery for complications

Specific operations such as stricturoplasty, drainage of abscess and small-bowel resections may be indicated (see 'Complications' below).

## Complications of IBD

 **In a nutshell ...**

**Ulcerative colitis**
- Toxic megacolon
- Perforation
- Haemorrhage
- Malignant change

**Crohn's disease**
- Small-bowel strictures
- Fistulation
- Perianal sepsis
- Perforation

### Toxic dilatation (megacolon)

- Acute severe UC can lead to toxic megacolon
- Such patients should be jointly managed by a physician and a surgeon
- Management involves daily review, medical treatment, nutrition, fluid and electrolyte replacement, and a treatment protocol if possible
- Sigmoidoscopy, biopsy and stool cultures are required
- Colonoscopy and barium enema are contraindicated
- Daily plain abdominal films assess degree of dilatation of the colon
- Toxic megacolon is suggested by colon diameter >6 cm
- Surgery is indicated in toxic megacolon

- Subtotal colectomy with ileostomy ± mucous fistula is the safest emergency option (see above, 'Principles of surgery for IBD')
- Left untreated, toxic megacolon leads to perforation, sepsis and high mortality

### Perforation

- Ideally, under close joint management, perforation should be avoided by early referral for surgery
- Perforation secondary to IBD has a high mortality
- Preoperative diagnosis and management of perforated large bowel is covered in detail in Section 6.2
- Again, a subtotal colectomy with ileostomy ± mucous fistula is the safest operation in UC, but more limited resections may be indicated in Crohn's disease

### Haemorrhage

- Bleeding can be acute or chronic with progressive anaemia
- It is more common in UC than in Crohn's disease
- Massive bleeding is rare and, when it occurs, the bleeding site is often in the rectum
- Emergency surgery is indicated in continued life-threatening bleed
- Severe recurrent anaemia may contribute to the indications for an elective colectomy

### Malignant change in UC

- There is a significant increase in the incidence of colonic carcinoma in patients with UC

- Compared with those in non-colitic bowel, these tumours are more likely to:
  - Affect a younger age group
  - Be anaplastic
  - Be multiple
  - Be masked by the symptoms of colitis
- The risk is greatest in:
  - Long-standing colitis
  - Continuous rather than episodic disease
  - Disease affecting the whole large bowel (pancolitis)
  - Patients affected since childhood
- Of patients with total colitis of 20 years' duration, 12% are likely to develop malignancy
- Patients with long-standing, active or widespread colitis should therefore have a regular colonoscopy to monitor for dysplasia and early invasive cancer
- These patients should also be considered for prophylactic surgery, especially as they also probably have more severe and debilitating symptoms

### Malignant change in Crohn's disease

- There is thought to be a very slightly increased risk of colon cancer in patients with Crohn's disease. However, prophylactic colectomy is not usually performed
- In long-standing Crohn's disease, adenocarcinoma may develop in the affected small bowel (the ileum in two-thirds of cases); this complication is rare and the prognosis is poor

## Strictures in Crohn's disease

- Strictures are more likely to occur in Crohn's disease than in UC due to its transmural pathology:
  - In **inflammatory** strictures causing small-bowel obstruction, steroids and low-residue diets may improve symptoms
  - In **fibrous** strictures surgery is indicated
- Stricturoplasty (Figure 1.61) overcomes obstruction while preserving intestine in patients with multiple short segments of disease
- Balloon dilatation of strictures is another bowel-preserving method of overcoming obstruction
- Resection of diseased small bowel and caecum is indicated in obstructed patients with poor response to medical management
- If surgery is delayed in such patients, fistulation may occur

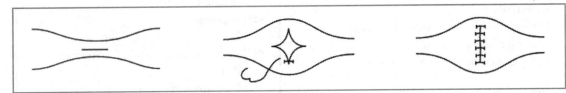

**Figure 1.61 Stricturoplasty in Crohn's disease**

## Fistulas in Crohn's disease

- Fistula formation is present in 15–30% of patients with Crohn's disease
- It is less common in UC because the ulceration is limited to the mucosa and is not transmural
- Types of Crohn's fistulas:
  - External (enterocutaneous)
  - Internal
  - Enterovesical
  - Enterovaginal
  - 'High–low' GI
- Contrast studies, including barium enemas, barium meals and sinograms, can identify the fistula
- Fistulas will occasionally respond to medical treatment, but surgical resection of the diseased bowel and fistula is usually required to achieve cure
- The principle of fistula surgery is to resect the diseased bowel and fistula en bloc and repair the secondary defect in the healthy organ or bowel
- Primary anastomosis should be performed under favourable conditions. In sepsis or malnourished patients, delayed anastomosis should be considered

## Perianal complications in Crohn's disease

- Up to 75% of patients with large-bowel Crohn's disease have an anal lesion:
  - Fissure
  - Anorectal sepsis (perianal abscess and fistulas)
  - Ulceration
  - Oedematous skin tags
  - Stenosis of the anorectal junction
  - Rectovaginal fistula

- Complex perianal abscesses and fistulas can be difficult to manage and supralevator abscesses may lead to proctectomy
- Operations on fistulas should be avoided
- Acute abscesses should be drained
- Long-term treatment with metronidazole reduces the number of exacerbations
- Occasionally, wide excision of the affected perineum, followed by skin grafting or flap repair, is performed once the acute sepsis has resolved
- Rectovaginal fistulas can be repaired successfully but some need proctectomy eventually
- Haemorrhoidectomy should be avoided in Crohn's disease if possible because it can be complicated by perianal sepsis

For IBD in children, see the Paediatric Surgery chapter in Book 1.

## 8.5 Benign colorectal tumours

 **In a nutshell ...**

### Classification of benign colonic tumours

**According to embryological origin**

*Epithelial*
- Adenoma (tubular, tubulovillous, villous)
- Metaplastic polyp

*Mesodermal*
- Lipoma
- Leiomyoma (GI stromal tumour or GIST)
- Haemangioma
- Other rare tumours

*Hamartoma*
- Juvenile polyp
- Peutz–Jeghers polyp

**Neoplastic or non-neoplastic**

*Neoplastic*
- Adenoma
- Benign lymphoma
- Lipoma
- Leiomyoma
- Fibroma
- Haemangioma

*Non-neoplastic*
- Metaplastic polyp
- Hamartomatous polyp
- Juvenile polyp
- Peutz–Jeghers polyp
- Inflammatory polyp

# Definitions

## Polyp

The term 'polyp' is very non-specific. A polyp is an abnormal elevation from an epithelial surface. It can be:

- Pedunculated (have a head and stalk)
- Sessile (no stalk but can be flat or villous)
- Acquired
- Inherited
- Symptomatic
- Non-symptomatic
- Part of a 'polyposis syndrome' (see 'Familial adenomatous polyposis', later in this section)
- Neoplastic
- Non-neoplastic
- Benign
- Malignant

Benign polyps can be classified according to embryological origin, or as neoplastic and non-neoplastic (see 'Nutshell' box above).

## Tumour

- The term 'tumour' is also very non-specific, meaning only 'swelling'
- It is often used interchangeably with 'neoplasm'

## Neoplasm

- A neoplasm is a new growth arising from uncontrolled and progressive cell multiplication
- It can be benign or malignant

## Cancer

- Cancer is the common term for all malignant tumours

## Malignant versus benign

- Often a difficult distinction to make but, in general, malignant tumours are non-differentiated, locally invasive and prone to metastasis (the rate of growth also helps to make the distinction)

# Non-neoplastic colorectal polyps

## Metaplastic polyps

These are also known as hyperplastic polyps.

- Most common type of polyp found in the rectum
- Polyps are 2–5 mm in diameter
- Usually flat-topped and the same colour as the mucosa

There is no evidence that they develop dysplastic or neoplastic change. Clinically they are seen and biopsied on sigmoidoscopy and, if large, may occasionally give rise to symptoms.

## Hamartomatous polyps

These are malformations in which the normal tissues of a particular part of the body are arranged haphazardly, usually with an excess of one or more of its components. There are two types of colonic hamartoma.

### Peutz–Jeghers polyps

- Found in patients with the rare familial Peutz–Jeghers syndrome
- Syndrome consists of pigmentation around the lips associated with characteristic intestinal polyps
- These polyps:
  - Occur most commonly in the small bowel, and occasionally in the colon

- Often present in childhood with intussusception or bleeding and are widespread (therefore hard to treat)
- Have very low-grade malignant potential

### Juvenile polyps
- Most common polyps in children
- Occur anywhere in the large bowel but usually in the rectum
- Occur in children aged <10 and present as prolapse through the anus or bleeding
- Are not premalignant and are easily treated by excision

## Inflammatory polyps
These are essentially normal mucosal tags in the colon of any patient suffering from a chronic inflammatory disease of the bowel. They occur commonly in UC and Crohn's disease.

## Benign neoplastic colorectal polyps

### Benign lymphoma
- Swelling arising from lymphatic tissue
- Most common non-epithelial benign tumour of the colorectum
- Usually a single reddish-purple polyp of varying size
- Differentiated from malignant lymphoma by the well-defined germinal centre on histology
- Treatment is by simple local excision

### Lipoma
- Relatively rare in large bowel
- Tends to present in caecum and right colon
- Variable size

- Can be multiple
- Tends not to undergo malignant change
- May cause intussusception or be confused with neoplastic tumour on contrast studies or colonoscopy
- Resection may be needed to make the histological diagnosis

### Leiomyoma (GIST)
- Rare smooth muscle tumour
- Histological differentiation between benign and malignant is very difficult

### Fibroma
- Rare colonic tumour arising from submucous layer
- Hard, mobile, pedunculated and covered by intact epithelium
- May contain muscle or glandular tissue
- Rarely undergoes malignant change

### Haemangioma
- Vascular lesions
- Need to be differentiated from angiodysplasia
- Can cause profuse rectal bleeding

### Adenomas
- Important because they are the most common neoplastic polyp of the large bowel
- Can develop into carcinoma

Adenomas are dealt with in more detail below.

# Adenomas of the colon and rectum

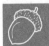

## In a nutshell ...

- Common benign neoplasm with malignant potential
- Can be tubular, tubulovillous or villous (the most premalignant)
- A dysplastic adenoma is not a cancer unless it transgresses the muscularis mucosa
- Once detected, a colonic polyp should be removed in case it is an adenoma in order to prevent the adenoma–carcinoma sequence
- If the polyp proves to be adenomatous, then imaging of the rest of the colon and follow-up endoscopy are indicated
- If the polyp is metaplastic or inflammatory, no follow-up is needed

## Pathology of large-bowel adenomas

An adenoma is a benign neoplasm of the large-bowel glandular epithelium. There are three microscopic categories of adenoma: tubular, villous and tubulovillous.

### Tubular adenomas

- Commonly multiple
- May coexist with a carcinoma
- Malignant potential is less than villous adenoma
- Can be pedunculated or sessile
- Usually small (<2 cm)

### Villous adenomas

- Often large and sessile with a shaggy frond-like surface
- May extend into a 'carpet-like' lesion
- More prone to malignant transformation
- Found more commonly in the rectum

### Tubulovillous adenoma

- An intermediate form, containing features of both morphological types

## Incidence of large-bowel adenomas

- About 33% of the population have an adenoma at postmortem examination
- M > F
- Of all sporadic (not familial adenomatous polyposis [FAP] or hereditary non-polyposis colorectal cancer [HNPCC]) colorectal adenomas, 66% occur distal to the splenic flexure
- This distribution is not the case in multiple polyposis coli syndrome or in elderly patients
- Adenomas occur at any stage, and increase with advancing age (typically present at 55–60 years)

## The adenoma–carcinoma sequence

- 'Dysplasia' refers to the following changes in the epithelial cells:
  - Increase in mitotic figures
  - Pleomorphism of the nuclei
  - Loss of polarity
  - Formation of several layers
- 60% of adenomas show mild dysplasia
- 30% show moderate dysplasia

- 10% show severe dysplasia (also called carcinoma in situ – CIS):
  - CIS is an adenoma still confined to the mucosa (not a cancer)
  - 'Malignant transformation' occurs when these abnormal epithelial cells invade through the muscularis mucosa to enter the submucosa
- Virtually all pathologists believe that adenomas go through the grades of dysplasia to frank malignancy – the so-called **adenoma–carcinoma sequence** – but the evidence is circumstantial

---

**Evidence of the adenoma–carcinoma sequence**
- Similar distribution on the left side of colon of adenomas and carcinomas
- High incidence of adenomas when a carcinoma is present
- Carcinoma patients with adenomas are twice as likely to develop another carcinoma as patients without adenomas
- Epidemiology of adenomas and carcinomas is similar
- Experimental carcinogens produce colorectal cancer and induce adenoma
- Histological examination of carcinomas shows elements of benign adenomas in many cases
- Histological examination of 'benign' adenomas show carcinomas in 3–4%
- FAP patients always develop carcinoma

---

## Clinical features of adenoma

Adenomatous polyps can present in a number of ways:
- Detected on routine screening
- Bleeding, fresh or altered depending on site
- Change in bowel habit (eg diarrhoea or mucus)

- Prolapse of rectal polyp
- Intussusception may present as colic or an acute abdomen
- Tenesmus, mucus and incontinence with large rectal polyps

## Diagnosis of adenoma

### Rectal examination
- Villous tumours are often difficult to feel because of their soft consistency
- Non-villous pedunculated lesions can be palpable
- Focal malignant invasion can be felt as areas of hardness within the polyp

### Endoscopy
- Rigid sigmoidoscopy detects polyps up to 25 cm from the anal verge
- Flexible sigmoidoscopy detects polyps up to 90 cm from the anal verge (detection is three times greater than with a rigid instrument)
- Colonoscopy detects polyps anywhere in the large bowel
- Dye spraying can enhance the pick-up rate

### Barium enema
- Adenomas can be detected on barium enemas, although the pick-up rate is lower than with endoscopy
- If an adenoma is detected by a barium enema, endoscopy and polypectomy/biopsy is indicated
- Subcentimetre polyps can be missed at barium enema, and biopsy/polypectomy may necessitate a second bowel cleansing, so endoscopy is preferred for polyp surveillance

After detection of an adenomatous polyp by whatever method, the rest of the large bowel must be examined by either colonoscopy or barium enema as far as the caecum.

## Management of rectal adenoma

Once a polyp has been detected it should be removed so that its histology can be determined, and to prevent the adenoma–carcinoma sequence.

### Endoscopic removal

- Best method for removing most rectal adenomas is via a sigmoidoscope using a diathermy snare
- Can be facilitated by injecting adrenaline and saline into the mucosa beneath the polyp to 'raise it up' if it is not on a stalk

### Endoscopic diathermy

- Not ideal because it may not destroy the whole tumour and does not allow histological analysis
- Can be the most suitable in certain cases

### Transanal excision

- Can be performed under regional anaesthesia or general anaesthesia via a Parks' self-retaining anal retractor
- Tumour is removed by sharp dissection and diathermy, taking care not to disrupt the underlying rectal muscle
- The mucosal defect is then repaired

### Transanal endoscopic microscopic surgery (TEMS)

- Technique used to remove lesions out of reach of transanal excision

### Laparotomy

- Can be necessary for large adenomas
- Resembles procedures used for low rectal carcinomas (eg abdominoperineal resection or proctectomy and coloanal anastomosis)

## Management of colonic adenoma

### Endoscopic removal

- Often possible via a colonoscope, but if a polyp is too large then colonic resection is necessary
- Diathermy snare is used for pedunculated polyps
- Piecemeal resections can be necessary for large sessile polyps

### Laparotomy

*Indications*

- Too large or sessile for endoscopic removal (usually >3 cm)
- Adenoma inaccessible to endoscopist
- Partially removed polyp which histology shows to be malignant

*Options at laparotomy*

- Surgical colonoscopic polypectomy (the surgeon helps colonoscopic removal of the polyp by manipulating the bowel through an abdominal incision; the bowel is not opened)
- Colotomy and polypectomy (the bowel is opened and the polyp removed; this is rarely indicated because colonic resection is usually safer if a tumour is too large to be removed endoscopically)
- Colonic resection (with primary anastomosis)

## Follow-up after polypectomy for adenoma

This is controversial.

### General principles of follow-up

- After adenoma removal, all patients must be followed up by endoscopy
- The whole colon must be visualised (if not possible on colonoscopy, a barium enema should be employed to exclude other polyps)
- If the polyp proves to be non-neoplastic (metaplastic or inflammatory) no follow-up is needed

- The surveillance interval for benign neoplastic tumours is under review; recent studies have suggested that 3 years is acceptable, then 5 years if the colon is clear
- Follow-up endoscopy should be more frequent if malignant features are seen on histology, several polyps >1 cm are seen or if the polyp is incompletely excised
- If symptoms develop before scheduled endoscopy follow-up, prompt investigation is indicated. Guidelines are regularly reviewed and updated by the British Society of Gastroenterology (BSG).
- Regular colonoscopy until colon is clear plus whenever symptoms develop

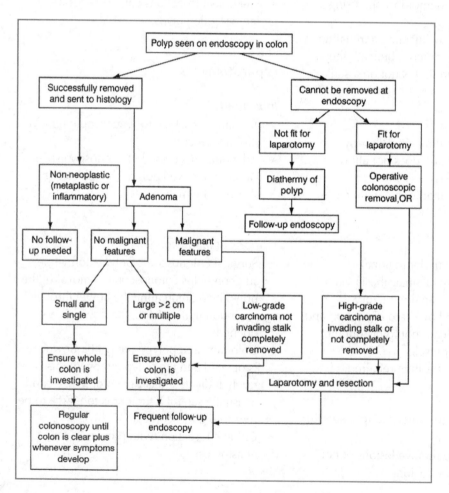

**Figure 1.62 Management of colonic adenoma**

## Complications of polypectomy

- Bleeding (2% have haemorrhage requiring transfusion)
- Perforation (occurs in <0.2% of polypectomies)
- Gas explosion (should not occur now that bowel preparation with mannitol has been abandoned)
- Overall mortality rate is about 0.05%

## Familial adenomatous polyposis

- FAP is a dominant inherited condition (the gene is carried on the short arm of chromosome 5)
- Characterised by multiple colorectal adenomas and sometimes typical extracolonic stigmata
- Affects 1 in 10 000 live births
- Usually hundreds or thousands of adenomas develop in the colon and rectum during the teenage years
- If left untreated, progression to colorectal carcinoma is inevitable within 20 years of adenomas developing
- FAP is responsible for 1% of all colorectal cancers

## Clinical features of FAP

- FAP is increasingly diagnosed by screening of children of affected individuals before symptoms can occur
- If not identified by screening, symptoms occur in the late teenage years or 20s
- Most common presentations are change in bowel habit, with loose stool, blood or mucus per rectum
- Patients may present with carcinoma of the colon or rectum

## Gardner syndrome

A subset of FAP in which the extracolonic manifestations, particularly desmoids, are a feature (see box 'Benign extracolonic manifestations of FAP'. This group also seems to have an increased incidence of other malignancies, especially of the stomach and duodenum.

## Investigating FAP

Screening in relatives of known FAP patients can be carried out in a number of ways.

### Ophthalmoscopy

Reveals congenital hypertrophy of the retinal pigment epithelium (CHRPE), which is highly specific for FAP before polyps develop.

### DNA screening

Identifies affected individuals with 95% confidence.

### Sigmoidoscopy

In children, until adenomas appear, sigmoidoscopy has largely been superseded by the above methods.

Diagnosis in new patients with new mutations and no family history is usually by sigmoidoscopy and biopsy after the adenomas become symptomatic. FAP is assumed in the presence of 100 or more adenomas. The rest of the bowel must be visualised to exclude carcinoma before management is decided on.

> ### Benign extracolonic manifestations of FAP
>
> - Hamartomatous polyps in the stomach
> - Dental cysts
> - Retinal pigmentation
> - Adenomas of the duodenum
> - Osteomas of the jaw
> - Epidermoid cysts
> - Desmoid tumours, usually in the abdomen

### Management of FAP

As a result of the inevitability of malignant transformation, surgery is indicated in all patients with FAP. There are three options for prophylactic surgery:

1. Panproctocolectomy and end-ileostomy
2. Colectomy and ileorectal anastomosis
3. Proctocolectomy with ileal pouch–anal anastomosis

#### Panproctocolectomy and end-ileostomy

- The advantage is that it removes all the affected bowel
- The disadvantage is a permanent stoma
- It is becoming less acceptable to this usually young group of patients

#### Colectomy and ileorectal anastomosis

- Rectum is spared so the patient retains relatively normal bowel function
- Main disadvantage is recurrence of disease
- Rectal adenomas may regress after surgery, but regular surveillance with removal of polyps endoscopically as necessary is rarely satisfactory
- Development of rectal cancer remains a risk which cannot be completely eliminated and which some patients and surgeons are not prepared to accept

#### Proctocolectomy with ileal pouch–anal anastomosis

- All the affected bowel is removed but permanent ileostomy is avoided
- Becoming the more popular option
- Disadvantages are poor functional results and risks of a large and complex operation

All FAP patients require long-term follow-up no matter which operation they have undergone because of the extracolonic manifestations, especially ampullary tumours of the duodenum.

## Other polyposis syndromes

Apart from FAP, other polyposis syndromes are rare and not as clinically significant.

> ### Classification of polyposis syndromes
> **Neoplastic**
> - Familial adenomatous polyposis
> - Turcot syndrome
> - Lymphosarcomatous polyposis
> - Leukaemia polyposis
>
> **Inflammatory**
> - Ulcerative colitis
> - Crohn's disease
> - Other inflammatory polyposis
>   - Amoebiasis
>   - Schistosomiasis
>   - Eosinophilic polyposis
> - Granulomatosis
> - Histoplasmosis
>
> **Hamartomatous**
> - Juvenile polyposis
> - Peutz–Jeghers syndrome
> - Neurofibromatous polyposis
> - Lipomatous polyposis
> - Cronkhite–Canada syndrome
> - Cowden's disease
>
> **Others**
> - Metaplastic
> - Pneumatosis cystoides intestinalis

## 8.6    Colorectal cancer

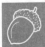 **In a nutshell ...**

The second most common cause of death from malignancy in the UK, colorectal cancers (CRCs) are usually moderately differentiated adenocarcinomas.

**Predisposing factors include:**
- Dietary factors
- Genetic factors (FAP, HNPCC)
- IBD

Seventy-five per cent of colon cancers are distal to the splenic flexure, so can be detected by flexible sigmoidoscopy.

**Classification** is historically by Dukes' staging or, more commonly, by the TNM staging system.

This common lethal cancer is the reason that, in most people, significant rectal bleeding should be investigated by a flexible sigmoidoscopy at least.

When investigating anaemia or change in bowel habit, colorectal cancer is excluded only by a full colonoscopy, a barium enema with rigid sigmoidoscopy or a CT pneumocolon.

**Complications** of CRCs include obstruction, perforation, fistulation and bleeding.

**Principles of surgery include:**
- Preop preparation
- In curable elective cases, aim for wide resection of tumour with regional lymphatics
- In obstructed emergency cases, aim for primary relief of the obstruction followed by elective surgery if necessary
- In incurable cases, aim to relieve present or potential obstruction and alleviate symptoms
- Postop care is vital

**Postop complications** include anastomotic leak, stricture, wound problems, adhesions, damage to the urinary tract, damage to the lumbosacral plexus nerves, problems with the colostomy and altered bowel function, and local or distal recurrence.

**Adjuvant chemotherapy** is of benefit to node-positive colorectal cancers and in some node-negative patients.

**Adjuvant radiotherapy** is not used routinely in colonic cancers but is used (usually preoperatively) in patients with rectal cancers who are at high risk of local recurrence due to circumferential resection margin involvement.

The aims of **follow-up** are to detect postoperative problems, local and distant recurrence, and for audit.

The 5-year survival rates vary according to stage and treatment from around 90% for Dukes' A (T1–T2, N0, M0) to less than 5% for Dukes' D (M1).

## Epidemiology of colorectal cancer

- The second most common cause of death from malignancy in the UK (after lung cancer)
- More common in western Europe and North America than in developing countries
- Less than 5% of patients are aged <40
- Peak incidence is in people aged 70–80 years
- F > M (marginally)

## Aetiology of colorectal cancer

The exact cause is unclear but both environmental and genetic factors are thought to be involved. Immigrants from an area of low incidence to an area with a high incidence soon become just as prone to develop the disease as the indigenous population. The following environmental factors have been implicated.

### Dietary factors and colorectal cancer

- **Lack of fibre:** it is thought that reduced speed of transit exposes gut mucosa to potential carcinogens
- **High-fat diet:** thought to favour bacterial flora which can degrade bile salts into carcinogens
- **High levels of bile acids:** bile salts have a direct effect on mucosa and are degraded into carcinogens
- **Previous cholecystectomy:** not proved

conclusively, but may lead to an increased production of degraded bile salts

### Genetic factors and colorectal cancer

- 75% of cases of colorectal cancer are sporadic
- 1% are in patients with pre-existing IBD (see Section 8.4)
- 24% are associated with genetic factors (Figure 1.63)

Some families have a higher incidence of colorectal cancer due to:
- FAP (Section 8.5)
- HNPCC
- Other familial colon cancer (essentially a diagnosis of exclusion of the first two conditions)

Several genes have been identified as contributing to hereditary colorectal cancer:
- Tumour suppressor genes (eg *APC*, *p53* and *DCC*)
- Oncogenes (eg *Ras*)
- Mismatch-repair genes (eg *hMSH2* and *hMLH1*)

It is unlikely that specific mutations are responsible for most cases of colonic cancer that run in families.

FAP and HNPCC are two hereditary cancers for which molecular genetic testing is available.

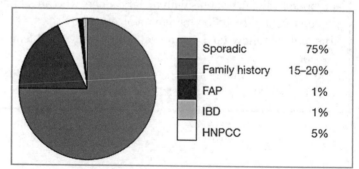

| Sporadic | 75% |
| Family history | 15–20% |
| FAP | 1% |
| IBD | 1% |
| HNPCC | 5% |

Figure 1.63 Risk factors associated with new cases of colorectal cancer

## Hereditary non-polyposis colon cancer

- An inherited colon cancer
- Accounts for 5% of new cases of colorectal cancer per year
- Mainly due to mutations in four different mismatch-repair genes, the products of which normally repair damaged DNA. HNPCC families have mutations in different mismatch repair genes:
  - *hMSH2* (31%)
  - *hMLH1* (33%)
  - *hPMS1* and *hPMS2* (5% between them)

### Characteristics of HNPCC

- Average age of diagnosis is 45 (or younger)
- It is more likely that these tumours will:
  - Develop in the proximal portion of the colon (unlike sporadic colorectal cancers)
  - Show rapid transformation from benign to malignant
  - Coexist with extracolonic cancers:
    - Endometrial cancer in 20–40%
    - Ovarian cancer in 10%
    - Gastric cancer in 6%
    - Biliary tract cancer in 4%
    - Urinary tract cancer in 2%
    - Brain tumours in 1%
    - Small-bowel cancers in 1%

Patients with a strong family history of colon cancer are likely to have HNPCC if they fit the so-called **Amsterdam criteria** as described in the box. Molecular genetic testing is the only way to properly classify the patient and family. Patients confirmed as having HNPCC should have regular colonoscopy and the rest of the family should be offered screenings.

---

**Amsterdam criteria for clinical diagnosis of HNPCC**

- Three or more family members with colorectal cancer
- Colorectal cancer extends over two generations
- One affected family member is a first-degree relative of the other two
- One or more affected before age 45
- Exclusion of FAP

---

Some patients with HNPCC also have an association with other cancers – typically of the ovary, endometrium, breast, stomach, transitional cell carcinoma (TCC) of the urinary tract and the pancreas (Lynch syndrome). These patients may need regular endometrial aspiration or ovarian screening.

## Inflammatory bowel disease

- Of patients with UC of 20 years' duration 12% are likely to develop malignant change
- Accounts for about 1% of all cases of colorectal carcinoma
- Can be a small (but not clinically significant) increase in the incidence of colorectal carcinoma in Crohn's disease

## Irradiation

- Pelvic irradiation increases risk of developing rectosigmoid carcinoma

## Ureterosigmoidostomy

- Technique for urinary diversion
- Less commonly performed now because carcinoma of the sigmoid develops more often in these patients

# Pathology of colorectal cancer

## Distribution of colorectal tumours

The distribution of carcinoma is shown in Figure 1.64:

- 75% of tumours are situated in the rectum and sigmoid colon (within reach of flexible sigmoidoscopy)
- Patients with familial colon cancer, FAP or HNPCC have a higher incidence of right-sided tumours
- Approximately 3% of patients with a primary carcinoma will have another (**synchronous**) tumour present at the time of presentation
- Approximately 75% of patients with a primary carcinoma will have associated benign adenoma
- Of patients with a successfully treated colon cancer, 3% will develop a further colorectal tumour within 10 years (**metachronous** tumour)

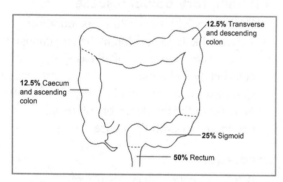

**Figure 1.64 Distribution of carcinoma within the large bowel**

## Classification of colorectal tumours

### In a nutshell ...

Of all cancers of the large bowel, 98% are adenocarcinomas. The other (rare) tumours of the large bowel are carcinoid, primary and secondary lymphomas and GISTs. This section deals only with adenocarcinomas, which are classified thus:

- Papilliferous
- Ulcerating
- Annular (circumferential, obstructing lesion)
- Diffuse infiltrating
- Colloid tumour (produce excess mucus)

## Grading of colorectal tumours

Colorectal tumours are graded histologically as I–IV according to the degree of differentiation of cells.

Grade I       Well differentiated (20%)
Grade II, III  Moderately differentiated (60%)
Grade IV      Anaplastic (20%)

## Spread of colorectal tumours

### Direct spread

- More common laterally than longitudinally
- A 2-cm longitudinal clearance is usually adequate (5 cm used to be recommended)
- Eventually involves adjacent viscera

The discovery that rectal tumours do not tend to spread any more distally than 2 cm was one of the factors that has helped to bring about an increase in low sphincter-sparing anterior resections, in cases that would previously have needed an abdominoperineal excision of rectum.

## Lymphatic spread

- Via lymphatics, which run with supplying arteries
- To regional lymph nodes, para-aortic nodes and thence to the thoracic duct
- Supraclavicular nodes can be involved in advanced cases
- Upward spread is more likely for rectal carcinomas than lateral spread or spread down to the lower lymphatics (this makes sphincter-saving operations more practicable)

## Blood-borne spread

- Portal vein spreads metastases to the liver
- 25% of patients have liver metastases at presentation; a further 25–40% will develop them subsequently
- Also to the lungs (5% of cases), adrenal glands, kidneys and bones

## Transcoelomic spread

- Produces deposits of malignant nodules throughout the peritoneal cavity

- Occurs in 10% of patients after resection
- Spread to the ovaries form metastatic deposits termed 'Krukenberg tumours'

## Implantation

- This method of spread is possible, but uncommon
- Recurrences occur in wounds, suture lines, colostomies and laparoscopy port sites

# Staging of colorectal cancer

## Pathological staging of colorectal cancer

Colorectal cancers are staged primarily on the pathological characteristics of the resected specimen. The Dukes' system, first described in 1932 by the pathologist Sir Cuthbert Dukes, was historically the accepted classification in the UK (although it was originally described only for rectal tumours). See the following table 'Dukes' pathological staging of colorectal cancer' for full staging details.

The TNM system has now superseded the Dukes' system and is used not only for postoperative pathological staging but for the all-important preoperative staging in multidisciplinary team (MDT) meetings to plan treatment. The prefix denotes the mode of staging: 'p' means that this is the pathological stage, and is the definitive staging; 'u', for example, indicates the staging as judged by ultrasonography.

## Dukes' pathological staging of colorectal cancer

| Dukes' stage | Extent of tumour | Frequency at presentation | 5-year survival rate |
|---|---|---|---|
| A | Confined to bowel wall | 11% | 83% |
| B | Through bowel wall Lymph nodes not involved | 35% | 64% |
| C | Lymph nodes involved No other metastases | 26% | 38% |
| $C_2$ | Highest node involved | | |
| D* | Distant metastases Long-term survival rare without liver resection | 29% | 3% |

*Not included in Dukes' original staging but often used.

## TNM clinical classification of colon and rectal tumours

| T | Primary tumour |
|---|---|
| Tx | Primary tumour cannot be assessed |
| T0 | No evidence of primary tumour |
| Tis | Carcinoma in situ: intraepithelial or invasion of the lamina propria |
| T1 | Tumour transgresses muscularis mucosa into the submucosa but not into muscularis propria |
| T2 | Tumour invades muscularis propria but does not go through the serosa |
| T3 | Tumour invades through muscularis propria into subserosa or into non-peritonealised pericolic or perirectal tissues |
| T4 | Tumour directly invades other organs or structures and/or perforates visceral peritoneum |
| **N** | **Regional lymph nodes** |
| Nx | Regional lymph nodes cannot be assessed |
| N0 | No regional lymph node metastases |
| N1 | Metastasis in one to three regional lymph nodes |
| N2 | Metastasis in four or more regional lymph nodes |
| **M** | **Distant metastasis** |
| Mx | Distant metastasis cannot be assessed |
| M0 | No distant metastasis |
| M1 | Distant metastasis |

## Comparison of the TNM and Dukes' staging systems

| TNM stage | T | N | M | Dukes' system |
|---|---|---|---|---|
| 0 | Tis | 0 | 0 | N/A |
| I | T1/T2 | N0 | M0 | A |
| II | T3/T4 | N0 | M0 | B |
| III | Any T | N1/N2 | M0 | C |
| IV | Any T | Any N | M1 | D |

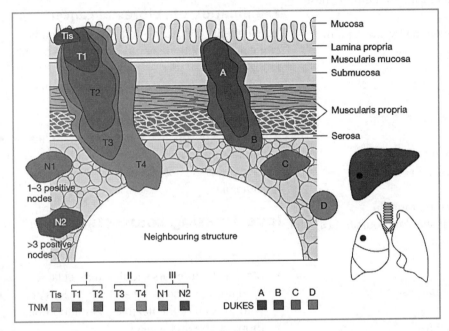

**Figure 1.65**
**Colorectal cancer staging: comparison of the TNM and Dukes' classifications**

## Clinical staging of colorectal cancer

There are three main prognostic groups following surgery:

1. **Incurable because of distant metastases:** as shown by histology or imaging
2. **Incurable because of residual local disease:** histological examination shows tumour at resection margin of specimen; specimen perforated or adherent to adjacent viscera. This is called an R1 resection, so a pathological report (as given to you in a pathology viva!) may read pT4, pN2, R1 indicating that the resection margin was involved, so tumour can be assumed to have been left behind. In the case of rectal tumours surgeons try to avoid this by giving preoperative chemoradiotherapy in order to downsize the tumour if preoperative imaging suggests that the circumferential margin may be threatened
3. **Curative operation:** in which all demonstrable tumour has been removed. This is called an R0 resection

# Clinical presentation of colorectal cancer

## General effects of malignant disease
- Anaemia
- Anorexia
- Weight loss
- Symptoms of secondary disease
- Liver metastases (jaundice; ascites; hepatomegaly)
- Lung metastases (incidental finding on chest radiograph; pleural effusion; recurrent chest infection)
- Others (eg lymphadenopathy, bone pain)

## Local effects

### Right colon tumours (usually proliferative, soft and friable)
- Change in bowel habit
- Altered blood per rectum
- Right-sided mass
- Abdominal pain and perforation
- More likely than left-sided tumours to be occult and symptomless

### Left colon tumours (usually annular and constricting)
- Change in bowel habit
- Constipation and obstruction
- Abdominal colic and perforation
- More overt bleeding and mucus per rectum
- 25–30% of patients with left colon tumours present as an emergency – usually obstruction or perforation

### Rectal tumours
- Bleeding is the presenting complaint in 60% of patients
- Change in bowel habit (including mucus)
- Tenesmus
- Palpable prolapsing mass
- Symptoms worse in the morning

Due to these early warning symptoms, rectal tumours are much less likely to present as an emergency. Spread to other pelvic organs is common and can cause fistulas, urinary tract symptoms or bone pain.

## Examination of colorectal cancer

In a patient with suspected colorectal cancer, clinical examination should concentrate on the following:
- Presence of a mass (either per abdomen or per rectum)
- Evidence of intestinal obstruction
- Evidence of spread (hepatomegaly, ascites, jaundice, supraclavicular lymph nodes)
- General effects of malignancy (weight loss, anaemia)

# Investigating colorectal cancer

## Sigmoidoscopy
- Most rectal tumours should be detectable on rigid sigmoidoscopy and most CRCs are within reach of the flexible sigmoidoscope. Biopsies should be taken
- The rest of the large bowel must be investigated in order to exclude adenomas or synchronous tumours

## Colonoscopy
- Complete investigation of the large bowel
- Biopsies may be taken
- Gold standard of large-bowel investigation for primary surgical pathology
- May not be possible to do a complete colonoscopy to the caecum, in which

case barium enema or CT pneumocolon is needed to complete the investigation
- May not be possible to traverse strictures

### Double-contrast barium enema
- Useful for visualising the right side of the large bowel
- Lesion is shown as a filling defect or 'apple-core' stricture
- Biopsies are not possible and small lesions may be missed

### CT colonography (CTC)
- An alternative to colonoscopy or barium enema which gives good bowel definition unlike standard CT
- In addition gives information about local spread and the presence or otherwise of distant metastases
- Biopsies cannot be taken
- Expensive

### Ultrasonography
- Good for characterising metastases in the liver pre- and postoperatively
- Transanal ultrasonography can be used in staging rectal tumours, especially early ones being considered for local excision

### Spiral CT scan
- Elective colorectal cancer patients usually have a staging chest, abdominal and pelvic CT scan to exclude distal metastases and give information about local tumour spread

### MRI
- Used for preoperative staging of rectal cancer
- Especially useful for identifying local lymph nodes + mesorectum to identify patients with a potentially involved circumferential resection margin (CRM)

- Also used to characterise suspected liver metastases and assess liver resectability

## Complications of colorectal cancer

### Obstruction
- More common in left colonic tumours, which tend to be annular and constricting
- Luminal contents are more solid than on the right, predisposing to absolute constipation
- Tumour may obstruct by acting as the apex for volvulus or intussusception
- Patients present with colicky, central lower abdominal pain, distension and absolute constipation

### Perforation
- May occur through a carcinoma or proximal to it
- Caecum is the most common area of perforation, especially in the presence of a competent ileocaecal valve
- Perforation may result in generalised faecal peritonitis or localised abscess
- Mortality is high and long-term surgical cure is much less likely in a perforated carcinoma

### Fistula formation
- Direct invasion of a colorectal tumour into a neighbouring organ (eg bladder or vagina) can cause a fistula
- Vesicocolic fistulas present with pneumaturia and recurrent urinary tract infections (UTIs)
- Rectovaginal fistulas present with faecal vaginal discharge
- Fistulas of the transverse colon and the stomach or duodenum may present with faecal vomiting
- Fistulas caused by colorectal cancer can be difficult to distinguish from those caused by diverticular disease

### Other complications

- Haemorrhage
- Appendicitis (secondary to caecal carcinoma)
- Colocolic intussusception (carcinoma causes 50% of all adult intussusceptions)
- Invasion into adjacent organs

## Surgical management of colorectal cancer

### In a nutshell ...

**Principles of surgery**
- Preop preparation
- In the curable elective cases, aim for wide resection of tumour with regional lymphatics
- In obstructed emergency cases, aim for primary relief of the obstruction preferably with a primary resection, but if not then follow by elective surgery if necessary
- In incurable cases, aim to relieve present or potential obstruction and alleviate symptoms
- Postop care is vital

### Preoperative preparation

- **Optimise fitness:** the patient's general condition influences choice of procedure; liaise with medical/anaesthetic staff. Respiratory function and nutritional status are especially important
- **Define extent of tumour:** the presence of distant metastases influences choice of surgical procedure. Patients should have a staging CT scan and any pathology, radiology, endoscopy results and clinical

features should be discussed at an MDT meeting before surgery to decide on optimal treatment, including pre- or postoperative adjuvant therapy

- **Imaging:** of the rest of the colon by actual or virtual colonoscopy or barium enema (essential to exclude synchronous pathology); of the lung and liver by spiral CT or MRI; of local anatomy (especially in rectal tumours) by MRI or endorectal ultrasonography (to assess local involvement). Neoadjuvant therapy (eg short-course radiotherapy or long-course chemoradiation) is often indicated depending on the local staging
- **Bowel preparation:** bowel lumen bacteria are thought to be the chief source of sepsis in bowel surgery. In elective cases, 1 day of liquid-only diet and two sachets of sodium picosulfate before surgery are a common regimen. This is becoming less popular as evidence has shown that bowel prep is not necessary, certainly in right-sided colon resections. In emergency obstructed cases, on-table lavage can be performed
- **Prophylactic antibiotics:** metronidazole and cephalosporin at induction and for at least three doses postoperatively
- **Counselling and consent:** diagnosis, results of investigations, planned procedures, possible outcomes, complications and risks of mortality are made clear to patients and, if they agree, their relatives. The chance of a stoma should always be explained and, if it is thought to be likely, and time permits, a stoma nurse should be involved in the preop counselling. Laparoscopic surgery should be offered in all suitable cases. Whether performed open or laparoscopically, the principles of surgery for bowel cancer are the same (see overleaf).

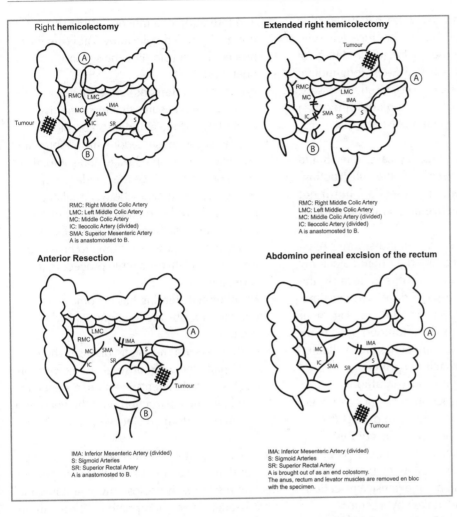

Figure 1.66 Large bowel resection for cancer. A is anastomosed to B in each case.

In the curable elective case, one should aim for wide resection of the tumour together with the regional lymphatics.

- **Non obstructed cancer of the right colon:** treated by right hemicolectomy and primary anastomosis (see Figure 1.66a) sparing the middle colic arteries
- **Non obstructed cancer of the transverse colon or splenic flexure:** treated by an extended right hemicolectomy taking the middle colic arteries (see Figure 1.66b)
- **Non obstructed cancer of the sigmoid colon, middle or upper rectum:** treated by an anterior resection taking the inferior mesenteric artery and its sigmoid and superior rectal branches
- **Operable low rectal and anorectal tumours:** treated by abdominoperineal excision and end colostomy taking the inferior mesenteric artery (see Figure 1.66d). Selected tumours maybe treated by transanal excision (see Section 8.6). The rectum, anus, sphincter and levator muscles are taken en bloc in an extralevator abdominoperineal excision of the rectum (ELAPE) which necessitates pelvic floor reconstruction with a mesh or myocutaneous flap.

The advent of stapling devices has meant that lower tumours are able to be resected with successful anastomoses. The discrediting of the 5-cm rule means that a 5-cm longitudinal clearance is no longer considered necessary, because tumours that have spread further than 1 cm usually have distant metastases.

**In the obstructed emergency case, one should aim for primary relief of the obstruction, preferably with a primary resection, but if not then followed by elective surgery if appropriate.**

Right-sided obstructing tumours are often suitable for an emergency right hemicolectomy and primary anastomosis – this is because the small bowel is not usually distended proximal to the ileocaecal valve. The management of obstructing left-sided tumours is more controversial. Several approaches are available:

- **Three-stage approach:** (1) primary decompression with a proximal-loop colostomy; (2) resection of tumour at a later date leaving the colostomy to protect the anastomosis; (3) closure of the colostomy. This has the advantage of a simple initial life-saving operation, allowing the patient to recover before the more extensive resection, which can be undertaken by a senior surgeon on an elective list. Unfortunately, cumulative mortality rate is about 20% and 50% of patients never have their colostomy closed
- **Hartmann's procedure:** primary resection with an end-colostomy. This approach achieves the dual objectives of relieving the obstruction and resecting the tumour while avoiding the potential complications of an anastomosis under suboptimal conditions. Reversal of Hartmann's procedure has a high complication rate and 10% mortality rate, so many patients end up with a permanent colostomy. Primary resection

and formation of a mucous fistula or double-barrelled colostomy (Paul Mikulicz's procedure) can simplify the second operation

- **Primary resection and anastomosis:** this approach ensures that the definitive operation is done at the first laparotomy but the anastomosis is done in suboptimal conditions. On-table lavage and subtotal colectomy can reduce the incidence of sepsis and discrepancy between dilated proximal bowel end and collapsed distal bowel end. A defunctioning loop ileostomy can give the anastomosis time to heal and involves a relatively simple procedure to reverse it
- **Endoluminal stenting** has become more common for obstructing tumours and is useful in:
  - Patients with metastatic disease who can be palliated without surgical intervention
  - Obstructed patients in whom a stent can relieve the obstruction until the operation can be performed electively

Obstructing rectal tumours are comparatively rare and may not be as curable, so primary decompression with a colostomy or endoluminal stent is often most appropriate until the tumour can be assessed and a management plan decided on.

**In the incurable case one should aim to relieve present or potential obstruction and alleviate symptoms.**

- Resection of the primary tumour offers the best palliation. It relieves obstruction, reduces the risk of future obstruction and reduces future metastatic spread
- A bypass procedure may be appropriate if the primary tumour is not resectable
- Defunctioning colostomy is less traumatic

and relieves obstruction in frail patients
- Radiotherapy and chemotherapy may give temporary alleviation. Radiotherapy is particularly useful in rectal tumours
- Stenting is becoming more widely practised in incurable obstructing lesions
- Local techniques for rectal cancer include electrocoagulation, contact irradiation, local excision or transanal resection of tumour (TART) with a cutting loop diathermy and laser treatment. TEMS is transanal endoscopic microsurgery

## Postoperative care after colonic or rectal resection is important.

- **Hydration and monitoring of electrolytes:** IV fluids needed until normal oral intake has resumed; hypokalaemia due to diarrhoea or high stoma output should be avoided to minimise ileus
- **Prophylactic antibiotics:** three postoperative doses of cefuroxime and metronidazole are often given
- **Analgesia:** patient-controlled analgesia, and epidural or regular opiates are important to minimise postoperative pain. Postoperative epidurals have been shown to reduce many major complications after abdominal surgery
- **Catheterisation:** to monitor urine output and avoid urinary retention in the postoperative period; beware the denervated bladder, which leads to more long-standing retention
- **Careful nursing and dressing of wound:** patients should be nursed in a low sitting position, except for after an abdomino-perineal resection, in which case they are nursed on the side. The wound should be carefully observed and kept clean and dry. Abdominal skin sutures usually can be removed at days 10–14
- **Physiotherapy:** chest physiotherapy to prevent atelectasis; early mobilisation to prevent urinary retention and deep vein thrombosis
- **Early enteral feeding** has shown significant benefit – the old 'nil by mouth for 10 days' adage is outdated
- **Deep vein thrombosis (DVT) prophylaxis:** subcutaneous heparin and anti-thrombo-embolic stockings
- **Care of colostomy:** initially an ileostomy drainable bag over the colostomy; stoma therapist must be involved to fit a permanent device; patients are taught how to care for stoma
- **Counselling and informing patients:** histology of specimen, what was done during the operation, plans for future surgery and prognosis should be explained to the patient and relative. Appropriate follow-up (and chemotherapy if appropriate) should be arranged

## Postoperative complications of colorectal cancer

### General complications
- Cardiorespiratory problems
- DVT
- Pulmonary embolism
- Postoperative renal failure

### Specific complications

#### Anastomotic leak
- Typically occurs 7–10 days postoperatively
- Along with cardiorespiratory problems, this is a major cause of postoperative mortality
- Risk is higher in low anastomoses
- The surgeon, male patient, preoperative radiotherapy and surgical technique are other major factors
- The results of anastomotic leak or dehiscence are pelvic abscess, peritonitis, fistulation or death

## Anastomotic stricture

- Caused by recurrence, fibrosis or ischaemia
- Tends to present later

## Wound infection and dehiscence

- As with any laparotomy the wound is less likely to heal if the patient is elderly with comorbidity and unwell at the time of surgery
- Risk of wound infection is higher in colorectal surgery and is minimised by preoperative optimisation of the patient, prophylactic antibiotics and meticulous technique
- Perineal wounds are especially prone to infection, abscess, pressure necrosis, and primary or secondary haemorrhage, especially after radiotherapy

## Intestinal obstruction

Due to:
- Herniation of small bowel through the lateral space
- Adherence of bowel to wound closure
- Adhesions between loops of bowel
- Oedema of colostomy
- Anastomotic stricture

## Urinary retention

Due to:
- Postoperative pain
- Prostatic obstruction
- Denervation of bladder

## Injury of urinary tract

- Ureteric injury leading to hydronephrosis, pyonephrosis, urinary fistula
- Bladder injury during anterior dissection

- Urethral injury during perineal dissection may lead to fistula or stricture

## Sexual dysfunction

- Erectile dysfunction due to injury of nervi erigentes more common after abdominoperineal excision than after anterior resection
- Failure of ejaculation due to damage to the presacral nerves
- Dyspareunia in females due to fibrosis around the vagina

## 'Phantom' rectum

- After abdominoperineal resection, this distressing sensation of an uncomfortable rectum occurs in up to 50% of patients

## Colostomy complications

Colostomies are discussed in Section 6.5:
- Bleeding
- Prolapse
- Retraction
- Stenosis
- Skin excoriation
- Parastomal hernia
- Fistulation

## Altered bowel function

- Bowel frequency and incontinence are more likely the lower the colorectal anastomosis
- 70% of patients with a coloanal anastomosis have normal continence
- Function tends to improve with time, up to 1 year after the operation

## Results of surgery for colorectal cancer

Of all colonic cancers, 70–80% are amenable to resection; 20–30% of patients have disseminated disease at presentation. The postoperative 5-year survival rate is 50–70% overall (but this varies depending on several factors). A worse prognosis is expected in the following:

- High Dukes'/TNM stage
- Emergency presentation (especially perforation)
- Young patients
- Short history of disease
- Development of complications
- Low rectal tumours
- Anaplastic tumours

**Local recurrence** is thought to be due to:

- Lateral spread beyond excision margin
- Spread into mesorectum
- Residual cancer in regional lymph nodes
- High Dukes'/TNM stage
- Low rectal tumours

Of local recurrence 80% occurs within 2 years postop, typically presenting as follows:

- Pelvic pain
- Leg pain
- Urinary symptoms
- Changes in bowel habit
- Seen at follow-up endoscopy

Distant metastases are most commonly seen in the liver (but also in the lungs).

## Management of liver metastases

- Some 15 000 patients die after colorectal cancer surgery every year
- In 20% of patients the liver is the first or only site of recurrence
- In recent years the trend has been to treat liver metastases more aggressively

- Studies have shown that patients with solitary resectable lesions survive longer if treated and 25% can be cured
- Multiple metastases in multiple segments of the liver are considered for resection so should be discussed with the liver surgeon if the patient is fit and willing
- Chemotherapy is also used in these patients

### Preoperative assessment of metastatic liver resection

- Ultrasonography
- CT
- MRI
- Hepatic angiography
- Laparoscopy
- Laparoscopic ultrasonography

Difficulties are presented by:

- Extensive adhesions
- Lesions close to the diaphragm
- Proximity to major vessels

It is important to exclude extrahepatic disease. Patients do better if:

- Primary was at an early stage
- They had a long disease-free interval
- There were fewer metastases
- Metastases were <8 cm (and low percentage of hepatic replacement)

The following are other prognostic factors:

- Extrahepatic disease
- Distribution of metastases
- Symptoms
- Sex (male)
- Age
- Resection margins and histological differentiation

## Results of resection

- 60–70% of patients develop recurrence after liver metastasis resection
- There are 25–30% long-term (5-year) survivors
- Surgery extends median survival by 14–20 months
- Postoperative mortality rates are <5%
- Adequate resection should improve long-term survival in at least 20% of patients

## Other treatment modalities for liver metastases

- Cryotherapy (can be used to blitz the margins of irresectable lesions intraoperatively)
- Radiofrequency ablation (one small study showed 46% 3-year survival rate)
- Laser interstitial therapy
- Microwave treatment

## Salvage surgery

In very advanced or even recurrent tumours an aggressive approach by an MDT of several specialties (eg colorectal surgeon, urologist, gynaecologist, orthopaedic surgeon) can result in up to 25% long-term salvage.

# Adjuvant therapy for colorectal cancer

## Radiotherapy

- Radiotherapy is used for rectal cancer rather than colonic cancer for two reasons:
  - There is a defined anatomical location
  - There is less risk of small-bowel injury
- Radiotherapy reduces local recurrence (by 40%) but does not affect distant metastases; it may lead to a 6% improvement in 5-year

survival in those patients going on to have curative resection
- Recent research has shown that **preoperative radiotherapy** should be used, unless the operating surgeon can demonstrate low baseline local recurrence rates (they show a smaller benefit). Debate continues about the timing, delivery and use of radiotherapy and chemoradiotherapy, but many centres would consider preoperative radiotherapy or chemoradiotherapy for a patient with a rectal cancer that appeared to be threatening the planned resection margin on preoperative investigations
- **Postoperative radiotherapy** should be reserved for patients who are judged after surgery to be at high risk of recurrence
- **Palliative radiotherapy** instead of surgery can be suitable for patients who are unfit for surgery and symptomatic (eg with pain, imminent obstruction, bleeding or mucus from a low rectal tumour)
- **Side effects** of radiotherapy include local effects (delayed wound healing, urinary and bowel dysfunction, nerve damage) and systemic effects (increased cardiovascular mortality)
- All decisions are taken through a structured MDT process

## Chemotherapy

Adjuvant chemotherapy is indicated in Dukes' C (TNM stage III) colorectal cancer but not in Dukes' A (TNM stage I). The benefit in Dukes' B (TNM stage II) cancer is not clear yet and often depends on the position of the tumour, grade of tumour, assessment of poor prognostic factors, surgery performed and fitness of the patient. Patients are discussed in an MDT on a case-by-case basis.

## Dukes' C (TNM stage III)

- Current UK guidelines suggest that fit patients with Dukes' C colorectal cancer should be offered either a:
  - 6-month course of 5-fluorouracil (5-FU) and folinic acid (FUFA), or a
  - 1-week course of 5-FU by continuous portal vein infusion
- This gives a 5-year survival benefit of around 6%

## Dukes' B (TNM stage II)

- The place of chemotherapy in the treatment of patients with Dukes' stage B cancer must be a matter for discussion between patients and oncologists
- Patients should be encouraged to become part of nationally coordinated randomised controlled trials (eg QUASAR and AXIS)

## Dukes' A (TNM stage I)

- Chemotherapy is not recommended
- Other methods of administering chemotherapeutic agents are being studied (eg intra-portal vein infusion at laparotomy [the AXIS trial] and hepatic artery infusion)

Other large, ongoing UK trials of chemotherapy for colorectal cancer include EPOC (chemotherapy ± cetuximab for bowel cancer with hepatic metastases) and FOxTROT (studying whether chemotherapy before surgery can reduce mortality and recurrence).

# Follow-up after surgery for colorectal cancer

## Short-term aims

- Check for postoperative complications
- Give emotional and practical support
- Assist with stoma management
- Ensure that patients who did not have preoperative colonoscopy or barium enema get one within 6 months of discharge
- Arrange appropriate adjuvant therapy
- GP follow-up has been found to be as effective as hospital follow-up

## Long-term aims

- Identify recurrence or metastatic disease
- Detect metachronous tumours
- Current follow-up practice varies widely, ranging from outpatient visits every 3 months to no follow-up at all
- In an effort to detect early cancer recurrence, surgeons may employ any of the investigations in the box opposite
- There is no clear evidence that any of these investigations allow earlier detection of recurrence than relying on patients presenting with symptoms; even if they did so, there is little evidence to show that subsequent treatment would result in improved survival (patients are currently being recruited for trials to examine the impact of various follow-up regimens)
- Re-colonoscopy within 3 years of removing a benign adenoma is the current recommendation, so many clinicians do at least this after resecting a colorectal cancer despite lack of evidence of the benefits
- It is essential to do a postoperative large-bowel investigation within 6 months of discharge if one was not performed preoperatively (more to complete the preoperative work-up, than as follow-up)

## Methods for identifying recurrence or metastatic disease

There are several methods for identifying recurrence or metastatic disease:

**Self-referral**

- Tell patients what to look out for and make sure that they understand how to come back if they develop symptoms
- 75% of recurrences produce symptoms between follow-up appointments even if they are scheduled 3-monthly

**Clinical review**

- Including questioning about bowel habit, pain, jaundice, etc, and examination of scar and abdomen for nodules, masses, ascites or hepatomegaly (this should be done but is not very sensitive)

**Endoscopy**

- Most common method, with regular colonoscopy recommended to detect recurrence or metachronous tumours
- Barium enema or CTC are alternatives. Evidence supporting an optimal postoperative interval between colonoscopies is weak

**CT**

- Imaging of the liver or pelvis by CT can detect local or distant metastases which may be suitable for surgical treatment

**Carcinoembryonic antigen (CEA)**

- This tumour marker can be used to predict recurrence
- Some centres recommend a 'second-look' laparotomy if CEA levels become raised after regular measurements

## Screening and surveillance for colorectal cancer

 **In a nutshell ...**

- **Screening** is testing an asymptomatic population to define a group for further investigation or treatment
- **Surveillance** is the regular re-examination of an at-risk population to diagnose disease at an earlier stage

Regular surveillance by colonoscopy is advocated in high-risk groups, such as patients with:

- Active long-standing UC
- Familial cancer syndromes, such as FAP and HNPCC, or strong family history
- Previous cancer of the colon
- Previous adenomatous polyps

Sporadic cancers account for about 90% of all cases of colorectal cancer, and it has been suggested that the general population should be screened over a certain age. The two methods now available for screening are **faecal occult blood test** (FOBT) and **flexible sigmoidoscopy**. It is generally thought that colonoscopy is too expensive with too low an acceptability to patients and high morbidity to be a good screening tool, so it is used as a second investigation, eg after a positive FOBT.

### Faecal occult blood testing

- Described in Section 8.3
- The National Bowel Screening Programme, which started in the UK in April 2006, screens members of the public between 59 and 69 years of age using FOBT. Those with

a positive FOBT (about 2%) are eligible for colonoscopy

- There are several types of FOBT, with various sensitivities and specificities
- Sensitivity is low generally; FOBT fails to detect 20–50% of cancers and 80% of polyps
- Specificity is also low; false-positive results are yielded by other conditions (eg haemorrhoids, peptic ulcer, anal fissures) and by ingestion of meat and some vegetables
- There is no associated morbidity but the test can be unacceptable to some patients
- Some studies have shown up to a 33% reduction in colorectal cancer-related mortality (although these have been FOBT with high false positives and, therefore, high negative colonoscopy rates)

### Flexible sigmoidoscopy

- Several studies are looking at the practicalities of using flexible sigmoidoscopy as a screening tool for colorectal cancer in the general population
- More expensive than FOBT, with lower patient acceptability, and low associated morbidity
- It only screens distal bowel, but 70% of colon cancers occur within the reach of a flexible sigmoidoscope
- Sensitivity is high (especially compared with FOBT)
- It can endoscopically remove polyps and biopsy tumours
- Other pathologies (eg IBD) can be diagnosed

The UK Flexible Sigmoidoscopy Trial concluded that flexible sigmoidoscopy offered once between the ages of 55 and 64 can reduce mortality by 43% and cumulative incidence by 50% (cancers of rectum and sigmoid colon) and 33% (bowel cancer overall).

## 8.7 Other colorectal conditions

### In a nutshell ...

- Vascular malformations:
  - Angiodysplasia
  - Haemangiomas
- Ischaemic disease of the large bowel
- Irradiation bowel disease
- Infective bowel disease

## Vascular malformations

Vascular malformations can cause colonic bleeding.

There are two main types of vascular malformations in the colon:
1. Angiodysplasia
2. Haemangiomas

### Angiodysplasia

- Colonic angiodysplasia consists of small, submucosal vascular swellings of unknown aetiology and unclear histology. They may occur sporadically, or in association with hereditary telangiectasia of the skin and mouth in Osler–Weber–Rendu disease. There is an association with aortic valve disease
- Bleeding per rectum can present as anaemia, positive FOBTs, recurrent small bleeds or a torrential acute bleed. The lesions are more common in the right colon *and* in elderly patients
- Diagnosis is by colonoscopy showing spider naevi-like lesions. In major haemorrhage selective mesenteric angiography shows a characteristic blush lesion

- Coagulation via colonoscopy may be curative for small lesions. Extensive troublesome areas of angiodysplasia may need resection

### Haemangiomas

These are usually cavernous or giant haemangiomas and involve the whole thickness of the bowel wall. They commonly occur in the rectum and present with bleeding per rectum. Colonoscopy or angiography can reveal the lesion. Electrocoagulation or sclerotherapy may control symptoms. Surgery may be required for more extensive lesions.

## Ischaemic disease of the large bowel

This is becoming more frequent with an ageing population. Causes are listed in the box below.

---

**Causes of ischaemic disease of the large bowel**

- Spontaneous arterial thrombosis (eg atheroma of IMA)
- Can be precipitated by embolus or low-flow states
- Small-vessel disease (eg polyarteritis, Buerger's disease, systemic lupus erythematosus [SLE], atheromatous disease, diabetes)
- Venous occlusion (eg extensive venous thrombosis – hypercoagulable state or idiopathic)
- Iatrogenic ischaemia (eg ligation of IMA at its origin during aneurysm repair or colonic surgery)
- Low-flow states (eg sepsis, heart failure, shock)
- Intestinal obstruction (eg obstructing carcinoma)
- Idiopathic infarction

---

### Subacute presentation

Patients can present with transient episodes of abdominal pain (clinically similar to diverticular disease or gastroenteritis) or with ischaemic strictures, usually near the splenic flexure. Treatment in mild cases is essentially supportive. Diagnosis is by barium enema or colonoscopy. Surgery is rarely needed unless the stricture causes an obstruction.

### Acute presentation

More typically a middle-aged or elderly patient presents with acute abdominal pain, rapid deterioration and shock. The clinical signs of generalised peritonitis (abdominal distension and systemic shock) usually indicate laparotomy at which the diagnosis will be made. Other investigations are notoriously non-specific:

- Abdominal radiograph may be normal at first and later show progressive dilatation
- Blood tests show leucocytosis, raised packed cell volume, metabolic acidosis, and raised amylase and transaminases
- Barium enema and angiography are of no value in these severe cases

Treatment in severe cases involves aggressive resuscitation and laparotomy with resection and exteriorisation of the bowel end. Primary anastomosis is contraindicated. There is a high mortality.

### Irradiation bowel disease

- Radiotherapy for uterine or bladder cancer can result in irradiation bowel disease, the effects of which are summarised in the box
- Rectal resection and coloanal anastomosis can be successful if the sphincter has not been damaged and recurrent tumour has been excluded

**Effects of irradiation bowel disease**
- Ulceration
- Fistula formation
  - Into vagina
  - Into bladder
- Stricture formation
- Radiation proctitis
- Bloody diarrhoea

# Infective bowel disease

Although strictly speaking a medical complaint, infective bowel disease can present as abdominal pain, change in bowel habit, diarrhoea and bleeding per rectum. It is, therefore, important to be aware of the differential diagnosis in order to avoid inappropriate surgery.

## Amoebic dysentery

Caused by the protozoon *Entamoeba histolytica*. The pathology is colonisation of the colonic wall, causing ulceration. The clinical presentation includes:
- Fluctuating, bleeding diarrhoea
- Chronic dysentery
- Amoebic appendicitis

Ulcers may be mistaken for carcinoma on colonoscopy. Fresh stool microscopy shows protozoa. Treatment is antibiotics and amoebicides.

## Bacillary dysentery (shigellosis)

This is caused by endotoxin-producing *Shigella* bacteria. The pathology is infection of the colon, leading to coagulopathy or haemolytic anaemia due to endotoxins. The clinical presentation includes the following:
- Abdominal pain and diarrhoea
- Systemic sepsis, coagulopathy and haemolytic anaemia

- Epidemic disease, usually with a contact history

Colonoscopy shows discrete ulcers, inflammation and formation of a membrane. Diagnosis is by stool culture. Treatment is supportive, with antibiotics reserved for severe cases.

## Schistosomiasis

This is caused by trematode worm *Schistosoma* which is carried by the freshwater snail. The trematode burrows into the skin, enters the blood supply and grows into egg-laying adults. Symptoms depend on the site of the eggs, which can be the bowel, lung, brain, spinal cord or urinary tract. Colonoscopy shows ulceration and barium enema shows an immobile, regular colon. Repeated stool microscopy may show the parasites. Rectal biopsy is often diagnostic. Treatment is with the drug praziquantel.

## Pseudomembranous colitis

This is caused by *Clostridium difficile* after the use of antibiotics, such as clindamycin, ampicillin or tetracycline. The pathology is overgrowth of the bowel with *Clostridium* infection which produces an inflammatory toxin. The clinical picture varies from diarrhoea to severe colitis. Colonoscopy shows epithelial necrosis and a white pseudomembrane. *Clostridium* toxin can be measured in stool. Rectal biopsy shows the characteristic histology of a pseudomembrane. Treatment is with vancomycin or metronidazole.

## Other colonic infections

*Campylobacter* enterocolitis and *Yersinia* enterocolitis predominantly involve the small bowel but may occasionally cause colitis. Intussusception is discussed in the Paediatric Surgery chapter of Book 1. Diverticulitis, large-bowel obstruction and caecal and sigmoid volvulus are discussed in Section 6.

# SECTION 9

# Perianal conditions

## 9.1 Anatomy and physiology of the rectum and anus

### Anatomy of the rectum

#### Gross anatomy of the rectum

The rectum commences at the level of the third piece of the sacrum where it is continuous with the sigmoid colon. It is about 13 cm long and ends where the longitudinal muscle coats are replaced by the sphincters of the anal canal (the anorectal junction) at the pelvic floor. There is a complete outer layer of longitudinal muscle over the rectum – the taenia coli coalesce. There are no appendices epiploicae.

#### The mesorectum

The rectum has no intraperitoneal mesentery. Peritoneum covers the upper third of the rectum at the front and sides, the middle third only at the front. The lower third is below the level of the peritoneum, which is reflected to form the rectovesical or rectouterine pouch. The mesorectum lies behind the rectum and so is largely retroperitoneal. It is removed intact during a low anterior resection of rectal cancer to reduce the chances of local recurrence (total mesorectal excision).

#### Relations of the rectum

Posterolateral relations at risk in rectal operations include the sympathetic trunk, pelvic and splanchnic nerves, the rectal vessels, and the anterior rami of the lower three sacral and coccygeal nerves.

#### Blood supply of the rectum

The blood supply is derived from the following:

- Superior rectal artery (the terminal branch of the inferior mesenteric artery)
- Median sacral artery (from the internal iliac artery)
- Middle rectal artery (from the internal iliac artery)
- Inferior rectal arteries (from the internal pudendal branch of the internal iliac artery)

All these vessels supply all layers of the rectum and anastomose freely. Veins correspond to the arteries and anastomose freely with each other; this is a portosystemic anastomosis.

## Lymph drainage of the rectum

Lymphatics run with the branches of the superior and middle rectal and the median sacral arteries. The three main groups of nodes are along:

- The median sacral artery in the hollow of the sacrum
- The middle rectal artery on the side wall of the pelvis
- The inferior mesenteric artery and upwards to the para-aortic nodes

## Nerve supply of the rectum

The sympathetic nerve supply is derived from branches from the hypogastric and coeliac plexus. The parasympathetic supply is from S2–S4 via the pelvic splanchnic nerves.

## Anatomy of the anus

### Gross anatomy of the anus

The anal canal is the last 4 cm of the alimentary tract. There are two layers of circular muscle making up the wall, an internal anal sphincter of smooth muscle, and an external anal sphincter of skeletal muscle. The intersphincteric groove is the area between the external and internal sphincters (Figure 1.67). It used to be called 'Hilton's white line'. The anorectal junction is at a 90° angle at the pelvic floor, where the puborectalis muscle forms a sling around the bowel and is continuous with the external sphincter. The mucous membrane in the anal canal forms horizontal folds called 'anal valves' above which submucosal anal glands secrete mucus. Infection in these glands produces anal abscesses and fistulas.

### The dentate line

The pectinate or dentate line is just above the level of the anal valves, some way above the intersphincteric groove (Figure 1.67). The colorectum is lined with columnar epithelium as far as the dentate line in the middle of the anal canal, where sensitive squamous epithelium takes over. The pecten is the area between the dentate line and the intersphincteric groove, where the epithelium is transitional. Above the dentate line the mucosa is derived from endoderm; below, it is derived from ectoderm. This is relevant for blood and nerve supplies and lymph drainage.

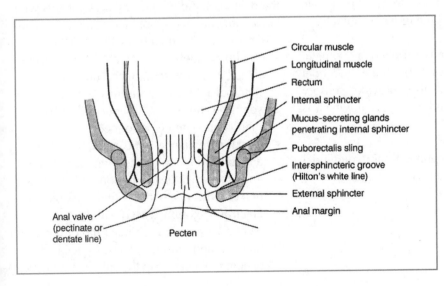

**Figure 1.67 Coronal section of the anal canal**

Circular muscle
Longitudinal muscle
Rectum
Internal sphincter
Mucus-secreting glands penetrating internal sphincter
Puborectalis sling
Intersphincteric groove (Hilton's white line)
External sphincter
Anal margin
Anal valve (pectinate or dentate line)
Pecten

## Blood supply of the anus

The blood supply is, as for the rectum, from the superior, middle and inferior rectal vessels and the median sacral artery. The veins correspond to the arteries and the site of the portosystemic anastomosis is in the upper third of the anal canal. The anatomy of the haemorrhoidal vascular cushions is discussed in Section 9.2.

## Venous drainage of the anus

The rectal venous plexus forms three cushions in the 3-, 7- and 11-o'clock positions which assist the sphincter in maintaining watertight closure of the canal. Haemorrhoids are varicosities at these sites.

## Lymph drainage of the anus

Lymph from above the dentate line drains to the internal iliac nodes and from below the dentate line to the palpable superficial inguinal group.

## Nerve supply of the anus

Sympathetic nerve fibres from the pelvic plexus cause contraction of the internal sphincter. Parasympathetic impulses from the pelvic splanchnic nerves relax the internal sphincter.

The external sphincter is supplied by somatic inferior rectal branches (S2) of the pudendal nerves. These nerves also provide sensory supply for the lower end of the canal, which is very sensitive.

For anatomy of the perineum and pudendal canal see Urological Surgery.

## Physiology of the rectum and the anus

### Defecation

The rectum is normally empty until left colonic motility is enhanced (eg by awakening or eating breakfast). Faeces enter the rectum and the person is called to stool. Anorectal sensation permits discrimination of solids from gas. Sitting or crouching straightens out the anorectal angle allowing faeces to be passed to the anal canal. The anal sphincter is under voluntary control with a normal pressure of 45–90 mmHg, which can be doubled voluntarily (squeeze pressure). If the passage of stool is not voluntarily stopped, faeces may be passed from as far as the splenic flexure. The diaphragm, abdominal wall and levator ani contract to aid defecation. The average daily volume passed is 150 ml. The rectum can accommodate 400 ml, while maintaining a low rectal pressure. Chronic tolerance of faeces in the rectum may be associated with severe constipation.

### Anorectal function tests

Assessment of anorectal physiology helps with the diagnosis and management of patients with faecal incontinence, sphincter injuries, rectal prolapse and abnormalities with defecation:

- **Anal manometry** uses an air-filled or water-filled balloon system to measure resting (internal sphincter) and squeeze (external sphincter) pressures; 24-hour ambulatory manometry can be performed
- **Rectal compliance** is measured by filling a rectal balloon and recording the volume and pressure at first sensation and noting the maximum capacity the patient will tolerate
- **Electromyography (EMG)** with fine electrodes assesses sphincter motor nerve function and muscle activity. Concentric needle EMG can map the sphincter muscle

in a traumatised anus. The rectoanal reflex test looks at the normal reduction in resting pressure when filling a rectal balloon, representing the reflex inhibition of sphincter contraction (absent in Hirschsprung's disease), rectal prolapse and incontinence. Anal sensation is measured by applying an electric current or thermal stimulus to the anal epithelium until the patient reports sensation. Loss of sensation may be present in incontinence or postoperatively

- **Proctography** with barium suspensions is used to measure the anorectal angle which may be obtuse in incontinent patients with pelvic floor weakness. Video-proctography records the expulsion of a thick barium suspension and can reveal prolapse, rectoceles and the function of ileoanal reservoirs
- **Colonic transit** is studied by ingestion of radio-opaque markers, which are viewed by serial abdominal radiographs
- **Endoanal ultrasonography** can identify defects in the sphincter

## 9.2 Haemorrhoids

### In a nutshell ...

Haemorrhoids are caused by enlargement and distal displacement of the normal arteriovenous anal cushions, which may prolapse through the anal canal. They are treated conservatively, by injection or banding in the outpatients clinic, or by a stapled or formal haemorrhoidectomy under general or regional anaesthesia. Other causes of rectal bleeding must be excluded, usually with a sigmoidoscopy, and underlying constipation corrected.

Even in a person with no haemorrhoids, three anal vascular cushions are found in the 3-, 7- and 11-o'clock positions consisting of redundant rectal mucosa, arterioles, venules and arterio-venular anastomoses. They are supported by elastic connective tissue and smooth muscle. They engorge during increased abdominal pressure, and theoretically assist the sphincter in maintaining watertight closure of the canal. They are mostly supplied by terminal superior rectal artery branches. They drain into the superior rectal veins which drain into the inferior mesenteric vein. Haemorrhoids occur when these vascular cushions enlarge and eventually prolapse through the anus.

'External haemorrhoids' is a non-specific term that should not be used. It is applied to several conditions:

- **Perianal haematoma** or **thrombosed perianal varices:** thrombosis of the external haemorrhoidal plexus beneath the skin of the distal anal canal below the dentate line
- **Sentinel pile:** a tag of skin at the outer edge of a fissure in ano
- **Perianal skin tags:** usually formed by resolved prolapsed internal haemorrhoids
- **Third- or fourth-degree (prolapsed) haemorrhoids**

## Classification of haemorrhoids

Different texts use different methods of classification but this is one common classification:

- **First-degree haemorrhoids:** confined to anal canal – may bleed but do not prolapse
- **Second-degree haemorrhoids:** prolapse on defecation, with spontaneous reduction
- **Third-degree haemorrhoids:** may prolapse spontaneously or with defecation and remain persistently prolapsed outside the anal margin unless digitally reduced
- **Fourth-degree haemorrhoids:** irreducible prolapse

---

**Factors predisposing to haemorrhoids**
- Idiopathic
- Pregnancy
- Cardiac failure
- Excessive use of purgatives
- Chronic constipation
- Portal hypertension

---

## Clinical features of haemorrhoids

### Symptoms of haemorrhoids
- Bleeding: painless; fresh blood; on paper or splash into pan; blood is seen around motion, not mixed in
- May cause anaemia, but this is rare and another cause should be sought
- Mucus discharge
- Pruritus
- Prolapse: on defecation; on exercise; needing digital replacement; permanently prolapsed
- Thrombosis
- Painful swelling

### Signs of haemorrhoids
- Skin tags may be present around anus
- Prolapsed haemorrhoids, or haemorrhoids prolapsing on straining: prolapsed haemorrhoids are usually at the 3-, 7- and 11-o'clock lithotomy positions. They often include tissue from above and below the dentate line, and are usually dark-red or purple, covered with pale areas of squamous metaplasia. It is important to differentiate haemorrhoids from a prolapsed rectum (see Section 9.8)
- On proctoscopy dark haemorrhoidal tissue is seen

- Haemorrhoids may flop into the lumen of the scope
- Abdomen should also be examined for pelvic mass or enlarged liver

## Differential diagnosis of haemorrhoids
- Fissure in ano
- Perianal haematoma due to trauma
- Perianal or ischiorectal abscess
- Tumour of the anal margin
- Prolapsing rectal polyp

## Management of haemorrhoids

### Exclusion of other pathology
Rectal bleeding or unexplained anaemia should not be attributed to haemorrhoids unless other, more serious causes are excluded. Depending on the symptoms and age of the patient, sigmoidoscopy, colonoscopy, gastroscopy or contrast studies may be appropriate. Predisposing causes, such as pelvic malignancy or an abdominal mass, should also be excluded by careful examination.

### Conservative treatment
Asymptomatic haemorrhoids should not be treated. First-degree haemorrhoids may respond to increasing fibre in the diet or to bulking agents. Patients may not want intervention once they are reassured that their symptoms are not due to anything more serious than haemorrhoids. Thrombosed strangulated haemorrhoids may be treated conservatively with analgesia, bedrest, elevated legs and an ice pack or by surgery.

# Injection sclerotherapy and rubber-band ligation

 **Procedure box: Injecting and banding haemorrhoids**

Banding or injection of a sclerosant via a proctoscope can be done as an outpatient in clinic on unprepared bowel.

## Indications

Symptomatic first- or second-degree haemorrhoids that have persisted despite medical intervention (asymptomatic haemorrhoids should not be treated).

Third- or fourth-degree haemorrhoids or above may be banded or injected in a patient reluctant or unfit to undergo surgery but the results will not be as effective. Banding is more effective than injections, but has more complications, such as pain or bleeding.

## Pre-procedure

The procedure and its risks and complications should be described to the patient. A per rectum examination and rigid sigmoidoscopy should be performed to exclude any other pathology that might cause anal canal-type bleeding. The patient lies in the left lateral position. This is not a sterile procedure, but gloves should be worn. The assistant drawing up the phenol should also wear gloves because it is highly irritant, and the injector should wear goggles.

- Do not inject phenol in almond oil if the patient is allergic to nuts.
- Do not band or inject if the patient is on warfarin, has a clotting disorder or is immunosuppressed.

## Procedure

A lubricated, illuminated proctoscope is inserted, the obturator is removed and the proctoscope slowly withdrawn to visualise the haemorrhoids.

The position and size of the haemorrhoids is noted as clock-face numbers, as if the patient were in lithotomy (ie anterior is 12-o'clock lithotomy, posterior is 6-o'clock lithotomy, right lateral is 9-o'clock lithotomy, left lateral is 3-o'clock lithotomy).

The proctoscope is then re-inserted with the obturator to above the dentate line.

- If injecting, a 3–4-ml aliquot of sclerosant (usually 5% phenol in almond oil) is injected submucosally (forming a thin-walled 'ballooning' of the mucosa immediately) above the dentate line in the position correlating with the most prominent haemorrhoids. A long-bevelled Gabriel or spinal needle is used for this because it is long enough to traverse the proctoscope. Do not inject anteriorly
- If banding, the mucosa is suctioned or grasped into the bander above the dentate line in the position correlating to the most prominent haemorrhoids and the band applied

No more than three haemorrhoids should be banded or injected at a single sitting. Between the applications, the proctoscope should be re-inserted, ensuring that another bit of mucosa is visualised and that the proctoscope is again positioned high above the dentate line.

If the patient feels sharp pain on insertion of the needle or grasping or suctioning the mucosa, the proctoscope should be repositioned before the sclerosant is injected or the bands applied.

**continued overleaf**

Other procedures aimed to produce mucosal adherence and prevent prolapse and bleeding include infrared photocoagulation, cryotherapy, bipolar diathermy, laser photocoagulation and direct-current electrotherapy.

### Intraprocedural hazards

- **Not applying the bands or injecting the sclerosant high enough:** often haemorrhoids prolapse below the dentate line into the perianal sensate area and so the procedure should be performed above the engorged, haemorrhoidal tissue into fairly normal-looking mucosa. If mucosa/skin below the dentate line is banded, the patient will feel immediate intense pain that will not be relieved unless the band is removed
- **Injecting sclerosant too deeply:** if the thin-walled mucosa does not immediately balloon out while injecting, pull back the needle. Deep injections anteriorly affect the adjacent prostate, urethra or vagina (see 'Complications' below)
- **Spilling sclerosant:** phenol is highly irritant and, if it is spilled or injected into the anal canal and runs out onto the perianal skin, it will cause pruritus and ulceration

### Postoperative management

- Review in outpatients in 6 weeks
- May need further treatments
- If heavy bleeds persist despite treatment or any worrying symptoms emerge, investigate the large bowel for other causes of bleeding
- If haemorrhoids do not regress and are still symptomatic, consider surgical options for treatment

### Complications of banding and injection of haemorrhoids

- **Recurrence of haemorrhoids:** avoid constipation. Repeat treatment may be necessary
- **Pain:** the procedure should be painless unless the band or sclerosant has been applied too low
- **Bleeding:** this is more likely with banding and can be torrential, requiring hospital admission. Advise the patient that some spotting is normal but to seek medical advice if it becomes heavy. Secondary haemorrhage may occur at 10 days after banding (when the bands slough off)
- **Deep injections of sclerosant:** can cause perirectal fibrosis, urethritis, vaginal or rectal oleogranulomas, pain, ulcers, haematospermia or impotence

## Lord's procedure – don't do it!

Manual dilatation of the anus under general anaesthesia involves the insertion of four fingers into the anal canal for 4 minutes. This procedure used to be used for haemorrhoids, fissures and proctitis fugax. It has fallen into disrepute due to the high incidence of subsequent incontinence of flatus or even faeces. It has no place in modern coloproctological practice.

## Surgery

Only about 5% of haemorrhoids need to be treated by haemorrhoidectomy. These are large, third-degree haemorrhoids that may straddle the dentate line or be too large to band. The most common method is the Milligan–Morgan haemorrhoidectomy, which involves dissection, transfixion and excision of the three main haemorrhoids, preserving the intervening skin and leaving the wounds open (see Op box). Thrombosed strangulated haemorrhoids that present as an emergency may be treated conservatively (see above) or by immediate haemorrhoidectomy. It should be noted that, although there is often pressure from the patient in pain to operate on thrombosed piles, they will almost always resolve with conservative treatment, and the risks of complications are increased in the acute haemorrhoidectomy. Acute perianal haematoma may be treated conservatively in the same way, or may be incised and evacuated under local or general anaesthesia. Modern methods of treating haemorrhoids are emerging, including the use of a circular stapling device. Results and complications of this method are being investigated.

---

## Op box: Formal haemorrhoidectomy

### Indications
Symptomatic haemorrhoids that have not responded to conservative or local management or are unsuitable for banding or injection of sclerosants. These are usually third- or fourth-degree haemorrhoids, haemorrhoids straddling the dentate line or long-standing haemorrhoids associated with anal skin tags.

A formal haemorrhoidectomy can also be performed for acutely thrombosed haemorrhoids as an alternative to conservative management, but complications are more likely.

### Preoperative preparation
The patient is fully consented and warned about the outcome, hazards and complications. The rectum is emptied by means of glycerine suppositories or a phosphate enema. The procedure is under general, regional or even local anaesthesia, and the patient is in the lithotomy position.

### Procedure
* Sigmoidoscopy is performed to exclude other causes of anal canal-type bleeding
* The perineum is prepped with antiseptic solution and the patient is draped
* The haemorrhoids are injected with 1% lidocaine plus adrenaline 1 in 200 000 to define tissue planes, reduce bleeding and assist analgesia during this short but painful op, making the general anaesthesia easier
* Place three Dunhill forceps on the junction between each of the haemorrhoids and the perianal skin (ie just distal to the haemorrhoidal cushion) including any tags. Traction on these will prolapse the haemorrhoids into view
* Place three Burkitt's forceps on the junction between each of the haemorrhoids and the normal anal mucosa (ie just proximal to the haemorrhoidal cushion)
* Starting with the lowest haemorrhoid to avoid blood in the surgical field, hold the other haemorrhoids out of the way and excise them one at a time
* To excise the haemorrhoid, place a forefinger into the anal canal under the prolapsed haemorrhoid and incise just the skin and mucosa with diathermy in an ellipse around the haemorrhoid (including any skin tag). Identify the white fibres of the anal sphincter before deepening the incision

**continued overleaf**

- The aim of dissection is to dissect the disc of prolapsed mucosa of the haemorrhoid off the sphincter, staying in a plane between the two. The pedicle will become evident and will need to be suture-ligated with a 2.0 Vicryl suture
- Before starting dissection on the remaining piles, ensure that an adequate skin bridge can be left between the incisions, thus avoiding anal stenosis. If it looks difficult, just excise the two most prominent haemorrhoids
- The final result should resemble a three-leafed clover, with triangular-shaped skin bridges between each excised pile
- The wounds can be left open or sutured with undyed Vicryl. They are dressed with Kaltostat that is tucked into the anal canal and folded out over the wounds

**Intraoperative hazards**
- Damage to the anal sphincter
- Incorporating the sphincter into the transfixion ligature (causing severe postop pain)

**Postop**
- Patient is sent home on metronidazole, lactulose and analgesia for 7 days
- Dressings are soaked off in the bath

**Complications**
- **Bleeding:** may be reactionary within 24 hours of the operation. Secondary bleeding, often due to infection, typically occurs on postop day 10. Bleeding may not be apparent externally if blood fills the rectum. The patient may need transfusion, examination under anaesthesia or packing of the anal canal
- **Acute retention of urine:** due to postop pain
- **Constipation:** avoided by postop analgesia and laxatives
- **Stricture:** occurs if the surgeon has failed to leave a bridge of epithelium between each excised haemorrhoid
- **Anal fissures:** due to poor healing

## 9.3 Anal fissures

 **In a nutshell ...**

Anal fissures (fissure in ano) are common, affecting males and females equally in people aged 30-50. The lesion is a longitudinal tear of the squamous-lined lower half of the anal canal from the anal verge towards the dentate line. Most fissures lie in the mid-line posteriorly, but anterior fissures are seen in women. Aetiology is unknown, both constipation and high sphincter pressures are more common in patients with an anal fissure, but these might be the result of the fissure rather than the cause. Fissures are the most common anal lesion in Crohn's disease and may often be multiple in these patients.

## Clinical features of anal fissures

- Pain on defecation (90% of patients) often lasting for 1–2 hours afterwards
- Minor bright-red bleeding on the paper after wiping
- Constipation, probably secondary to pain, in 20% of patients
- Pruritus occurs in 50% of patients
- Watery discharge in 20%

On inspection, the split in the anal canal can be seen when the skin is gently retracted. A sentinel pile occurs when the skin at the base of the fissure becomes oedematous and hypertrophied. Rectal examination may be impossible but it is useful to assess the degree of spasm.

## Management

- Glyceryl trinitrate (GTN) paste 0.2% has been shown to be a useful first-line treatment for anal fissures although recent evidence is contradictory
- Diltiazem cream 2% has been demonstrated to be effective and fewer patients report headaches compared with GTN
- Lateral sphincterotomy involves the division of the distal internal sphincter up to the dentate line lateral to the anal orifice, leaving the sphincter undisturbed; it can also lead to incontinence
- Long-term high-fibre diet should always be advised
- Botulinum A toxin can be injected into the sphincter to break the spasm–fissure cycle
- Rectal examination and proctoscopy to exclude an anal cancer is mandatory, and may necessitate a general anaesthetic if the fissure is still painful after initial treatment

## 9.4  Anorectal abscesses

the most common and most clinically important anorectal abscess is that caused by infection of the anal glands (Fig. 9.4a).

Other anorectal abscesses include the following:

- **Subcutaneous/perianal abscess:** results from infection of a hair follicle, sebaceous gland or perianal haematoma; the pus will grow skin flora and not enterococci
- **Submucous abscess:** results from an infected fissure or laceration of the anal canal or infection after injection of a haemorrhoid
- **Pelvirectal abscess:** caused by spread from a pelvic abscess; relatively rare

### Pathogenesis of anorectal abscesses

Apart from the abscesses described above, most anorectal abscesses are the result of infection of one of the 10–12 anal glands. As the gland body lies in the intersphincteric space, this is where the abscess usually starts. As the abscess expands, the pus may track longitudinally to present as a perianal, ischiorectal or supra-levator abscess (Fig. 9.4a).

Tracking can also occur circumferentially, leading to a horseshoe extension. This can be at the level of the intersphincteric space, the supralevator space or (most commonly) the ischiorectal space. A chronic intersphincteric abscess may occur if the cavity becomes walled-off by fibrosis.

### Clinical features of anorectal abscesses

- Pain: severe and worse on defecation
- Fever and inguinal lymphadenopathy
- Swelling and redness: may be absent

It may not be possible to do a rectal examination until the patient is under general anaesthesia. It is important to determine whether there have been any previous episodes, or if the patient has any associated conditions, such as inflammatory bowel disease (IBD), hidradenitis suppurativa or TB.

## Treatment of anorectal abscesses

An abscess should be incised and drained under general anaesthesia. Antibiotics are unlikely to abort the infection once the symptoms have been present for 24 hours. The procedure is performed as shown in the Op box.

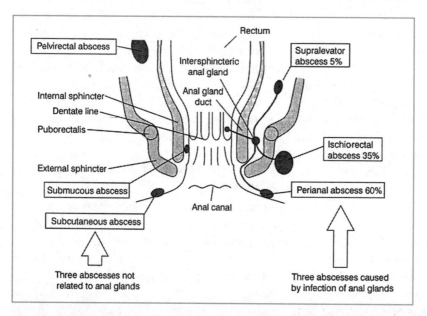

**Figure 1.68 Coronal section of the anal canal showing sites of anorectal abscesses**

## Op box: Incision and drainage of anorectal abscess

### Indications
A painful abscess pointing in the skin of the perianal area.

### Preoperative preparation
Note any history of previous abscess drainage, inflammatory bowel symptoms, diabetes or other immunocompromising conditions.

Consent for rigid sigmoidoscopy as well as incision and drainage, and describe the postop packing needed. For recurrent abscesses explain that postop follow-up and perhaps re-operation may be required to identify and deal with any fistula.

- Put the patient in lithotomy position under GA
- Hairy men should be shaved for comfortable change of dressings and avoidance of hair in the healing cavity
- Ensure diathermy is available

**continued opposite**

## Procedure
- Sigmoidoscopy is performed to exclude IBD and to check for pus in the lumen of the rectum
- Proctoscopy is performed to look for an internal opening
- Abscess is drained by an incision over the point of maximal tenderness (usually in the perineum)
- Pus is sent for culture and sensitivity
- Loculi are broken down with a finger
- Extent of the cavity is gently explored with a finger
- Cruciate incision is extended to the limits of the underlying cavity
- Corners of the cruciate incision are excised, deroofing the cavity by removing four triangles of skin; this prevents early closure of the wound
- Haemostasis is ensured using diathermy
- Cavity is then packed with a ribbon gauze, usually soaked in Betadine or Kaltostat

## Intraoperative hazards
- **Never use a probe:** it's inadvisable for a junior SHO to probe for, or lay open, a fistula at this stage because the anatomy may not be easily identified and a false passage may be created. This is best done at examination under anaesthesia 6 weeks after simple incision and drainage to relieve the abscess
- **Per rectal drainage:** if a large ischiorectal abscess has discharged into the rectum and pus can be seen on rigid sigmoidoscopy, senior advice should be sought. If the abscess is not pointing on the buttock, incising through the skin into the abscess would create a high rectocutaneous fistula. It may be more appropriate to drain the abscess through the rectum
- **Crohn's disease perineum:** these are complex areas of sepsis where radical deroofing is not appropriate. If the perineum looks grossly abnormal, there is a history of Crohn's disease or evidence of IBD at rigid sigmoidoscopy, senior advice should be sought

## Postop
- The first pack change is done on the ward at 12–24 hours, best done with analgesia after a soak in the bath. The patient can go home when he or she can tolerate the changes with oral analgesia
- The district nurse should change the packs regularly until healing has occurred. Kaltostat or some other non-adherent dressing is often more suitable for outpatient dressing
- Postoperative antibiotics are not usually required and should be given only to patients at high risk of infection, such as those with diabetes and immunocompromised patients, with significant cellulitis surrounding the cavity
- If a complex fistula is suspected, book a repeat examination under anaesthesia at 2 weeks
- Factors suggesting an associated fistula include:
  - A recurrent abscess
  - Growth of an enteric rather than a cutaneous organism in the pus culture
  - Pus draining from an internal opening seen on proctoscopy

## Complications
- Pain, bleeding, recurrence, delayed healing

## Chronic intersphincteric abscess

Chronic intersphincteric abscess is a separate pathological entity from anorectal abscess:

- Occurs when an intersphincteric abscess cavity becomes walled off by fibrosis and does not track to the exterior
- May remain dormant for long periods with acute exacerbations
- Clinical presentation is episodes of anal pain without evident discharge, redness or swelling
- Pain usually resolves spontaneously after a few days
- Internal opening lies posteriorly in the midline in 66% of cases

The abscess is identified on bi-digital palpation and is usually tender and about 1 cm in diameter. In cases where the internal opening is evident, a probe can be passed into the abscess, which can be laid open. Alternatively, the abscess can be dissected out.

## 9.5    Anorectal fistulas

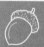

### In a nutshell ...

A fistula is an abnormal communication between two epithelialised surfaces.

- 80% of recurrent anorectal abscesses are associated with a fistula
- Most fistulas start as an abscess; others develop insidiously or are due to Crohn's disease, trauma, tuberculosis or carcinoma

## Pathology of anorectal fistulas

A fistula in ano has an internal opening (usually single) and an external opening (which may be multiple) connected by the primary track. The internal opening is usually at the level of the anal glands and, in 33% of cases, is tiny or stenosed. The track of most fistulas runs below the puborectalis and is more straightforward to treat. In complex fistulas, secondary tracks may run in the supralevator space or within the ischiorectal fossa. Fistulas with a main track running above the puborectalis are more difficult to treat.

## Clinical features of anorectal fistulas

- Intermittent acute abscess formation
- Discharge of pus from the external opening
- Rectal examination reveals induration around the tracks and abscesses
- The primary track is identified by the presence of the internal opening, usually felt as an area of induration at the level of the anal crypts
- In 66% of patients, the internal opening lies in the midline posteriorly
- In the remainder, the internal opening lies in the anterior quadrant

Lateral openings are very rare in fistulas not associated with Crohn's disease. Goodsall's rule (shown in Figure 1.69) usually applies. The presence of secondary tracks should be checked for by palpating the levator ani above the anorectal junction.

Features of a **complex fistula** include the following:

- Recurrent trouble after surgery
- Multiple external openings
- Induration felt above puborectalis
- Probe from external opening passes upwards instead of to anus

MRI is useful for delineating the anatomy of complex fistulas and has an increasing role to play in investigation.

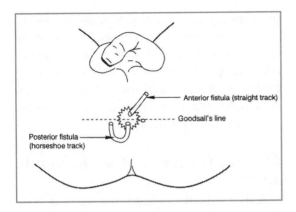

Figure 1.69 Goodsall's rule: an external opening lying anterior to Goodsall's line is usually associated with a straight tract, whereas an external opening lying posterior to it may not be.

## Treatment of anorectal fistulas

The principle of surgical management is to lay open the primary track and to drain any secondary tracks. It is important to maintain faecal continence by avoiding transection of the puborectalis muscle. The common **intersphincteric fistulas** lie well below puborectalis and can be laid open. The rarer **suprasphincteric** and high **trans-sphincteric fistulas** pass superior to the puborectalis and so should be treated by a Seton suture as immediate laying open has a high risk of incontinence (Figure 1.70).

Figure 1.70 Treatment of anorectal fistula.

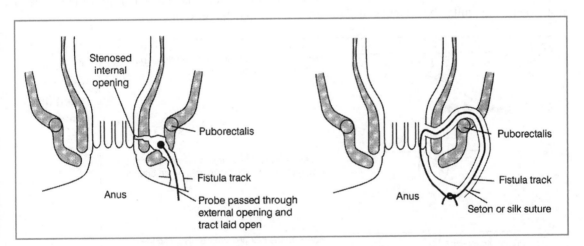

The Seton can be tied **tightly** with the aim of producing a slow division of the muscle over a period of weeks. Alternatively, a **loose** Seton drains any infection and allows healing to occur. It is then removed several weeks later, leaving a simple track which should heal. Treatment of complex fistulas with secondary tracks can be difficult, and MRI or intraoperative methylene blue can be helpful in defining the anatomy.

## Crohn's perianal fistulas

Seventy per cent of patients with Crohn's disease have perianal symptoms. Fistulas tend to be multiple, with more oedema, and may be less painful. Treatment is more conservative because surgical wounds tend to be slow to heal and the fistulas tend to be complex. Control of intestinal Crohn's disease medically is a priority.

## 9.6 Pilonidal sinus

A pilonidal sinus is a subcutaneous sinus that contains hair, and is most commonly found in the natal cleft associated with chronic inflammation and acute abscess formation. The condition is common and affects young adults. There are rare variants of the pilonidal sinus in other sites, eg the webs of barbers' fingers, the axilla, the lumbar region in children. The last are congenital and extend to the neural canal and dura.

### Pathology of a pilonidal sinus

Natal cleft pilonidal sinuses are thought to be an acquired condition, starting at the onset of puberty when the hair follicles become distended and inflamed (Figure 1.71). The sinus usually consists of a midline opening or openings in the natal cleft about 5 cm from the anus. The primary track (lined with squamous cell epithelium) leads to a subcutaneous cavity containing granulation tissue and usually a nest of hairs. Secondary openings can be seen, often 2.5 cm lateral to the midline pits.

### Clinical features of a pilonidal sinus

Patients are usually between the age of puberty and 40 years (75% male). Patients are often dark and hairy and may be obese; 50% present as emergencies with an acute pilonidal abscess. The rest have intermittent discomfort and discharge. Examination reveals the characteristic midline pit or pits that may have hair protruding. Lateral pits may be present.

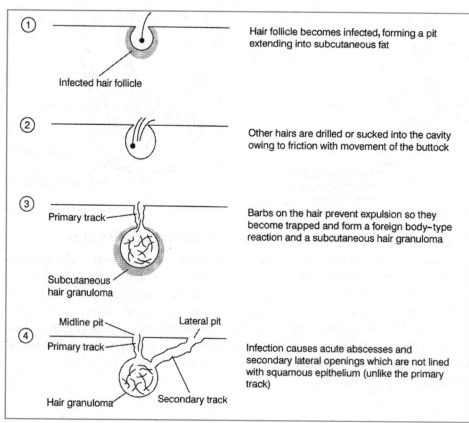

① Infected hair follicle — Hair follicle becomes infected, forming a pit extending into subcutaneous fat

② Other hairs are drilled or sucked into the cavity owing to friction with movement of the buttock

③ Primary track — Subcutaneous hair granuloma — Barbs on the hair prevent expulsion so they become trapped and form a foreign body–type reaction and a subcutaneous hair granuloma

④ Midline pit — Lateral pit — Primary track — Hair granuloma — Secondary track — Infection causes acute abscesses and secondary lateral openings which are not lined with squamous epithelium (unlike the primary track)

Figure 1.71 Formation of a pilonidal sinus

# Treatment of a pilonidal sinus

## Incision and drainage (acute)

An acute pilonidal abscess needs incision and drainage under general anaesthesia with follow-up. Later treatment of the pilonidal sinus may be required when the abscess cavity has healed if there are residual problems (33% of patients require further treatment).

## Excision of pits and laying open of sinus (elective)

This is usually done under general anaesthesia. The midline pits and lateral openings are excised with a small area of surrounding skin. The cavity is curetted and packed loosely with a gauze ribbon or Kaltostat. Frequent changes of dressing and close supervision are needed postoperatively. Regular rubbing with a finger avoids premature closure. Meticulous hygiene and shaving are important. Shaving may be stopped once the wound has healed.

## Excision with primary suture

Some surgeons recommend excision of the sinus with primary suturing of the defect. The advantages and disadvantages are shown in the box. The proportions of wounds healed at 2 months are similar for both forms of treatment. Attempts to reduce recurrence include primary closure with an off-centre scar, and rotation (Lindburgh) flaps.

## Recurrence of a pilonidal sinus

There is recurrence in up to 50% of excised pilonidal sinuses. Causes include the following:
- Neglect of wound care (eg shaving, packing)
- Persisting poorly drained tracks
- Recurrent infection of hair follicle
- Midline scars

---

**Advantages and disadvantages of laying open (vs primary closure) of pilonidal sinus**

**Advantages**
- Effective in most hands
- Shorter period in hospital
- Healing by secondary intention leaves broad, hairless scar that reduces recurrence

**Disadvantages**
- Slower healing
- Open wound delays return to work
- Active wound care with frequent wound dressing required

---

## 9.7 Pruritus ani

 **In a nutshell ...**

Irritation and itching around the anus (pruritus ani) is a common and frustrating symptom that can be difficult to treat. The symptoms can be caused by a variety of conditions which must be excluded, but most patients have no discernible cause.

## Clinical features of pruritus ani

- Men more commonly affected than women
- Symptoms worse at night and in hot weather
- Scratching affords short-term relief but worsens situation by causing excoriation

A full history, to exclude the general medical disease and skin disorders listed in the table, is essential. An anorectal examination may reveal anal tags, fissures, haemorrhoids or other potentially treatable causes. If the reddened skin has a clearly demarcated margin, fungal infection should be suspected (confirmed by microscopy of skin scrapings). Threadworms may be seen on examination of fresh stool.

## Management of pruritus ani

The principles of treatment are:

- Identify and treat secondary causes
- Give advice about personal hygiene
- Maintain patient's confidence
- Avoid frequent unproductive clinic visits

Symptomatic relief with local applications of soothing lotions, such as calamine lotion, or short courses of topical corticosteroids. In chronic cases, a dermatological opinion might be helpful. Deworming patients is a sensible precaution.

In intractable cases injecting methylene blue around the anus causes reversible sensory loss for 2–3 months and will break the itch–scratch cycle.

---

**Advice for patients with pruritus ani**

- Wash after defecation
- Use moist toilet tissue and dab rather than rub
- Wear cotton undergarments
- Wear cotton gloves at night to reduce the damage from subconscious scratching
- Avoid medicated or scented soaps
- Use only prescribed hypoallergenic ointments
- Avoid highly seasoned or spicy foods

---

Causes of pruritus ani

| | |
|---|---|
| Idiopathic (50%) | |
| General medical | Diabetes |
| | Myeloproliferative disorders |
| | Obstructive jaundice |
| | Lymphoma |
| Skin diseases | Eczema |
| | Psoriasis |
| | Lichen planus |
| Allergic eruptions | |
| Perianal disease | Fissure |
| | Carcinoma |
| | Crohn's disease |
| | Infection: fungal; yeast; worms |
| | Sexually transmitted infections (see Section 9.12) |
| Local irritants | Sweat |
| | Mucus (due to prolapse, polyp or cancer) |
| | Pus (eg in fistula) |
| | Faeces (eg diarrhoea, incontinence, poor anal hygiene) |
| | Chemicals (eg local anaesthetics or antibiotics) |
| | Psoriasis |
| | Lichen planus |
| | Allergic eruptions |

## 9.8 Rectal prolapse

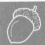

### In a nutshell ...

There are three main types of rectal prolapse (Figure 1.72):

- **Complete prolapse:** the full thickness of the rectum prolapses through the anus; the prolapse thus contains two layers of rectum with an intervening peritoneal sac that may contain small bowel
- **Incomplete prolapse:** the prolapse is limited to two layers of mucosa; this is often associated with haemorrhoids
- **Concealed prolapse:** there is an internal intussusception of the upper rectum into the lower rectum; this prolapse does not emerge through the anus

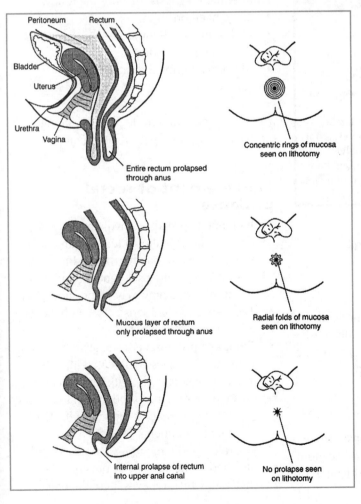

**Figure 1.72 Three types of rectal prolapse**

## Pathology of rectal prolapse

Incomplete prolapse can occur in children or adults. It is caused by excessive straining in children and is associated with haemorrhoids in adults (see table 'Causes of rectal prolapse'). Complete prolapse tends to occur in older adults (6F:1M) and is associated with weak pelvic and anal musculature or a floppy redundant sigmoid colon.

**Causes of rectal prolapse**

|  | Incomplete prolapse | Complete prolapse |
|---|---|---|
| Children | Excessive straining Constipation Cystic fibrosis | |
| Adults | Haemorrhoids After anal surgery Atony of anal sphincters | Idiopathic intussusception of rectum Lack of fixation of rectum to sacrum Weak pelvic and anal musculature Floppy redundant sigmoid colon |

## Clinical features of rectal prolapse

### In children

In children, prolapse is usually noticed by a parent after defecation. It is usually easily reduced and must be differentiated from colonic intussusception and prolapsing polyps.

### In adults

In adults, the presentation is of a prolapsing mass. Initially the prolapse is related to defecation; later it can occur on standing, coughing or sneezing. Initially it reduces spontaneously; later it may require digital replacement. Other symptoms include bleeding, mucus discharge and faecal incontinence.

On examination the prolapse may not be seen at rest but a patulous anus, large anal orifice or poor anal tone may be noted. The prolapse may be evident on straining. Complete rectal prolapse has concentric rings, whereas mucosal prolapse has radial folds (Figure 1.72). If >5 cm of bowel emerges, it will invariably be a complete prolapse.

**Differential diagnosis** includes the following:
- Large haemorrhoids
- Prolapsing rectal tumour
- Prolapsing anal polyp
- Abnormal perineal descent
- Anal warts

An acute, painful, irreducible or strangulated prolapse may present as an emergency.

## Management of rectal prolapse

- **Incomplete prolapse:** involving only the mucosal layer of the rectum, treatment is similar to that of haemorrhoids. Injection sclerotherapy, mucosal banding and formal haemorrhoidectomy may all be successful. The results are less satisfactory in patients with poor anal sphincters
- **Complete prolapse:** conservative treatment with bulk laxatives is indicated in patients too frail for surgery or with only occasional episodes of prolapse. Abdominal rectopexy (often laparoscopic) is the most effective treatment for patients fit enough for laparotomy. The rectum is mobilised and attached to the sacrum by prosthetic material, which relieves incontinence in

60% of patients but causes constipation in 60%. Other procedures are described in the box 'Operations for complete rectal prolapse'

- **Acute strangulated prolapse:** can usually be reduced with analgesia. Rarely, a patient presents with a gangrenous prolapse requiring urgent rectosigmoidectomy

## Managment in children
Dietary advice, toilet training and treatment of constipation will usually resolve the prolapse. An operation is rarely necessary.

---

**Operations for complete rectal prolapse**

**Perineal operations**
- **Perineal sutures:** this insertion of an encircling suture used to be popular in frail patients but has poor results
- **Delorme's procedure:** the rectal mucosa is excised and the underlying rectal muscle is plicated with sutures; long-term results are not very satisfactory
- **Perineal rectopexy/resection:** perineal rectosigmoidectomy (Altmeier's procedure) may be combined with a rectopexy and repair of pelvic floor and coloanal anastomosis

**Abdominal operations**
- **Abdominal rectopexy:** the treatment of choice in most patients well enough for laparotomy
- **Anterior resection rectopexy:** resection of the redundant sigmoid loop and upper rectum gives superior results but carries a significant morbidity risk
- **Laparoscopic rectopexy:** both rectopexy and anterior resection rectopexy can be done laparoscopically

---

## Solitary rectal ulcer
Solitary rectal ulcer is a chronic recurrent ulcer on the anterior wall of the rectum associated with bleeding, discharge of mucus and discomfort. There may be up to three ulcers, 7–10 cm above the anal verge, which are shallow with white, grey or yellow bases and surrounding hyperaemic mucosa. This rectal ulcer is believed to be caused by repeated mucosal trauma due to prolapse into the anal canal during straining and defecation and recent studies have suggested a link with nicorandil.

The anterior rectal mucosal prolapse can be shown by a defecating proctography (Figure 1.73). These patients usually use their fingers to aid defecation but this probably does not cause the ulcer. Principles of management include the following:

- Exclusion of other pathology (by biopsy if necessary)
- Treatment of constipation
- Conservative treatment if symptoms are tolerable
- Rectopexy may be effective if indicated
- Profuse haemorrhage may occur, necessitating urgent surgery

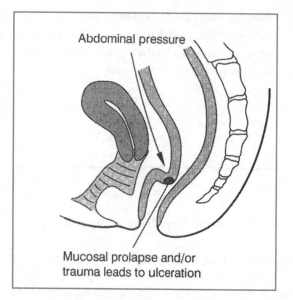

Abdominal pressure

Mucosal prolapse and/or
trauma leads to ulceration

**Figure 1.73 Possible aetiology of solitary rectal
ulcer**

## 9.9   Proctalgia fugax

This is a benign condition typically affecting
young men with anxiety:

- Attacks of pain in the rectum, perineum or
  urethra
- Not related to defecation; occurs at night
- Responds to smooth muscle relaxants, such
  as nitrates

**Management** involves:

- Exclusion of organic disease
- Explanation and reassurance
- Analgesics, antispasmodics
- GTN ointment

## 9.10   Faecal incontinence

Faecal incontinence is the involuntary loss
per anum of flatus or faeces. Patients find this
symptom distressing and embarrassing.

## Pathology of faecal incontinence

Maintenance of anal continence depends on:

- **Major factors:**
  - Anal sphincters with normal anatomy and
    function
  - An acute anorectal angle (maintained by
    the puborectalis)
  - A capacious and distensible rectum
  - Bulky and firm faeces
  - Intact rectal and anal sensation (mostly
    the pudendal nerve)
- **Minor factors:**
  - Vascular anal cushions above the dentate
    line
  - Cyclic retrograde propulsion (15/min)

The causes of faecal incontinence can thus
be classified as diarrhoea, neurological or
mechanical (as shown in the box).

---

**Causes of faecal incontinence**

**Diarrhoea**

- Inflammatory bowel disease
- Functional bowel disease
- Other causes (see section 8.1)

**Mechanical**

- Sphincter ring disruption:
  - Trauma
  - Congenital
- Fistula:
  - Extrarectal
  - Rectovaginal

**Neurological**

- General neurological diseases, eg MS
- Dementia
- Age
- Spinal trauma
- Pudendal nerve neuropathy
- Faecal impaction

---

# Clinical features of faecal incontinence

## History of faecal incontinence

Patients must be questioned directly and sensitively. The following are the factors to ask about:

- **Call to stool:** often altered in neuropathy
- **Urgency:** suggests voluntary muscle weakness
- **Consistency of stool:** excludes diarrhoea or impaction
- **Difficulty wiping:** indicates lax sphincter or prolapse
- **Leakage:** indicates low resting sphincter tone which suggests internal sphincter deficiency
- **Urinary incontinence:** usually coexists in obstetric damage to the pudendal nerve and pelvic floor
- **Obstetric history:** difficult deliveries often result in pudendal nerve damage
- **Anal surgery:** especially anal dilation or surgery for a fistula that may have damaged the anal sphincter

## Examination of faecal incontinence

The following are the factors to look for:

- Perianal soiling
- **Gaping of the anus:** suggests low resting sphincter tone and poor internal sphincter function
- **Descent of the anal verge below the ischial tuberosities:** suggests weakness of the pelvic floor
- Rectal prolapse
- **Scars:** indicating underlying muscle division

On digital rectal examination the following are the factors to look for:

- **Low anal tone:** on inserting a finger suggests poor internal sphincter tone

- **Anorectal angle:** formed by the puborectalis sling which is felt as a muscular sling
- **Squeeze test:** poor squeeze means damaged voluntary muscle either directly or due to pudendal neuropathy
- **Faecal masses:** impacted in the rectum may interfere with the anorectal mechanism
- **Tumours**

Endoscopy may reveal proctitis, which reduces rectal capacity and increases sensitivity, and causes diarrhoea.

# Investigating faecal incontinence

(See also Section 9.1.)

- Anal manometry
- Rectal compliance
- EMG
- Defecating video proctography
- Anal ultrasonography: gives an image of the anal sphincter and shows sphincter defects, such as scarring by obstetric or surgical trauma
- Barium enema or flexible sigmoidoscopy/colonoscopy: important to exclude tumours or proctitis

# Treatment of faecal incontinence

- **Conservative:** exclude causes of diarrhoea and bowel disorders, such as colitis, polyps or tumours. Solidify stools with drugs, such as codeine phosphate if stools are loose. Identify cause of incontinence
- **Physiotherapy:** if there is good muscle bulk and the voluntary contraction is shown to be weak, pelvic floor strengthening exercises can be useful (biofeedback)
- **Rectopexy:** if a rectal prolapse is identified, it should be repaired before any work is undertaken on the anal sphincter

- **Overlapping sphincter repair:** if direct obstetric or surgical trauma has caused identifiable scarring, sphincter repair can be curative in 85% of patients (Figure 1.74)
- **Post-anal repair:** if neuropathic damage has occurred, the pelvic floor is lax and the sphincter mechanism has descended, this will cause loss of the anorectal angle (which contributes to incontinence). Post-anal repair seeks to recreate this angle by opposing muscles behind the rectum, thus taking it upwards and forwards (Figure 1.74). It is successful in 50% of patients but

even good results deteriorate with time so this procedure is falling out of favour
- **Colostomy:** for a few patients, if other treatment has failed, a colostomy may be more acceptable than continued incontinence
- **Gracilis muscle transplantation:** work has been done on creating a new anal sphincter from the gracilis muscle of the thigh and an implanted nerve stimulator. This is mainly carried out in specialist centres
- **Artificial sphincter implant**

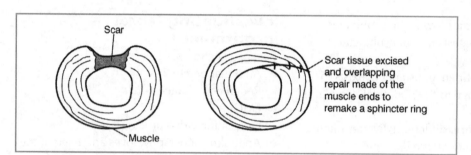

Figure 1.74 Overlapping sphincter repair

Scar

Scar tissue excised and overlapping repair made of the muscle ends to remake a sphincter ring

Muscle

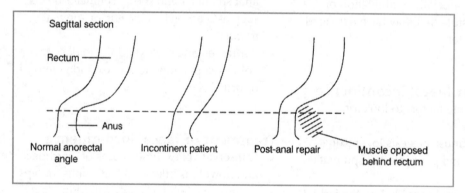

Figure 1.75 Post-anal repair

Sagittal section

Rectum

Anus

Normal anorectal angle

Incontinent patient

Post-anal repair

Muscle opposed behind rectum

# 9.11 Anal cancer

## In a nutshell ...

This accounts for only 10% of anorectal malignancies; 80% of anal cancers are squamous cell carcinomas, but malignant melanomas, lymphomas, Kaposi's sarcoma and anal gland adenocarcincomas can also occur. The two main types are **anal canal carcinomas** and **anal margin carcinomas**.

## Aetiology of anal cancer

Certain groups of people are predisposed to anal cancer:

- Male homosexuals
- People who practise anal sex
- People with a history of genital warts

It is postulated that human papillomavirus (HPV) predisposes to anal cancer as it does to cervical cancer. It is also now known to predispose to oropharyngeal cancers.

## Clinical features of anal cancer

- Patients are usually in their 50s or 60s
- Common presentations are bleeding, pain, swelling and ulceration around the anus
- Late cases can present with disturbed bowel habit, incontinence and rectovaginal fistulas
- Many patients have enlarged inguinal lymph nodes but only 50% of palpable glands contain tumour

Differential diagnosis includes:

- anal papilloma
- anal warts
- anal fissures
- haemorrhoids

Examination under anaesthesia is usually necessary in order to:

- determine if the tumour is arising from anal margin or anal canal
- determine if the tumour is ≥5 cm in diameter
- look for local spread to surrounding structures
- take biopsy specimens

### Anal margin cancers vs anal canal cancers

**Anal margin cancers**
- Arise below the dentate line
- Visible at the anus
- Tend to behave like basal cell skin carcinomas
- Spread to inguinal lymph nodes
- More common in men
- More likely to be treatable with local excision

**Anal canal cancers**
- Arise above the dentate line
- Not visible at the anus
- More locally invasive with a poorer prognosis
- Spread to internal iliac lymph nodes as well as superior haemorrhoidal lymph nodes
- More common in women
- More likely to be treated with radiotherapy

## Treatment of anal cancer

The principles of treatment for anal cancer have been changing as trials are carried out. The overall 5-year survival rate is about 50%. Generally, there are four main treatment strategies.

### Local resection

This is indicated in small tumours (<2 cm diameter) of the anal margin with no invasion of the anal sphincter. Less than 5% of anal cancers fulfil this criterion.

### Chemoradiotherapy

Radiotherapy has largely replaced radical surgery for first-line treatment in most anal cancers. The initial radiotherapy field includes the tumour and inguinal lymph nodes and the course lasts about 4–5 weeks. Women undergo artificial menopause and men become azoospermic. There is a temporary desquamation of the perineum. A radioisotope boost is given to the primary tumour under general anaesthesia. Fifty per cent of tumours are cured by radiotherapy, but some may need further surgery. Most treatment regimens combine chemotherapy with radiotherapy.

### Radical abdominoperineal resection

This surgery, which leaves the patient with a permanent colostomy, used to be the standard treatment for most anal cancers. This procedure is now usually reserved for cases in which radiotherapy fails or is contraindicated. Patients with obstructive cancers may benefit from a colostomy while they undergo radiotherapy.

### Chemotherapy

5-Fluorouracil (5-FU) and mitomycin have been used in combination with radiotherapy or surgery. Evidence supporting their use is controversial and side effects include thrombocytopenia and agranulocytosis. Chemotherapy is particularly useful in aggressively metastasising tumours, which may spread to the bones, abdominal lymph nodes or the brain.

## 9.12 Sexually transmitted anorectal infections

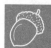 **In a nutshell ...**

These can affect women and heterosexual men, but are most commonly seen in homosexual men. Patients are best managed by a genitourinary physician but may present to a colorectal surgeon with anorectal symptoms. It is important to be able to differentiate these conditions from surgical disorders. In general, investigation of proctocolitis should include the features listed in the box below.

**Investigating proctocolitis**

**Test**
* Stool microscopy
* Rectal swabs
* Sigmoidoscopy and rectal biopsy

**Looking for:**
* Protozoa and bacteria, *Cryptosporidium* spp. and atypical mycobacteria
* Viruses (eg herpes simplex)
* Cytomegalovirus (CMV) and Kaposi's sarcoma

## Gonorrhoea

This is caused by *Neisseria gonorrhoeae*, a Gram-negative diplococcus. The organism is spread by anal intercourse and by contamination from the vagina to the anus in women. There is a 5- to 7-day incubation period.

It is asymptomatic in the majority. Symptoms can include the following:
* Pruritus ani
* Mucopurulent discharge
* Tenesmus
* Bleeding
* Joint pains
* Proctitis

Diagnosis is by anal swabs for microscopy and culture. Treatment is with amoxicillin for patient and partners. Eradication of infection should be confirmed after 2 weeks.

## Chlamydiasis

This is caused by *Chlamydia trachomatis*, an intracellular organism. The organism is spread by anal intercourse.

It is commonly asymptomatic. Symptoms can include the following:
* Mucopurulent discharge
* Bleeding
* Pain
* Tenesmus
* Fever
* Inguinal lymphadenopathy
* Proctitis

Diagnosis is by anal swab in special chlamydia culture medium. Treatment is with tetracycline or erythromycin for patient and partners. Rectal stricture is a rare complication.

## Syphilis

This is caused by *Treponema pallidum*, a spirochaete. The organism is spread by anal intercourse.

Symptoms include the following:
* **Primary syphilis** (2–6 weeks after infection): anal chancre (looks like a fissure); inguinal lymphadenopathy
* **Secondary syphilis** (6–8 weeks after primary chancre): condylomata lata (warty mass around anus); discharge; pruritus
* **Tertiary syphilis** (rare): rectal gumma (can be mistaken for tumour); tabes dorsalis; severe perianal pain; paralysis of sphincters

Diagnosis is by the VDRL (Venereal Disease Research Laboratory) assay, which is positive in 75% of patients with primary syphilis. Other serological tests are the fluorescent *Treponema* antibody test (FTA) and the *Treponema pallidum* haemagglutination assay (TPHA). Treatment is with intramuscular penicillin. Follow-up serological tests are repeated periodically for a year after treatment to confirm eradication.

## Herpes

Herpes is caused by herpes simplex virus (HSV); 90% of anal infections are due to HSV type 2 and 10% to HSV type 1. The organism is spread by anal intercourse. If the infection is ulcerative and lasts more than a month in an HIV-positive patient it is diagnostic for AIDS. There is a 1- to 3-week incubation period.

Symptoms include the following:
* Burning pain
* Mucoid or bloody discharge
* Malaise and fever
* Vesicles, pustules and ulcers around the anus

- Lesions too painful to be examined without general anaesthesia
- Proctitis and erythema on sigmoidoscopy

Diagnosis is by viral culture of vesicular fluid. Treat with aciclovir (oral or IV), which is continued until all mucocutaneous surfaces have healed. Partners should also be treated.

## Anal warts

Anal warts are caused by the human papillomavirus (HPV), usually types 6, 11 and 16. They are spread by anal intercourse, direct spread from genitals or may be sporadic with no history of anal intercourse.

It may be asymptomatic – patient notices warts and presents. Symptoms include the following:
- Itching and discomfort
- Discharge
- Bleeding

On examination, white, pink or grey lesions occur around the anus, perineum and inside the anal canal. There may be associated lesions on the penis or vulva. There may be a few scattered papillomas or bulky confluent lesions.

Proctoscopy should be performed and patients should be screened for other sexually transmitted infections (STIs). Diagnosis is clinical and treatments include the following:
- Chemical topical agents, eg podophyllin
- Surgical excision or diathermy

Partners should be treated. Papilloma infection is thought to predispose to anal cancer, but this is rare.

## HIV-associated anorectal problems

Patients with HIV infection are susceptible to anorectal problems such as:
- Haemorrhoids
- Fissures
- Perianal abscess
- Fistulas
- Kaposi's sarcoma
- Proctocolitis due to herpes, CMV, *Cryptosporidium*, isosporiasis, *Mycobacterium avium*, *Shigella* spp., *Campylobacter* spp., *Entamoeba histolytica*

# CHAPTER 2

# Breast Surgery

## Jenny McIlhenny and Ritchie Chalmers

# SECTION 1

# The breast

**CHAPTER 2**

## 1.1 Anatomy of the breast and axilla

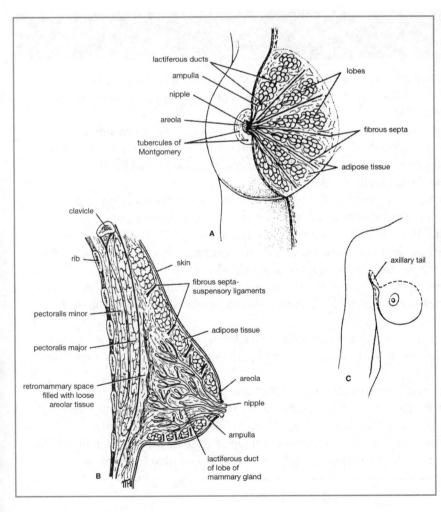

Figure 2.1 Anatomy of the breast. (A) Anterior view with skin partially removed to show internal structure. (B) Sagittal section. (C) The axillary tail, which pierces the deep fascia and extends into the axilla.

## Embryology of the breast

- The breast is a modified apocrine sweat gland
- Ectoderm gives rise to the epithelial lining of the ducts and acini
- Mesenchyme gives rise to the supporting tissue called the stroma
- There is downward growth of ectoderm into underlying mesenchyme at 4 weeks' gestation
- The breast develops from the mammary ridge (first seen at 5 weeks' gestation)

and this ridge develops from ectoderm at 5 weeks' gestation, extending from the axilla to the groin (milk line). In humans it regresses to leave a nipple with specialised epithelial cords which forms 15–20 lactiferous ducts

- At puberty the lactiferous ducts proliferate and the breast bud is formed (around age 10)
- Nipple development occurs at around 12 years

## Anatomy of the breast

### In a nutshell ...

- **Extent:** the breast extends from the second to the sixth rib, and from the midline to the midaxillary line. The axillary tail of Spence is a projection of the upper outer quadrant of the breast into the axilla.
- **Position:** the breast lies anterior to the muscles of the chest wall: medial two-thirds on pectoralis major and lateral third on serratus anterior; the inferior aspect of the breast base also rests on the upper aspects of the external oblique abdominis and rectus sheath. It is separated from these muscles by the deep fascia.
- **Structure:** the breast is composed of 15–20 lobules which open, via ducts, on to the nipple. Lobules drain into lactiferous ducts, which drain into lactiferous sinuses, the function of which is to store milk during lactation. The ducts of each lobule are lined with columnar or cuboidal epithelium, and the short excretory ducts (just beneath the nipple/areolar complex) are lined with squamous epithelium.
- **Suspensory ligaments:** anterior projections of the deep fascia form the suspensory ligaments of Astley Cooper which divide the breast into lobules and connect the deep fascia to the skin
- **Arterial supply:** lateral thoracic and thoracoacromial branches of the axillary artery, the internal thoracic (mammary) artery and the lateral perforating branches of the intercostal arteries
- **Venous drainage:** via the internal thoracic, axillary and posterior intercostal veins
- **Nerve supply:** intercostal nerves. Nipple sensation is from the fourth intercostal nerve
- **Lymphatic drainage:** >75% to axillary nodes, <25% to internal mammary nodes
- **The nipple** is anatomically in line with the fourth rib interspace (at the inframammary fold) but its position varies with increasing age as a result of glandular descent or ptosis.

## Arterial supply of the breast

There is considerable crossover of arterial supply and venous and lymphatic drainage across the breast.

### Lateral breast

Subclavian artery      → Axillary artery      → **Lateral thoracic artery**
     → **Thoracoacromial artery**

(Also the **superior thoracic** and **subscapular** branches of the axillary artery to a lesser extent.)
Lateral perforating branches of the **intercostal arteries**

### Medial breast

Subclavian artery      → **Internal thoracic (mammary) artery**      → Perforating branches (first to fourth intercostal spaces)

## Venous drainage of the breast

Lateral breast      → **Thoracoacromial vein**
     → **Lateral thoracic vein** → Axillary vein → Subclavian vein

Medial breast      → **Internal thoracic vein** → Subclavian vein

**Posterior intercostal vein**: the posterior intercostal veins also receive tributaries from the ribs and communicate with the vertebral venous plexus via a valveless system; hence metastatic cells from breast cancer can spread to the ribs and thoracic vertebrae with relative ease.

## Nerve supply of the breast

- Sensory supply via cutaneous branches of intercostal nerves of T4–6
- Also a sympathetic supply

## Lymphatic drainage of the breast

- Studies using radiolabelled tracers demonstrate that 75–97% of the lymphatic drainage of the breast drains to the axillary nodes
- Up to 25% drains to the internal mammary nodes through the second to fourth intercostal spaces
- There is free communication of lymphatic channels across the breast (lateral to medial and vice versa)
- There is an anastomosis of the lymphatics across the midline to the contralateral breast, and down the abdominal wall; therefore lymphatic spread of breast cancer can be to the opposite axilla, to the peritoneal cavity and liver and, rarely, to the inguinal nodes
- The sentinel lymph node or nodes are believed to be the first node(s) in the axilla to receive drainage from the breast (see Sentinel node biopsy)

## Anatomy of the axilla

The axilla is the space between the upper arm and the thorax. The surface markings are the anterior and posterior axillary folds, formed by pectoralis major and latissimus dorsi respectively. It is pyramidal in shape, with the base of the pyramid (the floor of the axilla) the most superficial, and the apex deep, towards the root of the neck (Figure 2.2). The axillary vessels and nerves pass through a space at the apex formed by the posterior clavicle, superior border of the scapula and lateral border of the first rib.

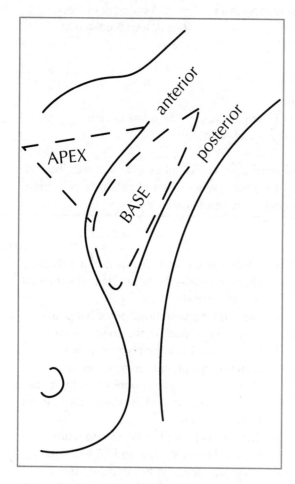

**Figure 2.2 The shape of the axilla**

 **In a nutshell ...**

### Contents of the axilla
- Brachial plexus
- Axillary artery
- Axillary vein
- Axillary fat pad, which contains 20–30 axillary lymph nodes
- Intercostal brachial nerves (sensory nerves to skin of axilla)
- Long thoracic nerve of Bell (motor nerve to serratus anterior)
- Thoracodorsal trunk (the artery, vein and motor nerve supplying latissimus dorsi)

### Boundaries of the axilla
- **Anteriorly:** pectoralis major and minor; subclavius at apex
- **Medial:** serratus anterior on the chest wall (and first four ribs)
- **Lateral:** coracobrachialis; short biceps tendon. These lie medial to the bicipital groove of the humerus (sometimes called the intertubercular groove, as it lies between the greater and lesser tubercles), where the anterior and posterior walls of the axilla converge
- **Posterior:** subscapularis superiorly; teres major; latissimus dorsi
- **Superior:** axillary vein
- **Apex:** clavicle; first rib; superior border of scapula
- **Floor (or base):** axillary fascia covers the axillary floor between serratus anterior, pectoralis major and latissimus dorsi, converging at a point to meet the deep fascia of the arm

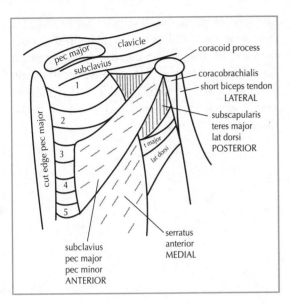

**Figure 2.3 The anatomical relations of the axilla**

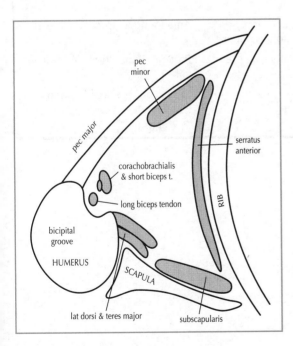

**Figure 2.4 The boundaries of the axilla**

## Blood vessels of the axilla

The **axillary artery** is a continuation of the subclavian artery. It begins at the lateral border of the first rib and becomes the brachial artery at the inferior border of teres major. It is invested in fascia – the axillary sheath – and divided into three parts by pectoralis minor: the first part is medial to pectoralis minor; the second part lies under pectoralis minor (and passes among the cords of the brachial plexus); and the third part is lateral to pectoralis minor.

### Branches of the axillary artery

First part: one branch:
→ superior thoracic artery (supplies both pectorals)

Second part: two branches:
→ thoracoacromial artery (supplies the clavicle, deltoid, pectorals, acromion and breast)
→ lateral thoracic artery (supplies both pectoral muscles and breast)

Third part: three branches:
→ subscapular artery (gives off thoracodorsal artery to supply latissimus dorsi)
→ anterior circumflex humeral artery (biceps and shoulder joint)
→ posterior circumflex humeral artery (deltoid, triceps and shoulder joint)

### The axillary vein

The **axillary vein** lies medial to the axillary artery and nerves and outside the axillary sheath. It is formed by the basilic vein and venae comitantes and starts at the lower border of the posterior axilla. It becomes the subclavian vein at the lateral border of the first rib.

*Tributaries to the axillary vein*

- First part: cephalic vein
- Second and third parts: tributaries correspond to the second and third part axillary artery branches

## Lymph nodes of the axilla

When describing a traditional axillary clearance, lymph nodes are classified according to their anatomical level:

- Level 1: lateral to pectoralis minor
- Level 2: posterior to pectoralis minor
- Level 3: medial to pectoralis minor

The supraclavicular nodes drain into the thoracic duct on the left, and into the right lymphatic duct on the right. These drain into the subclavian vein on each side. There is also an interpectoral node lying between pectoralis major and pectoralis minor which can be involved in heavy nodal disease.

*Classification of axillary lymph nodes*

| Lymph node group | Site | Drains |
|---|---|---|
| Lateral (brachial or humeral) | Lateral axilla, inferomedial to axillary vein | Upper limb |
| Anterior (pectoral) | Lie with the lateral thoracic artery on the lower border of pectoralis minor | Anterior upper trunk and breast |
| Posterior (subscapular) | Posterior wall of axilla along course of subscapular artery | Posterior upper trunk and axillary tail |
| Central | In the fat of the axilla | Lateral, anterior and posterior lymph nodes |
| Apical (subclavicular) | Apex of the axilla | All of the above |

# 1.2 Physiology of the breast

## In a nutshell ...

The main physiological changes to the breast occur at puberty, during pregnancy and breastfeeding, and at the menopause. Physiological effects are also seen in the male and female neonate, and during the menstrual cycle. Physiological changes are hormonally driven by oestrogen and progesterone.

**Neonate:** neonatal breast enlargement (in the male or female neonate) is caused by maternal oestrogens. It recedes within several days of birth. Can occasionally become infected (mastitis neonatorum).

**Puberty:** oestrogens stimulate the development and growth of the glandular tissue of the breast and the deposition of fat.

**Menstrual cycle:** during the follicular phase, oestrogen is secreted from the graafian follicle, leading to mammary duct proliferation and an increase in stromal tissue. In the luteal phase, a rise in progesterone leads to dilatation of the mammary ducts. At the onset of menstruation there is a drop in oestrogen and progesterone, and these changes reverse, causing involution of breast tissue.

**Pregnancy:** oestrogen levels remain elevated throughout pregnancy and the changes in the breast tissue are more sustained. Placental oestrogen causes proliferation and branching of the ductal system and further fat and stromal tissue are laid down. Progesterone causes lobular growth and aids in the development of the secretory function of the alveoli. In addition, capillary growth, vascular engorgement and myoepithelial cell hypertrophy occur. The breast weight can double, although some of this increase is due to fluid retention. An increase in nipple and areolar pigmentation is also seen.

**Breastfeeding:** milk production is inhibited during pregnancy by high levels of oestrogen and progesterone. Their levels drop sharply postpartum. Prolactin is released from the anterior pituitary and stimulates milk production and when this is unopposed by oestrogen lactation occurs. Colostrum, which is high in protein and IgA, is released for the first 2–4 days. If the mother is not breastfeeding, the prolactin levels decrease and return to normal within 2–3 weeks. Suckling of the baby leads to the release of oxytocin from the posterior pituitary. This causes contraction of myoepithelial cells and therefore milk ejection or 'let down'. Initially this is an endocrine process but gradually the expression of milk stimulates more milk production and the nutritional composition also changes to meet the changing demands of the child. A number of drugs can pass into breast milk, including alcohol, metronidazole, tetracycline and anticoagulants.

**Menopause:** involutional change starts at about 35 years with regression of breast tissues and their replacement with fat and fibrosis. The breast becomes less dense and easier to image with mammography. Reductions in oestrogen levels associated with menopause accelerate this process.

## 1.3 History and examination of the breast

### In a nutshell ...

**Examination of the breast and axilla**
- **Targeted history:** the most relevant features of the history are symptomatology and its history; patient age; duration and extent of oestrogen exposure; and the likelihood of the patient having a genetic component to her disease
- **Inspection:** general; breast-specific (sitting, raised arms; lying)
- **Palpation**
- **Diagnosis:** if breast lump present, complete triple assessment with imaging and pathology

If unilateral or bloodstained nipple discharge, complete with cytology slide of discharge

## Targeted history

### Presenting complaint
- Commonly palpable lump, breast pain, nipple discharge or itch, breast asymmetry
- A lump:
  - When did it appear? Suddenly or gradually?
  - How did you notice it?
  - Has it got bigger or smaller, or stayed the same?
  - Any trauma?
  - Any skin discoloration?
  - Any associated symptoms? Pain? Heat? Nipple discharge?
  - Any other lumps in breast or axilla?
  - Any treatment so far for this lump?
  - Has it persisted or changed after menstruation?
- Breast pain:
  - Is it cyclical?
  - Symptom onset sudden/gradual?
  - Any injury/event trigger?
- Nipple discharge:
  - Consider onset, volume, frequency, cyclicity, colour, blood, lump, pain, headaches, visual disturbances

### Past medical history
- Oestrogen exposure: age at menarche, parity, age at first pregnancy, breastfeeding, age at menopause, oral contraceptive pill (OCP)/depot oestrogen/hormone replacement therapy (HRT) use and duration
- Previous breast disease, previous breast imaging, participation in screening
- Any other conditions (eg diabetes predisposes to breast lumps)

### Family history
Breast cancer (especially first-degree relatives with breast cancer aged <50) and ovarian cancer (allows assessment of the genetic component of a patient's risk), other breast disease.

### Social history
Smoking predisposes to breast abscess and duct ectasia.

### Systemic enquiry
This should be targeted at a likely diagnosis. In malignancy ask about 'non-breast' symptoms of metastatic breast cancer, eg dyspnoea (in malignant effusion); abdominal swelling (in hepatic metastases or ascites); bone pain (if

bony metastases); upper limb lymphoedema (if axillary nodes infiltrated); weight loss (in advanced cancer); confusion/headaches (in brain metastases); skin deposits or distant lymphadenopathy. In galactorrhoea ask about visual disturbance (eg in pituitary prolactinoma). In sepsis ask about pyrexia, tachycardia, etc.

## Inspection

Chaperone. Patient sitting, undressed to waist, hands on hips.

### General

Weight loss, shortness of breath (SOB), pallor, hair loss if recent chemotherapy.

### Breast

- **Asymmetry**
- **Skin changes:** redness, puckering, peau d'orange, nodules, ulcer, previous radiotherapy causing telangiectasia and skin discoloration, or ink tattoo from radiotherapy treatment planning
- **Nipples and areolae:** retraction, eczema-type changes, asymmetry, discharge, accessory nipple (looks like a small skin tag usually in milk line, below breast)
- **Scars from previous surgery:** may be periareolar or located distant to the original disease process to improve cosmesis. Might relate to previous diagnostic surgery (lumpectomy), oncological surgery (wide local excision, mastectomy or oncoplastic resection, breast reconstruction) or to aesthetic surgery (reconstruction, reduction or augmentation). Evidence of reconstruction should also prompt you to look at the donor site scar (commonly on the abdomen or back but can be on the thigh)

## Axillae and arms

- **Scars** from previous node biopsy or clearance
- **Swelling** (lymphoedema): due to disruption of the lymphatics by previous surgery or infiltration by disease
- **Visible nodes** or skin changes
- **Muscle wasting**

Ask the patient to raise her arms above her head and inspect the breasts, axillae and inframammary fold (IMF) for tethering or dimpling during movement.

### Palpation of the breast

Ask the patient to point out sites of tenderness and lumps that she has noticed before you start palpation. Lie the patient at 45° with her hands behind her head (one arm at a time if she is elderly). It may be helpful to think of the breast as a clock face and work in from each 'hour' around the outside to the centre. Use flat fingers rather then the tips of your fingers. Start with the normal side to give yourself a point of reference and comparison. Examine all four quadrants of the breast, under the nipple and the axillary tail. Accessory breast tissue may lie laterally and in the axilla. Accessory nipples often lie on the chest wall in a vertical line with the nipple.

> **Describing a breast lump**
> - **General:** tenderness, site, size
> - **Define:** shape, surface, edges
> - **Composition:** consistency, fluctuance (rarely: pulsatility, compressibility, reducibility)
> - **Layer of origin:** skin, breast tissue, chest wall (muscle or bone)
> - **Relationship to surrounding structures:** mobility, fixity, tethering. Assess fixity to the pectoralis muscle by asking patient to put hands firmly on hips and assess infiltration of the overlying skin

### Palpation of the axilla

Palpate all four walls and the apex separately. Use the right hand to palpate the left axilla and vice versa. Take the patient's elbow with your other hand to lower the arm and relax the pectoral muscles as you palpate the apex. Note any palpable lumps/nodes, including number, tenderness, size, consistency and fixity. Look for lymphadenopathy in the **supraclavicular region** on both sides.

Note that small mobile axillary nodes are palpable in 30% of people without breast cancer, and impalpable in 40% of people with axillary node metastases.

If you suspect malignancy then **listen to the chest** (consider malignant pleural effusion) and **examine the abdomen** (hepatomegaly or ascites might be present in metastatic breast cancer).

## 1.4    Diagnosis of breast disease

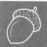 **In a nutshell ...**

**Triple assessment**

All discrete breast lumps should undergo triple assessment, which consists of:
1. Clinical examination
2. Radiological imaging: commonly by mammogram or ultrasonography but sometimes by MRI
3. Pathological diagnosis: cytology or histology

During triple assessment, each variable (clinical examination, imaging and pathology) is given a grade reflecting an index of suspicion from 1 (benign) to 5 (malignant):

- Clinical impression (P)
- Imaging (mammography M; ultrasonography U)
- Pathology (cytology C; core biopsy B)

1 Normal
2 Benign
3 Equivocal
4 Suspicious
5 Malignant

At each stage of assessment the level of suspicion is recorded independently. The examining doctor should record a clinical impression (P1–P5) in ignorance of the radiological or histological findings for a triple assessment to be effective. The radiologist records the mammographic and ultrasound findings as M1–M5 and U1–U5 and the pathologist grades the core biopsy as B1–B5. Cytology grading is slightly different, in that C1 means 'insufficient cells for diagnosis' (either an insufficient sample or a very acellular sample, eg from a lipoma). In addition core biopsy allows the pathologist to assess the tissue architecture and determine whether cancer cells are confined to the duct (DCIS) or invasive:

B5a        Carcinoma in situ (on histopathological core biopsy)
B5b        Invasive carcinoma (on histopathological core biopsy)

## Clinical assessment

Correlation of the three assessment techniques is very important to ensure accurate diagnosis. Clinical suspicion of malignancy (P3–P5) is as valid as mammographic or pathological suspicion, and should always prompt core biopsy.

## Imaging

Options for imaging include mammography, ultrasonography and magnetic resonance imaging (MRI). Breast cancers are sometimes diagnosed and staged with computed tomography (CT).

### Mammography

- A radiograph of the breast in two planes, mediolateral oblique (MLO) and cranio-caudal (CC), compressed between two plates. In some centres these are now obtained as more sensitive digital images
- Low radiation dosage (1.5 mGy), non-invasive and quick, but uncomfortable
- Relatively contraindicated in pregnancy but, if absolutely necessary, abdominal shielding can be used
- Used for diagnosis of a palpable lump, breast screening, stereotactic biopsy of impalpable lesions seen on screening/surveillance films, preoperative wire local-isation and postoperative surveillance
- Mammography is better for identifying malignant lesions than for characterising benign lesions
- Sensitivity of mammography is inversely related to breast density. Younger women have more dense breast tissue so <50% cancers are seen on a mammogram if the patient is <40; mammographic sensitivity increases as breast density decreases with

age and is 90–95% sensitive in patients >60
- First-line breast imaging for women aged >35; only occasionally used in women under this age (eg to image an abnormality that appears malignant on ultrasonography)
- Some cancers are mammographically occult, particularly ductal carcinoma in situ (DCIS) and lobular cancers can be difficult to see

### Ultrasonography

- Ultrasonography should be used as a targeted scan of a localised region of the breast (either a palpable lump or a mammographically detected abnormality); it is not useful as a screening or surveillance tool
- First-line imaging for breast lumps in women <35 due to dense breast tissue
- May be used to complement bilateral mammography in the characterisation of a lesion in women >35
- Ultrasonography is better than mammography at characterising lesions because it will differentiate between fluid-filled cysts and solid lumps. Cysts appear transparent. Benign solid lumps tend to have well-defined edges and homogeneous consistency. Cancers tend to have indistinct outlines and an acoustic shadow
- Ultrasonography can also be used for image-guided biopsy or aspiration of cysts and abscesses. The core biopsy needle can be seen as it penetrates the area of suspicion, reducing the risk of missing the lesion with the biopsy needle and ensuring that there is no residual mass lesion when a cyst is fully drained
- Ultrasonography is also used as the first line in staging the axilla, although its sensitivity for positive nodes is only 50–60%. It is then used to guide fine-needle aspiration (FNA) or biopsy of suspicious nodes

## MRI

- Specific MRI coils are required for breast MRI and it is therefore not universally available. Breast MRI is performed with the patient prone, allowing gravity to act on the breast
- It is very sensitive for invasive cancer but consequently has a high false-positive rate
- MRI is particularly useful for:
  - Screening high-risk young women with dense breasts
  - Imaging patients with implants
  - Assessing disease response to neoadjuvant treatments
  - Looking for disease recurrence
  - Excluding multifocal cancer (controversial)
  - Looking for spinal metastatic disease and cord compression
- Lobular cancers are more commonly mammographically occult and can be bilateral. The National Institute for Health and Clinical Excellence (NICE) guidelines of 2009 now recommend MRI for patients diagnosed with lobular cancers to delineate the extent of disease if the patient is to undergo breast-conserving surgery

---

### What to look for on the mammogram

Abnormalities are easier to detect if you compare the two sides as mirror images; respective regions (eg the upper pole) should look similar on the left and right. Look at both the MLO views together and then the CC views. Practice is essential and there are several good online resources (www.sprojects.mmi.mcgill.ca/mammography/index.htm is an interactive tutorial and www.rad.washington.edu/academics/academic-sections/mbi/education/mammoed/teaching-files has cases for practice [both last accessed August 2011]).

- Check patient name and date of study
- Look from a distance at first and note size, symmetry and composition (eg dense/fatty)
- Magnify small abnormalities and compare abnormalities with previous mammography if available

Mammographic appearances suggestive of malignancy include:

- **Mass lesion:** assess size, shape, edges (circumscribed, spiculated, ill defined or irregular), associated findings (skin tethering or distortion of nipple). Round and smooth lesions are more likely to be benign, but masses with spiculated or indistinct margins and distortion of surrounding breast architecture are more likely to be malignant
- **Asymmetrical density:** regional differences in density between the two breasts should be present on both views and may be normal or due to a developing mass or post-surgical scarring
- **Calcification:** round, large uniform calcification is usually benign but high-risk calcifications are either linear or clustered in groups of small, irregular and branching deposits (they look like the letters X, Y or Z) and are referred to as pleomorphic

Assess the position of the lesion in the breast by its relationship to the nipple – look at the MLO film; is the abnormality superior or inferior to the nipple? Look at the CC film; is the abnormality medial or lateral to the nipple? These distances can be measured directly on the film and transposed to the breast to give a rough idea of the position of the lesion but remember that the breast tissue is distorted by pressure during the mammogram.

## Other imaging

CT and bone scan are used for staging to detect metastases in women who are node positive or where there are signs or symptoms of advanced breast cancer. Positron-emission tomography (PET) can also be used to detect occult metastatic disease, especially in inflammatory cancers.

## Pathology

### In a nutshell ...

Pathological diagnosis is an essential component of the triple assessment. Methods of obtaining tissue for diagnosis include:

- **Cytology:** FNA of a solid lump, cytological assessment of suspicious cyst fluid
- **Histology:** core biopsy (gold standard), punch biopsy for breast skin, open surgical biopsy for diagnostically difficult, suspicious regions

Image guidance reduces the risk of inadvertently sampling the wrong bit of breast tissue. This may be under mammographic 'stereotactic', ultrasonographic or MRI control.

## Fine-needle aspiration cytology

- FNA provides cells for cytology, not tissue for histology. It requires specialist interpretation
- Cannot differentiate between in-situ and invasive disease
- It is the minimum pathology assessment for any lump in the breast, but, if a suspicious or malignant result is obtained, it must be supplemented with a core biopsy. Tissue architecture is important in diagnosis and so, in many units, FNA is gradually being replaced with up-front core biopsy
- It is usually performed by a doctor in a clinic, sometimes with ultrasound guidance
- A 21-G (green) needle on a 5- or 10-ml syringe is passed several times through the lesion while applying suction
- The cells are then expelled on to a slide, allowed to dry and sprayed with fixative
- At the gold-standard 'one-stop' clinic, a pathologist is present to report results immediately
- In the case of a cyst, the aspiration can be therapeutic. In rare cases where there is suspicion that a cyst is associated with a tumour, cyst fluid can be sent for cytology (see Breast cysts in Section 2.1.2)

## Op box: Fine-needle aspiration (FNA)

- Explain procedure to patient (verbal, rather than written, consent usually obtained).
- Offer local anaesthetic injection if desired (usually not needed).
- EMLA cream may be useful for the needle-phobic.
- Position patient – lying at 45°, hand behind head.
- You will need a dressing pack, green needle, 5-ml syringe and small dressing. Have two cytology slides ready.
- Use an aseptic technique (sterile gloves, chlorhexidine skin prep and small drape).
- Fix lump between your first finger and thumb, insert needle into the lump, apply suction.
- Maintaining suction, pass needle several times through the lump in different directions and angles (do not withdraw needle from skin until you have finished).
- After withdrawing needle, press firmly on biopsy site with a swab.
- Expel the syringe contents on to cytology slide and use both slides together to make a thin smear on each (in some units, if the pathologist is present, they might ask you to give them the syringe directly, and prepare the slides themself – ask the pathologist to show you how best to prepare the slides).
- Check for bleeding from the puncture wound and apply dressing.
- Label slides and request form and check details with the patient.
- One-stop clinics have an attending pathologist skilled at cytology, allowing immediate interpretation.

## Core biopsy

- Core biopsy (sometimes called Tru-Cut after a brand of core biopsy needle) provides a solid core of tissue for histology (14 G, 22-mm length)
- Preservation of the tissue architecture improves diagnostic accuracy (eg distinguishes between *in situ* and invasive disease. Remember that the diagnosis is still confined to a small piece of tissue, so in-situ disease can be present alongside a focus (or foci) of invasive disease and vice versa
- Can be performed freehand, using ultrasound guidance, or stereotactic biopsy
- More time-consuming than FNA, requires local anaesthetic injection, causes more discomfort and bruising afterwards, and carries more risk of damage to adjacent structures

- Results take several days as the tissue requires processing before interpretation
- Can give information about tumour type and oestrogen receptor status. Some pathologists will not assess grade because they consider the sample too small to be representative of the whole tumour
- Core biopsy of suspicious axillary nodes is indicated where these are palpable or detected on imaging. Axillary core biopsy should be performed under ultrasound guidance due to the risk of damage to the axillary vessels (or rarely the brachial plexus).

## Op box: Core biopsy

- This can be performed alone, but is easier with an assistant who can help reassure the patient, and also to press on the biopsy site in between cores to minimise bleeding and bruising. Make sure that you familiarise yourself with the length of the biopsy needle and biopsy gun beforehand. The gun must never be fired vertically down towards the chest wall.
- Prepare the patient as for FNA.
- You will need a dressing pack, scalpel (no. 11 blade is ideal), core biopsy gun, small pot of formalin and forceps, Steri-Strips and small dressing.
- Infiltrate the skin and tissue over the lump with local anaesthetic (1% lidocaine with adrenaline is sufficient). Use this interval to familiarise the patient with the loud 'click' that the biopsy gun makes.
- Make a small (2 mm) incision over the lump – place this to one side of the lump so that you can approach it at a shallow angle, virtually parallel to the chest wall, rather than having to fire the needle directly downwards.
- Fix the lump between your first finger and thumb, pass the core needle through the incision until you can feel it touching the lump.
- Obtain at least two to four cores from the lump, and put these straight into formalin. In general, though not as a rule, a core from a breast cancer or other solid breast lesion will sink to the bottom of the specimen pot whereas a core of fatty breast tissue will float.
- Keep pressure on the biopsy site with a swab in between cores and at the end of the procedure.
- Check that bleeding has stopped. Close incision with a Steri-Strip and apply dressing. Allow the patient to dress.
- Label specimen pot and form and check details with patient.
- Let patient know how long results will take and how they will be delivered (usually an appointment at a subsequent clinic is given). Recommend simple analgesic to be taken later that day if necessary.

**Complications:** bleeding (local pressure will almost always stop this); severe post-biopsy bruising (some bruising is inevitable); infection; and damage to adjacent structures such as ribs, lung and blood vessels (this risk is minimised with careful technique, but pneumothorax is not unheard of, and remember that the heart is also not far beneath the chest wall). There is a theoretical risk of cancer cells migrating along the core biopsy site to the skin and some surgeons excise the biopsy tract with a malignancy.

CHAPTER 2

## Punch biopsy of a skin lesion

Where there is a suspicious skin lesion on the breast or areola, this is a simple way of taking a small (3–4 mm) skin biopsy for histology using a specially designed circular cutting tool (similar to a tiny biscuit cutter). This is performed in the breast clinic under local anaesthetic, and a single suture is sufficient to close the defect.

## Open biopsy

If (rarely) a diagnosis cannot be achieved through core biopsy of a breast lump then an open biopsy may be considered. This is performed under general anaesthetic through a skin incision. This is a diagnostic rather than a therapeutic procedure so no more than 20 g of tissue should be excised.

Positive histology (with core biopsy, punch biopsy or open biopsy) is mandatory before proceeding to a cancer operation.

# SECTION 2

# Benign breast disease

## 2.1 Benign breast lumps

 **In a nutshell ...**

**Benign breast lumps**
- Fibrocystic disease
- Fibroadenoma and benign-spectrum phyllodes tumours
- Breast cyst
- Abscess
- Fat necrosis, haematoma
- Lipoma
- Granulomas: silicone, TB, sarcoid
- Other rare causes: blocked Montgomery's tubercles, Mondor's disease, galactocele

Many benign breast conditions are thought to occur as a result of the constant physiological changes affecting the breast throughout reproductive life. This concept has been referred to as an 'aberration of normal development or involution' or ANDI.

## 2.1.1 Fibrocystic breast disease

Fibrocystic breast disease is the most common cause of benign breast lumps (and lumpiness or nodularity) presenting to the breast clinic. It has also been described as fibroadenosis or fibrosclerosis, and is a benign condition rather than a 'disease'.

### Clinical features

- Each of the following may be present to a greater or lesser extent:
  - Nodular breast tissue – can have a 'cobblestone' texture
  - Discrete breast lumps – mobile, often tender, can enlarge and reduce cyclically
  - Breast pain and tenderness (usually cyclical)
  - Breast cysts
- Symptoms are often most pronounced in the upper outer quadrant of the breast
- There is frequently some cyclical variation in symptoms, with symptoms tending to peak at the end of the luteal phase, just before menstruation
- Incidence rises with age during the premenopausal years and symptoms improve after the menopause

## Pathological features

Various morphological changes are covered by the term 'fibrocystic disease'. These have been found post mortem in asymptomatic patients, supporting the theory that they are part of the normal spectrum of breast development and involution. As symptoms rarely begin before the age of 30, this is thought to be a cumulative process under hormonal influence.

Histological changes all affect the terminal duct lobular unit, and include stromal fibrosis, adenosis (an increase in glandular tissue), cyst formation (from microscopic to 5 cm or more), papillomatosis, and epithelial hyperplasia of ductal and lobular types. This type of epithelial hyperplasia carries no increased risk of malignancy; it falls into the premalignant category only when it shows atypia – see Section 3.2).

## Diagnosis

History taking plus triple assessment of any discrete lump. There may be no discrete lump but asymmetrical nodularity should also be assessed by pathology (using FNA or core biopsy).

## Treatment

- Reassurance and explanation
- Symptomatic treatment of pain (see Breast pain section)
- Aspiration of cysts as required
- Similar symptoms may be present in postmenopausal women on HRT whereas the OCP tends to improve symptoms in premenopausal women

## Outcome of fibrocystic disease

There is no evidence that fibrocystic disease carries an increased risk of breast cancer; however, in patients with very lumpy breasts, it may be more difficult to pick up an early cancer on clinical examination or imaging.

## 2.1.2 Breast cysts

Breast cysts occur as part of the range of histological changes of fibrocystic disease. They are thought to be due to duct obstruction.

## Clinical features

- Palpable cysts are usually between 1 cm and 5 cm in diameter (occasionally larger)
- Often multiple and bilateral
- Usually appear rapidly and can diminish after menstruation
- Smooth, round, discrete breast lump. May be fluctuant or tense
- Often tender
- May be bluish in colour ('Bloodgood's blue-domed cysts')
- Peak occurrence is between age 35 and 55

## Investigating breast cysts

- History taking and triple assessment
- Targeted ultrasonography if aged <35, mammography and targeted ultrasonography if aged >35
- Easy to identify on ultrasonography and appear as well-defined round opacities on mammography
- Note that impalpable microcysts seen on imaging are considered normal
- Needle aspiration: if clear fluid is aspirated the fluid is discarded. Provided the lump has resolved, no further treatment is necessary. Many centres offer aspiration under ultrasound guidance to ensure that there is no visible residual mass because this is more sensitive than palpation alone. If any abnormality remains or the aspirate was bloodstained, the aspirate should be sent

for cytological analysis, and a core biopsy performed of any residual mass. Cytology of cyst fluid is difficult and can be controversial

## Outcome of breast cysts

Cysts can recur but there is no significant association with breast cancer; however, it may be more difficult to pick up a small breast cancer clinically and on imaging in a patient with numerous cysts.

## 2.1.3 Fibroadenoma

This is the most common benign breast tumour in women and may affect up to 10% of the population. It typically affects women aged 15–40, most commonly late adolescence or early 20s. Its size may vary with the menstrual cycle. It is more common in women of Chinese and African origin. Incidence increases with exposure to oestrogens (eg OCP, ciclosporin use). It is a developmental aberration of the terminal lobular unit.

### Clinical features
- Smooth, firm, well-circumscribed breast lump
- More often left-sided and in the upper outer quadrant
- Diameter from <1 cm to <5 cm (those >5 cm are 'giant fibroadenomas' – see below)
- Often very mobile (hence the description 'breast mouse')
- Around 7% are bilateral; 7% are recurrent after excision

### Pathological features
- Polyclonal, arising from a single breast lobule: fibroadenoma can be considered an aberration of development rather than a tumour (as tumours are monoclonal, arising from a single cell)
- Growth of glandular and cystic tissue within network of fibrous stroma, enclosed by a well-defined capsule

### Investigating fibroadenoma
- Triple assessment using ultrasonography if aged <35 and mammography and ultrasonography if >35 (appears on mammogram as a well-defined mass, sometimes with some 'popcorn' calcification)
- Fibroadenoma is not distinguishable from phyllodes tumour on cytology, so core biopsy is preferred to confirm diagnosis

### Treatment options
- If confidently diagnosed by triple assessment, does not need to be excised as no increased risk of breast cancer
- Surgical excision: if fibroadenoma is large, at patient request, if there are diagnostic difficulties

### Outcome of fibroadenoma
- Ten per cent increase in size, the patient should be reassessed and the core biopsy repeated
- Thirty per cent decrease in size and may disappear

**Giant fibroadenomas** are fibroadenomas that are >5 cm in diameter and should be excised – there is some histopathological overlap with phyllodes tumours.

## 2.1.4 Phyllodes tumours
- Uncommon
- Most are >3 cm in diameter; often present with a recent and rapid increase in size

- Most common in women aged 40–50 (therefore occur in a different age group to fibroadenoma)
- Spectrum of disease: some benign and cured by excision; some recurrent; others malignant
- Similar to fibroadenoma, phyllodes tumours involve both fibrous and epithelial breast tissue, and can be well demarcated from the surrounding breast tissue
- The fibrous stroma in a phyllodes tumour shows more cellularity than that of fibroadenoma, and at the malignant end of the phyllodes spectrum the fibrous stroma is atypical and pleomorphic
- Malignant phyllodes tumours ('cystosarcoma phyllodes') behave in a similar fashion to sarcomas with a high risk of local recurrence, and metastatic spread to bone and lung
- Both benign and malignant phyllodes tumours tend to present as a rapidly enlarging painless breast mass
- Whether histologically benign or malignant, phyllodes tumour should be completely excised with a margin of normal breast tissue (as both benign and malignant tumours can exhibit local recurrence). Axillary surgery is not indicated for phyllodes tumours because they do not metastasise to the axillary lymph nodes

## 2.1.5 Fat necrosis and haematoma

### Fat necrosis

- Seen after blunt injury to the breast (eg road traffic accident [RTA] seat-belt injury) and after breast surgery or reconstruction
- More common in older women, about 50% of whom do not recall an injury
- Clinical features of fat necrosis may include: lump, skin dimpling and retraction

- Investigation is by triple assessment – where there is no history of trauma, there may initially be a high index of suspicion of breast cancer:
  - Mammography to exclude concurrent breast cancer. Fat necrosis may appear as focal calcification and scarring
  - Ultrasonography may show oil cysts
  - Core biopsy essential to confirm diagnosis
- Treatment of fat necrosis: may resolve over a 12-month period; excision biopsy if diagnosis is unclear, or persisting symptoms

### Haematoma

- Post-traumatic (eg from car seat-belts, core biopsy)
- Spontaneous (in patients on anticoagulants)
- Complicated by fat necrosis
- Treatment with aspiration and surgical evacuation if large

### Sclerotic lesions

Sclerotic lesions of the breast include sclerosing adenosis, radial scar and complex sclerosing lesions:

- Pathologically characterised by proliferation of the small breast ductules and fibrosis
- Important lesions because they are often detected on screening and they require biopsy to distinguish them from breast carcinoma
- These are benign lesions but 30% of radial scars may be associated with malignancy and therefore require a diagnostic excision biopsy in all cases
- As these lesions are usually picked up incidentally on mammography and are impalpable, they require a guided local-isation wire preoperatively to mark the area of abnormality
- Sclerosing adenosis is associated with a slightly increased risk of breast cancer

## 2.1.6 Other benign breast lumps

### Lipoma

Benign fatty tumour that is soft and compressible; lipomas are radiolucent and yield C1 (acellular) cytology on FNA. Once the diagnosis has been made confidently on triple assessment, the lipoma need not be excised. Note: differentiate between lipomas and the rare pseudolipoma (soft mass felt around breast cancer).

### Granuloma

Silicone granulomas may occur in patients with silicone breast implants due to rupture or silicone 'bleed' through the implant shell. Other granulomatous diseases (eg TB, sarcoid) can occur in the breast.

### Blocked Montgomery's tubercles

Blockage in the sebaceous glands of the areola; presents as periareolar lump; no treatment is necessary but they can be excised.

### Mondor's disease

This is a thrombophlebitis of a subcutaneous vein that occurs in the breast, anterior chest wall, and arms of men and women. It presents as tender skin dimpling or a groove on the breast with a palpable indurated cord. Treatment is with non-steroidal anti-inflammatory drugs (NSAIDs, eg ibuprofen 400 mg three times daily). In spontaneous cases investigate with mammography.

### Galactocele

This is a cystic lesion containing breast milk caused by the closure of a milk duct. It should be triple assessed and can be aspirated to dryness.

## 2.2 Nipple disease and discharge

### In a nutshell ...

**Nipple disorders**

Disorders of the nipple–areolar complex (NAC) are common and include:
- Structural problems such as inversion, adenoma or trauma during breastfeeding
- Skin conditions, eg eczema
- Manifestations of underlying malignant disease (Paget's disease, bloodstained discharge)

### Inverted nipples

Congenitally inverted nipples are normal (they often evert during development) but increasingly inverted nipples can be due to increasing breast ptosis (gradual, may be bilateral), breast cancer, duct ectasia (usually presents with a slit-like retraction), inflammatory breast disorders (eg periductal mastitis) and TB (rarely).

### Management

History and triple assessment. Mammography if aged >35. Ultrasonography of the NAC may also be helpful in younger women. Palpable lumps or radiological abnormalities should be biopsied.

### Treatment of inverted nipples

In the absence of a sinister cause, reassurance may be all that is required. Tethering of the nipple is often due to shortening of the ducts. Duct division is possible as a small procedure under local anaesthetic but leaves a scar and may result in a permanently erect nipple. Breast-feeding is not possible after duct division.

# Paget's disease of the nipple

Paget's disease of the nipple is eczematoid change of the nipple caused by either DCIS or invasive breast cancer growing along the ducts on to the nipple surface. It is a malignant condition.

## Clinical features of Paget's disease

- Presenting complaint in 1–2% of all breast cancers
- More common in elderly people
- Nipple lesion is scaly, unilateral and non-itchy
- There may be point bleeding, but nipple discharge is rare
- Can spread to the areola and destroy the nipple if left untreated

## Investigating Paget's disease

- Triple assessment
- History and examination
- Mammography
- Biopsy of underlying lesion (image-guided if impalpable)
- Biopsy of nipple (punch biopsy in clinic) is essential

If malignancy is found the surgical treatment of choice is usually mastectomy (as the underlying disease is usually extensive), with appropriate axillary staging and management.

## Itchy nipple

If there is no evidence of underlying malignancy after clinical assessment, and there is no visible skin complaint or palpable nipple adenoma, a short trial of treatment with topical cortico-steroids is appropriate. This should resolve dermatological causes of itch. If the condition does not settle, punch biopsy or incisional nipple biopsy should be repeated.

## Nipple discharge

Nipple discharge is a common complaint and is often physiological in nature. It accounts for 5% of all clinic referrals but only 5% of these patients have a malignancy. Discharge that is bilateral, from multiple ducts and not bloodstained, or that occurs only when expressed is rarely pathological.

### Comparison of Paget's disease of the nipple and eczema

|  | Paget's disease | Eczema |
|---|---|---|
| Laterality | Unilateral | Bilateral |
| Pruritis | No | Yes |
| Site | Nipple (may spread to areola) | Areola (infrequently affects nipple) |
| History of atopy | No | Yes, usually |
| Underlying breast disease | Yes – invasive cancer or ductal carcinoma in situ | No |

**Causes of nipple discharge**

**Physiological**

Usually bilateral and multiduct

- Clear or serous discharge is normal in premenopausal women
- Milky-white discharge: galactorrhoea is caused by hyperprolactinaemia (eg drug-induced, hypothyroidism, or in pituitary prolactinoma). Measure prolactin levels

**Inflammatory**

Usually more than one duct, can be bilateral. Multicoloured, opalescent (yellow, green, brown).

- Duct ectasia
- Periareolar abscess/mastitis (can be purulent, tender)

**Pathological**

Single duct, unilateral – usually signifies an intraductal lesion. May be watery or serosanguineous

- Intraductal papilloma
- DCIS/breast cancer
- Epithelial hyperplasia

## History of nipple discharge

- Colour of discharge
- Laterality: unilateral, bilateral, symmetrical/ asymmetrical
- Single or multiple ducts
- Ask about drugs that can cause hyperprolactinaemia (eg some psychotropic agents). If no cause is evident check prolactin levels to exclude prolactinoma
- Bloodstained or single-duct discharge should always be investigated further

## Investigating nipple discharge

- **Clinical examination:** examine both breasts; express nipple discharge, identifying colour, number of ducts (ie number of 'points' of discharge from the nipple), and quadrant of the trigger zone if possible. The trigger zone is the area of breast that yields nipple discharge when pressure is applied
- **Radiology:** mammography if >35 years; ultrasonography may show a small papilloma in the ducts just under the nipple
- **Pathology:** any mass identified on clinical examination or imaging must be biopsied. Diagnosis based on cytology of the nipple

discharge, ie looking for cancer cells, is controversial. The smear is difficult to assess (even for experienced cytologists) because frank clumping of malignant cells is very rarely seen and any epithelial cells in the sample look fragmented and abnormal. A negative smear does not exclude malignancy and so clinical concern should provoke surgical exploration to provide tissue for histopathology and to complete the triple assessment

- **Testing for blood:** Haemoccult and other commercial strips are not very accurate for nipple discharge. A smear preparation of duct discharge can be examined for red cells
- Some centres offer **ductoscopy**, which is endoscopic examination of the duct

## Management of nipple discharge

If there are **abnormal features** of the discharge (single duct, frankly bloodstained or red blood cells [RBCs] seen on cytology, papilloma seen on ultrasonography), then surgical excision of the affected duct (microdochectomy) should be performed. This is a diagnostic procedure and further treatment may be required depending on the results.

CHAPTER 2

If the discharge is **physiological** and clinical evaluation and imaging are normal, then the patient can be reassured. Troublesome discharges of a benign aetiology can be treated by total duct excision (Hadfield's procedure) but this will preclude breastfeeding in the future.

## Duct papilloma

This is a common benign polyp of the ductal epithelium, usually occurring within 2–3 cm of the nipple. They are rarely larger than a few millimetres. The most common cause of bloodstained nipple discharge, papillomas can be palpable. Usually single but may be multiple. Multiple papillomas are associated with an increased risk of breast cancer and solitary papillomas may be associated with DCIS in <5% cases.

## Op box: Microdochectomy

Microdochectomy is the removal of a portion of a diseased duct for pathological assessment. It results in disconnection of the affected duct, so it can also be used to treat troublesome single duct discharge of benign aetiology. It is performed under general anaesthetic.

**Indications:** bloodstained single duct discharge; troublesome benign single duct discharge; persistent periductal mastitis involving a single duct.

**Preop:** obtain informed consent – explaining that further treatment is required if the procedure leads to a diagnosis of carcinoma. Mark the side before the operation. Identify the trigger zone if possible. Do not express the discharge until the patient is on the table (and dissuade the patient from expressing the fluid in the weeks leading up to surgery because this will enable easier surgical identification of the duct).

**Position:** patient supine with ipsilateral arm abducted to 90° on an arm board. Prophylactic antibiotics at induction for patients with periductal mastitis.

**Procedure:** examine the breast, express the discharge to identify the duct immediately before incision and cannulate the duct with a lacrimal probe. Make a periareolar incision in the affected quadrant (not >50% of the areolar circumference to minimise risk of necrosis). Dissect down to the probe, and place a strong tie around it to secure it in the duct. Dissect out the duct with scissors, leaving a margin of breast tissue around the probe. Draw the breast tissue into view by pulling gently on the duct, and excise a generous cuff of the affected lobe at the end of the probe, en bloc with the duct. Use diathermy to ensure haemostasis. Send the specimen to histology, with the side and site recorded. It is important to close the defect in the breast tissue behind the nipple, leaving a flat bed for the nipple to sit on. Failure to do so will result in nipple distortion. Close with subcuticular suture.

**Postop:** usually a day case.

**Operative hazards:** excision of the wrong duct (if the discharge cannot be expressed in theatre it may be wise to postpone the surgery); failure to cannulate the duct, which may be blocked or stenosed (if the duct can be seen, a radial incision can be made over it and a wedge of tissue excised, ensuring that this includes the area that results in the discharge).

**Complications:** haematoma; infection; rarely, mammary duct fistula.

## Op box: Total subareolar duct excision (Hadfield's procedure)

**Indications:** multiple duct discharge; nipple inversion; recurrent periductal mastitis; mammary duct fistula; for diagnosis of cause of bloody or watery nipple discharge; treatment of galactorrhoea (if the patient has a normal prolactin and does not respond to anti-prolactin drugs).

**Preop:** obtain informed consent. Mark the side before the operation. Identify the trigger zone if possible. Do not express the discharge until the patient is on the table (and dissuade the patient from expressing the fluid in the weeks leading up to surgery because this will enable easier surgical identification of the duct).

**Position:** patient supine with ipsilateral arm abducted to 90° on an arm board. Prophylactic antibiotics at induction for patients with periductal mastitis.

**Procedure:** periareolar incision from the 3'o clock to 9'o clock position. Lift the nipple leaving a cuff of fat below it. Identify the confluence of ducts and place the artery forceps on the sheath of ducts just below the nipple.

If the operation is for galactorrhoea, ligate the ducts in the breast tissue and divide above the ligature. No tissue needs be excised or sent for histology.

If the operation is for multiple duct discharge, excise 1–2 cm of the ducts and send for histology (no deep ligation needed).

If the operation is for nipple retraction, take care to avoid button-holing of the inverted nipple by cutting through the skin. Excise 1–2 cm and send for histology (no deep ligation needed).

If the operation is for periductal mastitis all diseased ducts must be removed completely (not just 1–2 cm) and then sent for histology and microbiology. No deep ligation is needed. Carefully inspect the underside of the nipple and identify and divide any residual subareolar ducts.

Manually evert the nipple, dividing any tight bands or adhesions that prevent satisfactory eversion. Try not to use sutures on the back of the nipple (persistent erection of the nipple may result). Placing tissue glue as a dressing over the everted nipple bud at the end of the procedure maintains eversion while the wounds heal. Use diathermy to ensure haemostasis and close the defect in the breast tissue under the nipple. Subcuticular suture to skin.

**Operative hazards:** button-holing the nipple occurs when a wedge of skin is excised from underneath because of failure to appreciate how inverted the nipple is.

**Complications:** nipple necrosis, especially in reoperation (avoid this by limiting incision to 50% of the areolar circumference and avoiding dissection too close to the nipple or radial vessels); loss of nipple sensation, with greater risk in patients with periductal mastitis, where more extensive dissection is needed; recurrent nipple discharge or infection; mammary duct fistula (rarely).

CHAPTER 2

## Duct ectasia

Mammary duct ectasia is subareolar duct dilatation without marked inflammation. The duct is filled with cellular and secretory debris. It affects older women and is more common in smokers. Clinical features of duct ectasia include nipple discharge (often green or multicoloured) and sometimes nipple retraction. Troublesome discharge can be treated with duct excision.

## 2.3 Breast pain

### In a nutshell ...

Breast pain (mastalgia) may be cyclical or non-cyclical, unilateral or bilateral. It may originate within the breast itself or from the chest wall. It is a very common cause for referral, occurring at some point in up to 70% of women usually between the ages of 30 and 50.

### Cyclical mastalgia

Cyclical breast pain is usually seen in premenopausal women and may be associated with the benign lumps and nodularity of fibrocystic breast disease. It may present in postmenopausal women on HRT. It tends to respond better to treatment than non-cyclical mastalgia.

### Aetiology of cyclical mastalgia

No clear cause has been identified, but it is hormonally driven (trials have shown that it worsens with oestrogen-based HRT and improves with tamoxifen). Dietary deficiency in essential fatty acids has been suggested as a cause.

### Clinical features of cyclical mastalgia

- It usually affects the upper outer quadrant of the breast (as the breast is most glandular here)
- Usually bilateral, but may be unilateral or asymmetrical (ie worse on one side)
- Pain occurs 3–7 days before menstruation
- There is lumpiness, fullness and heaviness of the breast
- Symptoms improve after menstruation

### Treatment of cyclical mastalgia

- Explanation and reassurance
- Supportive bra at night-time
- Topical NSAID (eg diclofenac gel) is generally effective and well tolerated
- Simple oral analgesics, especially NSAIDs (eg ibuprofen 400 mg three times daily)
- Decreasing caffeine intake helps in some cases
- Using the OCP may help
- **Gamma-linolenic acid (GLA) 240 mg/day** (taken as 3 g evening primrose oil per day) was traditionally recommended for cyclical breast pain. Evening primrose oil contains GLA among other essential fatty acids, and GLA was thought to inhibit prostaglandins that may mediate breast pain. Recent systematic reviews of trials have failed to prove its benefit over placebo, and for this reason its UK prescription licence has been withdrawn and it is no longer recommended. It is still available over the counter

In severe, resistant cases:
- **Bromocriptine** (a dopamine agonist) introduced slowly to a maximum dose of 2.5 mg twice daily. Suppresses prolactin. Also causes nausea, dizziness, constipation and postural hypotension. Can be stopped gradually after 3 months
- **Low-dose danazol** is effective but carries side effects including voice deepening, weight gain and menorrhagia. It has androgenic effects on the fetus so must not be taken if pregnancy is possible. It can be gradually reduced after 3 months
- **Tamoxifen** 10 mg/day on days 10–25 of the menstrual cycle is also effective in cyclical breast pain (unlicensed indication). Tamoxifen carries a risk of venous thromboembolism and endometrial cancer, and should not be taken for more than 6 months for breast pain. It can also have teratogenic effects

- **Luteinising hormone-releasing hormone (LHRH) analogue (gonadorelin)** injection may be used in resistant cases. Its side effects include hot flushes and decreased libido

## Outcomes for cyclical mastalgia

- Eighty per cent are managed with conservative measures and reassurance
- Of the residual 20%, 80% will have relief of symptoms after a course of drug treatment
- Cyclical mastalgia symptoms will get better after the menopause
- Surgery is not used to treat breast pain under any circumstances

## Non-cyclical mastalgia

Non-cyclical mastalgia tends to affect older women (mean age 43 years) and is less common than cyclical mastalgia. It is also harder to treat. A careful history and clinical examination are required to define the cause.

## Investigations

- Mammography for patients aged >35 years
- Ultrasonography of a focal tender area for patients of any age
- Any other investigation indicated by the history, site and pattern of symptoms to look for non-breast cause (see box below).

## Treatment of non-cyclical mastalgia

- Supportive bra or sports bra
- NSAIDs – topical and oral
- Avoid surgical intervention

---

**Causes of non-cyclical mastalgia**

Pain from within the breast:

- Infection (periductal mastitis)
- Sclerosing adenosis
- Trauma and fat necrosis with inflammation
- HRT (may give non-cyclical as well as 'cyclical' pattern symptoms)
- Tumour (uncommonly); usually causes a focal area of pain rather than diffuse breast pain
- Idiopathic – commonly no cause is found

Non-breast causes of pain:

- Musculoskeletal chest wall pain
- Tietze syndrome (tender costochondral junctions). Usually self-limiting and viral in origin
- Cervical and thoracic spondylosis
- Bornholm's disease or 'devil's grip' (Cocksackie B virus)
- Lung disease
- Gallstones
- Exogenous oestrogens such as HRT
- Thoracic outlet syndrome
- Reflux oesophagitis
- Cardiac pain

---

## 2.4 Breast infection and abscess

Mastitis may occur in early life (neonatal), during breastfeeding (puerperal) or in non-lactating women. It is important to exclude abscess formation by imaging and the surrounding cellulitis must be distinguished clinically from inflammatory cancer.

### Mastitis neonatorum

- Seen in the first few weeks of life
- Presents as an infected enlarged breast bud
- Bacteria include *Staphylococcus aureus* and *Escherichia coli*
- Treatment with antibiotics (rarely needs incision and drainage)

### Puerperal mastitis and lactating breast abscess

Mastitis affects up to 30% of breastfeeding mothers, but fewer than 1 in 10 of these develop an abscess. Infection is usually seen in the first 6 weeks of breastfeeding. It can be severe and cause septicaemia. It arises when cracks in the nipple act as a port of entry for bacteria (usually *S. aureus*, *S. epidermidis* or streptococci).

### Clinical features of puerperal mastitis

- Pain, tenderness, erythema
- Swelling, fluctuance if abscess present
- Systemic symptoms of fever, rigors, malaise

### Treatment of lactating breast abscess

Traditionally, lactational breast abscess was treated with open incision and drainage, and placement of a wound drain under general anaesthetic. This is no longer appropriate because it is rarely necessary and can leave a disfiguring scar, as well as increasing the incidence of mammary duct fistula. Poor management of breast sepsis is an increasing reason for litigation:

- Antibiotics: flucloxacillin or co-amoxiclav (use erythromycin if penicillin-allergic). Avoid tetracycline, ciprofloxacin and chloramphenicol in breastfeeding patients
- Encourage emptying of the breast by continuing breastfeeding and/or use of a breast pump
- Simple analgesia and cold compress for pain
- Ultrasonography if abscess suspected and where mastitis does not settle after a course of antibiotics
- Aspiration of abscess under ultrasound guidance, with irrigation of sterile saline and local anaesthetic into the cavity, provides immediate relief and can be repeated at intervals of 2–3 days until resolved (send sample to microbiology for culture and sensitivity [C&S])
- If overlying skin is thin or necrotic, 'mini'-incision and drainage (I&D; through a very small incision) followed by regular irrigation at intervals of 2–3 days (again, send sample for C&S)
- Consider underlying diagnosis of inflammatory carcinoma if there is no response to treatment. Mammography, ultrasonography and core biopsy should be considered

## Non-lactating breast infection and abscess

Non-lactating breast abscesses can be periareolar or peripheral.

### Periareolar mastitis and abscess

- Periareolar infection is seen in women with an average age of 35
- More than 90% of patients are smokers
- Clinical features: periareolar inflammation (can be an associated lump); nipple discharge (yellow); nipple retraction
- Investigation: triple assessment
- Treatment: antibiotics; needle aspiration; subareolar duct excision if recurrent, although this carries a risk of creating mammary duct fistula
- Stop smoking

### Peripheral non-lactating breast abscess

- Associated with diabetes, rheumatoid arthritis, steroids, trauma, granulomatous lobular mastitis (rare recurrent peripheral abscesses in younger women)
- Commonly caused by *S. aureus*
- Treatment: antibiotics; aspiration or mini-I&D

Follow-up at breast clinic advisable for mammogram and clinical examination to ensure no remaining lump – to avoid missing underlying cancer.

### Mammary duct fistula

- Communication between a subareolar breast duct and the periareolar skin
- Complication of periareolar infection (usually non-lactational but may also complicate lactational breast abscess)
- Inadequate drainage (eg blockage of distal duct to nipple) leads to fistula formation
- Can occur after incision and drainage of a breast abscess, which creates a track to the skin
- Usually associated with a mixture of Gram-negative and Gram-positive, aerobic and anaerobic organisms
- Treatment is by excision of the diseased duct under antibiotic cover (in lactational abscess, once the infection has cleared mammary duct fistula may close spontaneously if there is no distal obstruction of the duct)
- Must stop smoking
- Total duct excision (Hadfield's procedure) can be considered

# SECTION 3

# Breast cancer

## 3.1 Breast cancer epidemiology

Breast cancer accounts for 31% of all new cancers in women in the UK. Its incidence is increasing, with the annual number of new cases in the UK having doubled between 1979 and 2008. The lifetime risk of developing breast cancer in UK women is 1 in 8, and 80% of these are diagnosed in women aged 50 or over.

Breast cancer is common in western Europe, but less so in Africa and Asia. Lifestyle and environment are strongly implicated, evidenced by higher rates of breast cancer in Asian immigrants to the west.

## 3.2 Pathology and classification

The histological changes from normal to malignancy represent a spectrum of cellular changes and there may be pathological debate about where hyperplasia with atypia ends and carcinoma in situ begins:

- Premalignant change: epithelial hyperplasia (ductal or lobular) with atypia

- Carcinoma in situ
  - Ductal carcinoma in situ (DCIS) – common
  - Lobular carcinoma in situ (LCIS) – less common, and not regarded as a cancer despite the name)
  - Cribriform subtype of DCIS (can also become invasive) – shows characteristic spaces between groups of tumour cells giving a 'Swiss cheese' appearance
- Invasive breast cancer:
  - Invasive ductal carcinoma (80%)
  - Invasive lobular carcinoma (15%)
  - Inflammatory breast cancer – poorly differentiated
  - Malignant phyllodes tumour
  - Rarer subtypes of invasive ductal carcinoma:
    - Mucoid carcinoma
    - Medullary carcinoma
    - Papillary carcinoma
    - Tubular carcinoma

## In a nutshell ...

**Classifying breast cancer**

Breast cancers may be classified by:
- Histopathological type
- Grade of cellular differentiation (1–3)
- TNM stage
- Receptor status (oestrogen, proges-terone and Herceptin)
- Pre- or postmenopausal

# Epithelial hyperplasia with atypia

Epithelial hyperplasia is a benign proliferative breast disease that falls into the spectrum of fibrocystic breast disease, with an increase in the number of cells lining the terminal lobular unit. It usually presents as a screen-detected mammographic lesion rather than as a lump. Simple hyperplasia carries no significant increased risk of breast cancer, but where cellular atypia is present there is a four to five times increased risk. Severely atypical epithelial hyperplasia is on a continuum with low-grade DCIS and LCIS and it can be difficult to distinguish histologically between atypical hyperplasia and carcinoma in situ.

Atypical hyperplasia, combined with a known family history of breast cancer, carries up to a 10 times increase in the risk of breast cancer, so family history follow-up and even risk-reducing surgery may be considered in this group.

# Carcinoma in situ

Carcinoma in situ is a proliferation of malignant cells that have not breached the basement membrane of the duct and do not therefore metastasise. The most common type in breast is DCIS, characterised by malignant cells in the ducts and ductules of the breast without invasion.

# Ductal carcinoma in situ

DCIS is a premalignant condition: forms the 'malignant' end of the spectrum with epithelial hyperplasia. More common in older women, DCIS has the same patient age group as invasive ductal cancer. It has increased in prevalence (from 2% to 30% of breast cancers) due to increased detection by mammographic screening.

DCIS is thought to be a precursor to invasive disease, with a latent period of usually more than 5 years. Follow-up of DCIS recurrence after excision in one of the EORTC (European Organisation for Research and Treatment of Cancer) trials shows similar biological profiles (grade and receptor expression) between the original DCIS and the recurrence, even when recurrence presents as invasive disease.

## Clinical features

DCIS may present as a palpable mass but is more commonly detected on mammographic screening. It accounts for 25% of all screen-detected cancer. It is confined within the ducts and so exhibits a typically branching structure, which may be more extensive than initial imaging suggests. Characteristic pleomorphic microcal-cifications may be seen on mammography. Often no abnormality is seen on ultrasonography and it is not always seen on MRI.

## Classification

DCIS is classified as low, intermediate or high grade. High-grade lesions are more likely to recur. The presence of large cells with pleomorphic nuclei and luminal necrosis is called 'comedo necrosis' and carries a worse prognosis.

## Treatment of DCIS

- **Wide local excision (WLE)** with 2-mm clear margins. Some units advocate the use of further cavity shavings (biopsies taken from the residual cavity) when excising DCIS. This is because the branching structure can make completeness of excision difficult to confirm and cavity biopsies randomly sample the surrounding breast region for more extensive disease
- **Consider adjuvant radiotherapy** after WLE, especially if lesion is large and/or high grade (studies have shown that this leads to a reduced rate of recurrence)
- **Mastectomy if DCIS is widespread** (>4 cm), multifocal or central. The introduction of oncoplastic reshaping techniques means that larger areas can be resected from the moderate or large breast and the upper limit of 4 cm may no longer lead to mandatory mastectomy
- **Consider sentinel node biopsy** if mastectomy being performed for large or multifocal high-grade DCIS, as foci of invasive carcinoma may well be found subsequently in the mastectomy specimen
- **Consider using adjuvant tamoxifen** for groups at higher risk of recurrence and in the premenopausal (the NSABP [National Surgical Adjuvant Breast and Bowel Project] B-24 trial showed decrease of 40% in recurrence in women aged <50 years using tamoxifen after resection)

## Lobular carcinoma in situ

Note that LCIS is not thought to be malignant (and is a misnomer) but it is a **marker of increased risk of breast cancer in either breast**.

LCIS develops in the acini of the lobules and, when the cells become very pleomorphic and abnormal, it is difficult to distinguish histologically from high-grade DCIS. It is often an incidental finding on histology because it is impalpable. It is often radiologically occult but may demonstrate calcification or architectural distortion. Often multifocal and can be bilateral in up to 50% of cases; most common in premenopausal women but rare in elderly women.

### LCIS as a marker of risk

- The detection of LCIS associated with radiological abnormality increases the risk of discovering a synchronous breast cancer to 30%
- The detection of LCIS without radiological abnormality (usually incidentally) acts as a predictor of risk for the development of a metachronous breast cancer. Approximately 30% of patients with incidental LCIS will develop invasive breast cancer: 20% of patients in the ipsilateral breast, 15% in the contralateral breast. There is a lag period of approximately 15 years to the development of a cancer. Subsequent invasive cancer can be either lobular or ductal
- The risk of developing a subsequent breast cancer is even higher if there is also a family history of breast cancer

### Management of LCIS

Management should be based on the individual risk and age of the patient. LCIS is a marker of increased risk but there is a lag to the development of subsequent cancer. Most young patients are placed under mammographic surveillance but this is probably not necessary in elderly women. If there is an additional family history, then the risk to the individual is significantly higher and risk-reducing mastectomy might be considered.

## Invasive carcinoma

### Invasive ductal carcinoma (IDC)

Macroscopically, invasive ductal breast cancers have a hard consistency and can contain areas of white necrosis and calcification. Subtypes of invasive ductal carcinoma include:

- **No specific type** – 80% of invasive breast cancers are invasive ductal carcinomas of 'no special type', or 'not otherwise specified' (NST or NOS)
- **Medullary ductal carcinoma** – this type of cancer is rare (3–5%). The tumour usually shows up on a mammogram and it does not always feel like a lump; rather it can feel like a spongy change of breast tissue. Often sizable (5–10 cm) but associated with a better overall prognosis than common invasive ductal cancers
- **Mucinous ductal carcinoma** – this occurs when cancer cells within the breast produce mucus. It is also called colloid carcinoma and is seen in 1–2% of cases. Pure mucinous ductal carcinoma carries a better prognosis than more common types of IDCs
- **Papillary ductal carcinoma** – this cancer looks like tiny fingers under the microscope. It is only in rare cases that this kind of cancer becomes invasive. Common among women aged 50 and older, this kind of cancer is treated like DCIS, despite being an invasive cancer
- **Tubular ductal carcinoma** – this is a rare diagnosis of IDC (2%). Tubular ductal carcinoma is more common in women >50 and is usually a small, oestrogen-receptor-positive cancer. The name comes from how the cancer looks under the microscope – like hundreds of tiny tubes

Although the breast is composed of both lobular and ductal elements, most breast cancer arises as an adenocarcinoma in the ductal elements. Malignant ductal cells are often dispersed within the fibrous stroma, leading to the appellation of scirrhous carcinoma. There are distinct histological criteria for classifying the subtypes of IDCs outlined above; these criteria must be met throughout the entire tumour. Histologically pure examples of these variant tumours are associated with a better long-term survival than ordinary-type IDC but, if the histology is mixed, the prognosis is similar to that of a non-specific IDC.

Invasive disease may coexist with areas of DCIS. This is not prognostically significant but may jeopardize the attempts at breast conservation as extensive DCIS may cover a wide area of the breast.

### Invasive lobular carcinoma

Invasive lobular carcinoma (ILC) arises from the lobular component of the breast and in most series accounts for approximately 10% of breast cancers. ILCs tend to be very poorly circumscribed and may feel less discrete than IDCs. They are characterised histologically by an 'Indian file' pattern – a single line of neoplastic cells within a fibrous stroma – or a 'bull's eye' pattern – neoplastic cells align around a normal acini. They are more likely to be mammographically occult than ductal carcinoma.

ILC is associated with a higher incidence of bilateral breast cancer reflected in almost every published series. The contralateral breast is involved either synchronously (3% of patients) or metachronously in up to 30% of patients.

CHAPTER 2

## Inflammatory breast cancer

Locally advanced breast cancer where invasion of the dermal lymphatics causes a warm, oedematous, erythematous breast is called inflammatory cancer. It can sometimes be clinically difficult to distinguish from cellulitis. It is usually treated by primary chemotherapy and then mastectomy and axillary clearance. It has a poor prognosis.

## Other cancers

Lymphomas, angiosarcomas (after radiotherapy) and metastasis from other cancers may also affect the breast.

## 3.3    Risk factors for breast cancer

### Risk factors for breast cancer

Most breast cancers occur in women with no specific risk factors. These are sporadic. However, calculating risk enables us to select the most appropriate management for each individual:
- Age and gender
- Genetics: personal and family history of breast or ovarian cancer (BRCA, TP53)
- Exposure to oestrogens:
  - Endogenous oestrogen: ages at menarche and menopause, timing and number of pregnancies, breastfeeding
  - Exogenous oestrogens: OCP or HRT use, obesity, lifestyle factors

## Age and gender

Incidence of breast cancer increases with age. Male breast cancer is uncommon and should prompt genetic investigation (<1% of all diagnoses).

## Personal and family history

### Personal history

Personal history of a risk lesion such as LCIS increases risk of synchronous or metachronous breast cancer as discussed above. The risks of tumour recurrence or new disease after a personal history of breast cancer or DCIS depend on the biology of the original cancer, as discussed below.

### Family history of breast cancer

The genetic risk of a breast cancer can be considered in terms of the genes that cause breast cancer which we know about and can test (eg BRCA, TP53) and the genes that cause breast cancer which we have not yet identified.

Five per cent of breast cancers are due to autosomal dominant high-penetrance genes and 20% of breast cancers in patients aged <30 are due to mutations in BRCA-1, BRCA-2 or TP53. BRCA genes are DNA-mismatch repair genes and are implicated in the development of breast and ovarian cancers.

**BRCA-1** (long arm of chromosome 17: autosomal dominant, associated with female breast cancer, ovarian cancer, prostate and colon cancer) – these breast cancers are generally high grade and oestrogen receptor/progesterone receptor (ER/PR) negative, with a well-circumscribed oval or round appearance.

**BRCA-2** (long arm of chromosome 13; associated with male and female breast cancer and also with ovarian cancer) – less well defined than BRCA-1 tumours and more commonly lobular in nature.

The lifetime risk of developing breast cancer in a BRCA-1 carrier is 70% and in BRCA-2 carriers the risk is 55%.

The lifetime risk of developing ovarian cancer in a *BRCA-1* carrier is 30–60% and in *BRCA-2* carriers the risk is 10–30%.

Mutation carriers who have developed a breast cancer have a 50% risk of developing a contralateral cancer.

Families with four or more members with early onset or bilateral cancers have a 50% chance of carrying a mutation in the *BRCA* genes. There are founder mutations in some ethnic groups, eg *BRCA-1* or *BRCA-2* gene mutations are carried by 1 in 40 Ashkenazi Jewish women.

## Other known mutations that increase breast cancer risk

- **Li–Fraumeni syndrome** (autosomal dominant mutation of gene on short arm of chromosome 17 that encodes for the tumour suppressor protein p53)
- **Peutz–Jeghers syndrome** (mutation of tumour-suppressor gene on chromosome 19)
- **Cowden syndrome** – multiple hamartomas

The importance of family history also lies in identifying those families who clearly carry an as yet unidentified gene mutation that puts them at increased risk.

---

### Which patients should be referred to a genetics clinic for breast cancer family history risk assessment?

Is there at least one of the following present in the family history? A tick in any box indicates requirement for genetics referral.

**If there are only female breast cancers in family:**
- Two first- or second-degree relatives* diagnosed before age 50 ☐
- Three first- or second-degree relatives* diagnosed before age 60 ☐
- Four relatives* diagnosed at any age ☐

*At least one must be a first-degree relative of the consultee.

**If there is a history of ovarian cancer in the family:**
One relative diagnosed with ovarian cancer at any age **and** on the same side of the family there is:
- One first- (including relative with ovarian cancer) or one second-degree relative diagnosed with breast cancer before age 50 ☐
- One additional relative diagnosed with ovarian cancer at any age ☐
- Two first- or second-degree relatives diagnosed with breast cancer before average age 60 ☐

**If there is a history of bilateral breast cancer in the family:**
- One first-degree relative with cancer diagnosed in both breasts before age 50 ☐
- One first- or second-degree relative diagnosed with bilateral breast cancer and one first- or second-degree relative diagnosed with breast cancer before average age 60 ☐

**If there is a history of male breast cancer in the family:**
One male breast cancer at any age **and** on the same side of the family there is:
- One first- or second-degree relative diagnosed with breast cancer before age 50 ☐
- Two first- or second-degree relatives diagnosed with breast cancer before average age 60 ☐

**CHAPTER 2**

## Management of genetic risk

Patients are assessed at a family history clinic and stratified into low-risk (same as general population), moderate-risk and high-risk categories. If the family history suggests a genetic mutation, specific genetic investigation may be offered. Not all mutations can be identified.

Patients in moderate- and high-risk groups are screened regularly. The approach varies throughout the country, but in general these patients should have annual examination and mammograms from age 35 (with annual examination starting younger if the family history includes a case under this age). Some women with dense breast tissue or under the age of 35 may be screened using MRI.

Some patients in high-risk groups, especially those with an identified mutation, may wish to consider bilateral risk-reducing mastectomy, with or without immediate breast reconstruction. This can be appropriate in carefully selected patients under the care of a multidisciplinary team.

## Oestrogen exposure

Incidence of breast cancer correlates with lifetime oestrogen exposure which may come from endogenous or exogenous sources.

### Endogenous oestrogens
- **Long reproductive life**, ie early menarche (<12) and/or late menopause (>50)
- **Late first pregnancy**/nulliparity

### Exogenous oestrogens
- **OCP:** associated with a small increase in incidence until the pill is stopped for 10 years

- **HRT:** The Women's Health Initiative and the Million Women Study are two large randomised controlled trials that have reported on the safety of HRT. Combined HRT preparations (oestrogen and progesterone) increase the risk of breast, ovarian and endometrial cancers, stroke and thromboembolic disease. The increased risk of breast cancer is apparent 1–2 years after starting HRT and 10 years of treatment results in an increase of 19 breast cancers per 1000 women. HRT does reduce the risk of osteoporosis and colorectal cancers. Women on HRT should attend their screening mammography and should be aware of the risks of long-term treatment
- **Lifestyle factors:** obesity, alcohol consumption and physical inactivity contribute to elevated levels of circulating oestrogen

## Environmental factors

### Irradiation
Multiple chest radiographs before age 30, and chest irradiation for Hodgkin's lymphoma. Women who had chest irradiation to treat Hodgkin's lymphoma as children/teenagers should enter a screening programme of annual examination and mammography similar to that for family history screening.

### Shift working
Night-shift workers have lower melatonin levels than the general population, and there is some evidence that low melatonin is associated with an increased breast cancer risk.

### Smoking
Unlike most cancers, smoking has not been conclusively proved to increase breast cancer risk.

## 3.4   Diagnosis of breast cancer

**Presenting signs and symptoms of breast cancer**

**Lump:**
- Breast lump – generally hard, irregular and non-tender, may be fixed to skin/muscle
- Axillary lump (primary tumour or lymphadenopathy)
- Infra-/supraclavicular lymphadenopathy

**Skin changes:**
- Skin tethering (where the ligaments of Astley Cooper are involved)
- Skin dimpling: peau d'orange – localised skin oedema
- Skin ulceration

**Nipple changes:**
- New nipple inversion
- Paget's disease of the nipple
- Bloodstained nipple discharge

**Pain** – rare, usually focal point rather than generalised

Swollen, painful, inflamed breast – inflammatory cancer (rare)

**Late presentation with metastases:**
- Weight loss
- Liver enlargement/ascites/jaundice
- Malignant pleural effusion
- Bone pain/pathological fracture
- Skin deposits
- Distant lymphadenopathy

**Asymptomatic presentation via screening**

## 3.5   Prognostic features and staging in breast cancer

**Prognostic features in breast cancer**

The most important indicators of prognosis in breast cancer are:
- Size of the primary tumour
- Tumour grade
- Nodal status

The Nottingham Prognostic Index (NPI) incorporates these three biological factors to score prognosis.

Tumour size and nodal status are also incorporated into all tumour staging systems.

Other prognostic indicators are:
- ER status (ER positive correlates with favourable prognosis)
- Her-2 status (poorer prognosis)
- Lymphovascular invasion (indicates poorer prognosis if present)

The **NPI scoring system** has been verified prospectively in a number of other centres and is widely used.

---

NPI = (0.2 × tumour size in centimetres) + tumour grade + lymph node status

Size is in centimetres, tumour grade is 1, 2 or 3. Lymph node status is:

1 if no nodes are involved
2 if 1–3 lymph nodes are involved
3 if ≥4 lymph nodes are involved

---

Patients with a high NPI score have a good prognosis (80% 15-year survival rate) and those with a low NPI score have a poor prognosis (13% 15-year survival rate). The NPI score is also useful to help predict which patients will benefit from chemotherapy.

### Tumour size

Tumour size reflects rapidity of growth and likelihood of vascular invasion and nodal spread.

### Grading breast cancer

Invasive ductal carcinomas are graded from I to III according to the degree of glandular formation, the degree of nuclear pleomorphism and the mitotic frequency (Bloom and Richardson grading system):

Grade I: well differentiated (better prognosis)
Grade II: moderately differentiated
Grade III: poorly differentiated (worse prognosis)

The grade is given based on the characteristics of the whole tumour and some pathologists will not assess grade on a core biopsy because more poorly differentiated areas may be found on resection of the tumour, effectively upgrading it. Grade III tumours are more likely to recur and more likely to metastasise.

## Staging the disease

Staging considers the extent of local (tumour), regional (lymph nodes) and distant disease (metastasis).

### Assessing local involvement: staging the tumour

Locally advanced tumours may be assessed by CT or MRI to exclude invasion of the chest wall.

### Assessing nodal involvement: staging the axilla

Axillary surgery is performed for two reasons:
* To stage the axilla (important for selection of adjuvant therapy, providing prognostic information and providing feedback on screening programmes)
* To treat axillary disease. Treatment aims are to achieve local disease control and prevent future recurrence. Clearance does not necessarily improve survival

Involvement of the axillary nodes may be identified by clinical examination or by imaging. The NICE guidelines of 2009 recommend that all patients with early breast cancer should have ultrasound evaluation of the axilla. Abnormal looking nodes should be biopsied under ultrasound guidance and the patient should proceed directly to axillary clearance if these biopsies are positive. If ultrasonography of the axilla is negative then the patient should have a sentinel node biopsy. Bear in mind that axillary ultrasonography is only 40–50% accurate at detecting positive axillary nodes.

## Sentinel node biopsy

The principles of a sentinel node biopsy are that all lymphatic drainage from the breast converges in the subareolar plexus and drains from here to the axillary and internal mammary nodes. There are a small group of nodes, the 'sentinel' nodes, that are the first to receive the lymphatics. There may be anywhere between one and seven sentinel nodes. Identification and removal of these nodes for histopathological examination indicates whether the tumour has spread to the axilla.

The nodes are identified by co-localisation of two techniques. First a technetium-99-labelled colloid solution is injected into the subareolar plexus. These large particles are carried to the sentinel node and trapped in its cellular filter. A hand-held gamma probe is used intraoperatively to locate the radiolabelled node(s). A second subareolar injection of blue dye (commonly Blue Patent V, unlicensed) is given in theatre. These small dye molecules travel quickly to the nodes and the blue colour is easily visualised against the yellow fat of the axilla. Axillary dissection can then be targeted by the sound of the gamma probe and colour of the target nodes.

The ALMANAC trial compared sentinel node biopsy with axillary clearance, and showed that sentinel node biopsy was safe and accurate, and caused less postoperative morbidity than the traditional treatment. Sentinel node biopsy is now the gold standard for staging the axilla.

---

 **Op box: Sentinel node biopsy**

**Obtain informed consent**, explaining procedure fully to patient – remember to warn her that she may still require axillary clearance later if the sentinel node is positive. Also warn patient (and relatives) that she may have a greyish hue to her skin on the evening of surgery, that her urine will be bright green for a day or so, and that the blue 'tattooing' of the breast may take more than 4–6 months to fade completely.

**Preop:** arrange subareolar injection of radioisotope by nuclear medicine. Under general anaesthesia inject 1–2 ml Blue Patent dye into the subareolar plexus (ask for anaesthetic consent before doing this because it can cause an artificial drop in the $O_2$ sats reading, and there is a very rare incidence of anaphylaxis).

**Positioning:** with patient supine, arm abducted at 90°, prep and drape the breast and axilla.

**Procedure:** use a hand-held Geiger counter to pinpoint the likely location of the first sentinel node in the axilla and make a small (2–3 cm) incision over this – ideally at the inferior edge of the axillary hairline. Try to place the incision in a sensible location to facilitate an axillary clearance should it be necessary in the future and don't extend it anteriorly over the border of pectoralis major.

Dissect down using the Geiger counter to guide direction – keep dissection and tissue handling to a minimum to avoid making subsequent axillary clearance difficult. If a blue lymphatic channel is found, follow this carefully because it may lead you to the sentinel node.

**continued oveleaf**

Excise each radioactive and/or blue-stained node until no further significant radioactivity is detected in the axilla – there may be one node only, or several. Use the Geiger counter to check that no lower nodes (ie nodes within the lower axilla or axillary tail of the breast) have been missed.

Close the wound with a subcuticular suture. No drain is needed.

Send the specimen to pathology (ideally fresh, or in formalin at the request of the pathologist).

### Assessing the node

Methods for rapid assessment of the sentinel node while the patient remains under anaesthesia include frozen section, touch imprint cytology and, more recently, the development of a machine based in theatre that uses a molecular biological technique (real-time polymerase chain reaction [PCR]) to identify cancer cells in the node tissue. Most centres do not have access to these facilities and, should the node prove positive on routine histopathology, the patient returns for an axillary clearance at a later date. In addition, frozen section has a high false-negative rate.

### What if the sentinel node is positive?

The current NICE recommendation (2009) is that patients with a positive sentinel node should undergo axillary clearance. This has become hotly controversial with the publication of the Z11 trial in New York, which randomised patients who were having wide local excisions for small cancers but who had a positive sentinel node to

clearance or no clearance. They demonstrated that the group who did not get an axillary clearance did not have a higher incidence of axillary or distant recurrence after 6 years of follow-up despite having a positive sentinel node. Some centres give axillary radiotherapy for a positive node rather than doing an axillary clearance, but there is little evidence to justify this approach at present. Axillary clearance can give further prognostic information as the proportion of nodes involved influences outcome. Clearance also aims to provide local disease control and so will be discussed further in the treatment section.

### Assessing distant disease: staging the spread

Locally advanced cancers and node-positive disease should prompt assessment of the likelihood of distant metastasis. CT and bone scanning are commonly employed to look for distant metastatic disease.

**TNM classification of breast cancer**

This is a means of formalising the stage of disease and allows comparison between patient groups and different centres.

Tis     carcinoma in situ
T1      primary tumour <2 cm
T2      2–5 cm
T3      >5 cm
T4      involving chest wall or skin
N0      no nodes involved
N1      palpable mobile ipsilateral axillary node involved
N2      fixed ipsilateral axillary node involved
N3      involved ipsilateral internal mammary node
M0      no distant metastases
M1      distant metastases, including distant involved nodes, eg supraclavicular or contralateral

**UICC staging**

Stage I      – tumour <2 cm, axillary node negative
Stage II     – tumour <2 cm, axillary node-positive and axillary node-negative tumours >2 cm
Stage III    – tumours of all sizes with positive axillary lymph nodes (matted together with extranodal spread)
             – tumours fixed to the skin or muscles of the chest wall
             – tumours with positive supraclavicular or internal mammary artery nodes
Stage IV     – metastatic disease

## Hormone receptor status

The expression of oestrogen receptor (ER) and, less frequently, progesterone receptor (PR) on the tumour should be measured routinely. These are nuclear steroid receptors identified by immunohistochemistry (the Allred score 0–8 quantifies the number of ER-positive cells and how strongly the receptor is expressed). There is a close relationship between ER status and nuclear grade. ER-positive tumours have a 75% chance of responding well to reduction in hormone levels (by tamoxifen or aromatase inhibitor).

## Her-2 status

The Her-2 protein is a growth factor receptor. Its levels in the tumour can be measured using immunohistochemistry and clarified using a gene amplification technique called fluorescence in situ hybridisation (FISH). Her-2-positive cancers that are node-positive have a poorer clinical outcome. Her-2-positive cancers do respond to chemotherapy and the development of the monoclonal antibody Herceptin has improved outcomes in this group.

## Lymphovascular invasion (LVI)

The direct invasion of tumour cells into vascular and lymphatic channels has a poorer prognosis because it correlates with node positivity and distant metastasis.

## 3.6    Treatment of breast cancer

### The multidisciplinary team meeting

All patients diagnosed with breast cancer should have their primary and adjuvant treatment discussed at a multidisciplinary team (MDT) meeting. Decisions about the most appropriate treatment are highly individualised and take into account: size and location of tumour relative to breast size, tumour stage, patient age and comorbid states, patient treatment preferences.

The MDT ideally consists of: surgeon (breast and plastics or oncoplastic breast surgeon), oncologist, radiologist, pathologist and specialist breast care nurse.

MDTs participate in clinical governance by recording details of all breast cancers for the regional managed clinical network for breast cancer. These networks contribute to the national cancer registry and statistics.

---

**Planning treatment**

It is helpful to think of planning treatment for each individual in a set way so that you don't miss an important aspect of her treatment. For example, in terms of:

**The breast:**
- Is the primary tumour operable?
- Is the patient fit for surgery?
- Is this patient suitable for breast conservation or does she need a mastectomy?
- In the event of mastectomy does she want to consider breast reconstruction?

**The axilla:**
- Is the axilla involved?
- Is the axilla operable?
- What does the ultrasonography ± biopsy show?
- Does this patient need a sentinel node biopsy for staging or a direct axillary clearance for disease control?

**Distant disease:**
- Is this advanced disease with distant spread?

**Adjuvant therapies:**
- Hormones:
  - Is the tumour ER-positive? If yes, is the patient pre- or postmenopausal?
- Radiotherapy:
  - Does the patient need adjuvant radiotherapy?
- Chemotherapy:
  - Would the patient benefit from chemotherapy?

---

# 3.6.1 Surgery to the breast

### In a nutshell ...

**Surgery for breast cancer**
Surgery is the first-line treatment for breast cancer. Breast conservation is often preferable but is not suitable for everyone.
**Breast conservation:** wide local excision, oncoplastic resection
**Mastectomy:** simple mastectomy, skin-sparing mastectomy, nipple-sparing mastectomy (envelope mastectomy)
**Reconstruction:**
* Timing → none, immediate, delayed
* Type → autologous tissue, implant-based

## Breast-conserving surgery

The advantages of breast-conserving surgery are: improved cosmesis, lower psychological morbidity and smaller procedure.

Although disease recurrence rates are slightly higher with breast-conserving surgery and mastectomy, there are no survival differences between the two techniques (note that this is true only if the patient has adjuvant radiotherapy after breast conservation; without adjuvant radiotherapy after breast-conserving surgery the recurrence rate is higher).

The most important factor to minimise disease recurrence is to achieve clear surgical margins. The only absolute indication for mastectomy is the inability to achieve clear margins with breast-conserving surgery. Failure to achieve clear margins (1 mm for invasive disease and 2 mm for DCIS) should prompt re-excision or completion mastectomy.

### Relative contraindications to breast-conserving surgery (and relative indications for mastectomy)

These indications are not absolute. The introduction of oncoplastic techniques has allowed the resection of larger volumes of breast tissue while still preserving an acceptable cosmetic result.
* Patient choice
* Large tumour (>4 cm), or high tumour:breast volume ratio (results in inability to preserve cosmesis due to resection of high proportion of the breast)
* Multifocal cancer or DCIS
* Centrally situated tumour (if the nipple must be removed to excise the tumour, it can be difficult to achieve a satisfactory cosmetic result with breast-conserving surgery although parenchymal rearrangement makes this easier to achieve)
* Male breast cancer
* Local recurrence after previous breast-conserving surgery
* If patient cannot receive adjuvant radiotherapy after wide local excision, eg due to previous irradiation
* Although older patients may be more willing to undergo mastectomy, age is not a criterion in deciding for/against breast-conserving surgery

### Important things to remember about breast-conserving surgery

Excision of more than 10% of the breast tissue results in a worse cosmetic result. Larger resections require rearrangement of the breast parenchyma.

Try to excise a cancer with a cuff of about 1 cm surrounding tissue. Most surgeons extend the posterior margin down to the pectoral fascia unless the lesion is very superficial.

Try to place the scar in a cosmetically acceptable place (eg circumareolar, inframammary fold) but, remember, the most important thing is to get the cancer out with clear margins!

---

 **Op box: Wide local excision of a breast cancer**

**Obtain informed consent:** ensure that the patient understands the procedure, the risks of bleeding, infection, requirement for re-excision in the event of involved margins, potential for change in breast shape and unpredictability of scarring.

**Preop:** make sure that the lesion is easily identifiable and palpable and corresponds to the lesion that has been biopsied for histopathology. Check the path report yourself. If it is difficult to feel the lesion, or it has been identified at screening and is impalpable, ask the radiologist to insert a guidewire into or bracketing the lesion.

**Procedure:** try to place your incision in a cosmetically forgiving place. Excise the cancer with a 1-cm cuff of normal tissue down to the pectoral fascia and orient the specimen with sutures or clips for the pathologist. Take a radiograph of the specimen if using a wire to guide excision or if there is concern as to the margin status of the excision. Additional cavity biopsies can be taken to assess disease extent (may be useful in DCIS). Mark the extent of the cavity with metal ligaclips to aid the radiologist in giving a radiotherapy boost to the tumour bed. Mobilise the skin flaps and parenchyma sufficiently to completely close the defect and oppose the breast tissue; otherwise it will form an unsightly depression after radiotherapy. Meticulous haemostasis is required. Close the skin with a subcuticular stitch.

---

## Mastectomy

**Simple mastectomy:** removal of breast tissue and its axillary tail with an ellipse of overlying skin including the nipple (no axillary surgery).

**Skin-sparing mastectomy:** removal of the breast and NAC through a periareolar incision.

**Subcutaneous mastectomy:** removal of breast tissue with skin and nipple left intact. This might be done for prophylactic bilateral mastectomy in high-risk patients with simultaneous reconstruction.

**Radical mastectomy:** removal of the breast tissue, overlying skin, nipple, pectoralis muscles and axillary contents.

**Modified radical mastectomy** (more commonly described as a simple mastectomy plus axillary clearance): removal of the breast tissue, overlying skin, nipple and full axillary clearance, but preserving the pectoralis muscles and their overlying fascia. This is a common operation in the UK.

**Patey modification of the radical mastectomy:** as for modified radical mastectomy but including division of pectoralis minor to assist with access to the axilla.

# Op box: Simple mastectomy

**Preop:** histology, radiology and clinical examination must have been discussed at an MDT meeting and the MDT decision of mastectomy must be documented. Patient must be fully consented and counselled, preferably with the help of a trained breast care nurse. Correct side must be marked.

**Position:** supine with ipsilateral arm abducted to 90° on an arm board, the surgeon must always examine the breast before incision. The arm should be prepped and wrapped so that it can be repositioned if necessary for axillary procedure.

**Incision:** incisions must be carefully planned to allow skin flaps to close neatly, but without tension. The incision is an ellipse centred along a line lying transversely across the chest (nipple and the areola lie within the ellipse). Priority is adequate clearance, so the incision must be away from any obvious tumour, even if this compromises closure.

**Procedure:** skin incision is deepened and a superior and inferior skin flap is raised following the mastectomy plane between subcutaneous fat and breast tissue, which is seen as a white line when tissues are placed under tension. There is no correct thickness for the flap; each patient is individual and the flap may not be of an even thickness. In young women breast tissue may reach the skin. Care must be taken to ensure that there is no breast tissue left on the flap but that the vascularity of the flaps is not compromised by cutting them too thinly. At the periphery of the breast take care to avoid dividing all the perforators that exit the chest wall and perfuse the skin. Dissect the breast free of the pectoral fascia, removing any portion of the pectoralis muscle that is involved by the tumour if necessary. The dissection of the axillary tail can be extended into the axilla if a clearance is indicated and the tissues removed en bloc.

A long non-absorbable tie should mark the highest extent of your axillary dissection on the specimen to orient it, or the breast should be marked with a recognised pattern of silk sutures prearranged with your pathologist. Insert fine suction drains to axilla and chest wound and ensure meticulous haemostasis because a large cavity can fill quickly with blood when there is no tamponade by surrounding tissues.

Close the dermis of the skin with 2.0 Vicryl and the epidermis with a subcuticular stitch. Avoid tension.

**Postop:** mobilise patient within 24 hours; remove drains when <40 ml approximately is drained in 24 hours after the first postoperative day (local surgeon preference applies). Early shoulder physiotherapy to prevent frozen shoulder.

Before discharge advise about prostheses, future reconstruction and follow-up appointments (preferably with the help of a trained breast care nurse).

Clinic appointment within 2 weeks to discuss histology and adjuvant therapy.

**Operative hazards:** flap necrosis from damage to perforating vessels medially and laterally or very thin dissection or tension. Button-hole damage to skin.

**Complications:** haematoma, seroma (may need aspirating), psychological trauma due to loss of breast and scarring, disease recurrence.

## 3.6.2 Surgery to the axilla

Nodal involvement in the axilla detected by ultrasonography and biopsy or after positive sentinel node biopsy (SNB) necessitates axillary clearance.

### Op box: Axillary clearance

**Obtain informed consent** including explanation of risks of lymphoedema, nerve damage, haematoma, seroma.

**Preop:** give antibiotics if there is already an axillary wound from previous SNB.

**Positioning:** supine with arm abducted at 90°. The arm may be draped separately to allow easier access to level 3 by rotation towards the patient's head.

**Procedure:** clearance can be completed through the lateral aspect of a mastectomy wound, or through a 4- to 5-cm (approximately) horizontal incision at the inferior aspect of the axillary hairline. Do not divide any structures until the vital anatomy of the axillary vein, thoracodorsal pedicle and long thoracic nerve has been demonstrated. Dissect initially along the borders of the latissmus dorsi and pectoralis major until you reach and open the axillary fascia. The soft axillary fat may be swept from the vital structures using a pledget until they have all been accurately and confidently identified. The anterior thoracic vein and tributaries and intercostobrachial nerves may then be divided. The inter-nerve tissues between the thoracodorsal nerve and the long thoracic nerve should not be missed from the dissection. Be careful to include the lymph nodes at the lower limit of your dissection because this is often significantly lower than the level of your incision.

Traditional axillary lymph node clearance was described as level 1–3 as follows. This classi-fication is no longer commonly used in UK centres. If axillary clearance is required, all accessible axillary tissue and nodes are removed, without dividing pectoralis minor:

> Level 1: axillary tissue and lymph nodes up to lateral border of pectoralis minor
> Level 2: axillary tissue and nodes up to medial border of pectoralis minor (ie the level 2 nodes are those sited behind pectoralis minor)
> Level 3: removal of all axillary tissue including the level 3 nodes which lie medial to pectoralis minor (traditionally this was accomplished by division of pectoralis minor if required)

A drain is left in situ at the end of the procedure and kept in place for 1–4 days until the volume of serous fluid abates to <50 ml per 24 hours – similar to mastectomy drain.

**Intraoperative hazards:** axillary vein, thoracodorsal trunk and long thoracic nerve. Do not dissect above the vein because this is the territory of the brachial plexus.

**Complications of axillary clearance:** lymphoedema of arm and breast; shoulder stiffness; numbness of inner arm due to division of intercostobrachial nerve (often divided routinely); risk of damage to thoracodorsal nerve (to latissimus dorsi) and long thoracic nerve of Bell (to serratus anterior), medial and lateral pectoral nerves.

## 3.6.3 Additional therapies

### In a nutshell ...

**Additional therapies** include hormonal therapies (tamoxifen, aromatase inhibitors, LHRH agonists), ovarian ablation, radiotherapy and chemotherapy
**Neoadjuvant therapy** is given before definitive surgery
**Adjuvant therapy** is given after definitive surgery

## Hormonal manipulation

### Primary hormone therapy

Patients who are elderly or unsuitable for a general anaesthetic and who have ER-positive breast cancer can be treated by primary endocrine treatment. An aromatase inhibitor or tamoxifen given alone may control disease progression and can have dramatic effects in strongly ER-positive tumours.

### Adjuvant hormonal therapy

Both normal and malignant breast cells contain ERs, but some tumours have very low levels and are thus effectively ER-negative. The presence of ERs in a cancer provides a further therapeutic opportunity to try to improve outcomes.

Hormonal therapy decreases the risk of local, regional and distant recurrence of breast cancer. It also reduces the risk of developing a contralateral breast cancer. The two classes of anti-oestrogen drugs most commonly used are selective oestrogen receptor modulators or SERMs (eg tamoxifen) and aromatase inhibitors.

Other options to reduce circulating oestrogen levels include LHRH agonists and ovarian ablation.

**Tamoxifen:** tamoxifen is an SERM that blocks the actions of oestrogen by binding to the oestrogen receptor. It was the original first-line adjuvant hormone treatment for ER-positive cancers, and the trials in the 1960s showed decreased disease recurrence (by 25%) and breast cancer-related deaths (by 17%) after tamoxifen treatment.

It is the first-line treatment for ER-positive cancers in premenopausal women. Five years of adjuvant treatment is recommended after the NSABP B-14 trial showed an increase in endometrial cancer in patients on extended treatment for 10 years. It may also be used as neoadjuvant therapy to downstage ER-positive tumours.

**Side effects of tamoxifen** include:
- Hot flushes (common)
- Increased risk of thromboembolic disease
- Vaginal dryness (common)
- Weight gain (common)
- Increased risk of endometrial carcinoma (very rare)
- Cataract (very rare)

**Aromatase inhibitors (AIs):** aromatase is an enzyme that converts circulating androgens to oestrogen. This occurs in peripheral fatty tissues, and is virtually the only source of oestrogen in postmenopausal women. In premenopausal women, the ovaries are the main source of oestrogen, and in this group AIs are contraindicated because they cause gonadotropin-mediated up-regulation of ovarian oestrogen production.

CHAPTER 2

Types of AI:

- Anastrozole (Arimidex)
- Exemestane (Aromasin)
- Letrozole (Femara)

The ATAC trial found that anastrozole reduced recurrence in ER-positive postmenopausal cancers with fewer side effects than tamoxifen. In addition, the BIG 198 trial compared tamoxifen with letrozole, demonstrating improved patient survival in this group. AIs are therefore the treatment of choice in postmenopausal women with ER-positive cancers.

**Side effects of AIs:** osteoporosis.

**Goserelin (Zoladex) LHRH agonist:** goserelin can be given to premenopausal women to induce a reversible 'chemical' menopause. Some trials have shown it to be as effective as standard chemotherapy regimens but with fewer side effects in women with ER-positive tumours. In these women an aromatase inhibitor can also be prescribed.

**Ovarian ablation:** ovarian ablation by surgery, radiotherapy or drugs can be used in premenopausal women to reduce recurrence and mortality from ER-positive tumours.

## Radiotherapy

All patients who have had breast conservation require **adjuvant radiotherapy** (as the NSABP B-06 trial demonstrated a reduction in the local recurrence rate from 30% to 10.4% when adjuvant radiotherapy is given after breast conservation).

Adjuvant radiotherapy after excision of DCIS also decreases recurrence.

Typically a total dose of 50 Gy is given over a period of 4–5 weeks, starting 2–3 weeks postoperatively, with or without a 'boost' radiation dose to the site of the primary tumour.

**Chest wall radiotherapy** may also be offered after mastectomy to patients with a high risk of local recurrence, eg:

- Grade III cancers that are multifocal or near to skin or muscle
- Larger cancers >4 cm
- Presence of lymphovascular invasion on histology
- Three or more positive axillary lymph nodes

**Axillary radiotherapy** may be given as an alternative to performing axillary clearance for patients who have had a positive sentinel node biopsy, if surgery is not desired.

Axillary recurrence may also be treated with radiotherapy if there has been no previous axillary radiotherapy, and surgery is not appropriate.

---

**Complications of radiotherapy**

- **Local skin reactions** (often permanent, although may diminish over time): erythema; telangiectasia; thickening; oedema; skin necrosis; skin more prone to cellulitis
- **Osteonecrosis** and delayed rib fracture
- **Radiation damage to heart and lungs** (rare) but may account for increased deaths from other causes in large population studies
- **Lymphoedema** of the arm from axillary radiotherapy (especially when combined with axillary surgery)
- **Distortion to breast** with thickening of tissue
- **Encapsulation of implants** if present

## Chemotherapy

Chemotherapy may either attempt to be curative or be palliative. Neoadjuvant chemotherapy is as effective as adjuvant treatment. Adjuvant chemotherapy reduces mortality from breast cancer in both pre- and postmenopausal patients, in hormone-positive and -negative tumours, and in both node-positive and node-negative disease.

The reduction in the chances of recurrence conferred by chemotherapy is small but constant. Thus the benefit of chemotherapy is greater as the prognosis worsens. In better prognosis groups, the number needed to treat to achieve a survival benefit is much larger. As chemotherapy carries significant morbidity of its own, this must be taken into account when discussing the perceived benefits.

### Indications for chemotherapy

* Young/premenopausal
* Lymph node positive
* ER negative
* Grade III
* Large tumour
* Lymphovascular invasion

Neoadjuvant chemotherapy is given for two reasons, particularly to younger/fitter women with high-grade cancers: to monitor the response of the tumour to chemotherapy and to allow optimisation of the chemotherapy regimen (this would not be possible after the tumour is excised) and to reduce the size of a tumour to allow breast-conserving surgery rather than mastectomy. A small group of women will have disease progression while on neoadjuvant chemotherapy, however, and the prognosis for this group is very poor.

NICE guidelines recommend an anthracycline and taxane-based regimen given in five or six cycles with one cycle every 2–3 weeks.

**Side effects of chemotherapy** include:
* Fatigue
* Hair loss
* Nausea and vomiting
* Induction of menopause (and infertility)
* Increased susceptibility to infection (including life-threatening neutropenic sepsis)
* Weight gain
* Diarrhoea
* Cardiotoxicity and congestive cardiac failure with anthracycline chemotherapy

## 3.7 Follow-up for breast cancer patients

Follow-up regimens vary between centres. Many review their patients yearly but there is now a trend towards enrolling women in mammographic screening programmes and running open-access clinics for them to attend only if they have new concerns. The NICE guidelines recommend discharge from clinic after just 2 years of follow-up. This creates difficulties in auditing outcomes for the department as patients can be lost to follow-up.

Patients who have had breast cancer are at risk of local, regional and distant recurrence, and are also at increased risk (about 10%) of a further breast primary on the contralateral side.

## 3.8 Oncoplastic breast surgery

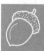 **In a nutshell ...**

**Oncoplastic breast surgery**
Oncoplastic surgery is the application of a range of plastic surgical techniques to the oncological resection of breast cancer. It includes techniques for parenchymal rearrangement after resection of large volumes of breast tissue, surgery to the contralateral breast to provide symmetry, and breast and nipple reconstruction.

## Oncoplastic remodelling for breast conservation

Techniques that have traditionally been employed for aesthetic breast reduction are capable of resecting large volumes of tissue from the breast while leaving a cosmetically acceptable result. There are numerous possibilities, allowing resection from any location within the breast. Examples include a Wise pattern skin reduction with inferior or superomedial pedicle carrying the nipple, Le Jour, Grissotti, Benelli, melon slice, tennis ball and dermoglandular rotation flaps.

Breast reduction in this context may also help delivery of a more even radiotherapy field to the treated breast. The disadvantage of these procedures is, however, that the original margins of the resection are often moved some distance from their original location by the rearrangement of the parenchyma. It is then very difficult to go back and excise an involved margin and difficult to explain where the obliterated cavity lies to the radiotherapist who wishes to give a boost of radiotherapy to the tumour bed. In addition the contralateral side usually requires surgery for symmetry.

## Breast reconstruction

The National Breast Reconstruction Audit and NICE guidelines suggest that reconstruction should be discussed with all patients who are undergoing mastectomy and are surgically fit.

Reconstruction can be performed as an immediate or as a delayed procedure using autologous tissues (myocutaneous or perforator flaps) or an implant-based technique.

Important considerations include the shape and size of the breast, body habitus and availability of autologous tissue (usually from the back or abdomen), and whether the patient will need adjuvant radiotherapy. Common donor sites for autologous tissue are the pedicled extended latissimus dorsi flap and free tissue transfer from the inferior epigastric artery perforator flap (DIEP). Autologous tissue is most resistant to radiotherapy damage and the latissimus dorsi flap is more resilient than free tissue transfer in this situation. There is a 75% capsular contracture rate for implant-based reconstructions that are subsequently irradiated. Some surgeons suggest delayed reconstruction if there is to be chest wall radiotherapy and the patient has insufficient tissue overlying latissimus dorsi to match the contralateral side. Implant reconstructions also require more maintenance surgery in the long term.

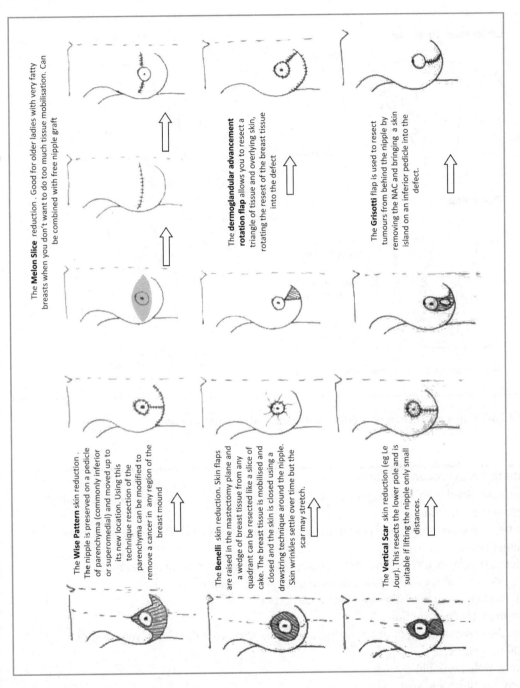

The **Melon Slice** reduction . Good for older ladies with very fatty breasts when you don't want to do too much tissue mobilisation. Can be combined with free nipple graft

The **dermoglandular advancement rotation flap** allows you to resect a triangle of tissue and overlying skin, rotating the resect of the breast tissue into the defect

The **Grisotti** flap is used to resect tumours from behind the nipple by removing the NAC and bringing a skin island on an inferior pedicle into the defect.

The **Wise Pattern** skin reduction . The nipple is preserved on a pedicle of parenchyma (commonly inferior or superomedial) and moved up to its new location. Using this technique resection of the parenchyma can be modified to remove a cancer in any region of the breast mound

The **Benelli** skin reduction. Skin flaps are raised in the mastectomy plane and a wedge of breast tissue from any quadrant can be resected like a slice of cake. The breast tissue is mobilised and closed and the skin is closed using a drawstring technique around the nipple. Skin wrinkles settle over time but the scar may stretch.

The **Vertical Scar** skin reduction (eg Le Jour). This resects the lower pole and is suitable if lifting the nipple only small distances.

**Figure 2.5: Oncoplastic techniques for resection.** You do not need to know these in detail for the exam, this diagram is simply to give you an idea of what can be achieved to improve cosmesis. If you see a cancer that lies in a cosmetically difficult place, like the lower pole, consider whether an oncoplastic procedure may be appropriate.

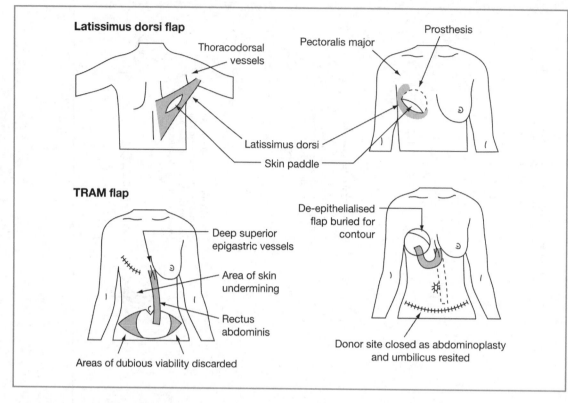

**Figure 2.6 Latissimus dorsi reconstruction and tram flap reconstruction**

---

**Immediate breast reconstruction**
- Often combined with a skin-sparing mastectomy to preserve the skin envelope; usually a single-stage procedure
- Can be a long procedure and postoperative complications can delay the delivery of adjuvant treatments
- Reduces psychological trauma of the change in body image after mastectomy
- No evidence that it increases rate of local or systemic relapse
- Radiotherapy and chemotherapy can be carried out

**Delayed breast reconstruction**
- Loses the cosmetic benefit of a skin-sparing mastectomy as more skin is removed during the initial procedure
- More widely available
- Needs a well-healed scar
- May utilise a two-stage reconstruction with expander, adjuvant treatment and then replacement of the expander with autologous tissue or an implant

**continued opposite**

## Tissue expansion
- Suitable if adequate skin flaps and good skin closure in small- to medium-sized breasts
- Silicone expander with a filler port is initially inserted (expander has saline injected weekly) under pectoralis major
- Should be over-expanded to produce ptosis
- Silicone expander is replaced with a permanent prosthesis, usually 6 months after surgery

## Implants
- Usually made of silicone or saline. New, anatomically shaped and textured implants offer much greater flexibility and improved cosmesis
- Complications of prostheses:
  - Fibrous capsules and contracture (reduced by textured prostheses)
  - Infection (5% of cases need removal; higher if radiotherapy given)
  - Implant rupture in 1% resulting in silicone leakage (contrary to media reports this has not been shown to increase incidence of carcinogenesis or autoimmune disorders)
  - Malposition

## Autologous tissues
- Preferable to expander-implant-based reconstruction where adjuvant radiotherapy is likely after mastectomy
- Suitable for importing a large volume of skin as well as breast volume, eg large skin defects or where there is doubtful skin closure and large breasts
- Used in delayed reconstruction if there has been previous radiotherapy
- May be combined with an implant under the flap to achieve adequate volume.
- Complications of myocutaneous flaps:
  - Flap necrosis
  - Infection
  - Abdominal hernias (in TRAM [transverse rectus abdominis myocutaneous] flaps)
  - Loss of entire flap
  - Donor site problems

## Nipple reconstruction
- Best done when the new breast mound is the correct size and shape (eg after 6 months)
- Nipple bud can be reconstructed using a local tissue flap, sharing the contralateral nipple or artificial adhesive nipple (worn for 1 month at a time)
- The pigmented areola is reproduced using a tattoo to match the contralateral side

## 3.9 Advanced breast cancer

Locally advanced breast cancer can represent either a primary tumour or a recurrence. Breast cancer that is locally advanced at presentation carries a poor prognosis. However, with modern oncology practice, patients with advanced, recurrent and indeed metastatic breast cancer may live for several years.

### Clinical features of locally advanced breast cancer

- Skin: tethering, ulceration, oedema (peau d'orange), erythema, 'satellite nodules' of tumour deposit on and around the breast
- Tumour fixed to skin or muscle
- Nipple retraction
- Palpable large, hard or fixed lymph nodes in axilla
- Infiltration of skin of chest, back and neck ('cancer en cuirasse')

### Treatment of locally advanced breast cancer

- Mastectomy (non-curative attempt to control ulceration/fungation; may require removal of a lot of skin and resurfacing of the chest wall with skin grafts or flaps)
- Radiotherapy (decreases bleeding from ulcerated tumour)
- Endocrine therapy if ER-positive (as effective as chemotherapy)
- Chemotherapy

### Recurrent and metastatic breast cancer

Breast cancer recurrence can be local (within the breast or on the chest wall), regional (involving the axilla or supraclavicular lymph nodes) or metastatic.

Of those who experience disease relapse, 50% do so in the first 2 years after primary treatment, and 85% within 5 years. However, breast cancer relapse can still occur after 10 years or more, although in these cases it can be difficult to separate diagnosis of relapse from a new primary cancer.

**Distant metastases** from breast cancer can involve the bones, liver, lungs, brain and adrenals, as well as non-regional lymphadenopathy, eg in neck or groin. The bones are the most frequent site for initial metastasis, followed by the lungs. Appropriate investigations for suspected metastatic disease include:

**Bone:** serum calcium and alkaline phosphatase, plain films, bone scan, MRI

**Liver:** liver function tests, ultrasonography, CT, aspiration of ascites for cytology, ultrasound/CT-guided liver biopsy

**Lung:** chest radiograph, CT, aspiration of pleural effusion for cytology

**Brain:** CT

Biopsy of any distant metastasis should be performed for confirmation, if the patient is well enough to be considered for further treatment. Once a patient has developed metastases her disease is probably incurable. Management may include hormonal therapy and chemotherapy.

**Palliation of symptoms** may additionally be achieved with:

- Blood transfusion for anaemia
- Bisphosphonates or radiotherapy for bone pain
- Orthopaedic fixation for pathological fractures
- Bisphosphonates for hypercalcaemia
- Pleurodesis for pleural effusion
- Analgesia

## 3.10 UK Breast Screening Programme

- The UK Breast Screening Programme started in the UK in 1988 following the Forrest Report and became fully operational in 1990
- Aims to reduce mortality from breast cancer by detecting and treating it early and before it has a chance to spread
- All women aged 50–70 are invited for mammography every 3 years (the upper age limit has recently increased from 65 years and it is planned to reduce the lower age limit to 47 years)
- Two-view mammography is performed on all screening visits
- Patients are recalled if an abnormality is detected and further imaging, FNA and/or core biopsy performed (under ultrasound or mammogram guidance if the lesion is impalpable)
- Compared with patients presenting with symptomatic cancers, breast screening tends to detect cancers that are smaller, less aggressive and node-negative. It is also more likely to detect in-situ disease (25% of screen-detected disease is DCIS)
- By the year 2003 the breast screening programme had detected 80 000 cancers, and it is estimated to save 300 lives per year

The drawbacks are anxiety (especially if the patient is recalled), increased radiation dose (although this is negligible) and unnecessary biopsy. It is also the case that in some patients the breastscreening programme detects disease (particularly in-situ disease) that would never have progressed to invasive cancer of any clinical significance. Treatment of screening-detected lesions in this group therefore causes morbidity by over-treatment.

**Interval cancers** – those that present symptomatically in the 3-year interval between breast screening visits – do occur (about 2.5 interval cancers occur in 3 years per 1000 women screened). Women in this group may also present later with symptoms, having been reassured by a normal result at their last screening appointment.

### Mammography screening

- NHS breast screening: from 50 years to 70 years. Two views every 3 years
- Moderate-risk family history: screening from 40 to 50 every year, then as for NHS Breast Screening Programme
- High-risk family history: screening from 30 to 50 every year, then as for NHS Breast Screening Programme

A Cochrane Review concluded that mammographic screening reduces the risk of dying of breast cancer by about 15%, at the expense of a 30% increase in diagnosis. About 2000 women need to be screened for 10 years to prevent a single death from breast cancer. Over the same period 10 women will be diagnosed with breast cancer that would otherwise have remained clinically occult, never to be diagnosed. However, despite the UK programme no consensus exists over the benefit of mammographic screening, and other analyses have concluded that mammography is more effective than the Cochrane review suggested, and these quote reductions in mortality of up to 35%. Across Europe and the USA no consensus exists on the age for starting screening or on frequency. Screening is therefore a topic of ongoing controversy.

# SECTION 4

# Male breast disease

## 4.1  Male breast cancer

Male breast cancer is rare. There are about 300 cases per year in the UK, mostly in men aged between 60 and 70.

**Risk factors:** bilateral testicular injury or bilateral undescended testis (cryptorchidism); Klinefelter syndrome (XXY karyotype causing hypogonadism, 50% increased risk of male breast cancer); irradiation; oestrogen exposure; *BRCA-1/-2*; cirrhosis; obesity.

Clinical presentation is similar to that of female breast cancer. Men should undergo triple assessment and MDT discussion in the same manner as women. Surgical treatment is mastectomy and axillary node clearance. Of male breast cancers 80% are ER/PR-positive and these patients are given adjuvant tamoxifen.

## 4.2  Gynaecomastia

Gynaecomastia is breast enlargement in males. It may be unilateral or bilateral, even where the cause is systemic (such as drug-related). It is almost always benign, and is usually reversible (although stopping the causative drug does not always lead to resolution).

Pathologically there is hyperplasia of the stromal and ductal tissue, usually due to increased circulating oestrogen and/or decreased testosterone.

Although gynaecomastia itself does not predispose to breast cancer, high levels of circulating oestrogens are associated with gynaecomastia and also predispose to male breast cancer.

### Investigation of gynaecomastia

- First exclude primary breast cancer and then identify the underlying cause if possible
- Careful history taking, including full drug history
- Examination of axillae and testes
- Complete triple assessment if discrete lump: ultrasonography or mammography; FNA/core biopsy
- Consider other imaging: testicular ultrasonography or chest radiograph
- Bloods (if any indication in history or examination that there may be a hormonal condition): U&Es, LFTs, TFTs, oestrogen, testosterone, FSH/LH, βhCG, α-fetoprotein, prolactin

## Treatment of gynaecomastia

- Treat the cause where possible
- Reassure – will often regress, especially pubertal gynaecomastia
- Drug treatment: danazol or tamoxifen
- Surgery (for cosmetic reasons): subcutaneous mastectomy (should be performed by experienced surgeon as good cosmesis can be difficult to achieve)

**Causes of gynaecomastia**

**Physiological**
- Neonatal, pubertal (juvenile), elderly

**Pathological**
- Liver cirrhosis (causes increased peripheral oestrogen synthesis)
- Hypogonadism (eg cryptorchidism, viral orchitis, Klinefelter syndrome)
- Renal failure and haemodialysis
- Hyper- and hypothyroidism
- Testicular tumour (eg oestrogen-secreting Leydig cell tumour)
- Lung tumour (eg human chorionic gonadotropin (hCG)-secreting lung tumours stimulate oestrogen secretion by testes)
- Adrenal tumours (may secrete oestrogen)
- Pituitary tumours (may secrete LH/FSH [follicle-stimulating hormone] or prolactin) can occur with acromegaly

**Drugs**
Most commonly, though by no means an exhaustive list:
- Cardiac: ACE (angiotensin-converting enzyme) inhibitors, $Ca^{2+}$ channel blockers, spirono-lactone, digoxin, amiodarone
- Anti-androgens, eg cyproterone for prostate cancer
- $H_2$-receptor antagonists/proton pump inhibitors (PPIs), eg cimetidine
- Antibiotics: metronidazole, ketoconazole
- Antiretrovirals
- Psychiatric/neurological: tricyclics, phenothiazines (eg chlorpromazine), methyldopa, diazepam
- Other: steroids, finasteride, metoclopramide

**Lifestyle**
- Anabolic steroids
- Cannabis
- Heroin
- Alcohol excess, particularly beer
- Obesity
- Lavender oil, tea tree oil topically

**Idiopathic**
- For many patients the cause is not identified

# SECTION 5

# Congenital and developmental breast abnormalities

Some breast asymmetry is normal.

**Amazia:** congenital absence of the breast.

**Athelia:** absence of a nipple (rare).

**Polythelia** – accessory nipple(s): these are found in 5% of the population and are twice as common in men as in women. These typically arise along the mammalian 'milk line' (from the embryological mammary ridge of the ectoderm) which runs from the axilla to the groin via the nipple on both sides.

**Polymastia** – presence of an accessory breast: also usually found along the milk line and can have an accessory nipple.

**Hypoplasia of breast:** the breast is absent but the nipple is present; 90% of patients have absent or hypoplastic pectoral muscles.

**Poland syndrome:** unilateral breast hypoplasia, absence of pectoralis major, shortening and webbing of the fingers on the ipsilateral side (brachysyndactyly), and sometimes other muscle, bone and organ deformities in the thorax, upper abdomen and upper limb. Males are more commonly affected, and the abnormal side is most commonly the right.

**Tubular breast** is a condition where constriction of the breast base results in long thin breasts with lower pole insufficiency and herniation of the tissue through the breast disc.

## Juvenile hypertrophy
- A disorder of breast development, with abnormal unilateral or bilateral breast enlargement in young women
- Prepubertal enlargement of one breast can occur and, if there are no other signs of sexual development, the patient can be reassured
- In most patients with juvenile hypertrophy, breast development begins in a normal fashion at puberty but uncontrolled growth then occurs and can be very rapid. It is not due to a hormonal abnormality
- Surgical breast reduction can be performed, but this should be delayed as long as possible (late teens, if possible) to allow complete breast development on both sides (the other breast may 'catch up', at least to some extent). If surgery is unavoidable, the patient should be fully counselled (ideally with parent/guardian if possible) about scarring, wound breakdown, asymmetry, risk of nipple loss, loss of nipple sensation and the possibility of being unable to breastfeed in the future. She should also be warned about the possibility of requiring further procedures for cosmesis/symmetry as she matures

# CHAPTER 3

# Cardiothoracic Surgery

**George Tse and Sai Prasad**

# SECTION 1

# Surgery for ischaemic heart disease

Ischaemic heart disease is one of the major causes of morbidity and mortality in the western world. Survival is slowly improving due to medical advances; however, worldwide prevalence is rapidly rising due to the westernisation of the developing world, with increased rates of diabetes, obesity and smoking. In the UK, 30% of patients who have a myocardial infarction (MI) never get to hospital.

## 1.1 Pathology of ischaemic heart disease

 **In a nutshell ...**

The majority of ischaemic heart disease is caused by atherosclerosis, with the steps of:
* Endothelial dysfunction
* Lipid accumulation (in subendothelial macrophages)
* Smooth muscle migration and fibroblast proliferation, resulting in intimal thickening
* Chronic inflammatory response, leading to calcification of the plaque

The vast majority of patients with coronary heart disease (CHD) have advancing occlusive coronary stenoses which, when sufficiently severe, erode the 'coronary reserve' and cause flow limitation on exercise, leading to exertional angina. Most myocardial infarctions (MIs) occur in the context of chronic atherosclerosis.

**Atherosclerosis** affects the epicardial vessels but not the intramyocardial coronary vessels (the proximal left anterior descending, circumflex and right coronary arteries are the worst affected). The internal thoracic (mammary) arteries (IMAs) are relatively spared from the disease and hence can be useful in revascularisation of the heart.

The pathological basis of atherosclerosis is still an area of research, but involves the following key steps:
* Endothelial cell injury and dysfunction due to several risk factors, most importantly hypertension, nicotine, immune mechanisms and hyperlipidaemia
* Low-density lipoprotein (LDL) accumulation form the plasma – plasma proteins carrying triglycerides and cholesterol. Leading to intimal thickening and atheroma formation
* Platelet adhesion to the surface of endothelial cells leading to microthrombi

formation and release of platelet-derived growth factor, which attracts monocytes to the area

- Low density lipoprotein (LDL) accumulation form the plasma – plasma proteins carrying triglycerides and cholesterol. Leading to intimal thickening and atheroma formation

- Monocytes/macrophages engulf cholesterol, becoming foam cells, and also secrete free radicals, which causes oxidation of circulating LDL

- Further oxidised LDL is taken up by macrophages via their scavenger receptors, leading to release of interleukin-1 (IL-1) and tumour necrosis factor (TNF), stimulating smooth muscle cell and fibroblast proliferation

- Fibroblasts lay down collagen and elastin which helps to form the mature athero-sclerotic plaque

- Smooth muscle cells migrate from the media to the intima and transform into secretory cells producing collagen, elastin and chemokines, which serve as important mediators of the process

- This chronic inflammatory response leads to calcification of the plaque

Initially, atherosclerotic plaques tend to bulge outwards and so the vascular lumen is maintained.

- Luminal loss of <50% can usually be tolerated without causing symptoms
- Obstruction of 75% is associated with exertional angina
- 90% stenosis causes angina at rest

In the progression of atherosclerotic plaques, there are two potential outcomes:

1. **Gradual progression of the plaque** causing increasing luminal stenosis and decreasing exercise tolerance

2. **Acute plaque rupture**, in which the endothelium becomes fissured, exposing the thrombogenic plaque contents (lipids, collagen and necrotic debris), and a clot forms on top of the plaque causing acute coronary obstruction, resulting in an 'acute coronary syndrome' (unstable angina, MI or acute coronary death)

The table opposite summarises the pathological and clinical features together with treatment options for stable and unstable angina and MI.

## 1.2 Indications for coronary artery revascularisation

 **In a nutshell ...**

When medical therapies are insufficient to adequately control angina symptoms, revascularisation may be attempted. This field is subject to rapid evolution as both percutaneous and surgical techniques improve.

As coronary vascular disease is primarily managed by cardiologists and **percutaneous coronary intervention** (PCI) has a lower risk of mortality and morbidity, surgery is largely offered when PCI options are exhausted. Hence the population undergoing **coronary artery bypass grafting** (CABG) is an older population, with more severe disease.

CHAPTER 3

## ISCHAEMIC HEART DISEASE: PATHOLOGY, CLINICAL FEATURES AND TREATMENT OF STABLE AND UNSTABLE ANGINA AND MYOCARDIAL INFARCTION

| Coronary syndrome | Stable angina | Unstable angina (crescendo angina, subendocardial infarction) | Myocardial infarction |
|---|---|---|---|
| **Pathology** | | | |
| Coronary | 'Fixed stenosis' Stable plaque | Acute plaque rupture or thrombosis | Acute plaque rupture or thrombosis |
| Myocardial | Reversible ischaemia | Reversible ischaemia or minor infarction in watershed areas, eg subendocardium | Full-thickness infarction |
| **Clinical features** | | | |
| Symptoms | Chest pain and shortness of breath on exertion Predictable exercise tolerance Symptoms relieved by nitrates and rest | Chest pain and shortness of breath on mild exertion Decreasing exercise tolerance Symptoms may or may not be relieved by rest or nitrates | Sudden death, 30 minutes of severe central chest pain and shortness of breath (except silent ischaemia, eg in diabetic patients) |
| ECG changes | ST depression in affected territory | ST depression in affected territory. May have deep T-wave inversion | ST elevation in affected territory, leading to Q waves |
| Enzyme rises | Nil | Rise of troponin I carries prognostic significance | Troponin I CK, LDH |
| Arrhythmias | Unlikely | VF or VT likely | VF or VT likely |
| **Management** | | | |
| Acute | GTN spray Rest | MONA (**m**orphine, **o**xygen, **n**itrates, **a**spirin) | MONA + clopidogrel |
| Medical | Aspirin Anti-angina agents: β Blockers Calcium channel blockers Long-acting nitrates Nicorandil Risk factor modification: Statin Stop smoking Control hypertension Lose weight Modify diet | Anticoagulation Enoxaparin Heparin infusion Abciximab GP IIb IIIa inhibitors Nitrates Nitrocine™ infusion GTN infusion Statin | PCI first line Thrombolysis if PCI not available within 90 minutes (streptokinase, rTPA) |
| PCI | If symptoms difficult to control medically | If anticoagulation and nitrates unsuccessful | First-line therapy |
| CABG | If anatomy unsuitable for PCI | If procedure unsafe for PCI | Rarely |

CABG, coronary artery bypass graft; GP, glycoprotein; GTN, glyceryl trinitrate; PCI, percutaneous coronary intervention; rTPA, recombinant tissue plasminogen activator; VF, ventricular fibrillation; VT, ventricular tachycardia.

CHAPTER 3

**Pros and cons of PCI and CABG**

|  | PCI | CABG |
|---|---|---|
| **Advantages** | Minimally invasive<br>Low morbidity<br>Acceptable to patients<br>Low immediate complication rates | Reliable revascularisation<br>Suitable for wide range of coronary lesions<br>Ability to perform simultaneous procedures, eg valve replacement |
| **Disadvantages** | Unsuitable for some coronary lesions (eg left main stem – LM)<br>Early re-occlusion of angioplasty sites and in-stent thrombosis<br>High rate of recurrence of symptoms<br>Poorer 'freedom from medication'<br>Requires cardiac surgical back-up in case of complications | Major procedure<br>Morbidity from sternotomy and conduit harvesting sites<br>Late graft failure (especially saphenous vein) |
| **Burgeoning technologies** | Drug-eluting stents<br>Wider range of suitable targets (LM) | Minimally invasive techniques<br>'Off-pump' techniques<br>Total arterial revascularisation |

# 1.3 Preoperative considerations and cardiac surgery

## In a nutshell ...

Usually performed in a pre-assessment clinic, preoperative work-up before cardiac surgery for ischaemic heart disease includes:
- History
- Examination
- Investigations
- Adjustment of medications
- Discussion of morbidity and mortality
- Discussion of treatment options

## History taking before cardiac surgery

Cardiac surgical procedures are major operations performed on patients who have high levels of comorbidity. Preoperative investigations allow physiological optimisation to reduce perioperative morbidity and mortality, either through alteration of medication or exclusion of other pathology. Therefore it is wise to see the patient in a pre-assessment clinic about 1 week before surgery.

CHAPTER 3

| The New York Heart Association (NYHA) SCORE | |
|---|---|
| **NYHA 1** | Patients with cardiac disease but without limitation of physical activity<br>Ordinary physical activity does not cause undue fatigue, palpitation or dyspnoea<br>Asymptomatic patients should be classified as class 1 |
| **NYHA 2** | Cardiac disease resulting in a slight limitation of physical activity<br>Patients are comfortable at rest<br>Ordinary physical activity results in fatigue, palpitations or dyspnoea |
| **NYHA 3** | Cardiac disease resulting in marked limitation of physical activity<br>Patients are comfortable at rest<br>Less than ordinary physical activity results in fatigue, palpitations or dyspnoea |
| **NYHA 4** | Cardiac disease resulting in an inability to conduct any physical activity without discomfort<br>Symptoms of cardiac failure may be present even at rest<br>If any physical activity is undertaken discomfort is increased |

**Things to think about when pre-assessing coronary cases**

- Higher rates of CVA due to smoking and other cardiovascular risk factors
- Higher risk of concurrent lung tumours or other neoplastic disease due to smoking
- Varicose veins (results in poor availability of conduit)
- Diabetes (exposes the patient to additional risk of infections at conduit harvesting sites and in the median sternotomy wound)

## Clinical examination before cardiac surgery

- Temperature (risk of endocarditis)
- Pulse and BP
- Auscultation of heart (valve disease)
- Auscultation of lungs (pneumonia, pulmonary oedema, chronic obstructive pulmonary disease [COPD])
- Examination of abdomen (aneurysmal disease)
- Neurology (documentation of preoperative function is very important in case of perioperative cerebrovascular accident [CVA])
- Carotids (carotid stenosis increases risk of CVA; patients with bruits need a duplex scan, and may require preoperative endarterectomy)
- For CABG, examination of lower limbs for varicose veins or examination and marking of radial artery
- Allen's test for harvesting radial artery for grafting (adequacy of ulnar collateral circulation)

## Investigations before cardiac surgery

### For diagnosis

- Coronary angiography for those undergoing CABG, and those with risk factors undergoing valve replacement who would benefit from surgical revascularisation during the same sitting
- Right heart catheterisation for complex valve and congenital cases

### For preoperative work-up

- ECG
- Chest radiograph for cardiac shadow, comorbid lung pathologies, and for comparison with postoperative films
- Lateral chest radiograph for re-do procedures to assess distance between front of right ventricle and back of sternum

403

- Pulmonary function tests (PFTs) to assess pulmonary reserve and ability to survive procedure
- Urea and electrolytes (U&Es)
- Full blood count (FBC)
- Glucose
- Coagulation screen (although this does not detect for effects of antiplatelet medications)
- Cross-match 4 units of packed cells for most procedures
- MRSA (meticillin-resistant *Staphyloccus aureus*) swabs

## Adjustment of medications before cardiac surgery

### Warfarin

Warfarin may need to be suspended for 72 hours, depending on the indication for its use. Patients may require systemic heparinisation where there is a high risk of clot formation (eg on an older-generation prosthetic valve).

### Platelet antagonists (coronary cases)

- **Aspirin:** cyclo-oxygenase (COX) inhibitor inhibits thromboxane $A_2$ production from arachidonic acid
- **Clopidogrel:** platelet ADP-receptor antagonist
- **Abciximab (and similar drugs):** infusible glycoprotein (GP) IIb and IIIa inhibitors

Oral antiplatelet drugs impair platelet function for the life of the platelet, whereas most infusible preparations have a half-life of hours, so, for platelet function to recover, it is conventional to stop oral medications 7 days preoperatively. Controversy persists over whether it is appropriate to stop platelet antagonists perioperatively, and unit policies differ on this issue; there is no doubt that aspirin increases rate of bleeding, but stopping it may cause a higher rate of acute coronary syndromes in the week

preceding surgery. Clopidogrel should be discontinued 5 days prior to surgery.

### ACE inhibitors

Angiotensin-converting enzyme (ACE) inhibitors are critical for long-term benefit in cardiac disease. However, patients treated with ACE inhibitors may experience severe perioperative vasodilation, which requires correction with vasoconstrictors. Occasionally it is not possible to salvage these patients, even with high doses of noradrenaline. Most units stop ACE inhibitors 1 week preoperatively.

## Discussion of surgical mortality and morbidity with patients and their families before cardiac surgery

Cardiac surgical procedures carry the risk of a wide range of complications and mortality. Most patients are terrified of dying from their surgery. Skill and thought are required to impart information about mortality and morbidity while simultaneously providing reassurance.

When a patient does die during surgery, remember that it is the relatives who are left behind (and who take legal action). It is wise to include them in discussions of perioperative risk.

The 1% rule is often used to decide which complications should be discussed with patients preoperatively in obtaining informed consent, although this is controversial.
- CVA: about 1% depending on risk factors
- Perioperative MI: 1% depending on risk factors
- Prolonged ventilation: 1% depending on risk factors
- Risk of re-intervention for bleeding: 2–6%
- AF: 25–40%

| EuroSCORE (Additive: percentage risk of mortality is given by the total of scores) | | |
|---|---|---|
| **Patient-related factors** | | **Score** |
| Age | Per 5 years or part thereof over 60 years | 1 |
| Sex | Female | 1 |
| Chronic pulmonary disease | Long-term use of bronchodilators or steroids for lung disease | 1 |
| Extracardiac arteriopathy | Any one or more of the following: claudication, carotid occlusion or >50% stenosis, previous or planned intervention on the abdominal aorta, limb arteries or carotids | 2 |
| Neurological dysfunctional disease | Severely affecting ambulation or day-to-day functioning | 2 |
| Previous cardiac surgery | Requiring opening of the pericardium | 3 |
| Serum creatinine | >200 µmol/l preoperatively | 2 |
| Active endocarditis | Patient still under antibiotic treatment for endocarditis at the time of surgery | 3 |
| Critical preop state | Any one or more of the following: VT or VF or aborted sudden death, preoperative cardiac massage, preop ventilation before arrival in the anaesthetic room, preop inotropic support, intra-aortic balloon counterpulsation, or preop ARF (anuria or oliguria < 10 ml/h) | 3 |
| **Cardiac-related factors** | | **Score** |
| Unstable angina | Rest angina requiring IV nitrates until arrival in the anaesthetic room | 2 |
| LV dysfunction | Moderate or LVEF 30–50% | 1 |
| | Poor or LVEF <30% | 3 |
| Recent MI | <90 days | 2 |
| Pulmonary hypertension | Systolic PA pressure >60 mmHg | 2 |
| **Operation-related factors** | | **Score** |
| Emergency | Carried out on referral before the beginning of the next working day | 2 |
| Other than isolated CABG | Major cardiac procedure other than or in addition to CABG | 2 |
| Surgery on thoracic aorta | For disorder of ascending arch or descending aorta | 3 |
| Post-infarct septal rupture | | 4 |

ARF, acute renal failure; LV, left ventricle; LVEF, left ventricular ejection fraction; PA, pulmonary artery.

- Overall infection risk 1–30%
- Wound infection: 1–10% depending on risk factors
- Other risks with respect to the individual patient

Scoring systems have been devised to estimate the risk of perioperative mortality for individual patients. The most commonly used is the logistic EuroSCORE (European System for Cardiac Operative Risk Evaluation).

## 1.4 Intraoperative considerations during cardiac surgery

### Anaesthesia

- Avoid respiratory depression
- Give regular medications on the morning of surgery (unless adjusted preoperatively – see above)
- Keep haemodynamics stable – avoid myocardial depression and increased afterload

### Patient monitoring

- **ECG:** checks for arrhythmias, ischaemia, confirms cardioplegia and pacing
- **Normal ventilatory monitoring:** pulse oximetry and end-tidal $CO_2$
- **Arterial line:** this monitors BP, allows regular blood gas measurement postoperatively. May need femoral line if peripheral vasospasm occurs due to core cooling
- **Pulmonary artery catheter (Swan–Ganz):** this is used to measure left ventricular preload and cardiac output
- **Core temperature measurement:** tympanic, oesophageal or rectal probes assess the adequacy of organ protection during hypothermic cardiopulmonary bypass. Nasopharyngeal for brain temperature
- **Intraoperative transoesophageal echocardiography (TOE):** this evaluates cardiac wall and valve function. Checks for air bubbles after cardiac closure and can monitor cardiac output

### Antibiotic prophylaxis

This is used for Gram-positive bacteria in normal cardiomyotomy cases, and for Gram-positive and Gram-negative bacteria in immunocompromised patients. Cefuroxime IV in 3 doses is the most commonly used antibiotic.

### Patient positioning

The patient should be supine for median sternotomy with chest and both groins prepped in case an intra-aortic balloon pump or femoral bypass is needed. Both legs and arms need to be prepped if harvesting is being done. Non-dominant arm is prepped if radial artery harvesting is planned.

## 1.5 The median sternotomy incision

 **In a nutshell ...**

This is the most frequently used approach to the heart. It offers excellent access to the epicardial coronary arteries, the ascending aorta, aortic valve, and mitral valve. Exposure of the pulmonary hila is much more limited, so it is not the incision of choice for lung surgery (see Figure 3.12).

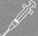

## Procedure box: Median sternotomy

**Position**
- Patient is placed supine on the operating table, with the neck extended

**Preop**
- Assessment and preparation as in Section 1.3
- Skin is prepared with iodine, and draped to expose the chest, abdomen and both groins
- Careful sterile technique is essential to avoid sternal osteomyelitis

**Incision**
- Incise from 2 cm below the sternal notch to the xiphoid, and deepen the incision through the fat using diathermy

**Procedure**
- Identify the midline by palpation of the intercostal spaces on each side. Mark it with diathermy
- When the midline is confidently identified mark the periosteum with diathermy
- Divide the suprasternal ligament with diathermy, taking care not to injure the underlying right brachiocephalic artery or the left brachiocephalic vein
- Divide the xiphoid with scissors, and finger-sweep the pericardium from the posterior surface of the sternum
- Use a pneumatic reciprocating saw to cut through the bone from one end to the other
- Retract the sternum using a sternal retractor. Haemostasis must be meticulous at this stage, because the patient will be anticoagulated on cardiopulmonary bypass (CPB). Bleeding from the marrow must be stopped with wax, and small bleeding points elsewhere controlled with diathermy
- Identify the midline of the thymus and sweep its two lobes to the sides
- Divide the pericardial fat and identify the brachiocephalic vein, taking great care not to injure it
- Open the pericardium with scissors between two pairs of forceps, to see the heart
- Place stay sutures in the pericardium to lift the heart into easier view

## Sternal closure

- Ensure excellent haemostasis within the chest
- Place drains as appropriate in the pericardium, right and left pleurae
- Steel wires or heavy sutures are placed through the sternum or the intercostal spaces and brought out anteriorly
- When wires are placed in the intercostal spaces, great care must be taken to avoid injuring the IMAs, which can bleed sufficiently to cause cardiac tamponade
- It is also essential to avoid injuring the coronary vein or IMA grafts that have been placed intraoperatively
- Haemostasis is rechecked, taking particular care over the entry points of the wires into the sternum
- The wires are twisted until they are sufficiently tight; the long ends are cut off and buried under subcutaneous fat
- The tissues are closed in layers

**CHAPTER 3**

## Complications of median sternotomy

- **Immediate complications:** vessel injury or chamber injury with the saw in redo cases (eg to right ventricle, or to the brachiocephalic artery and vein)
- **Late/delayed complications**
  - Sternal dehiscence
  - Sternal osteomyelitis or mediastinitis
  - Wire sinuses

## 1.6    Cardiopulmonary bypass

### In a nutshell ...

The first successful operation using CPB was performed in 1953. The introduction and development of this technique underpin all cardiac surgery. Over the last 30 years, CPB has made possible many cardiac surgical procedures that were previously unthinkable. It aims to divert the flow of blood away from the heart and lungs, while maintaining oxygen delivery to the rest of the body (See Figure 3.1). At first glance, the mass of pipes and pumps constituting a bypass circuit is overwhelming, so it is helpful to consider what the system aims to achieve:

- Pumping to replace the heart
- Oxygenation and $CO_2$ extraction to replace the lungs
- Total systemic cooling to reduce tissue $O_2$ consumption
- A bloodless field in which to operate
- A still heart on which to operate

## Components of the CPB circuit

In order to achieve the above aims, the CPB circuit consists of the following components:
- Venous cannula (sucks blood from the heart as it arrives)
- Venous reservoir
- Heat exchanger (cools and heats the blood)
- Pump
- Membrane oxygenator
- Aortic pipe (through which blood flows back into the arterial tree after oxygenation)

In addition, the circuit also contains:
- Cardiotomy suction: to recover 'spilt' blood from the surgical field back to the circuit
- Cardioplegia delivery: of cold blood with high potassium concentration to arrest the heart

It is necessary to anticoagulate patients with heparin to prevent clot formation within the circuit. Anticoagulation is reversed at the end of bypass using protamine.

## Physiological conditions of CPB

Most routine adult cardiac surgical procedures (eg CABG, atrial valve replacement, mitral valve replacement) are performed under the following conditions:
- **Non-pulsatile flow:** with a mean perfusion pressure of about 60 mmHg
- **Systemic cooling:** this is to about 30°–32°C. For more prolonged surgery it is possible to cool the circulation further. At very low temperatures surgery can be performed under **total circulatory arrest** (eg for aortic surgery)

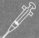

## Procedure box: Cannulation for cardiopulmonary bypass

### Aortic cannula
- A double purse-string suture is placed in the aortic root and rubber 'snuggers' are fitted. The stitches should penetrate the adventitia and muscularis layers of the aortic wall, but should not go full thickness because this can cause bleeding
- With a finger in place to prevent a fountain of blood, the aorta is incised with a pointed blade
- The clamped aortic cannula is placed into the hole; the 'snuggers' are tightened to keep it in place, and the whole assembly (cannula plus snuggers) is tied together to prevent slippage
- The cannula is connected to the bypass circuit very carefully to avoid bubbles that would cause CVA
- The whole assembly is fixed firmly in place, sometimes by sewing to the skin, to prevent any possibility whatsoever of it being pulled out

### Venous cannula
- A purse-string suture is placed in the right atrium
- An incision is made to admit the cannula
- A two-stage venous cannula is placed with its orifices in the right atrium and the inferior vena cava (IVC)

### Cardioplegia cannula
- This is normally placed in the aortic root, proximal to the aortic cross-clamp
- When the clamp has been applied, cardioplegia will be confined by the aortic valve and flow into the coronary orifices
- Alternative techniques are required when the aortic valve is incompetent

### Other cannulas
- Other cannulas (eg vents) may be required, such as a transmitral left ventricular (LV) vent in aortic valve replacement

CHAPTER 3

## Cardioplegia

The aims of cardioplegia are:
- Maintenance of a still surgical field
- Maintenance of myocardial energy stores by abolition of myocardial contraction

Cardioplegia achieves this by:
- Use of high-potassium cold cardioplegia solution which provokes cardiac arrest and minimises myocardial oxygen utilisation

The CPB circuit provides cold-blood cardioplegia.

## De-airing

When cardiac chambers are opened, air is entrained into the circulation. If that air travels to the brain, a CVA will ensue. Similarly, air in the coronary arteries can cause arrhythmias and MI, leading to cardiogenic shock. For this reason, de-airing is an important component of many cardiac procedures.

De-airing is performed from the **highest point** in any given chamber. It is performed **before removal of the aortic cross-clamp.**

Typical sites for de-airing include the aortic root, from a small needle placed in coronary bypass grafts, or with a large needle from the LV apex. The precise de-airing procedure depends on the exact operation that has been performed.

---

**Complications of cardiopulmonary bypass**

CPB may cause a host of complications, a few of which are listed here.

- **Coagulopathy** can result from platelet dysfunction and high doses of heparin and protamine
- **Inflammatory activation and vasodilatation** may result from exposure to 'foreign material' in the form of silicone tubing
- **CVA** can result from air embolus or dislodgement of calcium from the aortic cannulation site
- **Bleeding** can arise postoperatively from the various cannulation sites. It is worsened by coagulopathy
- **Cardiogenic shock** can result from failure of the patient's heart to resume an adequate cardiac output at the end of surgery, or from a sustained dysrhythmia (eg VF), or from cerebral dysfunction
- **Cognitive performance is impaired** transiently or permanently. It can result from microemboli and inflammatory activation

---

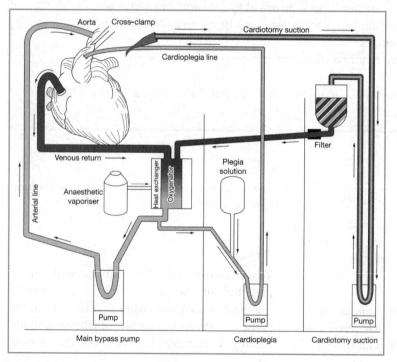

**Figure 3.1 Basic cardio-pulmonary bypass (CPB) circuit**

## Off-pump surgery

As a consequence of the wealth of complications arising from CPB, coronary artery bypass surgery is now sometimes performed on the beating heart using a stabilisation device. This surgery is more technically demanding than 'on-pump' surgery, and there is still strong debate about whether or not it is safer than conventional surgery or whether anastomotic patency is compromised.

## Intra-aortic balloon pump

This is indicated:

- Preoperatively for poor cardiac output or critical coronary stenosis
- Postoperatively when poor haemodynamics are seen or anticipated

### Suck and blow

The balloon is inserted via the femoral artery in the groin and is placed in the descending aorta. The balloon inflates in diastole, and deflates during systole.

- **Suck:** by deflating in systole a potential space is created in the aorta, decreasing the afterload (the pressure against which the ventricle must eject). This decreases myocardial work
- **Blow:** by inflating in diastole the balloon augments maximum diastolic pressure. This specifically increases coronary perfusion, which only occurs in diastole

## 1.7 Cardiac surgery procedures for ischaemic heart disease

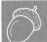

**In a nutshell ...**

For CABG surgery blood is diverted from the aorta or major division back to a coronary artery distal to the stenosis. There are two major divisions

1. Using harvested artery or vein anastomosed from the ascending aorta to a coronary vessel
2. Using an IMA and diverting flow by ligating the musculophrenic artery and anastomosing to a coronary artery

### Coronary artery bypass grafting

Coronary 'targets' are identified by coronary angiography, and a surgical strategy regarding on-pump or off-pump and the conduits is devised.

A 'standard' triple bypass involves grafting:

- The left internal mammary artery (LIMA) to the left anterior descending (LAD) artery
- A portion of the harvested long saphenous vein from the aorta to the circumflex artery
- A portion of the harvested long saphenous vein from the aorta to the distal right coronary artery

Recently, saphenous vein grafts are being replaced with radial artery grafts.

CHAPTER 3

## Principles of coronary artery bypass grafting

- The usual incision is a median sternotomy, although 'minimally invasive' procedures are sometimes performed via left anterolateral thoracotomy
- The IMAs are usually harvested before opening the pericardium
- The pericardium is opened, and stay sutures placed in order to lift the heart forwards
- The heart is cannulated for CPB in the standard way (see previous procedure box)
- CPB is initiated, an aortic cross-clamp applied and cardioplegia administered to stop the heart
- Previously planned coronary 'targets' are identified by direct examination of the coronary arteries
- Bottom-end anastomoses: conduits are anastomosed end to side on to the coronary targets using continuous 6/0 or 7/0 Prolene sutures. It helps to wear loupes for this procedure
- The aortic cross-clamp is removed, the heart rewarmed and weaned from bypass
- Top-end anastomoses: with the heart now beating, a side-biting clamp is applied to the ascending aorta and circular punches taken from it, to which the 'top ends' of the vein grafts are anastomosed
- De-airing: a small needle is placed into the grafts to enable trapped air to escape in order to prevent air-embolic MI
- Protamine is given and the heart decannulated
- Drains are placed in the pericardium, and the pleurae if open
- The median sternotomy is closed in the standard fashion, taking care to avoid entrapment of the new grafts

## Saphenous vein harvest

The long saphenous vein runs from anterior to the medial malleolus to its junction with the femoral vein in the groin.

The key surgical landmarks for saphenous vein harvesting are:
- **At the ankle:** the vein is immediately anterior to the medial malleolus. As it runs superiorly, in its first few centimetres, it becomes more posterior such that, at 5 cm above the superior margin of the medial malleolus, the vein lies at the midpoint of the medial malleolus in the anteroposterior (AP) plane

- **At the knee:** the vein lies approximately one handbreadth posterior to the medial border of the patella
- **At the groin:** the vein lies 1 cm medial to the midinguinal point

As the vein contains valves, when harvesting conduit it is essential to mark its ends so that it can be oriented correctly for blood to flow to the coronary anastomosis.

## Procedure box: Saphenous vein harvest

Make a small incision 5 cm proximal to the medial malleolus and at its midpoint in the AP plane (ideally, the incision is made after palpation of the vein, but this is not always possible); take great care not to puncture the vein itself with the skin incision.

Having identified the vein, extend the incision with scissors proximally up the leg; take care not to create a large flap of devitalised skin, which will increase the risk of wound infection. The amount of vein harvested will vary with the operative strategy. A rule of thumb is that one graft requires one scissor-length of vein. This may need to be altered if the heart is dilated. Bear in mind that the vein shrinks in length when harvested.

- Carefully dissect off the fine layer of fascia overlying the vein
- Carefully ligate each and every vein branch, however small, with fine silk (remember that ligatures will soon be exposed to arterial pressures)
- Handle vein graft very carefully throughout to avoid spasm
- When the required length has been exposed, and its branches divided, cannulate the distal end with a Hamilton–Bailey cannula (and tie it into place)
- Clamp the proximal end and excise the vein
- Flush the vein with heparinised blood
- Double-ligate the two vein ends remaining in the leg
- Close soft tissues in layers to obliterate dead space (can accommodate haematoma and lead to wound infections)

**CHAPTER 3**

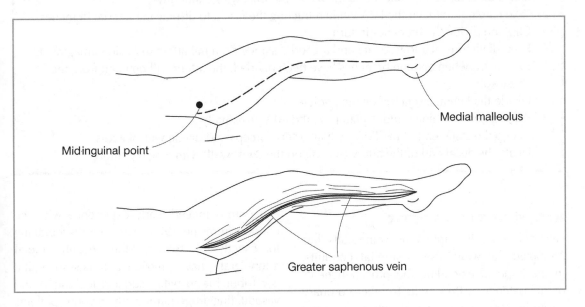

Midinguinal point

Medial malleolus

Greater saphenous vein

**Figure 3.2 Harvesting the long saphenous vein**

## LIMA harvest

- The LIMA–LAD artery graft is now almost ubiquitous in CABG surgery because the late patency and survival data are so compelling
- The LIMA harvest should be undertaken with care because the vessel is very easy to injure, and non-use of the vessel results in serious reduction of the patient's chance of survival

- The IMAs arise from the subclavian artery and run parallel and lateral to the sternum, giving off intercostal branches. The most superior is the superior intercostal branch, which supplies the first and second interspaces. The IMAs run anterior to the internal thoracic fascia

 **Principles of LIMA harvest**

It helps to wear magnifying loupes for this procedure.

**Procedure**
- Perform median sternotomy
- Insert a special retractor to lift the left hemisternum relative to the right hemisternum (IMA is viewed from the opposite side of the table as if the surgeon were peering through a letterbox)
- The details of the technique vary between surgeons, but most aim to create a pedicled (not a skeletonised) IMA graft, complete with associated fascia
- Take care not to injure the phrenic nerve as it crosses the IMA at the first rib
- Incise the internal thoracic fascia medial to the IMA with diathermy
- Take care not to touch the IMA while retracting the fascia to display the arterial branches
- Clip and divide the branches in turn
- Keep diathermy at a low setting and a good distance from the artery to avoid damaging it
- Eventually, when enough branches have been divided, the artery will be freed from the chest wall
- Divide the lateral fascia to free the pedicle
- Place a non-crushing bulldog clamp on the IMA proximally
- Clamp the distal end of the IMA with an artery forceps and divide with scissors
- Ligate the distal end of the artery (staying on the chest wall) with a heavy suture

## Radial artery harvest

Late occlusion in saphenous vein grafts has prompted the wider use of arterial conduits, in the hope of extending the proven benefits of late patency of IMA grafts to other coronary territories. The radial artery is extremely prone to spasm – indeed, early experience with the conduit from the 1970s was very discouraging for exactly this reason. More recently, radial artery grafts have enjoyed a renaissance that is attributable to better surgical technique and vasodilating drugs, particularly in young patients or those who have poor saphenous veins.

Patients are screened preoperatively with the Allen test (see box overleaf) to ensure adequate collateral ulnar flow. Patients with high functional requirements of their hands are usually excluded from radial artery harvesting. The non-dominant arm is normally used as the radial artery donor.

 **Radial artery harvest**

It helps to wear magnifying loupes to perform this procedure.

**Preparation**
- Place an oxygen saturation monitor on the index finger of the operated arm
- The arm, exposed from wrist to mid-upper arm, is prepared and draped on a board that is separate from the main operating table
- Landmarks are the **radial pulse** and the **brachial pulse**

**Incision**
- Make an incision from 2 cm distal to the brachial pulse to the radial pulse, and deepen through the subcutaneous fat, taking great care not to puncture the artery in its distal, subcutaneous part
- **Throughout the procedure, absolutely meticulous haemostasis is required in order to retain good views of the artery**

**Procedure**
- Divide the fascia overlying the brachioradialis medial to the lateral antebrachial nerve of the forearm. Retract the muscle laterally to reveal the radial artery
- Taking care not to touch the artery, handling it only via the associated fascia, divide the fascial covering of the radial artery on the lateral side. Ligate and divide the branches using titanium clips. Great care must be taken not to injure the superficial radial nerve which lies deep to the artery at this stage
- The medial border is then dissected free, ligating and dividing numerous branches
- Lift the artery from its bed, and ligate and divide the few posterior branches
- The procedure is almost complete. As a double-check of the preop Allen test (see overleaf) the artery is occluded between your fingers, and the trace from the oxygen saturation monitor on the patient's finger is watched. If this remains pulsatile, the artery may be safely removed
- Remaining ends of radial artery in the arms must be double ligated to prevent blood loss
- The artery is harvested and flushed with heparinised blood mixed with a vasodilator substance

**CHAPTER 3**

**The Allen test**

Aim: to assess the adequacy of the ulnar artery blood supply to the hand:

- The examiner's fingers press hard on both the radial and ulnar pulses so as to stop flow
- The patient opens and closes his hand in order to exsanguinate it (the hand becomes white)
- Pressure is released from the ulnar artery only
- If colour returns to the hand, the ulnar artery is likely to be adequate to supply the hand

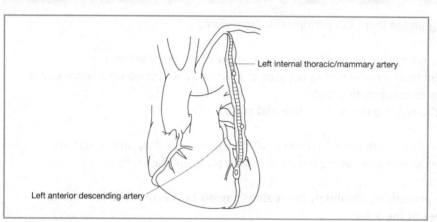

Left internal thoracic/mammary artery

Left anterior descending artery

**Figure 3.3 Left internal mammary artery (LIMA) to left anterior descending (LAD) artery single bypass graft**

## 1.8   Complications of CABG

### In a nutshell ...

**Immediate**
- Bleeding
- Low cardiac output syndrome
- Myocardial infarction
- Neurological complications

**Early**
- Pneumonia
- Sternal infections
- Leg infections
- Renal failure
- Atrial dysrhythmias
- Upper GI bleed and perforation

**Late**
- Recurrent stenosis

### Bleeding

Bleeding may be due to:

- **'Surgical' causes:**
  - Dehiscence of operative site
  - Ligatures falling off side branches of coronary grafts
  - Leakage from cannulation sites
- **'Non-surgical' causes:**
  - Coagulopathy arising from CPB, and clotting factor consumption
  - Generalised 'microvascular ooze'

When bleeding occurs within the confines of the pericardium, there is the potential for tamponade, even when the blood loss is relatively slow. Emergency re-opening of the thorax in the event of tamponade may be required to avoid cardiac arrest.

## Op box: Re-opening a sternotomy for bleeding

Judge the level of urgency of re-opening, and attempt to achieve a maximally controlled environment within the given timeframe. As re-opening predisposes to complications such as mediastinitis, best of all is an operating theatre with full sterile technique. It may be possible to temporise using fluid boluses and inotropes in order to re-open the patient in a controlled way, but in cardiac arrest situations a pair of sterile gloves may be the limit of preparation.

**Procedure**
- Re-open the skin and subcutaneous fascia using a scalpel
- Re-open the sternum by dividing the closure wires
- Place a self-retaining retractor. At this stage the haemodynamics may have improved simply by the alleviation of tamponade. For junior team members major bleeds can be controlled with a finger; smaller bleeds will await the arrival of the consultant. If cardiac arrest continues, or the BP is very low, gentle internal massage can be performed
- Inotropic and fluid support should be optimised
- Resolve the underlying problem as required
- Reclose the sternum, taking care not to provoke further bleeding

On occasions, the cardiac output cannot tolerate sternal reclosure, and the sternum must be left open under a bio-occlusive dressing.

## Low cardiac output syndrome

This is caused by:
- Poor ventricular function
- Incomplete revascularisation
- Inadequate myocardial protection

It is managed by:
- Maintenance of sinus rhythm (medically or with pacing)
- Optimised preload and afterload using fluid and monitoring (eg with pulmonary artery catheter)
- Maintenance of haematocrit of 30% (eg with packed red cell infusion)
- Optimised oxygenation and correct acidosis
- Inotropes (if all the above have been optimised and cardiac output is still poor)
- Vasodilators to reduce afterload
- Investigation with transthoracic echocardiography/TOE
- Intra-aortic balloon pump (to assist systolic emptying by reducing cardiac afterload while maintaining a mean arterial pressure for cerebral and coronary perfusion)

## Myocardial ischaemia and infarction

This is due to poor flow through the conduit, which is caused by:
- Tight anastomosis
- Arterial graft spasm
- Poor run-off (small distal coronary artery)
- Ventricular hypertrophy causing increased myocardial ischaemic watershed area

It is managed by:
- Optimised oxygenation, haematocrit and haemodynamics
- Nitrates
- Intra-aortic balloon pump

**CHAPTER 3**

# Neurological complications

Cognitive and psychological abnormalities may be detected in up to 40% of patients post-bypass. Most return to normal; 1% have a CVA.

## The risk of complications is increased by:

- Age >70
- Emergency cardiac surgery
- Arteriopathy (peripheral vascular disease, atherosclerosis, carotid occlusive disease, previous transient ischaemic attack [TIA] or CVA)
- Prolonged CPB
- Intraoperative or perioperative circulatory arrest
- Postoperative atrial fibrillation

## Neurological complications are caused by:

- Coexisting carotid artery disease
- Hypoperfusion (intraoperatively or perioperatively)

## They are managed by:

- Checking for carotid disease preoperatively
- Scheduling prior or simultaneous carotid endarterectomy if indicated
- Maintaining mean pressure of >80 mmHg while on bypass

Note that peripheral neurological complications are caused by conduit harvest (as shown in the table).

**Peripheral neurological complications caused by conduit harvest**

| Conduit harvest | Nerve damaged | Clinical deficit |
| --- | --- | --- |
| Internal thoracic (mammary) artery | Phrenic | Diaphragmatic paralysis |
| Radial artery | Superficial radial nerve Lateral antebrachial cutaneous nerve | Sensory loss over anatomical snuffbox Sensory loss over forearm |
| Long saphenous vein | Saphenous nerve | Sensory loss over front and medial leg |

# Pneumonia

## Pneumonia is related to:

- Preoperative smoking
- Preoperative lung disease

## It is caused by:

- Aspiration
- Prolonged artificial ventilation
- Inadequate analgesia/poor chest expansion
- Gram-negative rods or Gram-positive cocci (typical hospital-acquired pathogens)

## Management is by:

- Sputum culture and microbiologist involvement
- Broad-spectrum antibiotics then pathogen-targeted antibiotics
- Chest physiotherapy
- Bronchodilators
- Bronchoscopy in refractory cases

## Sternal infections

### Sternal infections are related to:
- Diabetes
- Peripheral vascular disease
- Obesity
- Bilateral IMA harvest
- Emergency re-opening
- Poor sterile technique

### Signs and symptoms are:
- Sternal click on movement or coughing
- Pain
- Sternal instability on examination (with a finger placed either side of the sternal wound ask the patient to cough. Movement between the two sides denotes instability)
- Discharge/wound breakdown
- Movement of wires on chest radiograph

### Sternal infections are caused by:
- Staphylococci (MRSA)
- Sometimes infection can spread by hand (eg from leg wounds)

### Management is by:
- Involvement of microbiologists
- Sternal debridement and rewiring
- Occasionally plastics involvement and flap placement
- Long-term antibiotics

## Leg infections

### Leg infections are related to:
- Diabetes
- Peripheral vascular disease
- Obesity
- Haematoma
- Poor sterile technique

### Leg infections are caused by:
- Staphylococci (MRSA)

### Management is by:
- Dressings
- Antibiotics, intravenous or oral, depending on the severity of the infection
- Incision and drainage of abscess areas

## Renal failure

There is usually underlying disease, with an acute insult:
- Pre-existing renal dysfunction due to hypertension
- Diabetes/small-vessel disease
- Low cardiac output states

### Management is by:
- Management of any underlying cause, eg low cardiac output
- Early renal team referral
- Depending on severity – just fluid management or haemofiltration or dialysis

## Atrial dysrhythmias

### Causes of atrial dysrhythmias include:
- Electrolyte imbalance
- Poor ventricular function
- Atrial distension by fluid overload
- Sepsis
- Drugs

### Atrial dysrhythmias are managed by:
- Correction of electrolytes
- Rate control
- Rhythm control

### Management of atrial fibrillation in cardiac surgery

**Question 1: Is the patient compromised?**
- If yes, then give acute life support/resuscitation as appropriate
- If no, ask the next question

**Question 2: Are the electrolytes normal?**
- Correct potassium to 4.5 mmol/l. Keeping potassium at this level prophylactically will prevent a lot of atrial fibrillation (AF) occurring in the first place
- Correct magnesium

**Question 3: Did the patient have preoperative atrial fibrillation?**
- If yes, then correct the rate only (eg digoxin or β blocker)
- If no, attempt to correct the rhythm

**Question 4: If attempting to revert to sinus rhythm, choose one of the following:**
1. Give IV amiodarone if:
   – On ventilator
   – Signs of right heart failure that may diminish oral drug absorption
   – BP <100 mmHg systolic
2. Give oral amiodarone if asymptomatic and mobile on ward
3. Use DC cardioversion if:
   – Acute onset and severely compromised
   – On ventilator

**Note:** don't forget to press the synchronise button (risk of VT)!
Don't forget to anticoagulate the patient first if they have been in AF for >24 hours due to risk of atrial/ventricular thrombus

## Upper GI bleed and perforation

**These are related to:**
- Surgical stress
- Prolonged intensive therapy unit (ITU) stay
- Past history of peptic ulcer disease
- Anticoagulation

**They are caused by:**
- *Helicobacter pylori*

**They are managed by:**
- Referral to a gastroenterology team (upper gastrointestinal [GI] bleed, for endoscopy) or to general surgeons (perforation, for laparotomy)
- Fluids
- Antibiotics
- Inotropes for sepsic shock

## 1.9 Percutaneous coronary interventions

Most coronary revascularisation is now performed via percutaneous access by cardiologists.

## Principles of the procedure

- A cannula is placed in the femoral artery or radial artery (usually the right)
- A guidewire followed by a fine cannula is passed from the artery around the aortic arch to the coronary ostia under fluoroscopy
- Dye is injected into the coronary ostia to visualise the right and left coronary systems and can be injected into the ventricle to obtain images of wall movement

After delineating any disease, a strategy is formulated for treating the lesions. Depending on the findings, the cardiologist can refer for CABG or perform percutaneous intervention.

## Types of percutaneous intervention

- **Angioplasty:** this involves inflation of a balloon at the site of a stenosis in order to flatten the intimal plaque and increase the coronary lumen. Treatment is often successful alone, but it can result in restenosis
- **Stenting:** an expandable metal stent mounted on a balloon may be deployed in the area of a stenosis. The balloon is inflated so that the stent irreversibly expands within the coronary lumen. This procedure decreases the risk of restenosis, but blood clot can accumulate within the stent ('in-stent thrombosis')

Both stenting and angioplasty can be performed in multiple vessels. For some patients this is an alternative to multivessel coronary artery bypass surgery.

## 1.10 Cardiac transplantation

**In a nutshell ...**

Cardiac transplantation is indicated in circumstances where cardiac function has decreased and is not amenable to other medical or surgical therapies.

- **Acute cases** are likely to require circulatory support in the form of intra-aortic balloon pumping or an LV assist device
- **Chronic cases** usually have an NYHA score of 3 or 4 and exertional dyspnoea on maximum medical therapy
- The **aetiology** of the disease is often cardiomyopathy or a congenital defect

The heart can be transplanted alone or en bloc with the lungs.

## Choice of donor

Certified brainstem-dead donors are matched against recipients for height and weight and blood group. An echocardiogram is performed on the donor heart to check for ventricular function, congenital defects and valvular defects.

**Principles of heart and lung harvesting for transplantation**

The procedure is usually performed jointly with teams harvesting the abdominal organs:

- An incision is made from the sternal notch to the pubis
- The aorta is cannulated for cardioplegia
- An aortic cross-clamp is placed
- The heart is perfused with cardioplegia solution
- The body is exsanguinated via the IVC
- The heart and lungs are removed en bloc by disconnection of the aorta (descending), the superior vena cava (SVC), IVC and trachea
- The organs are transported on ice to the recipient with maximum speed in order to minimise cold-ischaemic time

**Principles of cardiac transplantation**

This procedure is performed with maximum speed in order that the warm-ischaemic time is minimised. The transplant is orthotopic:

- The incision is median sternotomy
- CPB is established in the usual way, with venous cannulas in both SVC and IVC
- The heart is explanted, leaving a patch of left atrium posteriorly and both vena cavae
- The donor heart is implanted using a left atrial anastomosis technique rather than implantation of individual pulmonary veins
- The SVC and IVC are re-anastomosed
- The aorta is re-anastomosed
- The cross-clamp is removed and the new heart perfused
- If adequate cardiac output is achieved, the patient is weaned from CPB

**CHAPTER 3**

# SECTION 2

# Surgery of the heart valves

## 2.1 Aortic stenosis

 **In a nutshell ...**

Severe aortic stenosis occurs when the valve area is <1.0 cm² (normally it is 3–4 cm²). There is a transaortic pressure gradient (>50 mmHg is an indication for surgery) and a resistance to forward flow, causing increased LV work, LV mass and oxygen requirement. It is usually caused by aortic calcification or, less commonly, rheumatic disease.

The symptoms are given by the acronym SAD:

- **S**yncope
- **A**ngina
- **D**yspnoea

The surgery of choice is valve replacement, with either a bioprosthetic or a mechanical valve. The results of surgery are good. Mechanical and bioprosthetic valves have pros and cons.

## Pathology of aortic stenosis

The aortic valve is the main outflow valve from the heart. In the non-diseased state it is composed of three semilunar cusps of fine tissue (right and left anterior and posterior [non-coronary]); in approximately 1% it is bicuspid. Each cusp is associated with a sinus of Valsalva, and the left and right coronary orifices lie in two of these. The physiological aortic valve has an effective area of 3–4 cm². There is no resistance to forward flow and no transaortic pressure gradient when the left ventricle is contracting.

## Calcific aortic stenosis

Aortic stenosis is most commonly caused by heavy calcification in old age. The leaflets become ossified and stiff, causing outflow obstruction. An element of regurgitation may occur through failure of the inflexible leaflets to completely coapt.

**Risk factors for aortic stenosis**
- Old age
- Bicuspid valve
- Rheumatic fever
- Hypercalcaemia
- Congenital bicuspid valve (rarely unicuspic) which is asymptomatic until onset of the aortic stenosis

## Rheumatic aortic stenosis

This occurs in patients with a history of rheumatic fever (usually a group A β-haemolytic strepto-coccal pharyngeal infection). In these cases the valve is fibrotic, with fusion of the commissures. In these cases the aortic valve disease is rarely isolated, and other valvular lesions should be sought in the preoperative work-up.

## Physiology of aortic stenosis

Significant aortic stenosis is said to be:
- Mild when the valve area is >1.5 cm$^2$
- Moderate if the area is 1.0–1.5 cm$^2$
- Severe if the area is <1.0 cm$^2$

This equates to a peak gradient of 50 mmHg across the valve at rest (given normal cardiac output).

Resistance to flow through the aortic orifice causes LV hypertrophy (visible on the ECG as high-magnitude complexes in the chest leads). The increased LV mass and greater workload impose a greater requirement for myocardial oxygen. When combined with coronary disease, aortic stenosis confers a high risk of sudden death. Hypotension is particularly dangerous because it lowers coronary perfusion pressures to a hypertrophied myocardium.

## Indications for treatment

Risk–benefit analysis indicates that aortic stenosis should be operated on when the transaortic gradient exceeds 50 mmHg. The disease is often identified incidentally in asymptomatic patients. After developing symptoms, average survival without surgery is 2–3 years. Therefore, when present, symptoms indicate more severe disease and should prompt surgery with minimal delay.

## Preoperative preparation

This is as for coronary artery surgery (see Section 1.3). In addition, for valve surgery you must consider documenting coronary artery disease and consider a joint CABG/valve procedure if appropriate.

## Minimising the risk of endocarditis
- Dental examination
- Chest examination
- Urine dipstick
- Temperature

## Choice of valve type

Aortic valves are always replaced because there is no viable option for repair.
- Choose between mechanical and biopros-thetic valves
- Rarely, a cadaveric aortic homograft may be used

The principal indication is for active aortic valve endocarditis (native or prosthetic) with or without perivalvular tissue destruction (abscess cavity, fistula, detachment of the anterior mitral valve leaflet from the aortic annulus).

The main advantages and disadvantages are listed opposite. It is essential for patients to participate in the decision-making process regarding the type of valve implanted. Broadly speaking, young active patients without major comorbidities should receive mechanical prostheses, whereas elderly patients with risk of comorbidity and potential for poor compliance with medication should receive bioprostheses. Sometimes other reasons intervene, such as the young patient who wishes to drink heavily or whose occupation precludes taking warfarin.

## Pros and cons of mechanical prostheses and bioprostheses in any position

| Mechanical prosthesis | Bioprosthesis |
| --- | --- |
| Long life (up to and beyond 20 years or <65 years) | Shorter life (10–15 years or >65 years) |
| Requires warfarin | No need for warfarin |
| Noisy (metallic clicks) | Silent |

## Surgery for aortic stenosis

Surgery on the aortic valve is to replace the valve, because attempts at repair are unsuccessful.

CHAPTER 3

### Procedure box: Aortic valve replacement

- The aortic valve is almost always approached via a median sternotomy (as described previously)
- CPB is established, taking care to position the aortic pipe sufficiently far from the proposed line of aortic opening so that a cross-clamp can be positioned in between
- A vent is placed in the heart to maintain a dry operating field in the aortic root. Although there are many approaches, the common requirement is that the tip of the vent should be within the left ventricle
- Open the ascending aorta, taking care not to injure the coronary orifices (Figure 3.4)
- The native valve is excised and calcium deposits debrided (Figure 3.5). Take great care to wash out any residual debris, any of which could embolise to the brain or elsewhere as soon as ventricular ejection resumes
- Measure the valve orifice with a sizer to ensure a perfectly fitting valve. If the chosen valve is too small there is a risk of 'patient–prosthesis mismatch' which arises when the functional valve area is inadequate for the size of the patient. In this situation, a transaortic gradient may remain postoperatively. If the chosen valve is too large there may be technical difficulty in inserting it
- Place braided polyester pledgetted mattress sutures around the valve perimeter, and through the prosthesis sewing ring (Figure 3.6)
- Parachute the valve into position, tie sutures and cut to length
- Inspect the suture line to ensure that no spaces are present that could permit paravalvular leak
- Close the aorta using polypropylene suture
- De-airing is performed before the aortic cross-clamp is removed
- CPB is discontinued, haemostasis obtained and the chest closed

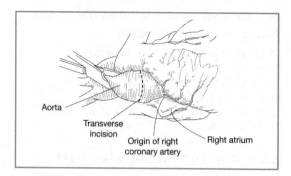

**Figure 3.4 Initial steps for aortic valve replacement**

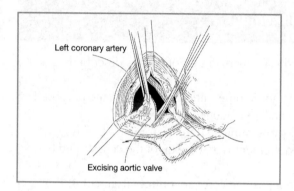

**Figure 3.5 Excision of aortic valve and debridement**

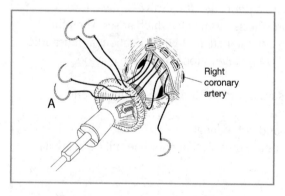

**Figure 3.6 Aortic valve replacement with mechanical prosthesis or stent-mounted bioprosthesis, interrupted suture technique**

# Outcomes and complications of aortic valve surgery

## Special postoperative considerations

- In aortic stenosis patients' perfusion pressures must be maintained high on the ITU in order that the hypertrophied myocardium is adequately oxygenated
- Warfarin must be introduced within 48 hours, and its dose titrated to the therapeutic international normalised ratio (INR)

## Results of surgery

These are good, with:

- Immediate improvement of symptoms
- Improved long-term survival

## Surgical mortality rate

This is 2–5%, with early complications similar to those of CABG (eg CVA, bleeding, arrhythmias, MI, pneumonia) (see Section 1.8). Late complications include infection leading to paravalvular leak or endocarditis.

Other complications depend on the type of valve used. Artificial valves lead to warfarin-related complications and thromboembolism. Tissue valves deteriorate faster than artificial valves but have a lower thromboembolism rate.

## Endovascular techniques

- Percutaneous transcatheter alternatives to standard aortic valve replacement have been developed with the aim of avoiding mortality and morbidity of surgery in patients in whom the risk is considered to be too high
- Transcatheter aortic valve implantation (TAVI) offers a minimally invasive approach by avoiding sternotomy and extracorporeal circulation. TAVI is performed under fluoroscopic and echocardiographic guidance

## Two approaches

The retrograde transfemoral (TF) or subclavian approach is performed using the Seldinger technique through the common femoral or subclavian/axillary artery, either prepared surgically or approached percutaneously.

The anterograde transapical (via the myocardium) approach concerns only the balloon-expandable prosthesis. It is performed through a left anterolateral mini-thoracotomy under general anaesthesia. However, this technology is in its infancy and long-term data are awaited.

## 2.2 Aortic regurgitation

 **In a nutshell ...**

Aortic regurgitation is less common than aortic stenosis and, if symptomatic at all, often presents as pulmonary venous hypertension.

It occurs as a consequence of rheumatic disease, Marfan syndrome, endocarditis or aortic dissection.

Surgery is indicated in the chronic situation for symptomatic patients or those developing LV dilatation, and in acute aortic dissection. Valve replacement is performed, as for aortic stenosis (see Section 2.1).

### Features of aortic regurgitation

**Symptoms**
- Frequently asymptomatic
- Most frequently related to pulmonary venous hypertension (back pressure)
- Dyspnoea
- Orthopnoea
- Paroxysmal nocturnal dyspnoea
- Pulmonary oedema
- Occasionally angina
- Syncope is rare

**Examination findings**
- Hyperdynamic apex
- 'Water-hammer' pulse
- Wide pulse pressure (eg very high systolic BP and very low diastolic BP)
- Early diastolic murmur at cardiac apex

**Investigations**
- **Chest radiograph:** LV enlargement. Aortic enlargement may be visible if there is an aneurysm. Signs of pulmonary venous hypertension may be present
- **ECG:** to confirm regurgitation and assess for other pathologies (eg other valvular lesions following rheumatic fever)
- **Coronary arteriography:** to exclude coronary stenoses in patients >40

## Pathology of aortic regurgitation

Aortic regurgitation is much less common than aortic stenosis, and it has a wider range of causes:
- **Rheumatic valve disease:** fibrosis in the valve leaflets causes the valves to shorten and fail in coaptation

- **Annuloaortic ectasia:** this is sometimes but not always associated with Marfan syndrome. The aortic root may become dilated, causing separation of the aortic cusps
- **Endocarditis:** this causes destruction of the aortic leaflets
- **Large-vessel vasculitis:** this is associated with a wide range of autoimmune diseases
- **Acute 'type A' aortic dissection:** this causes acute aortic regurgitation

### Natural history of aortic regurgitation

Mild and moderate aortic regurgitation has little effect on life expectancy. Severe incompetence causes progressive LV dilatation, which leads to hypertrophy. Patients with marked ventricular dilatation are at greatest risk of sudden death.

## Treatment of aortic regurgitation

- **Chronic presentations:** treatment is indicated for symptomatic patients or those developing LV dilatation
- **Acute presentations:** type A aortic dissection is a surgical emergency. It is always treated if the patient is deemed to have a chance of surviving the operation with a good quality of life

The preoperative preparation is as for any cardiac surgery. All patients undergo echocardiography.

Aortic valve replacement is the surgery of choice; the technique is as for aortic stenosis as described in Section 2.1, and the outcomes and complications are similar.

## 2.3   Mitral regurgitation

### In a nutshell ...

Mitral regurgitation is the second most common valvular lesion requiring surgery. The larger crescent-shaped posterior leaflet tends to prolapse. The cause of the valve regurgitating may be ischaemic damage to the papillary muscle, senile degeneration of the leaflets or ventricular dilatation due to ischaemia or cardiomyopathy. Mitral valves are repaired or (more commonly) replaced to prevent complications of regurgitation such as left atrial dilatation, pulmonary hypertension and atrial fibrillation.

- **Mitral valve:** this is located between the left atrium and the left ventricle. It is composed of an anterior and a posterior leaflet
- **Mitral valve leaflets:** these are prevented from prolapsing into the left atrium by the chordae tendineae attached to papillary muscles (which in turn arise from the myocardium of the left ventricle)
- **Chordae tendineae:** the primary chordae insert into the very edge of the valve leaflet. The secondary chordae insert further back

## Pathology of mitral regurgitation

Mitral regurgitation is the second most common valvular lesion requiring surgical intervention. The posterior leaflet is much larger than the anterior, and therefore it is much more prone to prolapse, and is much more commonly the cause of mitral regurgitation.

## Aetiology of mitral regurgitation

Mitral regurgitation occurs:

- **In disorders of the leaflet:**
  - The leaflet becomes stretched and baggy through senile degeneration
  - The excess leaflet tissue prolapses into the left atrium (parachute mitral valve)
- **In disorders of the papillary muscle and chordae tendineae:**
  - Chordal rupture allows the leaflet edge to prolapse freely into the left atrium
  - Papillary muscle dysfunction (usually ischaemic) fails to maintain valvular competence during systole
  - Papillary muscle rupture in MI causes acute, torrential mitral regurgitation
- **In disorders of the left ventricle:**
  - Ventricular dilatation (arising from chronic ischaemia or cardiomyopathy) causes distortion of mitral valve geometry and failure of leaflet coaptation

## Natural history of mitral regurgitation

Chronic mitral regurgitation leads to left atrial dilatation, raised pressures in pulmonary circulation and eventually pulmonary oedema. Left atrial dilatation causes atrial fibrillation.

## Surgical treatment of mitral valve regurgitation

Regurgitant mitral valves can be repaired, but are more often replaced using mechanical or bioprosthetic valves. **The preoperative preparation is as described for all cardiac valve surgery.** All patients require echocardiography including TOE to establish suitability for valve repair or replacement. All patients require examination of the coronary arteries to establish requirement for simultaneous CABG.

## Mitral valve surgery: intraoperative considerations

Many patients require intraoperative TOE to evaluate the outcome of mitral valve repair. Some patients fail to wean from CPB because of increased LV work caused by the loss of venting into the atrium.

## Mitral valve surgery: incisions

Mitral valves are most commonly approached via a median sternotomy. Alternative approaches are:

- Right thoracotomy: via the left atrium, for all types of mitral valve surgery
- Left thoracotomy: via the left ventricle, used for 'closed' mitral valvotomy

The right thoracotomy approach is particularly useful in re-do surgery when pericardial adhesions from previous median sternotomies create considerable difficulties and risk.

## Surgical options for mitral regurgitation

There are many procedures that may be performed on the regurgitant mitral valve, but essentially the choice is between mitral valve repair or replacement with a mechanical or biological prosthesis.

Repair is superior to replacement (when possible) because:

- The patient may avoid warfarin if not already on it for AF
- There is less prosthetic material to become infected
- The haemodynamics are superior

However, the anatomy of the regurgitant valve is often not suitable so replacement is more common.

**CHAPTER 3**

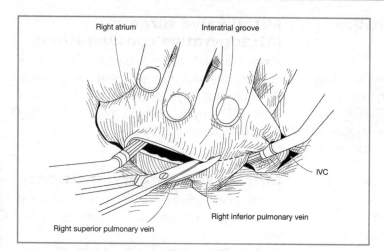

**Figure 3.7 Open mitral commissurotomy**

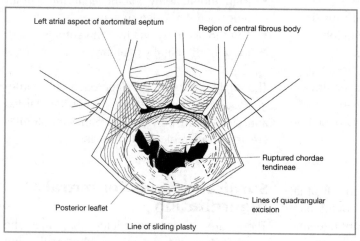

**Figure 3.8 Mitral valve repair for degenerative disease**

Important elements of the surgical technique to remember are:

- A careful suture technique avoids paraprosthetic leaks or injury to the circumflex coronary artery
- Meticulous asepsis and perioperative antibiotic policies are needed to avoid endocarditis
- Careful de-airing is important

## Mitral valve repair

In the most commonly used approach, the heart is cannulated in the usual way (as described previously in the section on preparation for CPB), frequently using a bicaval technique. CPB is always required for mitral valve repair and replacement, in order to create a bloodless field in which to operate. The interatrial groove is identified, and the left atrium is entered. The right atrium is retracted anteriorly to reveal the mitral valve.

One example of a mitral valve repair technique is a **sliding plasty**. A segment of the posterior valve leaflet is excised. The base of the valve leaflet is incised such that two 'flaps' of mitral valve are created. The free edges are re-approximated, and the valve base is sewn back onto

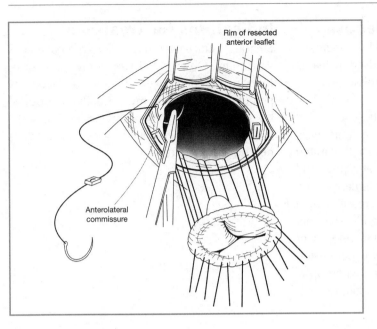

Rim of resected
anterior leaflet

Anterolateral
commissure

**Figure 3.9 Mitral valve
replacement**

the annulus. After this repair, valve competence is assessed using injection of saline into the left ventricle via the repaired valve (Figure 3.8).

## Mitral valve replacement

Mechanical and biological prostheses are available. Access to the mitral valve is as for mitral valve repair as described previously.

The diseased valve is excised. The valve orifice is measured for a valve using sizers. Pledgetted sutures are placed around the valvular orifice, and in the valve sewing ring. The valve is parachuted into place on the sutures which are tied down firmly to avoid paravalvular leak (Figure 3.9).

## Outcomes and complications of mitral valve surgery

Mitral valve surgery for regurgitation results in an improvement in both symptoms and postoperative survival.

Complications include those of CPB and median sternotomy. Late complications can include paravalvular leak and prosthetic valve endocarditis.

## 2.4   Mitral stenosis

   In a nutshell ...

Mitral stenosis is most commonly caused by rheumatic fever, and is often asymptomatic. Severe cases can result in left atrial hypertrophy, pulmonary oedema, and eventually right ventricular hypertrophy and secondary tricuspid regurgitation. The valve can be opened up by percutaneous valvotomy or it can be surgically replaced.

## Pathology of mitral stenosis

Mitral stenosis is often caused by rheumatic fever. Pathologically it is characterised by leaflet thickening and fusion of the commissures.

Many patients are asymptomatic, so mitral stenosis is found incidentally on examination. Greater resistance to flow through the mitral orifice leads to left atrial hypertrophy and a modest degree of left atrial enlargement. Pulmonary vascular pressures increase, which can lead to pulmonary oedema and exertional dyspnoea. In advanced cases that develop over a period of many years pulmonary hypertension can result in right ventricular hypertrophy leading to secondary tricuspid regurgitation.

## Indications for treatment

Stenotic mitral valves may undergo percutaneous valvotomy. Open mitral valvotomy for stenosis has in practice been largely replaced by percutaneous valvotomy, usually performed by cardiologists. When this is not feasible, mitral valve replacement may be indicated, as described in Section 2.3.

# SECTION 3

# Other cardiac surgical pathology

## In a nutshell ...

As well as ischaemic heart disease and valvular disease, you should be aware of the pathological basis and surgical treatment for the following:

**Myocardial and pericardial disease**
- Cardiomyopathy
- Restrictive pericarditis
- Pericardial effusions

**Congenital heart disease**
- Atrial septal defect (ASD)
- Ventricular septal defect (VSD)
- Patent ductus arteriosus (PDA)
- Tetralogy of Fallot
- Transposition of the great vessels

**Cardiac tumours**

**Cardiac trauma**

## 3.1 Myocardial and pericardial disease

## In a nutshell ...

**Cardiomyopathy**
- Dilated cardiomyopathy
- Restrictive cardiomyopathy
- Hypertrophic obstructive cardiomyopathy (HOCM)

**Restrictive pericarditis**
**Pericardial effusion**

## Cardiomyopathy

Cardiomyopathy is a disease of cardiac muscle that results in myocardial dysfunction.

### Dilated cardiomyopathy

This is defined by loss of ventricular function and increased ventricular volume. It may occur as the end-stage of a variety of disease processes (alcoholism, viral illnesses) or genetic predisposition. The prognosis is relatively poor, with a 80% mortality rate at 10 years.

Treatment is medical except for a few patients who undergo ventricular remodelling or cardiac transplantation.

### Restrictive cardiomyopathy

This usually results from amyloid deposition within the myocardium. It causes a loss of diastolic function arising from decreased ventricular compliance.

The clinical features resemble those of restrictive pericardial disease. The lifespan is reduced, with death occurring 5–20 years from diagnosis.

### Hypertrophic cardiomyopathy

This is characterised by ventricular hypertrophy (that may or may not obstruct ventricular outflow depending on whether the septum is involved). HOCM is well known for causing sudden death in young people. It is inherited as an autosomal dominant trait.

Symptoms are angina, dyspnoea, syncope and dizziness on exertion. Patients are treated with blockers and calcium antagonists.

Surgical treatments include septal myomectomy to relieve subaortic obstruction. If untreated, the mortality rate is up to 50% at 10 years.

### Restrictive pericarditis

Restrictive pericarditis is an inflammatory process that causes pericardial thickening leading to ventricular compression. A number of cases involve calcium accumulation, when a shadow can easily be seen on chest radiography. Cardiac output is diminished by limitation of diastolic filling.

Symptoms are fluid retention (ie leg swelling and abdominal distension due to right heart failure) and exertional dyspnoea.

Treatment is with pericardectomy, by either median sternotomy or left anterior thoracotomy. Care is needed not to injure the phrenic nerves, and to identify the plane between the myocardium and the thickened pericardium so that the ventricle is not entered.

### Pericardial effusion

Pericardial effusions result from acute or chronic inflammation of the pericardium stimulating accumulation of large volumes of fluid. Tamponade does not usually result because of the slow development of the fluid volume. Effusions may be caused by a variety of pathologies, including renal disease and malignancy.

Symptoms are variable; pain and shortness of breath can be features.

Treatment is by creation of a subxiphoid pericardial window to drain pericardial fluid into the abdominal cavity.

## 3.2 Congenital heart disease

### In a nutshell ...

Congenital heart defects are highly complex and variable. Only a few defects cause symptoms or are detected in infancy or childhood. Many defects are asymptomatic for life.

Due to the enormous range of lesions, only the major ones have been described here. These are:

- ASD
- VSD
- PDA
- Tetralogy of Fallot
- Transposition of the great vessels

### Atrial septal defect

The atrial septum develops from primum and secundum portions. In utero the foramen ovale is patent to allow blood to bypass the pulmonary circulation; failure of this hole to close is relatively common and results in a patent foramen ovale (PFO). An ostium secundum ASD is the most common type. Other defects occur, including: upper and lower sinus venosus defects and a defect involving the coronary sinus. A small number of these cause symptoms early in life.

**Symptoms** requiring intervention arise from:
- Left-to-right shunt causing pulmonary hypertension and exertional dyspnoea
- Atrial fibrillation or heart failure in later life
- Paradoxical embolus causing cerebral ischaemia

**Clinical signs** of ASD are:
- Parasternal heave
- Fixed splitting of the second heart sound
- Midsystolic flow murmur

**Investigations** should include:
- Echocardiography to delineate the extent and location of the defect, and to detect coexisting defects
- Coronary angiography in older patients to detect coronary disease that may benefit from simultaneous surgery

**Treatment** of ASD is with:
- Cardiologically: percutaneous closure
- Surgically: pericardial patch repair

### Ventricular septal defect

This is a hole of any size in the interventricular septum which is either congenital or acquired after an MI or bacterial endocarditis. The degree of left-to-right shunt is determined by the size of the hole.

Eighty per cent of VSDs occur in the membranous portion of the interventricular septum. Most patients with VSDs have other cardiac pathologies simultaneously.

The size of the VSD determines the progression of the disease and its presenting features:
- Large defects are likely to present neonatally
- Small defects may be asymptomatic into adulthood

**Clinical findings in infants** are:
- Tachypnoea
- Hepatomegaly
- Poor feeding/growth failure
- Cardiomegaly on chest radiograph
- Biventricular hypertrophy on ECG

**Clinical findings in older patients** are:
- Non-specific symptoms
- Systolic murmur
- Small shunts (may be asymptomatic)

**Disease progression** of VSD is as follows:
- Prognosis depends on the size of the defect
- 10% of infants with large defects die in the first year
- Eisenmenger syndrome describes pulmonary hypertension with reversal of the underlying left-to-right shunt

**Investigation** is with echocardiography, which delineates the defect and coexisting pathologies.

**Treatment** is by surgical pericardial patch repair and in some cases may be performed percutaneously.

## Patent ductus arteriosus

This is the abnormal persistence of a lumen in the ductus arteriosus, which connects the pulmonary artery with the arch of the aorta; it allows fetal blood to bypass the pulmonary circulation. The ductus arteriosus normally closes after birth to form the ligamentum arteriosum. It begins about 12 hours after birth due to loss of maternal prostaglandins, and it continues to close over the next few weeks.

**Clinical features** of PDA are:
- Tachycardia
- Tachypnoea
- Irritability
- Slow weight gain
- Pulmonary oedema leading to pneumonia
- Precordial thrill
- 'Machinery' continuous murmur
- Evidence of cardiac enlargement (thrusting apical impulse, jerky pulse)
- Hepatic enlargement

- Evidence of right ventricular (RV) enlargement on ECG
- Chest radiograph shows cardiomegaly or enlargement of pulmonary trunk and aorta
- Echocardiogram may visualise the PDA

**Disease progression** of PDA:
- Depends on the size of the PDA
- Prognosis correlates inversely with the degree of shunt leading to pulmonary hypertension, Eisenmenger syndrome, heart failure and death

**Treatment** of PDA:
- Non-steroidal anti-inflammatory drugs (NSAIDs) inhibit prostaglandin synthesis and may induce closure
- Percutaneous blockade of the PDA by interventional radiology
- Surgical ligation and division of the PDA

## Tetralogy of Fallot

This is a congenital malformation arising from diminished development of the pulmonary outflow tract. Four abnormalities make up the tetralogy:
1. VSD
2. Pulmonary stenosis
3. Over-riding aorta
4. RV hypertrophy

There is pulmonary stenosis together with mixing of oxygenated and non-oxygenated blood, so infants with this condition are cyanosed.

### Treatment of tetralogy of Fallot
- **Shunting procedure:** the degree of cyanosis depends on the degree of pulmonary stenosis. If it is very severe, the infant will be extremely hypoxic on minimal exertion. In this situation a shunting procedure may be warranted (eg a Blalock–Taussig

shunt), whereby a communication is made between the systemic and pulmonary arterial circulations in order to bypass the pulmonary stenosis and increase pulmonary blood flow and oxygenation

- **Definitive surgery:** this involves closure of surgical shunts, relief of pulmonary stenosis and patch repair of the VSD

## Transposition of the great vessels

In this condition the aortic root arises from the right ventricle, and the pulmonary trunk from the left. Unless there is a large ASD or VSD, the systemic and pulmonary circulations are in parallel, and the infant's life expectancy is very short due to hypoxia. The ductus arteriosus may remain open for a prolonged period, creating a physiological shunt.

### Treatment of transposition of the great vessels

- **Shunting procedures:** when there is minimal mixing of the systemic and pulmonary circulations, a communication is made between the systemic and pulmonary circulations
- **Arterial switch:** this definitive treatment involves division of the aorta and pulmonary trunk at their roots, and re-anastomosis with the LV and RV infundibula, respectively

## 3.3 Cardiac tumours

 **In a nutshell ...**

Of all primary cardiac tumours, 70% are benign. Atrial myxoma is the most common of these but still accounts for only half. The others are a collection of rarities.

## Atrial myxomas

Characteristically these are pedunculated tumours, most commonly arising from the interatrial septum in the left atrium. Symptoms arise from obstruction of flow, and embolisation of tumour fragments or adherent clot. Most are diagnosed on echocardiography. Excision is performed via median sternotomy, using CPB. Both atria are opened, the tumour excised and any resulting ASD repaired.

## Other rare tumours

Less common benign tumours of the heart include lipoma and cystic tumour of the atrioventricular nodal region.

Malignant tumours of the heart include rhabdomyosarcomas, angiosarcomas, myxosarcomas, fibrosarcomas, leiomyosarcomas, reticulum cell sarcomas, desmoplastic small round cell tumours and liposarcomas.

# SECTION 4

# Thoracic surgery for bronchogenic carcinoma

## 4.1 Pathology of bronchogenic carcinoma

**In a nutshell ...**

Bronchogenic carcinoma is one of the most common causes of cancer death in the UK. As a result of advanced disease at diagnosis, only about 10% of lung cancers are operated on in the UK. Although there is great variation in the pathological subtypes identified in lung tumours, in terms of surgical management the major division is between small-cell carcinoma (poor prognosis, rarely operated on) and non-small-cell carcinoma (surgery offered to those who fulfil certain patient and oncological criteria).

### Presenting features of bronchogenic carcinoma
- It may be asymptomatic
- It can be an incidental finding on radiology performed for another reason

The **symptoms and signs** that should indicate urgent chest radiography to investigate for bronchogenic carcinoma are:
- Cough
- Weight loss
- Chest/shoulder pain
- Dyspnoea
- Hoarseness
- Finger clubbing
- Cervical/supraclavicular lymphadenopathy
- Symptoms suggesting metastases (eg in brain, bone, liver or skin)

**Signs include:**
- Consolidation or other chest signs
- Signs of SVC obstruction
- Ptosis

**Chest radiograph shows:**
- Discrete opacity
- Lobar collapse
- Pleural effusion

Remember, opacities may be hidden behind the cardiac shadow or in the costophrenic angles. Consider this diagnosis if a smoker presents with recurrent chest infections.

## Small-cell carcinoma

### Histology of small-cell carcinoma shows:

- Poorly differentiated, small cells (oat cells)
- High mitotic rate
- Propensity to secrete neohormonal substances, leading to paraneoplastic syndromes

### The natural history:

- Rapid metastasis and micrometastasis can occur, so this is considered to be a 'systemic disease' at presentation
- Most patients have mediastinal lymph node involvement at presentation

### The prognosis of small cell carcinoma:

- In the order of months
- Surgery is almost never indicated, but occasional small-cell tumours that have not metastasised to the mediastinal nodes are found incidentally on pathological examination of lobectomy specimens
- Most patients receive palliative chemotherapy

## Non-small-cell carcinoma

The histology is according to broad grouping of different tumour types:

- **Adenocarcinomas** account for 30% of cases
- **Squamous cell carcinomas** account for 35% of cases, and are likely to be a cavitating lesion on chest radiograph or CT scan
- **Carcinoid tumours** are members of the neuroendocrine (amine precursor uptake and decarboxylation or APUD) group, with a propensity to recur very late after surgical resection
- Other rarer tumours

The natural history of non-small-cell carcinomas:

- They are usually much slower-growing and less aggressive than small-cell types

- Nevertheless, a large number present with locally advanced disease or lymph node metastases

---

### TNM staging of bronchogenic carcinoma

**Tumour stage**

| | |
|---|---|
| T1a | Tumour ≤2 cm |
| T1b | Tumour >2 but ≤3 cm with no invasion of visceral pleura or proximal to lobar bronchus |
| T2a | Tumour >3 but ≤5 cm |
| T2b | Tumour >5 but ≤7 cm **or** that invades visceral pleura **or** associated atelectasis/obstructive pneumonitis that extends to hilar region but not entire lung |
| T3 | Tumour >7 cm **or** any size of tumour with chest wall, diaphragmatic or mediastinal pleural involvement **or** tumour in main bronchus <2 cm from main carina **or** atelectasis/obstructive pneumonitis of entire lung |
| T4 | Any size of tumour that invades mediastinum, heart, great vessels, trachea, oesophagus, vertebral body **or** separate tumour nodules within ipsilateral lung |

**Node stage**

| | |
|---|---|
| N1 | Peribronchial or ipsilateral hilar nodes |
| N2 | Ipsilateral mediastinal or subcarinal nodes |
| N3 | Contralateral, scalene or supraclavicular nodes |

**Metastasis stage**

| | |
|---|---|
| M0 | No distant metastases |
| M1a | Local intrathoracic spread – malignant pleural/pericardial effusion |
| M1b | Disseminated (extrathoracic) spread |

## Surgical management of non-small-cell carcinoma

Surgery benefits only those patients who undergo complete resection of all disease. Survival in patients left with residual tumour is unaltered from those who undergo no intervention. Therefore surgery is offered only to those who fulfil certain patient criteria and oncological criteria.

### Patient factors

Patients must have:
- Adequate cardiovascular status to survive major surgery
- Sufficient lung function to be able to lose the required lung volume and still be left with forced expiratory volume in 1 s ($FEV_1$) >40% of predicted (see below)
- Adequate performance status (see box opposite)

### Predicting loss of lung function after lung resection

It is important to know that a patient will be left with enough functioning lung to survive after any planned surgery. Every patient has a 'predicted $FEV_1$' expected of a completely fit and well patient of that age and size.

---

### How to calculate estimated postoperative $FEV_1$

Calculate number of lung segments to be excised. There are 19 lung segments in total:
- Right upper lobe = 3
- Right middle lobe = 2
- Right lower lobe = 5
- Left upper lobe = 3
- Lingula = 2
- Left lower lobe = 4

Calculate estimated postoperative $FEV_1$ using the following formula:
- [Lung segments left after excision/Total number of functioning lung segments preoperatively] × Preoperative $FEV_1$ = Estimated postoperative $FEV_1$ (should not be <40% of predicted $FEV_1$)

---

### Oncological factors

- Tumour should not be disseminated within the thoracic cavity. Malignant effusion is an absolute contraindication
- Tumour must be amenable to resection with tolerable morbidity. Some T4 tumours may be fully resectable by an experienced surgeon, but others will not be
- There should be no metastases
- Patients should have no evidence of positive N2 or N3 staging lymph nodes

## Performance status

### Perioperative mortality
- Consider global risk score such as Thoracoscore

### Cardiovascular function
- Avoid surgery within 30 days of MI
- Optimise primary cardiac treatment and begin secondary cardiac prophylaxis as soon as possible
- Offer surgery if two or fewer risk factors and good cardiac functional capacity
- Cardiology review if active cardiac condition, three or more risk factors or poor cardiac functional capacity
- Consider revascularisation before surgery in stable angina
- Continue anti-ischaemic treatment in perioperative period. Discuss **anti**platelet treatment if patient has a coronary stent

### Lung function
- Perform spirometry, measure $T_LCO$ (CO transfer factor) if disproportionate breathlessness or other lung pathology, perform segment count and assess exercise tolerance
- Consider shuttle walk testing (cut-off 400 m) and cardiopulmonary exercise testing (cut-off 15 ml/kg per min) if moderate to high risk of postoperative dyspnoea
- Offer surgery if normal $FEV_1$ and good exercise tolerance or $FEV_1$ or $T_LCO$ <30% and patient accepts the risks of dyspnoea

Successful surgical resection depends on complete resection. If any disease remains, or surgical margins are positive, then survival is not improved beyond oncological treatment. Indeed if the tumour has spread into the pleural cavity then radiotherapy can be made much more difficult.

If mediastinal nodes are affected then surgical treatment does not improve survival. Thoracotomy is a painful incision and is not appropriate for 'palliative' incomplete resections.

### Surgery with curative intent for non-small-cell lung cancer
- Offer more extensive surgery (bronchoangioplastic surgery, bilobectomy, pneumonectomy) only when needed to obtain clear margins
- Perform hilar and mediastinal lymph node sampling or en-bloc resection for all patients undergoing surgery with curative intent
- For T3 non-small-cell lung cancer (NSCLC) with chest wall involvement, aim for complete resection by extrapleural or en-bloc chest wall resection
- Offer patients with NSCLC who are fit for surgery open or thoracoscopic lobectomy as the treatment of first choice. If complete resection is possible, consider segmentectomy or wedge resection for patients with smaller tumours (T1a–b, N0, M0) and borderline fitness

**CHAPTER 3**

## 4.2 Preoperative staging of bronchogenic carcinoma

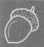

### In a nutshell ...

In view of the limited numbers of patients who benefit from surgical resection and the considerable morbidity of thoracotomy, accurate tumour staging is vital in order to maximise treatment effects.

**Clinical examination** looks for:
- Supraclavicular lymphadenopathy
- Evidence of hepatic metastasis
- Skin metastases

**CT chest (include liver, adrenals and lower neck)** looks for:
- Extent of primary tumour
- Surrounding atelectasis
- Intrapulmonary metastases
- Hepatic metastases
- Mediastinal lymphadenopathy (using mediastinal windows) – better viewed with positron-emission tomography (PET)/CT

**Further investigations** include:
- EBUS: endobronchial ultrasonography
- FNA: fine-needle aspiration
- TBNA: transbronchial needle aspiration
- EUS: endoscopic ultrasonography

## Bronchoscopy

Bronchoscopy is a procedure for examining the airways under direct vision. There are two major techniques: flexible bronchoscopy and rigid bronchoscopy.

### Flexible bronchoscopy
- Easier to perform
- Carries a low risk of trauma
- Small biopsies can be taken
- Visualisation of small airways

### Rigid bronchoscopy
- Preferred by some surgeons
- Gives direct feedback from the scope about tumour fixity
- Carries a higher risk of trauma to teeth and membranous trachea
- Does not allow visualisation of smaller airways
- Allows bigger biopsies

## Mediastinoscopy

Mediastinoscopy is a procedure that allows examination and biopsy of the paratracheal, tracheobronchial and subcarinal nodes.

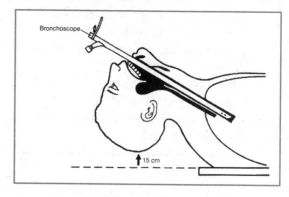

**Figure 3.10 Rigid bronchoscopy**

CHAPTER 3

## Procedure box: Mediastinoscopy

- Make a transverse skin incision 1 cm above the sternal notch and deepen through the platysma and between the strap muscles
- Lift the thyroid superiorly, and divide the pretracheal fascia
- Maintain a good view of the major vascular structures (in particular the right brachiocephalic artery) by ensuring perfect haemostasis throughout by careful blunt dissection
- Find a plane between the trachea and pretracheal fascia, and pass a finger to create a space
- The mediastinoscope is passed along the trachea and the lymph nodes are identified using gentle blunt dissection
- Biopsies are only taken after test aspiration with an epidural needle to ensure a vascular structure is not being entered

**Risks of mediastinoscopy**
- Injury to the brachiocephalic artery or other structures while gaining access to the trachea
- Injury to the trachea
- Oesophageal perforation
- Minor bleeding from perforation or biopsy of a bronchial artery
- Major bleeding from biopsy of azygos vein (may require thoracotomy)
- Torrential bleeding from biopsy of aortic arch or pulmonary trunk (may require median sternotomy or thoracotomy)
- Injury to left recurrent laryngeal nerve

## Indications for mediastinoscopy

The precise indications for mediastinoscopy are hotly debated by thoracic surgeons. Some perform it on all patients with mediastinal lymph nodes >1 cm in diameter demonstrated on CT scan. Others point out that CT-measured lymph node diameters do not necessarily predict tumour involvement, and perform mediastinoscopy in the preoperative assessment of every patient.

**CHAPTER 3**

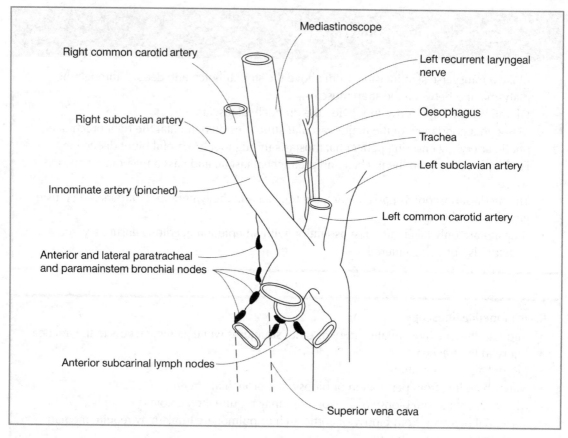

**Figure 3.11 Features that can be identified at mediastinoscopy**

## 4.3 Thoracic incisions

**In a nutshell ...**

- Anterolateral thoracotomy
- Posterolateral thoracotomy
- Chest drain insertion
- Video-assisted thoracic surgery (VATS)

### Anterolateral thoracotomy

This is the procedure of choice for emergency, resuscitation room procedures for management of cardiac or thoracic injuries, often in the context of major haemorrhage or cardiac arrest.

### Posterolateral thoracotomy

Although there are many variants on the thoracotomy, this is the most common incision through which elective thoracic procedures are performed.

## Procedure box: Anterolateral thoracotomy

Sterile technique is maximised within the limitations of speed.

**Position**

- The patient is supine

**Incision**

- Incise skin along the line of the rib aiming for the fifth interspace (below the nipple) from the lateral edge of the sternum laterally
- Use diathermy, if available, to incise the fat, and pectoralis and intercostal muscles. If not available, use a knife (and worry about haemostasis later)
- Avoid the IMA because it runs lateral to the sternal edge (it can cause substantial bleeding)

**Procedure**

- Open the pleura with suction ready, to obtain a good view
- Insert a self-retaining retractor
- Open the pericardium (if necessary)
- From here, it is possible to control cardiac bleeding: cross-clamp the descending aorta for abdominal injuries, or to control lung hilar or parenchymal bleeds

**Closure**

- See 'closure of thoracotomy'

## Closure of thoracotomy

- Place drains as required
- Avoid trauma to the intercostal bundles when placing heavy, braided nylon pericostal stitches in a figure-of-eight fashion around the two adjacent ribs
- Tie with slip knots so as to firmly close the chest
- Re-approximate serratus anterior and latissimus dorsi in layers
- Close the subcutaneous fascia
- Close the skin

## Procedure box: Chest drain insertion

Correct placement of chest drains is essential for management of pneumothorax, haemothorax and pleural effusions. Drains placed in the spleen, liver or left ventricle can be fatal. The following principles are invaluable.

**Chest drain insertion is painful**
- Always use plenty of local anaesthetic (LA) or, if there is time, ask an anaesthetist to place intercostal blocks
- Morphine may be used before the procedure as long as the patient does not have respiratory depression. **Pain kills**. Adequate analgesia is required to enable normal chest expansion and avoid respiratory tract infection, which can be fatal in elderly patients

**Size matters**
- Larger drains (28 Fr or 32 Fr gauge) are more effective for both fluid and air. Insert drains just anterior to the midaxillary line using an incision just large enough to admit your index finger. Deepen through the layers to the rib using a forceps

**Vertical mattress suture**
- Place a vertical mattress suture in the centre of the wound (to act as a purse-string when the drain is removed) and an anchoring suture at the end of the wound, both of heavy silk

**Over the rib**
- Gradually deepen through the intercostal muscles using a forceps. Stop and think when you reach the pleura

**Use a finger**
- Use a finger to break through the pleura. Can you feel anything on your fingertip? Can you feel the heart in front of you? Have you hit the liver? Is the lung tethered to the inside of the pleural cavity by adhesions? **If in doubt, STOP!**

**Place the drain**
- If your finger sweep has not revealed a contraindication
- Drains should be placed apically for pneumothoraces and basally for fluid
- **A** is for **a**ir and **a**pical
- **B** is for **b**lood and **b**asal

**Tie it in well**
- Throw the silk around the circumference of the drain twice. Place a surgeon's knot, and watch it tighten with a kink in the silicone tube. Lock the knot

**Check the position**
- Check the position on a chest radiograph

## Procedure box: Posterolateral thoracotomy

**Position**
- For right-sided thoracotomy, the patient is placed in the left lateral position, with the left (dependent) arm brought forward, and a pillow placed in the axilla
- The right (uppermost) arm is placed on an arm board so it is supported over the patient's head

**Preop**
- The skin is prepared and draped so as to expose the posterior midline (spinal column) posteriorly, the nipple anteriorly and the iliac crest inferiorly
- Superiorly, the drape should be placed above the midpoint of the scapula

**Incision**
The landmarks of the curved skin incision are:
- Halfway between the posterior scapular border and the spine, at the midpoint of the scapula
- 4 cm below the angle of the scapula
- Half way between the angle of the scapula and the nipple

**Procedure**
- Incise the skin and subcutaneous fat, using diathermy for haemostasis
- Divide latissimus dorsi with diathermy
- Anteriorly, divide serratus anterior with diathermy
- At this stage pass a hand under the scapula in order to count the ribs and identify the intercostal space to be entered
- Divide the external intercostal muscle by running the diathermy over the top edge of the appropriate rib, from back to front
- Divide the internal intercostal muscle by bringing the diathermy from front to back, again over the top of the rib
- The pleura is seen, and entered cautiously, bearing in mind the possibility of adherent lung (some surgeons resect a rib at this stage, believing that this will enhance exposure)
- Use a self-retaining retractor to spread the ribs

**Closure**
- See 'closure of thoracotomy'

**CHAPTER 3**

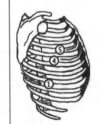
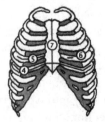
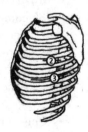
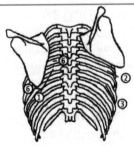

1. Posterolateral
2. Axillary
3. Lateral
4. Clamshell
5. Anterior
6. Thoracoscopy
7. Median sternotomy

**Figure 3.12 Posterolateral thoracotomy**

## Video-assisted thoracoscopic surgery

Many thoracic procedures can now be performed using minimally invasive video-assisted techniques. Such procedures aim to be essentially identical to their open counterparts with the exception of using smaller incisions.

### Principles of video-assisted thoracoscopic surgery

The principles of VATS are similar to laparoscopy but there are some differences:

- The precise location of ports depends on the operation being performed. In larger cases an **access port,** about 5 cm in length is used, as well as **instrument ports**
- The chest is relatively rigid, so $CO_2$ insufflation is not required. Ordinary instruments can be used without the requirement of air-tight seals

## 4.4 Thoracic procedures

### In a nutshell ...

Lung resection may remove:

- A whole lung: pneumonectomy
- A lobe: lobectomy
- A smaller piece of tissue: wedge resection

**Pleurodesis** is performed to fuse the pleural space.

Thoracic procedures of all sorts rely on **single-lung ventilation** using a **dual-lumen endotracheal tube**. Using this technique, the uppermost, operated lung can be deflated while the patient is oxygenated via the dependent, non-operated lung.

## Pneumonectomy

This is indicated for tumours that are centrally located or that impinge on the proximal bronchial tree.

### Procedure

- The resection is usually conducted via a posterolateral thoracotomy
- The lung is mobilised and any adhesions taken down
- Inspect the parietal pleura to exclude pleural metastases before proceeding
- Inspect the lung and hilum to ensure that no residual disease will be left after resection
- The hilum is circumnavigated, dividing the pleura overlying the pulmonary artery, veins and bronchus. Separate the lung from the oesophagus, and from the arch of the aorta on the left side
- Divide the hilar structures in any order, usually beginning with the pulmonary artery, then the pulmonary veins, then the bronchus. Ligate each structure with transfixion sutures or using a linear stapler
- Lymph node sampling may be performed
- Place a single basal drain in the pneumonectomy space
- The hemithorax is washed out thoroughly
- The thoracotomy is closed

### Complications of pneumonectomy

- **Bleeding** is a hazard:
  - Because of the huge vessels (pulmonary trunk, pulmonary veins) that are divided in the procedure
  - Because the pneumonectomy space is a huge cavity into which blood can be lost
- **Chest infection:** this can be lethal because of loss of pulmonary reserve. Patients should be informed of the need for aggressive

management of chest infections for the rest of their lives

- **Death:** this occurs in 6% of pneumonectomy patients

---

**Pneumonectomy spaces**

**Natural history**

- Pneumonectomy spaces fill with fluid over approximately 3 months. During this time, an air–fluid level is expected on the chest radiograph. When the space is completely obliterated, the space should be completely opaque on chest radiography

**Bronchopleural fistula**

- In the event that the bronchial stump breaks down, the pneumonectomy space becomes infected with respiratory organisms. In this event, an air–fluid level will be seen on the chest radiograph beyond the time when it should have been obliterated, or a new air–fluid level will appear

**Pneumonectomy space empyema**

- This may ensue from bronchopleural fistula and requires drainage

---

## Lobectomy

This is the most commonly performed lung resection. Each lobe is supplied by bronchial, pulmonary arterial and pulmonary venous branches. In addition there is a minor blood supply from the systemic circulation via the bronchial arteries. The precise technique differs for each of the lobes. Increasingly, lobectomies are performed using minimally invasive VATS.

## Procedure

- A posterolateral thoracotomy is usually performed
- Inspect parietal pleura for metastases
- Palpate the lung to determine location and extent of the tumour, and to ensure that lobectomy will be an adequate resection
- The hilum is circumnavigated to expose the relevant pulmonary artery, veins and bronchus. In the case of upper lobes, take great care to preserve the vessels supplying the lower lobes, which will remain after the resection
- The fissure is identified and developed using careful dissection with scissors and forceps. If the fissure is fully or partially fused, identify hilar landmarks and divide the lung parenchyma using a cutting linear stapler
- Divide pulmonary arterial, venous and bronchial branches and ligate them in order of convenience, usually the artery, then the vein, then the bronchus
- The specimen is removed. Haemostasis is obtained, and the remaining lobe re-inflated
- Lymph node sampling may be performed
- **B**asal (**b**lood) and **a**pical (**a**ir) drains are placed
- The thoracotomy is closed

## Complications of lobectomy

- **Bleeding:** this is usually tamponaded by the remaining lung, so is not often a problem
- **Chest infection:** this may result from poor chest expansion from poor analgesia, causing retention of secretions and pneumonia
- **Air leaks:** these can arise from parenchymal injury, or where excessively thick lung has been stapled. Prolonged air leaks can cause contamination of the pleural space with respiratory bacteria, and **empyema** can result

## Wedge resection, bullectomy and lung biopsy

These are largely the same from a technical point of view, differing only in their indication or the pathology excised. Wedge resections are normally performed for benign pathology. Apical bullectomy is performed for the removal of apical 'blebs' in young patients with recurrent pneumothoraces. Lung biopsy is performed for diffuse lung disease in order to provide tissue for definitive diagnosis.

These procedures are well suited to the VATS approach.

### Procedure

- Access is obtained via a posterolateral thoracotomy or using VATS
- Identify the target piece of lung and grab it with the Rampley sponge-holding forceps
- Excise the piece of lung using a linear stapler cutter
- Haemostasis is ensured
- If a **bullectomy** has been performed, pleurodesis may be achieved by insufflation of kaolin talc
- The lung is re-inflated
- Drains are placed apically and basally
- The chest is closed

Complications of wedge resection, bullectomy and lung biopsy are the same as those for lobectomy.

## Pleurodesis

In many thoracic conditions such as mesothelioma (see Section 5.1) or pneumothorax (see Section 5.3) it is desirable to 'glue' the pleurae together in order to eliminate the potential space. There are three techniques by which this can be achieved:

1. **Kaolin insufflation:** a 'snowstorm' of kaolin talc is pumped into the thoracic cavity in order to promote inflammation and adherence of the pleurae to one another (an alternative, for use on the ward, involves instillation of a **kaolin slurry** via a chest drain)
2. **Pleural abrasion:** the parietal pleura is abraded using emery paper to create a raw, inflamed surface
3. **Pleural stripping:** the parietal pleura is stripped off in order to create a raw surface

### Outcomes and complications

- **Postoperative pyrexia:** this results from an inflammatory reaction. It is deemed a sign of successful pleurodesis
- **Pain:** this is severe after pleurodesis procedures. It causes poor chest expansion, so may lead to **pneumonia** with high mortality in elderly patients with prior respiratory compromise

# SECTION 5

# Other thoracic surgical pathology

## In a nutshell ...

- Mesothelioma
- Empyema
- Pneumothorax
- Chronic obstructive pulmonary disease (COPD)
- Lung transplantation
- Thoracic aortic pathology

## 5.1  Mesothelioma

### In a nutshell ...

Mesothelioma is a lethal and largely untreatable cancer, which results from asbestos exposure. Initially, white fibrous **asbestos plaques** are formed, seen as pleural thickening on a chest radiograph. In a few patients these transform after many years into mesothelioma.

## Pathology of mesothelioma

Histologically, mesothelioma can be divided into **epithelial**, **sarcomatoid** and **mixed** subtypes. On light microscopy they can be difficult to distinguish from sarcomas and adenocarcinomas, although immunohisto-chemistry can make the distinction clearer. There are six different asbestos fibre types; the most commonly used are chrysotile (white curly fibres), amosite (brown needle-like fibres) and crocidolite (blue, needle-like fibres).

## Clinical presentation of mesothelioma

For most patients the first symptom is shortness of breath, caused by the presence of a pleural effusion, and relieved when the effusion is drained. As the disease becomes more advanced patients experience continuous chest discomfort. Tumour invasion of the chest wall results in more severe chest pain. In very advanced disease the pericardium and contralateral chest can be invaded.

## Diagnosis of mesothelioma

Histological diagnosis is made from pleural biopsy. Often a standard percutaneous biopsy is inadequate, and the patient is referred for formal rib resection, in which a mini-thoracotomy incision is made and a small section of rib excised to reveal a window of pleura. A 1-cm-square piece of thickened pleura is taken.

## Treatment of mesothelioma

In most cases, treatment is palliative. Only a few carefully selected patients undergo pleuropneumonectomy and adjunctive chemoradiotherapy with curative intent.

**Palliative pleurodesis** is performed to alleviate shortness of breath by preventing reaccumulation of the pleural effusion. When a formal histological diagnosis has been made, and no curative treatment seems possible, pleurodesis normally employs kaolin slurry (see Section 4.4).

## 5.2 Empyema

### In a nutshell ...

Empyema is defined as the presence of infected material within the chest cavity. It can occur as a complication of thoracic surgery of all kinds, or it can occur 'spontaneously' after pneumonia. In extreme situations the infected cavity can erode through the chest wall to point as an abscess. This is called **empyema necessitans**.

Of all empyemas, 40% are caused by streptococcal species.

## Pathology of empyema

When it follows pneumonia, empyema develops in the following stages:
- Accumulation of parapneumonic pleural effusion
- Invasion of microorganisms and fibrin deposition
- Organisation and fibrosis, forming a fixed **empyema cavity** and entrapping the lung within a fibrous rind

## Symptoms of empyema

Patients with empyema experience:
- Persistent fever
- Shortness of breath
- Pleuritic chest pain

## Clinical findings of empyema

- White cell count may be elevated
- CXR usually shows obliteration of a costophrenic angle
- Lateral CXR shows characteristic D-shaped shadow due to the loculated pus
- Chest CT reveals precise nature of the empyema allowing planning for a surgical approach

## Management of empyema

Successful management of empyema requires:
- Control of sepsis with appropriate antibiotics
- Removal of pus
- Obliteration of the empyema cavity

## Decortication of empyema

On some occasions, it is possible to clear the chest of pus, and mobilise the lung to permit re-expansion during the course of one procedure. In general, decortication is reserved for young fit patients with good respiratory reserve.

- A thoracotomy is performed
- The empyema cavity is broken down with a hand and pus is washed away
- The rind is picked off the visceral pleura in order to permit re-expansion of the lung
- Apical and basal drains are placed
- The chest is closed

**Complications** of empyema are **air leak** and **bleeding** from the raw visceral pleural surface.

## Rib resection

Often, prolonged drainage will be required for obliteration of the empyema cavity. It is essential to have at least lateral chest radiographs and probably CT scans available in theatre to plan the incision, which will often lie far posteriorly. The aim is to place a very large chest drain which will cause an **empyema track** to mature over the course of weeks or months so that the cavity is gradually obliterated. In general, rib resection is reserved for old or compromised patients who would not tolerate decortication.

---

 **Procedure box: Rib resection**

- Patients are placed on their side as for a posterolateral thoracotomy
- Location of the incision is checked by aspirating pus from the cavity using a syringe and large-bore needle
- A mini-thoracotomy incision is made over the empyema cavity
- Expose the rib, and ligate and divide the intercostal bundle lying on its inferior surface
- Use heavy rib shears to cut out a 1-cm section of rib
- Incise the pleura using a scalpel. Pus is collected for microbiological examination. Pus is sucked out, and the cavity washed out
- A skin incision is made beneath the mini-thoracotomy wound to admit the drain
- Place a very large (36 Ch) drain through the resected rib
- The chest wall is closed to skin

Postoperatively, if there has been no re-expansion of the lung on chest radiography, and if the drain is not swinging with respiration (implying that the empyema cavity is fixed), the drain can be cut to skin, and the pus drains into a gauze dressing.

## 5.3  Pneumothorax

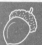

### In a nutshell ...

- Pneumothorax is the presence of air outside the lung and within the pleural space. It can be traumatic, iatrogenic or spontaneous:
  - **Traumatic pneumothorax:** may occur by blunt or penetrating trauma
  - **Iatrogenic pneumothorax:** caused by subclavian cannulation (pacemakers, central lines), percutaneous pleural or lung biopsy, barotrauma from artificial ventilation and a host of other interventions
  - **Spontaneous pneumothorax:** occurs most frequently in two groups of patients:
    - Elderly patients with bullous emphysema (COPD-related pneumothorax)
    - Young, tall (Marfan syndrome), thin, male smokers with apical 'blebs'

A one-off pneumothorax can be treated simply by observation with serial chest radiographs if the pneumothorax is small, or by placing a chest drain if it is >20% of lung volume.

- **Bilateral pneumothorax:** this is rare but it can be rapidly fatal
- **Tension pneumothorax:** this occurs when intrathoracic pressure rises so that the mediastinum is pushed to the contralateral side. It results in decreased cardiac output, tachycardia and sympathetic overdrive
- **Recurrent pneumothorax:** this is a frequent indication for surgical intervention. If the patient has had more than two pneumothoraces on one side, or pneumothoraces on both sides, or if there is an occupational hazard (eg pilots, oil platform workers, military personnel), then bullectomy and pleurodesis are performed

## Clinical features of pneumothorax

**Simple pneumothorax**

**Symptoms** (depend on the degree of collapse)
- Sharp chest pain
- Shortness of breath

**Signs**
- Loss of breath sounds
- Hyper-resonance

**Chest radiograph**
- Loss of lung markings

**Treatment**
- <20% 'observe' with serial chest radiographs
- 20–30% aspiration with Venflon and syringe
- >30% chest drain

---

**Tension pneumothorax**

**Chest radiograph findings** (should never be seen):
- Flattened diaphragm
- Mediastinal shift to contralateral side

**Treatment**
- If diagnosis suspected and patient in cardiac arrest, then large-bore Venflon in second intercostal space midclavicular line, followed by chest drain

---

## Surgical treatment of pneumothorax

Bullectomy and pleurodesis is increasingly performed using VATS:
- Access is obtained to the chest as described on pages 448–451
- The bulla (usually located apically) is excised using a linear cutter stapler
- The pleura is abraded, or stripped, or kaolin talc is insufflated
- Drains are placed
- The chest is closed

## Outcomes and complications of surgery for pneumothorax

- **Recurrence** of pneumothorax can occur, but it is rare after bullectomy and pleurodesis
- **Chest infection** may result from pain, poor chest expansion and retention of secretions
- **Death** ensues from chest infection in as many as 2% of elderly patients undergoing this procedure. It should not be done lightly

## 5.4 Chronic obstructive pulmonary disease

 **In a nutshell ...**

COPD is important in thoracic surgery because:
1. Many of the pathologies treated, such as bronchogenic carcinoma, coexist with COPD due to smoking
2. There are some indications for surgery in selected COPD patients

COPD is a constant companion of the thoracic surgeon because so many of the illnesses treated on a daily basis arise from cigarette smoking. Impaired lung function can markedly reduce a patient's suitability for and tolerance of surgery. COPD-related pneumothorax is discussed in Section 5.3.

Bullous emphysema can cause marked ventilation–perfusion mismatch, hypoxia and shortness of breath in those with advanced COPD. In highly selected patients, there can be some symptomatic benefit from **lung volume reduction surgery**. During this procedure particularly bullous areas of lung are excised to prevent compression of less affected areas of lung. As this procedure is performed on unfit patients with reduced respiratory reserve, it is associated with high morbidity and mortality. Therefore, candidates for surgery must be carefully selected and must be well motivated and well informed about the risks.

## 5.5  Lung transplantation

### In a nutshell ...

Lung transplantation has been performed successfully only for the last 20 years. Lungs can be transplanted singly, bilaterally or in combination with the heart.

### Indications and recipient selection

Typical indications for lung transplantation are as follows:

- **COPD:** in young patients with $\alpha_1$-antitrypsin deficiency. They may be suitable for single lung transplantation
- **Cystic fibrosis:** more likely to require bilateral lung transplantation in order to avoid spillage from a chronically infected 'bad' lung into the transplanted lung
- **Fibrosing lung diseases:** may be suitable for single lung transplantation
- **Congenital heart disease** leading to pulmonary vasculopathies such as Eisenmenger syndrome; may require heart and lung transplantation, or lung transplantation combined with correction of the cardiac defect

### Recipient selection

Lung transplantation carries a high risk of mortality, so it is offered only to patients with lung disease that is severe enough to limit their prognosis to a year or less. Often these patients need ambulatory oxygen preoperatively, and have an $FEV_1$ <15% predicted. As the risk to the recipient is so great, donor organs must be exceptionally carefully evaluated to ensure that the risk–benefit analysis is favourable.

The criteria for recipient selection are:
- Medical therapy is ineffective
- Activities of daily living are substantially limited
- Life expectancy is limited
- Cardiac function is adequate (if lung-only transplantation is planned)

## Donor organs and selection

### Shortage of donor organs

Lung transplantation is limited more than other transplantations by a shortage of donor organs, so much so that around a third of patients die on the waiting list. The problem is particularly acute because after brainstem death ventilated patients are very likely to aspirate, develop hospital-acquired pneumonia, or develop neurogenic pulmonary oedema.

There is ongoing research into ex-vivo lung perfusion (EVLP) to optimise harvested lungs before transplantation. EVLP involves connecting the pulmonary circulation to a machine and perfusing with fluid, with the aim of reducing inflammation. EVLP may allow the use of donors who do not fulfil the traditional criteria (see below).

### Donor selection

Donors are only suitable if:
- Age ≤55 years
- ABO-compatible
- Clear chest radiograph

CHAPTER 3

- $PaO_2$ ≥300 mmHg (39.9 kPa) on $FiO_2$ 1.0, 5 cmH$_2$O positive end-expiratory pressure
- Tobacco history ≤20 pack years
- Absence of chest trauma
- No evidence of aspiration/sepsis

- No prior cardiopulmonary surgery
- Sputum Gram stain: absence of organisms
- No purulent secretions at bronchoscopy

## Lung transplantation procedures

### Procedure box: Donor procedure (lung harvest only)

- The donor is opened from the suprasternal notch to the pubis by the abdominal organ retrieval team
- The lungs are mobilised and adhesions divided
- The venae cavae and aorta are mobilised, taking care not to injure the right pulmonary artery which runs behind
- The donor is heparinised
- Cannulas are placed in the ascending aorta and pulmonary trunk
- Pulmonary drugs that vasodilate may be injected into the pulmonary trunk at this stage
- An aortic cross-clamp is placed
- Cardioplegia fluid is run into the aortic root
- The cardioplegia fluid is vented into the pericardium via an incision in the IVC
- Divide both cavae, the aorta and the pulmonary trunk
- Incise the left atrium so as to leave a patch posteriorly joining the pulmonary veins
- The heart is explanted
- The left and right pulmonary arteries are separated
- Using scissors divide the posterior pericardium in a vertical direction between the left-sided and right-sided pulmonary veins
- The lungs are inflated by the anaesthetist and the two main bronchi are stapled off before division so that the lungs remain inflated in transit
- The lungs are placed on ice for rapid transit to the recipient

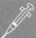

### Procedure box: Recipient procedure (single-lung transplantation)

- A posterolateral thoracotomy is performed
- The aorta and right atrium are cannulated for CPB
- The old lung is excised using clamps on the pulmonary artery, left atrium and bronchus
- The donor lung is placed in the thoracic cavity
- The artery, vein and bronchus are anastomosed
- Haemostasis is obtained, drains are placed and the chest is closed

## Outcomes and complications of lung transplantation

- **Bleeding:** from anastomotic lines
- **Bronchial stenosis:** at the site of anastomosis
- **Early graft dysfunction:** from ischaemic reperfusion injury
- **Rejection:** acute or chronic
- **Infections:** bacterial, fungal or viral. Predisposed to by immunosuppression
- **Death:** 20% at 1 year; 50% at 5 years

## 5.6 Thoracic aortic pathology

### Thoracic aortic aneurysm

> **In a nutshell ...**
>
> Thoracic aortic aneurysms are less common than abdominal aortic aneurysms and often arise in the context of connective tissue diseases such as Marfan syndrome.
> Classification is according to anatomical extent. Most patients are asymptomatic. Indications for surgery include symptoms, complications, size >5.5 cm or progressive enlargement.
> Surgery involves prosthetic graft replacement of the affected segment, and morbidity and mortality are high. Endovascular stent graft repair techniques have also been developed.

### Pathology of thoracic aortic aneurysms

- Congenital:
  - Marfan syndrome
  - Ehler–Danlos syndrome
- Degenerative:
  - Atherosclerotic
  - Cystic medial degeneration
- Traumatic
- Inflammatory:
  - Takayasu arthritis
  - Kawasaki syndrome
  - Behçet syndrome
  - Microvascular disorders
  - Infectious: bacterial, mycotic, spirochaetal, viral
- Mechanical:
  - Post-stenotic dilatation
  - Arteriovenous fistula aneurysms
- Pseudoaneurysm: infection, technical error

> **Classification of thoracic aortic aneurysms**
> 1. Ascending
> 2. Arch
> 3. Descending thoracic
> 4. Thoracoabdominal (four types – the Crawford classification):
>    – Extent I: descending aorta from left subclavian to renal arteries
>    – Extent II: descending aorta from left subclavian to beyond renal arteries
>    – Extent III: distal half of descending thoracic aorta and substantial segment of abdominal aorta
>    – Extent IV: level of diaphragm to aortic bifurcation

### Clinical features of thoracic aortic aneurysms

- Asymptomatic (detected incidentally)
- Symptomatic:
  - Chest pain

- Neck/jaw pain
- Aortic regurgitation
- Interscapular/back pain
- Abdominal/flank pain
- Wheeze, cough, pneumonitis, haemoptysis
- Ischaemia of gut or lower limbs
- Massive haematemesis/per-rectum bleed
- Sudden rupture and death

## Diagnosis of thoracic aortic aneurysms

- MRI + MR angiography
- CT
- Transoesophageal echocardiography
- Contrast aortography

---

**Indications for surgical management of thoracic aortic aneurysms**

- Symptoms
- Complications:
  - Acute proximal dissection
  - Rupture
  - Peripheral embolism
  - Aortic valvular regurgitation
- Large size: >5.5 cm in ascending aorta and 6.5 cm in the descending aorta (less in Marfan syndrome)
- Progressive enlargement (1 cm/year)

---

## Management of thoracic aortic aneurysms

- Direct operative repair by graft replacement
- Endovascular stent graft placement

The method of surgery depends on the location and extent of the aneurysm.

## Surgical outcomes

- Significant morbidity and mortality
- Worse in emergency surgery or if dissection is present
- Complications include:
  - Pulmonary complications
  - Bleeding
  - Neurological injury
  - Postoperative coronary insufficiency
  - False aneurysms
  - Graft infection

Descending aneurysms are more hazardous to replace, with a risk of mortality of about 10%.

# Aortic dissection

Aortic dissection is an acute event that begins when blood escapes from the aortic lumen via an intimal tear, and subsequently tracks outside the inner layers of the aortic media to create a **false lumen**. Rupture of the **vasa vasorum** causing intramural haematoma may also lead to aortic dissection. Where the aortic layers separate at the origins of vessels, those vessels may become occluded, resulting in ischaemia of the end-organ. Aortic dissection may occur anew. An aortic aneurysm is not always present before the acute event.

## Causes of aortic dissection

- Hypertension: associated with dissection
- Medial degeneration
- Aortitis: from syphilis or large-vessel vasculitis
- Connective tissue diseases, eg Marfan syndrome, Ehlers–Danlos syndrome
- Remember – many normal aortas dissect

**Classification of thoracic aortic dissection**
**De Bakey classification**
- Type I: intimal tear originates in ascending aorta and dissection propagates a variable distance distally to affect descending, abdominal and sometimes femoral vessels
- Type II: dissection confined to ascending aorta
- Type III: dissection arises in descending aorta and propagates distally

**Stanford classification**
- Type A: dissection affecting ascending aorta
- Type B: dissection affecting descending aorta

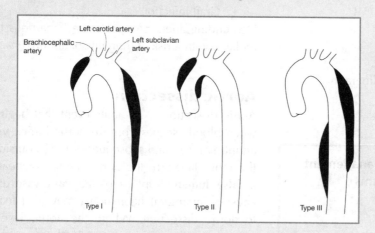

**Figure 3.13 De Bakey classification of thoracic aortic dissection**

## Presentation of aortic dissection

### Shock
- **Hypovolaemia** arising from **free rupture** of the dissection into the pleura or peritoneum (large effusion or haemothorax on chest radiograph; abdominal distension)
- **Tamponade** due to rupture into the pericardium (elevated neck veins, decreased BP)
- **Acute aortic regurgitation** from detachment of the aortic valve commissures (water-hammer pulse; widened pulse pressure; murmur)
- **Myocardial infarction** from dissection of the right coronary orifice (inferior ECG changes)

Depending on its severity, shock may cause **sudden death**, or hypotension on presentation. Some patients are not shocked on presentation.

### Pain
Pain begins suddenly, sometimes between the shoulder blades, but occasionally in the anterior chest, radiating into the arms or jaw, masquerading as myocardial pain. Indeed pain may be myocardial if it results from dissection of the coronary orifices.

### Symptoms of end-organ ischaemia
- Pulseless **cold legs** from femoral artery occlusion

CHAPTER 3

- **Oliguria** from occlusion of renal arteries
- **Paraplegia** from occlusion of the vertebral arteries

## Investigation of aortic dissection

- **Chest radiograph:** when the aortic arch or descending aorta is affected, the aortic shadow will be widened to the left. Pericardial effusion may cause cardio-megaly. In free rupture there may be (more often left-sided) pleural effusion
- **TOE:** may demonstrate intimal flap. Pericardial fluid, aortic regurgitation and wall-motion abnormalities of the ventricles may be detected. In conscious patients the procedure may cause gagging and raised BP, leading to worsening of the dissection
- **CT with contrast:** this may delineate the morphology of the dissection. CT cannot assess aortic regurgitation. In the non-acute setting CT may be augmented by MRI
- **Aortography:** this is the gold standard test, but it may not be as convenient to perform as CT

## Differential diagnosis of aortic dissection

The symptoms of aortic dissection are similar to those of acute MI. As it is possible to occlude the right coronary artery with aortic dissection, these patients will also have ST elevation on their ECG strips. Therefore, on rare occasions, patients with aortic dissection may be thrombolysed with disastrous consequences.

## Preoperative treatment of aortic dissection

- IV access
- Diagnostic investigations as above
- Intubation and ventilation if required
- Permissive hypotension with control of systolic BP to 90–100 mmHg using infusible β blockers or vasodilators

## Aims of surgery

- Alleviation of tamponade
- Prevention of further haemorrhage
- Restoration of blood flow to areas where arteries have been occluded
- In cases which affect the ascending aorta, correction of aortic regurgitation

## Repair of Stanford type A or De Bakey types I and II

This procedure aims to replace the ascending aorta with a synthetic tube graft. The aortic valve may be resuspended or replaced, often using a **composite graft** consisting of a valve and tube graft in one unit.

## Principles of repair of De Bakey type I and II aortic dissection

- The patient is placed supine on the operating table, prepped from legs to neck, and draped
- The femoral artery is exposed and cannulated for CPB
- A median sternotomy is performed
- A venous cannula is inserted into the right atrium
- CPB and systemic cooling are initiated
- Dissect the aorta free of the pulmonary trunk, taking care not to disrupt it
- Place a cross-clamp proximal to the innominate artery
- Incise the aorta longitudinally
- Give cardioplegia via the coronary ostia to induce cardiac arrest
- Depending on whether or not the aortic valve is to be replaced, the aorta can be transected above the valve, or the valve can be excised as well
- The coronary ostia are exposed and freed from the aortic root on 'buttons' of the aortic wall
- If there is aortic regurgitation, either resuspend the valvular commissures, or implant a prosthetic or bioprosthetic valve (often in the form of a composite graft)
- If the head and neck vessels are not affected by the dissection, replacement of the root is adequate. Alternatively, if it is deemed necessary to replace the aortic arch, the patient is cooled to below 20°C for total circulatory arrest
- If the patient is to undergo replacement of the arch, an island of aortic wall containing the brachiocephalic arterial ostia is retained and implanted into a similarly shaped defect in the tube graft
- The proximal end of the tube graft is implanted by buttressing the separated layers of the aortic wall together between two Teflon strips
- The coronary 'buttons' are re-implanted into the graft
- The top end of the graft is again anastomosed with the aorta using Teflon felt strips to buttress the layers together
- If the circulation has been arrested, it is restarted
- The patient is rewarmed
- Haemostasis is obtained
- The patient is weaned from CPB and decannulated
- The median sternotomy is closed

## Repair of Stanford type B or De Bakey type III aortic dissection

Many descending thoracic aortic aneurysms can be managed medically with BP control and serial follow-up imaging. Surgery is reserved for those at risk of rupture, or to correct end-organ ischaemia caused by dissection. The procedure outlined below aims to replace the affected part of the descending aorta with a synthetic graft. The descending aorta gives off vertebral arterial branches, so spinal cord ischaemia is a serious potential complication. Frequently, this procedure is performed using partial CPB in which a modified circuit takes oxygenated blood from the left atrium and pumps it back into the aorta distal to the aneurysm repair (eg by femoral cannulation).

### Principles of repair of De Bakey type III aortic dissection

- The anaesthetist passes a dual-lumen endotracheal tube to allow collapse of the left lung
- The patient is placed in the right lateral position for a left posterolateral thoracotomy
- If CPB is to be used, the left femoral artery is exposed and cannulated
- If a thoracoabdominal repair is to be attempted, extend incision anteriorly through the costal cartilages and into the abdomen. This incision provides a good view of the thoracic aorta and distal arch
- If bypass is to be used, the proximal aorta, left ventricle or left atrium can be cannulated
- Cross-clamps are placed just distal to the left subclavian artery, and below the level of the dissection
- Incise the aorta longitudinally, and identify the true lumen
- Buttress the layers of the aortic wall with Teflon felt
- Interpose tube graft between the two transected aortic ends. Clamps are removed above and below the graft
- Haemostasis is obtained
- Bypass cannulas are removed
- Drains are placed and the chest is closed

### Outcomes and complications of aortic dissection repair

- **Bleeding:** this may be severe, particularly if the patient had a major haemorrhage preoperatively (consumptive coagulopathy) or a prolonged period on CPB
- **Paraplegia:** this may result from spinal cord ischaemia in around 10%
- **CVA:** this can arise from emboli from the thoracic aortic manipulation

- **Infection:** of prosthetic material may occur
- **Pain:** this can arise from the thoracotomy wound
- **Chest infection:** this may occur secondary to poor chest expansion as a result of pain
- **Mortality:** around 10%
- **Renal failure:** especially when the dissection flap causes renal artery ischaemia. Can also be a result of prolonged CPB

## Thoracic aortic transection

Blunt chest trauma can result in life-threatening aortic injury. Often this is in association with injuries elsewhere (eg head trauma and hepatic laceration). In severe cases, aortic injury is rapidly fatal, but with more minor insults it can be survivable.

### Pathogenesis and morphology of thoracic aortic transection

At its superior end, the descending aorta is anchored to other chest contents by the ligamentum arteriosum, the exits of the brachiocephalic vessels and the vertebral arteries. When confronted with rapid deceleration, this part of the aorta decelerates with the thorax, whereas the adjoining portion of the aortic arch, full with blood, continues to move forward. Thus, the most frequent site of aortic transection is the interface of these two regions, 1 cm distal to the origin of the left subclavian, and just proximal to the ligamentum.

Depending on the force of deceleration, the transection can be complete, resulting in complete exsanguination into the pleura. In less severe cases, parts of the aortic wall, the mediastinal pleura and adventitia remain intact. In these cases, a more chronic, false aneurysm may result, which can gradually expand and rupture.

### Presentation of thoracic aortic transection

- **Haemodynamic instability:** many patients present with haemodynamic instability secondary to blood loss. They may be found to have a haemothorax on chest radiography and drain insertion, which then prompts a chest CT and definitive diagnosis
- **Pain:** this is a less common presenting feature

### Investigation of thoracic aortic transection

- **Chest radiograph:** shows left-sided pleural effusion or haemothorax from massive blood loss, upper mediastinal widening, and blurring of the aortic border
- **Chest CT:** this can be used to diagnose aortic transection. It is useful for investigation of simultaneous injuries, such as head trauma and abdominal trauma
- **TOE:** this is able to detect dissection flaps, disturbance of the aortic wall and periaortic haematoma. In the conscious patient it may raise BP and therefore worsen dissection. It may also prove more difficult if the cervical spine is immobilised
- **Aortography:** this has high specificity and sensitivity for aortic injury. However, its availability may be limited and it may impose a time delay on definitive treatment

### Treatment of thoracic aortic transection

Non-surgical and surgical treatment is similar to that used for non-traumatic aortic dissection, with the exception that in transection other injuries may require a modified approach.

#### Principles of treatment

- ABC (**a**irway, **b**reathing, **c**irculation); stabilisation of the cervical spine
- Control of systolic pressure to 90–100 mmHg using infusible β blockers or vasodilators
- Confirmation of diagnosis/imaging
- Definitive management

# CHAPTER 4

# Endocrine Surgery

**Nicholas E Gibbins and Sylvia Brown**

# SECTION 1

# Thyroid gland

## 1.1 Embryology of the thyroid

The thyroid gland first appears as an epithelial proliferation in week 4 of development, at the site of the foramen caecum in the base of the tongue (see Chapter 5, 'Embryology of the head and neck'). It descends to reach its final position by week 24 of gestation. It remains connected to the tongue by the thyroglossal duct, which later becomes solid and finally disappears.

Thyroglossal cysts can be found along this path of descent. They are cystic remnants of the thyroglossal duct. Accessory thyroid tissue can be found in the tongue, near the hyoid bone, deep to the sternomastoid muscle and in the superior mediastinum.

The thyroglossal tract may loop behind the hyoid. For this reason the central portion of the hyoid is usually excised with the tract in patients with thyroglossal fistula or cyst. It is important to recognise the fact that thyroglossal fistulae do **not** happen spontaneously but occur when an infected thyroglossal cyst is incised and drained in the mistaken belief that it is a simple abscess. Once incised they often do not heal and a fistula ensues.

## 1.2 Anatomy of the thyroid

 **In a nutshell ...**

The thyroid consists of two lobes connected by the thyroid isthmus. Each lobe has a lateral, a medial and a posterior surface. A pyramidal lobe is sometimes seen and is a remnant of the thyroglossal duct. The thyroid gland is surrounded by its own capsule and also by pretracheal fascia. The pretracheal fascia is attached to the larynx and trachea, both of which move upwards during swallowing – hence so does the thyroid gland.

### Blood supply of the thyroid
- **Superior thyroid artery:** first anterior branch of the external carotid artery
- **Inferior thyroid artery:** branch of the thyrocervical trunk from the first part of the subclavian artery (also supplies the parathyroid glands)

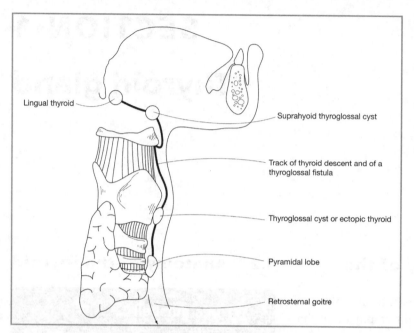

Lingual thyroid

Suprahyoid thyroglossal cyst

Track of thyroid descent and of a thyroglossal fistula

Thyroglossal cyst or ectopic thyroid

Pyramidal lobe

Retrosternal goitre

**Figure 4.1 The descent of the thyroid. Ectopic thyroid may occur anywhere along the path. The arrow shows the further descent of the thyroid which may take place retrosternally into the superior mediastinum**

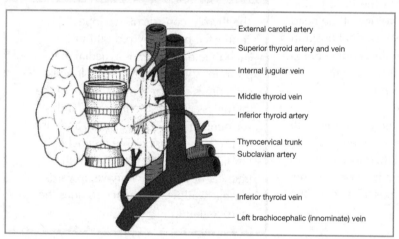

External carotid artery

Superior thyroid artery and vein

Internal jugular vein

Middle thyroid vein

Inferior thyroid artery

Thyrocervical trunk
Subclavian artery

Inferior thyroid vein

Left brachiocephalic (innominate) vein

**Figure 4.2 The thyroid and its blood supply**

- **Thyroid internal mammary artery** (IMA; present in only 3% of the population): it can be a branch from the brachiocephalic artery, the right common carotid artery or the aortic arch

## Venous drainage of the thyroid

- **Superior thyroid vein:** drains into the internal jugular vein either directly or via the facial vein
- **Middle thyroid vein:** drains into the internal jugular vein
- **Inferior thyroid vein:** forms a plexus inside the thyroid capsule which drains into the brachiocephalic vein (left more often than right)

CHAPTER 4

## Lymphatic drainage of the thyroid

- Upper pole: to the anterosuperior group of deep cervical nodes
- Lower pole: to the posteroinferior group of deep cervical nodes

Nodes in the central compartment of the neck (level 6) are removed along with the thyroid in patients with any well-differentiated carcinoma (papillary, follicular or medullary). For details of the levels of lymph nodes in the neck see Chapter 5, Head and Neck Surgery.

## Nerve supply of the thyroid

- **Sympathetic:** from the middle cervical ganglion (causes vasoconstriction)
- **Parasympathetic:** from the vagus (function is unknown)

## Recurrent laryngeal nerves

**The Beahr triangle** is the usual location of the recurrent laryngeal nerve:
- Superiorly: inferior thyroid artery
- Laterally: common cartoid artery
- Medially: trachea

Both the recurrent laryngeal nerves (RLNs) arise from the vagus, cranial nerve X.
- **Left RLN:** hooks around the ligamentum arteriosum under the arch of the aorta before ascending in the neck in the trachea–oesophageal groove
- **Right RLN:** hooks around the subclavian artery at the root of the neck. It ascends obliquely behind the common carotid artery to the trachea–oesophageal groove.

**Relations of the thyroid gland**

Lateral
- Strap muscles (sternothyroid, sterno-mastoid, sternohyoid)

Medial
- Recurrent laryngeal nerve
- External laryngeal nerve
- Larynx
- Pharynx
- Oesophagus
- Trachea

Posterior
- Parathyroid glands
- Carotid sheath and contents (contains internal carotid artery, internal jugular vein and the vagus nerve)
- Inferior thyroid artery
- Thoracic duct (on the left)

Isthmus
- Anastomosis between superior thyroid arteries
- Tributaries of the inferior thyroid veins
- Pyramidal lobe (remnant of the thyroglossal duct)

Both nerves ascend between the trachea and the oesophagus and pass behind the pretracheal fascia to lie next to the medial surface of the thyroid lobes.
- They are separated from the thyroid gland by pretracheal fascia
- They enter the larynx by approaching the cricothyroid joint from posteroinferiorly, curving anteriorly around it and dividing into its terminal branches
- Their relation to the inferior arteries is variable, but they can be located by identifying the Beahr triangle

**CHAPTER 4**

One per cent of right laryngeal nerves are 'non-recurrent', coming off the vagus in the neck. This is associated with an aberrant origin of the right subclavian artery.

Action of the RLNs:
- Motor supply to all the laryngeal muscles, except the cricothyroid, and sensation to the laryngeal mucosa from the vocal folds downwards
- Motor supply to the cricothyroid muscle is from the external laryngeal nerve (ELN), a branch of the superior laryngeal nerve, which is also a branch of the vagus nerve

## 1.3   Physiology of the thyroid

### In a nutshell ...

The thyroid is an endocrine gland which produces three hormones:
- Thyroxine ($T_4$)
- Triiodothyronine ($T_3$)
- Calcitonin

## Calcitonin

- Secreted from the parafollicular C cells of the thyroid gland
- This polypeptide inhibits resorption of calcium from bone when serum calcium concentrations become too high (see 'Hormonal control of bone activity' in Orthopaedic Surgery, Book 1)

- Medullary carcinoma of the thyroid is cancer of the parafollicular C cells (see Section 1.8) so medullary cancer of the thyroid produces calcitonin. Serum calcitonin can be measured to assess the presence, extent and recurrence of the disease

## Thyroxine and triiodothyronine

### Synthesis of $T_3$ and $T_4$

These hormones are iodine-containing amino acids. They are formed from the following:
- Dietary iodine in the bloodstream
- Tyrosine molecules bound to proteins in the colloid of the thyroid follicles

There are eight stages in the production of thyroid hormones (Figure 4.3).

### Actions of $T_3$ and $T_4$

Thyroid hormones stimulate oxygen consumption in most of the body's cells and increase the sensitivity of β receptors to catecholamines. Their actions are summarised in the table opposite.

Similar to most hormones, $T_3$ and $T_4$ exert their actions intracellularly by direct action on DNA expression and transcription of selected proteins. $T_3$ and $T_4$ are released from their plasma proteins, enter their target cells and are bound by intracellular proteins. Most $T_4$ is converted to $T_3$, which then binds to nuclear receptors.

CHAPTER 4

## Actions of T₃ and T₄ and their clinical implications

|  | Actions of T₃ and T₄ | Clinical effect in hyperthyroidism | Clinical effect in hypothyroidism |
|---|---|---|---|
| Catabolism | ↑ basal metabolic rate | Weight loss<br>Sweating<br>Heat intolerance<br>↑ appetite | Weight gain<br>Cold intolerance<br>↓ appetite |
|  | Lipolysis | Weight loss | Weight gain<br>Atherosclerosis |
|  | ↑ protein catabolism | Muscle wasting<br>Weakness<br>Weight loss |  |
|  | ↑ glycogenolysis | ↓ Diabetes mellitus control |  |
| Cardiovascular system | ↑ cardiac output due to:<br>↑ tissue metabolism<br>↑ pulse rate<br>Direct inotropic effect | Warm periphery<br>Vasodilatation<br>Wide pulse pressure | Cold peripheries |
|  | ↑ pulse rate due to action on β-adrenergic receptors | Tachycardia<br>Atrial fibrillation | Bradycardia |
| Gastrointestinal (GI) tract | ↑ GI motility and GI secretions | Diarrhoea | Constipation |
|  | ↑ glucose absorption | ↓ Diabetes mellitus control |  |
| Bone | ↑ bone resorption | Hungry bone disease<br>Hypercalcaemia |  |
| CNS | Aids normal development of CNS |  | Cretinism in children |
|  | Potentiates parasympathetic nervous system | Tremor<br>Anxiety<br>Brisk reflexes<br>Overactivity<br>Insomnia | Sluggishness<br>Apathy<br>Slowed reflexes<br>Tiredness |

CHAPTER 4

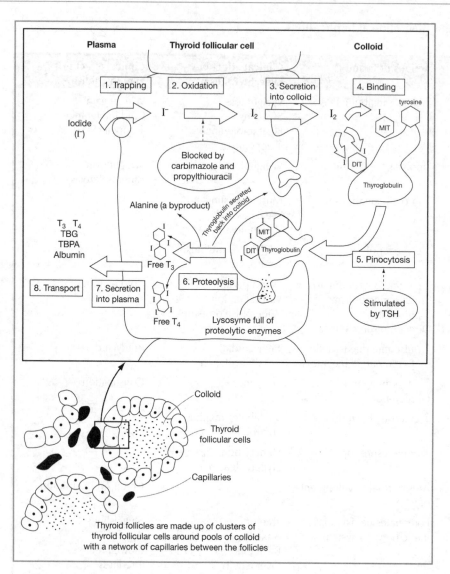

Figure 4.3 Synthesis of thyroid hormones

## Blood tests in thyroid disease

### Thyroid-stimulating hormone

- Normal serum range is 0.4–4.2 mU/l
- Often TSH is decreased in thyrotoxicosis and increased in hypothyroidism due to negative feedback (Figure 4.4). The exception occurs in pituitary tumours that secrete excess TSH and cause hyperthyroidism
- Iatrogenic suppression of TSH is achieved after thyroidectomy for malignancy by giving $T_4$ for life. Levels are measured in the postoperative clinic to ensure suppression. It is important to understand that $T_4$ is given for TSH suppression rather than replacement in this situation.

CHAPTER 4

## Explanation of the stages of synthesis of thyroid hormones shown in Figure 4.3

1. **Trapping:** iodide (I⁻) is absorbed from the plasma by the iodide pump, against its electrical gradient, into the thyroid follicular cell

2. **Oxidation:** iodide (I⁻) is converted to iodine (I$_2$) by the action of the enzyme thyroid peroxidase, with hydrogen peroxide accepting the electrons

3. **Secretion into colloid:** iodine is secreted out of the thyroid follicular cell in secretory droplets along with thyroglobulin, enzymes, and other thyroid secretions

4. **Binding:** tyrosine (an amino acid bound to thyroglobulin) is a large protein within the colloid. The iodination of tyrosine is catalysed by the enzyme iodinase. By addition of either one or two iodine molecules, tyrosine is converted to either monoiodotyrosine (MIT) or diiodotyrosine (DIT), respectively. These are precursors to the thyroid hormones and up to 2 months' supply of T$_3$ and T$_4$ can be stored in the colloid in this form. When the thyroid is inactive there are large pools of colloid

5. **Pinocytosis:** when there is a need for more plasma T$_3$ and T$_4$, the thyroid follicular cell transports the MIT and DIT into the thyroid follicular cell by pinocytosis. This process is stimulated by TSH

6. **Proteolysis:** enzymes are released into the reabsorption lacunae by lysosymes and free T$_3$ and T$_4$ molecules are released. Two DIT molecules form T$_4$ and a DIT plus an MIT molecule form T$_3$. The byproducts of this proteolysis are alanine, an amino acid, and the deiodinated thyroglobuin, which is secreted back into the colloid

7. **Secretion into plasma:** T$_3$ and T$_4$ can then be secreted into the bloodstream. The human thyroid secretes about 80 µg T$_4$ and 4 µg T$_3$ per day

8. **Transport:** 99% is bound to plasma proteins such as thyroid-binding globulin (TBG), thyroid-binding prealbumin (TBPA) and albumin. A tiny proportion of serum T$_3$ and T$_4$ is free. The actions of T$_3$ are about four times faster than those of T$_4$ because T$_4$ has a greater binding affinity for proteins. As a result of this high affinity, thyroid hormones are released slowly. The half-life of T$_3$ is 1 day and of T$_4$ about 7 days

## T$_3$, T$_4$ and thyroid-binding globulin

- Normal range for T$_3$ is 12–28 pmol/l
- Normal range for T$_4$ is 3–9 pmol/l

Ninety-nine per cent of T$_3$ and T$_4$ is carried in the plasma bound to proteins such as thyroid-binding globulin (TBG). Changes in the level of TBG can therefore affect total T$_3$ and T$_4$ levels, but the proportion of free T$_3$ and free T$_4$ should remain unchanged. TBG is increased in pregnancy and in patients on oestrogen therapy (eg combined oral contraceptive pill or OCP). It is decreased in liver disease, nephritic syndrome and systemic lupus erythematosus (SLE). This can lead to misleading serum measurements of thyroid hormone, eg in pregnancy measurements of total T$_3$ and total T$_4$ are increased because there is more TBG; however, the patient is euthyroid because free T$_3$ and free T$_4$ are within the normal range.

## Thyroglobulin

Used in the follow-up of well-differentiated thyroid cancers (see Section 1.8).

## Thyroid antibodies

- Anti-TSH receptor antibodies are detected in Graves' disease
- Anti-thyroid peroxidase (anti-TPO) antibodies (also known as antimicrosomal antibodies) are detected in Hashimoto's thyroiditis

## 1.4 Pathology of the thyroid

### In a nutshell ...

Thyroid disease may present as a swelling, a disordered metabolism or a combination; 7% of the world's population has a goitre, mostly as a result of iodine deficiency.

Thyroid swellings can be classified as follows:
- Diffuse goitre
- Multinodular goitre
- Solitary thyroid nodule

Patients may present with any combination of a normal or large thyroid coupled with hypo-, eu- or hyperthyroidism.

**Diffuse goitre**

See Section 1.5.

Usually this is non-toxic (ie euthyroid). Common causes are:
- Physiological: pregnancy, puberty
- Dietary: iodine deficiency or toxins
- Hereditary
- Treated Graves' disease

Rare causes include:
- Infection (TB, HIV, syphilis)
- Drugs (lithium, amiodarone, carbimazole)
- Amyloid deposits (this protein is characterised by β-pleated sheets which cannot be metabolised in humans) within the thyroid gland can cause goitre
- Congenital defects such as iodine transport defects, thyroglobulin synthesis defects and Pendred syndrome (congenital deafness in association with juvenile goitre)
- Drinking water contamination: high levels of *Escherichia coli*
- Fluoride

**Multinodular goitre**

See Section 1.6.

Most multinodular goitres are not thyrotoxic. **Non-toxic goitre** is caused by the following:
- Family trait
- Progression of diffuse goitre
- Sporadic multinodular goitre
- Pendred syndrome (a rare autosomal dominant condition)

**Toxic goitre** is caused by:
- Progression of diffuse goitre
- Graves' disease

**Solitary thyroid nodule**

See Section 1.7.

This may be a:
- Prominent nodule in a multinodular goitre
- True solitary nodule: eg an adenoma, cancer, cyst, fibrosis, thyroiditis
- Thyroglossal cyst

Thyroid swellings can also be classified as:
- **Goitre:** simple (non-toxic) or toxic; diffuse, nodular, multinodular or recurrent nodular
- **Neoplastic solitary nodule:** benign or malignant
- **Inflammatory goitre**
- **Rare goitre** (as above)

## 1.5 Diffuse goitre

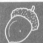 **In a nutshell ...**

Diffuse goitres may be toxic (producing hyperthyroidism) but more commonly are non-toxic (simple).

A diffuse non-toxic simple goitre diffusely involves the whole gland without producing nodularity and is not associated with hypothyroidism or hyperthyroidism. It is a compensatory hypertrophy and hyperplasia secondary to a reduction in output of $T_3$ and $T_4$. This reduction in output causes an increase in thyroid-releasing hormone and TSH, which in turn cause thyroid enlargement. The goitre may revert to normal, stay as a simple goitre or progress to a multinodular goitre (see below), which may be toxic or euthyroid.

## Causes of diffuse non-toxic simple goitre
- **Physiological goitre:** this is due to increased demands for thyroid hormone (eg in pregnancy and puberty)
- **Dietary iodine deficiency:** now this is uncommon in the UK, but traditionally it is the cause of goitres in areas far from the sea, such as the Alps, Himalayas and Andes, or even closer to home (eg Derbyshire neck)
- **Dietary goitrous agents:** these include uncooked brassicas (cabbage, turnips), calcium or fluoride in drinking water, *p*-aminosalicylic acid (PAS), lithium, phenyl-butazone and some drugs (eg thiouracil, carbimazole)
- **Hereditary congenital defects in thyroid metabolism:** these are very uncommon and do not usually require treatment, but may account for familial goitre. They include iodine transport defects, deiodinase deficiency, iodotyrosine coupling defects and thyroglobulin synthesis defects
- **Treated Graves' disease:** this is associated with a smooth, small or moderate-sized symmetrical goitre, hypervascularity, a bruit and typical facial signs (see Section 1.11). If untreated, Graves' disease is associated with hyperthyroidism
- **Other rare causes** of diffuse goitre: these are lymphoma, anaplastic carcinoma, autoimmune thyroiditis, de Quervain's thyroiditis and thyroid amyloidosis

## Treatment of diffuse non-toxic simple goitre

If small, no treatment is needed apart from reassurance and possibly iodine supplements. For cosmetic reasons or for pressure symptoms (if large), hemi- or total thyroidectomy may be required. Near-total thyroidectomy is no longer performed due to the risk of the residual thyroid enlarging, requiring repeated operations. Revision surgery would greatly increase the risk of complications, including RLN palsy.

## 1.6    Multinodular goitre

 **In a nutshell ...**

A multinodular goitre results from progression of the diffuse simple goitre to a larger (up to 2 kg) goitre with multinodular focal hyperplasia. Mostly these are euthyroid, but a proportion of them are hyperthyroid, and they may even be hypothyroid. Most of the toxic goitres that you see will be multinodular.

### Causes of multinodular goitre

- Progressive enlargement of diffuse goitre caused by any of the factors listed in Section 1.5
- Sporadic multinodular goitre predominantly affecting middle-aged women
- Previous radiation to the neck

### Pathological features of a multinodular goitre

- Follicles distended with colloid
- Inflammatory changes
- Areas of infarction
- Haemorrhage (may cause sudden or painful enlargement)
- Fibrosis
- Calcification (may be mistaken for malignancy)
- Cyst formation
- Hyperplastic nodules (may cause hyperthyroidism)

### Possible presentations of a multinodular goitre

- Cosmetic: unsightly swelling
- Discomfort, eg if enlargement was rapid, or there are areas of haemorrhage/infarction
- Irritating cough or biphasic stridor due to tracheal compression
- Dysphagia: less common because oesophagus is behind the trachea
- Patient/GP wishes to exclude malignancy
- Hyperthyroidism: see box on Plummer's disease below
- Hoarseness: from pressure on the larynx or RLNs. This is rare in non-malignant goitre

**Plummer's disease**

This is seen in patients over the age of 40. It is characterised by an autonomous hyperfunctioning nodule in a multinodular goitre. This leads to a mild hyperthyroidism which (unlike Graves' disease) is not associated with eye disease.

### Complications of multinodular goitre

- Local symptoms: stridor, superior vena cava (SVC) obstruction, dysphagia, cosmesis, retrosternal enlargement
- Toxicity: mild hyperthyroidism in the absence of Graves' disease, Plummer's disease
- Malignant change: 5% of untreated multinodular goitres
- Haemorrhage into a cyst: can lead to sudden, painful enlargement

## Treatment of multinodular goitre

Thyroxine will sometimes prevent progression but risks the side effects of thyrotoxicosis. Treatment should reduce TSH levels to zero.

**Indications for surgery** of a multinodular goitre:

- Local symptoms, eg significant or symptomatic retrosternal extension, dysphagia, tracheal deviation or stenosis
- Enlarging dominant nodule, unless unequivocally benign
- RLN palsy
- Cosmesis
- Hyperthyroidism

Surgery with hemithyroidectomy of the larger side or total thyroidectomy is the treatment of choice (see Section 1.13).

## 1.7    Thyroid nodule

### In a nutshell ...

Five per cent of the adult population will have a thyroid nodule. In 50% this is a **dominant nodule in a multinodular goitre**.

In 50% this is a **true solitary nodule** and of these:

- 80% are adenomas
- 10% are cancer (mostly papillary)
- 10% are cysts, fibrosis or thyroiditis

A thyroglossal cyst can be mistaken for a thyroid nodule (see Chapter 5, Head and Neck Surgery)

## Investigating a thyroid nodule

The two most sensible and universal thyroid investigations for you to mention in an exam situation are thyroid function tests (including autoantibodies) and ultrasound-guided fine-needle aspiration for cytology (FNAC).

- **Ultrasonography:** for anatomical information. One can see if the lump is a prominent nodule in a multinodular goitre, a solitary nodule or a cyst. Ultrasonography can also determine the size and nature of a mass but cannot say with 100% certainty whether it is benign or malignant. It is the most accurate method of diagnosing a multinodular goitre. In a cancer, it can help determine tumour size, assess the contra-lateral lobe, ascertain the nature of complex cysts and visualise abnormal lymph nodes in the neck
- **FNAC:** if a solitary thyroid nodule is seen, the next investigation is FNAC. FNAC is an excellent initial investigation of the solitary thyroid nodule with an overall diagnostic accuracy of >90% in specialist centres. If the results of FNAC are frankly malignant or suspicious the solitary nodule is treated surgically. If FNAC shows lymphoma, the patient should be further investigated by the haemato-oncology team (see box for classification of FNAC results)
- **Core biopsies:** these should be taken only from large or inoperable thyroid masses because they risk haemorrhage and damage to the surrounding structures, even when performed under ultrasound control. Core biopsies are being used increasingly in some specialist centres. Incisional biopsies are used only if lymphoma or anaplastic carcinoma is suspected (ie a rapidly growing mass)

**CHAPTER 4**

- Technetium-99m pertechnetate or iodine-123 **isotope scan** is indicated if the patient is clinically or chemically thyrotoxic. Isotope scans were previously used to determine if a nodule was 'hot' (ie functioning) or 'cold' (non-functioning). **Hot nodules** are almost invariably (>99%) benign and are typically caused by overactive tissue between the nodules of a multinodular goitre or by a hyperfunctioning thyroid adenoma. **Cold nodules** may be neoplastic. This investigation is used less commonly now because difficulties arose with 'warm' nodules that may or may not be malignant, and because of the fact that even a hot nodule should have FNAC to exclude neoplasia. In some centres this investigation has therefore been superseded by FNAC which should, in any case, be performed on all solitary thyroid nodules

---

**Classification of the FNAC result follows the Thy system:**

- Thy 1: insufficient for diagnosis
- Thy 2: benign (5% risk of malignancy)
- Thy 3: follicular lesion (unable to determine whether adenoma or carcinoma – 35% risk of malignancy)
- Thy 4: suspicious of papillary malignancy (75%)
- Thy 5: papillary malignancy (>95%)

If the result is **Thy 1**, the test is repeated and a core is considered.

**Thy 2** allows for reassurance, and if there are risk factors for cancer, re-scanning in 6 months' time.

A **Thy 3** result means that a diagnostic lobectomy should be performed with a warning to the patient that, if histology comes back as cancer rather than adenoma, a completion thyroidectomy with level VI dissection will need to be performed.

A **Thy 4** result is a grey area and depends on the surgeon with whom you work and the unit that you are in. Most will advocate a total thyroidectomy and level VI neck dissection but some will suggest hemithyroidectomy only in a similar way to a Thy 3 result.

**Thy 5** suggests that a total thyroidectomy is needed with level VI neck dissection.

Further treatment is advocated according to the type of cancer and is discussed later in the chapter.

---

## Preoperative assessment of the thyroid

Depending on the presentation, preoperative assessment may include:

- Flexible nasolaryngoscopy to assess vocal folds
- Chest radiograph to check for retrosternal extension and tracheal deviation
- Serum calcitonin if medullary carcinoma is suspected
- Barium swallow or endoscopy if the patient has dysphagia
- CT is now performed routinely preoperatively.

The sternum may need to be split in combination with the cardiothoracic surgeons if:

- There is extension into the posterior mediastinum
- Thyroid encroaches or wraps around the great vessels
- The thyroid is >30% of the volume of the thoracic inlet
- Isolated thyroid tissue in the thorax

## Management of a true solitary thyroid nodule

First do a full clinical assessment that includes:

- Thyroid function tests including anti-thyroid antibodies
- Ultrasonography
- FNAC

If FNAC shows that the lesion is malignant, treatment should proceed according to the particular cancer (see Section 1.8). If the lesion is benign and asymptomatic, the patient can be reassured.

If the lesion needs to be removed clinically (for pressure symptoms, cosmesis, patient wishes or FNAC suspicious of malignancy) a total lobectomy (which includes the isthmus) can be performed.

If patients are hyperthyroid they can be treated with drugs, radioiodine or surgery (see Section 1.13).

## 1.8 Thyroid cancers

### In a nutshell ...

- **70% papillary carcinoma:** affects young people; 95%+ survival
- **20% follicular carcinoma:** not able to diagnose on FNAC; 95%+ survival
- **5% medullary carcinoma:** C-cell multifocal cancer. May be part of MEN syndrome; genetic testing is required
- **<5% anaplastic carcinoma:** terrible prognosis. Seen in older patients
- **Lymphoma:** needs chemotherapy under the care of the haemato-oncologists. Good prognosis
- Other thyroid malignancy: rare

## Papillary carcinoma

- 70% of thyroid cancers are papillary carcinoma
- Often affects younger people. A history of irradiation to the neck should be sought
- Most papillary cancers are TSH-dependent
- Lymphatic spread to cervical lymph nodes

### Histology of papillary carcinoma

- No capsule
- May be multifocal
- Pale, empty-looking 'orphan Annie' nuclei
- Psammoma calcification, when seen, is diagnostic

### Treatment of papillary adenocarcinoma

**For lesions <1 cm:** this is controversial – for the exam answer, treat all papillary carcinomas as per lesions >1 cm. This approach is used only for young women with no lymphadenopathy and no high-risk factors, and only in certain institutions:

- Thyroid lobectomy
- $T_4$ for life (to suppress TSH and therefore recurrence; usually 125–150 µg/day)
- Annual thyroglobulin measurements and lifelong follow-up

**For lesions >1 cm** (including those with cervical metastases):

- Total thyroidectomy with neck dissection as appropriate
- Radioiodine ablation
- Lifelong TSH suppression with $T_4$
- Annual thyroglobulin (TG) measurements and lifelong follow-up

The 10-year survival is >90%.

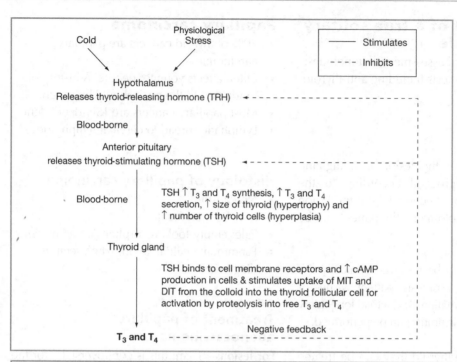

**Figure 4.4 Control of secretion of thyroid hormones**

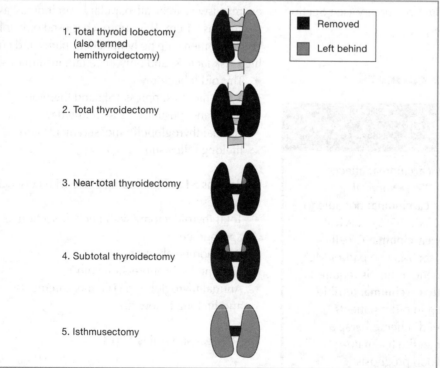

**Figure 4.5 Operations that can be performed on the thyroid to remove a cancer**

(Operations 3 and 4 are no longer employed. They are included purely for historical interest)

## Follow-up of papillary thyroid cancers

Follow-up comprises clinical examination and thyroglobulin (TG) levels. The most common presentation of recurrence is of a neck mass or an otherwise asymptomatic rise in the TG. Whole-body scintigraphy with iodine-131 is performed to detect local and distant metastases.

## Follicular carcinoma

- 20% of thyroid cancers are follicular carcinoma
- Usually unifocal
- Common in low-iodine areas
- Spreads via blood to lungs and bone

### Histology of follicular carcinoma

- Capsulated, but capsule breached = carcinoma
- Difficult to differentiate benign and malignant on FNAC alone
- May need to perform a thyroid lobectomy if preoperative investigations cannot determine whether the lesion is benign or malignant, and await the results of histology. If histology shows capsular transgression or vascular invasion, the other lobe must be removed surgically.
- Follicular adenomas look exactly the same as cancers on histology, but the capsule is not breached
- May see mixed papillary–follicular picture
- Treatment and follow-up are as for papillary carcinoma

## Medullary carcinoma

- 5% of thyroid cancers are medullary carcinoma
- Tumour of calcitonin-secreting parafollicular C cells (calcitonin is a biochemical marker

for these tumours). Other polypeptides such as carcinoembryonic antigen (CEA) can also be secreted
- Familial tendency can be part of the multiple endocrine neoplasia (MEN) syndrome (see Section 2.9)
- Can be multifocal
- May spread to lymph nodes

### Treatment of medullary carcinoma

- Treated by total thyroidectomy with routine neck dissection of nodes in the central compartment and on the affected side
- No value in postoperative radioiodine
- Follow-up is with clinical examination and calcitonin measurement. A rising calcitonin level is indicative of metastatic disease
- Recurrence can be treated surgically, but there is no evidence that this improves survival
- $T_4$ is given as a replacement but TSH does not need to be suppressed
- It is important to elicit a family history because affected relatives should be screened to exclude MEN or familial medullary carcinoma. In affected children prophylactic thyroidectomy is performed before school age

## Anaplastic carcinoma

- <5% of thyroid cancers are anaplastic carcinoma
- Seen in older patients
- Aggressive, undifferentiated tumour
- Spread is direct and via the lymph nodes
- It is thought to originate in pre-existing indolent tumours and there is sometimes a history of a long-standing goitre
- Diagnostic biopsy (core, needle or open) should be performed to exclude lymphomas, which can be treated successfully

## Treatment of anaplastic carcinoma

- Debulking surgery and palliative external-beam radiotherapy in selected cases
- Worst prognosis: 90% of patients are dead within a year (mean survival 6–8 months)
- Palliative care is usually involved. Tracheal stenting is sometimes an option

## Lymphoma in the thyroid

- Most commonly presents in elderly people but is also seen in younger age groups
- Rapidly expanding mass and obstructive symptoms
- Seen in patients with a long-standing history of Hashimoto's thyroiditis

- Core or open biopsy usually needed to make the diagnosis and distinguish it from anaplastic thyroid cancer (which presents similarly but has very different treatment and prognosis)
- Lymphoma is staged by CT

## Treatment of thyroid lymphoma

- Treatment is chemotherapy under the care of haemato-oncology
- Radiotherapy may be used in selected cases
- Thyroid surgery may be indicated in localised disease or for persistent disease
- Lymphoma patients have a good prognosis and 10-year survival rate

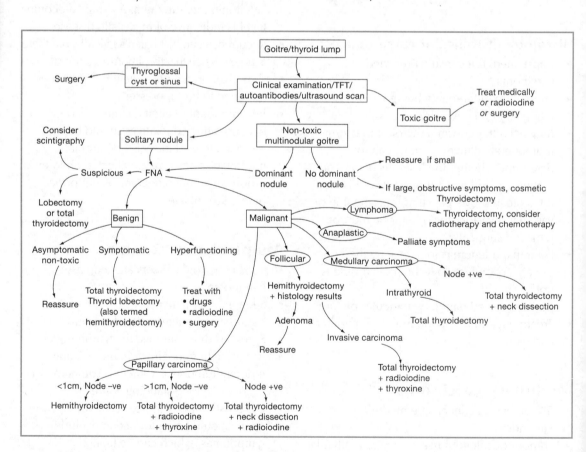

**Figure 4.6 The management of a thyroid nodule**

**Principles of thyroid cancer treatment**

**Surgical treatment of thyroid cancer**

**Total thyroid lobectomy (hemithyroidectomy):** the minimum operation for suspected thyroid malignancy (eg papillary and follicular cancers <1 cm). It is also used for unilateral multinodular disease and solitary nodule.

**Total thyroidectomy:** ideal for most other thyroid cancers, including those with cervical metastases and for patients with extensive benign disease. The parathyroids are spared if possible but no thyroid tissue is left behind.

**Isthmusectomy:** used for solitary nodules in the midline and for the relief of tracheal compression in anaplastic thyroid carcinomas or lymphomas.

**Routine neck dissection:** the thyroid gland drains to the lymph nodes in level VI in the middle of the neck. This region extends from the hyoid bone to the suprasternal notch and laterally to both internal jugular veins and the RLNs. The sternomastoid muscle and internal jugular veins are preserved, and the operation may have to be done through an extended thyroidectomy scar. This area should be routinely dissected in any cases of differentiated carcinomas that are node-positive and in all medullary thyroid cancers. Palpable disease more laterally will require lateral neck dissection and sacrifice of any surrounding structures that are involved.

**Non-surgical treatment of thyroid cancer**

**Thyroxine replacement therapy:** this suppresses TSH, which is a tumour growth factor. It reduces the risk of recurrence and is used as adjuvant therapy in papillary and follicular cancers.

**Radioactive iodine:** this is selectively taken up by well-differentiated thyroid cancers. It destroys the cells which take it up and is well tolerated. It is given to patients with papillary cancers >1 cm in size and/or node-positive and to patients with follicular carcinoma. If radioiodine is seen to be taken up postoperatively, a further dose is given 3–6 months later. To ensure good uptake of radioiodine, patients are rendered hypothyroid before its administration.

**Follow-up of thyroid cancer**

**Thyroglobulin measurements:** thyroglobulin is a protein that is unique to thyroid cells. Post-thyroidectomy levels should be <3 ng/ml. If levels increase, this is a sign of recurrent disease, and requires investigation and treatment. Thyroglobulin levels should be checked annually in the follow-up of papillary and follicular carcinomas. It is sometimes more difficult to interpret small changes in thyroglobulin levels after a lobectomy than after a total thyroidectomy.

**Whole-body scintigraphy with iodine-131:** after radioiodine, ablation is used in the follow-up of patients to detect local and distant metastases in well-differentiated thyroid cancers.

CHAPTER 4

## Other thyroid malignancies

- Sarcoma
- Metastases, typically from kidney, colon, breast or lung
- Lateral aberrant thyroid is no longer thought to exist. Detection of thyroid tissue lateral to the gland itself should be considered as metastatic thyroid cancer in a lymph node
- Hürtle cell carcinoma is a rare variant of follicular carcinoma. It may spread to nodes and may not take up radioactive iodine. The prognosis is a little worse than an equivalently sized follicular carcinoma

## 1.9 Thyroid adenoma

- Benign thyroid lesion (nearly all are follicular adenomas)
- Pathological features:
  - Discrete lesion with glandular or acinar pattern
  - Encapsulated
- Can 'hyperfunction' and cause hyperthyroidism
- Difficult to distinguish from malignancy as they are solid on ultrasonography, cold on isotope scanning and FNA/core biopsy cannot distinguish them from follicular carcinoma (the diagnosis depends on the presence or absence of vascular invasion)
- Usually diagnosed after excision (thyroid lobectomy) and the patient can be reassured

## 1.10 Thyroiditis

**In a nutshell ...**

- **Acute thyroiditis:** bacterial cause (usually streptococci)
- **Subacute thyroiditis** (de Quervain's thyroiditis): viral cause (Epstein–Barr virus [EBV], mumps, measles)
- **Chronic thyroiditis** (Hashimoto's thyroiditis): autoimmune cause

## Acute thyroiditis

Patients present with pain, tenderness and erythema over the thyroid gland. They are often systemically unwell with a fever, raised erythrocyte sedimentation rate (ESR) and raised white cell count (WCC). Thyroid function is normal. Infection can be caused by many organisms but is mostly due to streptococci, the natural flora of the oropharynx. Ultrasonography should be performed with an FNA and a sample should be obtained for MC&S (microscopy, culture and sensitivity). Treatment is with antibiotics and analgesia. Steroids are sometimes used.

## Subacute (de Quervain) thyroiditis

This is a granulomatous thyroiditis due to viral infection, mostly with EBV, mumps or measles. Patients present with a painful goitre and they classically have a period of hyperthyroidism followed by hypothyroidism, and then become euthyroid after 8 weeks, although a minority remain hypothyroid. ESR and WCC are elevated. Treatment is with aspirin and prednisolone for a 6- to 8-week period.

## Chronic (Hashimoto's) thyroiditis

This is an autoimmune disease seen most commonly in women. It is characterised by thyroglobulin antibodies and/or thyroid peroxidase antibodies. Pathologically, infiltration of lymphoid cells, which are organised in clumps and are associated with hyperplasia and fibrosis, is seen. The underlying immunological problem is thought to be a defect in suppressor T-cell function, which allows T-helper cells to be sensitised to thyroid antigens; thus B cells are stimulated to produce anti-thyroid antibodies.

Hashimoto thyroiditis tends to involve the whole thyroid diffusely, similar to Graves' disease, and presents with a firm, hard goitre. Although patients typically end up hypothyroid, they may be euthyroid or (rarely) even hyperthyroid in the initial stages of the disease. Treatment of Hashimoto's thyroiditis is with $T_4$, which usually improves the goitre. Surgery is sometimes required for pressure symptoms or to confirm the diagnosis of an indeterminate nodule.

## Riedel's thyroiditis

This is an idiopathic fibrosing condition (similar to retroperitoneal fibrosis) which can affect the thyroid among other areas. About 30–40% of patients end up hypothyroid and they may also have hypoparathyroidism. It is often difficult to distinguish this condition from malignancy, and FNAC often gives an acellular result, necessitating a core or open biopsy. Thyroid function tests and autoantibodies are normal. Treatment is palliative and surgery may be required if there is tracheal or oesophageal compression.

## 1.11 Hyperthyroidism (thyrotoxicosis)

### In a nutshell ...

Three causes account for 99% of cases:
- **Graves' disease** (autoimmune) accounts for 90% of cases
- **Toxic adenoma**
- **Toxic multinodular goitre** (Plummer's disease)

Other causes include:
- Drugs such as thyroxine (the Jod–Basedow effect is induction of thyrotoxicosis in a previously euthyroid individual by the over-treatment of multinodular goitre with iodine)
- Carcinoma (rare)
- Iodine-131 treatment
- Hyperfunctioning ovarian teratoma (struma ovarii)
- Subacute/acute thyroiditis
- TSH-secreting tumour (eg hydatidiform mole, choriocarcinoma, pituitary tumour)

Clinical features of hyperthyroidism are covered in Section 1.3.

### Graves' disease

Graves' disease is an immunological disorder of unknown aetiology characterised by stimulation of TSH receptors by immunoglobulins or antibodies. It is classically seen in women aged 20–40 years.

## Pathophysiology of Graves' disease

Thyroid-stimulating immunoglobulins or thyroid-receptor antibodies attach to TSH receptors on the surface of the thyroid follicular cell and cause excess secretion of $T_3$ and $T_4$.

## Clinical features of Graves' disease

- Hyperthyroidism
- 85% have eye signs (see box below)
- Diffuse goitre
- Thyroid acropachy (similar to clubbing)
- Pretibial myxoedema
- Thyroid bruit on auscultation due to increased vascularity

---

**Eye disease in hyperthyroidism**

Three-quarters of patients with Graves' disease have associated eye signs. Exophthalmos is due to:

- **Proptosis:** caused by increased retrobulbar orbital fat and enlarged intraorbital muscles infiltrated with lymphocytes and containing increased water and mucopolysaccharide
- **Lid retraction:** due to a direct effect of thyroxine on the orbital muscles
- **Orbital oedema**

Erythema of the conjunctiva is seen in association with the lid retraction. In severe cases, paralysis of the ocular muscles can lead to squint, diplopia and, rarely, optic nerve damage.

---

## Diagnosis of Graves' disease

- ↓TSH
- ↑ free $T_3$
- ↑ free $T_4$
- Thyroid-receptor antibodies
- Hot nodule on radioisotope scanning

## Treatment of Graves' disease

- Can be medical, with radioiodine, or surgical

### Medical treatment of Graves' disease

Propylthiouracil and carbimazole are thionamides that inhibit thyroid peroxidase and hence block the organification and coupling process in the thyroid follicular cell, and thus reduce thyroid hormone synthesis. Propylthiouracil also blocks peripheral conversion of $T_3$ to $T_4$ and is immunosuppressive. Standard treatment is for 18 months. Following this 20% patients remain in remission; those who relapse do so in the first 6 months. Patients put on carbimazole must be warned of the risks of granulocytosis.

---

**Advantages of medical treatment**
Rapid control
No permanent effects

**Disadvantages of medical treatment**
Side effects of drugs (dyspepsia, sensitivity, agranulocytosis, aplastic anaemia)
High risk of relapse

---

### Treatment of Graves' disease with radio-iodine (iodine-131)

This is given as a single oral dose. It causes direct radiation damage to the replicative mechanisms of the thyroid follicular cells. It is used in thyrotoxic patients with a small to moderate-sized goitre and no eye signs. It is contraindicated in patients who are pregnant, breastfeeding, very young, or who work with young children, and it is unsuitable for patients with a multinodular goitre or a toxic solitary nodule. Radioiodine also has adverse effects on the eye signs of Graves' disease, so may be avoided or used cautiously with steroid cover.

---

**Advantages of radioiodine treatment**
Cheap and easy to administer
Long-term safety

**Disadvantages of radioiodine treatment**
Late hypothyroidism
Restricted social contact in the short term

---

### Surgical treatment of Graves' disease

This is the treatment of choice for patients with a large goitre, multinodular goitre, solitary nodule, eye signs or those who are planning a possible pregnancy, and in those who have relapsed after medical treatment. Patients should be rendered euthyroid before surgery. A total or near-total thyroidectomy should be performed.

---

**Advantages of surgical treatment**
Effective and immediate

**Disadvantages of surgical treatment**
Hospital admission and general anaesthetic
Possible postoperative complications
Permanent hypothyroidism in about 5%

---

**Thyrotoxic crisis (thyroid storm)**
This serious clinical condition has a poor prognosis. It is seen when patients are not rendered euthyroid preoperatively or it can be triggered by infection or iodine administration. Patients develop fever, tachycardia, diarrhoea, jaundice and central nervous system (CNS) symptoms, from agitation through to delirium and coma. Patients should be treated on the intensive therapy unit (ITU) with careful fluid balance, cooling, β blockade, propylthiouracil and any supportive treatment necessary. Lugol's iodine, which acts by reducing the vascularity of the thyroid gland, can also be given to inhibit further release of thyroxine from the thyroid gland.

## 1.12 Hypothyroidism (myxoedema)

### Causes of hypothyroidism

- Iatrogenic causes (90% cases) include:
  - Post-iodine-131 therapy
  - Post-thyroidectomy
  - Post-radiotherapy
  - Drugs:
    - Carbimazole and propylthiouracil: used as treatment of hyperthyroidism to block thyroid peroxidase enzyme
    - Amiodarone: used as treatment for atrial fibrillation; contains iodine and can cause hyperthyroidism and hypothyroidism. Thyroid function tests (TFTs) should be checked every 6 months
    - Lithium: used as mood stabiliser in bipolar affective disorder

- Idiopathic myxoedema
- Autoimmune diseases:
  - Hashimoto's autoimmune thyroiditis (see Section 1.10)
  - Pernicious anaemia
  - Addison's disease
  - Rheumatoid arthritis
  - Sjögren syndrome
  - Ulcerative colitis
  - Lupoid hepatitis
  - SLE
  - Haemolytic anaemia
  - Diabetes mellitus
  - Graves' disease
  - Hypoparathyroidism
  - Patients with a long history of autoimmune disease are also at increased risk of developing lymphoma
- Iodine deficiency
- Hypopituitarism
- Tumour infiltration
- Subacute thyroiditis

**Myxoedema coma**

Elderly patients with undiagnosed hypothyroidism, or those who have not taken their medication, can present with altered mental status, coma, bradycardia, hypothermia and hypoglycaemia. TFTs should always be checked in patients with this clinical picture. Patients should be resuscitated on ITU with fluids, gentle rewarming, and $T_3$ and $T_4$ supplementation. Ventilation may be necessary.

## Clinical features of hypothyroidism

See table on actions of $T_3$ and $T_4$ and their clinical implications.

## Treatment of hypothyroidism

Oral $T_4$ for life. $T_4$ has a predictable biological activity and is cheap. It has a long half-life (1 week). The dose is usually 2 µg/kg (ie 100–150 µg/day). TFTs can be checked to ensure that the patient is euthyroid.

## 1.13 Thyroidectomy

 **Op box: Thyroidectomy**

**Preop**

All hyperthyroid patients should be rendered euthyroid preoperatively.

- **Propylthiouracil and carbimazole** inhibit thyroid peroxidase and thus prevent the organification and coupling process. They are also immunosuppressive and suppress TSH antibody production
- β **blockers** improve many of the symptoms of hyperthyroidism, particularly tremor, anxiety and tachycardia; β blockers also inhibit the peripheral conversion of $T_3$ to $T_4$
- **Iodine (Lugol's)** can also be used. If given for 7–10 days preoperatively it reduces thyroid vascularity and makes the gland firmer

**Procedure**

- GA (general anaesthetic), head ring, shoulder bolster to extend the neck
- Transverse incision 2 cm above sternal notch
- Skin, subcutaneous fat and platysma are incised transversely
- Investing fascia and connective tissue between the sternohyoid and sternothyroid muscles are incised vertically. As a rule the strap muscles are not divided, but this may be necessary, especially if the goitre is large. If they do need to be divided this should be done as high as possible (ie above the point of entry of the ansa cervicalis nerve branches) to prevent denervation and muscle wasting
- Pretracheal fascia around the thyroid is incised
- Thyroid lobe is mobilised
- RLN is identified
- Traditionally, the superior thyroid artery is tied off close to the thyroid gland (to protect the ELN) and the inferior thyroid artery is tied off laterally away from the thyroid (to protect the RLN). However, many surgeons now divide the branches of the inferior thyroid artery individually on the gland to protect the blood supply to the parathyroids
- If a parathyroid is excised, it can be cut up and implanted in the sternomastoid. The majority of these continue to function normally
- Thyroid gland is excised
- Haemostasis, suction drain, closure in layers (approximate strap muscles and platysma), clips to skin or beaded subcuticular monofilament such as Prolene

## Postoperative complications

These should be outlined when consenting patients.

- **Bleeding:** the expanding neck haematoma can lead to respiratory distress. This is an ENT emergency and is why thyroid incisions were traditionally closed with skin clips (and the editor of this book is old enough to remember a clip remover left by the bed of every thyroidectomy patient on the first postoperative night). In fact the haematoma usually collects deep to platysma and the strap muscles that are closed under the skin, so often these stitches also have to be cut. In any case, removal of the haematoma is not the whole story; the expanding haematoma obstructs venous drainage, leading to laryngeal oedema and airway obstruction. Thus, as always, the first priority is to manage the airway. The situation usually requires emergency evacuation of the haematoma in theatre
- **Nerve damage:** ELN and RLN damage (see later)
- **Thyroid crisis:** if patients are inadequately prepared for theatre
- **Hypothyroidism**
- **Temporary or permanent hypocalcaemia:** this is quite common. It can be due to 'bruising' of the parathyroids (which is temporary) and it can also be due to excision or ischaemia of the parathyroids (which is permanent). It can also occur as a result of reversal of thyrotoxic osteoporosis (hungry bone syndrome) so the bones mop up the calcium. Signs are paraesthesia, tetany and (if untreated) convulsions. It is treated by calcium tablets, or a slow infusion of intravenous calcium gluconate. In prolonged cases, oral vitamin D and alfacalcidol may be added
- **Stridor:** due to bilateral RLN injury (see 'Nerve injury in thyroidectomy' below) or laryngeal oedema due to haematoma. Unilateral vocal fold palsy does not usually give stridor, but the patient has a weak, breathy voice and a poor, bovine cough
- **Laryngeal oedema:** this may resolve with 48 hours of ventilation
- **Aspiration of vomit**
- **Tracheomalacia:** this is a rare complication in long-standing goitres, when tracheal wall collapses after the removal of its support. It is usually treated by ventilation for 48 hours and sometimes needs a tracheostomy or stenting
- **Pain**
- **Dysphagia**
- **Keloid/hypertrophic scar**

## What to do if a thyroidectomy patient gets postoperative neck swelling

Look out for:

- Discomfort
- Swelling under the incision
- Breathlessness
- Noisy breathing
- Agitation
- Confusion
- Reduced consciousness

} Signs of airway obstruction – proceed to next box!

Do not be misled by:

- Drains: they may be blocked
- Pulse oximetry: this may remain high until the patient is critically unwell

If there is slight swelling and no symptoms:

- Inform senior
- Review in 30 minutes

If there is significant swelling and mild symptoms:

- Seek senior help – anaesthetic and ENT
- Release skin sutures
- Evacuate any subcutaneous haematoma with sterile gloved finger
- If there is swelling beneath the strap muscles divide the Vicryl sutures, holding them together, and gently evacuate haematoma from this layer with sterile gloved finger
- You do not need to cut any skin or muscle or use any instruments apart from a finger to evacuate the clot

If there are signs of airway obstruction:

- See next box

## What to do if a thyroidectomy patient gets postoperative stridor

Bear in mind this can be due to RLN injury, wound haematoma or (rarely) tracheomalacia:

- High-flow oxygen by mask
- Ask your senior to come immediately
- Call senior anaesthetist urgently: an experienced anaesthetist may be able to perform laryngoscopy to check cord status and perform urgent re-intubation. Failed attempts at intubation should not be made by junior anaesthetists because this will cause further laryngeal oedema
- Send someone to get an emergency tracheostomy kit from ITU or theatre in case it is needed
- Proceed with evacuation of neck haematoma as in previous box if there is any sign of wound swelling
- Do not leave the patient until a definitive airway has been secured
- Inform consultant as soon as practicable

## Tracheostomy for post-thyroidectomy stridor

If an orotracheal airway is secured, either on the ward or in theatre, then a tracheostomy is usually not required. Even in the presence of tracheomalacia it is probably better to deal with any bleeding, put in fresh drains and send the patient for ventilation. The larynx can then be visualised by fibreoptic laryngoscopy and a decision made about when to extubate.

If intubation fails, then a tracheotomy on the ward or tracheostomy in theatre will be required urgently.

CHAPTER 4

# Nerve injury in thyroidectomy

## Recurrent laryngeal nerve

This is at risk where it crosses the inferior thyroid artery. It is imperative to identify the nerve before dividing or tying off any vessels. Incidence of injury is 1% on average. Injury to the RLN can be unilateral or bilateral and incomplete (neuropraxia) or complete (axonotmesis).

## External laryngeal nerve

This nerve is at risk when the superior pedicle is ligated and divided because it runs close to the superior thyroid artery. Double ties are usually placed proximally on the superior artery and vein together and a single tie distally, and they are divided with a scalpel over a metal guard close to the thyroid. The ELN is not usually seen during the course of the operation.

Damage to the ELN affects the cricothyroid muscle. The damage can go unnoticed but patients can complain of a weak voice when trying to sing or shout, which can be catastrophic for the professional voice user and can end careers.

For details of the sequelae of these injuries see Chapter 5, Head and Neck Surgery.

# SECTION 2
# Parathyroid glands

## 2.1 Embryology of the parathyroids

The superior parathyroid glands develop from the dorsal endoderm of the fourth branchial pouch. The ventral part of the fourth branchial pouch is fused to the developing thyroid gland.

Ninety per cent of superior parathyroid glands remain attached to the thyroid gland in adult life. The inferior parathyroid glands develop from the third branchial pouch – as does the thymus gland. As the thymus gland descends, the inferior parathyroids are carried down with it.

Both the superior and inferior glands migrate caudally during development and it is this migration which accounts for the numerous ectopic sites of the inferior parathyroid glands that have been described.

## 2.2 Anatomy of the parathyroids

 **In a nutshell ...**

Most people have four parathyroid glands – two on either side of the neck:
- 6% of the population have five glands
- 6% have only three glands
- 0.5% have six glands

The parathyroids are intimately related to the posterior aspect of the thyroid gland and each weighs 25–40 mg. They are brownish-yellow in colour.

### Site of the parathyroid glands
- The superior parathyroid glands lie at the level of the first tracheal ring at the level where the RLN crosses the inferior thyroid artery
- The inferior parathyroid glands are more variable in position but are found below the level of the inferior thyroid artery, usually at the inferior pole of the thyroid gland

- Due to the migration of the parathyroid glands during development, the location of the parathyroid glands is very variable and many ectopic positions are described in the neck and mediastinum

### Ectopic positions

- The superior parathyroid glands tend to be constant in their position but can be found between the thyroid and the oesophagus, behind the oesophagus or in the carotid sheath
- The inferior parathyroids can be found along the inferior thyroid veins, in front of the trachea or in the superior mediastinum, together with the thymus

### Blood supply of the parathyroid glands

- The blood supply comes almost exclusively from the inferior thyroid artery (branch of the thyrocervical trunk from the first part of the subclavian artery)
- Collateral supply can sometimes arise from the superior thyroid artery and aortic oesophageal branches

### Venous drainage of the parathyroid glands

- Blood drains to the thyroid venous plexus which drains in to the left brachiocephalic vein

### Histology of the parathyroid glands

Consist mainly of chief cells, with some oxyphil cells and water-clear cells. **Chief cells** have the following properties:

- Can be light (rich in glycogen), dark (secretory granules and water) or clear

- Usually contain intracellular fat
- Lie in extracellular areas of fat, which comprises up to 50% of the parathyroid glands

## 2.3 Physiology of the parathyroids

 **In a nutshell ...**

- The parathyroid glands produce parathyroid hormone (PTH)
- PTH increases serum calcium and decreases serum phosphate
- Along with vitamin D and calcitonin, PTH maintains calcium homeostasis
- Serum calcium exists as calcium bound to albumin (which is affected by albumin levels) and as free ionised calcium, which is physiologically active
- The serum calcium concentration should always be corrected with respect to the albumin level

The parathyroid glands produce parathyroid hormone which is involved in calcium homeostasis. PTH is released from chief cells (a type of epithelial cell) within the gland and is cleaved twice during the production of the active form:

Pre-pro-PTH (115 amino acids) → Pro-PTH (90 amino acids) → PTH (84 amino acids)

It has a half-life of 2–5 minutes and is degraded in the liver, circulation and kidney.

PTH acts on its effector cells in the bone, gut and kidney via cell surface receptors, and increases cAMP production. The overall effect on the body is to increase serum calcium and decrease serum phosphate in response to the decreased serum calcium level.

Most secretory cells increase their activity in response to high calcium, but chief cells increase their activity in response to low calcium levels. Low serum ionised calcium concentrations are sensed by two protein receptors in the membrane of the chief cell, and PTH secretion occurs in seconds as a result.

Calcium homeostasis is important because decreased serum calcium leads to neural excitability and eventually tetany. The effects of increased serum calcium are discussed later in this section.

## Serum calcium measurement

Serum calcium measurement is not a true measure of the physiologically active calcium in the blood as it measures bound calcium as well as free calcium.

Patients with high serum albumin levels may show high calcium readings, while those with low serum albumin may show low calcium readings, regardless of the level of ionised calcium in the serum. Once the figure is adjusted for the albumin level (corrected calcium) this gives a truer picture of the level of free calcium which is clinically significant.

> **Functions of calcium**
> - Muscle contraction
> - Conduction of nervous impulses
> - Enzyme cofactor (eg in blood clotting)
> - Constituent of bones and teeth
> - Intercellular adhesion
> - Cell division
> - Maintains permeability of cell membranes
> - Hormone release and action

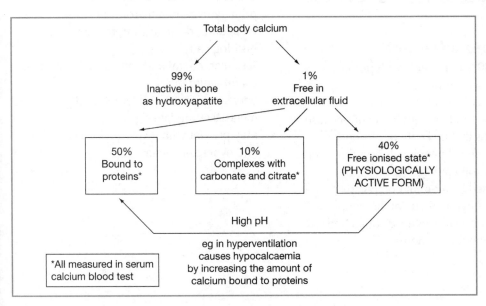

**Figure 4.7 Total body calcium**

**Hormones involved in calcium regulation**

| Hormone | Produced by | Effect on serum calcium levels | Acts on |
|---|---|---|---|
| PTH | Parathyroid gland | Increased | Kidney, bone, GI tract (indirectly) (Figure 4.8) |
| Vitamin D | Kidneys and liver | Increased | GI tract |
| Calcitonin | Parafollicular C cells of the thyroid | Increased | Bone and GI tract |

## 2.4 Pathology of the parathyroids

### In a nutshell ...

The main pathological processes that affect the parathyroid glands are:
- Adenoma
- Hyperplasia
- Carcinoma

The main presentation of these pathologies is hypercalcaemia due to primary hyperparathyroidism.

### Parathyroid adenoma

- Found in 80% of patients with primary hyperparathyroidism
- Consists of chief cells
- Monoclonal (and thought to occur because of mutations that make them respond to normal serum calcium levels as if they were low, ie by proliferation)
- Characterised by a rim of compressed normal parathyroid tissue at the periphery
- Often has a capsule with loss of fat and stroma within the adenoma

### Parathyroid hyperplasia

- Found in 12% of patients who have hyperparathyroidism
- Found in people with secondary hyperparathyroidism
- Consists of chief cells and occasionally water-clear cells
- Polyclonal (in contrast to adenoma)
- Little or no intracellular fat
- No rim of normal parathyroid tissue
- All four glands are affected

### Parathyroid carcinoma

- Found in 1–2% of patients who have primary hyperparathyroidism
- Difficult to distinguish from adenoma histologically
- Vascular, neural and soft-tissue invasion are useful hallmarks
- Local recurrence and lymph node metastases are late signs
- May present with a very high PTH (>1000) and hypercalcaemia

# 2.5 Hyperparathyroidism

## In a nutshell ...

**Primary hyperparathyroidism**
Spontaneous, excessive PTH production by a parathyroid gland, usually due to an adenoma, but can also be due to hyperplasia or carcinoma. Produces PTH regardless of calcium level.

**Secondary hyperparathyroidism**
Excessive PTH production by parathyroid gland in response to low calcium (eg in renal failure or malabsorption). Produces PTH only in the presence of low calcium.

**Tertiary hyperparathyroidism**
A parathyroid gland becomes hyperplastic due to secondary hyperparathyroidism and continues to overproduce PTH in the presence of normal calcium level (even after renal transplantation and after normal renal function is restored). Difficult to differentiate from severe secondary hyperparathyroidism.

**Persistent hyperparathyroidism**
Hypercalcaemia occurring within 6 months of parathyroidectomy, usually because of a missed adenoma, or mistaken diagnosis of adenoma in a hyperplastic gland, or residual supernumerary hyperplastic glands.

**Recurrent hyperparathyroidism**
Caused by hypercalcaemia that follows at least 6 months of normocalcaemia post-parathyroidectomy. This is due to regrowth of remnants of the hyperplastic gland or local or distant recurrence of a parathyroid cancer.

**Ectopic hyperparathyroidism**
Usually seen in patients with a tumour producing a PTH-like substance.

## Primary hyperparathyroidism

This is spontaneous, excessive PTH production by parathyroid glands, usually due to an adenoma, but can also be due to hyperplasia or carcinoma. It produces PTH regardless of the calcium level.

### Causes of primary hyperparathyroidism

- **Single adenoma (85%):** the other glands are suppressed by high calcium levels and are therefore smaller. Single and occasionally multiple adenomas have been described in association with the MEN 2 syndrome
- **Parathyroid hyperplasia (12%):** all four glands and any supernumerary glands are affected and produce excess PTH. Although most cases of parathyroid hyperplasia are sporadic, 95% of people with MEN 1 syndrome present with primary hyperpara-thyroidism due to four-gland hyperplasia (see Section 2.9 of this chapter); 5–20% of people with MEN 2 will also have parathyroid gland hyperplasia
- **Parathyroid carcinoma (1–2%):** again the other three glands will be suppressed if the carcinoma is over-producing PTH. This must be suspected if the PTH measurements are in the thousands
- **Multiple adenomas (rare):** if more than one gland is involved the true pathology may be hyperplasia with asymmetrical gland enlargement. Multiple adenomas have occasionally been described in association with MEN 2 syndrome

### Epidemiology of primary hyperparathyroidism

- 30 cases per 100 000 of population in the developed world

CHAPTER 4

- Peak age of presentation is 50–60 (20–40 in MEN 1 patients)
- Male:female ratio is 2:3.1 (1:1 in MEN 1 patients)
- Usually presents by chance blood test, renal calculi or vague symptoms (see table 'Signs and symptoms of primary hyperparathyroidism')

## Typical biochemistry in primary hyperparathyroidism

- Hypercalcaemia in the presence of normal or high PTH (diagnostic)
- Hypophosphataemia
- Hypochloraemia
- Mild acidosis
- Possible raised alkaline phosphatase
- Raised 24-hour urinary calcium secretion
- Normal vitamin D levels

# Secondary hyperparathyroidism

This is excessive PTH production by the parathyroid glands in response to low calcium (eg in renal failure or malabsorption).

Typical biochemistry in secondary hypo-parathyroidism may include:

- Normal calcium levels
- High phosphate levels
- Very high PTH levels

## Secondary hyperparathyroidism due to chronic renal insufficiency

This is the most common cause of secondary hyperparathyroidism. The reason for over-production of PTH in renal disease is complex, but is probably mainly due to four things:

1. Direct effect of high serum phosphate levels (one of the first biochemical abnormalities of renal disease), which stimulates PTH production even if the serum calcium is normal
2. Indirect effect of high serum phosphate levels, which reduces the activation (and therefore serum levels) of calcitrol; low serum calcitrol in turn stimulates PTH production
3. Failure to synthesise 1α-dihydroxyvitamin
4. Low serum calcium, which stimulates PTH production directly

Renal physicians have reduced the incidence of hyperplastic parathyroid disease secondary to renal failure in their patients by:

- Reducing phosphate content of the diet
- Prescribing 1α-dihydroxyvitamin D

## Secondary hyperparathyroidism due to calcium malabsorption syndromes

Calcium absorption, which mainly occurs in the duodenum, is reduced by:

- Increased dietary oxalates, phytates and phosphates (they chelate calcium and reduce its absorption)
- Vagotomy and gastrectomy (they reduce acid secretion and therefore reduce absorption)
- Steroids (they antagonise the effects of vitamin D on the gastrointestinal [GI] tract and reduce absorption)

---

**Familial hypocalciuric hypercalcaemia**
This is an autosomal dominant inherited disorder presenting with mild hypercalcaemia and often a slight elevation of serum PTH. It is asymptomatic, found incidentally and there is no need for surgery. A low 24-hour urinary calcium differentiates it from primary hyperparathyroidism.

---

# 2.6 Assessment of hyperparathyroidism

**Signs and symptoms of primary hyperparathyroidism**

| | Symptoms and signs | Reason |
|---|---|---|
| **Stones** (renal system) | Renal and ureteric stones<br>Nephrocalcinosis<br>Polyuria<br>Polydipsia<br>Renal failure | Due to increased urinary calcium and phosphate loss |
| **Bones** (musculo-skeletal system) | Pathological fractures<br>Osteoporosis<br>Osteoclastoma (brown tumour)<br>Bone pain due to resorption (ground-glass skull on radiograph)<br>Hungry bone disease (see box)<br>Subperiosteal bone resorption cysts (especially clavicles and phalanges)<br>Osteomalacia from calcitrol deficiency[a]<br>Renal bone disease with osteitis fibrosa cystica[a]<br>Aluminium bone disease due to dialysis[a]<br>Periarticular calcium deposits[a]<br>Periarticular amyloid from dialysis[a]<br>Loss of lamina dura around the teeth (pathognomonic)<br>Loss of tufts of terminal phalanx | Mostly seen in secondary hyperparathyroidism (only 5–10% of primary hyperparathyroidism patients have bone disease, due to early detection) |
| **Abdominal groans** (GI tract) | Abdominal pain<br>Constipation<br>Pancreatitis (acute and chronic)<br>Ulceration<br>Nausea, vomiting and weight loss | Hypercalcaemia can cause hypergastrinaemia, which can cause peptic ulceration |
| **Psychic moans** (neuropsychiatric confusion disorders) | Depression<br>Anxiety, paranoia, confusion<br>Dementia | |

[a]These are changes typical of hyperparathyroidism secondary to renal failure.

## Clinical features of primary hyperparathyroidism

The signs and symptoms are those of hypercalcaemia, and are summarised by the saying:

'stones, bones, abdominal groans and psychic moans'

**Hungry bone disease**

Hungry bone disease is seen when excess PTH causes leaching of the stores of calcium from the bones. When the PTH stimulus is removed (eg after surgery), the bones 'mop up' calcium, which can result in a temporary hypocalcaemia. This situation can also be seen after hyperthyroidism is treated (see Section 1, 'Thyroid gland').

CHAPTER 4

## Other presentations of primary hyperparathyroidism

### Asymptomatic primary hyperparathyroidism

- Detected on biochemical screening
- Family history screening
- Endocrine screening (eg MEN 1 or 2)

### Effects of hypercalcaemia

Hypercalcaemia can also cause hypertension, cardiac arrhythmia, left ventricular hypertrophy and short Q–T interval on ECG. Rarely, it can present as an emergency with a hypercalcaemic crisis (see box below).

---

**Hypercalcaemic crisis**

This is hypercalcaemia presenting as an emergency, characterised by:

- Drowsiness/acute confusion
- Loss of consciousness/coma
- Dehydration
- Weakness
- Vomiting
- Renal failure

Treatment is by:

- Rehydration with intravenous fluids
- Bisphosphonates (eg pamidronate), which prevent bone resorption
- Calcitonin (acts quickly but is effective for only 24–48 hours)

---

## Biochemistry of hyperparathyroidism

- **Biochemistry:** tests of renal function include serum urea, creatinine and electrolytes. Decreased renal function may alter calcium excretion. If renal impairment is suspected,

24-hour creatinine clearance should be measured

- **Serum calcium:** corrected for albumin. Ionised (active) calcium levels are optimal if available. Serum calcium:
  - Is elevated in 75% of primary hyperparathyroidism
  - May be the upper limit of normal
  - May be low or normal in secondary hyperparathyroidism
- **PTH:** 'intact' serum PTH levels. You must remember that an hour's worth of intact PTH is stored in the cells; it is cleaved into a biologically active fragment and a carboxyl terminal fragment in the circulation, liver and kidney – hence samples must be rushed to the lab on ice. High serum calcium in the presence of normal or high serum PTH is diagnostic of primary hyperparathyroidism:
  - 25% of patients with primary hyperparathyroidism will have a calcium level in the upper limits of normal
  - 13% of patients will have normal PTH levels

In the presence of hypercalcaemia due to other causes one would expect to see PTH levels suppressed

- **24-hour urinary calcium:** useful for differentiating familial hypocalciuric hypercalcaemia, FHH (see previous box) from primary hyperparathyroidism (FHH <200 mg calcium/24 h; primary hypothyroidism >300 mg calcium/24 h). Urinary phosphate will also be increased
- **Chloride:** a mild hyperchloraemic metabolic acidosis is seen as PTH increases renal bicarbonate loss
- **Alkaline phosphatase:** increased
- **Phosphate:** reduced
- **Bicarbonate:** decreased
- **Vitamin D:** low vitamin D levels my explain 'normocalcaemic' hyperparathyroidism in some patients

## Imaging in hyperparathyroidism

Localisation preoperatively is useful in re-operation or ectopic glands, but studies have not shown any advantage of imaging for locali-sation in straightforward first operations. No imaging method is perfect; many modalities are used.

- **Ultrasonography:** limited use in localisation
- **CT:** useful for identifying adenomas not found at operations and those in ectopic locations. It has 63% sensitivity for preoperative localisation. Malignancy outside the parathyroids is one of the most common causes of hypercalcaemia, so, if this is suspected, CT may be indicated. CT has been superseded by MRI in some centres
- **MRI:** this doesn't involve radiation or iodinated contrast so it is used instead of CT for localising ectopic glands and before re-operation. Sensitivity is 74%
- **Technetium–sestamibi scanning:** this is radionuclide imaging using agents that are selectively taken up by the parathyroids to localise the glands. Agents include thallium-201, technetium-99, pertechnetate (Tl–Tc subtraction scanning uses both of these) and $^{99m}$Tc–sestamibi. Problems include:
  - Thyroid uptake (especially in multinodular goitres and thyroid adenomas)
  - 'Mopping up' of the agents by the large parathyroid gland (making it difficult to see the others)
  - Poor anatomical detail
- **Selective venous catheterisation:** for PTH blood sampling is rarely done now as it is highly dependent on expertise

- **Angiography:** may be indicated in difficult cases, by cannulation of the internal thoracic (mammary) arteries and thyrocervical trunks. Common carotid angiography is a higher-risk procedure
- **Positron-emission tomography (PET) scanning:** available in some centres. Considered experimental

---

**Other causes to consider when investigating hypercalcaemia**

- Primary hyperparathyroidism and malignancy: account for 80% cases
- Addison's disease
- Drugs (thiazide diuretics, lithium)
- Milk-alkali syndrome
- Multiple myeloma
- Paget's disease
- Excess intake of vitamin D
- Familial hypocalciuric hypercalcaemia (FHH): an autosomal dominant condition characterised by hypercal-caemia with decreased calcium excretion in the urine (see box in Section 2.5)
- TB
- Phaeochromocytoma
- Sarcoidosis (due to production of 1,25-dihydroxy-vitamin D in sarcoid tissue)
- Prolonged immobility
- Thyrotoxicosis
- Ectopic PTH secretion (very rare)

---

**CHAPTER 4**

## 2.7 Management of hyperparathyroidism

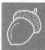

### In a nutshell ...

Treat hypercalcaemic crisis if necessary (see the box 'Hypercalcaemic crisis' above)

Ensure good hydration

Low-calcium diet (not much evidence to support this)

Surgery is the mainstay of treatment

## Parathyroid surgery

### Indications for parathyroid surgery

In asymptomatic patients, surgery remains controversial. However, it is the only cure for hyperparathyroidism, and should be performed before irreversible end-organ damage occurs; increased survival is seen in patients who undergo parathyroidectomy at an earlier stage. Laryngoscopy is used to exclude asymptomatic RLN injury in patients who have had previous neck surgery.

### Preoperative preparation

Preoperative localisation of the parathyroids can be done and depends on the surgeon's preference. Studies have shown no shorter operation time or lower recurrence rates if the parathyroids are localised preoperatively. It is, however, essential for re-exploration procedures.

Methods of localisation are outlined above, in 'Imaging in hyperparathyroidism'.

### Principles of parathyroid surgery

Most surgeons would explore both sides of the neck at the time of surgery to check for multiple adenomas and hyperplasia and findings/biopsy sites should always be clearly recorded. Some surgeons would advocate only a unilateral exploration with the advantage of decreased operating time and reduced morbidity. Bilateral exploration should always be performed in the following cases:

- If there is MEN 1 or 2A (see Section 2.9 of this chapter)
- If there is known bilateral disease
- If hyperplasia is seen in two glands on the same side of the neck
- If no abnormality is found on unilateral exploration

Immediate frozen section can be done to confirm that the tissue excised is parathyroid in origin if there is any doubt at surgery.

Newer approaches to parathyroid surgery include minimally invasive parathyroid surgery (MIPS) after localisation of the adenoma preoperatively. Several techniques have been described. The success of the procedure can be ascertained by intraoperative measurement of PTH levels.

CHAPTER 4

**Op box: Parathyroidectomy (standard technique)**

**Preop**
- Preoperative localisation of the parathyroids can be done and depends on the surgeon's preference
- Studies have shown no shorter operation times or better recurrence rates if the parathyroids are localised preoperatively. It is, however, essential for re-exploration procedures
- Methods of localisation are outlined above in 'Imaging in hyperparathyroidism'

**Position**
- GA, neck extended and head draped

**Incision**
- Transverse incision 2 cm above sternal notch

**Procedure**
- Lift skin and platysma flaps to the level of thyroid notch superiorly and the suprasternal notch inferiorly
- Divide the pretracheal fascia and strap muscles in the midline
- Retract strap muscles and expose thyroid lobes
- Identify recurrent laryngeal nerve and inferior thyroid artery
- Localise parathyroid glands and proceed as appropriate (see table 'Summary of parathyroid surgery options' overleaf)
- Take care to label each gland with its position and send each separately for histology
- Haemostasis, closure in layers (strap muscles, platysma), clips to skin

**Complications**
- As for thyroid surgery (see Section 1)
- Damage to RLN: risk is much less than in thyroid surgery
- Hypoparathyroidism and hypocalcaemia (see Sections 1 and 2.8)
- Bleeding/haematoma: threat to airway (see Section 1)
- Inability to identify all four glands
- Persistent hyperparathyroidism: mostly due to failed exploration. Check operation notes. Was a bilateral exploration carried out? How many glands were identified? Consider the possibility of an ectopic gland and perform localisation studies. Familial hypocalciuric hypercalcaemia should be considered

**Postop Management**
- As for thyroid surgery (see Section 1)
- Oral 1α-calcidol supplementation should be given after total and subtotal parathyroidectomy

**CHAPTER 4**

### Summary of parathyroid surgery options

| Finding | Action |
| --- | --- |
| Single adenoma | Remove the affected parathyroid and leave the three remaining glands |
| Multiple adenomas | Remove all affected glands |
| Hyperplasia | Excise three and a half glands. Mark the remaining gland in case future exploration is necessary, or remove and autotransplant the remaining gland into brachioradialis. Some surgeons now advocate total parathyroidectomy and 1α-calcidol supplementation |
| Carcinoma | En-bloc dissection with thyroid lobectomy and lymph nodes |
| Hyperparathyroidism in association with MEN 1 or 2A | Total parathyroidectomy and autotransplantation, transcervical thymectomy and exploration of the carotid sheath (there is a 20% incidence of supernumerary glands) |

### Autotransplantation

If the glands are hyperplastic, either from primary or secondary hyperparathyroidism, three and a half glands are removed. The residual tissue may be left in the neck, but if hyperparathyroidism recurs, re-operation is more difficult than the first operation, with a higher incidence of nerve injury and other complications. An alternative is to remove all the parathyroids and transplant one half of a gland into the forearm, where it can be easily located and removed if there is recurrence. The gland is sliced up and placed within the muscle belly of the sternomastoid, where it will hopefully 'take' and function as an autograft.

## 2.8 Hypoparathyroidism

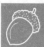

**In a nutshell ...**

Hypoparathyroidism is often iatrogenic but can be due to autoimmune or congenital causes. It presents with symptoms of hypocalcaemia and is treated by oral or intravenous calcium.

### Causes of hypoparathyroidism

*   Iatrogenic (following thyroid/parathyroid surgery or radical neck dissection)
*   Autoimmune
*   Pseudohypoparathyroidism (decreased sensitivity to PTH)
*   Congenital disorders (eg DiGeorge syndrome)

### Symptoms and signs of hypoparathyroidism

The symptoms and signs are those of hypocalcaemia:

*   Paraesthesia in lips (circumoral numbness) and fingers
*   Carpopedal spasm
*   Tetany
*   Convulsions (petit mal or grand mal)
*   Cramps
*   Dystonia
*   Psychosis
*   Chvostek's sign (twitching of facial muscles when facial nerve is tapped)
*   Trousseau's sign (spasm of fingers and wrist when the sphygmomanometer cuff is tightened around the arm for 3 minutes at 10–20 mmHg higher than the patient's systolic BP)
*   Prolonged Q–T interval on ECG

## Treatment of hypocalcaemia due to hypoparathyroidism

In symptomatic patients:
- 10 ml 10% calcium gluconate over 5 min
- Infusion of calcium gluconate at a maximum rate of 0.05 mmol/kg per hour if necessary
- Monitor calcium levels

In asymptomatic patients:
- Oral calcium preparations
- If the degree of hypocalcaemia is mild postoperatively, oral calcium supplementation and observation are adequate
- Check vitamin D levels are adequate or there is an increased risk of renal stones if high doses of calcium are given

---

**Other causes of hypocalcaemia**
- Acute pancreatitis
- Small-bowel disease (Crohn's disease, large resection)
- Post-vagotomy
- Massive blood transfusion
- Renal failure

---

## 2.9 Multiple endocrine neoplasia syndromes

 **In a nutshell ...**

MEN syndromes consist of rare clusters of endocrine tumours and have autosomal dominant inheritance. Most hyperparathyroidism is not associated with MEN but the diagnosis should be considered in any patient with an endocrine tumour.

### MEN 1 (Werner syndrome)
- Parathyroid hyperplasia (common)
- Pancreatic and duodenal endocrine tumours, such as Zollinger–Ellison syndrome, insulinoma, PPoma (where PP stands for pancreatic polypeptide) (common)
- Pituitary adenoma (prolactinoma, ACTHoma)
- Thyroid adenoma
- Adrenal adenoma or carcinoma
- Foregut or midgut carcinoid
- Lipoma

### MEN 2A (Sipple syndrome)
- Parathyroid hyperplasia
- Phaeochromocytoma (common)
- Medullary carcinoma of the thyroid (common)

### MEN 2B
- Phaeochromocytoma (common)
- Medullary carcinoma of the thyroid (common)
- Mucosal and ganglioneuromas
- Marfanoid appearance

### Screening for MEN

Screening for MEN 1 is biochemical and for MEN 2 genetic. The tests in patients suspected of MEN 1 should start at age 15 and should be repeated every 3 years. These tests are:
- Albumin-corrected total serum calcium
- Intact serum PTH
- Serum prolactin
- Fasting blood glucose
- Serum pancreatic polypeptide and gastrin
- Plasma chromgranin A

The *RET* mutation causes MEN II and can be screened for. Any patient found to have the *RET* mutation (even children) should have a thyroid-ectomy (because they will invariably develop medullary carcinoma). Family members should be screened from soon after birth. Prophylactic thyroidectomy is usually done before the child starts school.

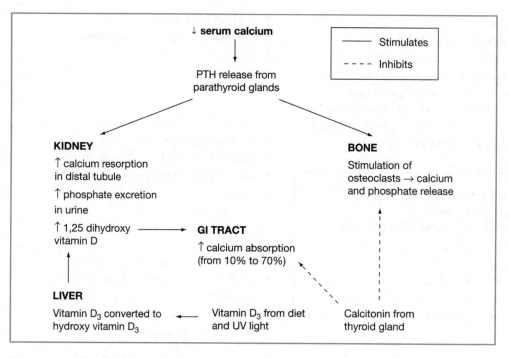

**Figure 4.8 Calcium homeostasis**

CHAPTER 4

# SECTION 3
# Adrenal glands

## 3.1 Anatomy of the adrenals

 **In a nutshell ...**

Each adrenal gland lies on top of the respective kidney. They are enclosed in the renal fascia but are separate from the kidney and are therefore undisturbed during a nephrectomy. The left adrenal gland lies more medially than the right and is crescentic in shape, whereas the right is pyramidal.

### Embryology of the adrenals

The adrenal gland originates from two different sources. The adrenal medulla arises from neural crest cells (ie it has an ectodermal origin), which also give rise to the ganglia of the sympathetic nervous system. The adrenal cortex arises from the mesoderm.

**Anatomical relations of the adrenal glands**

**Left adrenal gland**

Anteriorly
- Splenic artery
- Body of pancreas
- Lesser sac peritoneum

Posteriorly
- Left crus of diaphragm
- Left kidney
- Left inferior phrenic artery

Medially
- Coeliac ganglion
- Left gastric vessels

**Right adrenal gland**

Anteriorly
- Right lobe of liver
- Inferior vena cava (IVC)

Posteriorly
- Right crus of diaphragm
- Right kidney

Superiorly
- Bare area of liver

Medially
- Right inferior phrenic vessels

## Blood supply of the adrenals

The arterial supply comes from three main sources:

- Superior adrenal arteries (from inferior phrenic vessels)
- Middle adrenal arteries (direct branches from the aorta)
- Inferior adrenal arteries (from the renal arteries)

## Venous drainage of the adrenals

- Right adrenal vein drains into the IVC just superior to the renal vein
- Left adrenal vein drains into the left renal vein

## Histology of the adrenal glands

The different zones can be differentiated microscopically. The zona glomerulosa is characterised by small clusters of intensely stained cells, the zona fasciculata by parallel layers of large, pale cells and the zona reticularis by small cells arranged in a network. The medulla is positioned centrally and consists of cells containing basinophilic granules in the cytoplasm.

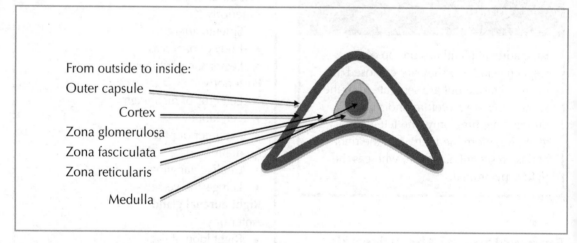

From outside to inside:
Outer capsule
Cortex
Zona glomerulosa
Zona fasciculata
Zona reticularis
Medulla

Figure 4.9 Zones of the adrenal glands

CHAPTER 4

## 3.2   Physiology of the adrenals

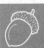 **In a nutshell ...**

**Cortex**
- **Zona glomerulosa:** produces mineralocorticoids (eg aldosterone)
- **Zona fasciculata:** produces glucocorticoids (eg cortisol)
- **Zona reticularis:** produces oestrogens and androgens (eg estradiol, progesterone, testosterone)

**Medulla**
- Produces catecholamines: 80% adrenaline/epinephrine, 20% noradrenaline/norepinephrine

# Synthesis of adrenocortical hormones

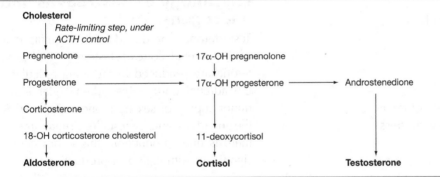

**Figure 4.10 Synthesis of adrenal hormones**

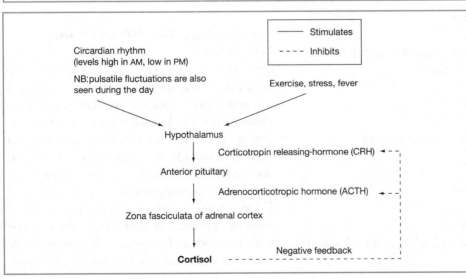

**Figure 4.11 Control of glucocorticoid secretion**

## Physiology of glucocorticoids (cortisol)

Glucocorticoids are not stored in the adrenal cortex. They are released on demand and are transported in the circulation bound to plasma proteins; 83% are bound to cortisol-binding globulin (CBG) and 17% to albumin. The half-life of cortisol is 90 minutes. Cortisol secretion is controlled by a negative feedback system.

## Actions of glucocorticoids

### Metabolism
- ↑ gluconeogenesis and glycogenolysis when fasting
- ↑ glycogen storage when feeding
- ↑ lipolysis
- ↑ protein catabolism

### CNS
- ↑ appetite
- ↑ psychological disturbances
- Role in coping with stress

### Bones
- ↑ bone resorption
- ↓ bone matrix
- ↑ risk of fracture, avascular necrosis (AVN) and growth retardation

### Stomach
- ↑ risk of peptic ulcer perforation

### Immune system
- Anti-inflammatory
- Immunosuppressive
- Inhibit fibroblasts, leading to thin skin and bruising

### CVS
- Vasoconstriction
- ↑ myocardial contractility
- ↓ capillary permeability
- ↑ blood volume

Deficiency of cortisol is known as Addison's disease and excess cortisol production Cushing syndrome.

## Physiology of mineralocorticoids (aldosterone)

See Figure 4.12 opposite.

## Physiology of oestrogens and androgens

Testosterone is produced by the zona fasciculata of the adrenal cortex. Oestrogens and progesterone are produced in the zona reticularis of the adrenal cortex. The adrenal glands are a minor supply of sex hormones compared with the gonads (ovaries or testicles). Therefore, when there is underproduction, this is not clinically significant, although over-production is.

## Physiology of the adrenal medulla

The adrenal medulla is often considered to be a part of the sympathetic nervous system. It is derived from neural crest cells which form chromaffin cells, and these produce adrenaline and noradrenaline. Both these hormones have a very short half-life of 3 minutes, so their effects are short-lived. Stimuli for their release are fear, stress, hypoglycaemia, anoxia, pain and haemorrhage. As with all parts of the sympathetic nervous system, preganglionic fibres come from the CNS and synapse with postganglionic neurones within the adrenal medulla. However,

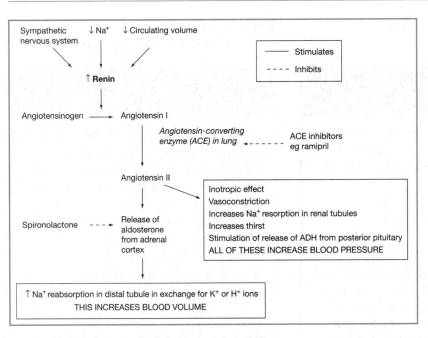

**Figure 4.12 The renin–angiotensin system**

CHAPTER 4

these postganglionic neurones – ie the chromaffin cells – release catecholamines directly into the bloodstream rather than directly leading to organs as other postganglionic fibres do.

Once synthesised (from dopamine via dopamine β-hydroxylase) both these hormones are stored in the chromaffin granules in the adrenal medulla. Catecholamine release into the bloodstream occurs by exocytosis of chromaffin granules.

The catecholamines act via α- and β-adrenergic receptors. The effects of stimulation of these are summarised below. These receptors have varying affinity for adrenaline and noradrenaline; physiologically, apart from $\beta_2$-receptors, the usual physiological agonist for these receptors is noradrenaline. Around 80% of the total catecholamine output of the adrenal medulla is adrenaline and 20% noradrenaline.

### Effects of catecholamines

| Catecholamine | Receptor | Site | Effect |
|---|---|---|---|
| Noradrenaline (norepinephrine) | α1 | Smooth muscle | Vasoconstriction<br>↑ sweating<br>↑ sphincter tone |
| | α2 | Smooth muscle<br>Fat<br>Platelets | Vasoconstriction<br>↓ insulin secretion<br>↑ sweating<br>↓ GI motility |
| | β1 | Cardiac tissue | ↑ myocardial contractility |
| Adrenaline (epinephrine) | β2 | Blood vessels<br>Bronchioles | Vasodilation<br>↑ glucagon<br>Bronchial dilation |
| | β3 | Fat | Lipolysis |

## 3.3 Pathology of the adrenals

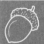

### In a nutshell ...

Disease of the adrenal gland is due to either hyperfunction or hypofunction.

**Syndromes/diseases characterised by hyperfunction:**

- Conn syndrome/aldosteronism: mineralocorticoid excess from the zona glomerulosa
- Cushing syndrome: glucocorticoid excess from the zona fasciculata
- Adrenogenital syndrome: sex hormone excess from the zona reticularis
- Phaeochromocytoma: catecholamine excess from the adrenal medulla

**Adrenocortical hyperfunction can be caused by:**

- Hyperplasia
- Benign tumour (adenoma)
- Malignant tumour
- Over-stimulation by pituitary pathology

**Syndromes/diseases characterised by hypofunction:**

- Adrenocortical insufficiency (Addison's disease)

**Adrenocortical hypofunction can be caused by:**

- Lack of tissue, eg post-adrenalectomy or Waterhouse–Friedrichson syndrome
- Lack of hormone production, as in autoimmune adrenal atrophy
- Lack of drive: in diseases which affect the hypothalamus or pituitary gland – this includes prolonged exogenous steroid use

## 3.4 Cushing syndrome (hypercortisolism)

### In a nutshell ...

Cushing syndrome is caused by an excess of circulating glucocorticoids. By far the most common cause is iatrogenic steroid use. When the increase in glucocorticoids is due to a pituitary tumour, this is Cushing's disease – this accounts for 60% of all cases of non-iatrogenic Cushing syndrome. It is a rare condition, seen more in women than in men (5:1).

### Causes of Cushing syndrome

Within the adrenal cortex:

- **Adrenal carcinoma** (the most likely cause in children)
- **Adrenal hyperplasia**
- **Adrenal adenoma**

Outside the adrenal cortex:

- **Iatrogenic:** due to steroid administration. This is by far the most common cause
- **Pituitary adenoma causing ACTH hypersecretion:** this is Cushing's disease (the next most common cause)
- **Ectopic ACTH secretion:** oat cell carcinoma, bronchial carcinoma, bronchial adenoma, thymic tumours, islet cell tumours, medullary carcinoma of the thyroid

---

**Clinical features of Cushing syndrome and their pathophysiological basis**

**Physical characteristics**
- Truncal obesity: increased protein catabolism leads to an accumulation of fat
- 'Buffalo hump': cortisol causes redistribution of fat to the trunk
- Muscle wasting and weakness: protein catabolism

**Effect on the skin**
- Striae: protein catabolism leads to reduced collagen in the skin
- Easy bruising: loss of collagen in capillary walls
- Skin pigmentation: high ACTH levels stimulate melanocyte-stimulating hormone (MSH)
- Poor wound healing: cortisol inhibits fibroblasts and is immunosuppressive

**Effect on other hormones**
- Diabetes mellitus: proteins are catabolised to glucose. Cortisol inhibits insulin
- Hirsutism/acne: increased adrenal androgens
- Amenorrhoea: cortisol suppresses pituitary gonadotropin

**Effects on the skeleton**
- Osteoporosis: the loss of protein from the bone matrix. Cortisol inhibits the action of vitamin D, which causes reduced calcium absorption from the gut
- Kyphosis: due to osteoporosis
- Pathological fractures: due to osteoporosis

**Effect on fluid balance**
- Hypertension: due to retention of sodium and water
- Oedema: due to retention of sodium and water

**Depression**
- Cortisol causes psychological disturbances

---

## Diagnosis of Cushing syndrome

- **Plasma cortisol measurements** (morning and midnight): raised, with loss of diurnal variation (note that these will also be raised in acutely ill patients)
- **24-hour urinary cortisol:** elevated
- **Dexamethasone suppression test:** administer 2 mg oral dexamethasone at midnight, which should inhibit ACTH production and morning cortisol levels. In patients with Cushing syndrome no decrease in the morning cortisol level is seen

- **Plasma ACTH levels:** should be checked to assess corticotropin function. Levels will be undetectable in primary adrenocortical tumours. Levels will be suppressed after administration of CRH in Cushing's disease (but not if the ACTH is ectopic)
- **Adrenal CT/MRI**
- **Pituitary CT/MRI:** only 10% of skull radiographs will show enlargement of the pituitary fossa (even CT will miss some microadenomas)
- **Chest radiograph, CT of the thorax:** to check for an ACTH-secreting tumour

CHAPTER 4

## Treatment of Cushing syndrome

Treatment depends on the underlying cause:

- **Pituitary disease:**
  - Trans-sphenoidal excision of the pituitary gland
  - External irradiation of the pituitary
  - Interstitial pituitary irradiation
- **Adrenal disease:** a bilateral adrenalectomy should be considered for patients who have bilateral adrenal hyperplasia or in those who have had unsuccessful treatment of pituitary disease. Nelson syndrome can occur when a bilateral adrenalectomy is performed for Cushing syndrome, and is characterised by hyperpigmentation, raised plasma ACTH and continued enlargement of the pituitary gland
- **Ectopic ACTH secretion:** surgical resection of the tumour may be possible

## 3.5   Addison's disease (adrenocortical insufficiency)

 **In a nutshell ...**

This is due to inadequate secretion of corticosteroid hormones from the zona fasciculata. The term 'Addison's disease' is generally used, whatever the cause.

**Causes of adrenocortical insufficiency:**

- Autoimmune
- Withdrawal of corticosteroid therapy (most common cause); exogenous steroids inhibit the production of ACTH and lead to adrenal cortical atrophy
- Post-adrenalectomy
- Drugs (ketoconazole, rifampicin, phenytoin)
- Infection (eg TB, HIV)
- Sarcoid
- Waterhouse–Friedrichson syndrome (meningococcal septicaemia causing bilateral adrenal haemorrhage and infarction; associated with disseminated intravascular coagulation (DIC)
- Metastatic deposits
- Amyloidosis
- Congenital adrenal hyperplasia
- Panhypopituitarism
- ACTH deficiency

**Symptoms and signs of adrenocortical insufficiency**

The presentation of adrenocortical insufficiency can be either acute or chronic.

**Acute**
- ↓ BP/shock
- Hypoglycaemia
- ↓ Na⁺
- Dehydration

**Chronic**
- Anorexia
- Postural ↓ BP (due to sodium and water loss – see Figure 4.12)
- Weight loss
- Muscle wasting
- Circumoral and skin pigmentation (because elevated levels of ACTH also act to stimulate MSH)

## Diagnosis of Addison's disease

Blood tests include:
- ↓ Na⁺
- ↑ ACTH
- ↓ cortisol
- Short Synacthen test: normally administration of Synacthen (an analogue of ACTH) causes an increase in plasma cortisol levels. In patients with adrenocortical insufficiency this increase is not seen

## Treatment of Addison's disease

If the patient presents acutely they should be fluid resuscitated and inotropic support commenced if necessary; intravenous (IV) hydrocortisone 100 mg 6-hourly should be given. If the underlying cause is not immediately obvious then tests for TB and sarcoid and imaging of the adrenals should be carried out.

## 3.6 Conn syndrome (primary aldosteronism)

 **In a nutshell ...**

Hyperaldosteronism may be primary or secondary. Primary aldosteronism is most commonly caused by an aldosterone-producing adenoma or carcinoma in the zona glomerulosa of the adrenal gland (Conn syndrome). Treatment is with surgery or spironolactone.

## Causes of aldosteronism

### Primary aldosteronism
- Aldosterone-producing adenoma (or, very rarely, carcinoma) in the zona glomerulosa causing Conn syndrome. The most common cause
- Adrenocortical hyperplasia
- Adrenal carcinoma
- Ovarian carcinoma
- Familial

### Secondary aldosteronism
- Congestive cardiac failure
- Liver cirrhosis

## Clinical features of aldosteronism
- ↑ BP due to sodium and water retention; accounts for 0.5% patients with 'essential' hypertension
- Tiredness
- Muscle weakness
- Thirst
- Polyuria/nocturia
- Headaches

## Investigating aldosteronism

### Blood tests
- ↑ aldosterone
- ↑ $Na^+$
- ↓ $K^+$ (hypokalaemic acidosis)
- ↓ plasma renin levels (due to negative feedback caused by ↑ BP and aldosterone)

### Imaging
- Should include CT/MRI of the adrenal glands (may show an adenoma)

## Treatment of aldosteronism
- Adrenalectomy for adrenal adenoma or carcinoma
- Aldosterone antagonists (eg spironolactone) for adrenocortical hyperplasia

---

**Adrenogenital syndrome (congenital adrenal hyperplasia)**

This is a rare syndrome and is due to a defect in the adrenal cortex. The most common cause is 21-hydroxylase deficiency, leading to decreased amounts of cortisol and aldosterone. This leads to an increase in the amount of ACTH and thus adrenal hyperplasia, and so to elevated production of testosterone. In females the clinical picture is of virilisation. In males it causes short stature and penile enlargement in childhood. The reduced aldosterone can cause wasting, vomiting and failure to thrive. Diagnosis is confirmed by radioimmunoassay of 17-hydroxyprogesterone, which is elevated. Treatment is with hydrocortisone and mineralocorticoid therapy.

---

## 3.7 Phaeochromocytoma

 **In a nutshell ...**

This is a rare tumour of the adrenal medulla, arising from chromaffin cells, which secretes excessive amounts of catecholamines. It presents in people aged 20–50 and is equally common in males and females. It most commonly presents as refractory hypertension and is diagnosed by the presence of high levels of catecholamines or their metabolites. It is the 'disease of 10%' in that:
- 10% are extra-adrenal (anywhere from the pelvis to the neck but mostly in the abdomen, usually in the region of the aortic bifurcation)
- 10% are bilateral
- 10% are multiple
- 10% are malignant
- 10% are familial (MEN 2A, MEN 2B, von Hippel–Lindau syndrome and neurofibromatosis)

## Causes of hypertension
- **Essential** (90% of cases)
- **Secondary** (10%)
- Renal causes:
  - Glomerulonephritis
  - Renal artery stenosis
  Coarctation of the aorta
- Endocrine causes:
  - Phaeochromocytoma: approximately 1 in every 400–800 patients with hypertension
  - Cushing syndrome
  - Conn syndrome
  - Acromegaly
- Hyperparathyroidism
- Drugs, eg oral contraceptive pill

## Clinical features of phaeochromocytoma

Most common features:

- Hypertension (can be sustained or paroxysmal)
- Palpitations
- Sweating
- Headache

Other features:

- Tachycardia
- Anxiety
- Weakness
- Tremor
- Epigastric pain
- Stroke
- Angina
- Pallor
- Nausea
- Shortness of breath/dyspnoea
- Psychological disturbances
- Diabetes due to anti-insulin effects of catecholamines; adrenaline also causes breakdown of glycogen in the liver, leading to hyperglycaemia

## Investigating phaeochromocytoma

- **Blood:** increased plasma levels of adrenaline and the metanephrines metadrenaline and normetadrenaline are highly sensitive for phaeochromocytoma
- **24-hour urine collection:** increased urinary levels of the metanephrines have been shown to be superior to increased urinary levels of the metabolite vanillyl mandelic acid (VMA) in the diagnosis of phaeochromocytoma. False-positive results for all of these plasma and urine tests may be due to medication such as tricyclic antidepressants
- **Radiology:**
  - CT/MRI to image adrenal glands: MRI is more sensitive

- Iodine-131-labelled MIBG scan to localise the phaeochromocytoma and detect extra-adrenal lesions

---

**Incidentalomas of the adrenal glands**

Incidentalomas are nodules found within the adrenal gland during routine abdominal imaging. It can be difficult to know how to manage these patients clinically:

- If the radiography is diagnostic, appropriate treatment should be instigated
- If there is a possibility that the lesion represents metastatic disease, PET may be diagnostic but FNA or core biopsy may be performed. A primary carcinoma source should be sought

Otherwise, the function should be checked:

- A hormonally active nodule should be excised, as should a lesion >4 cm
- Lesions <4 cm that are not hormonally active can be observed with repeat imaging in 6–18 months, because they are likely to be adenomas

---

## Treatment of phaeochromocytoma

Most phaeochromocytomas are treated surgically with adrenalectomy. Tight pre and post-operative control of blood pressure is essential.

### Adrenalectomy: management of blood pressure

#### Preoperatively

Severe intraoperative haemodynamic instability can occur if preoperative adrenoceptor blockade is not carried out.

- α block with phenoxybenzamine 20 mg three times daily 1 week preoperatively (doxazosin also used)
- β block with propranolol 40 mg three times daily 4 weeks preoperatively
- Insulin sliding scale if diabetic

### Perioperatively

- Preoperative loading with fluid
- Nitroprusside or phentolamine to stabilise blood pressure if necessary
- Early ligation of adrenal vein and minimal handling of tumour
- Fluids and dopamine infusion if necessary for circulatory support

### Postoperatively

- Monitor central venous pressure (CVP), arterial pressure, pulse rate, urine output and blood glucose
- Adequate fluid replacement

## 3.8  Adrenalectomy

 **In a nutshell ...**

Several surgical approaches to the adrenal glands have been described. These include:

- **Posterior extraperitoneal approach through ribs 11/12:** direct, atraumatic approach, not suitable for larger tumours (>5 cm)
- **Transabdominal approach via upper abdominal incision:** good exposure, used for malignancies and phaeochromocytoma
- **Laparoscopic technique:** associated with a smaller scar, shorter hospital stay and faster return to work. Considered the gold standard by most endocrine surgeons and can be extraperitoneal or transabdominal

 **Op box: Adrenalectomy**

**Preop**
- **Cushing syndrome:** control hypertension, cardiac failure, hypokalaemia and diabetes before surgery
- **Conn syndrome:** control hypokalaemia and hypertension
- **Phaeochromocytoma:** control hypertension with α blockers and arrhythmias with β blockers
- **Any adrenalectomy:** cross-match three units

**Patient position**
- Supine, table tilted to the right, head up. Consider lateral positioning

**Incision**
- Transverse subcostal

**continued opposite**

## Procedure
### LEFT adrenalectomy
- Divide lienorenal ligament. Some mobilisation of left colon may be necessary
- Retract spleen and tail of pancreas
- Identify lesion and mobilise adrenal gland
- During mobilisation, identify and ligate the adrenal arteries
- Divide the main vein LAST (to avoid venous engorgement and increased bleeding) on the medial side between clips or ties (except phaeochromocytoma)

### RIGHT adrenalectomy (trickier than left because IVC is a lot closer and liver obscures view)
- Divide peritoneum above hepatic flexure
- Retract hepatic flexure of colon downwards
- Retract kidney inferiorly and liver superiorly
- Identify IVC
- (It may be necessary to mobilise the right lobe of the liver to retract it medially and anteriorly)
- Divide the main vein **first** to avoid tearing the IVC
- Mobilise the adrenal gland
- Divide fascial attachments to the kidney last as the adrenal will spring superiorly out of view when released

### Closure
- No drains
- Close wound in layers with non-absorbable or PDS sutures
- Sutures or staples to skin

## BEWARE INTRAOPERATIVELY:
### Anatomical pitfalls:
- Extreme care must be made not to identify a renal vein wrongly as the adrenal vein
- Inadvertent entry may be made into pancreatic parenchyma during mobilisation

### Bleeding
- During mobilisation (especially carcinomas, phaeochromocytomas)
- IVC damage (if significant, pack and wait for blood before attempting repair)
- Damage to spleen or liver

### Phaeochromocytomas
- Continuous BP monitoring, gentle handling of gland, early ligation of vessels
- Hypertensive crisis (treat with IV nitroprusside or phentolamine)
- Arrhythmias (treat with propranolol and lidocaine)
- Expect hypotension after removal (treat with fluid replacement)

## Postop
- 30-minute BP observation until stable for 24 h
- Daily urea and electrolytes (U&Es)
- Postop steroids for Cushing syndrome and bilateral adrenalectomy
- Clips out at 7 days (10 days for Cushing syndrome)

### Later complications
- Acute circulatory failure (treat with fluids and maybe inotropes)
- Delayed wound healing in Cushing syndrome

Patients undergoing bilateral adrenalectomy require hydrocortisone during and after surgery. They should be given 100 mg intramuscular hydrocortisone preoperatively and then every 6 h for 2–3 days postoperatively. This should change to oral supplementation (20 mg in the morning and 10 mg at night) and long-term cover with oral fludrocortisone (100 µg daily). During elective surgery, illness or fever, doses of steroid should be doubled, and if patients are vomiting the steroids should be administered intravenously. Patients undergoing adrenalectomy for Cushing syndrome require intraoperative and postoperative steroids because the remaining adrenal gland will have been suppressed. In this case it may be possible to wean them off the steroids at a later date.

CHAPTER 4

# Chapter 5

# Head and Neck Surgery

**Nicholas E Gibbins**

CHAPTER 5

## 1.1 Embryology

### Branchial arches

Knowledge of how the head and neck develop in utero is essential for understanding its anatomy and its importance cannot be underestimated. Branchial comes from the Greek branchia meaning 'gill'. Examining gills of fish, each gill has a cartilage to give it shape, an artery to supply blood for oxygen exchange, muscles to move the gill and a corresponding nerve. As we all descend from a common ancestor you can extrapolate this to humans. Fish have seven to eight arches but humans have four (the fifth, seventh and eighth do not exist, and the sixth is rudimentary).

Once born, the gills have fused to form the head and neck but at a very early stage of development they are more easily seen (Figure 5.1).

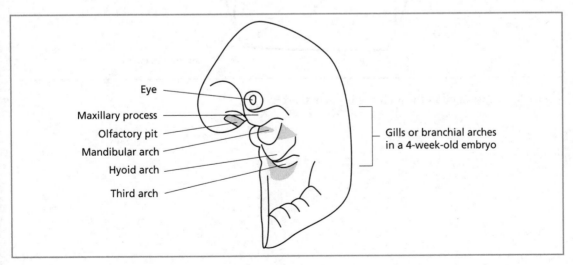

Eye
Maxillary process
Olfactory pit
Mandibular arch
Hyoid arch
Third arch

Gills or branchial arches in a 4-week-old embryo

**Figure 5.1 Lateral view of an embryo at 4 weeks**

These branchial arches grow forwards to meet their partners in the midline, forming a tube (the primitive pharynx), and superiorly and inferiorly to fuse with their neighbours.

These areas are called, variably, pharyngeal clefts, pharyngeal pouches, branchial pouches and pharyngeal arches, but they all refer to the same structures. For clarity and ease we refer to each gill as a branchial arch. It is separated from its neighbour by a branchial cleft on the outside (ectoderm) and a branchial, or pharyngeal, pouch on the inside (endoderm). Figure 5.2 highlights these relationships and also shows the tuberculum impar and the thyroid diverticulum, which are important landmarks in the formation of the tongue and the descent of the thyroid gland.

The table opposite shows the arrangements within each branchial arch. It can be seen that the arteries, nerves and muscles are aligned logically. The nerve of the first arch is the trigeminal, which supplies the muscles of mastication. The arch is also known as the 'mandibular arch' and is supplied by the maxillary and external carotid arteries. Extrapolating this from embryology to formed anatomy, it makes sense.

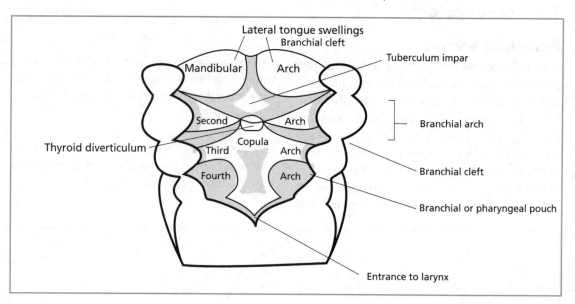

**Figure 5.2 Cross-section through the branchial arches**

## Branchial arches

| Arch | Cranial nerve | Artery | Skeletal component | Muscular component |
|------|---------------|--------|--------------------|--------------------|
| First (mandibular arch) | V – trigeminal | Maxillary External carotid | Maxilla Mandible Incus and malleus | **Muscles of mastication** Anterior belly of digastric Mylohyoid, tensor tympani, tensor veli palatini |
| Second (hyoid arch) | VII – facial | (Stapedial artery) | Stapes Styloid Lesser cornu of hyoid | **Muscles of facial expression** Posterior belly of digastric Platysma Stapedius |
| Third | IX – glossopharyngeal | Common carotid artery/internal carotid artery | Greater cornu of hyoid | Stylopharyngeus |
| Fourth | X – superior laryngeal | **Right: subclavian artery** **Left: aortic arch** | Thyroid cartilage Epiglottis | **Cricothyroid** Muscles of soft palate |
| Sixth | X – recurrent laryngeal | Pulmonary arteries | Cricoid cartilage Arytenoids | All intrinsic muscles of larynx except cricothyroid |

Important areas are in bold. Note the arteries of the fourth arch, around which the recurrent laryngeal nerves must pass before reaching their destination.

The nerve supply to the anterior and posterior bellies of the digastric should be noted, supplied by cranial nerves V and VII, respectively, but arguably the most important point is the relationship between the arteries and nerves of the fourth and sixth arches. Referring to the table above it can be seen that the arteries of the fourth arch (left aortic arch, right subclavian) arise in the neck, but during development the arch of the aorta descends into the thorax and the right subclavian descends to the thoracic inlet. Therefore the nerves 'below' them, the recurrent laryngeal nerves, are also forced to descend, to loop around their respective arteries before ascending towards their destination, the larynx.

It is this pattern of development that means that the recurrent laryngeal nerves are exposed and therefore at risk during thyroid surgery. It also means that intrathoracic pathology such as bronchial cancer can manifest itself as left vocal fold palsy.

## Face and palate

The paired maxillary and mandibular prominences are all part of the first branchial arch (and therefore the anatomy is supplied by the trigeminal nerve and the maxillary and external carotid arteries).

At the same time, within what will turn into the mouth, paired lateral palatine processes grow towards each other to meet in the midline, forming the secondary palate. The frontonasal prominence grows inferiorly to fill the gap between the

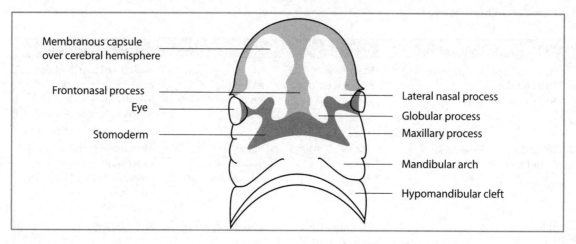

**Figure 5.3 Development of the face**

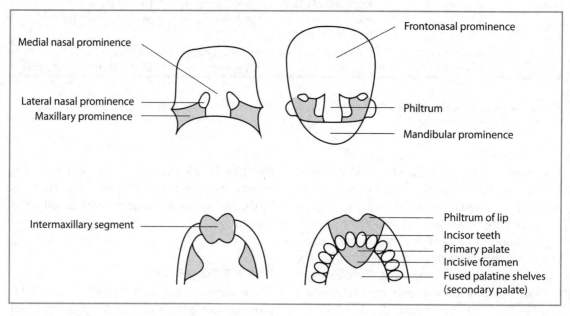

**Figure 5.4 Development of the palate and face**

maxillary prominences (anteriorly this will become the philtrum), and a medial palatine process grows posteriorly from here to fuse with the two lateral processes. The meeting point is the incisive foramen (Figure 5.4) and forms the primary palate. The combination of the primary and secondary palate makes the hard palate.

Malformations of the fusion process result in clefts, which can be unilateral or bilateral, and lip only, palate only or a combination. However, they all form along the fusion lines of the medial and two lateral palatine processes.

## Thyroid and parathyroid

The development of the thyroid is directly linked to the development of the tongue. If you look back at Figure 5.2, you can see two lateral tongue swellings from the first branchial arch and the copula from the third arch. They come together to form the tongue, with the epiglottis arising from the fourth arch. There is almost no contribution from the second arch. The tongue fuses along the line of the circumvallate papillae. The midpoint of this line is the foramen caecum, which marks the starting point of the descent of the thyroid gland into the neck.

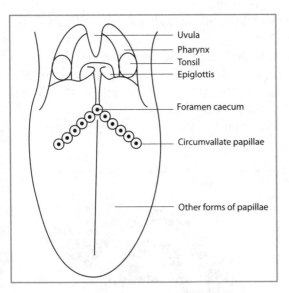

Uvula
Pharynx
Tonsil
Epiglottis

Foramen caecum

Circumvallate papillae

Other forms of papillae

**Figure 5.5 The tongue – upper surface**

The thyroid gland descends into the neck and comes to rest in its normal position in the anterior compartment just above the sternal notch. However, its route is circuitous because the tract along which it descends loops around the hyoid bone. Therefore surgery to remove a thyroglossal cyst, a remnant of this tract, must include removal of the middle third of the hyoid bone and tracing of the tract up to the mucosa of the tongue. Along with a wide cuff of tissue around the tract, this is known as a modified Sistrunk procedure.

The C cells, which secrete calcitonin and regulate calcium, are an important subset of cells within the thyroid. They arise from the fifth branchial pouch, as opposed to the thyroid, which arises from between the first and second branchial pouches (see Figure 5.2). As the thyroid descends, the C cells ascend and merge into the thyroid gland. This fact is important when considering the physiology and treatment of different thyroid cancers. In short, papillary and follicular cancers (derived purely from thyroid tissue) can be treated with surgery followed by radioactive iodine (RAI), whereas medullary thyroid cancer originating from the C cells is not affected by RAI and is treated by surgery only.

The parathyroid glands (PTGs) are divided into superior and inferior. The inferior PTGs are derived from the **third** branchial pouch whereas the superior PTGs are from the **fourth**. This results mainly because the third branchial pouch is also the origin of the thymus gland. As this descends in the neck, it pulls the PTGs with it, hence their inferior position in the neck. They may even be found in the intrathoracic compartment. This long descent also explains their widely variable position. The superior PTGs do not descend as far and thus their final position, intimately related to the posterior portion of the thyroid, is much more stable.

## 1.2    Anatomy of the head

### 1.2.1 The ear

#### Embryology of the ear

The ear is derived from the six hillocks of His (the same His as the one who described the bundles in the heart) which fuse to form the external ear. These hillocks are derived from the first two branchial arches, so a first branchial arch anomaly will affect the ear (some syndromes have these anomalies and patients often have microtia or even anotia). Similarly, a first branchial cleft anomaly arises from the ear canal.

## The external ear

- The auricle consists of elastic cartilage covered by skin
- The auricle has a medial and lateral aspect and bears a lobule which is a fibrofatty structure

The sensory supply to the auricle is derived from:
- **Auriculotemporal nerve:** innervates upper part of the lateral surface
- **Greater auricular nerve:** innervates entire medial surface and the lower part of the lateral surface

## External auditory canal

This is a 3-cm-long sinuous tube that develops from the first branchial cleft.

The lateral third is cartilaginous. Skin overlying this part of the canal contains hair follicles, sebaceous glands and cerumen wax-producing glands (modified sweat glands).

The medial two-thirds are bony. Skin overlying this part of the canal is thin and devoid of adnexal structures.

The sensory supply is from the:
- **Auriculotemporal nerve** (branch of the maxillary division of the trigeminal nerve)
- Auricular branch of the vagus
- **Facial nerve** via the tympanic plexus

The blood supply is from the:
- Posterior auricular artery
- Superficial temporal artery
- **Deep auricular artery** from the internal maxillary artery

## Tympanic membrane (eardrum)

The tympanic membrane (TM) separates the external auditory canal and the middle-ear cleft (MEC). Embryologically, the external ear is formed from the first branchial cleft. The eustachian tube, middle-ear cleft and its extension to the mastoid antrum are formed from the first branchial pouch. The TM is the only branchial membrane. Subsequently, one can understand why it has three layers:
- The outer ectodermal layer (squamous epithelium – skin-like)
- The inner endodermal layer (respiratory-like epithelium)
- The middle mesodermal layer (fibrous layer)

It is divided into the upper **pars flaccida**, or the attic, and the lower, larger **pars tensa** (Figure 5.6b). The TM is surrounded by the fibrous annulus, which anchors it into a groove in the tympanic part of the temporal bone, the tympanic annulus.

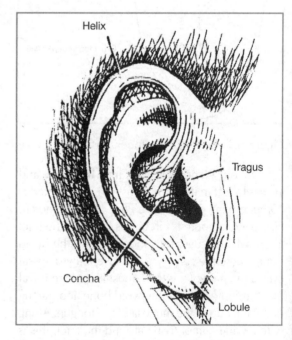

Helix

Tragus

Concha

Lobule

**Figure 5.6a The ear**

CHAPTER 5

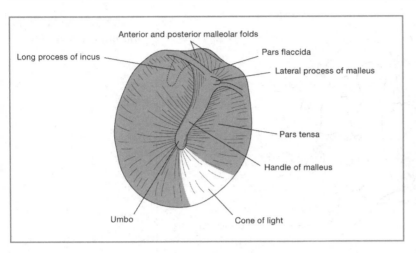

Anterior and posterior malleolar folds

Long process of incus

Pars flaccida

Lateral process of malleus

Pars tensa

Handle of malleus

Umbo

Cone of light

**Figure 5.6b The tympanic membrane**

The handle of the **malleus** sits visibly within the TM. It connects to the **incus** and then the **stapes** within the middle ear.

---

### External nerve supply
- Auriculotemporal nerve
- Vagus (cranial nerve [CN] X)
- Facial (CN VII)
- Glossopharyngeal (CN IX)

Note therefore that referred otalgia can come from any pathology affecting sites supplied by the facial, glossopharyneal and vagus nerves.

### Internal nerve supply
- Tympanic branch of the glossopharyngeal nerve (Jacobsen's nerve)

---

## The middle ear

The middle-ear cleft is a complex area with a great deal of important anatomy within it. It is best to think of it as an oblong, with the lateral surface being the medial wall of the TM, described above (Figure 5.7).

### Posterior wall

This contains the aditus ad antrum (mastoid antrum), which is the connecting passage between the MEC and the mastoid bone, which sits immediately behind. There is also a bony process, the pyramid, which attaches the stapedius tendon.

### Floor

A thin plate of bone that separates the MEC from the underlying jugular bulb (which descends into the internal jugular vein).

### Anterior wall

Contains the opening to the eustachian tube (which connects to the nasopharynx) and the tensor tympani muscle, which inserts into the malleus and helps protect the ear when a loud noise is expected. The muscle contracts, tenses the TM and prevents its excess movement, thus protecting the oval window from damage by the stapes. It is a thin layer of bone that separates the MEC from the internal carotid artery.

**CHAPTER 5**

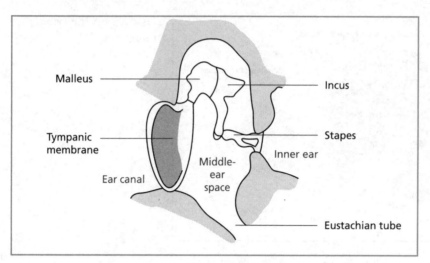

Figure 5.7 The auditory middle ear ossiscles

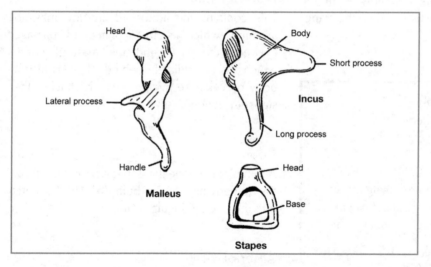

Figure 5.8 Ossicles

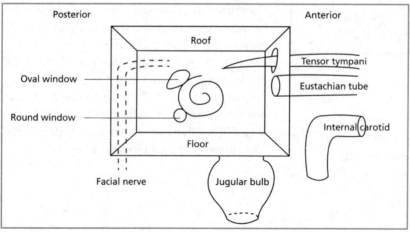

Figure 5.9 Schematic view of the middle ear

## Roof

A thin layer of bone, named the tegmen tympani, that separates the MEC from the dura of the middle cranial fossa.

## Medial wall

This houses most of the important anatomy of the MEC.

### Promontory

This is a bulge into the MEC formed by the basal turn of the cochlea. It is covered by the tympanic plexus (from the glossopharyngeal nerve – see inner surface of TM).

### The oval window

Lies superoposteriorly to the promontory. The stapes footplate sits within the oval window.

### The round window

Lies inferoposteriorly to the promontory and is the baffle port for the cochlea.

### The facial nerve

Enters the MEC anterosuperior to the promontory. It immediately forms the geniculate ganglion and turns posteriorly at this point – the first genu. It passes superior to the promontory and turns inferiorly at the second genu. At this point it passes posterosuperiorly to the oval window but anteroinferiorly to the lateral semicircular canal. This is discussed in depth later in the chapter.

> Therefore, from anteroinferior to postero-superior the following are found:
> Promontory → Oval window →
> Facial nerve at second genu →
> Lateral semicircular canal
> Once it has taken a 90° turn inferiorly it passes through the mastoid to exit the temporal bone via the stylomastoid foramen.

### Processus cochleariformis

Lies anteriorly and houses the tensor tympani muscle (which attaches to the medial surface of the malleus).

## Contents of the middle ear

### Ossicles

The malleus consists of a handle (both visible in the TM), a head, a lateral process and an articular surface to articulate with the incus.

The incus consists of a body (articulates with the malleus), a short process (projects posteriorly) and a long process that projects inferiorly. The tip of this is the lenticular process, which articulates with the stapes.

The stapes consists of a head that articulates with the lenticular process of the incus, two crura and a footplate. The footplate sits in the oval window.

All the joints are synovial.

### Nerves

*Chorda tympani*
- Branch of the facial nerve
- Arises from the descending portion of the facial nerve (in the mastoid)
- Passes posteriorly between the layers of the TM
- Exits the MEC through the petrotympanic fissure
- Joins the lingual nerve and supplies taste to the anterior two-thirds of the tongue

*Tympanic plexus*
- Formed from the glossopharyngeal and facial nerves
- Also has some sympathetic fibres from the internal carotid artery
- Forms Jacobsen's nerve (CN IX) which forms the lesser petrosal nerve as it exits the MEC
- Joins the auriculotemporal nerve and is the parasympathetic supply to the parotid gland

### Muscles

*Tensor tympani*
- **First branchial arch derivative** along with the malleus and half the incus
- Originates in the bony canal in the anterior wall of the MEC above the eustachian tube
- Inserts into the malleus via the processus cochleariformis
- Supplied by the medial pterygoid nerve (branch of the trigeminal nerve [V3], the nerve of the first branchial arch)

*Stapedius*
- **Second branchial arch derivative** along with the stapes and half the incus
- Originates from the pyramidal process on the posterior wall of the MEC
- Inserts into the neck of the stapes
- Supplied by the nerve to stapedius (branch of facial nerve, the nerve of the second branchial arch)

### Nerve supply of the middle ear
- Provided via the tympanic plexus
- Middle and external sections of the ear are supplied by cranial nerves V, VII, X and XI, **so pain in the ear (otalgia) may be referred to the larynx, pharynx, teeth and posterior part of the tongue** (referred otalgia – very important in identification of cancer)

### Arterial supply of the middle ear
- Tympanic branch of the maxillary artery
- Tympanic branch of the ascending pharyngeal artery
- Branches from the internal carotid artery
- Stylomastoid branch of the posterior auricular artery
- Petrosal branch of the middle meningeal artery

## The inner ear (labyrinth)

This develops from the otic placode of ectoderm at 3 weeks' gestation from 14 centres of ossification. It is the hardest bone in the body.
- It lies in the temporal bone and is divided into the bony and membranous labyrinth (the membranous labyrinth lies within the bony labyrinth). Think of blowing a balloon up within a tube. The balloon is the membranous labyrinth and the tube is the bony labyrinth

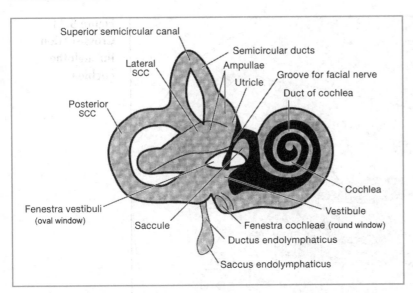

**Figure 5.10 The labyrinth with semicircular canals (SCC)**

Labels in figure:
- Superior semicircular canal
- Semicircular ducts
- Lateral SCC
- Ampullae
- Utricle
- Groove for facial nerve
- Duct of cochlea
- Posterior SCC
- Cochlea
- Fenestra vestibuli (oval window)
- Vestibule
- Saccule
- Fenestra cochleae (round window)
- Ductus endolymphaticus
- Saccus endolymphaticus

- The bony labyrinth is a bony shell surrounding the cochlea, vestibule and semicircular canals
- The membranous labyrinth consists of the cochlear duct, utricle and saccule, and the semicircular ducts

## Cochlea

The cochlea contains the cochlear duct (concerned with hearing). It spirals for two and a half turns around its centre or axis, which is called the modiolus.

The cochlear duct is separated into the scala vestibuli, scala media and scala tympani by Reissner's membrane and the basilar membrane. The scala media contains endolymph whereas the scala vestibuli and scala tympani contain perilymph. The scala tympani and scala vestibuli communicate at the helicotremma at the apex of the cochlear duct. The bony core around which the cochlea spirals is referred to as the modiolus and carries the cochlear nerve fibres. These come together at the base to form the cochlear nerve. Nerves coming from the semicircular canals join them to form the **vestibulocochlear nerve (CN VIII)**.

## Vestibule

The vestibule is a small oval chamber concerned with balance, which encases the saccule and utricle (sensitive to linear acceleration).

A small duct leads from both the saccule and the utricle to unite and form the endolymphatic duct, which projects to the posterior cranial fossa as the endolymphatic sac (where endolymph is absorbed).

## Semicircular canals

There are three semicircular canals: the anterior, posterior and lateral. These canals contain the semicircular ducts which are concerned with balance. They are at right angles to each other and occupy three planes in space. They open via their ampullae into the utricle.

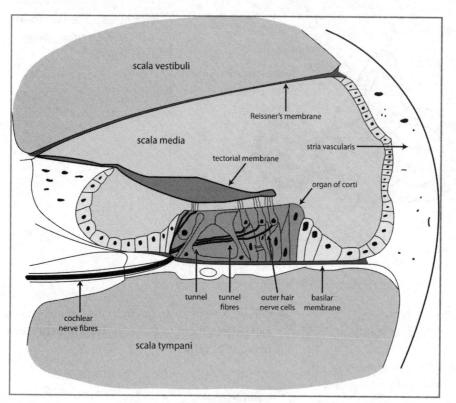

**Figure 5.11 Cross-section through the cochlea**

## Blood supply

The arterial supply of the inner ear is derived from the labyrinthine artery (a branch of the basilar artery) that accompanies the cochlear and vestibular nerves. A smaller contribution is from the stylomastoid branch of the posterior auricular artery. Venous drainage is via the labyrinthine vein, that drains into the inferior petrosal sinus.

### 1.2.2 The nose and paranasal sinuses

#### Functions

The main functions of the nose are respiration, olfaction and humidification. In addition, it is involved with vocal resonance and, to a limited degree, protection of the lower airway.

> REMEMBER: the nose and paranasal sinuses (and the middle ear) are part of the respiratory tree.

It is unclear why humans have paranasal sinuses. They make the skull only 1% lighter than if they were filled with bone and they have very few olfactory receptors, but it is known that only the higher primates (orang-utans, gorillas and humans) have ethmoid sinuses, and that the most primitive mammals (rodents) have only maxillary sinuses.

### External nose

Made of:
- Nasal bones:
  - Attach posteriorly to the maxilla

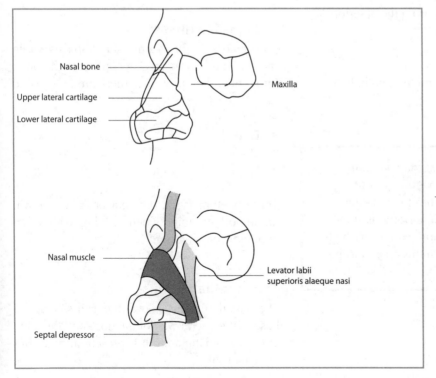

**Figure 5.12 The external nose**

Nasal bone

Upper lateral cartilage

Lower lateral cartilage

Maxilla

Nasal muscle

Levator labii superioris alaeque nasi

Septal depressor

CHAPTER 5

- Cartilage:
  - Upper lateral
  - Lower lateral
  - Sesamoid
  - Nasal septum
- Fibrofatty tissue
- Small muscles:
  - Septal depressor
  - Nasal muscle (scrunch nose)
  - Procerus
  - Levator labii superioris alaeque nasi (nostril flare)
- External lining: skin
- Internal lining: respiratory epithelium

### Blood supply

Arterial:

- Lateral nasal artery (branch of the facial artery)
- Nasal dorsal artery (terminal branch of the ophthalmic artery)
- External nasal artery (from the anterior ethmoidal artery)

Venous:

- Via the facial veins and the ophthalmic venous plexus

REMEMBER: the facial triangle drains posteriorly into the cavernous sinus, so sepsis in this area has the potential to spread and result in cavernous sinus thrombosis, a condition with a very high mortality. Infections in this area must be treated aggressively.

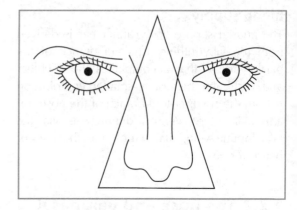

**Figure 5.13 The facial triangle**

### Nerve supply

- External nasal nerve (Va): supplies the dorsum and tip of the nose (branch of the anterior ethmoidal nerve, ie the ophthalmic nerve)
- Supratrochlear nerve (Va)
- Infratrochlear nerve (Vb)
- Infraorbital nerve (Vb)

## Paranasal sinuses

The paranasal sinuses are air-filled spaces within the skull and are named according to the bone into which they protrude. There are four paired paranasal sinuses:

- Maxillary
- Frontal
- Ethmoid
- Sphenoid

These pneumatise at different times after birth, an important point when dealing with nasal conditions in children.

## The maxillary sinus

The maxillary sinus is pyramidal in shape, the base at the lateral wall of the nose and the apex at the zygomatic arch. It is present at birth, but is a small slit.

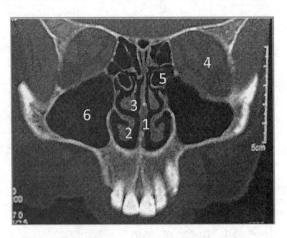

**Figure 5.14 Coronal CT through the maxillary and ethmoid sinuses**
1 – septum, 2 – inferior turbinate, 3 – middle turbinate, 4 – orbital contents, 5 – anterior ethmoid sinus, 6 – maxillary sinus

## Walls of the maxillary sinus

- **Anterior and posterior:** walls of the maxilla
- **Roof:** floor of the orbit
- **Floor:** alveolar part of maxilla
- **Medial wall:** lateral wall of the nose
- **Apex:** zygomatic process

## Arterial supply of the maxillary sinus

- This is derived from the facial, maxillary, infraorbital and greater palatine arteries
- The venous drainage is via the facial veins and pterygoid venous plexus

## Lymphatic drainage of the maxillary sinus

- Drainage occurs to the submandibular nodes

## Nerve supply of the maxillary sinus

This is from the superior alveolar nerves (posterior, middle and inferior), greater palatine and infraorbital nerves, which all originate from the maxillary nerve.

## Ethmoid sinuses

The ethmoid sinuses are similar to a honeycomb in that they comprise many interconnected cells. After attachment of the middle turbinate from anterior to posterior, it runs horizontally and then curves downwards. The curve inferiorly is the basal, or ground, lamella. All the cells anterior to this are the anterior ethmoid cells and those posterior are the posterior ethmoid cells. The basal lamella is an oblique plate of bone in the middle turbinate which is attached laterally to the lamina papyracea.

### Anterior ethmoid sinuses

These sinuses drain into the hiatus semilunaris within the middle meatus (anterior to the basal lamella).

> **Boundaries of anterior ethmoid sinuses (anterior to basal lamella)**
> - **Lateral:** lamina papyracea (antero-medial wall of orbit and paper-thin)
> - **Medial:** middle turbinate
> - **Roof:** frontal bone (may be asymmetrical)
> - **Posterior:** basal lamella (inferior deflection of middle turbinate)

**CHAPTER 5**

## Posterior ethmoid sinuses

These drain into the sphenoethmoidal recess within the superior meatus (posterior to basal lamella).

> **Boundaries of the posterior ethmoid sinuses**
> - **Lateral:** posteromedial wall of orbit
> - **Medial:** contralateral ethmoid sinus
> - **Roof:** frontal bone
> - **Posterior:** anterior wall of sphenoid sinus

*Arterial supply of the ethmoid sinuses*
- This is from both the internal carotid artery via the anterior and posterior ethmoidal and sphenopalatine arteries, and the external carotid artery via the supraorbital artery. Venous drainage is via the corresponding veins

*Lymphatic drainage of the ethmoid sinuses*
- This is to the submandibular and retropharyngeal nodes

*Nerve supply of the ethmoid sinuses*
- The ethmoid sinuses are innervated by the anterior and posterior ethmoidal nerves and orbital branches of the pterygopalatine ganglion

## Sphenoid sinus

This is located in the body of the sphenoid body and lies in front and below the pituitary fossa. The sphenoid sinus has important surrounding structures that must be considered when operating on it:

- **Superiorly:** the pituitary gland
- **Superolaterally:** the optic nerve
- **Inferolaterally:** the internal carotid artery
- **Inferiorly:** the pterygoid canal inferiorly (carries the nerve of the pterygoid canal, or vidian nerve)

> **Relations of the sphenoid sinus**
> - **Superiorly:** pituitary fossa, olfactory tracts, frontal lobes and optic chiasm
> - **Inferiorly:** roof of the nasopharynx
> - **Laterally:** cavernous sinus, internal carotid artery and abducens, oculomotor, trochlear, ophthalmic and maxillary nerves
> - **Medially:** septum of the sinus (this is often markedly asymmetrical)
> - **Posteriorly:** occipital bone, basilar artery, brainstem and pituitary fossa
> - **Anteriorly:** sphenoethmoidal recess and posterior ethmoidal cells

## Arterial supply of the sphenoid sinus
- This is from the posterior ethmoidal artery

## Nerve supply of the sphenoid sinus
- This is derived from the orbital branch of the pterygopalatine ganglion and the posterior ethmoidal nerve

## Lymphatic drainage of the sphenoid sinus
- The sphenoid sinuses drain to the retropharyngeal nodes

## Frontal sinus

This is not present at birth and appears in the second year. Its relations are the anterior cranial fossa and the orbit. It drains via the frontal recess into the anterior end of the hiatus semilunaris.

### Arterial supply of the frontal sinus
- This is derived from the supratrochlear, supraorbital and anterior ethmoidal arteries
- Venous drainage is via the diploic and superior ophthalmic veins

### Nerve supply of the frontal sinus
- The frontal sinus is supplied by the supraorbital and supratrochlear nerves

### Lymphatic drainage of the frontal sinus
- The sinus drains to the submandibular nodes and the overlying skin drains to the periauricular nodes

## 1.2.3 The oral cavity – mouth, tongue and the temporomandibular joint

### The oral cavity

The oral cavity extends from the vermillion border of the lips to the anterior tonsillar, or faucal, pillar. This pillar consists of the palatoglossus muscle. Therefore, the tonsils that lie between the anterior faucal pillar (palatoglossus) and the posterior faucal pillar (palatopharyngeus) are in the oropharynx, not the oral cavity.

It extends from the hard palate superiorly (and posteriorly to the junction of the hard and soft palates) to the floor of the mouth inferiorly. Laterally the oral cavity extends to the buccal mucosa.

---

### Contents of the oral cavity
- Tongue
- Hard palate
- Floor of mouth (Wharton's ducts from the submandibular glands open here)
- Lips
- Buccal mucosa (Stensen's ducts from the parotid glands open here)
- Upper and lower alveolar ridges (where teeth insert)
- Vestibule (space lateral to teeth)
- Retromolar trigone (mucosa behind last molar)

---

### Tongue

The sulcus terminalis divides the dorsum of the tongue into the anterior two-thirds and the posterior third. This is lined anteriorly with the **circumvallate** papillae (taste receptors). The other papillae present are the **filiform** (scattered, no taste receptors) and the **fungiform** (laterally placed, contain taste receptors).

The foramen caecum is the midpoint of the sulcus and is the remnant of the thyroglossal duct, the route of travel of the thyroid gland from its origin here to its resting place in the neck. This is discussed in Section 1.1 and in Chapter 4, Endocrine Surgery.

Posteriorly, the tongue is in continuation with the palatine tonsils laterally in an area known as the 'plica triangularis'. Further posteriorly, at its base, it attaches to the epiglottis in the midline via the aptly named 'glossoepiglottic ligaments'. The space between the base of the tongue and the epiglottis is the **vallecula**.

When performing direct laryngoscopy to intubate or gain direct visualisation of the larynx, the tip of the laryngoscope should lie in the vallecula. This pulls the tongue forwards and out of the way.

Due to its many muscle fibres running in all directions the tongue is very versatile but its functions are mainly:
- Speech
- Swallowing (oral phase of deglutition)
- Mastication
- Taste

**The anterior two-thirds of the tongue** (anterior to the circumvallate papillae and foramen caecum) are in the oral cavity. This part of the tongue is derived from the first branchial arch and, as such, the sensation is supplied by the first branchial arch nerve, the trigeminal (V) in the form of the lingual nerve. The chorda tympani (branch of the facial [VII]) runs with the lingual nerve and supplies taste to the anterior two-thirds of the tongue.

**The posterior third of the tongue** is derived from the third branchial arch and is therefore supplied by the nerve of the third arch, the glossopharyngeal (IX). Both sensation and taste are supplied by this nerve.

The muscles of the tongue are divided into intrinsic and extrinsic muscles.

**The intrinsic muscles** are ALL supplied by the glossopharyngeal nerve (IX). They are quite simply called:
- The longitudinal (superior and inferior)
- The transverse
- The vertical

**The extrinsic muscles** are supplied by the glosso-pharyngeal nerve (IX) EXCEPT palatoglossus,

which is on the border of the oral cavity and oropharynx. It is supplied by the pharyngeal plexus.

The muscles are all suffixed by -glossus:
- Genioglossus:
  - From the superior meatal spine
  - Protrudes the tongue
- Hyoglossus:
  - From greater cornu of hyoid
  - Rolls the tongue
- Styloglossus:
  - From the styloid process
  - Retracts the tongue
- Palatoglossus:
  - From palatal aponeurosis
  - Closes the oropharyngeal isthmus – the narrowest part – when swallowing

## Blood supply of the tongue

The lingual artery is the main source. It is the second anterior branch of the external carotid artery.

The venous drainage is directly to the internal jugular vein.

---

The relationship of the tip of the greater cornu of the hyoid, the lingual artery and the hypoglossal nerve in head and neck surgery is an important one because they lie just inferior and deep to the posterior belly of the digastric, known as the 'trainee's friend'. When tissue planes are destroyed in neoplastic disease, recognition of structural landmarks such as these allows dissection with confidence.

---

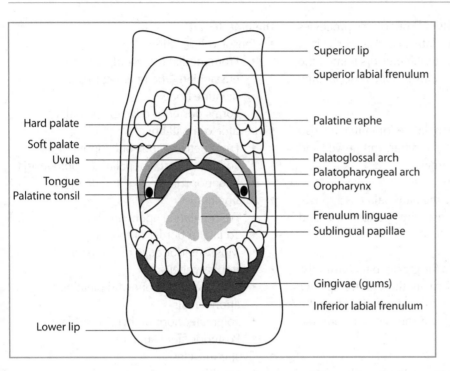

**Figure 5.15 The open mouth**

Superior lip
Superior labial frenulum
Palatine raphe
Hard palate
Soft palate
Uvula
Palatoglossal arch
Palatopharyngeal arch
Tongue
Oropharynx
Palatine tonsil
Frenulum linguae
Sublingual papillae
Gingivae (gums)
Inferior labial frenulum
Lower lip

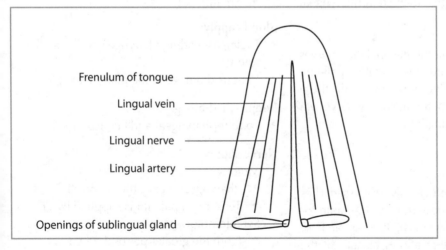

**Figure 5.16 Vasculature of the tongue**

Frenulum of tongue
Lingual vein
Lingual nerve
Lingual artery
Openings of sublingual gland

## Lymphatic drainage of the tongue

- The anterior two-thirds drain to the submandibular nodes (surgical level I)
- The posterior third drain to the deep cervical nodes (surgical level II)

This knowledge is important in the diagnosis and investigation of cancers in this area, when the initial presentation may be of a metastatic node in the neck.

## Hard palate

The hard palate is the roof of the oral cavity and consists of two palatal processes of the maxilla anteriorly and the two horizontal processes of the palatine bone laterally. Anteriorly is a foramen just posterior to the incisors named the incisive foramen. This transmits the nasopalatine nerve.

The greater and lesser palatine foramina are also seen, more posteriorly, and transmit nerves and vessels of the same names.

The mucosa overlying the hard palate is strongly adherent to the underlying periosteum and bone, which aids mastication.

**The blood supply** is via the greater palatine artery, which enters the oral cavity through the greater palatine foramen, traverses the soft tissues of the hard palate and exits via the incisive foramen into the nose.

**The lymphatic drainage** is to the retropharyngeal nodes.

**The nerve supply** is via the nasopalatine nerves (incisive foramen) and the greater palatine nerves (greater palatine foramina). All these nerves are from CN Vb, the maxillary nerve, via the pterygopalatine ganglion.

## Soft palate

The soft palate, as previously discussed, lies in the oropharynx (posterior to the anterior faucal pillar – palatoglossus). It is an arch of interlinking muscles that allows closure of the nasopharynx during swallowing and also pulls on the eustachian tube opening (torus tubaris) to open it when swallowing. This is one method of action that you can employ when trying to clear your ears – pinch your nose and swallow.

It is made of paired muscles that meet in the midline at an aponeurosis.

**The muscles** are:
- Tensor veli palatini:
  - From medial pterygoid plate and eustachian tube opening to the palatine bone
  - Forms posterior edge of soft palate
- Levator veli palatini:
  - From petrous apex of temporal bone
  - To nasal surface of palatine aponeurosis
  - Superior surface of soft palate
- Palatoglossus:
  - From palatine aponeurosis
  - To lateral border of tongue
  - Most anterior edge of soft palate
- Palatopharyngeus:
  - From palatine bone and palatine aponeurosis
  - To greater horn of thyroid cartilage
  - Posterior faucal pillar
- Uvular muscles:
  - Small!

**Blood supply:**
- Facial, ascending pharyngeal and maxillary artery
- Venous drainage to the pharyngeal plexus

**Lymphatic drainage:**
- To retropharyngeal and cervical nodes

**Nerve supply:**
- Motor:
  - Pharyngeal plexus (IX, X and XI)
  - Tensor veli palatini is supplied by Vc
- Secretomotor:
  - From the greater petrosal nerve (originally a branch of the facial in the middle ear, it picks up sympathetic fibres from the internal carotid artery plexus)
- Sensory:
  - Taste – greater petrosal nerve
  - Touch – lesser palatine nerve (Vb)

The ducts of the parotid and submandibular glands are dealt with later.

## The temporomandibular joint

The temporomandibular joint (TMJ) is the synovial joint of the mandible. It is so called because it articulates the mandible with the overlying temporal bone.

The important feature of the TMJ is the presence of an articular disc in the synovial joint – very unusual. This divides the joint into two parts:

- The lower part (articular disc and mandible) is concerned with **rotational** movements of the mandible, which is the first part of the mouth opening. There is no movement of the mandible with respect to the temporal bone
- The upper part (articular disc and temporal bone) is concerned with **translational** movements. This is when the jaw opens wide; the jaw glides forward with respect to the temporal bone. You can feel this on yourself by placing a finger on your own TMJ and slowly opening your mouth. Initially there is no movement of the TMJ, but at a certain point you will feel the condylar process move forwards

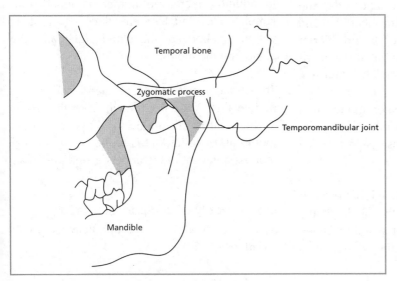

Figure 5.17 The temporo-mandibular joint (TMJ)

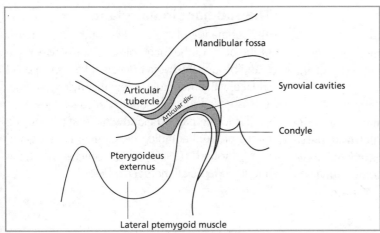

Figure 5.18 Relations of the TMJ

## 1.2.4 The salivary glands

There are three paired large salivary glands and hundreds of small salivary glands that open into the oral cavity.

The large salivary glands are:
- The parotid gland
- The submandibular gland
- The sublingual gland

### The parotid gland

The largest of the salivary glands, this overlies the ramus of the mandible on either side, and wraps around it medially to form superficial and deep lobes. It lies mainly anterior and inferior to the external auditory meatus but also extends posteriorly to the area behind the lobe of the ear.

Its bulk fills in the space between the external auditory meatus and the mandible. If someone has a parotidectomy, this mass is lost and a sulcus appears.

The parotid gland is variably sized, but extends from the zygomatic arch to the angle of the mandible. It can be thought of as a three-sided pyramid with the apex pointing down. It is covered by tough parotid fascia.

#### Function of the parotid gland

The parotid gland is made up almost entirely of serous acini which produce about 25% of the daily saliva.

Stimulation of the gland is mainly via the parasympathetics of the **lesser petrosal nerve** which is a branch of the glossopharyngeal nerve (IX). Stimulation produces a watery, amylase-rich saliva (sympathetic stimulation produces a thicker glycoprotein-rich saliva).

Secretion of saliva is part of the digestion process. Food boluses are coated in saliva in the oral cavity which starts to break down starches. In addition it aids in protection of the teeth.

#### Structures within the parotid gland

Three important structures traverse the gland: from lateral to medial they are the facial nerve (VII), the retromandibular vein (as it drains into the internal jugular vein) and the external carotid artery.

In addition there are numerous intraparotid lymph nodes and Stensen's duct, which starts within the body of the gland and drains the gland into the mouth.

The surface anatomy of Stensen's duct is the middle third of a line drawn from the tragus to the philtrum (Figure 5.20). It opens into the mouth at a papilla that is found on the buccal mucosa adjacent to the upper second premolar.

#### Blood supply of the parotid gland
- From the maxillary and superficial temporal arteries

### The submandibular gland

The submandibular gland lies partly under cover of the body of the mandible and sits between the mandible and the hyoid bone. It indents the medial surface of the mandible below the mylohyoid line. This is called the submandibular fossa. However, similar to the parotid gland wrapping around the ramus of the mandible, the submandibular gland wraps around the mylohyoid, which separates it into its superficial and deep lobes.

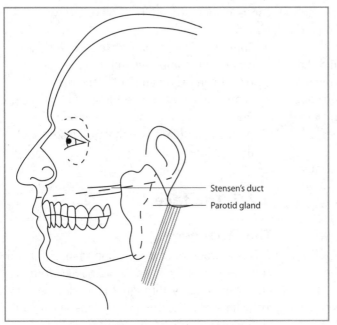

**Figure 5.19 Stensen's duct**

Stensen's duct
Parotid gland

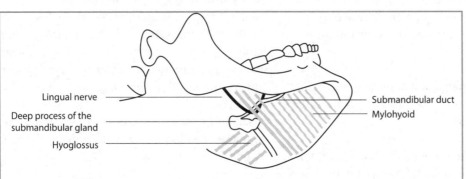

**Figure 5.20
The subman-
dibular gland**

Lingual nerve

Deep process of the
submandibular gland

Hyoglossus

Submandibular duct
Mylohyoid

The gland produces approx 70% of the daily saliva. It has both serous and mucinous acini, but the serous predominate.

**The superficial part of the gland** lies in the digastric triangle. It is separated posteriorly from the parotid gland by the stylomandibular ligament. Anteriorly lies the anterior belly of the digastric and, posteriorly, the posterior belly of the digastric. Medially lie the mylohyoid, the mylohyoid nerves and vessels, hyoglossus, and the lingual and hypoglossal nerves.

Laterally lies the mandible as already mentioned. It is also covered by the deep investing layer of cervical facia, platysma and skin.

**The deep part of the gland** extends forwards between the mylohyoid below and the hyoglossus and styloglossus above.

**Wharton's duct** runs in the plane of the deep lobe anteriorly under the mucous membrane of the floor of the mouth. It opens into the anterior floor of the mouth just lateral to the frenulum of the tongue at a small papilla.

As it is much longer and thinner than Stensen's duct, calculi are much more likely to form here.

**Important structures surrounding the gland** that need to be taken into consideration when contemplating excision include the facial artery and vein, the marginal mandibular nerve, and, deep to the gland, the lingual and the hypoglossal nerves.

The marginal mandibular nerve of the facial nerve (VII) runs on the deep surface of the platysma. It is variable in the distance where it drops below the body of the mandible, so to avoid injury to this nerve the following steps are taken:

- The incision is made 3–4 cm below the inferior margin of the mandible
- The platysma is incised at this low point
- The capsule of the gland is entered at its lowest point (for benign disease only – malignancy warrants an extracapsular excision)

In this way the marginal mandibular nerve does not even need to be found and can be safely retracted superiorly.

The lingual nerve is a branch of the mandibular nerve (Vc) arising in the infratemporal fossa. It is important in the anatomy of the submandibular gland because it is found intimately associated with Wharton's duct and gives the parasympathetic supply to the gland. As it runs anteriorly it first lies lateral, then inferior, then medial to Wharton's duct (Figure 5.21).

### The sublingual gland

The sublingual gland is the smallest of the three paired salivary glands. It lies beneath the mucous membrane of the floor of the mouth, either side of the midline. It contains serous and mucinous acini, the mucinous predominating.

These glands should be noted for two main reasons:

- Tumours of these glands are almost always malignant (compared with tumours of the parotid and submandibular glands)
- A ranula is a blocked sublingual gland (mucocele) in the floor of the mouth (a plunging ranula is one that prolapses through the mylohyoid)

## 1.2.5 The face

### The facial nerve

This is a structure of utmost importance in head and neck surgery because it passes from its brainstem origins through the middle cranial fossa (important for neurosurgeons and neuro-otologists), through the temporal bone and middle-ear cleft (important for otologists), and finally exits the skull and passes through the parotid gland to supply the muscles of facial expression (important for head and neck cancer surgery and facial plastic surgeons).

It is mainly a motor nerve but has a small sensory component within the external auditory canal.

### The course of the facial nerve

It arises from the facial nucleus (motor) and nervus intermedius (sensory) in the pons.

It enters the petrous part of the temporal bone through the internal auditory meatus. Once there it enters the facial, or fallopian, canal. It runs laterally above the vestibule to the medial wall of the middle ear.

Here it expands to form the **geniculate ganglion** and the first genu, or turn. Turning posteriorly, it passes over the promontory to the second genu which is positioned posterosuperiorly to the oval window and anteroinferiorly to the lateral semicircular canal.

At the second genu it turns inferiorly to pass behind the mastoid antrum, behind the pyramid (origin of stapedius) and through the mastoid to exit at the stylomastoid foramen.

It runs anteriorly and slightly inferiorly to enter the parotid gland, where it divides into its terminal branches.

## Branches of the facial nerve

| Branches | Type of nerve | Structure supplied |
|---|---|---|
| **First genu** | | |
| Greater petrosal | Parasympathetic | Lacrimal, nasal, palatine, pharyngeal glands |
| **Second genu** | | |
| No branches | | |
| **Descending portion** (through mastoid) | | |
| Unnamed nerve | Sensory | External auditory canal |
| Chorda tympani | Taste and parasympathetic | Taste anterior two-thirds of tongue |
| | | Parasympathetic to submandibular and sublingual glands |
| Nerve to stapedius | Motor | Stapedius muscle |
| **External branches (all motor):** | | |
| Posterior auricular | | Occipitofrontalis |
| Nerve to posterior belly of digastric | | Posterior belly of digastric |
| Nerve to stylohyoid | | Stylohyoid |
| Temporal | | Occipitofrontalis, orbicularis oculi |
| Zygomatic | | Orbicularis oculi |
| Buccal | | Buccinator, nasalis, levator labii superioris |
| Mandibular | | Mentalis, risorius |
| Cervical | | Platysma |

This table is not comprehensive. All muscles of facial expression are supplied by the facial nerve.

CHAPTER 5

## The muscles of facial expression (Figure 5.21)

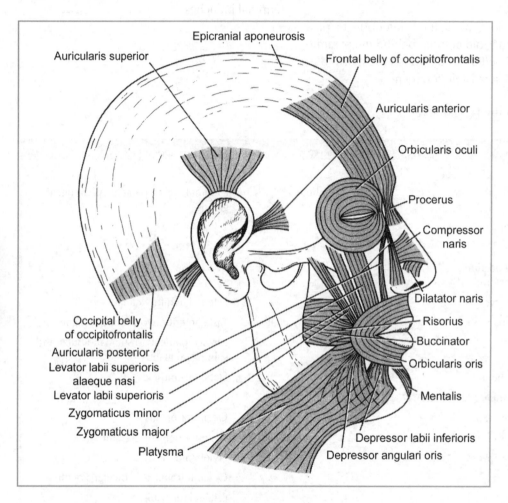

**Figure 5.21 The muscles of facial expression**

## Nerve supply to the muscles of facial expression

The motor supply to the muscles of the face is via the following branches of the facial nerve:

- Temporal
- Zygomatic
- Buccal
- Marginal mandibular
- Cervical

These muscles are derived from the mesoderm of the second pharyngeal arch and are members of the panniculus carnosus.

## Sensory supply of the face

The trigeminal nerve supplies the sensation to the face (Figure 5.22).

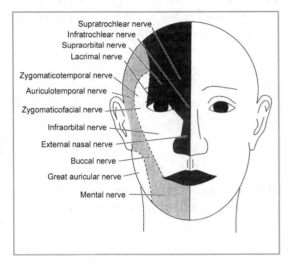

**Supratrochlear nerve**
**Infratrochlear nerve**
**Supraorbital nerve**
**Lacrimal nerve**
**Zygomaticotemporal nerve**
**Auriculotemporal nerve**
**Zygomaticofacial nerve**
**Infraorbital nerve**
**External nasal nerve**
**Buccal nerve**
**Great auricular nerve**
**Mental nerve**

**Figure 5.22 Sensory supply of the face**

| Divisions of the trigeminal nerve |
| --- |
| **Ophthalmic** |
| • Lacrimal |
| • Supraorbital |
| • Supratrochlear |
| • Infratrochlear |
| • External nasal |
| **Maxillary** |
| • Zygomaticotemporal |
| • Zygomaticofacial |
| • Infraorbital |
| **Mandibular** |
| • Auriculotemporal |
| • Buccal |
| • Mental |

## 1.2.6 The orbit and eyeball

The orbit is the space in which the eye sits. It is a pyramidal cavity with its apex situated posteromedially.

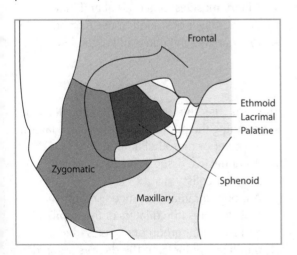

**Frontal**
**Ethmoid**
**Lacrimal**
**Palatine**
**Zygomatic**
**Sphenoid**
**Maxillary**

**Figure 5.23 The orbital bones**

The bony walls of the orbit are:
* **Roof:** the frontal bone
* **Lateral:** the zygoma and the greater wing of the sphenoid
* **Floor:** maxilla and the greater wing of the sphenoid
* **Medial:** maxilla, lacrimal, ethmoid and sphenoid bones

The orbits relations are:
* **Superiorly:** the frontal sinus and the anterior cranial fossa
* **Medially:** the ethmoid sinus air cells and the nasal cavity
* **Laterally:** the infratemporal fossa and skin
* **Inferiorly:** maxillary sinus
* **Posteriorly:** the middle cranial fossa

**CHAPTER 5**

> **Contents of the orbit**
>
> | Extraocular muscles | Blood vessels |
> |---|---|
> | Eyeball | Lymphatics |
> | Cranial nerves | Fat |
> | (II, III, IV, Va, Vb, VI) | |
>
> **Extraocular muscles**
>
> | Muscle | Nerve supply |
> |---|---|
> | Lateral rectus | Abducens (VI) |
> | Superior oblique | Trochlear (IV) |
>
> Reminder: the mnemonic LR6SO4
>
> | Medial rectus | |
> |---|---|
> | Inferior rectus | Oculomotor (III) |
> | Superior rectus | |
> | Inferior oblique | |

The eyeball has an incomplete fascial covering, the **fascia bulbi**, which facilitates movements of the eyeball. Within each eyelid, the **orbital septum** is thickened to form a **tarsal plate**, which is perforated by the **palpebral fissure**. The **lacrimal gland** is located at the superolateral angle of the orbit, its duct draining into the **conjunctival sac**. The **nasolacrimal canal** drains the **lacrimal punctum**, at the medial end of the lower lid, into the inferior meatus of the nose.

## The eyeball

The eyeball is about 2.5 cm in diameter and consists of:

- Anterior segment: transparent, prominent, anterior sixth of the sphere
- Posterior segment: opaque, posterior five-sixths of the sphere

The main structural features of the eye are the fibrous outer coat, vascular coat and neural coat. The contents of the eyeball are the lens, aqueous humour and vitreous body.

## Fibrous outer coat

The eyeball is encased in a fibrous outer coat with a transparent anterior cornea and opaque posterior sclera maintaining the shape of the eyeball, and receiving the insertion of the extraocular muscles.

## Vascular coat

The vascular coat is made up of the choroid, ciliary body and iris.

### Choroid

This is a thin vascular membrane lining the sclera, connected to the iris by the ciliary body.

### Ciliary body

This is made up of the ciliary ring, 60–80 ciliary processes and the ciliary muscles:

- **Ciliary ring:** a fibrous ring continuous with the choroid
- **Ciliary processes:** radiating from iris to ciliary ring and connected posteriorly to the suspensory ligament of the lens
- **Ciliary muscles:** outer radial and inner circular layer of smooth muscle responsible for changing the convexity of the lens

### Iris

The iris is the coloured contractile disc surrounding the pupil. It consists of four layers:

- An anterior mesothelial lining
- A connective tissue stroma containing pigment cells
- A group of radially arranged smooth muscle fibres (the dilators of the pupil) and a circular group of muscles (the pupillary sphincters). The dilators are under sympathetic control, the constrictors under parasympathetic control

- A posterior layer of pigmented cells continuous with the ciliary body

- A layer of ganglion cells whose axons form the superficial layer of optic nerve fibres

## Neural coat

This layer consists of the retina which is formed by an outer pigmented and an inner neural layer. The retina lies between the choroid and the hyaloid membrane of the vitreous, and has several features:

- **The ora serrata** is the anterior irregular edge
- **The optic disc** is the place on the retina where the nerve fibres on its surface collect to form the optic nerve. It is the blind spot
- **The macula lutea** is the site of central vision just lateral to the optic disc

The retina has:

- An inner receptor cell layer of rods and cones
- An intermediate layer of bipolar neurones

## The contents of the eyeball

Within the eyeball are the lens, aqueous humour and vitreous body:

- **The lens:** this is a biconvex laminated transparent disc placed between the vitreous and the aqueous humour just behind the iris. It functions to focus the image onto the retina by movements effected by the ciliary muscles
- **The aqueous humour:** this is a filtrate of plasma secreted by the vessels of the iris and ciliary body into the posterior chamber of the eye. From here it passes through the pupillary aperture into the anterior chamber and is absorbed into the ciliary veins by way of the sinus venosus sclerae (canal of Schlemm)

**CHAPTER 5**

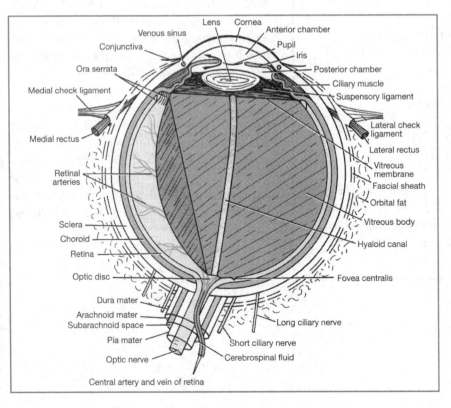

**Figure 5.24 The eye**

- **The vitreous body:** this is a thin transparent jelly encased in the delicate hyaline membrane. The vitreous body occupies the posterior 80% of the eyeball. The anterior part of the hyaline membrane is attached to the ciliary processes and gives rise to the suspensory ligament of the lens, which retains the lens in position and helps to change its convexity when the ciliary muscles contract

## Foramina of the orbit

There are three main foramina: the superior and inferior orbital fissures, and the optic canal; you should know the contents.

> **Contents of the orbital foramina**
> **Optic canal:**
> - Optic nerve (II)
> - Three layers of meninges
> - Cerebrospinal fluid
> - Ophthalmic artery
> - Central retinal vein
>
> **Superior orbital fissure:**
> - Oculomotor nerve (III)
> - Trochlear nerve (IV)
> - Abducens nerve (VI)
> - Lacrimal ⎫ nerves (all from
> - Frontal ⎬ ophthalmic branch
> - Nasociliary ⎭ of trigeminal [Va])
> - Superior and inferior ophthalmic veins
>
> **Inferior orbital fissure:**
> - Maxillary nerve (Vb)

## Anatomy of the light reflex

### Anatomy of the consensual pupillary light reflex

Some fibres of the optic tract synapse in the superior colliculus in the midbrain. These nuclei (bilaterally) synapse with cell bodies in the Edinger–Westphal nuclei on both sides. These in turn stimulate the ciliary ganglion and the sphincter pupillae bilaterally. Thus, a light shone in one eye will cause bilateral contraction of the pupils. If there is no effect on the contralateral pupil, one can determine the level of the intracranial lesion.

### Anatomy of the sympathetic pupillary pathway

Sympathetic innervation of the eye descends from the hypothalamus through the spinal cord via the anterior roots of C8 and T1 to the superior cervical ganglion. Postganglionic fibres ascend on the wall of the internal carotid artery to the ciliary ganglion, and thence to the eye and cranial nerves III, IV, V and VI.

This means that, if the sympathetic supply is disrupted, typically by an apical lung cancer, this affects pupillary dilatation (giving a small pupil – **miosis**), levator palpebrae superioris action (leading to a drooped eyelid – **ptosis**) and the vasoconstrictor fibres to the orbit, eye and face (leading to a lack of sweating – **anhidrosis**). This is classic Horner's triad.

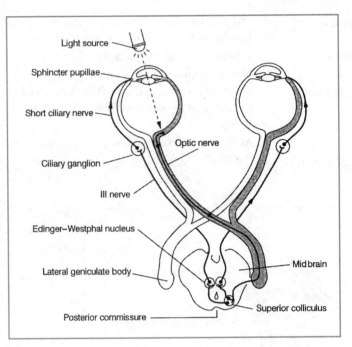

**Figure 5.25 Anatomy of the light reflex**

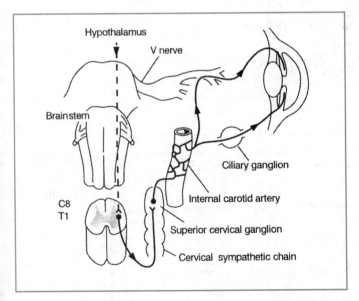

**Figure 5.26 Anatomy of the sympathetic light reflex**

CHAPTER 5

## 1.3 Anatomy of the neck

### 1.3.1 The anterior triangle

The neck is divided into the anterior and posterior triangles by the sternomastoid muscle.

**Sternomastoid muscle**

This is enclosed in the deep investing layer of cervical fascia:

- **Origin:** the clavicular and manubrial heads
- **Insertion:** the tip of the mastoid and the superior nuchal line of the occipital bone
- **Nerve supply:** the spinal part of the accessory nerve, ie C2 and C3 fibres from the cervical plexus (proprioceptive fibres only)
- **Action:** these rotate the head and protract the head when acting together

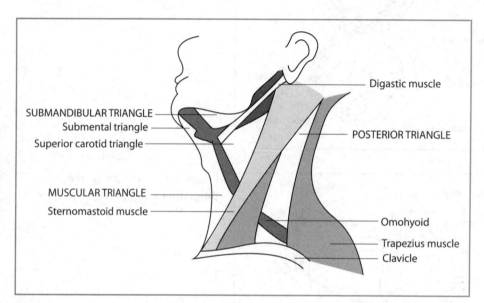

Figure 5.27
The triangles
of the neck

SUBMANDIBULAR TRIANGLE

Submental triangle

Superior carotid triangle

MUSCULAR TRIANGLE

Sternomastoid muscle

Digastic muscle

POSTERIOR TRIANGLE

Omohyoid

Trapezius muscle

Clavicle

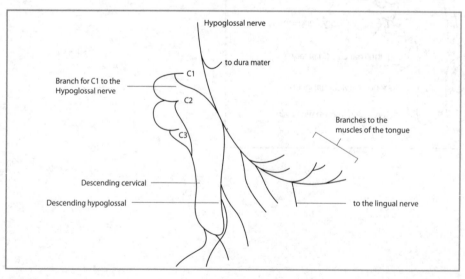

Figure 5.27a
The ansa
cervicalis

Hypoglossal nerve

to dura mater

Branch for C1 to the
Hypoglossal nerve

C1

C2

C3

Branches to the
muscles of the tongue

Descending cervical

Descending hypoglossal

to the lingual nerve

## Suprahyoid muscles

|  | Origin | Insertion | Nerve supply | Action |
|---|---|---|---|---|
| Digastric | Digastric notch on the mastoid process. It has an intermediate tendon attached to the lesser horn of the hyoid by a fascial sling, giving it anterior and posterior bellies | Digastric notch on the inner surface of the mandible | Facial nerve supplies anterior belly Nerve to mylohyoid supplies posterior belly | Depresses and retracts the chin and assists the lateral pterygoid in opening the mouth |
| Stylohyoid | Back of the styloid process | Greater horn of the hyoid | Facial nerve | Retracts and elevates the hyoid bone when swallowing |
| Geniohyoid | Inferior meatal spine | Upper border of the body of the hyoid | Branch from the hypoglossal nerve carrying C1 fibres only | Elevates the hyoid in swallowing |
| Mylohyoid | Mylohyoid line on the inferior surface of the mandible | Anteriorly it forms a midline raphe and posteriorly the body of the hyoid | Nerve to mylohyoid from the mandibular nerve | Supports the tongue and elevates the tongue and hyoid |

## Infrahyoid (strap) muscles

|  | Origin | Insertion | Nerve supply | Action |
|---|---|---|---|---|
| Sternohyoid | Inferior border of the hyoid | Back of the sternoclavicular joint | Branch from the ansa cervicalis (C1, C2, C3) | The strap muscles depress the larynx and prevent ascent of the hyoid against the digastric |
| Omohyoid | Inferior border of the hyoid | Transverse scapular ligament and the upper border of the scapula Bound along its length to the clavicle by a fascial sling, thus giving it a superior and inferior belly | Ansa cervicalis | |
| Thyrohyoid | Greater horn of the hyoid | Oblique line of the thyroid cartilage | C1 fibres from the hypoglossal nerve | |
| Sternothyroid | Posterior surface of the manubrium | Oblique line of the thyroid cartilage | Ansa cervicalis | |

**CHAPTER 5**

**Boundaries of the anterior triangle**
- **Medial:** the midline
- **Lateral:** the anterior border of sternomastoid
- **Superior:** the lower border of the mandible
- **Roof:** the investing fascia
- **Floor:** the prevertebral fascia

**Contents of the anterior triangle of the neck**
**Submental triangle**
- Submental lymph nodes
- Anterior jugular vein

**Carotid triangle** (note that all are contents of the carotid sheath)
- Common carotid artery
- Internal carotid artery
- External carotid artery and its branches
- Internal jugular vein and its tributaries
- Hypoglossal nerve and its descending branch
- Internal and external laryngeal nerves
- Deep cervical lymph nodes
- Accessory nerve
- Vagus nerve
- Ansa cervicalis

**Digastric (submandibular) triangle**
- Submandibular salivary gland
- Facial artery
- Facial vein
- Submandibular lymph nodes
- Hypoglossal nerve
- Hypoglossus muscle
- Nerve and vessels to mylohyoid
- Carotid sheath (see Carotid triangle above)
- Stylopharyngeus
- Glossopharyngeal nerve
- Parotid gland

**Muscular triangle**
- Sternohyoid muscle
- Sternothyroid muscle
- Structures underlying these muscles: thyroid gland, larynx, trachea, oesophagus

## The ansa cervicalis

The ansa cervicalis is a nerve loop that is embedded in the anterior wall of the internal jugular vein. Its anterior loop is from the nerve root of C1, which hitches a ride on the hypoglossal nerve (XII). When it branches off again, as the descendens hypoglossi, it runs inferiorly, giving off muscle branches.

The posterior loop originates from the nerve roots of C2 and C3. These come together as the descendens cervicalis and meet the descendens hypoglossi inferiorly.

In essence, the nerve branches given off by the ansa supplies all the strap muscles in the anterior neck except thyrohyoid.

## The thyroid gland

The thyroid and parathyroid glands are covered in depth in Chapter 4, Endocrine Surgery.

However, in brief, a normal thyroid gland is situated in the anterior triangle of the neck. It is an endocrine gland and lies on the anterior surface and around the larynx and trachea. Posteriorly, the thyroid lobes reach the carotid sheaths and the oesophagus.

It consists of two pyramid-shaped lobes connected by an isthmus that overlies the third and fourth tracheal rings. The size of the thyroid and the isthmus are highly variable but the weight will be between 18 and 60 g.

The superior and inferior parathyroid glands lie on the posterior surface of the two thyroid lobes. There are usually between four and six parathyroid glands.

## The larynx

The larynx in the adult is found between C3 and C6. It neonates it is situated at the base of the tongue (C2) to allow simultaneous feeding and respiration. The larynx drops into its adult position as the child grows. It connects the hypopharynx with the trachea. It extends from the tip of the epiglottis to the inferior border of the cricoid. It is divided into the supraglottis, glottis and subglottis.

Another important difference between the child and the adult larynx is that the narrowest point of the airway in a child is the subglottic region whereas in an adult it is the glottis (vocal folds). This is why adult endotracheal tubes have cuffs and those for children do not.

### Functions of the larynx

The larynx has three main functions:
* To protect the lower airway
* Valsalva's manoeuvre
* Phonation

Phonation, commonly cited as the main purpose of the larynx by students, is only the third purpose on the list. The first, and by far the most important, is protection of the lower airway. It can do this in two main ways: first, the cough reflex is stimulated by any substance making its way into the subglottic region and stimulating the tracheal wall (recurrent laryngeal nerve). This causes the vocal folds to clamp shut, thereby stopping any further leakage into the trachea and subsequently allows Valsalva's manoeuvre to occur.

The intrathoracic pressure builds dramatically and, at a certain point, the vocal folds open quickly. The intrathoracic air is expelled forcibly, removing the material within the airway and protecting the lower respiratory tree.

Valsalva's manoeuvre is also useful because it helps splint the shoulder girdle. It is involuntary, as anyone will discover when trying to lift a heavy object. Just as you are about to lift, you breathe in and hold your breath. This 'fixes' the chest wall and allows greater leverage of the upper limbs and subsequently a much greater force is generated.

Examples of this splinting action are highlighted by both the weightlifter who presents to the doctor with a hoarse voice because he or she has strained so hard that he or she has caused a haemorrhage of a vocal fold, and the patient who has had a laryngectomy and therefore has no vocal folds, who is unable to 'fix' the shoulder girdle and is subsequently unable to pick up any heavy objects and complains of feeling weak.

## The cartilages of the larynx

The larynx is formed from nine cartilages. Three are unpaired and three are paired.

| Unpaired | Paired |
|---|---|
| Thyroid | Arytenoid |
| Cricoid | Corniculate |
| Epiglottis | Cuneiform |

The hyoid is connected to the larynx but is not a part of it.

## The joints of the larynx

- **Cricothyroid:** synovial. Allows movement in the anteroposterior axis, ie the front of the cricoids and thyroid can move towards or away from each other. This stretches or contracts the vocal folds and changes the pitch of the voice

- **Cricoarytenoid:** synovial. Allows gliding and rotator movements of the arytenoids. This opens and closes the vocal folds for breathing, Valsalva's manoeuvre and speech

## The ligaments and membranes of the larynx

- Thyrohyoid membrane
- Cricothyroid ligament (laryngotomy is made through this as an emergency airway)
- Cricotracheal ligament
- Quadrangular membrane

The **false vocal folds** (vestibular folds) are the lower border of the quadrangular membrane.

The **true vocal folds** extend from the vocal process of the arytenoids to the thyroid laminae.

Phonation is produced by the vocal folds being held together and blown apart by discrete jets of air.

## The muscles of the larynx

There are many muscles that have some action on the larynx. You do not need to know these in detail, but there are a few that it is important to know.

| Intrinsic muscles | Extrinsic muscles |
|---|---|
| **Cricothyroid** | Thyrohyoid |
| **Posterior cricoarytenoid** | Sternothyroid |
| Lateral cricoarytenoid | Omohyoid |
| **Transverse cricoarytenoid** | Inferior constrictor |
| Oblique cricoarytenoid | Digastric |
| **Vocalis** | Stylohyoid |
| **Thyroarytenoid** | Mylohyoid |
| | Geniohyoid |
| | Hyoglossus |

- PCA: this is the only muscle to open the vocal cords
- CT: lengthens vocal cords ($\uparrow$ pitch)
- V and TA: these muscles run parallel to each other just lateral to the vocal ligament and form the body of the vocal cords

With regard to the intrinsic muscles, motor supply to them all is from the recurrent laryngeal nerve, except for the cricothyroid which is supplied by the superior laryngeal nerve (external branch). These muscles either change the shape of the vocal folds or alter the size of the laryngeal inlet.

The extrinsic muscles of the larynx either elevate or depress the larynx. This is primarily to elevate the larynx during deglutition and allow food to pass laterally into the piriform fossae, then into the postcricoid space and the oesophagus.

Sensory supply to the larynx above the vocal folds is from the superior laryngeal nerve (internal branch). Below the vocal folds it is supplied by the recurrent laryngeal nerve.

### Blood supply and lymphatic drainage of the larynx

|  | Blood supply | Lymphatic drainage[*] |
|---|---|---|
| Above vocal folds | Superior laryngeal branch from STA | Upper group of deep cervical nodes of the superior thyroid artery |
| Below vocal folds | Inferior laryngeal branch of the inferior thyroid artery | Lower group of deep cervical nodes |

[*]Lymphatic drainage also occurs to the pretracheal and tracheobronchial nodes.

The vocal folds are the embryological meeting point of the fourth and sixth branchial arches. This is why the blood supply and nerve supply are different below and above the vocal folds. In addition, and of great importance in the treatment of laryngeal cancer, it also means that the lymphatic drainage here is poor. It is not unusual to see a patient with a T4 cancer of the larynx with no lymph node spread in the neck. It is extremely unusual to see the same situation in cases of oropharyngeal cancer, where the lymphatic drainage is very good and patients often present with a metastatic lymph node as a first sign.

## The pharynx and oesophagus

The pharynx is situated behind the nose and mouth and above the oesophagus and larynx. The junction of the oral cavity and the oropharynx is the palatoglossus muscle (anterior faucal pillar). The posterior choanae separate the nasal cavity from the nasopharynx. The oropharynx and nasopharynx are separated by the soft palate.

## The nasopharynx

The nasopharynx is the most cephalad part of the pharynx. It contains the eustachian tube orifices (torus tubarius) and the pharyngeal tonsils, otherwise known as the adenoids. It stretches from the skull base to the upper part of the soft palate. The recess behind the eustachian tube orifice and the posterior wall of the nasopharynx is known as the *fossa of Rosenmüller* (pharyngeal recess), and is an important landmark because it is the point at which most nasopharyngeal carcinomas arise.

CHAPTER 5

559

## Waldeyer's ring

The adenoids are part of a ring of lymphoid tissue that encircles the pharynx. It includes the pharyngeal tonsils (adenoids), tubal tonsils (around the eustachian tube), palatine tonsils and lingual tonsils (on the tongue base).

They produce IgA and are theorised to be the first line of defence against airborne pathogens.

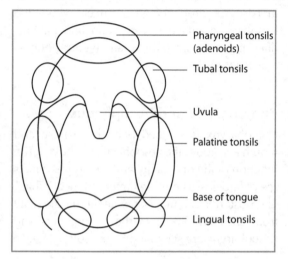

**Figure 5.28 Waldeyer's ring**

## The oropharynx

This extends from the underside of the soft palate to the level of the hyoid bone. It opens anteriorly into the oral cavity. The borders are:
- **Superiorly:** soft palate
- **Inferiorly:** hypopharynx (below level of hyoid)
- **Anteriorly:** palatoglossus (anterior faucal pillar), tongue base and vallecula
- **Laterally:** tonsil, tonsillar fossa, palato-pharyngeus (posterior faucal pillar), lateral pharyngeal walls
- **Posteriorly:** posterior pharyngeal wall

## The hypopharynx

This is the most caudal part of the pharynx. It connects the oropharynx to the start of the oesophagus and the larynx.

The hypopharynx divides around the larynx into the two pyriform sinuses which are connected posteriorly by the postcricoid region. This lies immediately superior to the opening of the oesophagus.

It contains the epiglottis and it runs up to the borders of the larynx, which are:
- **Posteriorly:** the arytenoids
- **Laterally:** the aryepiglottic folds
- **Anteriorly:** the petiole of the epiglottis

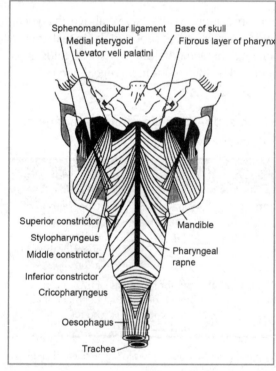

**Figure 5.29 The anatomy of the pharynx**

CHAPTER 5

**Figure 5.30a The anterolateral view of the larynx**

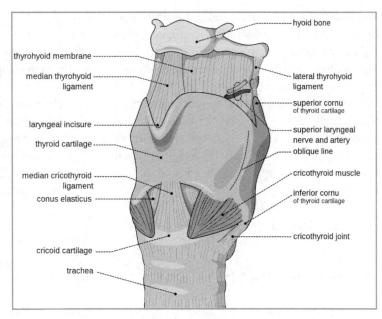

hyoid bone

thyrohyoid membrane

median thyrohyoid ligament

lateral thyrohyoid ligament

superior cornu of thyroid cartilage

superior laryngeal nerve and artery

laryngeal incisure

thyroid cartilage

oblique line

cricothyroid muscle

median cricothyroid ligament

conus elasticus

inferior cornu of thyroid cartilage

cricothyroid joint

cricoid cartilage

trachea

**Figure 5.30b The larynx viewed from above**

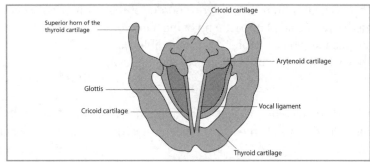

Cricoid cartilage

Superior horn of the thyroid cartilage

Arytenoid cartilage

Glottis

Cricoid cartilage

Vocal ligament

Thyroid cartilage

**Figure 5.30c The muscles of the larynx**

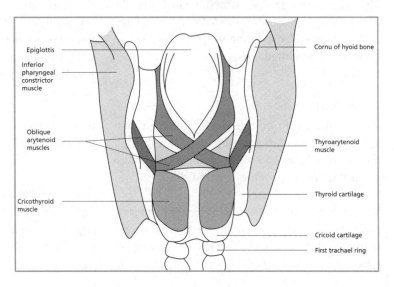

Epiglottis

Inferior pharyngeal constrictor muscle

Cornu of hyoid bone

Oblique arytenoid muscles

Thyroarytenoid muscle

Cricothyroid muscle

Thyroid cartilage

Cricoid cartilage

First trachael ring

The whole of the pharynx is surrounded by layers of muscle that are all striated, compared with the muscle of the oesophagus, which is smooth. The reason for this is that, during deglutition, respiration ceases until the food bolus is passed into the oesophagus and no longer represents a threat to the airway. To pass the bolus into the oesophagus as quickly as possible, the lining of the pharynx is striated muscle, which is much faster-acting than the smooth muscle of the oesophagus.

The muscle layers of the pharynx are as follows.

### External circular layer

#### Superior constrictor
This originates from the posterior border of the medial pterygoid plate to the tip of the hamulus, pterygomandibular raphe and mandible just above the attachment of the pterygomandibular raphe.

It inserts into the pharyngeal raphe and tubercle and extends down to the level of the vocal folds.

The gap between the superior and middle constrictors is plugged by the back of the tongue and is traversed by stylopharyngeus, and glosso-pharyngeal and lingual nerves.

#### Middle constrictor
This originates from the angle between the stylohyoid ligament and the greater horn of the hyoid. It inserts into the midline raphe and extends to the level of the vocal folds.

The gap between middle and inferior constrictors is plugged by the thyrohyoid membrane, which is pierced by the internal laryngeal nerve and superior laryngeal vessels.

#### Inferior constrictor
This consists of two parts, thyropharyngeus and cricopharyngeus:
- **Thyropharyngeus** originates at the oblique line of the thyroid cartilage and the fibrous arch spanning the cricothyroid, and inserts on the pharyngeal raphe
- **Cricopharyngeus** forms a ring and extends from one end of the cricoid cartilage to the other; there is no pharyngeal raphe at this level (it is closed except in deglutition)

### Killian's dehiscence
This is a potentially weak area between thyropharyngeus and cricopharyngeus.

A diverticulum of mucosa may protrude through this dehiscence to produce a pharyngeal pouch. This is a pulsion diverticulum.

### Inner longitudinal layer

#### Palatopharyngeus
This is internal to the superior constrictor within the pharynx. It arises from the anterior head on the horizontal plate of the palatine bone and the posterior head on the upper surface of the palatine aponeurosis. It passes downwards to pass lateral and behind the tonsil and inserts into the posterior part of the thyroid lamina and its horns.

It acts to elevate the larynx and pharynx and to depress the soft palate.

#### Salpingopharyngeus
This arises from the lower part of the cartilaginous part of the auditory tube and runs downwards to blend with palatopharyngeus.

## Stylopharyngeus

This arises from the styloid process and after passing medial to the middle constrictor it inserts on the posterior border of the thyroid lamina.

## Arterial supply to the pharynx

The pharynx receives branches from the following arteries:

- Ascending pharyngeal
- Ascending palatine
- Lingual
- Tonsillar
- Greater palatine
- Artery of the pterygoid canal
- Superior and inferior laryngeal

## Venous drainage of the pharynx

This is chiefly via the pharyngeal venous plexus, which drains to the pterygoid venous plexus or directly to the internal jugular vein. The lower part drains to the inferior thyroid veins.

## Lymphatic drainage of the pharynx

Lymph drains to the upper and lower deep cervical nodes, either directly or through the retropharyngeal nodes.

## Nerve supply of the pharynx

### Motor nerve supply of the pharynx

The motor supply of the pharynx is complex. The pharyngeal plexus provides motor supply to all the pharyngeal musculature except stylopharyngeus, which is supplied by the glossopharyngeal nerve. The pharyngeal plexus is formed from the union of pharyngeal branches of the vagus, glossopharyngeal nerve and cervical sympathetic chain.

In addition, cricopharyngeus may be supplied by the recurrent or external laryngeal nerves.

### Sensory nerve supply of the pharynx

The sensory supply of the nasopharynx is provided by the pharyngeal branch of the pterygopalatine ganglion. The oropharynx is largely supplied by the glossopharyngeal nerve and the internal laryngeal nerve, which supplies the valleculae. The remaining pharyngeal mucosa is innervated by the internal and recurrent pharyngeal nerves.

The pharynx is attached via the superior constrictor to the skull base at the pharyngeal tubercle in the midline. The gap between the skull base and the superior constrictor as it hangs down like a tent is the pharygobasilar fascia, which is dense and fibrous.

## The oesophagus

The oesophagus is a muscular tube approximately 25 cm long extending from the pharynx to the stomach. It starts posterior to the cricoid cartilage at the level of the sixth cervical vertebra. This is where cricopharyngeus is situated. It is a circular muscle and is closed at rest. The oesophagus begins in the midline but tends to the left within the neck. Once in the thorax it becomes more left-sided. The intrathoracic description of the oesophagus is in Chapter 1 Abdominal Surgery.

## Blood supply of the oesophagus

In the neck the supply is from the inferior thyroid arteries. Venous drainage is into the inferior thyroid veins.

## Lymphatic drainage of the oesophagus

The deep cervical nodes.

## Nerve supply of the oesophagus

From the recurrent laryngeal nerves (X) and the sympathetic trunks.

CHAPTER 5

## The trachea

The total length of the trachea is 10 cm. It extends from the level of C6 in continuity with the larynx. It is made up of C-shaped hyaline cartilage rings, trachealis muscle posteriorly and a fibroelastic membrane.

### Blood supply of the trachea

- Inferior thyroid artery

---

**Relations of the trachea**

**Anteriorly**

- Inferior thyroid vein
- Anterior jugular venous arch
- Thyroid IMA artery
- Isthmus of the thyroid gland (second, third and fourth rings)

**Posteriorly**

- Oesophagus
- Recurrent laryngeal nerve (RLN)

**Laterally**

- Carotid sheath
- Thyroid lobes (down to the level of the sixth ring)

---

### Lymphatic drainage of the trachea

- Posteroinferior group of deep cervical nodes

### Nerve supply of the trachea

- Parasympathetic supply from the vagi and RLNs (supply pain sensation)
- Sympathetic supply from the upper ganglia of the sympathetic trunk (supplies smooth muscle and blood vessels)

## 1.3.2 The posterior triangle

Boundaries of the posterior triangle:

- **Anterior:** sternomastoid

- **Posterior:** trapezius
- **Base:** middle third of clavicle
- **Roof:** investing fascia
- **Floor:** prevertebral fascia overlying prevertebral muscles (splenius capitis, levator scapulae, scalenus, anterior, middle and posterior)

The three trunks of the brachial plexus, subclavian artery and cervical plexus lie deep to the prevertebral fascia.

---

**Contents of the posterior triangle**

Accessory nerve
Lymph nodes
Occipital artery
Inferior belly of omohyoid
External jugular vein
Transverse cervical and suprascapular vessels
Cutaneous branches of the cervical plexus:

- Lesser occipital (C2)
- Greater auricular (C2, C3)
- Transverse cervical (C2, C3)
- Suprascapular (C3, C4)

---

## Surface marking of the accessory nerve

It runs (roughly) from the junction of the proximal third and the lower two-thirds of the posterior border of sternomastoid to the junction of the proximal two-thirds and distal third of the anterior border of trapezius.

The nerve runs across the posterior triangle, where it lies on levator scapulae. The deep investing layer of cervical fascia and the pretracheal fascia merge here, so the nerve is in a very superficial position. Excision of neck masses in this area needs to performed carefully, with full awareness of the potential risks.

Note: the accessory nerve emerges from the posterior border of the sternomastoid approximately 1 cm below the point (Erb's point) where the great auricular nerve emerges.

> If you are ever asked to excise a subcutaneous neck lump in your SHO minor ops list – DO NOT DO IT! Instead refer the patient to an ENT surgeon for full assessment.
> If you excise an enlarged lymph node with metastatic disease you may seriously compromise a potentially curative neck en-bloc dissection by cutting across the planes and disturbing the lymphatic drainage.
> A much safer approach is to arrange for ultrasound-guided fine-needle aspiration cytology (FNAC) as a first-line investigation and then act on the results appropriately.

## Levels of the neck

Levels of the neck are not to be confused with triangles of the neck. The levels of the neck are a way of categorising the lymph node distribution of the neck. This becomes vital in the diagnosis and treatment of head and neck cancers.

A neck lump in level I may indicate an intraoral pathology, whereas a lymph node in level V may indicate a nasopharyngeal pathology. In the treatment of cancers, neck dissections are performed as part of the treatment of some cancers and are also categorised by the levels that are removed. A supraomohyoid neck dissection removes levels II and III (± I), and a modified radical neck dissection removes I–V.

There are surgical and radiological levels, but for the purposes of the surgical exam we shall stick to the surgical levels.

**Levels of lymph nodes in the neck**

| | |
|---|---|
| Level I | Submental and submandibular nodes |
| Level II | Upper jugular from skull base to hyoid |
| Level III | Middle jugular from the hyoid to the cricoid cartilage |
| Level IV | Lower jugular from the cricoid cartilage to the clavicle |
| Level V | Posterior triangle nodes |
| Level VI | Anterior compartment nodes from the hyoid bone to the suprasternal notch, bounded laterally by the medial border of the carotid sheath |
| Level VII | Nodes in the superior mediastinum |

If you look closely there are some features of note:

- First there is no room in these levels for parotid or retropharyngeal lymph nodes
- Second, levels I–IV and VI are in the anterior triangle. However, the lymph nodes are often situated **deep** to sternomastoid. Here, levels and triangles differ; the anterior triangle stops at the anterior border of sternomastoid whereas levels II–IV run deep to, and all the way to the posterior edge of, sternomastoid. Level V starts at the most lateral border of the muscle

**CHAPTER 5**

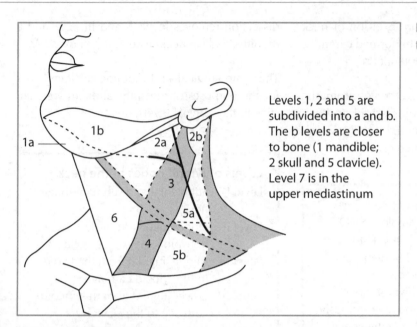

Levels 1, 2 and 5 are
subdivided into a and b.
The b levels are closer
to bone (1 mandible;
2 skull and 5 clavicle).
Level 7 is in the
upper mediastinum

**Figure 5.31 The levels of
the neck**

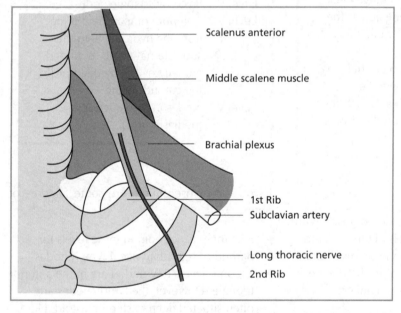

Scalenus anterior

Middle scalene muscle

Brachial plexus

1st Rib
Subclavian artery

Long thoracic nerve
2nd Rib

**Figure 5.32 The
relationship between
anterior scalene and the
subclavian artery**

This difference is important to realise. Lymph nodes hidden by sternomastoid are officially in neither anterior nor posterior triangles, but are described by their correct level.

## Thoracic inlet

The thoracic inlet, or the root of the neck, is the area of the neck immediately above the inlet into the thorax. It can be thought of, but not accurately described as, the area within and just above the circle formed by T1, the first ribs and the manubrium.

The first ribs are angled inferiorly so that the root of the neck lies at an oblique angle. The most posterior part is the T1 vertebra, but the most anterior part, the manubrium, is at the level of T3. Note that this is only just superior to the apex of the arch of the aorta, which is at the level of T4.

The structures that pass through the root of the neck from neck to thorax (or vice versa) are:

---

**Vasculature**
Subclavian artery (2)
Subclavian vein (2)
Thoracic duct (1)

**Viscera**
Trachea (1)
Oesophagus (1)
Pleura of the lung (2)
Sympathetic plexus (2)

**Nerves**
Vagus (2)
RLN (2)
Phrenic (2)

---

Subsequently, surgical procedures in the inferior part of the anterior neck are to be undertaken with caution because the great vessels are easily within reach and damaging them is potentially life-threatening.

The subclavian artery, subclavian vein, brachial plexus and scalene muscles are intimately related in the region of the lateral border of the thoracic inlet. It is important to understand this relationship. The subclavian vein runs anterior to scalenus anterior where it attaches to the first rib, the artery posterior. As well as the artery, the brachial plexus emerges through this space to descend into and supply the upper limb.

The subclavian artery is divided into three parts, according to where it is in relation to the anterior scalene muscle: first part medial, second part posterior and third part lateral to the muscle.

**CHAPTER 5**

---

**Branches of the first part of the subclavian**

| Name | Route |
|------|-------|
| Vertebral artery | Ascends between longus colli and scalenus anterior |
| | Passes in front of transverse process of C7 |
| | Ascends through foramina of C6–1 |
| | Passes posteriorly in through dura mater |
| | Enters the skull through foramen magnum |
| Thyrocervical trunk | Gives off three branches: inferior thyroid, superficial cervical and suprascapular arteries |
| Internal thoracic artery | Enters thorax behind first costal cartilage in front of pleura |

**Branches of the second part of the subclavian**

| | |
|------|-------|
| Costocervical trunk | Runs backwards above pleura to the neck of the first rib |
| | Gives off superior intercostals and deep cervical arteries |

There are no branches of the third part of the subclavian artery

---

## The thoracic duct

The duct begins within the abdomen at the upper end of the cysterna chyli. It enters the thorax through the aortic opening in the diaphragm and ascends, inclining to the left. At the root of the neck it is found on the left lateral border of the oesophagus until it reaches the transverse process of C7. Here it curves behind the carotid sheath and in front of the vertebral vessels. At the medial border of scalenus anterior it curves inferiorly to drain into the root of the brachio-cephalic vein. It may join a little more laterally (subclavian vein) or superiorly (internal jugular vein). This is important to know as the thoracic duct drains the foregut. Malignancy in the foregut may therefore present with an enlarged left supraclavicular lymph node (Virchow's or Trossier's sign).

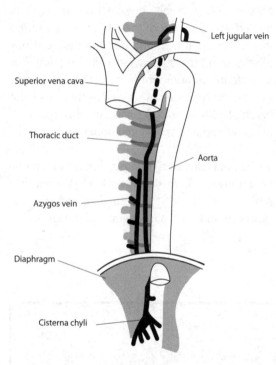

**Figure 5.33 The thoracic duct**

Labels: Left jugular vein, Superior vena cava, Thoracic duct, Aorta, Azygos vein, Diaphragm, Cisterna chyli

# Layers and spaces of the neck

## Fascial layers of the neck

### Deep investing layer of cervical fascia

- This extends from the base of the skull and lower border of the mandible to the spine of the scapula, lateral part of the clavicle and sternum
- It splits into two layers to form the parotid fascia and also forms the stylomandibular ligament

### Prevertebral fascia

- This lies in front of the prevertebral muscles and covers the muscles forming the floor of the posterior triangle
- The accessory nerve lies superficial to this fascia

## Pretracheal fascia

- This splits to enclose the thyroid gland and provides a slippery surface for the trachea to move on during swallowing
- It blends with the carotid sheath laterally

## Carotid sheath

- This surrounds the internal jugular vein, common carotid artery and vagus nerve
- It is loose areolar tissue that allows expansion of the internal jugular vein
- The surface marking of the carotid sheath in the neck is from the sternoclavicular joint to the greater cornu of the hyoid

## Potential spaces in the neck

> Infections in any of the following potential spaces can be life threatening and must be treated aggressively.

## Prevertebral space

- This is posterior to the prevertebral fascia overlying the prevertebral muscle
- Infection from the cervical vertebrae can lift up the fascia down to the level of T3 but cannot expand further without perforating the fascia

## Retropharyngeal space

- This is a potential space between the prevertebral space and the buccopharyngeal membrane that surrounds the outer wall of the pharynx
- The retropharyngeal space extends from the base of the skull to the diaphragm

- Infection here can pass into the posterior mediastinum
- Infection can be seen in children and may present with neck stiffness, pyrexia and stridor

## Parapharyngeal space

- This is the lateral extension of the retropharyngeal space and is bounded laterally by the pterygoid muscles and the parotid sheath
- Tonsillitis and quinsies (peritonsillar abscess) can lead to parapharyngeal abscesses

## Submandibular space

- This space is bounded by the investing fascia between the hyoid bone and mandible and the mucous membrane of the floor of the mouth
- The space contains the submandibular, mylohyoid and sublingual glands
- Infection in this space is termed 'Ludwig's angina' and can lead to respiratory distress

## 1.4 Management of the airway

## The larynx and the airway

### Laryngeal structures

The structures palpable in the anterior neck are the hyoid bone, thyroid cartilage and thyroid notch, and cricoid, descending in that order.

The thyroid notch is the superior end of the thyroid and is the most prominent part. It is commonly known as the Adam's apple and is more prominent in postpubertal males. It is a starting point to orient oneself with respect to the neck structures.

In a dire emergency a mini-tracheostomy can be inserted through the cricothyroid membrane. In the out-of-hospital scenario, this is the 'steak knife and biro' situation. In the elective situation this is to be avoided because the cricothyroid membrane is only just inferior to the vocal folds (deep to the thyroid cartilage) and the cricoid is the narrowest part of the adult airway. Traumatising it increases the risk of subglottic stenosis.

A tracheostomy, on the other hand, is placed through the second or third tracheal rings. This avoids possible damage to the subglottis within the cricoid.

## Emergency airway problems

### Stridor
'Bovine-like' inspiratory noise associated with laryngeal obstruction is more common in children.

### Management of stridor
- **Remove** false teeth and secretions

**In emergency situation:**
- Endotracheal (ET) tube
- Laryngotomy (cricothyroidotomy)
- Jet insufflation

**If there is time:**
- Laryngoscopy for removal of foreign body
- ET tube if intubation required for few days
- Tracheostomy for longer period of intubation

---

**Causes of stridor**

**In adults**
- **Extraluminal causes:**
  - Neurological (eg motor neurone disease)
  - Iatrogenic (eg thyroidectomy)
  - Trauma
- **Mural causes:**
  - Angioneurotic oedema
  - Granuloma
  - Malignancy
  - Laryngomalacia
- **Luminal causes:**
  - Tuberculosis (TB)
  - Foreign body

**In children**
- **Extraluminal causes:**
  - Trauma
  - Mediastinal tumours
  - Anomalous blood vessels
  - Vagal or recurrent laryngeal nerve paralysis
- **Mural causes**
  - Angioneurotic oedema
  - Laryngeal web
  - Subglottic stenosis
  - Laryngotracheobronchitis (croup)
  - Laryngeal papilloma or haemangioma
  - Acute laryngitis/acute epiglottitis
- **Luminal causes:**
  - Foreign body

CHAPTER 5

# Tracheostomy

## Indications for tracheostomy

**Relief of airway obstruction**

- Congenital (eg laryngeal cysts, subglottic stenosis, tracheo-oesophageal anomalies)
- Trauma to larynx and trachea
- Infection (eg acute epiglottitis, laryngotracheobronchitis)
- Tumour (eg tongue, larynx, pharynx, thyroid)
- Trauma (le Fort II and III fractures, haemorrhage)
- Bilateral vocal fold paralysis
- Foreign body
- Sleep apnoea syndrome

**Temporary or permanent protection of the tracheobronchial tree**

- Neurological diseases (eg myasthenia gravis, multiple sclerosis)
- Trauma (burns to the face and neck)
- Coma (eg drug overdose, head injury)
- Head and neck surgery (supraglottic laryngectomy, oropharyngeal resection)

**Treatment of respiratory insufficiency**

- Tracheostomy reduces upper airway dead space by 70%

**Chest injury (flail chest)**

**Pulmonary disease**

## Op box: Performing a tracheostomy

**Indications**
- See previous box

**Preop**
- General anaesthesia (GA) and intubation
- Local anaesthesia (LA; in emergency)

**Position**
- Head extended on a head ring; sandbag under shoulders

**Skin incision**
- Transverse incision midway between the cricoid cartilage and suprasternal notch

**Procedure**
- Separate strap muscles
- Divide thyroid isthmus
- Cut circular disc from second/third tracheal rings (injury of the first ring leads to subglottic stenosis)
- Vertical incision in children (do not remove cartilage because this can lead to tracheal collapse); stay sutures taped to the chest
- Aspirate trachea
- Insert tube and withdraw ETT
- Inflate tracheostomy tube cuff

**Closure**
- Skin edges closed
- Tapes tied to secure tube

**Postop**
- Nurse upright
- Regular suction
- Humidified $O_2$ with 5–7% $CO_2$ to prevent apnoea
- Chest radiograph to exclude pneumothorax if necessary

**CHAPTER 5**

## Complications of a surgical tracheostomy

### Early complications
- Asphyxia
- Aspiration
- Haemorrhage or haematoma
- Obstruction
- Subcutaneous emphysema
- Pneumothorax
- Pneumomediastinum
- Malpositioned tube
- Injury to cricoid cartilage

### Late complications
- Cellulitis
- Subglottic stenosis
- Vocal fold palsy
- Tracheocutaneous fistula
- Tracheo-oesophageal fistula
- Delayed haemorrhage
- Displacement of tube
- Atelectasis and pulmonary infection
- Tracheomalacia
- Dysphagia
- Difficult decannulation
- Tracheal stenosis

### Types of tracheostomy tubes

Tracheostomy tubes can be:
- Metal tubes, eg Negus, Chevalier–Jackson, Durham, Koenig
- Synthetic tubes, eg Portex, Shiley, Franklin, Great Ormond Street. Synthetic tubes may have a cuff for protection of the airway
- Speaking tubes

Both synthetic and metal tubes may have an inner tube to facilitate cleaning, and may be fenestrated (hole in the upper part of the shaft) to allow airflow through the larynx and thus speech.

## Acute epiglottitis

This is a bacterial infection of the throat characterised by progressive acute laryngitis that affects all the supraglottis, but predominantly the loose connective tissue of the epiglottis.

### Aetiology of acute epiglottitis
- *Haemophilus influenzae* type b (Hib) is usually the causative organism
- Staphylococci, β-haemolytic streptococci and pneumococci have been implicated, particularly in adults
- The incidence of acute epiglottitis in children has been declining, which may be due to Hib vaccine administration

### Clinical features of acute epiglottitis
- Usually occurs in children aged 2–7 years
- Initially the child complains of a sore throat which rapidly progresses to inspiratory stridor
- Pyrexia (temperature of 38–40°C)
- Child tends to lean forwards and drools

**Do NOT attempt to examine the throat of a child with acute epiglottitis because this may precipitate laryngospasm.**

### Management of acute epiglottitis
- The child's airway must be secured
- An experienced paediatric anaesthetist and otolaryngologist must be in attendance
- Child and parent are moved to an induction area with operating facilities adjacent
- Anaesthesia is induced by inhalation
- An endotracheal tube is passed and a cherry-red epiglottis will be seen

- Rigid bronchoscopy can be used to intubate if initial attempts at intubation fail
- Tracheostomy is rarely required
- Intravenous access, blood cultures and throat swabs are performed after the airway has been secured
- Patients respond quickly to intravenous antibiotics (eg chloramphenicol) and usually can be extubated after 24–48 hours
- Steroids may be of value before decannulation to reduce oedema

The incidence of acute epiglottitis in children has been declining, which is due to administration of Hib vaccine.

# The vasculature of the neck

## Middle meningeal artery

The middle meningeal artery is a branch of the first part of the maxillary artery (the three parts being named with regard to its relationship with the lateral pterygoid – posterior, within or anterior to the lateral pterygoid muscle).

It passes from the infratemporal fossa superiorly through the foramen spinosum within the greater wing of the sphenoid into the cranial cavity. It runs superiorly and anterolaterally on the inner surface of the temporal bone in its own groove.

It divides into anterior and posterior branches. The anterior branch curves posteriorly up to the anteroinferior angle of the parietal bone.

> As it passes superiorly on the parietal bone over the pterion it is at risk of damage after a blow to the head.

Damage to the artery can cause an extradural haemorrhage. A classic history is the young cricketer who is hit on the side of the head by a cricket ball. He has initial loss of consciousness for between a few seconds and a few minutes, but regains full consciousness and normal Glasgow Coma Scale (GCS) score. An hour later his GCS score slowly drops, at first becoming confused and incoherent and later becoming unconscious. Unless the bleed is identified and the haematoma evacuated via craniotomy, death may ensue.

## Carotid artery and jugular vein

The great vessels of the neck are intimately associated within the carotid sheath in the neck but their relationship changes as they pass through the neck. Superiorly, the common carotid artery (CCA) is medial to the internal jugular vein (IJV) but, as we move inferiorly down the neck, the IJV moves more anteriorly to the CCA.

Placement of a central venous catheter in the internal jugular vein is easier inferiorly in the neck because the IJV is more anteriorly placed.

### Central venous catheter placement

The patient is placed supine in a 15° head-down position to distend the neck veins and prevent air embolism. The head is turned to the contralateral side (usually left for a right-handed person) and the position of the IJV is identified by placing two fingers of the left hand on the CCA. The IJV will lie slightly anterior and lateral to this. An alternative insertion point in the neck is between the sternal and clavicular heads of the sternomastoid muscle. (See Critical Care, Book 1 for more detail.)

## 1.5 Imaging for the head and neck

It is vital to know your surface anatomy to avoid damage to structures lying just beneath the skin. However, bear in mind that many diseases change or distort the normal anatomy to such a degree that even detailed knowledge of the surface anatomy may be rendered useless.

Imaging helps to differentiate tissues, stage disease and elucidate anatomy. In the head and neck, you should be familiar with the use of common imaging modalities such as radiographs, ultrasonography, computed tomography (CT), magnetic resonance imaging (MRI), positron-emission tomography (PET) and angiography.

### Radiographs of the head and neck

These are used only in very specific situations. The most common is to identify inhaled or swallowed foreign bodies, which is most common in children. In addition, a chest radiograph is performed to ascertain the position of a central line or nasogastric tube placement.

### Ultrasonography

Ultrasonography of the head and neck is extremely useful and used very regularly. As ultrasound technology has improved, so the detail of the structures seen has improved. The higher-frequency ultrasound machines (20 MHz) can delineate individual nerves and are being used to identify nerves before some operations. Machines with such high frequencies can image only a very short distance under the skin and so are of limited help.

The more usual ultrasound machines are 10 MHz and are used to determine the nature of head and neck lumps. This is commonly combined with FNAC, which can give an accurate diagnosis approximately 90% of the time. As the procedure is quick, relatively painless, well tolerated and cheap, it has become the mainstay of primary investigation for head and neck masses.

You will not need to be able to decipher an ultrasound image, but will need to know when it is appropriate to request one.

### CT

CT can give a great deal of information about the deep structures of the head and neck. Within the cranial vault, mass effect lesions, hydrocephalus and haemorrhages are readily seen. In the face, a CT clearly delineates the sinus anatomy and is the investigation of choice in someone with chronic rhinosinusitis. In the neck, with regard to the thyroid or cervical lymphadenopathy, CT scans are used to investigate the extent of disease or to stage cancerous lesions. It is a very good imaging tool for looking at bone.

When interpreting CT scans it is important to know the following:

- Is the name and date of birth correct?
- The time of day that it was performed (4am suggests an emergency!)
- The plane of the image
- Whether contrast was used

The three planes are as follows.

| Aide-mémoire | |
|---|---|
| Axial | Head chopped off with an AXe |
| Coronal | Placing CROWN on your head |
| Sagittal | SAGITER in Latin is arrow. Imagine the direction of being shot with an arrow |

CHAPTER 5

Axial is the most commonly used plane in the head and neck. Remember that when looking at a CT or an MR scan it is as if you are standing at the foot of your patient's bed looking up at them.

Coronal sections are used particularly in sinus investigations.

Sagittal sections are least commonly used but are sometimes evaluated for posterior pharyngeal and intracranial pathology.

Contrast is used to highlight specific areas so that the tissues are more visible. In the head and neck this is restricted to the vasculature but in the abdomen includes the liver and kidneys. It is injected intravenously and contains iodine, so patient allergies must be ascertained before administration. In addition, many units now request a glomerular filtration rate (GFR) blood test.

## MRI

MRI is primarily used to investigate soft-tissue lesions. Whereas, with CT, fluid, tissue, tumour and pus are all grey, MRI gives great definition between these different tissues and substances.

The most common types of MR scan are T1-and T2-weighted, although there are many more (diffusion-weighted, spin density-weighted, etc). An easy way to remember what colour water is in these scans is the simple phrase 'one and two, black and white'. In a T1-weighted scan water is black and in a T2-weighted one it is white.

In the head and neck they are commonly used for evaluation of patients with oral, oropharyngeal and hypopharyngeal cancers.

## PET

PET is a nuclear medicine technology that images metabolic activity. It is very useful for the investigation of a cancer of unknown origin (the unknown primary) and is regularly used in the follow-up of cancer patients after chemoradiotherapy.

It works by measuring the levels of fludeoxy-glucose (FDG), a glucose analogue, which in turn gives information about metabolic activity of the tissue. In cancer tissues, metabolic activity is very high, with quick cell turnover, and is highlighted with this scan.

PET can be combined with other scans (typically CT) to give a combination of anatomical (CT) and metabolic (PET) information on one image.

## Angiography

Angiography in the head and neck is used to look at the carotid arteries within the neck and the four major vessels supplying the intracranial structures (two internal carotid arteries and two vertebral arteries, forming the circle of Willis).

This may be done in the case of intractable arterial bleeding of unknown origin (eg epistaxis), when there is a suspicion of aneurysm, or to assess cerebral circulation when there is a suspicion of intracranial bleeding or thrombosis.

It is performed by inserting a catheter into the femoral artery, feeding the catheter up the aorta into the common carotid arteries, and injecting dye (typically iodine-based).

The risks of an angiogram include allergy, thrombosis formation, bleeding and a 2–3% chance of a cerebrovascular accident.

CHAPTER 5

# SECTION 2

# Surgery to the head and neck

## 2.1 Benign masses of the neck

### 2.1.1 Congenital masses in the neck

Congenital masses in the neck include:
- **Thyroglossal cyst:** this is discussed in Chapter 4, Endocrine Surgery
- **Branchial cyst:** branchial cleft cysts are congenital epithelial cysts, occurring laterally due to failure of obliteration of the second branchial cleft in embryonic development. They may be asymptomatic or become tender, enlarged or inflamed, or they may develop abscesses
- **Cystic hygroma:** this is a cystic lymphatic lesion that occurs in the posterior triangle of the neck. Most present at birth or before the age of 2 years

### 2.1.2 Benign acquired neck masses

The most common acquired benign neck masses are:
- Ranula
- Laryngocele
- Pharyngeal pouch

### Ranula

A ranula is a type of mucocele in the floor of the mouth originating from the sublingual glands. There are two types:
- A blocked duct causing a swelling of the normal duct
- A ruptured cyst that leads to extravasation of mucin

Usually, these are contained within the floor of the mouth. If they push through the mylohyoid (floor of the mouth), they are termed 'plunging ranulas'.

Treatment is by surgical excision, which must include excision of the sublingual gland.

### Laryngocele

A laryngocele is an air pocket that arises from the deepest point of the laryngeal ventricle. An air-filled cyst can bulge internally into the larynx, externally into the neck or be combined (where the connection is through the thyrohyoid membrane).

Treatment is by surgical excision.

## Pharyngeal pouch

This is an acquired diverticulum, which is a pouch caused by protrusion of mucosa through muscle layers of the wall of pharynx. It most commonly occurs through Killian's dehiscence in the pharynx, which is an area of dehiscence between thyropharyngeus and cricopharyngeus.

There are two types of diverticulum: pulsion and traction. A pulsion diverticulum is one that is formed by internal luminal pressure forcing mucosa outwards. A traction diverticulum is one where external scarring (eg by tubercular lymphadenopathy in the mediastinum) 'pulls' the mucosa outwards. A pharyngeal pouch is a **pulsion diverticulum**.

- Incidence is 5 per million
- It tends to occur in people aged >50
- Sex ratio is 2 male:1 female

The true aetiology is unknown but it may involve increased cricopharyngeal tonicity due to gastro-oesophageal reflux. Neuromuscular incoordination may also play a part.

---

**Clinical features of pharyngeal pouch**
- Dysphagia
- Regurgitation
- Weight loss
- Hoarseness
- Aspiration pneumonia
- Swelling on the left side of the neck which gurgles on palpation (Boyce's sign)
- Halitosis
- Recurrent sore throat
- Lung abscesses
Eventually these may lead to a malnourished patient with weight loss.

---

The **Lahey classification** of pharyngeal pouches is as follows:
- **Type I:** small mucosal protrusion
- **Type II:** definite pouch (the oesophagus and hypopharynx are in line on barium swallow examination)
- **Type III:** large pouch (the hypopharynx and pouch are in line the lateral view on barium swallow; the oesophagus is pushed forwards)

### Investigating pharyngeal pouch
- Full blood count (FBC)
- Plain neck radiograph (there may be a triangular lucency in the prevertebral tissue and/or fluid level)
- Barium swallow
- Careful endoscopy

### Treatment of pharyngeal pouch
- Pouches can be excised endoscopically or externally.

## Op box: Open excision of pharyngeal pouch

- **Endoscopic stapling/diathermy:** endoscopic resection is much less invasive, it avoids many of the postoperative complications seen with an external excision (see box below) and it is often the only option in elderly high-risk patients. Opponents of the endoscopic method claim an increased rate of recurrence compared with external excision (6–7%), and the chance of missing a malignancy in the pouch which cannot be sent for histology

**External approach:** this is best done by a one-stage diverticulectomy

**Indications**
- Symptomatic pharyngeal pouch

**Preop**
- Starve patient overnight preoperatively
- Beware of inhalation during induction of GA (Mendelson syndrome)
- Examine pouch transorally and pack pouch with proflavin ribbon for easy identification
- Pass nasogastric (NG) tube after intubation if not possible preoperatively

**Incision**
- Make incision at level of the cricoid at the anterior border of the left sternomastoid

**Procedure**
- Retract sternomastoid and carotid sheath laterally to expose the packed pouch
- Remove pack via the mouth
- Excise or invert pouch, then oversew or staple
- Perform cricopharyngeal myotomy (to try to prevent recurrence)
- Send pouch for histological examination (1% risk of carcinoma in a pouch)

**Postop**
- Keep patients nil by mouth and feed via NG tube

**Complications**
- *Immediate complications*
  - Haemorrhage
  - Pneumothorax
  - Surgical emphysema
- *Early complications*
  - Secondary haemorrhage
  - Recurrent laryngeal nerve palsy (hoarseness, stridor)
  - Wound infection
  - Fistula
  - Mediastinitis
  - Aerocele in the superior mediastinum
- *Late complications*
  - Persistent hoarseness
  - Recurrence
  - Stricture

**CHAPTER 5**

**Infective and inflammatory masses of the neck**
Infection may be present in the lymph nodes or tissues of the neck.
**Infective causes**
**Viral**
- Epstein–Barr virus (EBV)
- HIV

**Bacterial**
- TB
- Actinomycosis
- Cat scratch disease
- Brucellosis
- Atypical mycobacteria
- Ludwig's angina (infection of the submental and submandibular triangles bilaterally; can lead to airway compromise)

**Parasitic**
- Toxoplasmosis

## 2.1.3 Salivary stone disease

The essential history of a patient with stones in the salivary gland (sialolithiasis) includes:
- Acute painful swelling of one major salivary gland (if it is symmetrical other causes must be excluded)
- Symptoms that are much worse after eating
- Swelling reduces over 1–2 hours after meals
- A stone may be felt in either Stensen's duct (parotid) or Wharton's duct (submandibular)
- Swellings may be recurrent

### General points
- 80–90% are in the submandibular gland, 10–20% in the parotid gland
- Can occur at any age
- Slight male preponderance

### Risk factors
- Dehydration
- Gout
- Diabetes
- Hypertension

Most stones are made of hydroxyapatite (abundant in saliva). They form around a nidus of mineralised deposits within the salivary duct. As Wharton's duct is much longer than Stensen's duct, and due to the higher content of mucin and calcium and phosphate in the submandibular saliva, stones in the submandibular duct are much more common.

Due to the high content of calcium in the submandibular duct stones, 85% are radio-opaque and can be seen on a radiograph. Parotid saliva has a much lower concentration of calcium and only 10–15% of these are radio-opaque.

### Imaging
As described above, not all stones are visible on a radiograph, so floor-of-the-mouth and occlusal radiographs are no longer routinely used.

More regularly, ultrasonography of the gland is used. This can highlight most stones, but also gives anatomical details of the intraglandular

**CHAPTER 5**

ducts and the dimensions of the duct. This will show up stones, stenoses and intraglandular duct dilatation.

Sialography is the most accurate imaging method to detect calculi but is more invasive than ultrasonography and is contraindicated in those with an iodine allergy.

CT and MRI also give useful information when the diagnosis is in doubt. The high calcium content of submandibular duct stones means that CT gives excellent images of the anatomy.

More recently submandibular gland duct endoscopy has been used in specialist centres to enter the duct and remove the stone using an adapted Dormier basket, similar to those used in urology.

This can only be used when the stone is mobile (seen on ultrasonography or sialography). If it is fixed in the duct, or if it rolls back into the gland then endoscopic removal is not possible.

## 2.2 Cancers of the head and neck

Cancer of the head and neck is a vast topic and there are many books written on this subject alone.

These malignancies can simply be divided into cancers of mucosal surfaces (oral cavity, pharynx, larynx and nasal cavity and sinuses) and those of the head and neck viscera (submandibular glands, thyroid and parathyroids).

Cancers of the thyroid and parathyroids are discussed in Chapter 4, Endocrine Surgery. Cancers of the salivary glands are discussed here.

## 2.2.1 Cancers of the mucosal surfaces

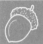 **In a nutshell ...**

Of cancers of the mucosal surfaces 95% are squamous cell carcinomas (SCCs).
SCCs of the head and neck are classified anatomically. These are:
- Oral cavity
- Oropharynx
- Nasopharynx
- Hypopharynx
- Larynx
- Nasal cavity and sinuses

Investigations are centred around:
- Histological diagnosis (with FNAC, or core, incisional or excision biopsy)
- Staging by means of ultrasonography, CT, MRI or PET

Treatment options include conservative management, surgical treatment, radiotherapy and chemotherapy. Treatment can involve combinations of these. Treatment of the primary site and the neck can be considered as two separate treatment plans, eg treatment of a cancer of the oral cavity with a neck node can be broken down as:
- **Primary cancer:** surgical excision, radiotherapy, chemotherapy, surgical excision with postoperative radiotherapy
- **Neck disease:** neck dissection, radiotherapy, chemotherapy, chemoradiotherapy (CRT), neck dissection with postoperative radiotherapy

Recently, evidence has shown that cancers of the internal mucosal surfaces of the head and neck especially of the oropharynx that are associated with human papillomavirus (HPV) infection have a much better outcome with CRT than those not associated with HPV. Therefore when investigating cancers of the head and neck, tissue typing for HPV is now performed.

## 2.2.2 Cancers of the oral cavity

Of oral tumours 85% are SCCs. Other types of tumour in the oral cavity include:
- Minor salivary gland tumours (benign and malignant)
- Lymphoma (Hodgkin's and non-Hodgkin's)
- Sarcoma
- Fibrosarcoma
- Melanoma
- Haemangioma
- Granular cell myeoblastoma

## Risk factors for SCC of the oral cavity
- Smoking and alcohol
- Betel nut chewing
- Leukoplakia
- Dental caries
- Chronic glossitis
- Malnutrition
- Cirrhosis
- HIV

**CHAPTER 5**

## Assessment of suspected oral cavity tumours

- Clinical examination
- Examination under anaesthetic (EUA) and biopsy
- Panendoscopy (to exclude a second primary):
  - Oral cavity
  - Postnasal space
  - Pharynx
  - Oesophagus
- Trachea and bronchus
- Plain radiography to assess mandibular involvement
- CT (sometimes MRI) to assess extent and nodal status

The T of the TNM classification roughly runs along the lines of tumour <2 cm, tumour between 2 and 4 cm and tumour >4 cm. There are of course variations between each anatomical area.

---

**TNM classification of malignant oral cavity tumours**

**Primary tumours**
- TX: Primary tumour cannot be assessed
- Tis: Carcinoma in situ
- T0: No evidence of primary tumour
- T1: Tumour <2 cm
- T2: Tumour 2–4 cm in diameter
- T3: >4 cm diameter
- T4: Lip: invades adjacent structures (eg cortical bone, skin of face, inferior alveolar nerve)
- T4a: Oral cavity: invades adjacent structures (eg cortical bone, muscles of tongue, maxillary sinus, skin of face)
- T4b: Masticator space, pterygoid plate, skull base or internal carotid artery

**Nodal classification of metastatic sites** (this is the same for all head and neck sites except nasopharynx and thyroid malignancies)
- NX: Nodal status cannot be assessed
- N0: No lymph node metastases
- N1: Metastasis in a single ipsilateral node, <3 cm in diameter
- N2a: Single ipsilateral node 3–6 cm
- N2b: or multiple ipsilateral nodes <6 cm
- N2c: or bilateral or contralateral nodes <6 cm
- N3: Metastasis in a lymph node >6 cm

---

## Management of oral cavity cancers

Note that treatment options should always be discussed with the local head and neck multidisciplinary team (MDT).

### Management of early-stage oral cavity cancers

Smaller T1 and T2 tumours <3 cm are usually treated by single modality, ie surgery or radiotherapy if the patient is unfit for surgery.

## Management of large-volume T2, T3 and T4 oral cavity cancers

These are treated with a combination of surgery and postoperative radiotherapy. Surgery includes resection (eg hemiglossectomy) and primary closure or reconstruction. Reconstruction may involve local skin flaps, skin grafts or composite flaps (eg fibula flap, medial forearm flap).

## Management of oral cavity cancers with neck metastases

- N0: there is a debate about whether the neck should be treated in this situation. Currently the neck is treated with either surgery or radiotherapy; however, some advocate the use of sentinel node biopsy before making a decision about the neck
- N1–3: patients require either modified radical or extended neck dissection

It should be remembered that lesions near the midline and anterior lesions can metastasise bilaterally, and this should be considered when treating the neck.

Oral tongue lesions metastasise more frequently to levels II and III than level I and may metastasise and skip to level IV. Therefore, a selective neck dissection including levels I–IV may be indicated in these cases.

There is a rough rule of thumb which is that you can draw a line from the angle of the jaw to the medial canthus. Cancers anterior to this spread to level I first and those behind spread to level II or III. Although not entirely accurate it is a good rough guide.

## Oropharyngeal cancer

Primarily SCC of the oropharynx; 8% of SCCs have distant metastases at presentation and 30% have a synchronous second primary, or will develop a metachronous primary within 10 years.

### Risk factors for squamous cell carcinoma of the oropharynx

- Smoking
- Alcohol
- Betel nut and tobacco chewing
- Dental sepsis
- Ionising radiation
- HPV infection (types 8 and 16)
- Submucosal fibrosis of the palatine arch
- The male:female ratio is 5:1

### Clinical features of oropharyngeal carcinoma

- 20% present with a neck lump (level II, IV, V or retropharyngeal)
- Sore throat
- Odynophagia
- Trismus
- Ulceration
- Leukoplakia or erythroplakia
- Otalgia
- 'Hot potato' speech

### Investigating suspected oropharyngeal carcinoma

- FNAC of neck node
- Panendoscopy and bilateral tonsillectomy
- CT of neck and chest (staging CT) and MRI or PET–CT
- Liver ultrasonography if metastases suspected

> ## TNM staging of SCC of the oropharynx
> - TX: Tumour cannot be assessed
> - Tis: Carcinoma in situ
> - T0: No evidence of tumour
> - T1: Tumour <2 cm in maximum diameter
> - T2: Tumour 2–4 cm diameter
> - T3: Tumour >4 cm diameter
> - T4: Tumour extends beyond the oropharynx
> - T4a: Tumour invades the mandible, larynx, medial pterygoid, hard palate, deep or extrinsic muscles of the tongue
> - T4b: Tumour invades the lateral pterygoid plate, pterygoid plates, skull base, nasopharynx or carotid artery
>
> Nodal classification is as for malignancies of the oral cavity (see above).

## Management of oropharyngeal carcinoma

**SCC and minor salivary gland tumours** are treated with a combination of surgery and radiotherapy.
**Base of tongue lesions** are treated with:
- T1: radical radiotherapy
- T2–4: either chemoradiotherapy or resection with free flap reconstruction and bilateral neck dissection with postoperative radiotherapy (PORT). This choice depends on the head and neck MDT, the patient's comorbidities, HPV status and their wishes

**Carcinoma of the soft palate** is treated by:
- T1–2: resection (± $CO_2$ laser) or radical radiotherapy
- T3–4: resection with reconstruction

**Posterior pharyngeal wall carcinomas:**
- T1–2: resection or radical radiotherapy
- T3–4: resection with postoperative radiotherapy

**Carcinoma of the tonsil:**
- T1–2: transoral surgery or radical radiotherapy to site and neck
- T3–4: radical resection with neck dissection and reconstruction. Reconstruction may involve the use of a pectoralis major flap or free radial flap. If a segment of the mandible is taken, a fibula flap may be required

## Treatment of the neck in oropharyngeal squamous carcinoma

- **N0** (node-negative patients): midline tumours (eg palate, posterior pharyngeal wall, tongue base) can metastasise to both sides of the neck, so, when treating the T1–2 primary tumour, radiotherapy or surgery (depending on the primary treatment) to level I–III nodes should be considered. For larger lesions, level IV should be treated
- **N1** (metastasis in a single ipsilateral node of diameter <3 cm): a selective or modified radical neck dissection should be carried out, but radical radiotherapy may be appropriate in early lesions
- **N2–3** (more extensive nodal involvement than in N1): a modified radical neck dissection is indicated. If the IJV, accessory nerve and sternomastoid are involved by the cancer, a radical neck dissection may be indicated

Postoperative radiotherapy is indicated if more than one node is involved or if there is extracapsular spread.

## 2.2.3 Hypopharyngeal carcinoma

As described above, the hypopharynx is divided into subsites: the postcricoid region, pyriform sinuses, and posterior and lateral hypopharyngeal walls.

Pyriform fossa tumours are the most common, but postcricoid tumours are seen more frequently in women.

### Risk factors for hypopharyngeal carcinoma

- Smoking
- Alcohol
- Plummer–Vinson syndrome (hypopharyngeal web, iron deficiency anaemia)
- Pharyngeal webs and strictures
- Chemicals (asbestos, nickel)
- Previous radiotherapy

### Pathology of hypopharyngeal carcinoma

Most tumours are SCCs, but sarcomas, leiomyosarcomas, adenoid cystic carcinomas and lipomas have been described.

### Clinical features of hypopharyngeal carcinoma

- Dysphagia
- Weight loss
- Otalgia
- Foreign body sensation
- Lymphadenopathy (level II)
- Hoarseness (advanced disease due to vocal fold fixation)

### Investigating hypopharyngeal carcinoma

- EUA and biopsy
- Panendoscopy
- Chest radiograph
- Staging CT of neck and chest (± MRI)
- Thyroid function tests

---

**Classification of hypopharyngeal tumours**

- T1: Tumour <2 cm and limited to one subsite of hypopharynx
- T2: Tumour invades more than one subsite of the hypopharynx of an adjacent area
- **or** tumour 2–4 cm without fixation of the hemilarynx
- T3: Tumour >4 cm
- **or** tumour with fixation of the hemilarynx
- T4a: Tumour invades the thyroid or cricoid cartilages, hyoid bone, strap muscles, oesophagus or thyroid gland
- T4b: Tumour invades the prevertebral fascia and mediastinal structures, or envelopes the carotid artery; 60–75% have lymphadenopathy at presentation (levels II–IV) and 5% have bilateral lymphadenopathy

---

### Management of hypopharyngeal carcinomas

#### T1–2 tumours

- Partial pharyngolaryngectomy, CRT or endoscopic resection

#### T3–4 tumours

- **Surgery**
  - Partial pharyngectomy
  - Total laryngectomy and partial pharyngectomy

CHAPTER 5

- Total pharyngolaryngectomy
- **Reconstruction:** can take the form of jejunal flap, radial forearm flap, gastric transposition or myocutaneous flap
- **Primary radiotherapy:** can be used for patients who are unsuitable for surgery or for small hypopharyngeal tumours
- **Postoperative radiotherapy:** should be given with T1–2 and N0 tumours if there is:
  - Positive margin perineural spread
  - Vascular invasion
  - Extracapsular spread
  - No neck dissection

*Treatment of the neck in hypopharyngeal carcinoma*

Metastases occur in level II–IV nodes and to level VI with postcricoid and apical pyriform fossa tumours. It is recommended that the neck be treated in the same modality as the primary tumour, with either neck dissection or radiotherapy.

## 2.2.4 Nasopharyngeal tumours

Nasopharyngeal carcinoma is most common in Chinese and Hong Kong populations and commonly presents in the fourth decade. It presents in the sixth decade in non-Chinese populations.

A typical 'exam' presentation is of the 35-year-old South-East Asian man with a neck lump, nasal blockage, epistaxis and ipsilateral middle-ear effusion.

Aetiology of nasopharyngeal tumours
- Genetic predisposition:
  - HLA-A2
  - Positive family history

- EBV infection
- Salt-preserved fish (nitrosamines)
- Vitamin C deficiency
- Male preponderance

Clinical features of nasopharyngeal tumours
- Epistaxis
- Nasal obstruction
- Neck lump (70% have a neck node metastasis at presentation)
- Otalgia
- Otitis media with effusion (anterior spread)
- Posterolateral spread causes:
  - Mandibular nerve palsy
  - Cranial nerve IX, XII palsies
  - Horner syndrome
  - Cranial nerve III, IV, V (ophthalmic and maxillary) palsies

Investigating nasopharyngeal tumours
- FBC and erythrocyte sedimentation rate (ESR) (lymphoma)
- EBV antigen and viral capsid antigen
- Audiogram and tympanogram
- Visual fields
- CT (nasopharynx, neck, chest, abdomen)
- MRI if intracranial extension suspected
- Angiography if angiofibroma suspected:

Pathology of nasopharyngeal tumours
- 85% are SCCs
- Lymphoma, adenocarcinoma, adenoid cystic carcinoma and melanoma also present in the nasopharynx
- Rhabdomyosarcoma can present in children, whereas nasopharyngeal angiofibroma must be suspected in adolescent males presenting with epistaxis

Classification of nasopharyngeal tumours

*WHO classification of nasopharyngeal tumours*
- Type 1: keratinising (well-differentiated) SCC
- Type 2: non-keratinising carcinoma
- Type 3: undifferentiated carcinoma

---

**TNM classification of nasopharyngeal tumours**
- T1: Tumour confined to nasopharynx
- T2: Tumour extends to soft tissues
- T2a: Extension to oropharynx and/or nasal cavity without parapharyngeal extension
- T2b: Parapharyngeal extension
- T3: Extension to bony structures or paranasal sinuses
- T4: Cranial nerve, intracranial involvement, or extension into hypopharynx, masticator space, orbit or infratemporal fossa

The classification of nodal involvement of nasopharyngeal carcinoma is different from other head and neck sites:
- NX: Nodes cannot be assessed
- N0: No nodal involvement
- N1: Unilateral metastasis <6 cm diameter, above the supraclavicular fossa
- N2: Bilateral metastasis <6 cm diameter, above the supraclavicular fossa
- N3: Metastasis in a lymph node
- N3a: >6 cm diameter
- N3b: Into the supraclavicular fossa

---

Management of nasopharyngeal tumours
- **Nasopharyngeal carcinoma:** CRT. (Surgery has no place in the treatment of nasopharyngeal carcinoma)
- **Lymphoma:** referral to haemato-oncology for chemotherapy
- **Rhabdomyosarcoma:** referral to centralised sarcoma MDT for chemotherapy plus radiotherapy
- **Nasopharyngeal angiofibroma:** surgery

## 2.3 Cancers of the neck viscera

Cancers of the thyroid and parathyroid glands discussed in Chapter 4, Endocrine Surgery.

### 2.3.1 Tumours of the salivary glands

These salivary gland neoplasms can be divided into benign and malignant tumours, and malignant tumours can be primary or secondary tumours:
- 80% of all salivary gland tumours are in the parotid gland
- 80% of parotid tumours are benign (80% of these are pleomorphic adenomas)
- 50% of tumours arising in the submandibular gland are benign
- 10% of sublingual tumours are benign
- <1% of minor salivary glands are benign

CHAPTER 5

Salivary gland lesions are grouped as follows.

**Adenomas**
- Pleomorphic adenoma
- Adenolymphoma (Warthin's tumour)
- Myoepithelial
- Basal cell adenoma
- Ductal papilloma
- Cystadenoma

**Carcinomas**
- Mucoepidermoid carcinoma (most common malignancy in children and adults)
- Actinic cell carcinoma
- Adenoid cystic carcinoma
- Carcinoma ex-pleomorphic adenoma
- Squamous cell carcinoma
- Undifferentiated carcinoma
- Rarities

**Non-epithelial tumours**
- Haemangioma (most common tumour in children)
- Lymphangioma
- Lipoma

**Malignant lymphomas**
**Secondary tumours**
**Unclassified tumours**
**Tumour-like conditions, eg sialometaplasia, sialoadenitis**

## Salivary adenomas

- **Pleomorphic adenomas** account for 80% of benign parotid gland tumours. They occur most frequently in the fifth decade, equally in men and women. They have a pseudo-capsule and arise from myoepithelial cells and intercalated duct cells. They present as a painless enlarging smooth mass. Treatment is with excision because there is a 2% per year malignancy transformation rate

- **Adenolymphomas (Warthin's tumours)** are seen mainly in men (7M:1F) aged 60–70 years. They usually arise in the parotid tail from lymphoid tissue. One in ten patients has bilateral tumours, but these rarely occur synchronously. They can be treated conservatively but, if cosmetic appearance is distressing, they can be removed

## Salivary carcinomas

- **Mucoepidermoid tumours** arise mainly in the parotid gland. These tumours metastasise to lymph nodes and can spread to the lungs and brain. They are the most common salivary neoplasms in both children and adults

- **Adenoid cystic carcinoma** is a slow-growing tumour that often spreads along nerve sheaths. It occurs more frequently in minor rather than major salivary glands. Patients may present with facial pain and facial nerve or trigeminal nerve palsy. Tumours do not metastasise early and lymph node metastasis is uncommon but, due to perineural spread, these cancers are often treated over many years and re-present many years later with new lesions

- **Adenocarcinomas** make up 3% of parotid tumours and 10% of submandibular and minor salivary gland tumours; 20% of patients have nodal disease at presentation

- **Carcinoma ex-pleomorphic adenoma** is a malignancy arising within a pre-existing benign pleomorphic adenoma. The incidence of malignant change is estimated to be 2% per year in an adenoma that has been present for >10 years

CHAPTER 5

Staging of salivary gland neoplasms

---

**The AJC system (American Joint Committee) staging of malignant parotid tumours**

- T0: No clinical evidence of tumour
- T1: <2 cm diameter, without extra-parenchymal extension
- T2: 2–4 cm diameter, without extra-parenchymal extension
- T3: 4–6 cm diameter, and/or extra-parenchymal extension
- T4a: Invasion of ear canal, skin, mandible or facial nerve
- T4b: Base of skull, nerve VII involvement and/or >6 cm

---

A parotid lump with facial nerve palsy is cancer until proved otherwise.

Investigating salivary gland neoplasms
- MRI helps to assess relation of tumours to anatomical structures (eg facial nerve)
- FNAC

## 2.3.2 Parotid gland surgery
This aims to resect tumour with a margin of macroscopically normal tissue and preservation of the facial nerve.
- **Superficial parotidectomy:** excision of the superficial lobe only is known as superficial parotidectomy – but tumours extending to the deep lobe require **total parotidectomy** (deep and superficial lobes removed)
- **Total conservative parotidectomy** preserves the facial nerve

- **Total radical parotidectomy** sacrifices the facial nerve (if sacrificed, this is known as a total radical parotidectomy)
- **Extended parotidectomy** involves excision of additional structures (eg TMJ, mandible, zygoma or sternomastoid)
- **Facial nerve resection:** adenoid cystic carcinomas may require parts of the facial nerve to be resected if they are infiltrated by tumour
- **Neck dissection** is indicated in nodal disease and may be indicated in high-grade tumours (eg a high-grade mucoepidermoid cancer with an N0 neck will still get a neck dissection. A similarly sized low-grade tumour may not)

Postoperative radiotherapy is indicated for:
- Residual disease
- If there is evidence of extracapsular spread in lymph nodes
- High-grade tumours with high risk of local recurrence
- Surgery for recurrent disease
- Adenoid cystic tumours
- Perineural disease

Palliative radiotherapy alone can be offered for inoperable cases.

## 2.4 Neck dissection
The original description of a neck dissection by Crile in 1906 involved en-bloc removal of the lymph nodes of the neck along with the internal jugular vein, sternomastoid muscle and the accessory nerve.

There are different incisions that can be used for the surgery which will either be satisfactory for the neck dissection or enable surgical removal of the primary disease and the neck dissection.

**CHAPTER 5**

The indications for neck dissection are:
- Operable metastatic neck disease
- Access before reconstruction

Neck dissection should not be performed in those patients:
- Who are unfit for surgery
- With an inoperable neck
- With inoperable primary disease
- With distant metastases

> **Neck dissection**
> The original operation has been modified over the years and now there are different classifications of neck dissection:
> - Radical neck dissection
> - Modified radical neck dissection
> - Selective neck dissection
> - Extended radical neck dissection
>
> Cervical node groups I–VI are removed, but non-lymphatic structures may be preserved:
>
> **Type 1** Accessory nerve preserved; IJV and sternomastoid removed
>
> **Type 2** Accessory nerve and IJV preserved; sternomastoid removed
>
> **Type 3** Accessory nerve, IJV and sterno-mastoid preserved

## Selective neck dissection

This comprises removal of certain lymph node groups, but preservation of some lymph node groups and the accessory nerve, IJV and sternomastoid.

**Lymph node groups removed in selective neck dissection**

| Type of selective neck dissection | Lymph node group(s) removed |
|---|---|
| Supraomohyoid | I–III, submandibular gland |
| Extended supraomohyoid | I–IV, submandibular gland |
| Lateral | II–IV |
| Posterolateral | II–IV, with postauricular and suboccipital nodes |
| Anterior | VI |
| Superior | VII |

## Extended radical neck dissection

The structures that may be removed during a radical neck dissection, depending on the extent of the surgery include:
- IJV
- Accessory nerve
- Sternomastoid muscle
- Parotid nodes and parotid gland
- Level I–VI lymph nodes
- Retropharyngeal nodes
- Mandible
- Tip of mastoid

**Op box: Neck dissection (modified radical type 1)**

**Position**
- Supine, shoulder bolster and head ring to give neck extension and a stable head. Head turned to the contralateral side to allow maximum exposure

**Incision**
- The standard incision used today begins at the tip of the mastoid process in a curvilinear fashion, two finger breadths below the angle of the mandible, and extends onto the tip of the hyoid bone and medially to the midline of the chin

**Procedure**
- The skin flaps are raised
- The sternomastoid is divided at its lower end
- The IJV is divided at its lower end
- The omohyoid is divided
- The lymph node groups of the anterior and posterior triangle are dissected 'en bloc' (according to the type of neck dissection)
- The upper end of sternomastoid is divided
- The IJV is ligated and divided
- The hypoglossal nerve should be identified and preserved
- The submandibular gland is dissected and removed after ligating the duct
- The wound is closed and two drains are inserted (away from the carotid artery)

**Intraoperative hazards**
- Bleeding
- Chylous leak (thoracic duct damage)
- Nerve injury to the:
    - Brachial plexus
    - Phrenic nerve
    - Marginal mandibular nerve (branch of the facial nerve)
    - Sympathetic trunk
    - Vagus nerve
    - Hypoglossal nerve
    - Lingual nerve

**Complications**

Early:
- Cerebral oedema
- Wound breakdown or infection
- Facial oedema
- Carotid artery rupture

Late:
- Frozen shoulder
- Recurrence of tumour

# CHAPTER 6

# Neurosurgery (Elective)

**Paul M Brennan**

CHAPTER 6

# SECTION 1

# Elective neurosurgery

## In a nutshell ...

In this section the basic anatomy, physiology, pathologies and principles relating to elective neurosurgery are covered. Emergency neurosurgery and traumatic brain injury are covered in Trauma, Book 1.

## 1.1 Neuroanatomy

## In a nutshell ...

- Scalp
- Skull
- Structure of the brain
- Meninges
- Blood supply
- Venous drainage
- Cerebrospinal fluid (CSF)

## The scalp

The scalp is made of five layers, denoted by the acronym **SCALP**:

**S**kin
**C**onnective tissue (dense)
**A**poneurotic layer (galea)
**L**oose connective tissue
**P**ericranium

The aponeurotic layer is where frontalis (anterior), occipitalis (posterior) and temporalis (lateral) merge.

## Blood supply to the scalp

- External carotid artery (superficial temporal, posterior auricular and occipital branches)
- Internal carotid artery (supratrochlear and supraorbital branches of the ophthalmic artery)
- Free anastomosis between the vessels supplying the scalp
- Vessels run in the dense connective tissue layer of the scalp, and therefore bleed profusely if cut (cannot easily retract or go into spasm)

## Nerve supply to the scalp
- Supratrochlear and supraorbital branches of Va (to vertex anteriorly)
- Posterior rami of C2 and C3 (to vertex posteriorly)
- Auriculotemporal branch of Vc (laterally)

## The skull

### Cranial vault
Key features of the cranial vault:
- Inner table and outer table of cortical bone, with a layer of trabecular bone sandwiched between (diploë)
- Venous lakes in the diploë
- Suture lines at fibrous joints between skull bones limit extension of extradural but not subdural haematoma, defining the characteristic lenticular shape of the former. **Sutures:** coronal (between frontal and parietal bones), metopic (between frontal bones) and lambdoid (connects parietal and temporal with occipital bones)
- Thinnest part of the skull is at the pterion inferolaterally, at the junction of the frontal, parietal, temporal and sphenoid (greater wing) bones – site of middle meningeal artery, hence easy injury in trauma causing extradural haematoma

### Skull base
The skull base is stepped into three cranial fossae.

### Anterior fossa
- Floor is level with upper margin of the orbit
- Contains the frontal lobe
- Extends posteriorly to the lesser wing of the sphenoid bone
- Formed primarily by the orbital part of the frontal bone
- Cribriform plate and crista galli in midline. Site of olfactory bulbs. Susceptibility to injury in trauma

### Middle fossa
- Floor approximately level with the zygomatic arch
- Contains the temporal lobe and pituitary
- Extends posteriorly to the upper border of the petrous temporal bone at the insertion of the tentorium cerebelli
- Formed primarily by the greater wing of the sphenoid bone and the squamous and petrous parts of the temporal bone
- Sella turcica in the sphenoid in the midline (containing the pituitary)

### Posterior fossa
- Contains cerebellum and brainstem
- Lies beneath the tentorium cerebelli which limits its volume, making any additional tumour or blood masses particularly dangerous

# Major skull base foramina

| Site | Foramen | Transmits | Notes |
|---|---|---|---|
| Anterior fossa | Cribriform plate | Olfactory nerve (I) | Nerves arise from respiratory epithelium in roof of nasal cavity, synapse in olfactory bulb, and pass via olfactory tract to para-amygdaloid cortex of temporal lobe (primary olfactory cortex) |
| Middle fossa | Optic canal | Optic nerve (II) | Nerve arises from retina and passes to optic chiasma, where nasal fibres decussate. Ipsilateral temporal fibres and contralateral nasal fibres then pass via optic tract to lateral geniculate nucleus in the thalamus, and thence via the optic radiation to occipital (visual) cortex |
| | Superior orbital fissure | Lacrimal nerve | Branch of ophthalmic nerve (Va) to supply conjunctiva. Gains secretomotor fibres from zygomaticotemporal nerve to innervate lacrimal gland |
| | | Frontal nerve | Branch of ophthalmic nerve (Va) to supply forehead |
| | | Trochlear nerve (IV) | To supply superior oblique. Arises from the posterior surface of the midbrain. Runs in lateral wall of cavernous sinus before exiting skull |
| | | Oculomotor nerve (III) | To supply sphincter pupillae and muscles of eye movement except superior oblique (IV) and lateral rectus (VI). Arises from the anterior midbrain and runs along the free edge of the tentorium, where it is vulnerable to compression by uncal herniation or posterior communicating artery aneurysms. Runs in lateral wall of cavernous sinus before exiting skull |
| | | Nasociliary nerve | Branch of ophthalmic nerve (Va) to supply skin of bridge of nose, ethmoidal and sphenoid air cells and lacrimal sac. Supplies motor fibres to dilator pupillae via long ciliary nerves |
| | | Abducens nerve (VI) | Supplies lateral rectus. Arises from the inferior border of the pons and runs upwards to enter the lateral wall of the cavernous sinus before running into the superior orbital fissure. Downward movement of the brainstem can cause traction on the nerve – a false localising sign. Runs in lateral wall of cavernous sinus before exiting skull |
| | | Ophthalmic artery | |
| | Inferior orbital fissure | Maxillary nerve (Vb) | Supplies sensation to skin of cheek and nose. Also supplies secretomotor fibres to the lacrimal gland via zygomaticotemporal nerve branch to lacrimal nerve. Maxillary nerve arises from trigeminal ganglion and passes through foramen rotundum into pterygopalatine fossa, and enters orbit from here via the inferior orbital fissure |
| | Foramen rotundum | Maxillary nerve (Vb) | See 'Inferior orbital fissure' (above) |
| | Foramen ovale | Mandibular nerve (Vc) | Supplies motor supply to the muscles of mastication. Supplies sensation to the anterior two-thirds of the tongue, floor of the mouth and skin over the mandible, tragus and temporal areas. Also distributes chorda tympani nerve fibres from the facial nerve to provide secretomotor supply to sublingual and submandibular salivary glands and taste to the anterior two-thirds of the tongue. Arises from the trigeminal ganglion |

CHAPTER 6

| Site | Foramen | Transmits | Notes |
|---|---|---|---|
| | Foramen lacerum | Nothing (internal carotid traverses the upper third) | Not a true foramen. No significant structures cross its fibrocartilage |
| | Carotid canal | Internal carotid artery | With ascending cervical sympathetic plexus. Canal joins foramen lacerum at its upper third |
| | Foramen spinosum | Middle meningeal artery | Branch of external carotid. The artery may remain intraosseous as it courses laterally across the floor of the middle fossa, as far as the pterion. Fractures of the pterion can cause laceration of the artery and acute extradural haematoma |
| Posterior fossa | Internal acoustic meatus | Facial nerve (VII) | Supplies muscles of facial expression, stapedius and secretomotor fibres via chorda tympani nerve to Vc. Small sensory root (nervus intermedius) supplies anterior two-thirds of the tongue with taste sensation (also via chorda tympani). Arises from the pontomedullary junction and passes laterally upwards to enter the meatus. Exits petrous bone at the stylomastoid foramen |
| | | Vestibulocochlear nerve (VIII) | Arises from the pontomedullary junction and passes laterally upwards to enter the meatus. Fibres pass centrally to brainstem nuclei and cerebellum (vestibular part), and to the medial geniculate body, the inferior colliculus and thence to the auditory cortex of the superior temporal gyrus (cochlear part) |
| | | Labyrinthine artery | Branch of the basilar |
| | Jugular foramen | Inferior petrosal sinus | To join jugular vein immediately below the base of the skull |
| | | Glossopharyngeal nerve (IX) | Supplies sensation to middle ear, oropharynx, palatine tonsil and posterior third of the tongue (including taste). Innervates the carotid sinus. Motor supply to stylopharyngeus and secretomotor fibres to the parotid, via the lesser petrosal nerve to Vc. Arises from the side of the medulla oblongata between the olive and the inferior cerebellar peduncle |
| | | Vagus nerve (X) | Motor supply to the muscles of the pharynx, larynx, soft palate and oesophagus. Parasympathetic and sensory supply to abdominal and thoracic viscera. Arises below glossopharyngeal nerve from the side of the medulla |
| | | Accessory nerve (XI) | Cranial root arises below vagus nerve from the side of the medulla and joins with spinal root. Cranial root fibres exit the nerve just below the base of the skull and join the vagus nerve. They supply the striated muscle of the viscera, being distributed with the vagus |
| | | Internal jugular vein | Draining transverse sinus |
| | Foramen magnum | Spinal cord | |
| | | Ascending (spinal) portion of accessory nerve (XI) | Motor supply to sternomastoid and trapezuis. Arises from the lateral surface of the upper six segments of the cervical cord and passes up through the foramen magnum to join with the cranial portion |
| | | Vertebral artery | |
| | | Spinal arteries | |
| | Hypoglossal canal | Hypoglossal nerve (XII) | Motor supply to the muscles of the tongue. Arises from the anterior surface of the medulla, between pyramid and olive |

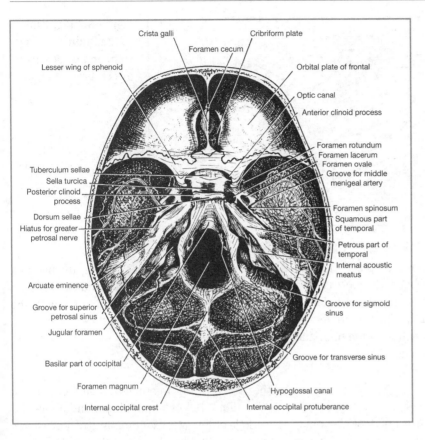

Crista galli
Cribriform plate
Foramen cecum
Lesser wing of sphenoid
Orbital plate of frontal
Optic canal
Anterior clinoid process
Foramen rotundum
Foramen lacerum
Foramen ovale
Tuberculum sellae
Groove for middle
Sella turcica
menigeal artery
Posterior clinoid
process
Foramen spinosum
Dorsum sellae
Squamous part
Hiatus for greater
of temporal
petrosal nerve
Petrous part of
temporal
Internal acoustic
meatus
Arcuate eminence
Groove for superior
petrosal sinus
Groove for sigmoid
sinus
Jugular foramen
Basilar part of occipital
Groove for transverse sinus
Foramen magnum
Hypoglossal canal
Internal occipital crest
Internal occipital protuberance

**Figure 6.1 Internal surface of the base of the skull**

## Structure of the brain

A detailed description of neuroanatomy is beyond the scope of this book, but you should appreciate the arrangement of the main parts of the brain. The brain is that part of the central nervous system (CNS) that lies within the cranial cavity. It is best considered as consisting of three parts: the forebrain, midbrain and hindbrain. The hindbrain is continuous with the spinal cord through the foramen magnum. Each part of the brain is arranged around ventricles, cavities filled with cerebrospinal fluid (CSF) which are continuous with the central canal of the spinal canal.

### The forebrain

The forebrain consists of the cerebrum and the diencephalon.

### Cerebrum

The cerebrum is the largest part of the brain and is divided into two cerebral hemispheres connected by a mass of white matter called the corpus callosum. The cerebral hemispheres each have a central cavity called the lateral ventricles, which communicates with the third ventricle through the interventricular foramina. The lateral ventricles are separated from each other by the septum pellucidum, which may be absent. The cerebral hemispheres have a wrinkled surface of prominent gyri. Gyri are separated by grooves called sulci. Prominent sulci divide the cerebrum into lobes which are associated with certain brain functions (Figure 6.2).

CHAPTER 6

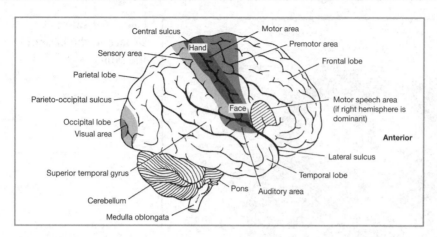

Figure 6.2 Right side of the brain showing some important areas of cerebral function

### Diencephalon

The diencephalon is almost completely hidden from the surface of the brain. It consists of a dorsal **thalamus** and a ventral **hypothalamus** and the cavity within it is the third ventricle. The optic chiasma is at the junction of the floor and anterior wall of the third ventricle.

### The midbrain

The midbrain is the narrow part of the brain that passes through the tentorial notch. It has two main sections: the cerebral peduncle and the tectum. The cavity within the midbrain is the cerebral aqueduct, which connects the third and fourth ventricles.

### The cerebral peduncles

Containing the crus cerebri, substantia nigra and the tegmentum, the cerebral peduncles are two lateral halves of the midbrain.

### The tectum

This is the part of the midbrain posterior to the cerebral aqueduct. It bears four surface swellings, the colliculi, and a small glandular structure called the pineal body, which can become calcified.

### The hindbrain

The hindbrain consists of the pons, the medulla oblongata and the cerebellum, and encloses the fourth ventricle, which is continuous with the central canal of the spinal cord.

### The pons

The pons is on the anterior surface of the cerebellum, below the midbrain and above the medulla oblongata. It is composed of nerve fibres connecting the two halves of the cerebellum. It also contains some of the cranial nerve nuclei.

### The medulla oblongata

The medulla oblongata connects the pons to the spinal cord. On its anterior surface it bears the pyramids, which contain bundles of nerve fibres originating in the cerebral cortex. Many of these fibres cross over to the opposite side of the medulla, forming the decussation of the pyramids.

### The cerebellum

The cerebellum lies beneath the tentorium cerebelli and consists of two hemispheres connected by a median 'vermis'.

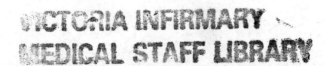

CHAPTER 6

- Superior cerebellar peduncles – connect the cerebellum to the midbrain
- Middle cerebellar peduncles – connect the cerebellum to the pons
- Inferior cerebellar peduncles – connect the cerebellum to the medulla

The cerebellum controls muscle tone and coordination of muscle movement.

## Meninges

### Dura mater

- Thick and fibrous
- Folds of dura form the falx cerebri and the tentorium cerebelli
- Inner layer projects down into spinal canal as the spinal dura
- Intracranial venous sinuses contained within folds of dura
- Extradural space (a potential space) separates dura from skull, and is limited by suture lines. Meningeal vessels run in potential dural space
- Subdural space (a potential space) separates arachnoid from dura; nothing lies in the subdural space normally (except for a thin film of lymph)

### Arachnoid mater

- Delicate impermeable membrane, in contact with the dura
- Arachnoid villi project through dura into dural venous sinuses, emptying CSF into the circulation
- Subarachnoid space contains CSF and delicate meshwork of arachnoid strands
- Subarachnoid space traversed by cranial nerves, arteries and veins
- Subarachnoid cisterns: larger pools of CSF at the base of the brain, formed because of the different shape of the brain and skull base,

eg cisterna magna (around cerebellum), basal cisterns (around brainstem and pons)

### Pia mater

- Invests brain and spinal cord tissue
- Runs deep into fissures
- Highly vascular

## Blood supply

See Figures 6.3 and 6.4.

### Internal carotid artery

- Arises from the common carotid
- No branches in the neck
- Passes through skull base in the carotid canal
- Immediately enters cavernous sinus
- Tortuous course in the sinus and on exiting it ('carotid siphon')
- Intracranial branches:
  - Ophthalmic artery
  - Branches to hypophysis and meninges
- Ends with a division into anterior and middle cerebral arteries

### Vertebral artery

- Arises from the subclavian artery
- Runs upwards through the foramina transversaria of C6–1 (arches laterally to gain access to C1 foramen)
- On exiting C1 foramen, turns sharply medially to pierce atlanto-occipital membrane and dura
- Passes upwards through foramen magnum
- Intradural branches are:
  - Anterior and posterior spinal arteries
  - Posterior inferior cerebellar artery
- Joins opposite vertebral to form **basilar artery** (runs up anterior to pons, on the clivus)

**CHAPTER 6**

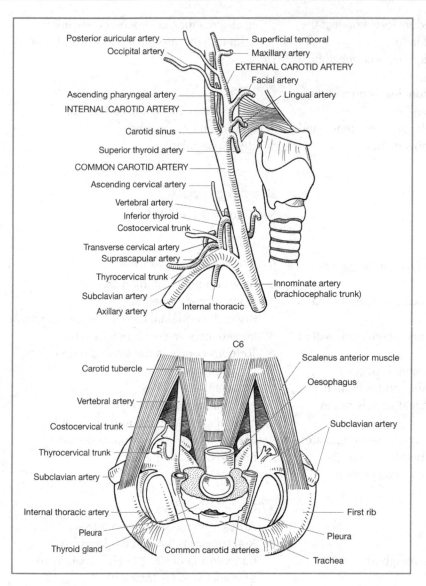

Figure 6.3 The arterial supply to the brain showing internal carotid (above) and vertebral arteries (below)

- Branches of the basilar are:
  - Anterior inferior cerebellar artery
  - Pontine and labyrinthine branches
  - Superior cerebellar artery
- Ends with a division into the posterior cerebral arteries

## Circle of Willis

The circle of Willis (Figure 6.4) is an anastomosis at the base of the brain between the internal carotid and vertebral arterial supply. It is variable ('normal' arrangement seen in <50% of brains).

- The posterior communicating artery connects the middle and posterior cerebral arteries

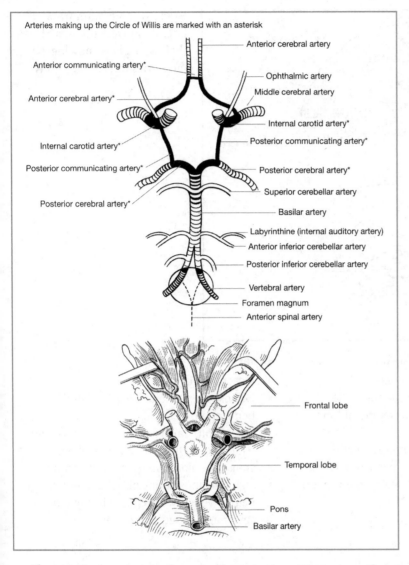

Arteries making up the Circle of Willis are marked with an asterisk

- Anterior cerebral artery
- Anterior communicating artery*
- Ophthalmic artery
- Middle cerebral artery
- Anterior cerebral artery*
- Internal carotid artery*
- Internal carotid artery*
- Posterior communicating artery*
- Posterior communicating artery*
- Posterior cerebral artery*
- Superior cerebellar artery
- Posterior cerebral artery*
- Basilar artery
- Labyrinthine (internal auditory artery)
- Anterior inferior cerebellar artery
- Posterior inferior cerebellar artery
- Vertebral artery
- Foramen magnum
- Anterior spinal artery

- Frontal lobe
- Temporal lobe
- Pons
- Basilar artery

**Figure 6.4 The circle of Willis: schematic representation (above) and relationship to the base of the brain (below)**

CHAPTER 6

- The anterior communicating artery connects the left and right anterior cerebral arteries
- Allows equalisation of blood flow around the brain should one vessel fail (eg internal carotid blockage at bulb)
- Tiny perforating branches from circle of Willis enter the anterior and posterior perforated substance at the base of the brain to supply the basal ganglia, thalamus and internal capsule (thalamostriate, lenticulo-striate, recurrent artery of Hübner)

## Patterns of arterial supply

The arteries of the brain are end-arteries. There is little anastomosis between the territories, so there are predictable deficits should a given vessel fail (Figure 6.5):

- **Anterior cerebral artery:** supplies medial frontal and parietal lobe (the motor and sensory areas for the leg)
- **Middle cerebral artery:** supplies lateral frontal and parietal lobe, superior temporal lobe – the motor and sensory areas for face

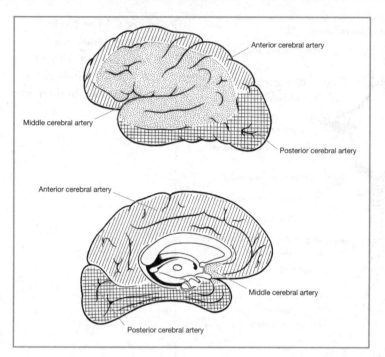

Figure 6.5 The brain from lateral (above) and medial (below) aspects showing territories of arterial supply

and arm and (in the dominant hemisphere) the auditory and speech areas

- **Posterior cerebral artery:** supplies the occipital lobe, the inferior temporal lobe – the visual areas
- **Basilar artery:** supplies brainstem and cerebellum. Occlusion of this vessel causes severe functional deficit due to interruption of brainstem functions

## Venous drainage

### Cerebral hemispheres

Veins run in the subarachnoid space and drain into the dural venous sinuses (superior sagittal sinus, transverse sinus, and cavernous sinus – Figure 6.6). Rupture of a vein as it passes through the arachnoid into a dural sinus can cause subdural haematoma.

### Superior sagittal sinus

- Lies in falx cerebri
- Drains superolateral surface of the hemisphere
- Drains into transverse sinus (right usually) which lies in the tentorium cerebelli
- Transverse sinus drains into the sigmoid sinus
- Sigmoid sinus drains into the internal jugular vein, by which it exits the cranial cavity at the jugular foramen

### Cavernous sinus

- Lies on the lateral surface of the body of the sphenoid, within which the pituitary gland sits
- Drains lateral surface of the hemisphere, pituitary, orbital contents and deep facial structures
- Connected with opposite cavernous sinus via circular sinus around the pituitary gland
- Drains into sigmoid sinus via superior and inferior petrosal sinuses

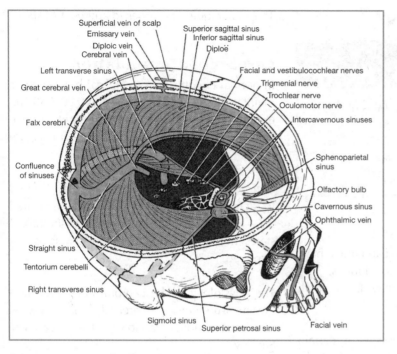

**Figure 6.6 Interior of the skull, showing the dura mater and its contained venous sinuses**

## Deep venous drainage

- **Internal cerebral vein:** drains thalamus, caudate, choroid plexus and corpus callosum
- Joins its opposite fellow to form the **great cerebral vein** (the vein of Galen)
- **Basal veins:** drain into the vein of Galen from lower basal ganglia
- **Straight sinus** (in tentorium cerebelli) formed at confluence of the Galen vein and inferior sagittal sinus. Drains into transverse sinus (usually the left)

## Cerebrospinal fluid

This is produced primarily by the choroid plexus in the lateral, third and fourth ventricles. Flow is from the lateral ventricle to the third ventricle, along the midbrain aqueduct to the fourth ventricle and then either:

- Down the central canal of the spinal cord
- Through the foramen of Magendie (midline) or Luschka (laterally) in the roof of the fourth ventricle into the cisterna magna

(thence over the surface of brain and spinal cord in the subarachnoid space)

CSF is absorbed back into blood (an active process) via arachnoid villi, projecting into the superior sagittal sinus.

## Production of CSF

- 0.3 ml/min
- 18 ml/h
- 500 ml/day

## Volume of CSF

The normal volume of CSF is 130 ml:

- 30 ml is in the ventricles
- 25 ml is in the other cranial CSF spaces
- 75 ml is in the spinal CSF spaces

Hence CSF is replaced about four times a day, and blockage of CSF flow can cause rapid increases in intracranial CSF volume and intracranial pressure (ICP).

## 1.2 Neurophysiology

### In a nutshell ...

You should understand principles of:
- The blood–brain barrier
- Intracranial pressure
- Cerebral perfusion pressure
- Cerebral autoregulation

### The blood–brain barrier

Endothelial cells of cerebral capillaries have many tight junctions (zona occludens) and few pinocytic vesicle channels. Even small molecules cannot cross (eg mannitol at 180 Da).

Active mechanisms allow passage of certain molecules. Lipophilic molecules cross easily. Cells of the immune system cross with difficulty – the CNS is an immunoprivileged site.

### Intracranial pressure

Normally this is 10–15 mmHg when supine. It decreases on sitting or standing. It increases with straining, or with increasing intracranial volume caused by:
- Blood/haemorrhage
- Tumour
- Hydrocephalus
- Oedema

### Cerebral perfusion pressure

Cerebral perfusion pressure (CPP) is the difference between the mean arterial pressure (MAP) and intracranial pressure (ICP):

$$CPP = MAP - ICP$$

Normally this is >50 mmHg. CPP should be maintained in parallel with reducing ICP.

This may require inotropes to augment MAP.

### Cerebral autoregulation

In normal circumstances cerebral blood flow is maintained relatively constant at 700–750 ml/minute (about 13% of cardiac output) despite changes in cerebral perfusion pressure (Figure 6.7).

In normal circumstances blood flow is diverted to active areas of the brain. This is called flow–metabolism coupling. In pathological states normal autoregulatory mechanisms are impaired.

The physiology of the cerebral circulation and the measurement of cerebral blood flow is discussed in more detail in Chapter 12, Vascular Surgery.

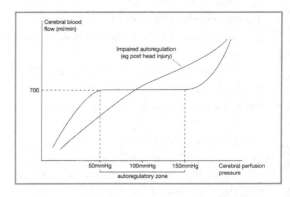

**Figure 6.7 Autoregulation of cerebral blood flow:** progressive vasoconstriction in arteriolar resistance vessels between cerebral perfusion pressures (CPP) of 50 and 150 mmHg maintains cerebral blood flow relatively constant. Outside this range cerebral autoregulation fails and cerebral blood flow falls (or rises). In pathological states (eg head injury) autoregulation fails and decreased CPP can result in significant drops in cerebral blood flow

CHAPTER 6

# 1.3 Cerebrovascular accident

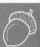

## In a nutshell ...

Stroke or cerebrovascular accident (CVA) is an abrupt onset of a new neurological deficit; 95% of CVAs are vascular in origin. The remainder are due to seizure or tumour, or are functional.
Of this 95%:

**85% are ischaemic** in origin:
- Mostly unknown cause
- 20% lacunar (small artery/arteriole)
- 15% cardiogenic embolus (eg atrial fibrillation, ventricular wall aneurysm)
- 10% large-artery lesion (eg carotid atheroma)

**10% are haemorrhagic:**
- Intracerebral haemorrhage
- Subarachnoid haemorrhage

Most ischaemic CVAs are managed without input from neurosurgical teams. Very occasionally an area of ischaemic brain may be resected if it is causing pressure effects, such as occurs when swelling cerebellar infarction presses directly on the brainstem. HAMLET, DECIMAL and DESTINY trials have failed to generate compelling evidence for the role of decompressive craniectomy in malignant stroke (where swollen infarcted brain compromises the Glasgow Coma Scale [GCS] score).
Chronic subdural haematoma is also covered in this section although it is technically a traumatic brain injury.

# Intracerebral haemorrhage

## Primary intracerebral haemorrhage
Usually this is into the basal ganglia. Other sites are the cerebellum and brainstem.

Risk factors include:
- Age (incidence doubles with each decade >40 years)
- Gender – male
- Ethnicity – African-Caribbean
- Previous CVA
- Hypertension (this is controversial because the incidence of hypertension is high in the age group affected by intracerebral haemorrhages)

Primary intracerebral haemorrhage is caused by rupture of microaneurysms of Charcot–Bouchard on the perforating arteries supplying the basal ganglia.

## Secondary intracerebral haemorrhage
This is bleeding due to identifiable other pathology, such as:
- Haemorrhagic transformation of pre-existing ischaemic CVA
- Haemorrhagic contusion after trauma
- Bleed into a tumour
- Ruptured arteriovenous malformation (AVM)
- Ruptured berry aneurysm (if aneurysm is adherent to brain, bleeding is intracerebral rather than subarachnoid)
- Amyloid angiopathy
- Post-surgical

**CHAPTER 6**

607

**Intracranial pressure and its relationship to intracranial volume**

The Monro–Kellie hypothesis states that the sum volume of all intracranial contents is constant and an increase in one must be offset by a decrease in another if ICP is not to rise. Compensatory mechanisms can cope with about 20 ml of increased intracranial volume before ICP begins to rise significantly. Rapid changes in volume are tolerated less well. If the ICP is already elevated, small changes in volume can cause large changes in ICP (Figure 6.8).

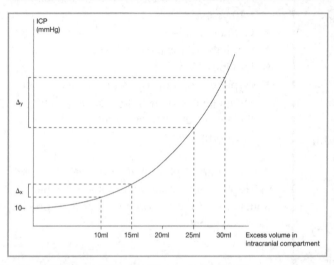

**Figure 6.8 The Monro–Kellie hypothesis:** increasing intracranial volume produces an increase in intracranial pressure (ICP). At higher ICP (or intracranial volume) an equal further increase in intracranial volume produces a much larger rise in ICP (compare 5 ml increase from 10 ml [Δx] with 5 ml increase from 25 ml [Δy]). ICP starts to increase more rapidly above 20 ml of excess intracranial volume as compensatory mechanisms start to fail

**Non-surgical interventions to control ICP**

Enhance venous outflow: head up at 30°, neck straight, consider loosening cervical collar (if intubated and depending on fracture) or tight tracheostomy tape. Cervical spine stabilisation can be maintained with sandbags.

Anaesthetise, paralyse and ventilate.

Mannitol or hypotonic saline boluses (repeated mannitol boluses will increase serum osmolality. Aim to keep serum osmolality <320 mmol/kg).

Optimise $PaCO_2$. Hyperventilate (only to $PaCO_2$ 30–35 mmHg [4.00–4.66 kPa]) if other ICP control measures fail to manage acute exacerbations (peak effect is at about 10 min). Hypocapnia decreases intracranial blood volume by vasoconstriction but can induce hypoxia.

Hypothermia (target temperature controversial; some say 'cool' to normoxia).

GABAergic burst suppression with thiopental (GABA is γ-aminobutyric acid).

**Surgical interventions to control ICP**

Remove space-occupying lesion (eg haematoma).

Drain CSF (external ventricular drain, lumbar puncture if **not** contraindicated).

Decompressive craniectomy – remove part of skull vault to allow brain to swell (current focus of RESCUEicp study; DECRA trial did not support its use).

CHAPTER 6

## Clinical features of intracerebral haemorrhage

Compared with embolic CVA, haemorrhagic CVA usually has the following features:

- Headache and/or vomiting as a pronounced symptom
- Association with depression of conscious level
- Neurological deficit that deteriorates over minutes or hours, as opposed to ischaemic CVA, where the deficit is maximal at presentation

## Role of surgery for intracerebral haemorrhage

Although studies have shown that survival is improved with surgery in some subgroups of patients with primary intracerebral haemorrhage (ICH), morbidity remains high (compared with medical management). Patients who survive are rarely independent at discharge. The STICH II study is asking whether a subgroup of patients with more superficial non-traumatic ICH benefits from surgery.

Surgery cannot reverse a focal neurological defect resulting from damaged brain tissue. Surgery simply removes haematoma, decreases ICP, and thereby hopes to reduce the risk of secondary damage to the rest of the brain and subsequent death.

Factors to consider are:

- **Age**
- **Site of haematoma:** for deep haematomas surgical access requires going through undamaged brain tissue, with the potential to cause more functional deficit. Superficial or surfacing haematomas are easier to evacuate without damaging normal brain tissue
- **Side:** dominant hemisphere haematomas carry a worse prognosis than non-dominant haematomas, because of the important structures already damaged; Broca's and Wernicke's areas are on the dominant side
- **Initial presentation and conscious level:** initial minor deficit and deterioration of conscious level thereafter suggests that ICP is a major problem and evacuation of the clot may be of benefit. Severe deficit or coma from the outset suggests that primary brain damage caused by a bleed is a major problem and evacuation of the clot is unlikely to be helpful
- **Comorbidity**
- **Wishes of the patient** (if expressed) and family
- **Presence of other treatable pathology** such as an AVM or aneurysm that needs clipping, or tumour that needs biopsy/debulk, in a patient who would otherwise not need surgery simply for the haematoma

## Subarachnoid haemorrhage

 **In a nutshell ...**

Note that the most common cause of subarachnoid blood seen on CT is trauma; history is crucial.

Of spontaneous subarachnoid haemorrhage:

- 75% are due to ruptured intracranial aneurysm
- 5% are due to AVM

There are rare causes:

- Vasculitis
- Clotting disorder
- Pituitary apoplexy
- Extending carotid dissection

No cause is identified in about 20%.

## Epidemiology of aneurysmal subarachnoid haemorrhage

- Incidence is about 1 in 10 000 per year
- Postmortem prevalence of intracranial aneurysms is about 1 in 20 (5%)
- Not all aneurysms will rupture (so screening is problematic)

**Risk factors** include:
- Hypertension (especially transient episodes)
- Smoking
- Substance abuse (especially cocaine)
- Polycystic kidney disease (**not** polycystic ovary)
- Connective tissue disorders:
  - Marfan syndrome
  - Ehlers–Danlos syndrome type IV
  - Neurofibromatosis type 1

## Pathology and aetiology of subarachnoid aneurysms

- There is less smooth muscle and less elastin in the media and adventitia of intracranial vessels
- The vessels lie free in the subarachnoid space so they are less supported
- Aneurysms tend to arise at branch points and at areas of haemodynamic stress (hence the high incidence in the circle of Willis)
- They may not grow smoothly but in fits and starts, perhaps associated with transient elevations of BP (hence association with cocaine use)

Other causes:
- Direct trauma to the vessels
- Infection (mycotic aneurysms occur in 3–10% of patients with infective endocarditis; often multiple)

## Presentation of subarachnoid haemorrhage

- Sudden onset of headache is the cardinal feature
- Beware: 30% of subarachnoid haemorrhage (SAH) occurs during sleep and the history may not be characteristic
- Meningism (neck stiffness, photophobia)
- Focal neurological deficit and/or depressed conscious level in some

## Investigation of subarachnoid haemorrhage

- **CT:** modern scanners will detect 95% of subarachnoid haemorrhages
- **Lumbar puncture:** there are equal numbers of red cells in tubes 1 and 3. CSF xanthochromia (red cell breakdown products in the CSF) is diagnostic but may not occur for 6–12 hours after symptom onset. With a bloody tap it is important to spin down CSF immediately and decant off the supernatant to test for xanthochromia (otherwise in-vitro red cell breakdown can cause a false-positive result)
- **Angiography** (digital subtraction, MR or CT): defines the anatomy of any aneurysm

## Complications of subarachnoid haemorrhage

- **Rebleeding:**
  - Often more severe than initial bleed (80% mortality rate)
  - 3% risk in the first 24 hours after the initial bleed
  - 1% per day thereafter for about a month
  - Purpose of surgery is to prevent rebleeding

- **Hyponatraemia:**
  - Loss of sodium in the urine after SAH (cerebral salt wasting)
  - May be due to rise in natriuretic peptides
  - Usually associated with hypovolaemia
  - Treated with 'triple H' therapy (see box on page 612)
- **Vasospasm:**
  - Called 'delayed ischaemic deficit'
  - Major cause of residual disability after SAH
  - May be due to breakdown products of blood in the CSF
  - Usually occurs between 3 and 10 days after a bleed
  - Treated with calcium channel

antagonists (nimodipine) and 'triple H' therapy (see box page 612)
- **Hydrocephalus:**
  - Blood in the subarachnoid space interferes with CSF flow through the ventricles and over the brain convexity
  - May also affect CSF resorption at arachnoid granulations
  - May be transient or chronic after SAH
  - Transient headache can be treated temporarily with analgesia. Lumbar puncture, external ventricular drain or ventriculoperitoneal shunt in chronic cases
- **Seizures**
- **Cardiac abnormalities:** arrhythmia and ECG changes may be seen

---

**Surgery for subarachnoid haemorrhage**

Surgery aims to prevent rebleeding.

**Clipping of aneurysms**

Titanium clips are applied around the neck of the aneurysm, via a craniotomy. This requires brain retraction to access vessels at the base of the brain, with risk of damage to important perforating blood vessels and neurological deficits.

**Coiling of aneurysms**

Platinum coils (GDC) are inserted into the lumen of the aneurysm via an endovascular technique, to encourage the aneurysm to thrombose.

- Recent trials show coiling results in less morbidity
- Some aneurysms are not coilable; some are not clippable
- Long-term follow-up required (Do coiled aneurysms recur? Clipping considered definitive)

**Clips, coils and MR scanners**

There is a case report of an aneurysm clip being moved by the magnetic field of a magnetic resonance (MR) scanner with fatal consequences.

If a patient has an intracranial clip or coil in situ it must be assumed that they are not safe to enter an MR scanner until the exact nature of the clip or coil (and its MR compatibility) is known with certainty. This may involve contacting the manufacturer. An inventory of MR-compatible implants is available.

Most modern clips and coils are made of titanium or platinum and are safe in an MR scanner, but any metal object will interfere with the local field strength in the scanner and cause artefact and signal loss (drop-out) in the region of the object. This may seriously limit the diagnostic utility of the scan.

**CHAPTER 6**

> **'Triple H' therapy for subarachnoid haemorrhage**
>
> 'Triple H' therapy consists of:
> - Hypervolaemia
> - Hypertension
> - Haemodilution
>
> This involves use of aggressive fluid resuscitation to keep the intravascular compartment well filled, thereby preserving flow through any spastic vessels. Physiological (0.9%) saline is used to prevent hyponatraemia from cerebral salt wasting. Usually at least 3 litres 0.9% saline per day is given, and often more is needed. Despite the sodium load, iatrogenic cardiac failure in a patient with SAH is rare.
>
> Inotropes or vasopressors are used if signs of vasospasm persist despite adequate volume expansion. This requires a high dependency unit (HDU) setting because accurate fluid balance measurement and close monitoring of neurological observations is needed. Intensive therapy unit (ITU) and anaesthetic input may be needed.
>
> **Note:** care must be taken if the patient has an untreated aneurysm, because elevating the blood volume and pressure can precipitate rebleeding. This is an argument for treating/ securing aneurysms early.

## Outcome after subarachnoid haemorrhage

- 10% die before arriving in hospital
- 30-day mortality rate is 40–50%
- 30% of survivors have moderate or severe disability after an SAH
- 35% have mild or no deficit

# Chronic subdural haematoma

This is, strictly speaking, a traumatic brain injury, but it often presents (50%) with no history of trauma. It is a common referral for semi-elective neurosurgery.

## Aetiology of chronic subdural haematoma

- Usually occurs in the context of pre-existing brain atrophy
- Risk factors:
  - Age
  - Alcohol
  - Dementia
- In atrophy, cerebral veins are tented across the subdural space
- Minor head injury causes a vein tear and leak into the subdural space
- Causes in the young adult: intracranial hypotension, vascular malformations, haematological malignancies causing thrombocytopenia, solid tumour dural metastases, infection, hypervitaminosis, coagulopathy
- The leak is at low pressure, so may not cause symptoms initially
- The inflammatory response causes clot lysis and membrane formation in the subdural space
- The balance of rebleeding and exudation from, and resorption into, capillaries in the membranes determines whether the clot is resorbed or enlarges

## Presentation of chronic subdural haematoma

- Patients are usually elderly
- Mild headache
- Confusion
- Coma
- Less often, gradual onset of focal neurological signs
- May present acutely if large rebleed into pre-existing subdural haematoma

Symptoms may fluctuate.

## Management of chronic subdural haematoma

- Burr hole drainage of subdural space (see the box below)
- 25% symptomatic recurrence. May need re-do surgery

---

**Burr hole drainage of chronic subdural haematoma**

Can be performed under local or general anaesthetic (LA or GA), with antibiotic prophylaxis. Usually two burr holes are required. Common positions are posterior frontal and posterior parietal, although exact positions are chosen using CT as a guide. Care must be taken to avoid the course of the middle meningeal artery and the dural venous sinuses.

Burr holes are made with a brace and bit or an automatic burr. Care must be taken to avoid plunging the burr into the cranial cavity once the inner table has been breached.

The dura is incised and the chronic haematoma is irrigated using copious quantities (litres) of warm saline. The saline should flow between the two burr holes and should run clear at the end of the procedure.

Re-expansion of the brain into the space occupied by the haematoma is a good sign. If the brain does not re-expand there is more chance that the subdural haematoma will re-collect and require repeat surgery. Re-expansion may be prevented by persistent clot membranes. Expansion of the brain can be facilitated (under GA) by asking the anaesthetist to perform a Valsalva manoeuvre and bring up the $PCO_2$.

A recent study has supported the use of burr hole drains at the end of the procedure. The galea and skin are closed as separate layers. The dependent hole is closed first and any cavity left behind filled with saline before closing the upper hole.

**Potential complications**
- Infection
- Bleeding (requiring craniotomy)
- Recurrence
- Technical success but no impact on neurology
- GA risks

## 1.4　Brain tumours

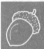

> **In a nutshell …**
>
> **Cerebral metastasis** (the most common brain tumour)
> **Gliomas** (50% of primary brain tumours)
> - Glioblastoma multiforme (GBM)
> - Anaplastic astrocytoma (AA)
>
> **Meningiomas**
> **Pituitary tumours**

### Presentation of brain tumours
- Progressive onset of neurological deficit (compared with CVA): usually the deficit is motor
- Signs of raised ICP (mass effects) from tumour or oedema
- Seizure (consider especially in a new seizure disorder in an adult)
- Sudden onset of symptoms: if presentation is due to a bleed into a tumour

### Cerebral metastasis
The most common brain tumour is metastasis from outside the CNS:
- 30–50% of brain tumours are metastases
- 15% of patients with malignancy present with a brain metastasis as the presenting symptom
- 50% of brain metastases are solitary on CT (30% on MRI)
- They seed at the interface of grey and white matter

**Common origins** are:
- Lung
- Breast
- Bowel
- Melanoma
- Renal cell

### Investigating cerebral metastasis
Search for a primary, using at least the following investigations:
- Thorough history and examination (including breast and skin)
- Chest radiograph
- Markers: liver function tests, bone profile, faecal occult blood (FOB)
- Consider also abdominal/pelvic CT, endoscopy and/or bone scan

If no primary is found you need to get a tissue diagnosis, using:
- Stereotactic brain biopsy
- Excision biopsy

### Management of cerebral metastasis
See also 'Management of primary brain tumours' on page 617.
- **Corticosteroids** (reduce oedema and associated mass effect):
  - Dexamethasone 4 mg orally four times daily
  - Usually with gastric protection such as ranitidine or proton pump inhibitor
- **Anticonvulsants** – if symptomatic with seizures
- **Chemotherapy**
- **Radiotherapy:**
  - Of whole brain
  - To lesion only (stereotactic radiosurgery)
- **Excision** ('metastasectomy') is only suitable if:
  - Patient is fit
  - Symptomatic lesion is in an accessible location
  - There is a good prognosis of the primary (extracerebral) lesion

> **Metastasectomy**
> This can be performed through a small incision and 'mini-craniotomy'. It requires **accurate localisation of the lesion in theatre** to allow accurate siting of the incision and craniotomy.
> This is facilitated by:
> - 'Neuro-navigation' devices which allow surgical instruments to be tracked relative to the lesion's position in real time during surgery
> - Stereotactic frame

## Primary brain tumours

The existing classification based on putative cell lineage of origin is problematic because we don't fully understand the origin of brain tumours. It serves as a starting point, however:

- Glial cell origin ('glioma'):
  - Astrocytoma
  - Oligodendroglioma
  - Ependymoma
- Non-glial cell origin:
  - Mesenchymal tumours (meningioma)
  - Pituitary lesions
  - Nerve sheath tumours (schwannoma, neurofibroma)
  - Haematopoietic tumours (primary cerebral lymphoma)
  - Germ-cell tumours (germinoma, teratoma)
  - Neuronal tumours
  - Others, including craniopharyngioma

This is by no means an exhaustive list!

The most common forms of primary brain tumour are:
- **Glioma** (50% of primary brain tumours): three-quarters are high grade (GBM or AA – see below)

- **Meningioma** (15% of primary brain tumours)
- **Pituitary lesions** (5% of primary brain tumours)

## Glioblastoma multiforme

This is the most common form of primary brain tumour: WHO grade IV.

Survival after optimum treatment is:
- Approximately 35% at 1 year
- Approximately 10% at 2 years
- Median 14.6 months

Tumours are non-resectable because of tumour cell migration. Malignant cells may be found at a distance from the lesion in otherwise normal brain tissue. Some cases of GBM arise anew, others from de-differentiation of low-grade astrocytomas.

The macroscopic appearance is of:
- Greyish ill-defined mass
- Areas of necrosis and haemorrhage

Histology is variable (hence 'multiforme'):
- Regional heterogeneity within a single lesion
- Highly anaplastic glial cells
- Vascular proliferation and thrombosis (diagnostic)
- Necrosis (diagnostic)

## Anaplastic astrocytoma

This is also known as 'malignant astrocytoma': WHO grade III. It is the second most common primary brain tumour after GBM.

Survival (after optimum treatment) is:
- 65% at 1 year
- 45% at 2 years
- Median 2 years

CHAPTER 6

615

It is non-resectable, for the same reason as GBM. The macroscopic appearance is of:

- White ill-defined mass, sometimes expanding into a gyrus

Histology shows:

- Diffusely infiltrating astrocytes
- Nuclear atypia
- **No** microvascular proliferation or necrosis (seen only with GBM)

## Meningioma

Meningioma arises from arachnoid cap cells. It is usually benign (WHO grade I) and slow growing. It may be found incidentally on imaging for unrelated symptoms. Meningiomas can more rarely be higher grade or even anaplastic.

Complete resection is usually curative. Small asymptomatic meningiomas generally do not need surgery.

Macroscopic appearance is of:

- Rubbery, round, lobulated mass
- Firmly attached to dura

Histology shows:

- Many types (meningothelial, fibroblastic, transitional, and many more)
- Calcification, not uncommon (psammoma bodies)
- Whorls and lobules of cells in some types
- Sheets of spindle-shaped cells in others
- Histological type does **not** correlate with prognosis

## Diagnosis of primary brain tumours

### Imaging

- **CT** – pre-contrast and post-contrast scans usually required:
  - Lesion enhancement with contrast is possible only if there is a defect in the blood–brain barrier in the lesion
  - Some lesions are relatively homogeneous and show quite uniform enhancement with contrast (eg meningioma)
  - Some lesions are heterogeneous with areas of increased attenuation (whiter) and areas of decreased attenuation (darker), and show non-uniform enhancement (eg GBM)
  - CT scan (even with contrast) may miss small lesions
- **MRI:** more sensitive than CT. Smaller lesions can be identified. Commonly used sequences are:
  - T1-weighted: CSF low signal (dark)
  - T2-weighted: CSF high signal (white)
  - FLAIR: selective suppression of water signal (for periventricular lesions)
  - STIR: selective suppression of fat signal (often shows pathology very conspicuously)
- Stereotactic brain biopsy

## Stereotactic brain biopsy

The **stereotactic frame** consists of three parts:

- Base ring
- Reference frame with CT- or MRI-visible reference markers (fiducials)
- Biopsy (adjustable) frame with a guide that directs biopsy needle to its centre

### Procedure

The base ring is firmly pinned to the patient's skull and the reference frame is attached to it. The patient's head is scanned within the reference frame. Target points within the lesion are chosen (with the mouse).

The scanner software calculates $x$, $y$ and $z$ coordinates of the target relative to the base ring. The reference frame is removed and replaced with the adjustable frame. The centre of the adjustable frame is set to the target point by moving the adjustable frame relative to the base ring according to these x, y and z coordinates.

A needle is passed through the needle guide to the centre of the adjustable frame (ie to the target). The needle guide can be moved such that the centre of the frame (target) can be approached from any trajectory. This allows the surgeon to avoid passing the needle through eloquent areas of the cortex.

It is accurate to within 2 mm.

### Risks

- Inconclusive sample <5%
- Death (haemorrhage) <1%

## Management of primary brain tumours

- **Surgery:** biopsy is necessary for diagnosis, particularly to exclude non-glioma pathologies such as lymphoma that might require other treatment strategies. Debulking is not curative – see box 'Debulking surgery for primary brain tumours' below
- **Radiotherapy:** this is mainly used for malignant neoplasms. It is the standard adjuvant therapy for treatment of most high-grade gliomas. Radiotherapy has more impact on survival than the type of surgery (debulking versus biopsy)
- **Stereotactic radiosurgery:** this is high-dose radiation therapy from multiple trajectories converging on the target tumour tissue. Maximises treatment to the target, minimises effect on normal tissue. The target is identified with a modified stereotactic frame. The target needs to be small (<3 cm). Stereotactic radiosurgery can be done as a one-shot day case or a fractionated course. Accepted indications are:
  - AVM – useful for lesions not amenable to clipping or coiling, or as part of a combined procedure
  - Vestibular schwannoma (acoustic neuroma)
  - Metastasis

## Adjuvant therapies

- **Chemotherapy:** this is routine for high-grade gliomas (AAs and GBM) in all but the most unfit/elderly. It also has a role in other tumours such as lymphoma, and in some childhood tumours. Chemotherapy can be administered either intravenously (temozolomide) or via wafers left in the operative bed at the end of debulking surgery (carmustine, Gliadel)

**CHAPTER 6**

617

- **Corticosteroids:** these reduce oedema and the associated mass effect. Give dexamethasone 4 mg orally four times daily, usually with gastric protection
- **Anticonvulsants:** give as necessary to control symptoms

Sometimes a watch-and-wait policy is indicated, especially if symptoms can be controlled by other means (eg low-grade gliomas causing seizures that can be controlled with anticonvulsants). It is uncertain how to predict if and when a low-grade tumour will convert into a higher-grade lesion.

---

**Debulking surgery for malignant primary brain tumours**

Curative resection is not possible for GBM and AA. Debulking (cytoreductive) surgery increases median survival (but not drastically) in younger, fitter patients. Surgery may also be justified to decrease mass effects for symptom relief, to reduce ICP, or to remove a lesion causing motor symptoms due to local pressure/oedema effects.

In other patients, especially those aged >65 years, the benefit of debulking surgery over other treatments is minimal. The aim is to prolong **quality survival**.

---

# 1.5 Pituitary disease and other endocrine abnormalities

 **In a nutshell ...**

Endocrine abnormalities can be associated with neurosurgical conditions. Pituitary disease, syndrome of inappropriate antidiuretic hormone secretion (SIADH) and diabetes insipidus should be understood by the neurosurgeon.

## Pituitary anatomy

The pituitary lies in the sella turcica of the sphenoid bone. The sella is roofed in by a fold of dura (diaphragma sella) through which the pituitary stalk passes, connecting the pituitary with the hypothalamus.

The pituitary consists of two anatomically distinct parts:
1. **Adenohypophysis (anterior lobe):** endocrine tissue; embryologically derived from a bud of ectoderm from the posterior wall of the oral cavity (Rathke pouch)
2. **Neurohypophysis (posterior lobe):** nervous tissue; an inferior extension of the median eminence of the hypothalamus

**Important relationships** of the pituitary are:
- Superiorly:
  - Hypothalamus
  - Optic chiasm (hence enlarging pituitary tumours can impinge upon the decussating nasal retinal fibres of the optic chiasm, causing a characteristic visual field defect – bitemporal hemianopia)

CHAPTER 6

- Optic tract: more posteriorly – pressure from tumours on the optic tract can cause a contralateral homonymous hemianopia
- Inferiorly:
  - Sphenoid sinus (allows trans-sphenoidal surgical access to the pituitary)
- Laterally:
  - Cavernous sinus and its contents, including the internal carotid artery and cranial nerves III, IV, Va, Vb and VI

## Blood supply of the pituitary

The pituitary blood supply is a portal system whereby blood passes through two sets of capillary beds before draining into the veins. This arrangement allows close control of pituitary function by the hypothalamus.

## Arterial supply of the pituitary

- This is from the meningohypophyseal trunk
- The trunk arises from the common carotid and gives off inferior and superior hypophyseal branches
- The inferior branch supplies the posterior pituitary
- The superior branch enters the capillary bed of the hypothalamus. The capillaries drain into the sinusoids that run down into the adenohypophysis. The sinusoids divide in the adenohypophysis to form a second capillary bed around endocrine cells here

## Venous drainage of the pituitary

- This is via venules directly into the cavernous sinus (thence by the petrosal sinuses to the jugular vein)

## Pituitary physiology

The hypothalamus and pituitary gland are the dominant controllers of the endocrine system.

The blood–brain barrier is absent in the pituitary. This allows hormones in the bloodstream easy access to cells of the pituitary, facilitating feedback loops (see below).

### Anterior pituitary

Releasing and inhibiting hormones are stored in neurosecretory granules in the nerve terminals of the hypothalamic neurones.

On release these hormones travel through the portal venous system to the endocrine cells of the anterior pituitary, where they stimulate or inhibit release of pituitary hormones.

The function of the anterior pituitary is, therefore, largely controlled by the hypothalamus (but see 'Negative feedback' below – feedback loops also affect hormone release).

### Posterior pituitary

These hormones are synthesised in the hypothalamus. They travel down the axons of hypothalamic nerve cells to nerve terminals in the posterior pituitary, where they are stored in neurosecretory granules.

The hormones are released directly into the bloodstream, bypassing the portal venous system. The following table summarises pituitary hormonal control and the peripheral actions of the pituitary hormones.

CHAPTER 6

## PITUITARY HORMONAL CONTROL AND PERIPHERAL ACTIONS OF HORMONES

| Site of release | Pituitary hormone | Controlling hormones (from hypothalamus) | Target organ | Effect |
|---|---|---|---|---|
| Anterior pituitary | ACTH | CRF | Adrenal cortex | Corticosteroid release from adrenal |
| | TSH | TRF | Thyroid | Thyroxine release ($T_3$ and $T_4$) |
| | GH | GHRH, GHIH | Widespread: liver, muscle, bone, adipose tissue | Anabolic action and growth |
| | FSH | GnRH | Ovaries and testes | Follicle development (female) and spermatogenesis (male) |
| | LH | GnRH | Ovaries and testes | Oestradiol and testosterone production (male and female) Progesterone production and control over ovulation (female) |
| | Prolactin | PIF, PRF | Breast | Breast hyperplasia (in pregnancy) and milk production |
| Posterior pituitary | ADH | None | Distal tubule and collecting ducts of kidney Arteriolar smooth muscle | Water resorption Vasoconstriction |
| | Oxytocin | None | Uterus Myoepithelial cells of the breast | Uterine contraction Breast milk expression |

### Negative feedback

In general, control of the various endocrine secretions of the pituitary is under negative feedback. This often occurs at multiple levels:

- Short loop: from the pituitary back to the hypothalamus
- Long loop: from the target organ to the hypothalamus and pituitary

For example, in control of the adreno-corticotropic axis:

- ACTH inhibits corticotropin-releasing factor (CRF) release (short loop)
- Cortisol inhibits CRF and ACTH release (long loop)

Negative feedback also occurs at the level of the physiological endpoint of a hormone's effect, eg in ADH production decreased plasma osmolality inhibits antidiuretic hormone (ADH) secretion.

Negative feedback helps to maintain a constant hormonal milieu, but some hormone levels show variation overlaid on this background milieu:

- **CRF, ACTH, cortisol:** these show diurnal variation (peaking at about 5–6am) and release is increased in stressful situations
- **Gonadotropin-releasing hormone (GnRH):** pulsatile release (every few hours on average)

- **Follicle-stimulating hormone (FSH), luteinising hormone (LH), sex steroid hormones:** change with menstrual cycle in women

## Positive feedback

Positive feedback loops are also seen, especially where a large surge in a hormone level is required. Positive and negative feedback loops are delicately balanced to allow complex patterns of hormonal release, eg the LH surge that occurs mid-menstrual cycle in females is positive feedback from oestradiol.

## Pituitary tumours

Pituitary tumours are best managed by a multidisciplinary team consisting of endocrinologists, radiotherapists, neurosurgeons and ophthalmologists.

## Classification of pituitary tumours

### Functional tumours

- These tumours secrete hormones (usually in excess)
- Usually present with symptoms attributable to excess hormone production, such as:
  - Acromegaly (excess of growth hormone) – see Chapter 4, Endocrine Surgery
  - Cushing's disease (excess of ACTH) – see Chapter 4, Endocrine Surgery
  - Galactorrhoea (milky nipple discharge) and infertility in women (excess of prolactin)
  - Hyperthyroidism (excess of thyroid-stimulating hormone) – rare

### Non-functional tumours

- These tumours do not secrete hormones

- Usually present with local symptoms of mass effect:
  - Visual field defects or deteriorating visual acuity
  - Headache
  - Cranial nerve palsy/proptosis (if invading cavernous sinus)
- May present with symptoms of hormone underproduction due to compression of normal glandular tissue in the sella

Alternatively, tumours can be classified according to their cell of origin or size:
- Microadenomas are <10 mm
- Macroadenomas are >10 mm

Five per cent of pituitary tumours are locally invasive. Distant spread (CSF or blood-borne) is rare.

## Investigating pituitary tumours

- Assessment of vision
- Endocrine tests
- Imaging
  - MRI: the investigation of choice
  - CT or plain films: may show an enlarged sella
- Petrosal sinus sampling: to lateralise a functional tumour not seen on imaging

## Treatment of pituitary tumours

Treatment depends on the presentation and type of tumour.
- **Surgery** is recommended for:
  - Non-functional tumours presenting with mass effects
  - Cushing's disease
  - Acromegaly
  - Acute visual deterioration
  - Pituitary apoplexy

- **Medical therapy** is for:
  - Prolactinomas: most will shrink with dopamine agonists
  - Patients in whom surgery is impossible, is declined or has failed
- **Radiotherapy** is primarily used for residual or recurrent tumour after surgery

---

**Surgery for pituitary tumours**
- Trans-sphenoidal approach to sella
- Alternatives are transcranial or transethmoidal
- Complications include hormonal imbalance, CSF leak, infection, hydrocephalus

---

## Pituitary apoplexy

- This is due to a bleed in the sella, usually into a pre-existing tumour
- It presents with sudden-onset headache with or without visual disturbance and deterioration in conscious level (much like SAH)
- It causes acute panhypopituitarism and patients can go into acute addisonian crisis
- Acute surgery is indicated if there is rapid deterioration in visual acuity or fields

## Endocrine abnormalities associated with other neurosurgical conditions

### Syndrome of inappropriate ADH secretion (SIADH)

#### Associations of SIADH

- Raised ICP:
  - Head injury (5%)

- Intracranial tumour
- Bronchogenic tumours:
  - Paraneoplastic phenomenon
  - Does not necessarily imply cerebral metastasis

#### Features of SIADH

- Confusion, lethargy, nausea and vomiting (differential diagnosis includes cerebral space-occupying lesion and a CT of the brain may be needed to exclude this)
- Hyponatraemia and low serum osmolality
- Inappropriately concentrated urine
- Hypervolaemia or euvolaemia

#### Treatment of SIADH

- Fluid restriction (<1 litre/day)
- Monitor sodium

**Note:** it can be difficult, clinically and biochemically, to differentiate between SIADH and cerebral salt wasting. Both produce hyponatraemia and intercurrent treatment may make assessment of volaemic state and urinary osmolality problematic.

As a rule of thumb, **SIADH is very rare after SAH**, and hyponatraemia after SAH should be treated with triple-H therapy. Fluid and salt restriction after SAH can be extremely dangerous (precipitating vasospasm).

### Diabetes insipidus (DI)

There are two types of diabetes insipidus.

#### Central/neurogenic type

- Levels of ADH are low
- Seen most commonly after pituitary surgery: 85% of posterior pituitary must be lost before DI occurs

- Usually transient: due to swelling in the pituitary fossa associated with the surgery

## Nephrogenic type
- ADH is normal or high, but kidneys are unresponsive to it

## Features of DI
- Hypernatraemia and high serum osmolality
- Large output of inappropriately dilute urine
- Thirst (if alert)

## Treatment of DI
- Instruct patient to drink if alert
- Give subcutaneous. DDAVP (desmopressin, an ADH analogue)
- Infuse fluid: 0.9% saline, which is **hypotonic** relative to the patient's plasma; dextrose may drop sodium too quickly
- Closely monitor urine output and plasma and urine sodium and osmolality. Usually requires HDU care

# 1.6 Hydrocephalus

 **In a nutshell ...**

Hydrocephalus presents with symptoms and signs of raised ICP (see Section 1.2). It can present extremely acutely (over minutes) or chronically (over weeks).

## Classification of hydrocephalus
There are two main subgroups of hydrocephalus, communicating and non-communicating.

### Communicating hydrocephalus
- CSF resorption at the arachnoid granulations is arrested or slowed, eg secondary to SAH
- All CSF spaces are increased in volume

### Non-communicating (obstructive) hydrocephalus
There is a block to CSF flow proximal to the arachnoid granulations. A distinction between the two can be made on CT or MRI. This distinction is important because:
- Lumbar puncture is therapeutic and can be life-saving in communicating hydrocephalus
- Lumbar puncture can precipitate tonsillar herniation, coning and death in non-communicating hydrocephalus

## Other types of hydrocephalus

### 'Normal pressure' hydrocephalus
- Clinical triad of dementia, gait dyspraxia and incontinence
- Ventriculomegaly is seen on CT (but could be caused by atrophy, hence *hydrocephalus ex vacuo*)
- Some cases may improve with a ventriculo-peritoneal shunt
- Ascertaining which patient will benefit form treatment is difficult

## Causes of hydrocephalus
- Acquired lesions:
  - Post-meningitis (communicating)
  - Post-SAH, including traumatic or aneurysmal (communicating)
  - Space-occupying lesions that obstruct CSF flow, eg tumours, vascular malformations (non-communicating)

- CSF-producing lesions (choroid plexus papilloma)
- Congenital malformations (non-communicating)

## Treatment of hydrocephalus
- Lumbar puncture in communicating hydrocephalus
- Surgery (see box below). The options are external ventricular drain, ventriculoperitoneal (VP) shunt or third ventriculostomy

---

**Surgical options for hydrocephalus**

**External ventricular drain**

This is only for control of acute hydrocephalus. It is not a long-term solution.
- Insert through a right (non-dominant hemisphere) frontal burr hole
- Pass through the right frontal lobe into the anterior horn of the right lateral ventricle
- Tunnel subcutaneously in the scalp to reduce infection risk
- Connect to a closed drainage system that allows accurate measurement of drainage and will only drain if the ICP exceeds a chosen pressure

**VP shunt**
- The ventricular catheter (usually) inserts into the occipital horn of the lateral ventricle via the burr hole
- Tunnel the peritoneal catheter subcutaneously and insert into the peritoneal cavity at the costal margin
- Connect the two catheters with the valve, which only drains CSF above a certain pressure (to prevent overdrainage and CSF siphoning into the peritoneum)
- Variable-pressure valves are available

***Complications of VP shunt***
- Infection with *Staphylococcus epidermidis* and *S. aureus* primarily (ie skin commensals, usually introduced at time of surgery)
- Blockage (choroid plexus, protein, infection)
- Disconnection/kinking

**Third ventriculostomy**

This is used in non-communicating hydrocephalus. It allows CSF to drain from the ventricles, bypassing a more distal obstruction (eg aqueduct stenosis). It needs good preoperative delineation of anatomy (high-resolution MRI) to avoid damage to adjacent structures.

It is performed endoscopically in the following way:
- Endoscope is inserted into the anterior horn of the lateral ventricle (via burr hole)
- It is navigated into the third ventricle
- Fenestration is made in the floor of the third ventricle (laser, balloon or diathermy)

***Complications of ventriculostomy***
- Uncontrollable bleeding from basilar artery
- Cardiac arrest
- Hypothalamic injury

---

# 1.7   Surgical CNS infections

## Cerebral abscess

### Source of cerebral infection

### Haematogenous spread from another source
- Bronchiectasis
- Bacterial endocarditis
- Dental abscess and caries

### Local spread from an anatomically adjacent source
- Middle-ear infection (especially cholesteatoma)
- Frontal and sphenoid sinusitis
- Usually associated with bone erosion of skull base to allow infection access to cranial cavity

### Pathogens in cerebral abscess
- Streptococci primarily
- Atypical organisms in immunocompromised (especially *Toxoplasma* sp.)

### Presentation of cerebral abscess
- Symptoms of raised ICP
- Seizure
- Focal neurology

### Management of cerebral abscess
- Needle drainage (usually stereotactic)
- Antibiotics

### Prognosis of cerebral abscess
- Low mortality (5–10%) but worsens if empyema develops
- High morbidity with epilepsy, visual impairment, hemiparesis

## Subdural empyema
- Source: usually local spread from paranasal sinuses
- Requires surgical drainage: burr hole or craniotomy

Other intracranial infections are covered in Chapter 5, Head and Neck Surgery.

**CHAPTER 6**

# CHAPTER 7

# Transplant Surgery

**Karen S Stevenson**

CHAPTER 7

# SECTION 1
# Transplantation

## 1.1    Chronic kidney disease

 **In a nutshell ...**

This is a permanent loss in renal function that occurs over a period of several months.
Defined by a glomerular filtration rate (GFR) <60 ml/min per 1.73 m² for 3 months or more.
**Causes of chronic renal failure** are:
- Diabetic nephropathy (34%)
- Hypertension (29%)
- Glomerulonephritis (14%)
- Polycystic kidney disease (14%)
- Chronic pyelonephritis (10%)
- Obstructive/reflux nephropathy

Classification of chronic kidney disease (CKD)

| Stage | Description | GFR (ml/min per 1.73 m²) | Action plan |
|---|---|---|---|
| 1 | Kidney damage with normal or elevated GFR | ≥90 | Diagnosis and treatment, treatment of comorbid conditions, interventions to slow disease progression, reduction of risk factors for cardiovascular disease |
| 2 | Kidney damage with mildly decreased GFR | 60–89 | Estimation of disease progression |
| 3 | Moderately decreased GFR | 30–59 | Evaluation and treatment of disease complications |
| 4 | Severely decreased GFR | 15–29 | Preparation for kidney replacement therapy (dialysis, transplantation) |
| 5 | Kidney failure | <15 (or dialysis) | Kidney replacement therapy if uraemia is present |

## Clinical features of chronic kidney disease

- **Systemic upset:** this is common and often occurs first (symptoms include fatigue, lack of energy, insomnia, anorexia, nausea and vomiting)
- **Anaemia:** caused by relative lack of erythropoietin
- **Platelet dysfunction** (impaired coagulation): occurs in 60% of patients
- **Pericarditis:** caused by high blood urea levels (indication for immediate dialysis)
- **Neuropathy** (peripheral): caused by loss of myelin from peripheral nerves; 'restless legs' a common symptom
- **Encephalopathy:** this is due to high urea levels
- **Renal bone disease 'osteodystrophy':** caused by various factors (eg secondary hyperparathyroidism and vitamin D deficiency)
- **Erectile dysfunction and amenorrhoea:** secondary to hyperprolactinaemia
- **Acquired cystic disease:** particularly common in patients on dialysis (an important predisposing factor for renal carcinoma)
- **Cardiovascular disease:** mortality from cardiovascular disease is 10–20 times greater than in the general population

## Treatment of chronic renal failure

This is a complex subject. Specialist medical advice should be sought. Several features are relevant to surgery:

- Anaemia can be treated with rHu-EPO (recombinant human erythropoietin)
- Protein restriction reduces the accumulation of nitrogenous waste products
- Potassium should also be restricted
- Fluid intake should be made to equal daily urine output + 500 ml for insensible losses
- Acidosis should be treated with sodium bicarbonate
- Dialysis and haemofiltration are ways of replacing the excretory functions of the kidney (see below)

## Dialysis

Dialysis is used in patients with renal failure to replace the excretory functions of the kidney. It relies on two principles:

- **Diffusion:** this relies on a concentration gradient between blood and dialysis fluid
- **Ultrafiltration:** this relies on a pressure difference between blood and dialysis fluid

### Haemodialysis

In this method the blood is pumped from the patient into an extracorporeal dialysis circuit, where it is separated by a semipermeable membrane from the dialysis fluid running in a countercurrent direction. This removes solutes by diffusion. A pump is used to generate a pressure difference for ultrafiltration to remove fluid accumulated during the interval between dialysis sessions.

Large-bore vascular access is required, which can be obtained temporarily through a percutaneous cannula in a central vein; however, most patients require formation of an **arteriovenous fistula** (see section on surgical fistula, below).

An adult requires 4–5 hours of haemodialysis three times a week.

### Peritoneal dialysis

This is performed by introducing fluid into the peritoneal cavity. Solute removal occurs by diffusion across a concentration gradient from extracellular fluid into the peritoneal dialysate. Ultrafiltration is achieved by increased osmotic pressure within the dialysis fluid. This is usually produced by the addition of dextrose; 1500 ml to 3 litres of dialysate is instilled and allowed to remain in situ for several hours before draining and being discarded. The two types of peritoneal dialysis are:

- Continuous ambulatory peritoneal dialysis (CAPD)
- Intermittent peritoneal dialysis (PD)

The lower rates of solute removal by PD are offset by more prolonged treatment times.

---

**Continuous ambulatory peritoneal dialysis**

**CAPD is suitable for patients who:**
- Are mobile and self-caring (to retain independence and continue work)
- Have poor arm veins
- Have extensive atheroma
- Have a needle phobia
- Are children

**CAPD is unsuitable for patients who:**
- Have extensive previous abdominal surgery (intra-abdominal adhesions)
- Have poor dexterity
- Have diabetes with poor glycaemic control on CAPD

---

**Advantages of peritoneal dialysis:**
- Portable
- Can be carried out by the patient at home
- Does not require anticoagulation
- Patients generally feel better on it

PD requires surgical insertion of an indwelling peritoneal catheter (Tenchkoff catheter), placed through a lower midline abdominal incision and held in place by two cuffs (one in the peritoneum and one just under the skin) or laparoscopically.

The most important complication is peritonitis (may require laparotomy and abdominal lavage).

Recurrent peritonitis leads to reduced capacity of the peritoneum to act as an exchange membrane for dialysis (recurrent peritonitis leads to scarring and long-term peritoneal dialysis leads to glycosylation of the peritoneal membrane).

Sclerosing peritonitis is a complication of long-term peritoneal dialysis characterised by diffuse fibrous thickening of the peritoneal membrane, which can lead to encapsulation and subsequent small-bowel obstruction.

## Haemofiltration

This is used mainly on an intensive therapy unit (ITU) for short-term management. Blood is driven through a filter using the patient's BP to allow ultrafiltration. It is simpler than haemodialysis because a pump is not required.

It is very useful for removing large volumes of fluid in fluid-overloaded patients.

**CHAPTER 7**

| Advantages | Disadvantages |
| --- | --- |
| **Haemodialysis** | |
| Shorter treatment time<br>Efficient small-solute removal (K$^+$)<br>Community and close follow-up at dialysis unit | Requires heparinisation<br>Requires vascular access (central vein cannula or arterio-venous fistula)<br>Large fluid shifts<br>Blood pressure control more difficult<br>Need to attend treatment centres regularly<br>To perform at home requires a willing carer and training |
| **Peritoneal dialysis** | |
| Biochemical changes less marked (steady state achieved)<br>Higher haematocrit<br>Self-care form of therapy<br>Efficient large-solute removal | Peritonitis<br>Hernia formation |

## Arteriovenous fistula

These are created for vascular access in patients with renal failure who need regular haemodialysis. It avoids the need for a long-term percutaneous central venous catheter, which carries risks of infection, central venous stenosis and thrombosis.

## Types of arteriovenous fistula

* **Autologous:** direct joining of a vein with a neighbouring artery, usually end vein to side artery, using the principles of the Brescia–Cimino technique
* **Autologous bridge:** a vein and an artery are joined using a separate vein graft (eg saphenous vein)
* **Synthetic loop grafts:** an artery and vein are joined by a loop of graft tunnelled subcutaneously

## Sites of arteriovenous fistulae

In order of preference these are: radiocephalic, brachiocephalic, brachiobasilic, forearm loop, thigh loop graft using long saphenous vein or synthetic Gore-Tex graft. The non-dominant hand and more distal sites are usually considered first.

## Preoperative issues that you should consider

* Which is the patient's dominant hand?
* Were there any previous attempts at access and reasons for failure?
* Examine the forearm veins, if necessary using a proximal tourniquet (40 mmHg)
* Aim for an autologous fistula, but warn the patient of the risks of synthetic bridges in case the veins aren't good enough
* Perform the Allen test (see Chapter 3, Cardiothoracic Surgery) to evaluate potential arterial inflow sites. Non-palpable pulses should not be used. Increasingly preoperative planning using duplex ultrasonography is used to identify aberrant anatomy or unsatisfactory-calibre vessels
* Exclude local or systemic infection

## Postoperative complications

- Nerve injury: especially radial and median
- Thrombosis: usually due to poor flow, kinking or compression by haematoma
- Steal phenomenon: claudication symptoms due to inadequate perfusion. Treated by ligating artery just distal to the graft, except in proximal fistulae which require bypass
- Infection: especially in synthetic grafts
- False aneurysm
- Venous hypertension
- Cardiac failure (high-flow fistulae only)

## 1.2 Principles of transplantation

### In a nutshell ...

In the event of organ failure, transplantation is an option. Most commonly performed in the kidney, liver, heart and lung; other organs are increasingly being transplanted. Donors may be dead or alive.

**Dead (cadaveric)**
- Donors after brainstem death (DBD)
- Donors after circulatory death (DCD)

**Alive**
- Related
- Unrelated
- Altruistic

Issues to be addressed when discussing any organ transplantation are consent, compatibility, immunosuppression and rejection.

### Organs commonly used for transplantation
- Blood (transfusion)
- Kidney – see below
- Liver – see below
- Heart ± lung
- Pancreas – see below
- Bone
- Small bowel – see below
- Skin (for treatment of burns)

## Cadaveric donors

### Donors after brainstem death

Donors who meet the criteria for brainstem death, usually after trauma or intracranial bleed, who continue to be ventilated on the ITU, are classified as brainstem-dead donors. Organs (usually multiple) are retrieved in the operating theatre, where ventilation is ceased.

### Donors after circulatory death

Donors after circulatory death are classified by the Maastricht criteria.

### Maastricht category

| | |
|---|---|
| I | Dead on arrival (uncontrolled) |
| II | Unsuccessful resuscitation (uncontrolled) |
| III | Awaiting cardiac arrest (controlled) |
| IV | Cardiac arrest while brain-dead (controlled) |

The time from functional warm ischaemia to organ retrieval is crucial to the quality and usability of organs retrieved in these cases.

## Cadaveric surgical organ retrieval

There are three stages of cadaveric organ retrieval from DBD donors.

## The warm ischaemic time

In the warm phase the heart is still beating and the major vessels are cannulated (thoracic vessels for retrieval of the heart, abdominal aorta and portal system for intra-abdominal organs).

## Perfusion of the organs

Perfusion of the organs with ice-cold perfusion solution and cessation of ventilation heralds the start of the cold ischaemic time. Perfusion solutions (eg University of Wisconsin or Marshall solution) contain:

- Impermeable solutes (minimise cellular swelling)
- Buffers (for pH balance)
- Free radical scavengers and inhibitors
- Membrane stabilisers
- Adenosine (for ATP synthesis)

## The cold ischaemic time

In the cold phase the organ is removed from the body cavity and packaged in ice for transport. In general, kidneys are transplanted within 24 hours and livers within 12 hours.

In donors after circulatory death the vessels are cannulated after spontaneous cardiac arrest; organs are therefore exposed to a longer warm ischaemia time due to the peri-arrest period of hypotension.

---

**In organ retrieval from donors after circulatory death**

**Primary warm ischaemic time** is the time from cessation of mechanical cardiac function to the perfusion of the organs with cold preservation solution in situ.

**The functional (or true) warm ischaemic period** commences when the systolic blood pressure has a sustained (ie at least 2 min) fall to <50 mmHg (or the haemoglobin oxygen saturation <70%) and extends up to the onset of cold in situ perfusion.

---

## Live donors

There are increasing numbers of live donors who are either related or non-related. Live related donors are usually first-degree relatives whereas unrelated donors include spouses and, in some cases, 'altruistic' donors.

In order to maximise the number of patients who can benefit from live donation of kidneys in the UK, a system allows paired organ donation between two or three pairs of donor/recipient combinations who alone are incompatible.

CHAPTER 7

## Evaluation of a live donor

- Complete history and examination
- Psychological examination
- Evaluation of BMI (body mass index)
- Blood pressure measurements on three separate occasions
- Blood tests – FBC (full blood count), coagulation screen, U&Es (urea and electrolytes), LFTs (liver function tests), bone profile , fasting blood sugar, fasting cholesterol and triglycerides
- Timed urine collection to measure creatinine clearance or measurement of GFR using radiolabelled filtration marker
- 24-hour urine collection to measure protein
- ECG
- Viral serologies: HIV, hepatitis B and C, HTLV-1, cytomegalovirus, Epstein–Barr virus
- VRDL (Venereal Reference Disease Laboratory)
- Renal imaging: CT angiogram or MR angiogram, renal ultrasonography
- Independent assessment by approved person authorised by the Human Tissue Authority

## Kidney donation

There is an increasing frequency of live kidney donation at multiple UK centres, and live renal transplantation now accounts for 40% of transplantations. Donor work-up includes recipient cross-match, screening for transmissible disease, MR angiography and isotope renography (the donor keeps the kidney with a greater functional percentage). Donor nephrectomy is open via loin incision or laparoscopic (total or hand-assisted). Donors usually have normal renal function post-transplantation but can develop mild hypertension and proteinuria later in life.

There has been an increase in the use of kidneys from expanded criteria donors (ECDs) to meet the growing need for donor organs.

## Living ECD criteria

1. Age >60 years or 50–59 years
2. Pre-existing hypertension
3. Estimated GFR (eGFR) <70 ml/minute

## Cadaveric ECD criteria

1. Age 50–59 years plus 2 of the following:
2. Pre-existing hypertension
3. eGFR <70 ml/minute
4. Death from cerebrovascular accident

## Liver donation

Programmes for live donation of liver tissue are up and running in the USA and are being incorporated into the UK transplant programme, eg:

- Left lateral segment from adult to child
- Right hepatectomy specimen from adult to adult

A small number of cases of living donation of lung segments, pancreatic tail and small-bowel segments have been reported.

# Contraindications for organ and tissue donation

## Contraindications for organ donation

- HIV-positive
- Creutzfeldt–Jakob (CJD) positive
- Solid organs are rarely retrieved in donors aged >80

## Contraindications for tissue donation

- HIV, hepatitis B, hepatitis C, HTLV, syphilis or risk factors for these infections
- CJD or family history of CJD
- Progressive neurological disease of unknown pathophysiology, eg multiple sclerosis, Alzheimer's disease, Parkinson's disease, motor neurone disease
- Leukaemia, lymphoma, myeloma
- Active TB
- Untreated bacterial infection
- Previous transplant requiring immunosuppressive treatment
- Systemic malignancy (except for cornea transplantation)

## Consent issues in organ transplantation

The process for organ donation in cadaveric patients is complex and requires a multidisciplinary approach (Figure 10.1). The consent of a live donor involves detailed counselling and it is the clinician's responsibility to ensure that the donor appreciates the short- and long-term implications of organ donation on his or her own health, as well as the risks of failure of the transplant.

### Consent issues for the live donor

Immediate risks

- Mortality risk (0.03%)
- Re-operation rate (<1%)
- Blood transfusion (1.5%)

Postoperative complications

- Wound infection
- Pneumonia
- Deep vein thrombosis
- Pulmonary embolism
- Cardiac event

Long-term risks

- Chronic kidney disease
- Hypertension
- Consequences if require future treatment for as yet unknown disease

## Donor–recipient compatibility

Ideally there should be:

- Similarity in donor and recipient age – particularly at extremes of age
- ABO blood group matching
- HLA matching: HLA-A, HLA-B and HLA-DR are the most important, with the best matches having all six alleles the same
- Antibody cross-matching: recipient serum is tested against donor B and T cells to ensure no cross-reactivity with preformed anti-human leucocyte antibodies in the serum. These antibodies arise in response to blood transfusions, pregnancy or previous failed transplants

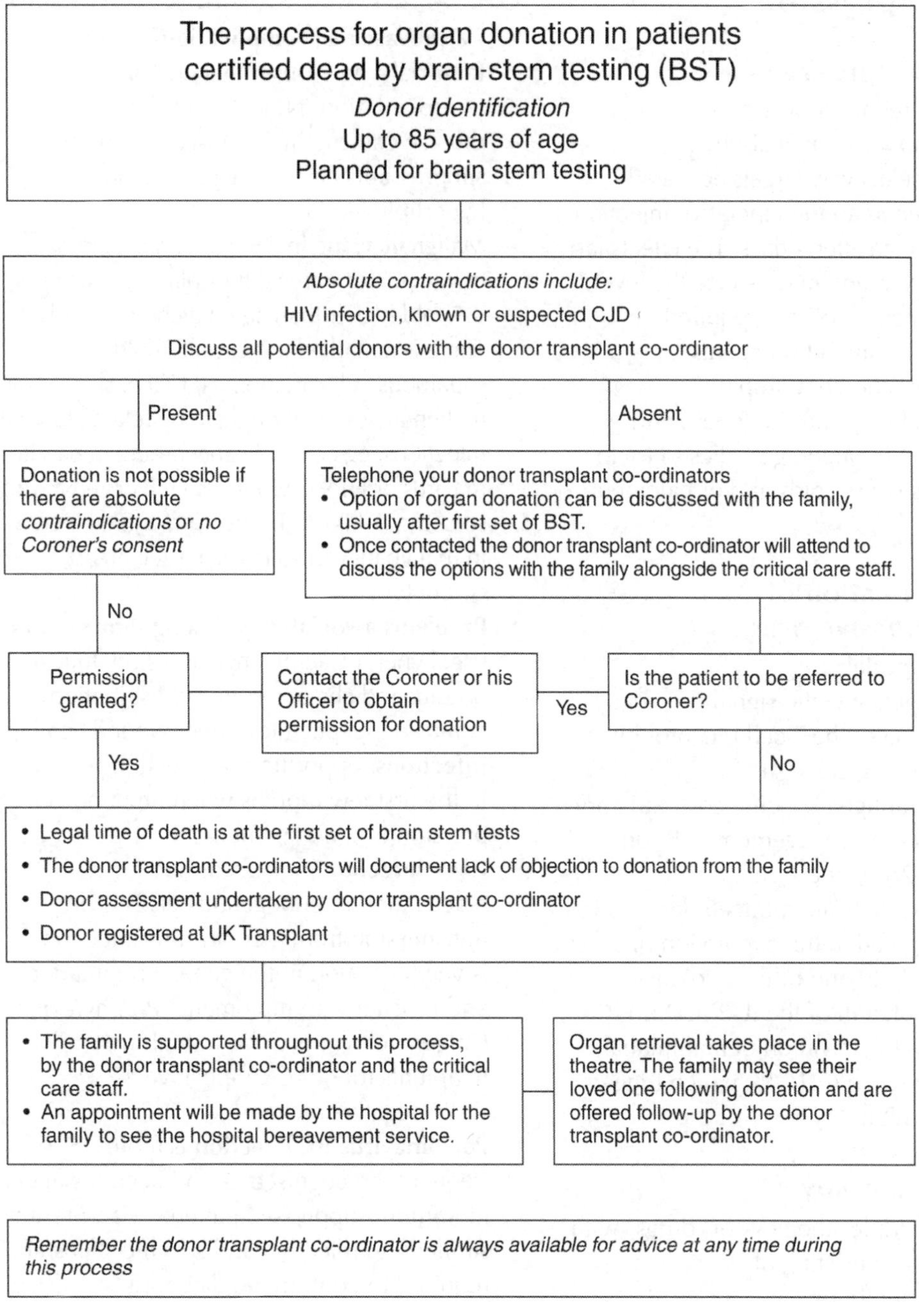

## The process for organ donation in patients certified dead by brain-stem testing (BST)

*Donor Identification*
Up to 85 years of age
Planned for brain stem testing

---

*Absolute contraindications include:*

HIV infection, known or suspected CJD

Discuss all potential donors with the donor transplant co-ordinator

Present | Absent

Donation is not possible if there are absolute *contraindications* or *no Coroner's consent*

Telephone your donor transplant co-ordinators
- Option of organ donation can be discussed with the family, usually after first set of BST.
- Once contacted the donor transplant co-ordinator will attend to discuss the options with the family alongside the critical care staff.

No

Permission granted? | Contact the Coroner or his Officer to obtain permission for donation | Yes | Is the patient to be referred to Coroner?

Yes | No

- Legal time of death is at the first set of brain stem tests
- The donor transplant co-ordinators will document lack of objection to donation from the family
- Donor assessment undertaken by donor transplant co-ordinator
- Donor registered at UK Transplant

- The family is supported throughout this process, by the donor transplant co-ordinator and the critical care staff.
- An appointment will be made by the hospital for the family to see the hospital bereavement service.

Organ retrieval takes place in the theatre. The family may see their loved one following donation and are offered follow-up by the donor transplant co-ordinator.

*Remember the donor transplant co-ordinator is always available for advice at any time during this process*

CHAPTER 7

Figure 7.1 Identifying an organ donor

## Immunosuppression

### At the time of surgery
- Give methylprednisolone 1 g.
- Anti-CD25 monoclonal antibody (eg basiliximab) selectively targets activated T cells. It is given as an intraoperative injection, which is repeated after 4 days. The effects last for several weeks and may reduce the level of ciclosporin or tacrolimus required.
- More aggressive induction agents include alemtuzumab (Campath), anti-thymoglobulin and rituximab, and are the subject of ongoing studies to try to reduce the use of steroids and/or calcineurin inhibitors.

### Mechanism of action of immunosuppressive drugs
The three signal model:
- Signal 1: antigen-specific signal provided by the triggering of the T-cell receptor by antigen-presenting cells (APCs)
- Signal 2: non-antigen-specific costimulatory signal provided by engagement of B7on APC with CD28 on the T cell.
- Signals 1 and 2 activate intracellular pathways that lead to the expression of interleukin 2 (IL-2) and other cytokines
- Signal 3: stimulation of the IL-2 (CD25) receptor leads to activation of **m**ammalian **t**arget **of r**apamycin (mTOR), which triggers T-cell proliferation

### Maintenance therapy
Most units use triple therapy of drugs with synergistic effects, consisting of:
- A calcineurin inhibitor
- An antiproliferative agent
- A steroid (prednisolone)

Other immunosuppressants used are mTOR inhibitors such as sirolimus or everolimus.

## Complications of immunosuppression
- **Cardiovascular complications (multi-factorial):** new-onset diabetes after transplantation (NODAT), underlying disease causing hypertension, immuno-suppressants causing hypertension, hyperlipidaemia
- **Malignancy:** the incidence of non-skin malignancies in renal transplant recipients is 3.5-fold higher than age-matched controls. There is a marked increase (65-fold) in squamous cell carcinoma (SCC) of skin. Some malignancies are thought to be related to viral infections, eg cervical cancer (human papillo-mavirus or HPV), lymphoma (EBV) and Kaposi sarcoma (HHV-8). There is a marginal increase in malignancy of solid organs (eg breast, colon, lung)
- **Problems associated with long-term steroid use:** hyperglycaemia, hypertension, thin skin, obesity and characteristic fat distribution, confusion, peptic ulcer, poor wound healing
- **Infections:** opportunistic infections occur in the first few months when immunosup-pression is at a maximum
- **CMV infection** may occur due to reactivation of endogenous disease or transmission from a donor; this infection is very common in the general population, and is usually asymptomatic. Prophylaxis (valganciclovir) is given to high-risk recipients (donor CMV-positive to CMV-negative recipients)
- **Polyomavirus BK infection** is more frequently recognised as an infectious agent in immunosuppressed patients. Can present similarly to rejection and specific stains are required to confirm the diagnosis.

## Rejection of transplanted organs
Patients at higher risk of rejection include those who have received previous transplants

**CHAPTER 7**

or multiple blood transfusions, had previous rejection reactions, and African-Caribbean people and children.

There are several mechanisms of transplant rejection.

## Hyperacute rejection

- Due to presence of recipient antibodies against the donor kidney
- Occurs within minutes of revascularisation
- Kidney swells and becomes discoloured
- There is clumping of red blood cells (RBCs) and platelets, fibrin is deposited and

interstitial haemorrhage occurs
- Rarely seen because of antibody cross-reactivity testing (see 'Donor–recipient compatibility' above)
- Transplant nephrectomy is required

## Acute rejection

- Defined as an acute deterioration in allograft function that is associated with specific pathological changes in the graft. The two principal forms of rejection are acute cell-mediated rejection and acute antibody-mediated rejection

| Immunosuppressant class | Mechanism of action | Side effects |
|---|---|---|
| **Calcineurin inhibitors** | | |
| Ciclosporin | Inhibits production of IL-2 and tumour necrosis factor α (TNF-α) by binding to cyclophilin protein and inhibiting calcineurin | Nephrotoxicity, hyperkalaemia, hypomagnesaemia, gingival hyperplasia, hyperlipidaemia, glucose intolerance, hypertension |
| Tacrolimus | Inhibits production of IL-2 by helper T cells, by binding calcineurin to tacrolimus-binding protein | Nephrotoxicity, neurotoxicity, glucose intolerance, prolonged Q–T (rare) |
| **Antiproliferative agents** | | |
| Mycophenolate mofetil | A prodrug. The active compound is mycophenolic acid, which inhibits the enzyme inosine monophosphate dehydrogenase (required for guanosine synthesis); impairs B- and T-cell proliferation selectively because of the presence of guanosine salvage pathways in other rapidly dividing cells | Nausea diarrhoea, leucopenia, anaemia and thrombocytopenia |
| Azathioprine | A derivative of 6-mercaptopurine. It functions as an antimetabolite to inhibit DNA and RNA synthesis | Leucopenia, thrombocytopenia, gastrointestinal disturbance, cholestasis, alopecia |
| **Steroids** | Reduce IL-1–3, IL-6 and TNF-α production and inhibit T-cell activation Impairment of dendritic cell function (important APCs) | Glucose intolerance, bone disease (osteoporosis, avascular necrosis) Cataracts Cushingoid appearance Infection Poor wound healing |
| **mTOR inhibitors** (sirolimus/everolimus) | TOR is a regulatory kinase. Inhibition reduces cytokine-dependent cellular proliferation at the G1–S phase of the cell cycle | Hyperkalaemia, hypomagnesaemia, hyperlipidaemia, leucopenia, anaemia, impaired wound healing, joint pain |

CHAPTER 7

Rejection is classified based on pathological findings using the Banff classification system.

---

**Banff classification (revised 2007)**

1 Normal
2 Antibody-mediated rejection (acute/ chronic subtypes)
3 Borderline changes
4 T-cell-mediated rejection (acute and chronic subtypes)
5 Interstitial fibrosis and tubular atrophy without evidence of specific aetiology (previously called 'chronic allograft nephropathy')
6 Other changes not the result of acute or chronic rejection

---

## Cell-mediated rejection

- Common in first 2 weeks but can occur up to 6 months after transplantation
- Mononuclear cell infiltration in interstitium and subsequently in vessel walls
- Treatment with high-dose steroids (often reversible)
- Difficult to distinguish clinically from acute tubular necrosis (ATN) or drug nephrotoxicity

## Antibody-mediated rejection

Diagnosis of AMR is provided by the presence of at least three of the following four criteria:
- Graft dysfunction
- Histological evidence of tissue injury
- Positive staining for C4d
- Presence of donor-specific antibody

## Differential diagnosis

Acute rejection must be differentiated from other causes of graft dysfunction and/or similar biopsy findings, eg post-transplant lymphopro-liferative disorder (PTLD) or polyoma BK virus because these may necessitate reduction rather than increase in immunosuppression.

# 1.3 Renal transplantation

 **In a nutshell ...**

In the UK during 2010–11, 1502 people received a cadaveric renal transplant and 1020 received a live renal transplant, with 6597 still waiting. The indication for renal transplantation is end-stage renal failure. In the UK the incidence of end-stage renal failure patients commencing renal replacement therapy is $109/10^6$ people. It affects more men than women, and more African-Caribbean people than white people.

## Patient selection for renal transplantation

### Indications for renal transplant
Renal transplantation is usually done for chronic renal failure (see Section 1.2). The advantages of renal transplantation over continued dialysis are:
- Improved quality of life (requirement for dialysis reduced or eliminated)
- Increase in patient survival rate compared with dialysis (note that selection of fitter patients for surgery may introduce bias)
- Cost-effective in the long term

## Patient assessment for renal transplantation

### Risk of recurrent disease in the transplanted kidney
- Will recurrent disease cause graft failure and, if so, how quickly?
- There is a high risk of recurrences in focal segmental glomerular sclerosis, amyloidosis, IgA nephropathy and haemolytic uraemic syndrome
- Renal transplantation may be inappropriate for live related donors with high recurrence risk of primary disease

## Technical considerations

- Atheromatous iliac vessels in patients with arteriopathy
- Bladder dysfunction (neurogenic bladder or outflow obstruction)
- Pretransplantation nephrectomy of a native kidney
- Adult polycystic kidney disease (APKD): bleeding or infection in cystic spaces
- Large and bulky kidneys with little space for the transplant
- Uncontrollable hypertension
- Renal calculi
- Persistent anti-glomerular antibodies

## Additional investigations

- ABO and HLA typing
- Virology (hepatitis B, hepatitis C; CMV may require treatment pretransplantation)
- Urinalysis and culture
- Consider effects of common comorbidities (hypertension, diabetes)
- Cardiovascular assessment:
  - High mortality rate from cardiovascular disease in renal transplant recipients
  - ECG ± stress test ± echocardiography
  - Exclude peripheral vascular disease
- Psychological issues and compliance with lifelong immunosuppressive medication

## Contraindications for renal transplantation

- Active malignancy (cancer-free for at least 2 years)
- Active infection: exclude dental sepsis and gallstones (risk of cholecystitis)
- Advanced atheromatous disease (relative contraindication)

## Renal transplantation procedure
### Anatomy of the transplanted kidney

- The kidney is placed extraperitoneally in the right or left iliac fossa, usually on the right side (dictated by existing scars or previous transplants)
- Renal vessels are anastomosed (end to side) to the recipient's external iliac vessels
- The ureter is taken down into the pelvis where it is anastomosed to the bladder mucosa, either directly (extravesical approach) or by threading it through a submucosal tunnel and suturing from inside the bladder through a separate incision in the bladder wall (intravesical approach)
- The ureter is stented (reduces stricture formation) and the stent is removed by cystoscopy after 6 weeks

### Length of renal vessels

- The right renal vein is anatomically shorter than the left because of the right-sided position of the inferior vena cava (IVC; may make transplantation of the kidney more difficult in a large recipient)
- Cadaver kidneys are retrieved with a cuff of tissue taken from the aorta and IVC at the end of the normal renal vessels
- Live donor kidneys do not have this extra tissue and so the renal vessels are shorter (occasionally this necessitates end-to-end arterial anastomosis with the internal iliac artery)

### Ureteric blood supply

- Upper third comes from the renal artery
- Middle third comes from the gonadal vessels
- Lower third comes from the common iliacs

It is important not to strip the adventitial tissue from around the ureter because this contributes to its blood supply from the renal artery (other sources of supply ligated at retrieval).

CHAPTER 7

**Op box: Renal transplantation**

**Indications**
- End-stage renal failure

**Preop**
- Ensure all cross-matching has been performed and is optimum
- Give broad-spectrum prophylactic antibiotics
- Start immunosuppression just before surgery in cadaveric organ recipients. In live donor recipients it may be started a week before surgery
- The bladder is washed out or filled with approximately 150 ml antiseptic solution

**Procedure**
- An oblique Gibson incision is made in the iliac fossa. The rectus is preserved
- Generally the renal vein is anastomosed at the external iliac vein and the renal artery (with patch) to the external iliac artery
- During the anastomosis the donor kidney is kept cool on ice or wrapped in a swab soaked with cold saline
- The ureter is usually anastomosed to the bladder using an extravesical technique. It is tunnelled submucosally in order to prevent reflux. A ureteric stent is placed between the kidney and the bladder (it is removed by cystoscopy at 6 weeks)

**Postop**
- Careful fluid balance is required (usually urine output + 30 ml/h)
- In situations where the patient remains oliguric or anuric a Doppler scan will assess blood flow and ultrasonography will rule out urinary extravasation or hydronephrosis
- ATN is associated with increased ischaemia time and may lead to delayed graft function. Renal biopsy may be performed to confirm this and exclude rejection

**Complications**
- Vascular: renal artery or vein thrombosis, renal artery stenosis
- Urological: urethral stricture or obstruction
- Lymphocele: due to failure of ligation of lymphatics (can be aspirated)

## Surgical complications of renal transplantation

### Early complications
- Delayed graft function – the requirement for dialysis in the first postoperative week:
  - Most commonly due to ATN (but thrombosis and acute rejection must be considered)
- Associated with long cold ischaemic time, warm ischaemic time and reperfusion injury
- Requires good patient hydration and supportive management with dialysis (haemodialysis or PD)
- Usually diagnosed by cortical biopsy
- Occurs in approximately 25% of transplants

- Vascular complications:
  - Anastomotic bleed
  - Vessel kinking or arterial / venous thrombosis
- Urine leak
- Lymphocele
- Infections: commonly wound, urinary or respiratory tract

### Late complications

- Ureteric stricture
- Reflux nephropathy
- Renal artery stenosis: due to atherosclerosis and hyperlipidaemia

## Non-surgical complications of renal transplantation

- Complications of immunosuppression (see Section 1.2)
- Primary non-function of unknown cause
- Rejection (see Section 1.2)

## Prognosis after renal transplantation

Prognostic factors include:

- Primary diagnosis
- Previous graft failures
- Episodes of rejection
- Kidney total ischaemic time
- Donor factors (eg age)

The 1-year graft survival rate is about 94% in live related transplants and 88% in cadaveric transplants. The 10-year graft survival rate for first grafts is 70–80%. In general, live related recipients fare better than cadaveric recipients.

# 1.4   Liver transplantation

## In a nutshell ...

In the UK during 2010–11, 668 people received a cadaveric liver transplant and 21 received a lobe from a live donor. The most common indication is chronic liver failure, although some transplantations are performed for acute liver failure. Before reading this section you may need to refresh your memory by reviewing the following:
- Normal anatomy of the liver (in the Liver and spleen section of Chapter 1, Abdominal Surgery)
- Pathology of the liver (below)
- Portal hypertension

## Patient selection for liver transplantation

Chronic liver failure is the most common reason for liver transplantation.

Patients are usually in a Child's C category disease and life-threatening complications (eg varices); these patients often have significant multiple comorbidities and require very careful evaluation and work-up.

Early transplantation has improved survival rates in this group over the last 10 years.

## Indications for liver transplantation

### Chronic liver failure

- Primary biliary cirrhosis
- Primary sclerosing cholangitis (often associated with ulcerative colitis)
- Alcoholic liver disease (abstain from alcohol for at least 6 months)
- Hepatitis B and hepatitis C
- Budd–Chiari syndrome

- Metabolic disease (eg Wilson's disease, $\alpha_1$-antitrypsin deficiency, haemochromatosis)
- Paediatric conditions: 10–15% of transplants (eg congenital biliary atresia)

Transplantation is considered in cirrhotic patients if they have a complication of portal hypertension or a manifestation of insufficient synthetic function (MELD score).

### Acute liver failure

- Refers to the rapid development of severe acute liver injury with impaired synthetic function and encephalopthy in a person with previously normal or well-compensated liver function
- Fulminant liver failure can be defined as the development of encephalopathy within 8 weeks of the onset of symptoms in those with a previously normal liver or the appearance of encephalopathy within 2 weeks of developing jaundice in a patient with underlying liver dysfunction
- There may be spontaneous recovery. It may be fulminant and rapid
- It requires intensive care with cardiorespiratory and renal support
- There are strict criteria for supra-urgent listing for transplantation as an emergency

**Causes of acute liver failure:**

- Drug-induced (eg from paracetamol or rifampicin overdose)
- Metabolic disease (eg Wilson's disease)
- Viral hepatitis

### Liver tumours

- Primary or secondary hepatocellular carcinoma (HCC)
- Secondary neuroendocrine tumours
- Cholangiocarcinoma (very rare and only if there is intrahepatic disease without extrahepatic disease)

HCC (either primary or on a background of cirrhosis) is the most common tumour to be treated with transplantation (primary tumours of <4 cm diameter with no more than two foci of disease).

## Contraindications for liver transplantation

- Patient unlikely to survive the procedure (cardiopulmonary comorbidity)
- Extrahepatic malignancy (individually assessed, but must be cancer-free for 2 years)
- Portal vein thrombosis (relative contraindication)
- Active generalised sepsis
- Psychosocial reasons (eg continued alcohol/drug abuse)

## Liver transplantation procedures

### Types of graft

There are a limited number of donors, so a variety of techniques have been developed to help optimise the number of transplants available.

### Whole graft

- Conventional transplant: total native hepatectomy plus grafting
- Accessory transplant 'piggyback': partial native hepatectomy, preserving segments 1–3 with grafting of transplanted liver to the side of the native IVC (a new technique, used as a supportive measure for reversible causes of acute liver failure when native liver is expected to recover from the aetiological insult and regenerate). Immunosuppression may be withdrawn after recovery of liver function, whereupon graft is rejected, becoming small and fibrosed. Less liver tissue is required, so it can be performed with specimen from split graft

## Split graft

- A whole graft can be divided on the basis of its blood supply. Split graft is usually used for two recipients (often an adult and a child)

## Live related graft

- An example is a left lateral segmentectomy specimen from an adult to a child
- Rapid regeneration occurs in the donor
- Transplanted segment grows with the child
- Live related grafts are becoming part of the transplant programme in the UK

### Principles of liver transplantation

- **Mercedes or roof-top incision**
- **Hepatectomy**
  - Often this is technically challenging due to intra-abdominal varices and adhesions
  - It may be performed with the patient on veno–veno bypass (femoral vein to internal jugular)
  - The IVC (above and below liver), portal vein and hepatic artery are divided
- **Vascular anastomoses**
  - IVC (above and below liver)
  - Portal vein
  - Hepatic artery
- **Biliary reconstruction**
  - Direct anastomosis of recipient to donor common bile duct (CBD)
  - Roux loop for diseased recipient CBD

# Surgical complications of liver transplantation

## Vascular complications

- Haemorrhage: common, due to multiple vascular anastomoses, coagulopathy and thrombocytopenia
- Vessel thrombosis: due to low-flow states or small-diameter vessels (eg accessory arteries)
- Anastomotic stricture: late

## Biliary tree complications

- Leak
- Anastomotic stricture
- Ischaemic cholangiopathy

# Non-surgical complications of liver transplantation

- **Primary non-function** occurs rarely but is a very serious complication. There is a climbing prothrombin time and deteriorating clinical condition in first 24–48 hours with coagulopathy, oliguria, hypoglycaemia and central nervous system (CNS) changes. This may require re-grafting
- **Early rejection** is fairly common (up to 30%). It is diagnosed by deteriorating LFTs and confirmed on biopsy, and it responds to high-dose steroids
- **Chronic rejection** occurs months after transplantation with progressive deterioration of graft function. Retransplantation is required

## Infections

- General: eg wound infection, respiratory infection
- Viral: eg CMV

## Long-term

- Malignancy risk – skin, PTLD
- NODAT
- Chronic renal failure
- Recurrence of primary liver disease/infection

**CHAPTER 7**

## Prognosis after liver transplantation

The primary diagnosis, comorbidity and stage of disease impact on outcome measures. Patients are given individually tailored outcome measures based on risk assessments by a multidisciplinary team (hepatologist, surgeon and transplant anaesthetist).

Transplantation for chronic liver failure has the highest survival rates.

## 1.5   Transplantation of other organs

### Pancreas transplantation

In 2010–11, 156 pancreas/kidney transplants and 13 islet cell transplants were performed in the UK.

#### Indications

- The main indication for pancreatic transplantation is diabetes mellitus in young patients with brittle disease (lack of hypoglycaemic awareness) and end-stage nephropathy. It may be done in conjunction with kidney transplant (simultaneous pancreas/kidney [SPK] transplant)
- Less commonly, pancreas after kidney (PAK) transplants or pancreas transplants alone (PTA) are performed

#### Technique

- In whole-organ transplants the arterial supply of the pancreas is reconstructed using the donor iliac bifurcation
- Exocrine drainage is by means of anastomosis of the duodenal segment to the small intestine (80%) or bladder (20%)

### Complications

- Vascular thrombosis, a common cause of early graft loss:
- Haemorrhage
- Pancreatitis
- Rejection that is difficult to diagnose (increased blood glucose is a relatively late indicator)
- Infection (patients are very susceptible)

## Small-bowel transplantation

### Indications

- Intestinal failure with nutritional failure

### Graft rejection

- The small bowel is a highly immunological organ requiring high-level immunosuppression. Graft rejection is common and may cause bacterial translocation and sepsis

## Multi-visceral transplantation

- May involve transplantation of any combination of kidney, liver, pancreas and small bowel
- Success rates are low but are improving

## Other transplant material

**Cardiac and lung transplantation** is covered in Chapter 3, Cardiothoracic Surgery.

**Skin grafting** is covered in Plastic Surgery, Book 1.

**Bone grafting** is covered in Orthopaedic Surgery, Book 1.

**Blood transfusion** is covered in Book 1.

# CHAPTER 8

# Urological Surgery

Mary M Brown

CHAPTER 8

648

# SECTION 1

# Clinical features and investigation of the urinary tract

## 1.1 Urological symptoms

 **In a nutshell ...**

Pathology in the urological tract may be asymptomatic, present as a systemic illness (eg weight loss, fever) or present with any of the following urological symptoms:
- Pain
- Lower urinary tract symptoms
- Urinary incontinence
- Urinary retention
- Haematuria
- Pneumaturia

### Pain

Pain from the renal tract can be felt anywhere from the renal angle to the genitalia:
- Renal angle pain: kidney
- Flank/loin pain: upper and mid-ureters, non-urological causes (eg abdominal aortic aneurysm)
- Suprapubic pain: bladder (eg retention)

- Perineal/genital pain: lower ureters, epididymis, testes
- Urethral pain: usually infection

**Obstructive pain** is dull in nature and exacerbated by fluid intake. It is due to distension of the renal pelvis or renal capsule. Chronic progressive obstruction is usually painless.

**Colicky pain** is due to passage of a calculus or blood clot and is intermittent, severe and often associated with vomiting. It is due to ureteric spasm and peristalsis. It may classically radiate 'from loin to groin' and into the genitalia (these structures all share a common innervation at T11–12). Differential diagnosis includes any cause of an acute abdomen but, most importantly, leaking or ruptured abdominal aortic aneurysm (AAA) must be excluded.

### Lower urinary tract symptoms

Lower urinary tract symptoms (LUTSs) include storage symptoms and voiding symptoms:
- **Storage symptoms:** these include frequency, nocturia, urgency, dysuria and/or pyrexia). Commonly idiopathic but may be due to:
  - Infection
  - Malignancy

- Reduced functional bladder capacity (inflammation, fibrosis, oedema of the bladder wall)
- Calculi in the distal ureter (causes trigonal irritation) or the bladder
- **Voiding symptoms** include hesitancy and/or straining, poor stream and terminal dribbling. These symptoms are commonly due to urethral stricture in young men, and to prostatic hypertrophy or malignancy in older men. As bladder outflow obstruction progresses the detrusor muscle thickens and is less controllable, causing urgency and frequency.

## Urinary retention

Urinary retention can be acute, acute on chronic or chronic.

- **Acute retention** is very painful. It may occur on a background of chronic bladder outflow obstruction or be precipitated by constipation, infection, or around the time of surgery due to location of pain (eg inguinal hernia repair) or use of anaesthetic and analgesic agents
- **Chronic retention** is usually due to bladder outflow obstruction and is usually painless with gradually increasing residual volumes. It may present with overflow incontinence

## Urinary incontinence

Urinary incontinence can be subdivided into stress incontinence, urge incontinence and continuous incontinence.

- **Stress incontinence** occurs during raised intra-abdominal pressure and is due to weakness of the external urethral sphincter
- **Urge incontinence** is often neurological in origin and is due to spasmodic loss of control of the detrusor muscle

- **Continuous incontinence** is usually due to an anatomical abnormality

For further details see Section 2.3.

## Haematuria

This is a common urological symptom and will always need some form of investigation. Although it has a multitude of causes the priority is to exclude neoplasms of the kidney (renal cell carcinoma) or of the transitional epithelium (mostly bladder cancer). Both of these conditions are covered in Section 7 'Urological malignancy'.

### Clinical presentation of haematuria

Haematuria may be macroscopic (visibly discoloured urine) or microscopic (picked up on dipstick testing). The timing may give an indication as to the site of bleeding:

- Blood early in the stream suggests a urethral/prostatic cause
- Blood at the end of the stream is more indicative of a problem at the bladder neck
- Blood mixed throughout the stream is probably coming from the higher renal tract

The colour of the blood should be noted. Darker blood ± clots is likely to have come from higher up in the renal tract. Urinary discoloration may also occur due to certain drugs (eg rifampicin, allopurinol, laxatives) and ingestion of certain foodstuffs (eg beetroot).

Underlying urological malignancy exists in:

- 20% of patients with macroscopic haematuria
- <5% of patients with microscopic haematuria

The pick-up rate for malignancy is higher in patients who smoke.

## Investigating haematuria

Urgent investigation (within 2 weeks) in the context of a haematuria clinic is suggested for:
- All patients with macroscopic haematuria
- All patients aged >50 with microscopic haematuria

This is usually a one-stop clinic where patients receive:
- Flexible cystoscopy
- Ultrasonography of the kidneys
- CT intravenous urogram or intravenous urography IVU (alternatively called CT KUB [kidneys, ureters and bladder])
- Plain film of the abdomen
- Urinary cytology
- Digital rectal examination (DRE) of prostate in men
- Urine culture

## Management of haematuria

Patients with negative investigations in whom haematuria resolves can usually be reassured. If haematuria persists and suspicion for malignancy is high (eg more elderly patients) further investigations should be performed, including:
- CT IVU (if only ultrasonography had been performed previously)
- Retrograde studies of ureters
- Rigid cystoscopy and/or biopsy

In younger patients with persistent microscopic haematuria, nephrological referral is warranted.

## Pneumaturia

Air in the urine is due to fistulation of any part of the urinary tract with the bowel (commonly the bladder). It is often associated with chronic urinary infection due to passage of enteric bacteria. Common causes include diverticulitis, inflammatory bowel disease, and tumour of the bowel or bladder wall. Full investigation of the bowel is required and, although the fistula is rarely visualised directly at endoscopy, the site of fistulation may be identified by radiological contrast studies, usually barium enema.

# 1.2   Urological investigation and imaging

### In a nutshell ...

**Urological investigation**
- Urinalysis
- Blood tests
- Urinary flow rates
- Urological imaging

**KUB**
- Contrast studies
- Ultrasonography
- Angiography
- CT and MRI
- Radioisotope imaging of the renal tract
- Isotope bone scanning
- Ureteroscopy/retrograde studies

## Urological investigations

### Urinalysis

Urinalysis is performed on a midstream (or clean-catch) urine sample. Tests on urine include:
- **Urine dipstick (eg Multistix) testing:** initial bedside analysis. Sensitive for blood, protein, leucocytes, ketones, glucose and nitrites

- **Urine microscopy:** further laboratory analysis looking for red blood cells (RBCs), organisms, cellular casts (which imply renal disease), and crystals such as oxalate or uric acid (which imply stone disease)
- **Urine culture:** for organism and antibiotic sensitivity. Significant growth is considered to be >10$^5$ organisms/ml
- **Urine cytology:** looking for abnormal transitional epithelial cells. This warrants further investigation for malignancy

### Blood tests
- **Urea level:** this is a very insensitive indicator of renal function. Levels are affected by hydration, metabolism and protein intake, as well as glomerular and tubular function
- **Creatinine level:** this is determined by muscle mass and glomerular filtration. It is a more sensitive indicator of renal clearance when used as creatinine clearance measurement
- **Electrolytes:** sodium, potassium and hydrogen (acidosis) and bicarbonate ions give direct evidence of renal-concentrating dysfunction

### Urinary flow rates
These are used for quantifying bladder outflow obstruction. Normal flow rates are >15 ml/second.

## Urological imaging

### Plain film KUB
This radiograph is angled to image the entire length of the urinary tract. Look for the renal outlines (T12–L2) and any visible renal mass. Follow the anatomical path of the ureters into the bladder, looking for calcification or opacities that could be calculi, although this is relatively insensitive because it will identify only 50% of ureteric calculi.

### Contrast studies
- **IVU:** intravenous (IV) injection of contrast media is followed by radiological examination at subsequent time points. This demonstrates the baseline or delayed renal excretion because the contrast is filtered by the kidney, giving the renal outline, including any masses. It shows the renal pelvis and ureters, including any filling defects (eg stone or tumour) that can be compared for location with calcification visible on the KUB. The bladder-filling and post-voiding films also give an idea about the degree of bladder emptying. This has largely been superseded by CT IVU
- **Retrograde urogram:** retrograde injection of contrast is used at cystoscopy to visualise ureters
- **Urethrography:** this is useful if traumatic disruption of the urethra is suspected. The meatus only is cannulated and contrast media is introduced. The urethra is visualised by radiography
- **Micturating cystogram:** this is used for demonstrating fistulation, vesicoureteric reflux, urethral strictures and functional bladder studies

### Angiography
Selective renal arteriography is used to visualise renal arterial anatomy, arterial stenoses or aneurysms, in staging of renal tumours (for invasion of the renal vein), and for persistent haemorrhage after trauma.

## CT and MRI

- CT is useful for diagnosis and staging of malignancy, and for abscess and cyst drainage
- Non-contrast CT (CT KUB) is increasingly the standard investigation for urinary calculi and contrast-enhanced CT (CT IVU)
- MRI takes longer than CT but avoids the need for radiation. It is more sensitive than CT for staging and detection of lymph node metastases in prostate cancer. It is also used for diagnosing vertebral metastases and spinal cord compression

## Ultrasonography

> **Ultrasonography of the genitourinary system**
>
> Ultrasonography is important for visualisation and guided biopsy at many levels of the renal tract.
>
> - **Renal ultrasonography:** assesses renal size and cortical thickness, renal masses (cystic/solid), calculi and hydronephrosis. Also guides nephrostomy insertion and renal biopsy. The latter carries a small risk of haemorrhage and arteriovenous (AV) fistulation
> - **Bladder ultrasonography:** residual volume, filling defects (stone, tumour), bladder wall thickness
> - **Testis ultrasonography:** masses, blood flow (eg torsion)
> - **Prostate ultrasonography:** transrectal ultrasound (TRUS) is used to guide prostate biopsies or drain prostatic abscesses

## Radioisotope imaging of the renal tract

Nuclear imaging can determine the individual components of glomerular and tubular renal function. Renal excretion or glomerular filtration rate (GFR) is imaged using a compound filtered by the glomerulus, eg [$^{99m}$Tc]DTPA ($^{99m}$Tc-labelled diethylenetriaminepentaacetic acid) and split functioning of the individual kidneys (eg before nephrectomy) can be assessed using [$^{99m}$Tc]DMSA ($^{99m}$Tc-labelled dimecaptosuccinic acid), which is taken up by the proximal tubules and retained there with only a small amount excreted. [$^{99m}$Tc]MAG-3 ($^{99m}$Tc-labelled mercaptoacetyltriglycine) is predominantly excreted by tubular secretion with a minimal amount filtered by the kidney and can therefore be used to assess degree of renal obstruction.

### Isotope bone scanning

Radioisotope uptake in the bone correlates with vascularity. It shows metastatic deposits as areas of increased activity. It is used for staging of malignancy (particularly prostate).

### Ureteroscopy

Two forms of ureteroscopy may be performed at cystoscopy.

#### Rigid/semi-rigid ureteroscopy

- Scopes vary from 4.5 Fr to 9.5 Fr
- In theory they can reach the whole ureter but it is difficult to access the upper third
- In men large prostates can make manoeuvring difficult

#### Flexible ureteroscopy

- Scopes vary from 6.2 Fr to 9.3 Fr
- They are introduced over a wire or through a specially designed access sheath
- They give much better access to the upper ureter and can be used within the renal collecting system

- A narrow working channel reduces the range of instrumentation available
- Flexible scopes are expensive and easy to damage

### Indications for ureteroscopy

- **Ureteric stones:** rigid ureteroscopy and stone fragmentation are a good treatment for lower and midureteric stones; extracorporeal shockwave lithotripsy (ESWL) is an alternative but may not be successful with these if over bony landmarks. Flexible ureteroscopy is good for upper ureteric stones that are not adequately treated by ESWL
- **Renal stones:** flexible ureteroscopy may be useful for small stones where the drainage does not favour ESWL
- **Haematuria:** ureteroscopy is useful for diagnosing filling defects seen on IVU and biopsies may be obtained

## Procedure box: Ureteroscopy

**Preop**
- Urinary infection should be excluded with a midstream specimen of urine (MSU)
- Appropriate imaging should be available to aid orientation during the procedure
- In cases of stone disease antibiotics are given to reduce the risk of sepsis (eg intravenous gentamicin and amoxicillin)
- X-ray fluoroscopic imaging is required during the procedure

**Procedure**
- Patient in lithotomy position
- Initial retrograde ureterogram is usually performed
- Dilation of the ureter can be performed using balloon or graduated dilators
- The rigid ureteroscope is usually inserted alongside a guidewire or flexible scope over a wire, or through a specially designed access sheath
- Methods for stone destruction include Holmium laser and pneumatic lithoclast
- A JJ stent may be left in the ureter to ensure adequate drainage, especially after prolonged procedures, or where residual fragments remain

**Postop**
- Patients with uncomplicated stones (no infection or obstruction) can often go home on the same day
- Stent removal is by flexible cystoscopy (under local anaesthetic [LA])
- Plain KUB film will confirm stone clearance in most cases

**Complications**
- **Failure to reach stone:** leaving a JJ stent in the ureter for a short period often allows easier access subsequently
- **Urinary tract infection (UTI)/septicaemia:** septicaemia is a risk when operating on patients with UTI or infected stones. It's important to monitor these patients closely postoperatively because this situation can be life-threatening
- **Ureteric injury:** small perforations are managed by stenting. Major injuries are rare but may require open re-implantation/replacement with ileum

# SECTION 2

# Bladder dysfunction and incontinence

## 2.1 Anatomy of the bladder

### In a nutshell ...

The bladder is a hollow organ with a capacity of 500 ml in adults. The empty bladder lies within the pelvis and is pyramidal in shape with the apex anteriorly, a base posteriorly, a superior surface and two inferolateral surfaces.

## Anatomical relations of the bladder

### Superior

- The apex is joined to the anterior abdominal wall by the median umbilical ligament (remains of urachus)
- The superior surface is covered by peritoneum and related to coils of ileum or sigmoid colon. With distension, the bladder rises out of the pelvis and separates the peritoneum from the anterior abdominal wall, allowing suprapubic catheterisation to be performed without risk of entry into the peritoneal cavity

### Inferolateral relations

- These surfaces are related anteriorly to a retropubic pad of fat and the pubic bones, and posteriorly to the obturator internus muscle above and levator ani below

### Base of the bladder

- The base of the bladder faces postero-inferiorly and is triangular in shape. The two superolateral angles are joined by the ureters and the inferior angle gives rise to the urethra
- In females the base of the bladder lies lower because of the absence of the prostate
- In males the seminal vesicles lie behind the base of the bladder, along with the vasa deferentia. Above these is a pouch of peritoneum – the rectovesical pouch
- In females the vagina separates the bladder from the rectum, with the uterovesical pouch superior to this
- The puboprostatic ligaments in the male and the pubovesical ligaments in the female support the neck of the bladder where it enters the urethra

### The trigone relations

- This is the internal surface of the base of the bladder. Like the rest of the bladder it is lined by transitional cell epithelium. Unlike the rest of the bladder the mucosa here is firmly adherent to the underlying muscle and therefore does not form folds
- The ureters enter the trigone at its superior angles. They enter the bladder obliquely with an intramural part that is important in preventing vesicoureteric reflux

### Blood supply of the bladder

Superior and inferior vesical arteries (both are branches of the internal iliac arteries). In addition to these branches the bladder may be supplied by any adjacent artery arising from the internal iliac.

### Venous drainage of the bladder

The vesical venous plexus communicates below with the prostatic plexus in males and drains into the internal iliac vein.

### Lymphatic drainage of the bladder

This is to the external and internal iliac and obturator nodes.

### Nerve supply of the bladder and sphincter mechanism

There are three sources of nerves to the bladder and the sphincter:

1. Parasympathetic autonomic nerves (S2–4) are autonomic efferents that arise from the inferior hypogastric plexus
2. Sympathetic nerves originate from T10–L2 and run on the presacral fascia into the pelvis. These nerves are at risk during pelvic surgery, especially anterior resection of the rectum
3. Somatic nerves are derived from S2–4 which are transmitted to the urethra in the pudendal nerves. These originate in a region called the Onuf nucleus

## 2.2 Physiology of micturition

The normal lower urinary tract should be able to store urine and expel it completely at an appropriate time. This relies on several factors.

### Storage of urine depends on the bladder having adequate capacity

**Compliance** is the term for the ability of the bladder to increase in volume (to 400–500 ml) with only minimal increases in pressure. It is crucial to normal bladder function and is mediated by relaxation of the detrusor muscle as the bladder fills (due to tonic inhibition of the parasympathetic nerves). At volumes >500 ml the pressure rises sharply and stretching of the detrusor muscle causes reflex contraction.

### Continence and expulsion of urine requires competent sphincters

There are two **urethral sphincters**: an internal smooth muscle sphincter in the bladder neck (sympathetically innervated) and an external striated muscular sphincter (in the male membranous urethra, and midurethra in the female) under voluntary motor control via the pudendal nerves. During filling, sacral reflexes increase urethral pressure and maintain continence. The urethral sphincter mechanism should act as a valve for the control of continence and open appropriately during voiding.

## Timing of micturition is under the control of the pons

The centre for coordinating bladder and urethral function lies within the pons and is known as the **pontine micturition centre**. This gives descending input to those centres in the cord that are involved with innervating the muscle of the bladder and sphincter. To commence micturition, the inhibitory input from the higher centres is silenced and this is transmitted via the sympathetic and pudendal nerves, allowing the urethra to relax and decrease intraurethral pressure.

## Completeness of micturition depends on parasympathetic nerve supply and detrusor contraction

The parasympathetic nerves stimulate detrusor muscle contraction. All of the detrusor smooth muscle contracts simultaneously, directing the pressure towards the urethra. Intravesical pressure therefore exceeds intraurethral pressure and voiding occurs.

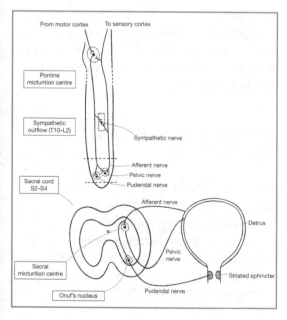

**Figure 8.1 Neural pathways in micturition**

# 2.3 Urinary incontinence

**In a nutshell ...**

Incontinence is defined by the International Continence Society as a condition in which involuntary loss of urine is a social or hygiene problem and is objectively demonstrable.

**Urine loss can be urethral or extraurethral**

- Extraurethral loss is secondary to abnormal anatomy (eg ectopic ureter, vesicovaginal fistula). It presents as constant incontinence
- Urethral loss is usually classified into stress incontinence (sphincter failure) and urge incontinence (bladder dysfunction)

**Evaluation of urinary incontinence**

- History
- Examination
- Investigations
- MSU
- Ultrasonography
- Cystoscopy
- Urodynamic testing

**Management of stress incontinence**

- Conservative/lifestyle modification
- Midurethral tapes
- Colposuspension
- Sphincter reinforcement

**Management of urge incontinence**

- Behavioural modification, eg bladder retraining
- Antimuscarinics
- Intrathecal Botox
- Tricyclic antidepressants
- Cystoplasty or ileal conduit

**CHAPTER 8**

# Classification of urinary incontinence

Frequently patients will have the picture of mixed incontinence, eg many women with stress incontinence also have symptoms of urgency.

## Stress incontinence

Characteristically this produces symptoms of involuntary loss of urine from the urethra during raised intra-abdominal pressure (eg coughing, sneezing, laughing or physical exertion). It can be demonstrated by the Valsalva manoeuvre. Stress incontinence is essentially due to hypermobility of the urethra and/or intrinsic sphincter deficiency.

Causes include:
- Pressure denervation of the pelvic floor post-pregnancy and post-childbirth
- External sphincter damage (eg post-TURP – transurethral resection of the prostate)
- Trauma to posterior urethra (eg pelvic fracture)
- Hormonal status (postmenopausal), constipation and obesity

## Urge incontinence

This is the involuntary loss of urine associated with a sudden strong desire to void (urgency). It occurs on a background of normal bladder anatomy and increases with age. It is associated with organic brain damage in elderly people (eg stroke, Parkinson's disease) and is a common cause of incontinence in this group. It is a component of the overactive bladder syndrome.

Causes include:
- Idiopathic detrusor instability (irritable bladder syndrome)
- Infection (bladder wall irritability)

- Loss of cortical control, where the bladder fills to capacity and empties spontaneously (eg dementia, paraplegia, multiple sclerosis [MS])

## Continuous incontinence

Constant incontinence can result from:
- Overflow incontinence: this occurs in men with chronic urinary retention. There is chronic loss of urine particularly at night
- Bladder fistulae (eg vesicovaginal)
- Anatomical abnormality (eg ectopic ureter, epispadias)

## Functional incontinence

In this situation lower urinary tract function is essentially normal but patients are unable to void appropriately because of limitations of mobility or confusion.

## Post-void dribbling

This is not true incontinence, but reflects pooling of urine in the bulbar urethra and is common in elderly men.

## Nocturnal enuresis

Involuntary loss of urine during sleep. Childhood enuresis can be divided into primary (never been dry) and secondary (have been dry for at least 6–12 months).

# Evaluation of urinary incontinence

## History of urinary incontinence

Important features in the history are:
- Storage or voiding symptoms
- Gynaecological/obstetric history in women
- History of any neurological symptoms
- Drug history
- Previous surgery or radiotherapy

A relatively quick onset of urge incontinence symptoms should alert the clinician to the possibility of bladder irritation by infection, stone or tumour.

## Examination for urinary incontinence

Abdominal examination should be performed, together with rectal examination in men (to assess the prostate) and pelvic examination in women (which may objectively demonstrate stress incontinence and signs of pelvic floor weakness). Neurological examination should also be performed if indicated from the history.

## Investigating urinary incontinence

- **Initial tests** should include MSU, ultrasonography to assess post-void residual, and possibly cystoscopy. Bladder diaries and questionnaires are useful
- **Urodynamic testing** is not required in all patients. Essentially it measures the pressure–volume relationships of the bladder during filling (cystometry) and then the pressure–flow relationships during voiding. A catheter in the bladder allows measurement of bladder pressure and also filling. As bladder pressure consists of both abdominal and detrusor pressures, abdominal pressure is measured separately by an intrarectal pressure sensor and subtracted. Video-urodynamics can be performed if the bladder is filled with contrast material. This allows visualisation of the bladder neck to look for hypermobility or sphincter problems. As well as being useful in diagnosing the cause of urinary incontinence, urodynamics has a large role to play in the assessment of bladder outflow obstruction (see Section 6.3 'Urinary tract obstruction')

# Management of urinary incontinence

It is important to begin with conservative measures before progressing to pharmacological or surgical treatment. First exclude a urinary tract infection (UTI), diabetes, constipation, diuretic use and atrophic vaginitis.

## Stress incontinence

### Conservative measures

- Weight loss, smoking cessation and pelvic floor exercises help many women
- Biofeedback mechanisms can improve the results of pelvic floor exercises

### Surgical techniques

These aim to either lift the bladder or supplement the sphincter:

- **Burch colposuspension:** this is the traditional operation which involves elevation of the bladder neck and urethra through a lower abdominal incision
- **Needle suspension of the bladder neck (Stamey procedure):** this is a relatively minimally invasive procedure that gives good initial results, but in the long term it is not as good as colposuspension
- **Pubovaginal slings:**
  - Autologous – using rectus fascia
  - Synthetic – tension-free vaginal tape which is commonly inserted via the obturator foramen (TVT-O). This has good results, with 80% improvement. Complications include bladder injury, erosion, new overactivity, voiding disorders and bleeding
- **Periurethral bulking agents:** these increase sphincter resistance in intrinsic sphincter deficiency
- **Artificial sphincter implantation:** this is a last-resort measure because there is a high complication rate

CHAPTER 8

### Urge incontinence

- **Conservative measures:** bladder retraining, behavioural changes, eg decreasing caffeine
- **Antimuscarinic agents:** these act on the detrusor muscle (eg oxybutynin, tolterodine, solifenacin)
- **Intravesical Botox:** botulinium toxin A (BTX-A) inhibits release of acetylcholine at the neuromuscular junction. It is very useful in neuropathic overactivity but is now also used when medical therapy fails in idiopathic detrusor overactivity
- **Tricyclic antidepressants:** these have an anticholinergic effect and may also have central effects
- **Surgery:** this is a last resort in these patients; options include cystoplasty, which involves augmenting the overactive detrusor with bowel, or, in extreme cases, urinary diversion with an ileal conduit

### Overflow incontinence

This is usually due to failure of the detrusor muscle, which is irreversible. Men sometimes undergo TURP but the success rate is not high. Intermittent self-catheterisation is an option but if this is not feasible then long-term permanent catheterisation is required. This may also be a symptom of high-pressure chronic retention.

## 2.4 Neurological bladder dysfunction

 **In a nutshell ...**

There are several neurological diseases that affect the function of the bladder. Neurological dysfunction may lead either to overactivity or underactivity of the bladder or sphincter and possibly a combination of these.

The balance between the bladder and the sphincter dysfunction will determine the following:

- **Pressure in the bladder:** if this is high it may have implications for renal function because of transmission of this high pressure to the renal pelvis
- **Effectiveness of bladder emptying:** this may manifest as either incontinence or incomplete emptying, with recurrent UTIs

### Diseases above the brainstem (eg cerebrovascular disease)

Cerebral disease may result in **detrusor hyper-reflexia**. The bladder is hyper-reflexic but retains normal coordination of voiding and sensation. Symptoms are frequency, urgency, nocturia and urge incontinence (often due to loss of cortical control). Immediately after a cerebrovascular accident (CVA) there may be a period when the detrusor becomes atonic (cerebral shock); the reason for this is unclear and it usually recovers.

# Spinal cord injury

The spinal cord ends at the level of L2 and becomes the cauda equina. In the initial period after a spinal cord injury there is a period of spinal shock, which is associated with suppression of autonomic and somatic nerve activity, and the bladder becomes acontractile and areflexic. This usually results in urinary retention and requires catheterisation. What happens subsequently depends on the level of the spinal cord injury.

## Lesions above the sacral spinal cord

- These lead to interruption of fibres passing from the sacral cord to the pontine micturition centre
- Subsequently there is lack of coordination between the detrusor and the sphincter, in a condition known as **detrusor sphincter dyssynergia** (DSD)
- The bladder will contract against a closed sphincter and develop high pressure
- These patients are prone to renal damage

## Lesions of the sacral cord and cauda equina

- These tend to produce paralysis of the detrusor, so patients have problems with retention because they are unable to empty their bladders

Almost three-quarters of patients with MS have spinal cord involvement leading to bladder dysfunction. These patients usually complain of urgency secondary to detrusor hyper-reflexia.

# 2.5 Urinary fistulae

 **In a nutshell ...**

A fistula is an abnormal connection between two epithelial-lined surfaces. Causes of urinary fistulae include:

**Obstetric/gynaecological**
- Birth injury (most common in developing countries)
- Iatrogenic
- Malignancy

**Gastrointestinal (GI) disease**
- Diverticulitis (50%)
- Malignancy (25%)
- Crohn's disease (10%)

**Trauma**
- Pelvic fractures

## Types of urinary fistulae

- Vesicovaginal
- Vesicocolic
- Vesicocutaneous
- Ureterovaginal or ureterourethral

## Symptoms of urinary fistulae

- Recurrent UTI
- Pneumaturia
- Passive incontinence

**CHAPTER 8**

## Investigating urinary fistulae

- Examination: a per vaginam examination may detect a vesicovaginal fistula (VVF)
- Cystogram or CT IVU
- Cystoscopy and/or retrograde studies
- Dye test: if a VVF is suspected blue dye is instilled into the bladder, and the patient wears a tampon while walking about for an hour. The dye will be seen on the tampon if there is a fistula
- CT of pneumocolon or Gastrografin enema
- Sigmoidoscopy

## Treatment of urinary fistulae

- Conservative: a catheter and course of antibiotics may heal a small fistula
- Excision of the fistula and bladder repair or ureteric re-implantation
- Bowel resection and/or temporary colostomy may be needed

# SECTION 3

# Urinary tract anatomy

## 3.1 Anatomy of the kidney

### In a nutshell ...

The kidneys lie on the posterior abdominal wall in a retroperitoneal position. They are largely under the cover of the costal margin. The right kidney lies slightly lower than the left because of the large size of the right lobe of the liver. The renal hila lie just above and below the transpyloric plane, 5 cm from the midline. The average male kidney weighs 150 g and the average female kidney 135 g. The normal size of the kidney is vertically 10–12 cm, transversely 5–7 cm and anteroposteriorly 3 cm approximately.

### Coverings of the kidneys

The kidneys are covered (from inside to out) by:
- Fibrous capsule
- Perirenal fat
- Perirenal or **Gerota fascia** (dense connective tissue layer surrounding kidneys and adrenal glands and continuous laterally with the fascia transversalis)
- Pararenal fat

## Kidney structure

On the medial border of each kidney is the **renal hilum**. This opens into the renal sinus space in the central portion of the kidney occupied by the urinary collecting structures and the renal vessels. The hila lie at the level of the transpyloric plane, just lateral to the midline (right hilum lower than the left). The order of the structures at the hilum is (anterior to posterior): renal vein, renal artery and ureter. Other structures that pass through the hilum are lymph vessels and sympathetic nerve fibres. The kidneys are divided into an outer **cortex** and

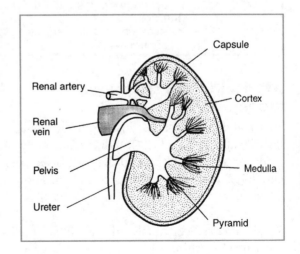

Figure 8.2 Anatomy of the kidney

an inner **medulla**. The medulla is divided into a dozen renal pyramids, each with their base oriented towards the cortex, and a **renal papilla** at the apex. Renal papillae project into the **renal calyces**. Minor calyces fuse to become major calyces (of which there are usually two or three). These then coalesce to form the **renal pelvis** (Figure 11.2).

## Anatomical relations of the kidney

The peritoneal reflection almost completely separates the upper pole of the right kidney from the liver. This appears to help prevent direct spread of renal tumours to the right lobe. The peritoneum between the Gerota fascia and the inferior splenic capsule is called the **lienorenal** or **splenorenal ligament**. Traction on this during left nephrectomy may cause tears in the spleen and necessitate splenectomy.

| ANATOMIC RELATIONS OF THE KIDNEY | | |
|---|---|---|
| | **Anterior** | **Posterior** |
| **Left kidney** | **Superior**<br>Stomach<br>Spleen (with lienorenal or splenorenal ligament)<br>**Medial**<br>Pancreas<br>**Inferior**<br>Left colon | **Superior**<br>Diaphragm covers upper third<br>Costodiaphragmatic recess<br>**Inferior**<br>Twelfth rib crosses lower pole<br>Iliohypogastric nerve<br>Ilioinguinal nerve<br>**Medial**<br>Psoas muscle |
| **Right kidney** | **Superior**<br>Adrenal gland<br>Right lobe of liver<br>**Medial**<br>Second part of the duodenum<br>**Inferior**<br>Right colon (retroperitoneal)<br>Small bowel | **Lateral**<br>Quadratus lumborum and transversus abdominus muscles |

## Arterial blood supply of the kidney

The paired renal arteries arise from the aorta laterally at the level of L2. The right renal artery is longer as it passes behind the inferior vena cava (IVC). Multiple renal arteries on both sides are not uncommon.

Renal arteries commonly divide into five segmental branches:
- One posterior branch supplies most of the posterior part of the kidney

- Four anterior branches are called the apical, upper, middle and lower anterior segmental arteries

All these arteries are end-arteries without any collateral circulation (occlusion will produce ischaemia and infarction of the corresponding renal parenchyma). Segmental arteries divide into lobar arteries, to supply a single renal pyramid. Subsequently, interlobar arteries give off the arcuate arteries, and these give off several interlobular arteries (eventually becoming the afferent glomerular arterioles).

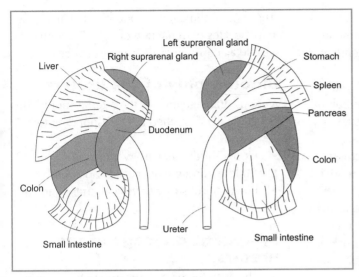

**Figure 8.3 Anterior relations of the kidney**

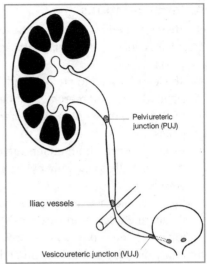

**Figure 8.4 Sites where stones tend to get impacted in the urinary tract**

## Venous drainage of the kidney

Unlike the arteries, renal venous tributaries anastomose freely. Renal veins both drain directly into the IVC:

- The left renal vein is generally three times longer than the right (6–10 cm) and crosses anterior to the aorta. It typically receives the left adrenal vein superiorly, the left gonadal vein inferiorly and a lumbar vein posteriorly
- The right renal vein is shorter than the left (2–4 cm) and usually has no tributary

## Lymphatic drainage of the kidney

This is to the para-aortic nodes around the origin of the renal vessels.

## Nerve supply of the kidney

- Sympathetic input is from T8–L1
- Parasympathetic input is from the vagus nerve. The main function of the nerves appears to be vasomotor

- Complete denervation of the kidney as in transplantation appears to have little effect on renal function

## 3.2 Anatomy of the ureters

The ureter represents the tubular extension of the renal collecting system which courses downwards to connect the kidney to the bladder.

- Ureters vary in length from 22 cm to 30 cm
- The ureter is lined by transitional cell epithelium contiguous with that of the bladder

## Anatomical relations of the ureters

The position of the ureters is very important because they are at risk of surgical injury in a wide number of abdominal procedures.

**CHAPTER 8**

### Anterior relations

- The right ureter is related to the terminal ileum, caecum, appendix and ascending colon
- The left is related to the descending colon, sigmoid and their mesentery. It lies behind the sigmoid mesocolon as it enters the pelvis
- As they descend both ureters are crossed from medially to laterally by the gonadal vessels anteriorly
- In the female they are crossed anteriorly by the uterine arteries and are closely related to the uterine cervix, so they are at risk of injury during gynaecology procedures such as a hysterectomy
- Within the pelvis in the male the vas deferens crosses anterior to the ureter just before it enters the bladder

### Posterior relations

- The ureters on both sides are related to the psoas muscles that separate them from the lumbar transverse processes
- As they enter the pelvis the ureters cross the bifurcation of the common iliac artery

## Narrowings in the ureter

Classically three points are described at which the ureter is particularly narrow. These are:

1. The pelviureteric junction
2. At the bifurcation of the iliac vessels where the ureter enters the pelvis
3. The vesicoureteric junction

These are clinically important, because they may be sites of impaction of calculi and may be visible as narrowings on contrast studies.

## Blood supply of the ureters

Venous drainage mirrors the arterial supply. This is classically described as corresponding to:

- Upper third: renal artery and vein
- Middle third: gonadal artery and vein
- Lower third: superior vesical artery and vein

## Lymphatic drainage of the ureters

- This is to the para-aortic and pelvic lymph nodes

## Nerve supply of the ureters

- Autonomic nerves are sympathetic from T10–L2 spinal segments and parasympathetic from S2–4 segments. Pain fibres leave with the sympathetic nerves and the resulting visceral pain is referred to somatic distributions that correspond to these spinal segments. Pain is therefore produced over the distributions of the subcostal, iliohypogastric, ilioinguinal and/or genitofemoral nerves, resulting in flank, groin or scrotal (or labial) pain

## 4.1  Pathogenesis of urological infections

> **In a nutshell ...**
>
> Most acute infections are due to a single organism (usually *Escherichia coli*). Chronic infections are often due to multiple organisms and may be related to the presence of a foreign body (eg an indwelling catheter) or underlying pathology.
> Infection is dependent on bacterial and host factors.

- **Bacteriuria:** the presence of bacteria in the urine. It is subject to the possibility of contamination, and the risk varies according to the technique used for detection. Suprapubic aspiration is the gold standard
- **Pyuria:** the presence of white blood cells in the urine
- **UTI:** involves the invasion of urothelium by bacteria. It is usually associated with bacteriuria and pyuria

- **Sterile pyuria:** this is pyuria without bacteriuria. It warrants evaluation for tuberculosis (TB), stones or cancer
- **Recurrent UTI:** defined as more than three infections in a year. Causes include re-infection (95% of all recurrent infections in women) and bacterial persistence (more common in men). It may also be due to an underlying urological abnormality (eg reflux) or the presence of calculi (eg staghorn). It is common in patients with indwelling catheters
- **Uncomplicated UTI:** this is an infection in a healthy patient with a structurally and functionally normal urinary tract
- **Complicated UTI:** an infection in a patient with a structural or functional abnormality of the urinary tract or infection associated with immunosuppression or a foreign body

### Microbiology of urological infections

Most acute infections are due to a single organism. Chronic infections are often due to multiple organisms and may be related to the presence of a foreign body (eg an indwelling catheter) or underlying pathology.

CHAPTER 8

### *Escherichia coli* infection

*E. coli* causes 90% of community-acquired infections. In hospitals 50% of infections are caused by *E. coli* (usually from a faecal source).

### Other pathogens

- Enterobacteria: eg *Streptococcus faecalis*, *Proteus* spp., *Klebsiella* spp. These are less common causes of acute uncomplicated UTIs in both sexes and at all ages
- *Pseudomonas* spp.: presence of *Pseudomonas* indicates a foreign body, eg a catheter
- *Proteus* spp.: hydrolyse urea to produce ammonia, which increases urinary pH and predisposes to stone formation
- *Staphylococcus saprophyticus*: especially in sexually active women
- *Staphylococcus aureus*: occurs after surgery on or instrumentation of the urinary tract

### Rare causes of chronic infection

- TB: this is becoming increasingly common, especially in HIV patients, and may cause a diffuse interstitial picture or localised caseating lesions
- Schistosomiasis
- Hydatid disease

## Aetiology of urological infections

Infection is dependent on bacterial and host factors.

### Bacterial factors in urological infections

These are thought to be related to the bacterium's adherence to the transitional epithelium. Only a select number of *E. coli* strains possess sufficient fimbriae to allow urinary infection. Different forms of fimbriae allow organisms to colonise different areas of the urinary tract (eg upper vs lower urinary tract) and an organism can adapt and change its fimbriae type, allowing infection to progress upwards.

### Host factors in urological infections

The urinary tract has several defence mechanisms:

- Acidic urine
- High levels of urea
- High osmolality
- Antibacterial secretions, eg:
  - Tamm–Horsfall protein secreted in the loop of Henle
  - Prostatic antibacterial factor
  - Urinary immunoglobulins
- Repeated voiding: prevents urinary stasis

Conditions predisposing to urinary tract infections usually alter or impair defence mechanisms, such as:

- **Female sex** – woman are at greater risk of UTIs than men because:
  - Shorter urethra allows transfer of faecal flora
  - Transfer of vaginal flora occurs during sexual intercourse
  - Hormonal changes cause changes in urine composition during pregnancy and the menopause
- **Diabetes** – this predisposes to UTI because of:
  - Increased glycosuria
  - Immunosuppression
- **Obstruction** – if this occurs in any part of the urinary tract it causes urinary stasis, which predisposes to infection
- **Foreign bodies,** eg catheter, calculi, predispose to UTI

## 4.2 Lower urinary tract infections

### In a nutshell ...

Lower urinary tract infections include:
- Acute bacterial cystitis (commonly referred to as a UTI)
- Epididymo-orchitis
- Prostatitis

Fournier's gangrene is a serious complication that can result from a lower UTI, especially in an immunocompromised patient. It needs urgent surgical debridement and is a life-threatening surgical emergency.

UTIs in children are covered in Paediatric Surgery , Book 1.

### Acute bacterial cystitis

Fifty per cent of women experience at least one attack during their lifetime. Acute bacterial cystitis may also be a cause of confusion and sepsis in elderly people, with minimal symptoms.

Remember that procedures performed when the urinary tract is infected can cause severe generalised sepsis, and should be performed under antibiotic cover (eg single-dose gentamicin before catheter insertion).

### Clinical features of acute bacterial cystitis

- Frequency and urgency of micturition
- Dysuria ± haematuria

### Investigations of acute bacterial cystitis

#### Urine culture

It is arguable whether this is needed in all women with symptoms suggestive of acute cystitis and no complicating factors, because treatment is often completed before results are available, and it markedly increases the cost of treatment. A dipstick positive for pyuria, haematuria or bacteriuria is usually sufficient. Some dipsticks detect nitrites (produced from nitrate by bacterial degradation) and these are more sensitive for infection.

You should obtain urine culture:
- For all men with suspected cystitis
- For women when symptoms persist or if there are recurrent infections
- For women who are elderly, if they are diabetic, or are pregnant (because in these situations pathogens may not be typical)

Typical findings from MSU culture in a UTI include bacterial growth and pyuria. Causes of a sterile pyuria include:
- Inadequately treated infection
- Atypical organisms (eg TB)
- Inflammation in or near the urinary tract (eg calculi, tumour, chemical or radiation cystitis, interstitial nephritis, prostatitis, appendicitis)

The degree of symptoms may not be related to the findings of MSU

#### Further investigations

Further investigations are required in all men and women with severe recurrent UTIs:
- Tests include: renal function, ultrasonography (to check kidneys for scarring and assess adequate bladder emptying), plain abdominal film (to exclude renal calculi)

CHAPTER 8

- CT IVU
- Patients with haematuria require a cystoscopy

## Treatment of acute bacterial cystitis

- Several studies suggest that 3 days of antibiotics are adequate in uncomplicated cystitis in women. Empirical treatment is usually with trimethoprim
- All women should be given general advice about hygiene, adequate fluid intake and regular bladder emptying (including after intercourse)
- Recurrent UTIs may necessitate prophylactic antibiotics, taken either every night or only after intercourse
- In elderly women hormone replacement therapy (HRT) may be used to treat atrophic vaginitis, which predisposes to UTI
- Evidence of outflow obstruction requires treatment of its cause

---

**Beware UTIs**
- **In children:** see Paediatric Surgery, Book 1
- **If planning urological instrumentation:** may cause sepsis, so cover with antibiotics
- **With obstruction:** needs urgent decompression
- **With *Pseudomonas*:** look for foreign bodies
- **With *Proteus*:** look for stones
- **With sterile pyuria:** look for TB

---

# Epididymo-orchitis

## Clinical features of epididymo-orchitis

- Acute onset of testicular pain with swelling of the scrotum
- Symptoms of UTI may be present
- Occasionally patients are systemically unwell

## Pathogenesis of epididymo-orchitis

- Epididymitis is most common (usually bacterial)
- Orchitis is less common (often viral, eg mumps, coxsackievirus)
- In older men epididymitis is nearly always related to Gram-negative infection of the urine (usually *E. coli*). This is most often due to bladder outflow obstruction
- In younger men sexually transmitted infections (STIs) are more common (causative organisms include *Chlamydia* spp. and *Neisseria gonorrhoeae*)

## Differential diagnosis of epididymo-orchitis

- In younger men **torsion of the testis** (see Section 8). If there is any suspicion of this, exploration of the scrotum is mandatory
- About 10% of testicular tumours present with acute symptoms

## Investigating epididymo-orchitis

- Urinalysis often reveals abnormalities such as pyuria or bacteriuria
- Ultrasonography is useful to exclude an abscess

## Treatment of epididymo-orchitis

- Symptomatic treatment includes bedrest, scrotal support and analgesia
- Antibiotics are also given:
  - In elderly men ciprofloxacin is sufficient
  - In younger men doxycycline should be added to cover *Chlamydia* spp.
- In older men, formal assessment for bladder outflow obstruction should be undertaken

## Prostatitis

Prostate inflammation is often related to bladder outflow obstruction. In some cases no bacterial cause is found; this chronic pelvic pain syndrome (CPPS) is difficult to treat.

### Clinical presentation of prostatitis

- Usually presents with similar symptoms to cystitis
- Acute bacterial prostatitis patients may be systemically unwell, with fever, purulent discharge, tender prostate, pain on ejaculation and haemospermia

### Investigating prostatitis

- Blood culture
- Urine culture
- TRUS, to exclude and treat abscess formation

### Treatment of prostatitis

- Antibiotics appropriate to the organism
- In CPPS there is some evidence for the use of non-steroidal anti-inflammatory drugs (NSAIDs) and α blockers

## Fournier's gangrene

Fournier's gangrene is a form of **necrotising fasciitis** of the male genitalia and surrounding areas.

> If you ever diagnose Fournier's gangrene (eg if you feel crepitus in an infected perineum) you must act quickly. This is a urological emergency and an experienced urologist capable of debriding the perineum should see the patient **within minutes** of diagnosis. Every minute that the patient is not in theatre means another few centimetres of tissue necrosis. Death can occur within hours. In the few minutes that you are waiting for the urologist you should give fluids, give personally (not just prescribe) broad-spectrum antibiotics and book an emergency theatre.

### Clinical presentation of Fournier's gangrene

- Generally occurs in older patients and is particularly common in men with diabetes
- Cellulitis of the external genitalia with swelling, erythema and necrotic areas
- Crepitus can often be elicited on examination
- Pain is prominent and there is marked systemic upset
- Infection may extend to involve the groin and suprapubic areas

### Investigating Fournier's gangrene

- Cultures often reveal multiple organisms. This is a classic anaerobic/aerobic synergistic infection
- Typical organisms include *Pseudomonas* spp., β-haemolytic streptococci, *E. coli* and *Clostridium* spp.

### Treatment of Fournier's gangrene

- Prompt diagnosis essential

**CHAPTER 8**

- IV antibiotics and rehydration should be followed by **early surgical debridement**

**Mortality rate is high** (10–75%) and reflects the pre-existing morbidity.

## 4.3 Upper urinary tract infection

### In a nutshell ...

Infection of the renal pelvis and kidneys is referred to as pyelonephritis.

**Acute pyelonephritis**
- Presents with pyrexia, loin pain and rigors on a background of UTI
- Ultrasonography or IVU is useful to exclude an infected obstructed system
- Treatment is antibiotics

**Chronic pyelonephritis**
- Usually radiologically diagnosed small kidney atrophied by chronic bacterial infections
- Investigations aim to assess the damage with ultrasonography, IVU and tests of kidney function
- Treatment is aimed at the underlying cause (eg vesicoureteric reflux [VUR]) and antibiotic prophylaxis
- Nephrectomy may be needed

## Acute pyelonephritis

### Clinical features of acute pyelonephritis
- Classically presents with pyrexia and loin pain and rigors
- Occasionally presents with septic shock

- May be preceding or concurrent symptoms suggestive of UTI
- Alternatively, infection may occur via haematogenous spread from another source

### Investigating acute pyelonephritis
- Urine should be tested by dipstick and sent for urine culture
- Blood culture should be taken from all patients with suspicion of septicaemia
- Plain film (KUB) may show stone disease
- Ultrasonography is used to exclude obstruction
- IVU may show enlargement of the kidney and poor urinary concentration

### Treatment of acute pyelonephritis
- Antibiotic therapy is the mainstay of treatment in uncomplicated acute pyelonephritis
- Initial empirical therapy with broad-spectrum antibiotics (eg amoxicillin, gentamicin) can be changed to specific antibiotics when cultures become available
- 14-day course of antibiotics is recommended

### Complications of acute pyelonephritis
- **Pyonephrosis (pus in the renal collecting system):** this may result from pyelonephritis associated with distal obstruction. It requires prompt drainage, usually with percutaneous nephrostomy
- **Perinephric abscess (pus around the kidney):** this may rupture and reach adjacent organs. It requires surgical or ultrasound-guided percutaneous drainage

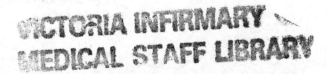

# Chronic pyelonephritis

## Clinical features of chronic pyelonephritis

- Usually a radiological diagnosis
- Refers to a small, contracted, atrophic kidney that results from a chronic bacterial infection
- Although patients may present with recurrent UTIs, the disease may present at an advanced stage when chronic renal failure (CRF) is present
- These patients are susceptible to hypertension, renal impairment and stone formation

## Investigating chronic pyelonephritis

- Ultrasonography will confirm a scarred kidney
- IVU will demonstrate loss of renal parenchyma, especially over the renal poles and overlying the calyces
- **VUR** is often associated with chronic pyelonephritis. This diagnosis can be made by **micturating cystourethrogram**

## Treatment of chronic pyelonephritis

- Deal with any predisposing cause
- Antibiotic prophylaxis is often required
- For severely diseased kidneys with minimal function, nephrectomy may be appropriate

Chronic inflammation may cause a granulomatous mass that is difficult to distinguish from a renal tumour (called chronic xanthogranulomatous pyelonephritis).

# 4.4 Inflammatory conditions of the bladder

## Interstitial cystitis

- Causes pain, frequency and urgency
- Characterised by mucosal ulceration and fissures
- Histologically shows chronic inflammatory change
- Exclude carcinoma in situ (CIS)

## Radiation cystitis

- Radiation damage to blood supply and bladder wall ischaemia
- May present acutely with severe bleeding
- May cause fistulae and fibrosis in the long term

# 4.5 Bladder diverticula

## Congenital diverticula

- True diverticula (full-thickness wall)
- Tend to occur in urachus and paraureteric, contributing to reflux

## Acquired diverticuli

- Usually false diverticuli (mucosal outpouching only)
- High vesical pressures associated with obstruction cause trabeculation of bladder wall and formation of diverticula
- May cause:
  - Stasis with infection
  - Stasis with stone formation
  - Voiding inefficiency

CHAPTER 8

## 4.6 Antibiotic prophylaxis in urology

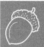

**In a nutshell ...**

Patients undergoing endoscopic surgery, open surgery or prostatic biopsies require antibiotic prophylaxis.

### Endoscopic surgery

Any patient undergoing endoscopic surgery to the urinary tract is at risk of bacterial infection.

Preoperative antibiotic prophylaxis required:
- Before instrumentation of upper urinary tract
- Where the risk of infection is greater due to the presence of potentially infected urine (eg presence of a catheter, urinary stone disease)
- In patients with increased risk

### Patients at increased risk
- Known UTI
- Indwelling catheter
- Congenital cardiac abnormality
- Cardiac valve disease
- Diabetes
- Immunocompromised
- Implanted prosthetic materials (joint, heart valve, pacemaker)

### Current antibiotic practice
- Check with your local guidelines
- A preoperative dose of gentamicin or a cephalosporin is usually adequate
- At-risk patients should be covered with a combination of antibiotics (eg amoxicillin and gentamicin) when having catheters removed

### Open surgery

Antibiotic prophylaxis for open surgery is as for general surgery, with a broad-spectrum gentamicin plus metronidazole if bowel is used (eg cystectomy).

### Prostate biopsy

All patients undergoing transrectal prostate biopsies should receive prophylaxis to minimise the risk of potentially fatal sepsis. Oral ciprofloxacin is usually given (some units add a dose of IV antibiotic at the time of biopsy).

# SECTION 5

# Urinary stone disease

## 5.1 Pathology of urinary stones (calculi)

### In a nutshell ...

Stones in the urinary tract are a common urological problem and the prevalence is estimated at 2–3% in the developed world (one in eight white people have stones by the age of 70). Stones commonly affect men aged <65 years. Eighty per cent of urinary tract stones are calcium-based. Stone formation is encouraged by supersaturation and the presence of a nucleus, and is inhibited by citrate and magnesium.

Metabolic abnormalities that predispose to stone formation:
- Hypercalciuria
- Hyperoxaluria
- Hyperuricuria
- Cystinuria
- Hypocitraturia
- Infection

**Risks factors for urinary tract stones**
- Higher in carnivores (higher protein intake)
- Increased incidence in relatives of sufferers
- Warm climate
- Metabolic abnormalities (see below)
- Dehydration
- Previous stones: risk of recurrence is 35–75% at 10 years

The treatment of stones has been revolutionised over the last 20 years with minimally invasive techniques, meaning that very few patients now require open surgery for management of their stone disease. The specialty of endourology has developed around these techniques and also encompasses some non-stone disease and laparoscopy.

### Aetiology of urinary tract stones

Composition of the most common urinary stones is shown in the table overleaf. Most (80%) are based on calcium.

**CHAPTER 8**

| COMPOSITION OF URINARY STONES | | |
|---|---|---|
| Calcium oxalate | 35% | Hard, brittle, irregular in shape |
| Calcium phosphate | 10% | |
| Mixed calcium oxalate and phosphate | 35% | |
| Magnesium ammonium phosphate (struvite) | 10% | Soft, white<br>Fill renal pelvis<br>Associated with infection (eg *Proteus*) |
| Uric acid | 8% | Radiolucent<br>Yellow with fine projections |
| Cystine | 1% | Hard, white stones |
| Others (eg xanthine) | 1% | |

Stone formation takes place only when urine is supersaturated (solubility product of that particular solute has been exceeded), but in the normal state many stone components in urine are supersaturated (aided by mucoproteins and alanine), and a nucleus is probably needed for further crystal deposition. This may be a small crystal, a protein, a foreign body or sloughed papilla.

Urine contains natural inhibitors of stone formation, including citrate and magnesium.

## Metabolic abnormalities in stone formers

### Hypercalciuria

Of patients with calcium oxalate-based kidney stones 30–60% have increased calcium in the urine. The main causes are:

- **Absorptive hypercalciuria:** this is when increased absorption of calcium in the gut takes place in response to vitamin D
- **Renal hypercalciuria:** the kidneys are unable to reabsorb calcium, increasing its concentration in the urine
- **Resorptive hypercalciuria:** this is rare; there

is hyperparathyroidism in most cases, due to increased calcium resorption from bones (associated with hypercalcaemia)

Calcium metabolism is covered in more detail in Chapter 4, Endocrine Surgery.

### Hyperoxaluria

- **Primary hyperoxaluria** is a rare genetic disorder
- **Secondary hyperoxaluria** results from any cause of small-bowel malabsorption (eg small-bowel resection) or bowel-intrinsic disease (eg Crohn's disease). The reason is increased colonic permeability to oxalate as a result of exposure of the colonic epithelium to bile salts. Increased intake (eg of tea) is another cause

### Hyperuricuria

Most commonly caused by excessive dietary purine intake (eg meat) and contributed to by dehydration. Predisposes to urate stones and calcium oxalate stones. Other causes include ileostomy, chronic diarrhoea, myeloproliferative disease and gout.

Purine metabolism is covered in more detail in Section 2.3, Chapter 7, Orthopaedics Surgery.

## Cystinuria

This inherited autosomal recessive condition involves a defect in amino acid transport in the intestine and kidneys.

## Hypocitraturia

As stated above, citrate is thought to be an inhibitor of stone formation. A low citrate contributes to formation of urinary stones in up to 60% of patients.

## Infection stones

These account for 10% of all urinary stones. They are often large, filling the pelvicalyceal system, giving a characteristic staghorn appearance. Chemical composition is of magnesium ammonium phosphate (struvite).

They usually arise in response to chronic infection with organisms such as *Proteus*, *Pseudomonas* and *Klebsiella* spp. These are urea-splitting organisms that alkalinise urine by production of ammonia and cause deposition of calcium and other ions.

## 5.2 Clinical presentation of stone disease

 **In a nutshell ...**

The usual presentation of stones in the urinary tract is acute ureteric colic. Other modes of presentation include:
- UTIs
- Haematuria
- An incidental findings during imaging for other symptoms

## Ureteric colic

This is the result of a stone impacting in the urinary tract and causing obstruction behind it. The ureter undergoes spasm and hyperperistalsis.

Stones impact at sites of narrowing in the ureter, which can be pathological narrowings (eg stricture) or anatomical narrowings:
- At the pelviureteric junction (PUJ)
- In the pelvis where the ureter crosses the iliac vessels at the sacroiliac joint (SIJ)
- At the VUJ

### Clinical features of ureteric colic
- Abrupt onset
- Severe pain from the flank: this radiates laterally from the flank, around the abdomen, to the groin and genitals (common innervation of referred pain)
- Patients writhe with pain: they find it impossible to be still. In contrast, patients with peritonitis tend to lie still as movement exacerbates pain
- Lower urinary tract symptoms: these are caused when the stone nears the bladder and irritates the trigone
- Nausea and vomiting: this is common because the autonomic nervous system transmits visceral pain and the coeliac ganglion serves both kidneys and stomach. Other GI symptoms can lead to confusion in the diagnosis
- Tachycardia: this is common
- Pyrexia: obstruction leads to stasis, which leads to infection
- Loin tenderness: note that the abdominal examination may be normal
- Haematuria: this can be macroscopic or microscopic. It occurs in about 90% of patients

### Differential diagnosis of ureteric colic

- Appendicitis
- Diverticulitis
- Ectopic pregnancy
- Salpingitis
- Torsion of ovarian cyst
- Biliary colic
- Ruptured AAA
- Pyelonephritis
- PUJ obstruction

## 5.3  Investigating stone disease

### In a nutshell ...

The aims of investigation in urinary stone disease are to:
- Confirm diagnosis
- Elucidate whether infection is present
- Determine location and size of stones
- Determine degree of obstruction
- Determine renal function, both overall and relative for each kidney
- Identify underlying abnormalities that may have caused stone formation (metabolic or anatomical)

### Intravenous urography

Half of all stones are radio-opaque and visualised on the control KUB film (urate stones are radiolucent). Ideally an IVU will confirm the presence of a stone, its size and location, and also the degree of renal obstruction.

Films can sometimes be difficult to interpret if there is a lot of bowel gas or faeces. Some centres advocate bowel prep before elective IVU.

IVU should be used with caution in patients with poor renal function because it is nephrotoxic – ensure that patients are well hydrated pre- and post-procedure – and in patients with diabetes who are on metformin (stop 24 hours before the procedure). It is contraindicated in patients with a history of adverse reaction to contrast media.

### Ultrasonography

This is excellent for determining if there is acute obstruction; it will also detect stones within the kidney. However, it is unreliable for detecting ureteric calculi.

### Non-contrast computed tomography

This technique has superseded the use of IVU in some centres. It is rapid to perform, requires no contrast media, and identifies both radio-opaque and radiolucent stones. The main disadvantage is the increased radiation dose administered. CT will not allow assessment of the degree of obstruction or of renal function and it is not as easy to interpret anatomical location or detailed pelvicalyceal anatomy.

### Metabolic studies

This is not usually relevant in the acute situation, but if any stones are passed then analysis will allow targeted future treatment if applicable. Metabolic screening usually involves serum levels of calcium and urate and a 24-hour urine collection, which, in addition to measuring these ions, also measures citrate, oxalate and phosphate.

# 5.4 Management of stone disease

## In a nutshell ...

Stones <5 mm mostly pass spontaneously over a 6-week period. Stones >6 mm rarely pass spontaneously.

Options for treatment depend on:
- Site of the stone
- Size of the stone
- Any associated infection

Modalities include:
- Watch and wait ± medical expulsive therapy (eg α blockers)
- ESWL
- Ureteroscopy and stone extraction
- Percutaneous nephrolithotomy (PCNL)

## Acute management of ureteric colic

- **Supportive treatment:** with analgesia (diclofenac is the drug of choice if the renal function is normal), antiemetics and rehydration. There is evidence that α blockers increase the rate of stone passage
- **Drainage:** if there are signs of sepsis (pyrexia, rigors, raised WCC), immediate drainage is required because the risk of renal damage is high. The preferred method is percutaneous nephrostomy under LA. An alternative is retrograde placement of a ureteric stent, but this can be difficult and carries an increased risk of septicaemia
- **Conservative approach:** use this if there is no evidence of sepsis. Patients may experience further pain (ensure adequate analgesia). Sieve urine to identify the stone. Follow-up with regular KUB until the stone is passed (up to 6 weeks)

The likelihood of a stone passing spontaneously depends on its size and position:
- 90% of stones are <4 mm and in the lower ureter, and are likely to pass
- 5% of stones are >6 mm and in the upper ureter, and are unlikely to pass

## Management of ureteric stones

For patients with large stones or persistent pain or who fail conservative management there are two main options: ESWL and ureteroscopic stone destruction.

## Extracorporeal shock wave lithotripsy

- This uses an external energy source that is focused accurately on the stone, causing it to shatter. It relies on accurate localisation of the stone by a radiograph or ultrasonography, which may be difficult if the stone lies over a bony landmark such as a transverse process or over the pelvis
- ESWL is indicated for all stones with diameter <2 cm
- Complications include colic due to fragments from large stones, haematuria, failure to shatter harder/larger stones and renal trauma (rarely)
- Contraindications are pregnancy, aortic aneurysm, urosepsis and uncorrected coagulopathy

## Ureteroscopy

With modern ureteroscopy most ureteric stones are accessible nowadays. Results are better for lower ureteric stones. Details of ureteroscopy are given in Section 1.2.

CHAPTER 8

# Management of renal stones

There are several management options for renal stones.

## Conservative treatment of renal stones

- Can be used for asymptomatic patients with small renal calculi (<5 mm)

## ESWL

- Good results can be obtained for stones <2 cm
- Ensure that the renal anatomy is appropriate to allow drainage of the fragments
- For larger stones place a ureteric stent to prevent steinstrasse or 'stone street' (a column of obstructing stone fragments in the ureter)

## Percutaneous nephrolithotomy

- Access is gained to the renal collecting system percutaneously with dilation of a track to allow insertion of a nephroscope
- Stones are then broken by various methods including electrohydraulic lithotripsy and ultrasonography
- PCNL is the preferred method for larger stones (eg staghorn calculi)

## Flexible ureterorenoscopy and laser lithotripsy

- This is ideal for small stones in the renal collecting system that are unfavourable for ESWL because of poor anatomical drainage
- It is the method of choice for patients who have both ureteric and renal calculi

## Open surgery

- **Open nephrolithotomy:** this is very rarely required because of increasing expertise in endoscopic techniques. It may be combined with pyeloplasty in patients with PUJ obstruction and secondary stones
- **Nephrectomy:** this should be considered in patients with symptomatic renal stones and a kidney contributing <15% of overall function (assuming overall renal function is normal)

# Bladder stones

These are fairly rare except in certain geographical areas.

## Causes of bladder stones

- Bladder outflow obstruction and urinary stasis
- Chronic infection
- Foreign body (eg non-absorbable suture)
- Renal calculus

## Presentation of bladder stones

- Pain, frequency and haematuria
- Infection
- Chronic irritation of urothelium and increased risks of transitional cell carcinoma

## Management of bladder stones

- Usually radio-opaque
- Can be removed by lithoclast fragmentation but require open surgery if >5 cm

# SECTION 6

# Urinary tract obstruction and benign prostatic hyperplasia

## 6.1 Anatomy of the prostate

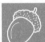 **In a nutshell ...**

The prostate lies inferior to the bladder and surrounds the prostatic urethra. It is roughly conical in shape, with the base superiorly.
- Weight of the normal prostate is about 20 g
- Length of the normal prostate is 3 cm

### Anatomical relations of the prostate

- **Superior relations:** the base of the prostate is continuous with the neck of the bladder. Smooth muscle passes continuously from one organ to the other
- **Inferior relations:** the apex of the prostate lies on the urogenital diaphragm. The urethra leaves at this point to become the membranous urethra (see page 682). Anteriorly here the prostate is related to the symphysis pubis and separated from it by extraperitoneal fat in the retropubic space.

The puboprostatic ligaments connect this surface of the prostate to the pubic bones
- **Posterior relations:** the prostate is separated from the rectum posteriorly by the **fascia of Denonvilliers**
- **Lateral relations:** the pubococcygeal portion of levator ani cradles the lateral surfaces of the prostate

### Structure of the prostate

The prostate is composed of 70% glandular elements and 30% fibromuscular stroma. It has a discrete zonal anatomy, with zones being distinguished by both their location and their differing propensity for pathological lesions.
- **Transition zone:** this surrounds the urethra proximal to the ejaculatory ducts; this is the area where benign prostatic hyperplasia (BPH) occurs
- **Central zone:** this surrounds the ejaculatory ducts and projects under the bladder base to the seminal vesicles
- **Peripheral zone:** this constitutes the bulk of the apical, posterior and lateral aspects of the prostate; 75% of prostate cancers arise in this zone
- **Anterior fibromuscular stroma:** this is a variable amount of prostatic tissue anteriorly

Clinically the prostate is described as having two lateral lobes separated by a central sulcus that is palpable on rectal examination. A middle lobe is often present in older men and projects into the bladder. These lobes do not correspond to any histologically defined structures.

## Blood supply of the prostate

- Branches of the inferior vesical and middle rectal arteries

## Venous drainage of the prostate

The veins form the prostatic venous plexus, which receives the deep dorsal vein of the penis and drains with the vesical venous plexus into the internal iliac vein. Drainage also occurs into the vertebral venous plexus and this may be a route of metastasis to the lumber vertebrae for prostate carcinoma cells.

## Lymphatic drainage of the prostate

This is to the internal iliac nodes.

## Nerve supply of the prostate

Autonomic supply is as with the bladder. Sympathetic nerves with $\alpha_1$-adrenergic receptors cause contraction of prostatic smooth muscle and are targeted therapeutically in men with BPH.

## 6.2 Anatomy of the urethra and perineum and the female genital tract

### Anatomy of the male urethra

The male urethra is about 20 cm long. It extends from the neck of the bladder to the external urethral meatus. It is divided into four parts:

1. **Prostatic urethra:** as described above, 3 cm long and is the widest and most dilatable portion of the urethra
2. **Membranous urethra:** a 2-cm portion of the urethra that pierces the urogenital diaphragm
3. **Bulbar urethra**
4. **Penile urethra** (see below)

### Anatomy of the pelvic diaphragm

The perineum is separated from the pelvic cavity by a transverse sheet of muscle and covering fascia called the pelvic diaphragm (formed by the slings of the levator ani and coccygeus muscles). Levator ani has two parts: posteriorly the iliococcygeus and anteriorly the pubococcygeus. The anterior portion of the sacrospinous ligament also has a muscular component (the coccygeus muscle) which contributes to the pelvic diaphragm.

### Iliococcygeus

This joins the muscle of the contralateral side by interdigitating at the anococcygeal raphe. It extends from the coccyx to the anorectal junction.

## Pubococcygeus

This divides into three parts:

1. **Posterior relations:** it interdigitates at the anococcygeal raphe
2. **Anterior relations:** it forms the anorectal sling around the anorectal junction; this contributes to formation of the anorectal angle and is important in continence. The fibres also blend with the deep part of the external anal sphincter
3. **The puboprostaticus or pubovaginalis:** this is a small portion running in front of the anorectal junction behind the prostate or vagina

## Anatomy of the perineum

The perineum has a diamond-shaped outline. This region can be divided into two triangular areas by drawing a line that links the anterior ends of the ischial tuberosities.

## The anal region

This is delineated by the coccyx posteriorly and the ischial tuberosities laterally. It contains the anal canal as a midline structure, and laterally on each side there is a space called the 'ischioanal fossa' which extends superiorly in continuity with the ischiorectal fossa. These are packed with fat and are huge potential spaces for the collection of pus and abscess formation; they can be accessed by an incision in the skin of the buttock.

Borders of the ischioanal and ischiorectal fossae are:

- Medially, the anus and rectum
- Superiorly (the roof), the levator ani
- Laterally, the medial surface of the obturator internus
- Inferiorly (the floor), the skin of the buttock

The pudendal nerve and internal pudendal vessels pass along the lateral wall of the fossa in a fascial pudendal canal. The pudendal nerve supplies the external anal sphincter and skin of the perineum. The internal pudendal artery, a branch of the internal iliac, gives rise to the inferior rectal artery and branches to the penis or to the labia and clitoris.

See Chapter 1, Abdominal Surgery for the anatomy of the anal canal and sphincters, and for discussion of perianal sepsis.

**Figure 8.5**
**Ischiorectal fossa**

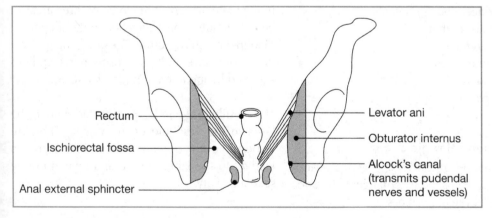

Rectum

Ischiorectal fossa

Anal external sphincter

Levator ani

Obturator internus

Alcock's canal (transmits pudendal nerves and vessels)

**CHAPTER 8**

## The urogenital region

This is an area delineated by the symphysis pubis anteriorly and the ischiopubic rami of the pubic bones laterally. The urethra (and vagina in the female) pass through the incomplete anterior portion of the pelvic diaphragm.

Anterior to the pelvic diaphragm lies the urogenital diaphragm. This has two muscular and fascial layers attached to the margins of the pubic arch laterally and the perineal body posteriorly. Anterior to these layers just under the skin lies the superficial perineal pouch. Between these layers is enclosed the deep perineal pouch.

### Male urogenital region

See also the anatomy of the penis (Section 8.2). Contains the penis and scrotum.

The **superficial perineal** pouch contains:
- The root of the penis (the bulb is attached to the urogenital diaphragm and the crura are attached to the pubic bones on either side)
- Muscles covering the root of the penis that also originate in the superficial perineal pouch (bulbospongiosus and ischiocavernosus)

The **deep perineal pouch** contains:
- Membranous urethra
- Sphincter urethrae
- Bulbourethral glands
- Internal pudendal vessels
- Dorsal nerve of the penis

### Female urogenital region

See also 'Anatomy of the female genital tract' (below). This contains the external genitalia and the urethral and vaginal orifices.

The **superficial perineal pouch** contains:
- Structures forming the root of the clitoris (bulbospongiosus and ischiocavernosus)

The **deep perineal pouch** contains:
- Part of the urethra
- Part of the vagina
- Sphincter urethrae
- Internal pudendal vessels
- Dorsal nerve of the clitoris

## Anatomy of the female genital tract

### Urethra

The female urethra is much shorter than the male urethra (around 3.5 cm in length) and extends from the bladder into the vestibule. The meatus lies a couple of centimetres below the clitoris.

### Vulva

The female external genitalia include the labia majora and minora, the clitoris, the vestibule of the vagina (the area enclosed by the labia minora) and the vestibular glands.

The clitoris has a structure similar to the penis in the male. Its root is made up of three areas of erectile tissue, a bulb attached to the urogenital diaphragm and two crura. The body and glans of the clitoris have multiple sensory nerve endings supplied by the internal pudendal nerve.

The vestibular glands are located under the labia in the vestibule of the vagina. They are responsible for secreting mucus into a groove leading to the labia minora and hymen during sexual activity.

# Vagina

The muscular tube of the vagina is approximately 7–8 cm long, with the upper half lying in the pelvis in close proximity to the rectum (separated by a fold of peritoneum which is called the pouch of Douglas). The vagina passes through the pelvic diaphragm where it is supported by the pubovaginalis muscle and the attachment of the posterior wall to the perineal body. The lower half of the vagina lies in the perineum. The cervix of the uterus opens into the vault of the vagina on the anterior surface, encircled by the vaginal walls. The vaginal vault can be divided into anterior, posterior and lateral fornices. Of particular importance is the close passage of the ureters to the lateral fornix of the vagina (these can be injured during hysterectomy).

## Anatomical relations of the vagina

Anteriorly:
- Uterine cervix
- Base of bladder
- Urethra

Posteriorly:
- Pouch of Douglas
- Rectum
- Perineal body
- Anal canal

Laterally:
- Ureter (superior to lateral fornix)
- Pelvic diaphragm

## Arterial supply of the vagina
The uterine, vaginal, middle rectal and internal pudendal arteries form a vascular anastomosis.

## Venous drainage of the vagina
A venous plexus drains into the internal iliac veins.

## Lymphatic drainage of the vagina
Upper two-thirds drains to the internal and external iliac nodes. Lower third drains to the superficial inguinal nodes.

# Uterus

The uterus is a hollow pear-shaped organ that is divided into three anatomically distinct areas: the fundus (above the fallopian tubes), body, and neck or cervix. The cervix pierces the anterior wall of the vagina and therefore has two parts: the supravaginal and vaginal parts of the cervix. The cervical canal connects the uterine and vaginal cavities and the ends of the canal are referred to as the 'internal os' and the 'external os'. The walls of the uterus are thick and muscular and lined with endometrium, which is continuous with the lining of the fallopian tube.

## Anatomical relations of the uterus

Anteriorly:
- Uterovesical pouch and bladder
- Anterior fornix of vagina

Posteriorly:
- Pouch of Douglas

Laterally:
- Fallopian tubes
- Broad ligaments
- Uterine artery and vein
- Ureter

CHAPTER 8

### Arterial supply of the uterus

This is from the uterine artery (from the internal iliac).

### Venous drainage of the uterus

The uterine vein drains into the internal iliac vein.

### Lymphatic drainage of the uterus

The fundus drains to the para-aortic nodes. The body and cervix drain to the internal and external iliac lymph nodes.

### Ligaments of the uterus

The **round ligament** is the remains of the gubernaculum and thus follows the same pathway through the deep or internal inguinal ring and along the inguinal canal to the labia majora. It maintains the anteverted uterine position but is not essential.

The **broad ligament** is a fold of peritoneum extending from the uterus to the lateral pelvic walls. It forms a mesentery, with the fallopian tube running along the superior border. Part of the medial aspect of the broad ligament forms the suspensory ligament of the ovary.

The uterus is supported within the pelvic cavity by the levator ani muscles and three ligaments formed from condensations of pelvic fascia: the transverse cervical ligament, pubocervical ligament and sacrocervical ligament. The round and broad ligaments do not have any supportive function. The uterus usually sits at 90° to the top of the vagina pointing anteriorly (an anteverted position). In some women, however, it may lie pointing posteriorly into the pouch of Douglas, in a retroverted position.

### Fallopian (uterine) tubes

The fallopian or uterine tubes lie in continuity with the cavity of the uterus and extend laterally for approximately 10 cm. They run along the superior border of the broad ligament and have a free opening near to the ovary. This opening is called the ostium and is surrounded by fimbriae. The tubes have a double layer of muscle fibres (inner circular and outer longitudinal) which cause peristalsis. The mucosal lining also has cilia and secretes mucus to aid passage of the fertilised ovum to the uterine body.

## 6.3 Urinary tract obstruction

 **In a nutshell ...**

The most common causes of upper urinary tract obstruction are stones, malignancy and PUJ obstruction.
The most common causes of lower urinary tract obstruction are BPH and urethral stricture.
Urinary tract obstruction is usually characterised by dilatation of the renal tract (hydronephrosis), although there are other causes of hydronephrosis that are not all associated with obstruction.

## Hydronephrosis

Obstruction of the renal tract usually results in dilatation. Hydronephrosis is defined as a dilatation of the renal pelvis. It is important to remember that there are causes of renal tract dilatation other than obstruction (eg vesico-ureteric reflux and congenital megaureter).

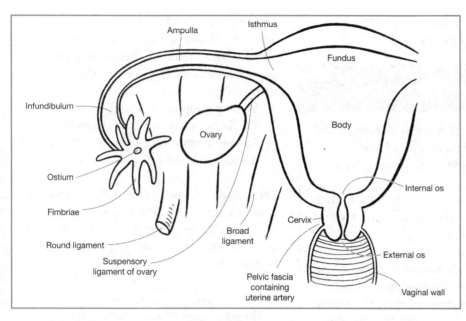

**Figure 8.6 Female reproductive tract**

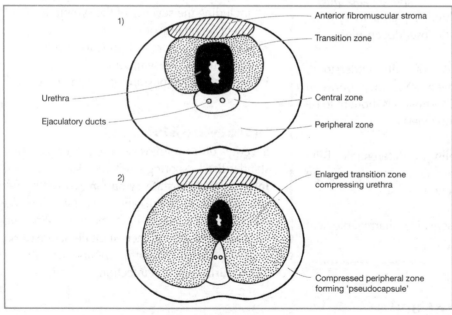

**Figure 8.7 Transverse sections of the prostate: 1) normal and 2) benign prostatic hypertrophy**

Urine leaves the kidney by gravity, aided by the peristaltic action of the pelvis and upper ureter. If the collecting system is obstructed the pressure in the renal pelvis quickly rises. A compensatory decrease in muscular tone of the renal pelvis allows a reduction in pressure back towards normal levels and this is followed by a reduction in GFR and impairment of the concentrating ability of the renal tubules.

Obstruction of the renal tract is confirmed by renal excretion studies, usually a MAG-3 scan.

**CHAPTER 8**

# 6.4 Benign prostatic hypertrophy

## In a nutshell ...

This pathological condition is characterised by an increase in both stromal and glandular elements of the prostate gland.

It is very common, affecting 50% of men aged >50, and having almost universal prevalence by age 80.

It occurs in the transition zone of the prostate (the area surrounding the urethra). As the transition zone enlarges, the urethra becomes compressed and the peripheral zone becomes thinner, eventually forming what is known as a 'pseudocapsule'.

The **aetiology** is not fully understood, but local androgen imbalance between testosterone and oestrogen is thought to be important in pathogenesis.

**Investigations** aim to differentiate BPH from other pathologies and to quantify the degree of obstruction.

**Treatment** is conservative, pharmacological or surgical (TURP).

## Presentation of BPH

- Asymptomatic
- Lower urinary tract symptoms
- Acute urinary retention or chronic urinary retention

## Evaluation of LUTSs

The term 'lower urinary tract symptoms' was coined because of problems associated with previous terms such as 'prostatism'. LUTSs are divided into:

- **Voiding symptoms**, eg hesitancy, poor stream, straining, terminal dribbling
- **Storage symptoms**, eg frequency, urgency, nocturia, incontinence

There may also be symptoms associated with complications of BPH, including retention (acute or chronic), infection, bladder diverticula and stones, and renal impairment due to hydronephrosis.

The major goals of evaluation are:

- To get an overall assessment of the patient, including the severity of the symptoms and effect on quality of life
- To perform objective testing to document the cause of the symptoms
- To exclude serious urological pathology

## History of BPH

Severity of symptoms can be judged using standardised scoring systems such as the **International Prostate Symptom Score** (IPSS). A voiding diary is useful when discussing lifestyle measures to improve symptoms. Specific symptoms of importance include **haematuria** (mandates investigation for urinary tract cancer) and **dysuria** (suggests infection).

## Physical examination in BPH

Abdominal examination will detect a distended palpable bladder if present. Examination of the external genitalia should be done to exclude meatal stenosis. Rectal examination will allow identification of any prostatic abnormalities and also a rough estimate of size.

# Investigating benign prostatic hypertrophy

## Urinalysis

- Should be performed in all patients to exclude a UTI
- Detection of haematuria mandates its investigation

## Renal biochemistry

- Measurement of serum urea and creatinine are mandatory for all patients with LUTSs
- Abnormal results warrant investigation of the upper urinary tract to exclude obstructive uropathy

## Prostate-specific antigen

- This is not a specific test for LUTSs, but many of these men will be concerned about prostate cancer so it is reasonable to perform this test after appropriate patient counselling. Prostate-specific antigen (PSA) is also thought to be a surrogate indicator of prostatic size

## Uroflowmetry

- Simple test of the rate and pattern of urine flow. At least 100 ml needs to be voided to make the test valid
- Obstruction is unlikely in men with a maximum flow ($Q_{max}$) >15 ml/s. A $Q_{max}$ of <10 ml/s is compatible with obstruction

## Ultrasonography for post-void residual volume

- Often performed after uroflowmetry
- A residual of >300 ml indicates chronic urinary retention

## Formal urodynamic studies

- Performed where there is a strong possibility that symptoms are not due to bladder outflow obstruction (eg equivocal flow rate of 10–15 ml/s, neurological disease such as diabetic neuropathy, men aged <60, men who have had previous surgery)
- Normograms are available in order to accurately define whether obstruction is present. These are useful in counselling patients before prostatic surgery

# Management of BPH

It is important to appreciate that not all men require medical treatment. Some may simply be reassured if prostate cancer is excluded. In others, simple lifestyle measures may suffice, such as decreasing fluid at night and reducing caffeine intake. In those in whom this is not sufficient, pharmacological or surgical treatment may be appropriate.

## Pharmacological treatment of BPH

- **Adrenergic antagonists (eg alfuzosin, tamsulosin):** these act on $\alpha_1$-receptors within the prostatic and bladder neck smooth muscle. It is thought that about 50% of bladder outflow obstruction caused by prostatic enlargement is due to prostate smooth muscle tone (which is how these drugs have their effect). Their main side effect is postural hypotension and retrograde ejaculation
- **5α-Reductase inhibitors (eg finasteride, dutasteride):** these block the enzyme 5α-reductase and hence conversion of testosterone to dihydrotestosterone (its active metabolite). They are effective in men with large prostates (>40 g) and reduce the likelihood of acute urinary retention or surgery. Twenty-five per cent report improved symptoms but the drugs can take

CHAPTER 8

6–9 months to take effect. These inhibitors reduce serum PSA by about 50% and it is important to appreciate this if there are concerns about prostate cancer

- Studies have shown that patients with PSA > 1.4 benefit from continuation of these two groups of drugs

## Op box: Transurethral resection of the prostate

**Indications**
- Moderate to severe LUTSs
- Complications of BPH, eg bladder stones, UTI, acute urinary retention and chronic urinary retention
- Failure of medical therapy
- Renal impairment due to LUTSs

**Preop**
- Exclude or treat UTI
- Group and save (5% require transfusion)
- Broad-spectrum antibiotic prophylaxis with gentamicin
- Thromboembolic deterrent stocking (TEDS) for deep vein thrombosis (DVT) prophylaxis; most do not use subcutaneous heparin
- Spinal (preferable) or GA

**Procedure**
- Patient in lithotomy position
- Initial cystoscopy to exclude urethral stricture or bladder pathology
- Urethral dilation is normally performed before insertion of resectoscope (24–28 Fr)
- Irrigation fluid is glycine 1.5% which allows electrocautery
- Resection of prostatic tissue is performed to capsule, from bladder neck proximally to verumontanum distally (to mark level of the external sphincter)
- Chips of prostate tissue removed with an Ellik evacuator
- Haemostasis is secured and a three-way irrigating catheter placed in the bladder

**Postop**
- Irrigate for 24–48 hours until urine is clear
- In larger resections check haemoglobin and electrolytes postoperatively

**Complications**
- **Bleeding:** primary, secondary and reactive haemorrhage may occur causing haematuria ± clot retention
- **Infection** leading to septicaemia
- **TURP syndrome**
- **Failure to void:** causes include hypotonic bladder or incomplete resection
- **Incontinence:** sphincter damage or pre-existing detrusor overactivity
- **Urethral stricture or bladder neck stricture:** occurs in 2–5% and requires incision
- **Impotence:** occurs in up to 20%. Warn patients and document existing function
- **Retrograde ejaculation:** occurs in >80% due to resection of bladder neck

## Surgical treatment of BPH

Surgery is indicated in patients who do not have adequate symptom relief on pharmacological therapy. Men who have recurrent infections or bladder stones or who present with acute urinary retention also require surgery. Standard surgery is TURP, as described in the operation box.

Several minimally invasive therapies (eg laser or microwave ablation of the prostate) have been proposed in order to reduce the morbidity associated with TURP but none has so far replaced it as the gold standard operation. Tissue ablative techniques prevent histological examination of the tissue removed, which can be important for excluding malignancy.

In patients with very large prostates (>90 g) open retropubic prostatectomy may be required.

## TURP syndrome

This syndrome develops during or post-TURP surgery due to absorption of large volumes of irrigation fluid through the prostatic venous plexus. It causes electrolyte disturbances (hyponatraemia) and high nitrogen load, hypervolaemia, cerebral oedema and hypothermia. It can cause visual disturbance, nausea, vomiting, mental confusion, seizures, hypertension and bradycardia. It has been observed in 2% of post-TURP patients.

Treatment is with supportive measures (including ITU if necessary), fluid restriction and diuretics.

It is associated with high mortality. The syndrome can be avoided by minimising surgical time (to <1 hour) and reducing irrigation pressures.

---

**Urethral stricture**

Injury to the urethral mucosa will heal as a circumferential scar with subsequent fibrosis. This can cause bladder outflow obstruction.

**Causes of urethral stricture**

- Traumatic (eg catheterisation, pelvic fracture)
- Neoplastic (eg bladder, penile and prostatic cancer)
- Inflammatory (eg urethritis, gonococci)

**Management of urethral stricture**

- Repeated dilation
- Urethrotomy with stricture excision and/or stenting
- Open reconstruction may be required

---

# 6.5   Acute urinary retention

 **In a nutshell ...**

This is an acute painful inability to micturate. It is ten times more common in men than women.

## Causes of acute urinary retention

Acute urinary retention is caused by:

- Any cause of bladder outflow obstruction (commonly BPH in elderly men, but also prostate carcinoma and urethral strictures)
- Neurological diseases leading to detrusor dysfunction or non-coordination between detrusor contraction and sphincter relaxation (see Section 2 'Bladder dysfunction and incontinence')

CHAPTER 8

**Predisposing factors** include:
- Constipation
- Urinary infection
- Postoperative factors (pain, immobility, drugs, anaesthetic factors)
- Drugs with an anticholinergic effect (eg antidepressants)
- High fluid intake and bladder over-distension (eg high alcohol intake)

It is likely that in most cases there is a combination of prostatic oedema (eg infection) and detrusor dysfunction (eg due to over-distension or drugs).

Caution should be exercised in young patients who present with retention because this may indicate cauda equina syndrome. Acute retention in women is uncommon and requires further investigation with pelvic ultrasonography.

## Presentation of acute urinary retention

Patients present acutely with an inability to pass urine and severe lower abdominal discomfort. The bladder is usually palpable and tender.

## Management of acute urinary retention

- **Urgent catheterisation:** either per urethra or suprapubically. This is initial emergency treatment. The residual volume should be accurately recorded because it may predict the likely success of trial without catheter (TWOC). Subsequent management depends on the patient's prior symptoms, residual volume and fitness for surgery
- **TWOC:** in the past TURP was considered standard treatment for acute urinary retention. But in modern practice many patients will be allowed a TWOC, which has much more chance of success if a recognised predisposing factor had been treated (eg constipation, UTI) and with small residual volumes (<800 ml). Patients with deranged renal function and hydronephrosis due to chronic high-pressure retention will always require surgery and TWOC is therefore not required in this group
- **TURP:** patients who have a successful TWOC should be followed up, because a significant number will still come to surgery eventually. However, elective rather than acute surgery has fewer complications
- **Long-term indwelling catheterisation:** may be required by some patients

 **Procedure: Insertion of a urinary catheter**

This is probably the most common urological intervention but is still associated with many problems. The two main forms of catheterisation are urethral or suprapubic.

**Urethral catheterisation**
Various catheters are available:
- Two-way catheters come in a variety of sizes, the most commonly used being 12–16 Fr
- They can be made of latex rubber for short-term use only (for up to 4 weeks) or of silicone for long-term catheterisation (12 weeks between changes)
- Three-way catheters are available in sizes up to 22 Fr in order to allow bladder washout of blood or debris

continued opposite

When inserting a urethral catheter in a male it is important to remember that the urethra takes a fairly sharp bend anteriorly at the level of the bulbar urethra. If this fact is not appreciated it is easy to create a false passage posteriorly. Once a false passage has been created the catheter will naturally head in this direction and it is very difficult to perform subsequent catheterisation.

**The most common causes of difficulty or failure to catheterise are:**

- Urethral stricture
- Prostate hypertrophy/bladder neck hypertrophy
- Sphincter spasm

In the case of urethral stricture it is unwise to try to force a catheter and either suprapubic catheterisation or cystoscopy, with or without urethrotomy, should be performed.

For large prostates or bladder neck hypertrophy a catheter introducer can be used to negotiate the prostatic urethra. This should be done only by someone with experience.

Sphincter spasm is common and may be eased by lidocaine gel but often it is just patience that allows the catheter to be passed when the spasm temporarily relents.

## Suprapubic catheterisation

At the bedside this can only be performed in patients with an easily palpable bladder. It is increasingly performed under ultrasound guidance.

### Procedure

- The lower half of the abdomen is prepared with antiseptic solution and LA is infiltrated at a point 2 or 3 fingerbreadths above the pubic symphysis in the midline
- As the anaesthetic is infiltrated more deeply the urine can often be aspirated and the catheter should not be inserted if urine cannot be aspirated
- After a small skin incision the catheter can be inserted percutaneously
- Several methods are available for introducing the catheter percutaneously. The most common involves using a trocar and plastic sheath to introduce a standard 16 Fr catheter

### Contraindications to suprapubic catheterisation

- Previous abdominal surgery that may have resulted in small-bowel adhesions to the anterior abdominal wall
- History of transitional cell carcinoma of the bladder – because of the risk of seeding into the tract
- Any bleeding tendency

Recent evidence suggests that all suprapubic catheters should be inserted under radiological guidance due to the high incidence of morbidity related to this procedure.

**CHAPTER 8**

## 6.6    Chronic urinary retention

### In a nutshell ...

The strict definition is a residual volume >300 ml; however, patients often present with residuals much greater than this.

## Presentation of chronic urinary retention

- Patients often have no pain
- Low-pressure retention may present with overflow incontinence
- High-pressure retention often presents with renal failure

## Management of chronic urinary retention

- **Catheterisation:** this is the standard treatment
- **Monitor diuresis:** patients with renal dysfunction need to be monitored closely because they will have a postobstructive diuresis. Diuresis is physiological and represents offloading of salt and water that was retained while the patient was in renal failure. Careful observation and fluid balance are required and IV fluid replacement is usually necessary initially
- **No TWOC:** in contrast to patients with acute urinary retention, patients who have had an episode of high-pressure chronic urinary retention should **not** have a TWOC
- **TURP:** this is the standard treatment after stabilisation of renal function, although success rates in terms of voiding are lower than in patients with acute urinary retention (70% vs 90%)
- **Intermittent self-catheterisation (ISC):** an option in patients with detrusor failure secondary to chronic obstruction

# Urological malignancy

## 7.1   Renal tumours

 **In a nutshell ...**

The table 'Classification of renal tumours' shows many different causes of a tumour in the kidney, but if a mass is identified in the kidney it can rarely be identified until a pathological specimen is obtained.

Thus a mass in the kidney is treated as if it is a renal carcinoma (ie with a radical nephrectomy) unless:

- It can be shown to be benign (eg the diagnostic CT appearance of angiomyolipoma)
- It is <2 cm and does not enlarge on annual CT

Thus a benign mass may be removed with a radical nephrectomy rather than risk missing a cancer.

**Classification of renal tumours**

|        | Benign | Malignant |
|--------|--------|-----------|
| Solid  | Angiomyolipoma[a] | Renal cell carcinoma (adenocarcinoma) |
|        | Oncocytoma[b] | Wilms tumour (nephroblastoma) |
|        |        | Metastatic deposits |
|        |        | Transitional cell carcinoma (renal pelvis) |
|        |        | Renal sarcoma |
| Cystic | Simple cyst | Cystadenocarcinoma (cystic renal cell carcinoma) |
|        | Polycystic kidney | Cystic necrosis of renal carcinoma |

[a]Although most are clinically benign, they may occasionally be locally invasive.
[b]Oncocytoma can metastasise.

**CHAPTER 8**

The **Bosniak classification** grades cysts from I to IV according to their CT appearance (calcification, septa, wall thickness, etc). Grade I cysts are almost always benign and grade IV cysts are almost always malignant.

## Renal cell adenocarcinoma

Also known as renal cell carcinoma or hypernephroma, renal cell carcinoma is a common malignant solid cancer accounting for 3% of all adult malignancies. The incidence is increasing (mainly due to incidental diagnosis) and there is a sex ratio of 2M:1F.

Renal cell carcinoma arises from cells of the proximal renal tubule, commonly at the pole of the kidney. It is yellowish (full of fat) and very vascular.

**Spread** is by:
- Direct extension:
  - Perinephric fat and fascia
  - Wall and lumen of renal vein/IVC
- Metastasis
  - Cannonball metastases to lung, bone and brain

### Aetiology of renal cell carcinoma

Two per cent of renal cell adenocarcinomas are familial, and these are associated with:
- Von Hippel–Lindau syndrome (70% risk by age 60 years)
- Haemangioblastomas of the cerebellum and spine
- Retinal haemangiomas
- Phaeochromocytomas
- Islet cell tumours

Risk factors for non-familial renal cell carcinoma include:
- Acquired renal cystic disease (90% of dialysis patients) – have a 17% risk of renal cancer
- Smoking
- Exposure to cadmium, lead, asbestos, polycarbons

### Histology of renal cell carcinoma
- Clear cell adenocarcinomas (well over half all cases)
- Papillary (18% of cases)
- Chromophobe (5% of cases)

Papillary and chromophobe carcinomas carry a slightly better prognosis. Collecting duct-type carcinomas have a significantly worse prognosis. Grading of renal tumour is by the Fuhrman system, using a scale of 1–4.

### Clinical features of renal cell carcinoma

Classic triad of pain, mass and haematuria is now seen in <10% patients. Commonly an incidental finding (>50%).

May present with paraneoplastic syndromes due to secretion of renin, erythropoietin or a parahormone. This may result in hypercalcaemia, hypertension, polycythaemia, fever and night sweats, or Stauffer syndrome (hepatic dysfunction).
- Renal vein involvement in 20%
- IVC involvement in 10%

### Investigating renal cell carcinoma

Ultrasonography is the usual initial diagnostic investigation. CT scan of the chest and abdomen with IV contrast is used for staging and is very sensitive, picking up:
- Renal vein involvement (91% sensitivity)
- IVC extension (97% sensitivity)

- Perirenal extension (79% sensitivity)
- Lymph node metastases (87% sensitivity)

---

**Staging of renal cell carcinoma**

**Tumour staging**

| | |
|---|---|
| T1 | Tumour <7 cm, limited to kidney |
| T1a | Tumour <4 cm |
| T1b | Tumour 4–7 cm |
| T2 | Tumour >7 cm, limited to kidney |
| T3 | Tumour extends outside kidney but within the Gerota fascia |
| T3a | Tumour invades adrenals or perinephric tissues |
| T3b | Tumour extends into renal vein or IVC below the diaphragm |
| T3c | Tumour extends into the IVC above the diaphragm |
| T4 | Tumour invades beyond Gerota fascia |

**Lymph node staging**

| | |
|---|---|
| Nx | Cannot be assessed |
| N0 | No nodes involved |
| N1 | Metastasis in a single node |
| N2 | Metastasis in more than one node |

**Metastasis staging**

| | |
|---|---|
| Mx | Cannot be assessed |
| M0 | No distant metastases |
| M1 | Distant metastases present |

---

## Management of renal cell carcinoma

### Localised disease

- **Radical nephrectomy:** this is the gold standard (see Op box)
- **Laparoscopic radical nephrectomy:** this is the preferred approach for T1 and some T2 tumours
- **Partial nephrectomy:** this should be offered to all patients with T1a disease if appropriate, particularly those with a single kidney, poor renal function or multifocal tumours

IVC involvement does not affect prognosis of the cancer, although it may need cardiac bypass during surgery and this has associated morbidity.

### Metastatic disease

Thirty per cent present with metastases and another 30% develop them.

- **Nephrectomy:** this may be palliative for haematuria. There is a small increase in short-term survival with nephrectomy despite distant metastasis
- **Embolisation:** this can be effective
- **Chemotherapy/radiotherapy:** results with these alone are poor
- **Tyrosine kinase inhibitors (eg sorafinib, sunitinib):** these have shown promising results in patients with metastatic disease

**CHAPTER 8**

697

**Op box: Nephrectomy**

### Indications

Radical nephrectomy is indicated for localised renal carcinoma. It involves removal of the kidney with the surrounding Gerota fascia. Simple nephrectomy is indicated in cases of non-functioning kidneys.

### Preop

- Exclude or treat UTI
- Cross-match 2–4 units of blood
- DVT prophylaxis with TEDS and subcutaneous heparin
- Ensure adequate imaging to confirm side of operation and anatomy
- The side of surgery should be marked

### Procedure

- Both lateral loin approach (extraperitoneal) and transabdominal approaches are used. In the loin approach, the operating table is 'broken', allowing flexion, with patients lying on their side, to maximise exposure
- In the loin approach, the abdominal wall muscles are divided and the incision continues above the level of either rib 11 or rib 12 in order to avoid the neurovascular bundle
- In both approaches, dissection allows exposure of the renal hilum. The renal artery is tied before the vein to prevent renal congestion
- On the right, the renal vein is short and care is needed
- On the left, undue traction should be avoided to prevent splenic injury. The tail of the pancreas is also at risk

### Postop

- IV fluids are required until ileus resolves (longer with the transabdominal approach)
- Chest physiotherapy and early mobilisation are important

### Complications

- Bleeding
- Chest infection: particularly in smokers and those with pre-existing chest disease
- Pain: pain from the incision prevents adequate chest expansion and leads to pulmonary collapse so adequate analgesia and chest physiotherapy are vital
- DVT/PE (pulmonary embolism)

## Prognosis of renal cell carcinoma

This is influenced by tumour grade, degree of local invasion, venous invasion and distant metastasis.

The 5-year survival rate is approximately:

- 90% for T1 disease
- 60% for T2–3 disease
- 0–20% for distant metastasis

CHAPTER 8

# Other malignant renal tumours

## In a nutshell ...

Apart from renal cell carcinomas, the other important malignant tumours of the kidney are:

- Renal nephroblastoma (Wilms tumour). See Section 4 of Paediatric Surgery, Book 1
- Transitional cell carcinoma (TCC) of the renal pelvis (see Section 7.2)
- Renal sarcoma
- Metastasis to the kidney

## Renal sarcoma

This accounts for 1–2% of renal neoplasms. This tumour is commonly a leiomyosarcoma. It presents in the fifth decade with flank pain and weight loss. Treatment is with radical nephrectomy.

## Metastatic deposits in the kidney

The kidney can be affected by metastasis from the lung (20%), breast (12%), stomach (11%) and lymphoma (rare).

# Benign renal tumours

## Angiomyolipoma

An angiomyolipoma is a benign hamartoma consisting of fat (approximately 80%), blood vessels and smooth muscle. It is rare, accounting for 0.5% of renal tumours.

Of angiomyolipomas 20–50% are associated with tuberous sclerosis, a syndrome of learning disabilities, epilepsy and adenoma sebaceum, but most commonly angiomyolipoma is asymptomatic. Haemorrhage into the tumour can result in flank pain and hypotension.

Angiomyolipoma may be confidently diagnosed by CT due to diagnostic appearance of a high fat content.

**Treatment options** include:

- Conservative if <4 cm
- Consider enucleation or partial nephrectomy for symptomatic lesions or those >4 cm
- Treatment of acute bleeding requires embolisation or nephrectomy

## Oncocytoma

Accounting for 3–7% of solid renal masses, oncocytoma is a solid benign tumour of the kidney. It is a neoplasm of the intercalated cells of the collecting duct, and is usually well circumscribed, encapsulated and rarely metastasises.

Eighty per cent are asymptomatic and discovered incidentally.

Unfortunately it cannot be accurately distinguished from renal adenocarcinoma radiologically, so radical nephrectomy (see Op box) is the standard treatment.

CHAPTER 8

## 7.2 Bladder cancer and urothelial tumours of the urinary tract

### In a nutshell ...

Bladder cancer is most commonly a transitional cell carcinoma (TCC), which is a urothelial tumour of the type that affects the entire urinary tract.

Of urothelial tumours 95% affect the bladder; 5% affect the upper tract. One urothelial tumour in one area of the renal tract increases the risk of another (unstable urothelium).

The grade and stage of the tumour varies widely. Superficial disease, although often recurrent and needing repeated treatment, has a very good prognosis. In aggressive metastatic disease patients are unlikely to survive a year.

### Epidemiology and pathology of urothelial cancers and bladder TCC

The renal tract is lined with transitional cell urothelium from the renal pelvis to the urethra. TCCs may therefore occur at any point along this tract, including in the kidney.

- Bladder TCC is the second most common urological malignancy
- Incidence is gradually increasing
- Sex ratio is 3M:1F
- Affects older patients (peak incidence at 65)
- There are geographical variations
- Of these cancers >90% are TCCs, 5% are SCCs and the rest are adenocarcinomas. Sarcoma is rare. Benign tumours are uncommon

Patterns of bladder TCC include:
- Papillary
- Solid invasive
- CIS (may be ulcerated)

### Risk factors for bladder and urothelial cancers

- Smoking: major risk factor in the developed world
- Occupational factors: historically important for workers in the rubber, dye, leather and textile industries
- Chronic inflammation, eg stone disease, long-term catheters, recurrent infections, bilharzia
- Congenital anomaly, eg remnant of urachus

### Presentation of bladder and urothelial cancers

- 80–90% present with painless macroscopic haematuria
- Microscopic haematuria in patients aged >50 also requires investigation for bladder cancer
- Irritative bladder symptoms may be a presenting feature (a third will have a persistent chronic urine infection)
- 5% present with metastatic disease

### Investigating bladder and urothelial cancer

- Diagnosis is usually by flexible cystoscopy
- All patients with haematuria should have an investigation of the upper urinary tract
- Occasionally diagnosis is made on ultrasonography or IVU when a filling defect in the bladder is demonstrated

## Staging of bladder cancer
### Tumour staging
| | |
|---|---|
| Tis | Carcinoma in situ (CIS) |
| Ta | Papillary non-I–IV carcinoma |
| T1 | Tumour invades subepithelial connective tissue (through lamina propria) |
| T2 | Tumour invades muscle |
| T2a | Tumour invades superficial muscle (inner half) |
| T2b | Tumour invades deep muscle (outer half) |
| T3 | Tumour invades perivesical tissue: |
| T3a | Microscopically |
| T3b | Macroscopically (extravesical mass) |
| T4 | Tumour invades adjacent structures |
| T4a | Invades prostate, uterus or vagina |
| T4b | Invades pelvic or abdominal wall |

### Lymph node staging
| | |
|---|---|
| Nx | Cannot be assessed |
| N0 | No nodes involved |
| N1 | Single node metastasis <2 cm |
| N2 | Single lymph node 2–5 cm or multiple nodes but none >5 cm |
| N3 | Lymph node metastasis >5 cm |

### Metastasis staging
| | |
|---|---|
| Mx | Cannot be assessed |
| M0 | No distant metastases |
| M1 | Distant metastases present |

The major distinction is between 'superficial' bladder cancer (Tis, Ta and T1), which accounts for 80% of all tumours, and muscle-invasive bladder cancer.

Histological grading of bladder tumours is:
| | |
|---|---|
| G1 | Well differentiated |
| G2 | Moderately differentiated |
| G3 | Poorly differentiated |

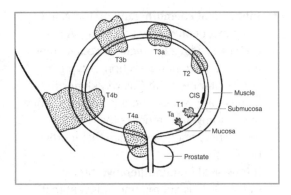

Figure 8.8 Bladder cancer staging

# Management of superficial bladder cancer

'Superficial' bladder cancer is a term that covers stages Ta, T1 and CIS. It covers a wide range of tumours, and these may have quite different clinical behaviours.

Most tumours are managed by **transurethral endoscopic resection (TURBT) with a single shot of mitomycin C intravesically**, but there is a risk of progression to muscle-invasive disease so more radical therapy may be required (see below). Risk of progression depends predominantly on the stage and grade:
- G1 pTa tumours have a very good prognosis; <5% will progress
- CIS or G3 pT1 tumours are G3 tumours confined to the urothelium; up to 50% progress and so all patients with G3 disease should be re-resected at 6 weeks
- All patients with superficial bladder cancer should undergo regular check cystoscopies (intervals determined by cystoscopic and histological findings). Significant numbers of patients develop a further tumour (even if disease free for a long time). High-risk patients and those with multiple tumours or frequent recurrences should be considered for intravesical therapy. Both chemotherapy and immunotherapy are used

**CHAPTER 8**

- **Intravesical chemotherapy:** mitomycin C is the most commonly used drug. A single dose can reduce the recurrence rate after initial transurethral resection. A typical course of mitomycin C is weekly instillations for 6 weeks. There is good evidence that mitomycin C reduces the risk of recurrence, but no evidence that it prevents progression
- **Intravesical immunotherapy:** intravesicular BCG is an immune adjuvant that upregulates the host immune response against the tumour. Also given as a 6-week course and is standard therapy for G3 pT1 tumours and CIS. More effective than mitomycin C at preventing recurrence and may have some impact on progression (but this is controversial). Maintenance therapy with further shorter courses improves results. Toxicity is greater than with mitomycin C. Irritative bladder symptoms are common and occasional systemic upset can occur

Patients with high-risk disease who have recurrence despite intravesical therapy are considered for radical therapy (invasive bladder cancer is discussed below).

## Management of invasive bladder cancer

This tumour has invaded into the detrusor muscle of the bladder and therefore cannot be completely excised by endoscopic measures.

Before trying curative treatment it is important to exclude extravesical spread or metastatic disease. Prognosis of invasive bladder cancer is poor, with a 5-year survival after surgery and radiotherapy of 30–50%.

- **Staging** is vital to planning treatment if invasion of the muscle is suspected. CT of chest, abdomen and pelvis should be performed. Occasionally a bone scan will be required to exclude distant metastases
- **Radical cystectomy** has been the standard treatment for patients with T2–3 non-metastatic bladder cancer. Urinary diversion is needed and is most commonly obtained by formation of an ileal conduit. Patients are increasingly being offered bladder reconstruction using small bowel
- **Radical radiotherapy** is also an option for attempted cure. It has been used particularly for patients who are unfit for cystectomy. An advantage is that the bladder is preserved; however, there may be symptoms of radiation cystitis and proctitis. Check cystoscopies are required and, if the tumour recurs, salvage cystectomy may be an option
- **Neoadjuvant cisplatin-based chemotherapy:** this has been shown to confer a 5% survival benefit compared with cystectomy alone

## Treatment of metastatic disease

- Platinum-based chemotherapy for patients with metastatic disease who are fit enough to tolerate its toxicity
- In many patients only palliative care is appropriate
- Prognosis is poor, with survival about 1 year from diagnosis

**Op box: Radical cystectomy**

### Indications
- Invasive bladder cancer
- Recurrent bladder cancer after radical radiotherapy
- High-grade superficial bladder cancer resistant to local treatment

### Preop
- The patient should see a stoma nurse to discuss living with an ileal conduit, and the position should be marked. This should happen even for patients where bladder reconstruction is planned
- Bowel prep may be given
- DVT prophylaxis with subcutaneous heparin and TED stockings is required
- Broad-spectrum antibiotic prophylaxis is given
- 4–6 units of blood should be cross-matched

### Procedure
- The patient should be supine and catheterised
- Lower midline incision
- A full laparotomy is performed
- Initial dissection involves mobilising the urachal remnant (median umbilical ligament) because this should be excised en bloc with the bladder
- Bowel mobilisation of the caecum and ascending colon on the right and descending colon on the left allows packing of colon and small bowel into the epigastrium The ureters are mobilised and divided close to the bladder
- A full lymph node dissection is performed to include the obturator lymph nodes, the internal iliac, external iliac and common iliac nodes as far as the aortic bifurcation. As well as providing important staging information, this gives good dissection of the vascular anatomy before cystectomy
- The bladder is dissected free. Prostate is also removed in men. Particular care is needed with the dorsal venous complex and while dissecting the prostate and bladder neck from the rectum
- In patients with urethral tumours the urethra is dissected through a separate perineal incision and removed en bloc with the bladder and prostate
- The standard method of urinary drainage is an ileal conduit, as a loop of small bowel proximal to the terminal ileum is resected and this needs to be long enough to reach the abdominal wall (approximately 25 cm). Once the loop has been isolated, small-bowel anastomosis is performed to restore continuity of the remaining ileum
- Various methods exist to anastomose the ureters to the ileal loop; they can either be anastomosed to the end of the loop or through separate incisions. Stents are placed across the anastomosis
- A stoma is formed with a spout to ensure urine does not directly drain onto the skin surface

**continued overleaf**

CHAPTER 8

- If continent diversion is planned, various forms of ileal neobladder exist
- A tube drain is inserted into the abdomen

**Postop**

- Patients often need high-dependency care immediately postoperatively
- Nasogastric (NG) drainage should continue until bowel activity returns
- Epidural anaesthesia is the optimum method of ensuring that patients are pain-free and for reducing the risk of chest infections
- Chest physiotherapy should be given
- Tube drains should be left for at least 48 hours
- Ureteric stents can be removed after 10–12 days

**Complications**

Perioperative complications:

- Bleeding
- Rectal damage

Early complications:

- Prolonged ileus
- Chest infection, DVT or PE
- Urine leak
- Pelvic abscess formation (usually follows pelvic haematoma)
- Problems related to the bowel anastomosis such as leakage
- Wound infection

Late complications:

- Hernias of the wound or stoma
- UTIs or urinary stones
- Stenosis of the conduit
- Upper tract deterioration is common and electrolytes should be monitored

## Other (non-urothelial) tumours of the bladder

### Squamous cell carcinoma of the bladder

This is common in the Middle East and Egypt. It presents late and infiltrates, and may be a complication of chronic inflammation with stone disease or bilharzias. It is treated by resection.

### Adenocarcinoma of the bladder

This accounts for about 1% of bladder tumours. It may develop in the vault at the site of a urachal remnant and the tumour itself grows outside the bladder. It is managed with surgery and chemotherapy.

### Bladder sarcoma

This has a poor prognosis apart from liposarcoma.

## Urothelial tumours of the ureter and renal pelvis

These account for 5% of all TCCs. Renal pelvis tumours are three times more common than ureteric tumours and account for 8% of all kidney cancers. Risk factors are similar to those for TCCs in the bladder. These tumours are commonly superficial.

Importantly, the risk of a bladder TCC after an upper tract TCC is about 50% (it represents a field change within the urothelium). The risk of upper tract TCC after TCC bladder is low (<2%).

### Presentation of urothelial tumours of the ureter and renal pelvis

- As in renal cell carcinomas, painless haematuria is again the most common presentation
- Ultrasonography is not good for detecting upper tract TCCs, so IVU is recommended for patients with persistent haematuria in whom ultrasonography and cystoscopy are normal

### Treatment of urothelial tumours of the ureter and renal pelvis

- Staging to exclude metastatic disease is as for bladder cancer
- If metastases are excluded, curative treatment with **nephroureterectomy** is the gold standard
- More conservative treatments for patients with a solitary kidney or renal impairment (eg ureteroscopic and percutaneous resection)

All patients should have follow-up cystoscopies because of the high risk of subsequent bladder cancer.

## 7.3  Prostate cancer

### In a nutshell ...

This is the most common urological malignancy and the second most common cause of cancer death in males.

### Epidemiology of prostate cancer

This is a disease of advancing age, and incidence is increasing with increasing life expectancy. Postmortem studies show that microscopic foci of prostate cancer are present in up to 80% of men aged 80. This incidence seems to be the same worldwide, and is thought to represent 'latent' cancer, most of which is clinically insignificant. However, the risks of prostate cancer as a cause of death is about 3% (men are more likely to die with the disease than because of it).

The incidence of 'significant' prostate cancer is far more common in the developed world. The reasons for this are not clear.

**Risk factors for prostate cancer**
- Environmental factors (eg diet, saturated fats, phyto-oestrogens)
- Genetic factors (family history)
- Geography/race (more common in people of African origin and less common in people from Asia)

## Pathology of prostate cancer

Ninety-five per cent of prostate cancers are adenocarcinomas. The rest consist of TCCs, SCCs and lymphomas. Most (75%) arise in the peripheral zone of the prostate, unlike BPH, which affects the transition zone.

Commonly well differentiated with slow growth in response to androgen, or occasionally poorly differentiated with rapid metastasis. Arises from the epithelium of the prostatic duct acini and preceded by intraepithelial neoplasia.

### Gleason grading system

- Used for histological assessment of prostate cancer
- Correlates with prognosis
- Takes into account the heterogeneous nature of the disease by grading the two predominant areas of a tumour
- An individual area may have a Gleason grade of 1 (well differentiated) to 5 (poorly differentiated), leading to a sum score of 2–10 when the scores of the two areas are combined

### Presentation of prostate cancer

- **Asymptomatic:** localised prostate cancer often produces no symptoms

- **Incidental finding:** many of these men will also have BPH and present with LUTSs. The prostate cancer is diagnosed on digital rectal examination (hard, craggy prostate, asymmetry and loss of median sulcus) or by testing for prostate-specific antigen (PSA)
- **Bladder outlet obstruction (BOO):** locally advanced disease may present with ureteric obstruction due to local infiltration and renal failure
- **Symptoms of distal disease:** metastatic disease may present with bone pain, pathological fracture or spinal cord compression

## Prostate-specific antigen

This is a proteolytic enzyme produced specifically by the prostate that has a role in the liquefaction of the ejaculate. Large amounts are secreted into the semen and small quantities escape into the bloodstream.

The PSA level is elevated in prostate cancer but it can also be elevated by BPH, a UTI or urethral instrumentation such as catheterisation or cystoscopy.

The likelihood of diagnosis of prostate cancer rises with the level of PSA (as shown in the table below). As PSA increases with increasing age (probably due to BPH), age-related values have also been defined.

Predictive value of PSA and digital rectal examination (DRE) for a biopsy diagnosis of prostate cancer

| PSA level (ng/ml) | ≤0.5 | 0.6–1.0 | 1.1–2.0 | 2.1–3.0 | 3.1–4.0 | 4.1–10.0 | ≥10 |
|---|---|---|---|---|---|---|---|
| DRE normal (%) | 6.6 | 10 | 17 | 24 | 27 | 27 | >50 |
| DRE abnormal (%) | NA | 15 | 15 | 30 | 30 | 45 | >75 |

# Diagnosis and investigation of prostate cancer

Diagnosis of prostate cancer is usually obtained by **prostatic biopsy** performed during **transrectal ultrasonography** (TRUS). Random biopsies are taken (usually 10–12) to get a representative sample of prostate gland. Abnormal areas are sometimes seen (classically **hypoechoic** areas on ultrasonography) and these should be biopsied although they are not specific for prostate cancer. Because the biopsies are transrectal, infection is a major risk and all patients should have prophylactic antibiotics.

# Staging of prostate cancer

This is based on the TNM system.

## Tumour staging

T1      Clinically unapparent tumour not palpable or visible by imaging

T1a     Incidental finding at TURP (<5% of tissue resected involved)

T1b     Incidental finding at TURP (>5% of tissue resected involved)

T1c     Identified by needle biopsy (eg because of elevated PSA)

T2      Tumour confined to prostate (palpable or visible on imaging)

T2a     Involving half of one lobe or less

T2b     Involving more than half of one lobe, but not both lobes

T2c     Involving both lobes

T3      Tumour extends through prostatic capsule

T3a     Extracapsular extension

T3b     Extension into seminal vesicle(s)

T4      Tumour fixed or invading adjacent structures other than seminal vesicles (eg bladder neck, external sphincter, levator muscles or pelvic sidewall)

## Lymph node staging

Nx      Cannot be assessed

N0      No nodes involved

N1      Lymph nodes involved

## Metastasis staging

Mx      Cannot be assessed

M0      No distant metastases

M1      Distant metastases present

M1a     Non-regional lymph node metastasis

M1b     Metastasis to bone

M1c     Metastasis to other sites

## Localised and advanced disease

- T1 or T2 disease is considered localised and therefore potentially curable
- T3 disease is locally advanced and therefore unlikely to be cured
- T4 disease and metastatic disease are advanced disease

In clinically localised disease where curative treatment is proposed, an MR scan will give information on localised tumour stage and lymph node involvement in the pelvis.

The most common site of distant spread after the lymph nodes is the bony skeleton. Bone scan is a sensitive method of detecting skeletal metastases.

# Management of localised prostate cancer

It is important to realise that not all prostate cancer requires treatment. Many men with this cancer die of other causes, and do not benefit from treatment (but will be put at risk of any side effects or complications). One of the great challenges in urology at the present time is to identify groups of patients who are likely to have 'aggressive disease' with a high risk of mortality, who therefore require intervention.

CHAPTER 8

There are three main options for men with localised prostate cancer:

1. Active surveillance
2. Radical prostatectomy
3. Radical radiotherapy or brachytherapy

### Active surveillance of localised prostate cancer

Ideal for men with well-differentiated tumours and relatively low PSA levels. Morbidity associated with radical treatment is avoided. Monitoring is with regular PSA test and repeat prostatic biopsies. Usually offered to men with a life expectancy >10 years.

### Radical prostatectomy of localised prostate cancer

Radical prostatectomy is the removal of the prostate with re-anastomosis of the bladder neck to the urethra. Pelvic lymph node dissection may also be carried out. The traditional approach has been retropubic via laparotomy, but laparoscopic and perineal approaches are also used.

This is a major operation with significant complications (eg bleeding and PE). In the long term 70% have erectile dysfunction and there is a 5% incontinence rate.

### Radical radiotherapy of localised prostate cancer

A 6-week course of daily treatments avoids a major operation for localised prostate cancer. Modern conformal therapy is associated with minimal complications, but bladder and bowel toxicity can occur. There are no clinical trials showing a difference in efficacy between radical prostatectomy and radical radiotherapy, but these trials suffer from bias because of differences in patient selection. There is evidence that neoadjuvant hormone therapy improves the results of radiotherapy and some men are offered adjuvant hormone therapy for 3 years post-radiotherapy.

Monitoring patients with radical radiotherapy can be difficult because PSA levels do not always fall to zero.

### Prostate brachytherapy

This method of treating localised disease involves implantation of radioactive seeds into the prostate. Results are comparable with surgery, and complication rates are lower, but there are only a few centres in the country with a long experience of this technique.

Cryotherapy is usually reserved for patients who have local recurrence after radical radiotherapy.

## Management of advanced/ metastatic prostate cancer

### Locally advanced disease

Radical prostatectomy is not usually indicated in this group of patients although there may be a role for surgery in a small proportion of these patients. Active monitoring is an option in asymptomatic men. Good 5-year survival figures are obtained with palliative radiotherapy, which is often used in combination with hormonal therapy.

### Metastatic disease

Most of these patients require systemic palliative treatment because evidence suggests that, in metastatic disease, early institution of hormonal treatment may prevent complications such as spinal cord compression and pathological fractures.

## Hormonal treatment

The aim of all these treatments is to prevent the action of testosterone on prostate cancer cells. Initial response is normally excellent but eventually prostate cancer cells will become androgen-independent and at that time hormonal therapy is ineffective. Once this occurs median survival is only 6 months.

### Luteinising hormone-releasing hormone agonists

- These act on the pituitary to prevent the release of LH. This is because normal stimulation of LH is by pulsed release of LH-releasing hormone (LHRH) by the hypothalamus and continuous stimulation leads to inhibition
- Lack of LH means that testosterone is not produced by the Leydig cells in the testes
- Hence this is a form of medical castration

- Side effects include lack of energy, loss of libido and hot flushes

### Bilateral orchidectomy

- Before the development of LHRH agonists this was the standard treatment for prostate cancer
- Very effective
- Cheaper than medical therapy
- Avoids repeated injections
- Rarely used in modern practice

## Anti-androgens

These drugs compete with testosterone at the androgen receptor and examples include cyproterone acetate, flutamide and bicalutamide. They are not as effective alone as LHRH agonists but may sometimes be used in combination with LHRH agonists. Anti-androgens do have fewer side effects than LHRH agonists.

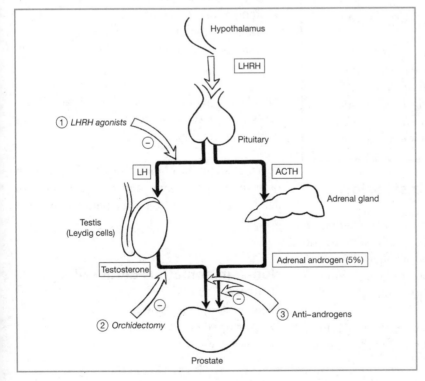

**Figure 8.9 Hormonal control of the prostate and mechanisms of action of hormonal therapies**

CHAPTER 8

## Management of hormone-escaped prostate cancer

Various chemotherapy regimens have been tried in this situation but prognosis is poor and palliative care alone is usually appropriate. Addition of diethylstilbestrol or prednisolone may provide some benefit. Localised radiotherapy to bone metastases is an excellent form of pain control. Randomised studies have also shown a median survival benefit of 3 months in patients treated with docetaxel.

## 7.4 Testicular cancer

 **In a nutshell ...**

Testicular cancers are the commonest solid tumours in young men. There are two main types:
- Seminomas
- Non-seminomatous germ cell tumours (NSGCTs)

Radical orchidectomy is the treatment of choice in both tumours. Seminomas are usually treated by irradiation with or without chemotherapy. NSGCTs may need chemotherapy or (rarely in the UK) retroperitoneal lymph node dissection.

## Epidemiology of testicular tumours

Testicular tumour is the most common tumour in boys and men aged 15–35, and it is increasing in incidence. It is reported to affect 7 men in 100 000, and is four times more common in white people; 2.5–5% are bilateral.

A history of undescended testis leads to a 10-fold increased risk, even if orchidopexy has been carried out. The contralateral, normally descended testis is also at risk in these patients, with a 5% risk of CIS, a premalignant condition.

## Pathology of testicular tumours

**Germ cell tumours:** 95% are germ cell tumours such as seminoma and NSGCTs.

**Stromal tumours:** these may arise from Leydig or Sertoli cells. They are rare and about 10% are malignant.

Lymphomas occur in older men.

### Seminoma
- Accounts for about 50% of germ cell tumours
- Divided into classic (85%), anaplastic and spermatocytic subtypes
- Tend to occur in men in their 30s
- Typically tumours have a homogeneous macroscopic appearance. They consist of sheets of clear cells

**Anaplastic seminoma** is a more aggressive subtype and accounts for 30% of all patients dying with seminoma.

**Spermatocytic seminoma** tends to occur in older men with nearly half occurring in men aged >50. It appears to have a particularly good prognosis.

### Non-seminomatous germ cell tumours

There are four main types:
1. Embryonal carcinoma
2. Yolk sac tumour

3. Choriocarcinoma

4. Classic teratoma

Most (60%) have a mixed pattern, containing some or all of these histological subtypes.

## Presentation of testicular tumours

- Most men present with a painless testicular lump
- 10–20% may have pain, often described as a heaviness or an ache
- Testis may feel firm and bosselated, with thickening of the cord (due to infiltration) and a small hydrocele
- Occasionally men present with metastatic disease (eg abdominal mass due to lymph nodes, respiratory symptoms, bone pain)

- Gynaecomastia occurs in about 5% of patients and is related to human chorionic gonadotropin ($\beta$-hCG) production

## Investigating testicular tumours

- Scrotal ultrasonography confirms the diagnosis and excludes abnormalities in the other testis
- Chest radiograph excludes pulmonary metastases
- Testicular tumour markers (as shown in the table) are used for diagnosis, staging, monitoring response to treatment and predicting prognosis

### Testicular tumour markers

| | |
|---|---|
| $\alpha$-Fetoprotein (AFP) | Normally undetectable after the first year of life<br>Elevated in non-seminomatous tumours only (eg teratoma, yolk sac) |
| Human chorionic gonadotropin ($\beta$-hCG) | Normally produced by the placenta during pregnancy<br>Produced by all non-seminomatous tumours containing choriocarcinoma elements and 40–60% containing embryonal carcinoma elements<br>5–10% of patients with pure seminoma have low levels of hCG detectable |
| Lactate dehydrogenase (LDH) | This is a ubiquitous enzyme and therefore non-specific<br>It is secreted by seminomas and in non-seminomatous disease and seems to be a marker of tumour bulk |
| Placental alkaline phosphatase (PLAP) | Detected in 65% of seminomas and may be a sensitive marker for metastatic seminomatous disease |

## Staging of testicular tumours

The UICC (Union Internationale Contrele Cancer) 2002 staging system is unique in that, in addition to the TNM categories, there is an 'S category' for serum tumour markers – see overleaf.

CHAPTER 8

**Tumour staging (based on pathological information after radical orchidectomy)**

Tis Intratubular germ cell neoplasia (CIS)

T1 Tumour limited to testis/epididymis without vascular/lymphatic invasion or tumour may invade tunica albuginea but not tunica vaginalis

T2 Tumour limited to testis/epididymis with vascular/lymphatic invasion or tumour extends through tunica albuginea with involvement of tunica vaginalis

T3 Tumour invades spermatic cord with or without vascular/lymphatic invasion

T4 Tumour invades scrotum with or without vascular/lymphatic invasion

**Regional lymph node staging**

Nx Cannot be assessed

N0 No nodes involved

N1 Lymph node mass <2 cm or multiple nodes, none >2 cm

N2 Lymph node mass 2–5 cm or multiple nodes, none >5 cm or pathological extranodal extension

N3 Lymph node mass >5 cm

**Metastasis staging**

Mx Cannot be assessed

M0 No distant metastases

M1 Distant metastases present

M1a Non-regional lymph node(s) or lung

M1b Other sites

**Serum tumour markers**

Sx Serum markers not available

S0 Serum markers within normal limits

S1–S3 Serum markers outside normal limits (as shown in the table below)

**Serum tumour markers levels for staging**

|    | LDH (mIU/ml) | hCG (mIU/ml) | AFP (ng/ml) |
|----|---|---|---|
| S1 | 1.5 × normal level and | <5000 and | <1000 |
| S2 | 1.5–10 × normal level or | 5000–50 000 or | 1000–10 000 |
| S3 | >10 × normal level or | >50 000 or | >10 000 |

## Treatment of testicular tumours

### Orchidectomy

- Initial definitive treatment is **radical inguinal orchidectomy**. This provides a pathological diagnosis and will cure about 80% of patients

- Further treatment depends upon histology and staging of CT scans of chest and abdomen to look for metastatic disease

## Op box: Radical inguinal orchidectomy

**Indication**
* Testicular tumour

**Preop**
* It is important to have measured tumour markers preoperatively
* Testicular prosthesis should be offered

**Operative procedure**
* Patient is placed supine
* Inguinal approach similar to that for an inguinal hernia repair is used
* External oblique upper aponeurosis is opened from the external to the internal ring
* Aspermatic cord is mobilised and clamped at the deep ring
* Testis is mobilised in the scrotum and delivered into the inguinal incision
* Cord should be transfixed with a heavy non-absorbable suture and then divided at the deep ring. Suture should be left long so that it can be identified at retroperitoneal lymph node dissection, should this be required, and haemostasis ensured before allowing the cord to retract
* If a prosthesis is to be inserted this can now be sutured to the most dependent part of the scrotal skin

**Postop**
* Patients can often go home on the same day

**Complications**
* Scrotal haematoma
* Wound infection

## Postoperative management of seminomas

### Seminoma confined to the testis

This may be managed by surveillance alone; 20% of patients relapse. However, surveillance does require repeated CT scans. A single shot of carboplatin should be offered to patients to decrease the risk of relapse.

### Seminoma with lymph node metastases

Treated by radiotherapy. Seminoma with large lymph node metastases (N3) or metastatic disease is usually treated initially with **combination chemotherapy**.

## Postoperative management of NSGCTs

### NSGCTs confined to the testis

Treatment varies in the USA and the UK.

Around 20% have disease in the retroperitoneal lymph node that is not picked up on imaging, so in the USA the recommended treatment is **retroperitoneal lymph node dissection** (RPLND) which has a cure rate >90%. As RPLND is over-treatment for many patients, the UK approach is for close surveillance.

Patients with high-risk tumours may be given two cycles of chemotherapy.

CHAPTER 8

Metastatic NSGCTs

These are best treated with combination chemotherapy. A standard regimen is bleomycin, etoposide and cisplatin (BEP).

Residual masses in the retroperitoneum may be resected by RPLND.

## Prognosis of testicular tumours

Prognosis depends on the stage but the overall 5-year survival rate is now >90%. Men with stage 1 testicular cancer of either type should have a 100% 5-year survival rate.

## 7.5 Penile carcinoma

### In a nutshell ...

This is a rare squamous cell cancer, representing 1% of male cancers. It is more common in the developing world and in elderly people.
Surgical excision and chemotherapy are the main treatment options.

## Aetiology of penile carcinoma

**Chronic irritation:** penile cancer is almost unheard of in men circumcised at a young age. It is associated with an unretractable phimosis and it is thought that chronic irritation with smegma and balanitis are contributory factors.

**Human papillomavirus (HPV):** incidence is higher in men who have been infected with HPV-16, -18 and -31. It is higher in men whose sexual partners have cancer of the uterine cervix.

## Pathology of penile carcinoma

Squamous cell carcinoma is the most common penile tumour. It is seen as an erythematous indurated area, wart or ulceration.

## Presentation of penile carcinoma

Usually presents with a lesion on the glans, prepuce or foreskin. Most lesions are not painful (may account for the long delay in seeking attention).

Up to 50% of patients delay seeking medical attention for more than 1 year. Fifty per cent have palpable inguinal nodes at the time of presentation (these may be inflammatory due to balanitis rather than neoplastic).

## Diagnosis and staging of penile carcinoma

With small lesions or those involving the foreskin, diagnosis is usually combined with treatment. Staging is by the TNM system (see opposite).

## Treatment of penile carcinoma

### Local disease

- **Circumcision** or local biopsy may be adequate for T1 lesions with favourable histology
- **Glansectomy and split-skin reconstruction** is an option for more extensive lesions
- **Topical chemotherapy** with, for example, 5-fluorouracil (5FU)
- **Partial or total amputation of the penis** is recommended for poorly differentiated T1 lesions or for lesions at a more advanced stage. Partial amputation is suitable if a 2-cm margin of palpably normal shaft can be retained (so patients can micturate while standing)

## Management of the lymph nodes

The most important predictor of outcome is the status and management of the regional lymph nodes.

Fifty per cent have palpable adenopathy at presentation, but less than half of these have histological evidence of tumour in the lymph nodes. In the remainder it is thought to be caused by infection or inflammation.

Consider sentinel node biopsy for clinically node-negative G2 or above and observation for G1pT1.

In patients with palpable nodes after antibiotic treatment, bilateral **radical inguinal lymphadenectomy** with en-bloc dissection is recommended (the glans penis drains bilaterally). Inguinal lymphadenectomy is associated with significant morbidity in terms of lower limb swelling, wound infection, and wound necrosis.

## Prognosis in penile carcinoma

The 5-year survival rates are:
- Localised disease without metastases 60–90%
- Inguinal node involvement 30–50%
- Iliac node involvement 20%

---

**Staging of penile cancer**

| | |
|---|---|
| Tis | CIS |
| Ta | Non-invasive verrucous carcinoma |
| T1 | Tumour invades subepithelial connective tissue |
| T2 | Tumour invades corpus spongiosum or cavernosum |
| T3 | Tumour invades urethra or prostate |
| T4 | Tumour invades other adjacent structures |

**Regional lymph node staging**

| | |
|---|---|
| Nx | Cannot be assessed |
| N0 | No nodes involved |
| N1 | Single superficial inguinal node involved |
| N2 | Multiple or bilateral superficial inguinal nodes |
| N3 | Deep inguinal or pelvic node involvement |

**Metastasis staging**

| | |
|---|---|
| Mx | Cannot be assessed |
| M0 | No distant metastases |
| M1 | Distant metastases present |

# SECTION 8

# Disorders of the scrotum and penis

## 8.1 Anatomy of the scrotum and testis

 **In a nutshell ...**

The testes are tough, mobile organs lying within the scrotum. The scrotum is an outpouching of the lower part of the anterior abdominal wall. It contains the testes, epididymes and lower part of the spermatic cords.

### Layers of the scrotum

1. **Skin**
2. **Superficial fascia:** this is divided into the superficial and deep layers and contains the dartos muscle. The deep layer of superficial fascia is called Colles' fascia and is continuous with the membranous fascial layer of the anterior abdominal wall (scarpa fascia). Posteriorly it is attached to the perineal body and the posterior edge of the perineal membrane

3. **Spermatic fasciae:** these are derived from the muscles of the anterior abdominal wall:
   - **External spermatic fascia:** derived from the external oblique
   - **Cremasteric fascia:** derived from the internal oblique. The cremaster muscle fibres are supplied by the genital branch of the genitofemoral nerve, which gives rise to the 'cremasteric reflex' allowing elevation of the testes for warmth and protection
   - **Internal spermatic fascia:** derived from the fascia transversalis
4. **Tunica vaginalis:** originally an evagination of the peritoneal cavity, this becomes shut off from the processus vaginalis as it closes just before birth. If it remains patent it can be filled with water (infantile hydrocele) or intraperitoneal contents (indirect hernia)
5. A tough capsule, the **tunica albuginea**, surrounds each testis. Extending inwards from this are a series of fibrous septa that divide the organ into lobules, and within each lobule are coiled seminiferous tubules. The tubules open into channels called the 'rete testis' and small efferent ductules connect this to the epididymis

Normal spermatogenesis requires that the testes are maintained at a lower temperature than the abdominal cavity. This lower temperature is achieved by:

- Location outside the abdomen in the scrotum (3° lower than the body temperature)
- Dartos muscle
- Countercurrent heat exchange between testicular arteries and the venous pampiniform plexus

## Arterial supply of the scrotum and testis

Testicular artery is a branch of the abdominal aorta and follows the embryological descent of the testis down the posterior abdominal wall, into the deep ring, through the inguinal canal, out via the superficial ring, and into the scrotum. Significant anastomosis between this artery and the epididymal, cremasteric and vasal arteries.

## Venous drainage of the scrotum and testis

Testicular veins form several anastomotic channels around the testicular artery, the **pampiniform plexus**. It is thought that this allows counter-current heat exchange and contributes to keeping the testicles cool. The left testicular vein drains into the left renal vein, the right directly into the IVC.

## Lymphatic drainage of the scrotum and testis

This is to the para-aortic nodes at the level of L1.

## Epididymis

- Lies posteromedial to the testis
- Has an expanded head, body and inferior tail

- Structurally it is a coiled tube about 6 m long, embedded in connective tissue
- The tail is in continuity with the vas deferens, which exits from the medial side

The epididymis has three functions:
1. Sperm storage
2. Sperm maturation
3. Fluid resorption

## Vas deferens

- This tube of about 40 cm conveys sperm to the ejaculatory ducts
- It arises in continuity with the tail of the epididymis and passes superomedially up through the scrotum and through the inguinal canal to the deep inguinal ring to enter the abdominal cavity
- As it enters the abdomen it hooks around the inferior epigastric artery
- It crosses the ureter at the level of the ischial spine and passes inferiomedially on the posterior surface of the bladder towards the seminal vesicle

## Seminal vesicles and ejaculatory ducts

- Seminal vesicles are lobulated organs, 5 cm long, lying on the lower posterior aspect of the bladder
- These coiled tubes embedded in connective tissue function to produce nourishing secretions that are added to sperm in the ejaculate
- Ducts of the seminal vesicles join the vas deferens medially and become the ejaculatory ducts, which pierce the posterior part of the prostate and enter the urethra close to the prostatic utricle

**CHAPTER 8**

## 8.2 Anatomy of the penis

### In a nutshell ...

The penis has a fixed **root** and a **body** that hangs free.

The right and left **crura** are attached to the inferior pubic rami and perineal membrane. They continue anteriorly as the corpora cavernosa, each surrounded by a tough fascial sheath, the **tunica albuginea.** Each crus is covered on its outer surface by the **ischiocavernosus** muscle.

The **bulb** is attached to the centre of the perineal membrane and surrounded by the **bulbospongiosus** muscle. The forward continuation of the bulb is the corpus spongiosum, which surrounds the penile urethra. Distally the corpus spongiosum expands to form the **glans** penis.

The body of the penis is essentially composed of these three cylinders of erectile tissue enclosed in a tubular sheath of fascia (**Buck's fascia)**.

### Arterial supply of the penis

The common penile artery is the terminal branch of the internal pudendal artery. It terminates in three branches to supply the erectile bodies.

### Venous drainage

The **dorsal vein** of the penis runs in a groove between the corporal bodies and eventually drains into the prostatic venous plexus.

### Nerve supply of the penis

This is via the pudendal nerve and pelvic autonomic plexuses.

### Lymphatic drainage of the penis

This is to the inguinal and eventually the iliac lymph nodes. The primary route of spread of penile carcinoma is via the lymphatic channels and therefore knowledge of these is important in its management.

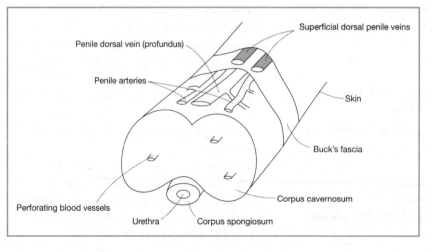

**Figure 8.10 Anatomy of the penis**

**CHAPTER 8**

## 8.3 Physiology of the male reproductive system

### Testicular function and androgen secretion

The normal hypothalamic–pituitary–gonadal axis has been alluded to in the section on prostate cancer (see Section 7.3).

The pituitary produces both LH and FSH in response to the pulsatile release of LHRH.

- **LH** is responsible for stimulating Leydig cells of the testis to produce testosterone
- **FSH** is important in spermatogenesis and acts on the Sertoli cells in the testis

The Sertoli cells are contained within the seminiferous tubules and surround the developing germ cells (nutritive and supportive role). Tight junctions between the Sertoli cells create an effective blood–testis barrier. Sertoli cells secrete inhibin which acts as negative feedback on FSH secretion via the pituitary.

Spermatozoa are derived from spermatogonia via several stages in which meiosis occurs (Figure 11.11).

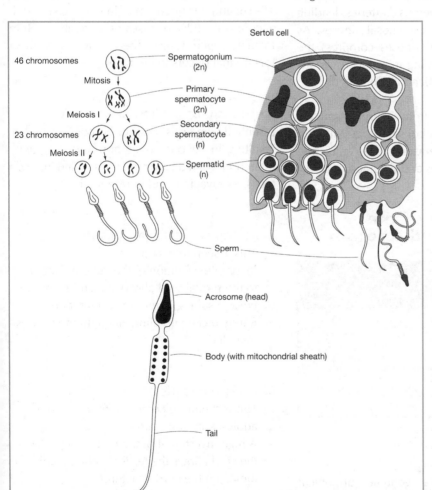

**Figure 8.11 Spermatogenesis**

CHAPTER 8

## Physiology of normal erection

Branches of the **pudendal nerves** containing autonomic fibres from T12–L2 (sympathetic) and S2–4 (parasympathetic) innervate the cavernosal artery smooth muscle.

Stimulation of parasympathetic nerves leads to the release of neurotransmitters including **nitric oxide** and **prostaglandin**. This causes activation of guanylyl cyclase and adenylyl cyclase, increasing local concentrations of **cGMP** and **cAMP**.

These bring about smooth muscle relaxation and dilatation of the cavernosal arteries, leading to blood flow into the cavernosal sinuses. As they fill, the cavernosal sinuses compress the subtunical venules resulting in reduced venous outflow, so the corpora become engorged.

Decreased stimulation from neurotransmitters coupled with the metabolism of cGMP and cAMP by **phosphodiesterases** leads to relaxation of the cavernosal arteries and detumescence.

## 8.4  Disorders of the testicle and scrotum

### In a nutshell ...

- Testicular torsion
- Hydrocele
- Epididymal cyst
- Varicocele
- Vasectomy

## Testicular torsion

Testicular torsion is a genuine urological emergency. Surgery should be underway within 1 hour of diagnosis so the role of the admitting senior house officer (SHO) is crucial – he or she must recognise and confirm a queried torsion, ensure that the operating surgeon sees it, inform acute theatres and the on-call anaesthetist, and arrange consent (including for orchidectomy) and transport of the patient straight to theatre (not to the ward!), all within minutes of the patient being referred. Irreversible ischaemia occurs within 6 hours of the torsion first occurring.

### Epidemiology of testicular torsion

This occurs most commonly in boys aged 10–16, and it is uncommon in men aged >30. It accounts for 90% of cases of an acute scrotum in males aged 13–21. There is a rare form of torsion that occurs in neonates.

### Aetiology of testicular torsion

Essentially the testis twists on its cord structures, resulting in venous congestion and eventually infarction. Testicular torsion is classified into two types, extravaginal and intravaginal.

#### Extravaginal testicular torsion
- This is seen in neonates
- Incomplete fixation of the gubernaculum to the scrotal wall allows the entire cord to twist, resulting in testicular infarction
- Rarely picked up clinically until the testis is infarcted

#### Intravaginal testicular torsion
- This is the more common form, found in adolescents and adults
- A high investment of the tunica vaginalis on the cord allows the testis to rotate within the tunica on the cord structures

## Presentation of testicular torsion

Typically patients present with an acutely painful tender hemi-scrotum. There may be some swelling. Occasionally pain radiates to the groin and even the loin, reflecting the embryological origin of the testis.

- Vomiting can occur
- There may be previous episodes of the pain, suggesting intermittent torsion
- On physical examination the testis is extremely tender
- Classically the testis lies horizontally and slightly higher (bell-clapper testis), although neither of these signs is specific

## Differential diagnosis of testicular torsion

- Epididymo-orchitis
- Trauma
- Neoplasia
- Inguinoscrotal hernia
- Torsion of hydatid of Morgagni
- Referred pain from ureteric calculus at the VUJ

The main differential is epididymo-orchitis (covered in Section 4, 'Urological infections'). Presentation is generally less acute and usually there are urinary symptoms, although not always.

**Torsion of the hydatid of Morgagni** can also mimic testicular torsion although there is normally less swelling. This small appendicular attachment to the testis can become twisted and gangrenous in the presence of a completely normal, viable testis. Usually this diagnosis is made at surgery because it is never possible to exclude torsion completely in this situation.

## Investigating testicular torsion

If torsion is suspected no investigations are required; indeed time is at a premium so exploration should not be delayed.

## Treatment of testicular torsion

Scrotal exploration should be carried out as soon as possible if testicular torsion is suspected (this is the case in almost all young men with an acutely painful testis). Irreversible ischaemic changes can occur within 6 hours of torsion so surgery should be performed within 1 hour of presentation. At operation the testis is approached trans-scrotally:

- If torsion is discovered, the testis is untwisted
- If the testis remains dusky after de-torsion it should be wrapped in warm saline-soaked swabs for 15 minutes

If there is still doubt about its viability, then perform **orchidectomy**. This should be included in the patient consent. If viable the testis should be fixed in the scrotum (**orchiopexy**), as should the contralateral testis.

## Hydroceles

This is a common cause of scrotal swelling in all age groups. It represents a collection of fluid around the testis within the tunica vaginalis.

## Aetiology of hydrocele

In children this is caused by a **patent processus vaginalis** (see Paediatric Surgery, Book 1) and it is a primary hydrocele. In adults they may be primary or, rarely, secondary hydroceles due to chronic infection, trauma (and damage to lymphatics) or testicular tumour.

CHAPTER 8

### Clinical presentation of hydrocele

This is with painless scrotal swelling. It should be possible to palpate the spermatic cord above the swelling; if this is not possible it may be a hernia. Classically, hydroceles **transilluminate** although this is not always the case.

### Investigating hydrocele

Perform US in young men to exclude testicular tumours. Not necessary in elderly men.

### Treatment of hydrocele

- **None:** do not treat unless they are causing discomfort
- **Aspiration** can be carried out but carries a risk of infection and the hydrocele almost invariably recurs within a few weeks
- **Open repair** is the gold standard treatment. The tunica vaginalis may be plicated as in the Lord repair or turned 'inside out' as in the Jaboulay repair

---

 **Op box: Hydrocele repair**

**Indication**
- In adults hydrocele repair is indicated only in large hydroceles that are causing significant symptoms. Pain is not a characteristic feature of hydroceles and patients should be counselled that it will not always resolve after hydrocele repair

**Preop**
- In younger patients, preoperative ultrasound scan should be performed to exclude a testicular tumour as the cause of the hydrocele

**Procedure**
- Either a transverse incision or a median raphe incision can be used. There are two well-described methods for hydrocele repair: the Jaboulay repair and the Lord repair

**Jaboulay repair**
- The tunica is dissected free from the dartos and delivered out of the scrotum together with the testicle
- The tunica is then divided longitudinally and sutured behind the cord
- If the hydrocele is very large some of the tunica may need to be excised

**Lord repair**
- The incision through skin and dartos is continued through the tunica and the hydrocele is emptied
- The tunica is then plicated by using several sutures

**Postop**
- Wear supportive underwear until recovered
- Expect some bruising and swelling initially
- Home when patient is comfortable and has passed urine

**Complications**
- Scrotal haematoma
- Wound infection
- Recurrence

## Epididymal cysts

These fluid-filled scrotal masses are thought to arise from congenital diverticula of the epididymal tubules.

## Presentation of epididymal cysts

Cysts may be multiple and are usually tense, spherical and transilluminable. The testis can be felt separately (which is how epididymal cyst is differentiated from hydrocele).

## Treatment of epididymal cysts

* **None:** if no symptoms, no treatment is required
* **Surgical excision** if there is pain. However, the patient should be warned that further cysts might arise and that scarring may affect fertility. Removing the cyst does not always remove the pain and the patient needs to be aware of this

## Varicoceles

A varicocele is a varicose dilatation of the pampiniform venous plexus that runs within the spermatic cord. Incidence is 15%. It is more common on the left, where the testicular vein drains into the renal vein (the system with the higher pressure).

## Presentation of varicocele

Most are asymptomatic. Occasionally there is an aching pain, especially after prolonged standing.

They may be detected during investigation of infertility because they are related to male subfertility (due to increased temperature).

## Classification of varicocele

Grade 1:    subclinical but detectable using Doppler ultrasonography
Grade 2:    palpable when the patient is standing
Grade 3:    visible as a scrotal swelling and palpable when the patient is lying

## Investigating varicocele

Renal ultrasonography is indicated in older patients because occasionally renal cancer presents with varicocele if the renal vein is involved.

## Treatment of varicocele

* **Surgical treatment** by ligation of the veins in the groin. Clearly the higher the veins are ligated the fewer tributaries there will be
* **Laparoscopic ligation** of the veins within the pelvis is effective
* **Embolisation** is an effective treatment that avoids surgery

This may recur or persist (in 20%) due to collateral circulation or incomplete venous ligation.

## Vasectomy

Vasectomy is a procedure performed for contraception. Both vasa deferentia are ligated in the scrotum. The procedure can be performed under LA or GA. Vasectomy is a common cause of medicolegal problems in urology and careful counselling must be performed before the procedure.

Patients must be aware of the following:
* Vasectomy is considered irreversible
* Late recanalisation of the vas deferens occurs in 1 in 2000 patients and can lead to fertility being regained

CHAPTER 8

- The results of vasectomy are not immediate because sperm will continue to appear in the ejaculate for several months. Alternative contraception is essential until consecutive semen analyses show no sperm
- Wound infection or scrotal haematoma may occur
- Chronic scrotal pain is a recognised complication

The procedure should be carried out under GA if the patient is very anxious or has had previous scrotal or groin surgery.

## 8.5  Disorders of the penis and foreskin

**In a nutshell ...**

Peyronie's disease
Erectile dysfunction
Priapism
- Phimosis
- Paraphimosis

## Peyronie's disease

This is a fibromatosis of unknown aetiology that affects focal areas of the tunica albuginea of the corpus cavernosum.

### Epidemiology of Peyronie's disease
- Incidence is estimated at 1%
- Average age at onset is 53
- Associated with a Dupuytren contracture and a plantar fascial contracture

### Aetiology of Peyronie's disease
- Uncertain
- Repeated minor trauma in association with vascular insufficiency is postulated to lead to scarring

### Presentation of Peyronie's disease
- Symptoms usually start with penile pain on erection
- Gradually deviation of the erection progresses, occasionally reaching a stage where sexual intercourse becomes impossible
- Pain usually resolves within 6–9 months

### Treatment of Peyronie's disease
Conservative treatment is appropriate for the first year because it takes this long for the disease to stabilise. Various potential drug therapies have been suggested but none has been proven in randomised controlled trials.

**ESWL** has been used to soften or destroy the penile plaque. This shows promising early results although long-term follow-up is not available.

**Surgery:** after 1 year, if the deformity has made sexual intercourse impossible, surgery can be offered. There are three main surgical options:
1. **Nesbit operation** (or variation) in which plication with or without excision of the tunica albuginea on the opposite side to the plaque is performed; this procedure is inevitably associated with penile shortening
2. **Plaque excision and patching** with a graft such as saphenous vein; this is purported to produce less penile shortening but can lead to problems associated with softer erections
3. **Implantation of a penile prosthesis** can be used to straighten the penis in men who have existing erectile dysfunction

# Erectile dysfunction

Erectile dysfunction is defined as the persistent inability to obtain and maintain an erection sufficient for sexual intercourse. The prevalence of complete erectile dysfunction varies from 5% at age 40 to 15% at age 70.

## Classification of erectile dysfunction

- Broadly this is classified as **psychogenic** or **organic**
- About 50% of men fall into each group, although organic impotence is more common in older men (see box)

> **Causes of organic erectile dysfunction**
> - Vascular disease
> - Neurogenic, eg MS, spinal injury
> - Trauma, eg pelvic surgery, prostatectomy, pelvic fracture
> - Drugs, eg antihypertensives, antidepressants, alcohol
> - Hypogonadism (pituitary or gonadal)
> - Peyronie's disease
> - Chronic illness, eg diabetes, renal failure

## Evaluation of erectile dysfunction

- **History:** useful for distinguishing psychogenic from organic impotence. Nocturnal erections suggest psychogenic cause. Drug history is important
- **Examination:** should include external genitalia and digital rectal examination
- **Examination of the peripheral pulses:** should be carried out to detect generalised atheromatous disease

- **Urine analysis:** may reveal diabetes
- **Serum testosterone and prolactin:** indicated if hypogonadism is suggested
- **Further tests:** such as Doppler sonography and cavernosography may be indicated but are not applicable in the vast majority of men

## Treatment of erectile dysfunction

### General measures

- Patients are advised to stop smoking and to reduce alcohol consumption
- Drugs may be adjusted
- Psychosexual counselling may help in psychogenic erectile dysfunction

### Oral drug therapy

- **Phosphodiesterase-5 inhibitors**, eg sildenafil/Viagra, which maintain high concentrations of cGMP in the cavernosal smooth muscle and facilitate maintenance of an erection. More than 70% of erectile dysfunction responds to these drugs. Contraindicated in patients taking nitrates
- **Dopamine agonists**, eg apomorphine. These act on the paraventricular nucleus in the brain (centre that controls sexual drive)

### Local pharmacotherapy to the penis

**Prostaglandin E$_1$** can be administered by intracorporeal injection or as a urethral pellet. It increases the concentration of cAMP in the cavernosal smooth muscle. An erection is produced in 80% of patients, but:
- Pain at the injection site can be a problem
- Priapism occurs in 1% of all patients on injection therapy (see below)

**CHAPTER 8**

### Vacuum pump

- Although this is effective it is considered unnatural and is not popular

### Penile prostheses

- These are usually reserved as a last resort
- They can be either solid or inflatable
- Both mechanical failure and infection are problems
- They are expensive

## Priapism

This is a prolonged, painful erection that is not associated with sexual desire. It is classified as low-flow (veno-occlusive) or high-flow (which is rare, and usually due to AV malformation).

### Pathophysiology of priapism

The corpora are rigid because of sludging of blood. Ischaemia and hypoxia lead to pain.

- After 3–4 hours there is pain
- After 12 hours there is interstitial oedema
- After 24–48 hours there is smooth muscle necrosis
- After >1 week there is fibrosis and erectile dysfunction

### Causes of priapism

- Therapy for erectile dysfunction: causes 20% of cases, which is common if administered by injection, but rare with oral therapies
- Haematological diseases: due to the hyperviscosity in sickle cell disease/trait, in other haemoglobinopathies, leukaemia, erythropoietin (EPO) therapy or cessation of anticoagulation

- Malignant infiltration by solid tumours, eg bladder, prostate, renal
- Neurological disease, eg lumbar disc disease, CVA
- Drugs, eg antihypertensives, paroxetine, fluoxetine, trazodone

### Management of priapism

- Conservative, eg exercise, ice, ejaculation
- Aspiration (corporal) and irrigation with warm saline
- Oral medication, eg terbutaline 5–10 mg, 36% response
- Intracavernosal medication, eg phenylephrine – note close monitoring of BP is essential
- Surgical intervention; this includes:
  - Glans–cavernosal shunt
  - Cavernosal–spongiosum shunt
  - Cavernosal–saphenous shunt

### Prognosis of priapism

Increasing duration results in a higher probability of subsequent impotence:

- <24 hours leads to impotence in about 43%
- >24 hours leads to impotence in about 90%

## Phimosis

Phimosis is simply non-retraction of the foreskin. It is quite normal at birth because of preputial adhesions (see Paediatric Surgery, Book 1).

True pathological phimosis occurs secondary to scarring of the foreskin, most commonly due to **balanitis xerotica obliterans** (BXO), which is a fibrosing condition of unknown aetiology. BXO can also affect the urethra, causing problems with voiding.

Pathological phimosis is an indication for circumcision.

## Paraphimosis

This is a urological emergency caused by retraction of a tight foreskin. If the foreskin is not replaced it causes constriction of the glans, leading to swelling, which makes it more difficult to reduce.

## Treatment of paraphimosis

- Aims to reduce swelling using ice-packs and squeezing the oedematous tissue

- Reduction can then be attempted
- LA (penile block or ring block) can be administered
- Occasionally it is necessary to drain the oedematous fluid using a needle
- GA is sometimes required for reduction
- Circumcision (see Op box) is recommended in all these patients to prevent the problem recurring

---

 **Op box: Circumcision**

**Indications**
- Phimosis
- Paraphimosis
- Recurrent balanitis
- Penile tumour

**Preop**
- Treat any active infection

**Procedure**
- Administer GA or LA with penile nerve block
- Mark the incision with the penis on stretch (some use artificial erection) to avoid taking too much or too little skin
- Various methods exist to remove the two layers of foreskin. Most surgeons do it in two layers although some take both together and a knife or scissors can be used
- Avoid monopolar diathermy because there is a risk of damage to end-arteries and subsequent necrosis. Bipolar diathermy or ties are used for haemostasis
- Use absorbable sutures for closure

**Postop**
- This is a day-case procedure
- Patient can go home as soon as he is comfortable and has passed urine
- Avoid sexual intercourse for 2–3 weeks

**Complications**
- Bleeding (if immediately postoperatively, return to theatre is usually necessary)
- Urinary retention
- Wound infection
- Change in gland sensation
- Urethral damage
- Excessive skin removal

# CHAPTER 9

# Vascular Surgery

**Sam Andrews**

## 1.1 Principles of vascular surgery

 **In a nutshell ...**

Vascular disease includes:
- Arterial disease: occlusive, aneurysm, carotid, trauma
- Venous disease: thromboembolic, varicose veins, leg ulcers
- Lymphatic diseases

Also included are miscellaneous conditions traditionally treated by vascular surgeons:
- Vasospastic disorders
- Thoracic outlet syndrome
- Hyperhidrosis
- Amputations
- Vascular trauma (see Book 1 of this series)

Arterial interventions are performed:
- To improve or restore arterial flow (eg angioplasty, stenting, bypass)
- To prevent vascular catastrophe (eg carotid endarterectomy, aneurysm surgery)

The main principles of arterial surgery are to first gain proximal and distal control of flow and then correct the vascular abnormality. These principles can be applied equally well to peripheral vascular disease (PVD), carotid surgery, aneurysm or vascular trauma. Vascular physiology is covered in Chapter 3, Book 1 of this series.

CHAPTER 9

## 1.2 Vascular investigations

### In a nutshell ...

**General vascular investigations**, eg blood tests, chest radiograph, etc
**Specific vascular investigations:**
- Ankle–brachial pressure index (ABPI)
- Duplex Doppler ultrasonography
- Angiography
- Digital subtraction angiography
- CT and MR angiography
- Venography
- Lymphoscintigraphy
- Radio-isotope imaging

## General vascular investigations

As vascular disease is a multisystem disorder, all vascular patients require a general work-up with modification of vascular risk factors. In addition, those requiring complex vascular procedures may need other specific investigations:
- Full blood count (FBC), looking for:
  - Anaemia
  - Polycythaemia
  - Concurrent infection
- Clotting:
  - Especially if anticoagulated
  - Excludes prothrombotic states
  - Baseline before heparinisation or warfarinisation
- Urea and electrolytes or U&Es (for renal function)
- Erythrocyte sedimentation rate or ESR (for vasculitides)
- Random or fasting blood glucose (to exclude diabetes)
- Fasting lipids
- Urinalysis
- Chest radiograph (often smokers)
- ECG (coexisting cardiovascular disease is common in patients with arteriopathy and has implications for surgery)
- Echocardiography or exercise ECG in high-risk cardiac patients
- CPEX (cardiopulmonary exercise testing): this is an increasingly used, non-invasive, multimodal tool for preoperative assessment of vascular patients

## Specific vascular investigations

### Ankle–brachial pressure index

Ankle–brachial pressure index (ABPI) is used to assess the blood supply to the lower limb. It is simply a measure of BP in the foot, which is usually roughly equal to that of the arm. Hence, this absolute pressure in the foot can be compared with the brachial systolic BP to provide the ABPI.

$$\text{ABPI} = \frac{\text{foot artery occlusion pressure}}{\text{brachial systolic pressure}}$$

## Procedure box: How to perform an ABPI

- Place a BP cuff around the calf.
- Use a hand-held Doppler probe to find the dorsalis pedis or posterior tibial artery signal.
- Inflate the cuff, noting the pressure at which the signal stops.
- Release the pressure, confirming that the signal returns at the pressure noted. This is the occlusion pressure.
- Take the blood pressure at the brachial artery in the normal way.
- Compare the systolic BP recorded in the arm with the occlusion pressure recorded in the foot. If they are the same, the ABPI is 1 (normal ABPI is 0.9–1.1).
- If the peripheral circulation in the lower limb is reduced, the BP in the foot is low and the ABPI is low.

ABPI may be used to confirm the presence of PVD and as a baseline measure before treatment.

The following ABPI values imply:

>1.1: calcified or incompressible vessels (eg in diabetes or renal failure)

0.7–0.9: mild ischaemia

0.4–0.7: moderate ischaemia

<0.4: severe peripheral (critical) ischaemia

## Duplex Doppler ultrasonography

Duplex Doppler ultrasonography (US) is used for:
- Assessment and monitoring of arterial blood flow
  - Carotid disease
  - PVD
  - Graft surveillance
- Abdominal aortic aneurysm (AAA)
  - Assessment

- Monitoring
- Screening
- Renal disease
  - Renal artery stenosis
- Venous disease
  - Demonstrates reflux in varicose veins (with reverse flow in veins after calf compression)
  - Useful to mark varicose vein perforators
  - Diagnosis of DVT (veins non-compressible with Doppler probe)
  - Used for cannulation and positioning in endovenous laser surgery and endovenous radiofrequency ablation

There are two aspects to duplex Doppler US (bimodal system):
- **Grey-scale US:** visualises the vessel, vessel wall, plaque and lumen and measures degree of stenosis in millimetres
- **Doppler US:** uses the Doppler principle to measure the blood velocity, which is proportional to the degree of stenosis of the vessel

**Duplex Doppler US as an investigation for vascular disease**

**Advantages of duplex Doppler US**

- Cheap
- Non-invasive
- Accurate measurement of stenosis
- Colour image shows direction of blood and turbulent flow

**Disadvantages of duplex Doppler US**

- Operator-dependent
- Views may be obscured by bowel gas
- Poor images in calcified vessels
- Not good for near-occlusions

## Contrast angiography

Traditional contrast angiography is performed by introducing a radio-opaque dye into a vessel and taking X-ray images. BEWARE: contrast is nephrotoxic. Most radiology departments have a protocol for a renal protection regimen based on the patient's creatinine level or glomerular filtration rate (GFR). In pre-existing severe renal impairment, imaging may be performed using a stream of small bubbles of carbon dioxide. This protects renal function but compromises the quality of the images obtained.

### Uses of contrast angiography

- Assessment of arterial disease in most areas (especially upper and lower limbs, abdomen and thorax)
- Emergency assessment of vascular crises, such as:
  - Acute ischaemia
  - Lower limb embolus
  - Brachial artery occlusion
- Differentiates mesenteric ischaemia due to arterial occlusion (will show abrupt cut-off in superior mesenteric artery circulation) from vein thrombosis (will show delayed contrast passage)
- Renovascular disease:
  - Renal artery stenosis
  - Fibromuscular hyperplasia
- Calibrating angiograms to assess suitability of AAA endovascular repair

## Classification of contrast angiography

- By method of administration (eg intra-arterial, intravenous)
- By route of administration (eg translumbar, transfemoral, transbrachial)
- By area to be imaged (eg carotid, visceral, femoral)
- By method of image processing (eg traditional, digital subtraction, CT, MR)

In intra-arterial angiography, the contrast is introduced by direct arterial puncture via a catheter which is directed to the area to be imaged (eg femoral puncture to release contrast into the aorta to image the iliac and femoral vessels).

## Digital subtraction angiography (DSA)

Digital subtraction is a process that enhances the images obtained with contrast angiography. The pre-angiography image without contrast is subtracted from the post-angiography image with contrast to leave just an outline of the lumen of the vessel. This can be via intra-arterial (IADSA) or intravenous (IVDSA) injection of contrast (rarely used). IADSA is the most accurate investigation for imaging the arterial system.

---

**Intra-arterial angiography**

**Advantages of intra-arterial angiography**

- Small volume of contrast required
- Good-quality images (especially below knee where Doppler imaging is less useful)
- Allows concurrent treatment (angioplasty or stenting)

**Disadvantages of intra-arterial angiography**

- Arterial wall damage (can cause bleeding, bruising, false aneurysm, dissection)
- Contrast reactions (including anaphylaxis)
- Distal embolisation
- Groin haematoma

---

**CT and MR angiography**

**Advantages of CT and MRA**

- Quick
- Non-invasive
- No radiation dose for MR

**Disadvantages of CT and MRA**

- Relatively expensive
- Operator-dependent
- MR not possible in patients with metal implants
- Picture degeneration in CT of patients with metal implants
- Does not allow concurrent angioplasty and stenting
- Variable image quality

---

## CT and MR angiography

Multislice computed tomography (CT) and magnetic resonance angiography (MRA) are now becoming the mainstays of vascular investigation. Computer-generated, three-dimensional images can be produced, and detailed image reconstruction performed. MRA is a specific application of MRI, producing angiogram-type images utilising blood flow through the vessel to create images.

## Venography and MR venography

**Venography** uses contrast to image the venous system, either ascending venography (contrast injected into foot vein) or descending venography (contrast injected into groin, ie femoral vein). The technique has been largely replaced by Doppler ultrasonography. However, it is occasionally used to differentiate primary from secondary venous insufficiency, or to diagnose below-knee deep vein thrombosis (DVT), when ultrasonography cannot adequately demonstrate the calf veins.

**Magnetic resonance venography** (MRV) is a specific application of MRI that can be performed with or without gadolinium contrast. It is effective for evaluating diseases of larger veins (identification of obstruction, or occlusion of the brachiocephalic, subclavian and jugular veins, venous sinus thrombosis, pelvic circulation). MRV has not been established as superior to duplex ultrasonography for diagnosis of DVT.

## Imaging of the lymphatics

Lymphoscintigraphy is now the main investigation to image the lymphatic system. Radiolabelled colloid is injected into the web spaces between the second and third toes and images obtained with a gamma camera.

## Radio-isotope imaging

Radiolabelled fibrinogen is occasionally used in the diagnosis of thrombotic venous disease (eg DVT). Radiolabelled white cell scans may be used for assessing graft infection.

# SECTION 2

# Aneurysms

## In a nutshell ...

An aneurysm is a pathological dilatation of an artery to >1.5 times its normal diameter. In the western world arterial aneurysms are usually due to athero-sclerosis. Aneurysms have clinical implications because of their ability to rupture, leak or embolise.

Rupture of abdominal aortic aneurysm (AAA) is a common cause of sudden death and the risk of rupture increases with the size of the aneurysm. For this reason surgery is considered for all symptomatic AAAs, for those >5.5 cm in diameter and those that are expanding at a rate of >1 cm/year.

Other arteries may become aneurysmal but this is less common.

## 2.1    Arterial anatomy

## In a nutshell ...

**Two types of artery**
- Elastic
- Muscular

**Three histological layers**
- Tunica intima
- Tunica media
- Tunica adventitia

### Structure of arteries

There are two types of arteries:
- **Elastic** conducting arteries (eg aorta) which expand to take the forward blood flow of systole and use this stored energy to recoil during diastole (this provides constant blood flow)
- **Muscular** distributing arteries (eg femoral artery) which taper as the media thins down to a few layers of vascular smooth muscle cells and become arterioles

Microscopically, arteries consist of three layers:

- **Tunica intima:** innermost layer; composed of a single layer of endothelial cells which are oriented in the direction of flow and have a role in both coagulation and vasomotor tone
- **Tunica media:** middle layer; composed of elastin and collagen fibres with vascular smooth muscle cells which function either to control vasomotor tone or to synthesise the structural proteins of the vessel wall
- **Tunica adventitia:** outermost layer of connective tissue

Elastic arteries have a high amount of elastin and collagen in the media, with relatively fewer smooth muscle cells (which predominate in muscular arteries). The media is an important structure in the arterial wall, and abnormalities within the media of the vessel are pathological in aneurysmal disease.

## Anatomy of the aorta

The aorta has thoracic and abdominal components. Aortic wall histology changes rapidly as the aorta descends past the renal arteries, with the thoracic aorta having >30% elastin compared with <20% in the abdominal section.

## Thoracic aorta

The **ascending thoracic aorta** is 5 cm long, beginning at the aortic valve. The sinuses of Valsalva are three bulges in the wall of the ascending aorta just above the aortic valve – these give rise to the right and left coronary arteries.

The **aortic arch** starts behind the right margin of the sternum and gives rise to the brachiocephalic, left common carotid and left subclavian arteries. It ends at the level of T4.

The **descending thoracic aorta** lies in the posterior mediastinum, extending between T4 and T12. It gives branches to pericardium, lungs, bronchi, oesophagus, intercostal and phrenic arteries.

For a detailed discussion of the pathology and surgery of the thoracic aorta see Chapter 3, Cardiothoracic Surgery.

## Abdominal aorta

The abdominal aorta enters the abdomen between the diaphragmatic crura anterior to T12, as a continuation of the thoracic aorta. It descends on the vertebral bodies until its bifurcation at the level of the body of L4, where it bifurcates into the common iliac arteries, with a small median sacral artery between. It is crossed anteriorly by the splenic vein, body of the pancreas, third part of the duodenum and the left renal vein. On its right lie the inferior vena cava (IVC), the right ureter and the azygos vein. On its left lie the left sympathetic trunk and the left ureter.

### Branches of the abdominal aorta

Three paired visceral branches
- Suprarenal (adrenal)
- Renal
- Gonadal

Three unpaired visceral branches
- Coeliac axis
- Superior mesenteric artery (SMA)
- Inferior mesenteric artery (IMA)

Parietal branches
- One pair inferior phrenic
- Four pairs lumbar (usually), plus median sacral artery (variable)

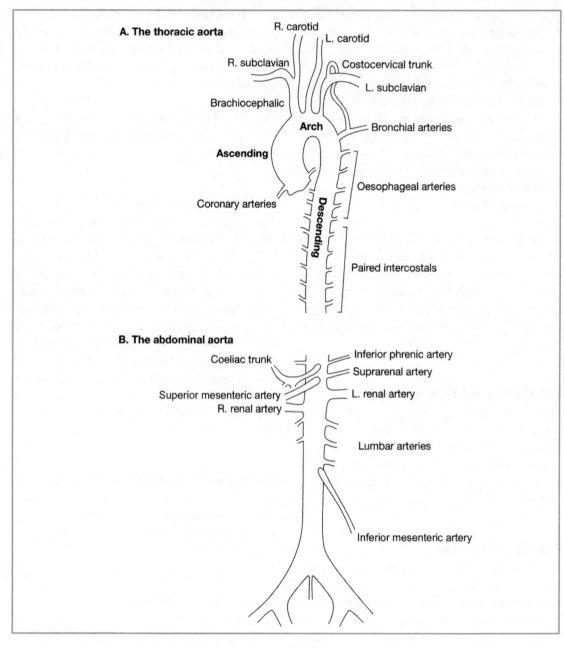

Figure 9.1 The aorta

(Note that the artery of Adamkiewiecz arises from lumbar arteries as the main blood supply to the spinal cord; high aortic surgery can cause spinal cord ischaemia).

## 2.2 Pathology of aneurysms

### In a nutshell ...

An aneurysm is a pathological dilatation of an artery to >1.5 times its normal diameter. The upper limit of the normal aorta is considered to be 2 cm, ie it is aneurysmal at 3 cm. Mechanical factors are very important in progression of an aneurysm. According to **Laplace's law**, any increase in vessel diameter will increase wall tension, causing continued arterial dilatation and eventually rupture.

Aneurysms may be classified as the following:
- **True aneurysms:** dilatation of an artery involving all layers of the arterial wall
- **False aneurysms:** pulsatile, expansile swelling due to a defect in an arterial wall, with blood outside the arterial lumen,

surrounded by a capsule of fibrous tissue or compressed surrounding tissues

True aneurysms may be **fusiform** (spindle-shaped) or **saccular** (bag-like weakness in part of the arterial wall).

Other descriptions of abnormal arteries:
- **Tortuous:** increase in length of an artery causing curvature between two fixed points
- **Arteriomegaly:** generalised dilatation or lengthening of arteries

### Aetiology of aneurysms
- **Degenerative (atherosclerotic):** this is the most common cause, due to inflammation and proteolysis in the substrata of the tunica media
- **Inflammatory:** possibly a more severe form of degenerative AAA. It is characterised by variable degrees of inflammation in the aneurysm wall, causing adhesion to adjacent structures (especially duodenum,

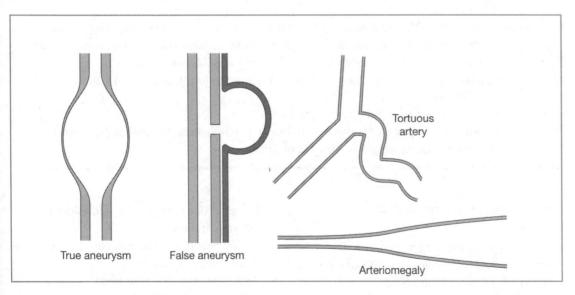

**Figure 9.2 Types of aneurysm**

small bowel, ureters), and it is related to (sometimes associated with) retroperitoneal fibrosis (with symptoms of ureteric obstruction and chronic renal failure). Usually it presents with abdominal pain, weight loss and a raised ESR. Management is conventional or endovascular repair but surgery may be more challenging due to inflammation and fibrosis

- **Congenital:** eg berry aneurysms of the cerebral circulation
- **Mycotic:** these can be from endogenous sources (eg infected emboli in endocarditis) or from exogenous causes (eg from infected needles in intravenous drug abuse)
- **Infective:** these are most common in

syphilitic aneurysms (often affecting the arch of the aorta and descending aorta). Syphilitic aortitis is rare now because of increased use of antibiotics in primary and secondary syphilis

- **Traumatic:** damage to the arterial wall can be from blunt or penetrating injury (including iatrogenic) and can result in true or false aneurysm formation
- **Connective tissue disorders:** tend to present young at 40–50 years or with a family history, eg Marfan syndrome, Ehlers–Danlos syndrome, tuberous sclerosis, Takayasu's arteritis
- **Post-stenotic:** due to altered vessel haemodynamics

## 2.3 Abdominal aortic aneurysm

### In a nutshell ...

The infrarenal abdominal aorta is the commonest site for atherosclerotic aneurysm. A ruptured AAA is the thirteenth most common cause of death in the western world.
- Size is the most important risk factor for rupture, although rate of expansion is also significant.
- Seventy-five per cent present as an asymptomatic incidental finding on imaging.
- Symptomatic aneurysms are usually expanding rapidly or leaking and need prompt repair.
- Treatment is surgical replacement with a graft or endovascular stenting.
- Elective repair has a mortality rate of 5% and is offered to fit patients with an aneurysm of >5.5 cm diameter.
- Elective surgery aims to avoid future rupture.
- Most patients with ruptured aneurysms die before reaching hospital, and of those operated on, 50% will die during or within 30 days of surgery.

### Demographics of AAA

- 6M to 1F
- Affects 1 in 20 (5%) men aged >65
- Incidence increases with age (6% of men aged 65–74; 9% of men >75)

- Risks include smoking, hypercholesterolaemia, male sex
- Family history (12-fold increased occurrence in first-degree relatives)
- 95% infrarenal; 5% suprarenal
- 30% involve iliac arteries

## Natural history of AAAs

The natural progression of an AAA is to expand and rupture.

Size is the most important risk factor for rupture. An increase in size by 10% per year or more also significantly increases risk. Smaller aneurysms expand more slowly than larger aneurysms. Not all growth is linear and there may be periods where expansion accelerates or stops altogether.

Rates of rupture taken from a non-operated series are:
- <4% per year if <5 cm
- 7% per year if 5–6 cm
- >20% per year if >6 cm

There may be some value in risk factor modification to reduce growth rate (eg decrease BP, prescribe statins).

## Presentation of AAAs

- **Asymptomatic:** usually incidental finding on clinical or radiological examination; 75% present this way
- **Pain:** this is central abdominal and may radiate to the back. This is a sign of expansion or, if sudden and acute, rupture
- **Rupture:** this is the most devastating presentation. There is a 95% mortality rate overall, and 50% mortality rate in those who reach hospital alive. The patient typically presents with a hypotensive episode or collapse, associated with severe central abdominal pain radiating to the back and the flanks. An aneurysm commonly ruptures the posterolateral wall, causing a retroperitoneal haematoma. This may be seen as bruising in the flanks or it may track down into the scrotum. Occasionally rupture may form a temporarily contained haematoma. Coexisting chronic obstructive pulmonary disease (COPD) is a known risk factor for aneurysm rupture

**CHAPTER 9**

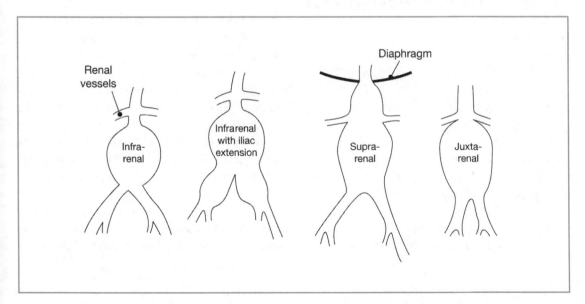

**Figure 9.3 Types of abdominal aortic aneurysm. All AAAs can extend into the iliac vessels. Suprarenal AAAs can extend into the chest as a thoracoabdominal aneurysm**

- **Shock**
- **Embolisation:** thrombus/atheroma from the aneurysm may give rise to acute limb ischaemia or small areas of distal infarction (trash foot)
- **Others:** AAAs can rarely present with acute thrombosis or fistulation into surrounding structures (eg IVC, duodenum, terminal ileum)

## Screening for AAAs

This is currently being rolled out across England and Wales. Some areas have been screening for AAAs for many years. The NHS AAA screening programme offers men an abdominal ultrasound examination during the year that they are 65. Patients with AAAs >5.5 cm are offered open or endovascular repair. Patients with smaller aneurysms are offered ongoing ultrasound surveillance to monitor aneurysm growth.

## Preoperative investigations for AAA repair

- **Bloods:**
  - FBC
  - U&Es (for concurrent renal failure)
  - Blood sugar
  - ESR (may be elevated in inflammatory aneurysms)
  - Cross-match
- **ABPI:** to assess coexisting PVD and document preoperative state in case of trash foot postoperatively
- **Chest radiograph**
- **ECG and echocardiogram**
- **Lung function tests:** to aid anaesthetic assessment

- **Ultrasonography:** usually used as a screening tool
- **CT:** this is mandatory for elective aneurysm surgery, allowing assessment of proximal neck anatomy, iliac extension, inflammation and other possible intra-abdominal pathology (these patients are often elderly and an occult tumour is occasionally found)
- **Arteriography:** this is not currently part of standard elective AAA work-up, but is necessary before endovascular repair
- **CPEX testing** (cardiopulmonary exercise testing)

In ruptured AAAs there is often insufficient time for full preoperative investigations. Minimal requirements for an emergency aneurysm repair include intravenous access × 2, basic bloods, cross-match 10 units and portable chest radiograph. A CT scan may be required to confirm the diagnosis but bear in mind that unstable patients should not be taken for CT.

## Elective open repair of AAAs

Elective repair is offered to patients whose aneurysms have a maximum diameter of >5.5 cm and who are fit enough to withstand surgery, to prevent continued expansion and rupture. Following the recommendations of the **UK Small Aneurysm Trial**, surveillance screening is offered to patients with asymptomatic small aneurysms <5.5 cm. Surgery is considered for all symptomatic AAAs and those >5.5 cm.

Elective infrarenal aneurysm repair has a mortality rate of about 5%. Emergency aneurysm repair has a mortality rate of around 50%.

**Op box: The principles of open abdominal aortic aneurysm repair**

**Indications**

Elective repair if diameter >5.5 cm; urgent repair if the aneurysm is undergoing rapid expansion or the patient presents with pain; emergency repair for rupture.

**Preop**

Appropriate preoperative assessment and management (eg antihypertensives, smoking cessation).

General anaesthetic with an endotracheal (ET) tube, central line, arterial line, epidural catheter and urethral catheter.

Prophylactic antibiotics and thromboprophylaxis.

Consent, with complications and hazards in mind.

**Positioning**

Supine.

**Incision**

Usually midline longitudinal incision. Some use a transverse incision.

**Procedure (summarised)**

- Enter abdominal cavity, retract bowel and duodenum to right
- Divide posterior peritoneum and dissect aneurysm
- Define proximal neck of aneurysm and distal extension (may be into iliacs)
- Administer intravenous heparinisation
- Apply aortic clamps (distal then proximal) and secure before opening aneurysm sac
- Over-sew lumbar arteries and IMA if they are patent
- Repair with either inlay tube graft or Y-graft (trouser) if iliac arteries involved
- Achieve haemostasis; close aneurysm sac over the graft

**Intraoperative hazards**

Beware abnormal anatomy affecting the renal vessels; duodenum and ureters lie close to an aneurysmal sac (and may be involved if inflammatory aetiology).

**Closure**

Standard abdominal closure for laparotomy.

**Postop instructions**

ITU for postoperative care.

## Complications of open AAA repair

Elective perioperative mortality rate is 3–5%.

### Immediate complications of AAA repair

- Haemorrhage (primary)
- Distal embolisation (ischaemic leg, trash foot)

### Early complications of AAA repair

- Haemorrhage (reactive, secondary)
- Myocardial infarction (MI)
- Renal failure (especially if proximal clamp above renal vessels)
- Multiorgan failure, disseminated intravascular coagulation (DIC), acute respiratory distress syndrome (ARDS)
- Colonic ischaemia
- Pneumonia, ARDS
- Stroke
- DVT, pulmonary embolism (PE)
- Paraparesis due to spinal ischaemia (lumbar vessels over-sewn)

### Late complications of AAA repair

- Late graft infection (causing graft thrombosis, false aneurysm formation or rupture)
- Aortoenteric fistula
- Anastomotic aneurysm

## Endovascular AAA repair (EVAR)

EVAR is an alternative modality of treatment of AAAs. A prosthesis consisting of a vascular graft with an integral metallic stent is introduced via a catheter through a femoral arteriotomy. It is advanced over a guidewire under fluoroscopic control into the aneurysm. The 'stent–graft' is then positioned such that, when the stents are expanded (usually by balloon catheters), the aneurysm is excluded from the circulation and thus is no longer at risk of rupture.

In **conventional EVAR** the aneurysm needs to have a proximal neck of at least 5 mm above the aneurysm and below the renal arteries, which is not too conical in shape and does not have thrombus within it. The better the quality of the proximal neck, the better the graft fixation and lower the risk of complications.

Aneurysms without a suitable proximal neck can be treated by **fenestrated EVAR** (FEVAR). Here, the fixation is above the visceral vessels, with side branches within the graft for visceral artery extensions. These grafts currently have to be custom-made and are very expensive.

Distal fixation can be in the distal aorta, but is usually in the iliac arteries. Thus an aneurysm with iliac extension can also be treated.

Thoracic aneurysm can be repaired with **thoracic EVAR** (TEVAR) devices.

After the EVAR there is a need for ongoing surveillance because there are many late complications. These include endoleaks, continued sac expansion, stent–graft failure, stent–graft migration and late rupture. Surveillance is usually performed by annual CT.

Late complications can often be treated by further endovascular surgery – the insertion of so-called extension devices or cuffs.

## Advantages of endovascular repair

- Avoids large chest/abdominal incisions
- No aortic cross-clamping and physiological insult
- Reduced blood loss
- Potentially shorter anaesthetic

## Disadvantages and complications of endovascular repair

- High cost
- Long-term results unclear (device failure possible)
- Endoleak
- Distal embolisation
- Stent–graft migration
- Femoral false aneurysm (at groin puncture site)
- Renal failure (as large volume of contrast required)

## Classification of endoleaks

- **Type I** – leak from stent–graft attachment site:
  - Ia – from proximal attachment
  - Ib – from distal attachment
  - Type I endoleaks usually require treatment
- **Type II** – leak due to retrograde flow through visceral or lumbar arteries into aneurysm sac. This is the most common type of endoleak, and can often be managed conservatively
- **Type III** – this is due to structural failure of the stent–graft, due to holes, disintegration of the structural components or junctional separation of the different parts of the endograft. These usually require treatment
- **Type IV** – this is due to graft porosity and usually settles in time
- **Type V** – this is when the aneurysm sac continues to expand with time, but no leak is identified (so-called 'endotension'). It is usually due to occult type I, II or III, which becomes more apparent with time

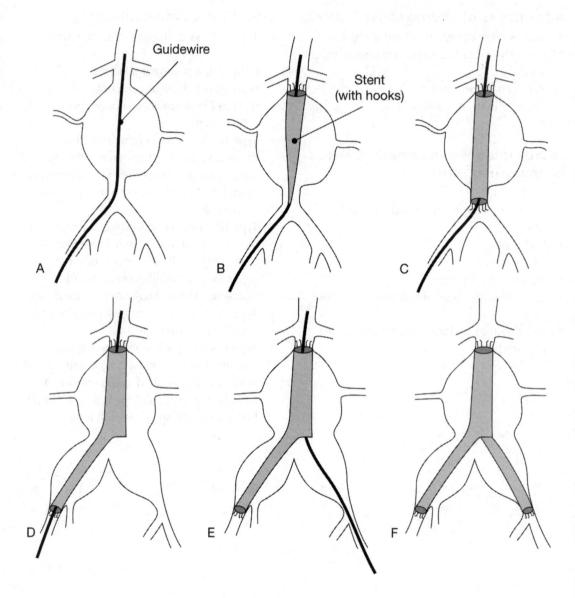

**Figure 9.4 Deployment of conventional EVAR**

(A) A guidewire is passed from a femoral puncture site through the common iliac artery and across the lumen of the AAA to the infrarenal aorta of normal diameter. (B) The proximal end of the stent is deployed by balloon angioplasty. (C) The distal end of the stent is deployed by balloon angioplasty. (D) If a bifurcated graft is required the first component is inserted through the right femoral puncture over a guidewire. (E) A second guidewire is introduced through the left femoral artery and navigated into the lumen of the first stent. (F) The second component of the graft is deployed.

## 2.4 Peripheral aneurysms

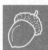
**In a nutshell ...**

- Popliteal aneurysms
- Femoral aneurysms
- Iliac aneurysms
- Visceral artery aneurysms
- Splenic aneurysms

## Popliteal aneurysms

- The popliteal artery is the second most common site of atherosclerotic aneurysms
- Popliteal aneurysms account for 70% of peripheral aneurysms
- Occasionally they present with expansile swelling, but more commonly with aneurysm thrombosis or distal emboli leading to peripheral ischaemia
- Rupture is rare
- Diagnosis confirmed by US/CT or arteriography (also assesses distal vasculature)
- Repair by ligation and vein bypass graft or endovascular stent–graft
- More than 30% of patients with a popliteal artery aneurysm will also have an AAA (remember to request a screening abdominal US in this group)

## Femoral aneurysms

- These can occur in isolation but are usually part of a generalised arterial dilatation
- Most femoral aneurysms are false, occurring after arterial groin puncture
- Often they are asymptomatic and rupture rarely
- Occasionally they are a source of distal emboli and may thrombose

- Repair is by insertion of prosthetic graft or reversed saphenous vein
- Infected chronic femoral aneurysm due to intravenous drug abuse is becoming more common and is difficult to treat because prosthetic grafts invariably become infected

## Iliac aneurysms

- The majority of these are found associated with an AAA
- Isolated aneurysms are rare (2%) and most of these involve the common iliac
- Rupture can occur

## Visceral artery aneurysms

- Aneurysms can also occur in the renal, coeliac or mesenteric arteries
- Often they are asymptomatic but may present with rupture

## Splenic aneurysms

Splenic aneurysms represent 60% of visceral artery aneurysms. The prevalence is 1–10% in postmortem studies. They are usually saccular, isolated, and found in the middle or distal splenic artery. They are most common in middle-aged women but 10% are associated with AAAs.

### Presentation and treatment

- 80% asymptomatic; 20% cause left upper quadrant pain; 2–10% rupture
- Signet-ring calcification may be seen in the left upper quadrant on plain abdominal radiograph
- Treatment options include simple ligation, resection with bypass, embolisation or covered stent

# SECTION 3

# Lower limb ischaemia

**CHAPTER 9**

## 3.1 Anatomy of the lower limb arteries

**In a nutshell ...**

Knowledge of the vascular anatomy of the lower limb is important for both diagnosis and reconstructive surgery.

- Iliac arteries
- Femoral artery
- Femoral triangle (see Chapter 1, Abdominal Surgery)
- Popliteal artery
- Anterior tibial artery
- Posterior tibial artery
- Peroneal artery

## Iliac arteries

### Common iliac artery

- The aorta divides into the common iliac arteries to the left of the midline at the level of the body of L4
- The common iliac arteries pass downwards and laterally to bifurcate into external and internal iliac arteries in front of the sacroiliac joint
- There are usually no branches of the common iliac artery
- The ureter passes in front of the common iliac artery at the level of the bifurcation

### External iliac artery

- Commencing at the bifurcation of the common iliac artery, the external iliac artery travels downwards and laterally to pass under the inguinal ligament at the midinguinal point, where it becomes the femoral artery
- The branches are the inferior epigastric and the deep circumflex iliac artery

### Internal iliac artery

- Commencing at the bifurcation of the common iliac artery, the internal iliac runs inferiorly to lie opposite the upper margin of the greater sciatic notch, where it divides into an anterior and posterior trunk
- The internal iliac artery lies between the internal iliac vein (posteriorly) and the ureter (anteriorly)
- The anterior and posterior trunks of the internal iliac artery supply the pelvic organs, perineum, buttocks and anal canal

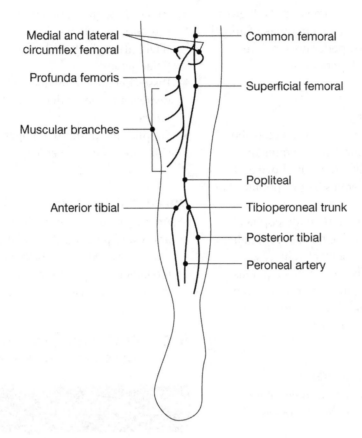

Figure 9.5 Arterial supply of the lower limb

## Femoral artery

- Arises from the external iliac artery
- Crosses the inguinal ligament and enters the thigh at the midinguinal point (halfway between symphysis pubis and anterior superior iliac spine)
- Lies in femoral triangle, lateral to femoral vein, medial to femoral nerve where it gives off the following branches:
  - Superficial circumflex iliac
  - Superficial epigastric
  - Superficial and deep external pudendals
  - Profunda femoris
- Descends almost vertically through the femoral canal to enter the adductor canal

- The adductor canal is also known as the subsartorial or Hunter's canal. It is an important landmark for bypass grafting because it contains the femoral artery and vein, saphenous nerve and nerve to vastus medialis. The boundaries of the adductor canal are:
  - Vastus medialis
  - Adductor muscles
  - Sartorius (the roof)
- The femoral artery then enters the popliteal fossa via the adductor hiatus in the adductor magnus, to become the popliteal artery
- The profunda femoris is the largest branch of the femoral artery. It arises posteriorly or posterolaterally before descending medially

to enter the adductor compartment. It gives off the medial and lateral circumflex femoral branches then three perforators, before ending as the fourth perforator

## Popliteal artery

- Arises from femoral artery as it enters the popliteal fossa (bounded by semimem-branosus and semitendinosus above and medially, gastrocnemius below, popliteus in floor)
- It is the deepest structure in the popliteal fossa (tibial nerve is the most superficial)
- Lies medial to the popliteal vein
- Ends at the lower border of the popliteus muscle by dividing into anterior tibial and tibioperoneal trunk (gives rise to posterior tibial and peroneal arteries)

## Anterior tibial artery

- Enters the anterior compartment of the leg via an opening in the interosseous membrane
- Descends with the deep peroneal nerve
- Enters the foot under the extensor retinaculum to become the dorsalis pedis artery
- Extensor hallucis longus (EHL) tendon lies medial, and the extensor digitorum longus (EDL) tendons lie laterally
- Surface markings: from midway between the tibial tuberosity and fibular head to midway between medial and lateral malleolus

## Posterior tibial artery

- Passes deep to soleus and gastrocnemius
- Tibial nerve is initially medial but crosses posteriorly to lie on the lateral side

- Passes through tarsal tunnel (with tibialis posterior muscle, flexor digitorum longus [FDL], flexor hallucis longus [FHL] and tibial nerve)
- Passes behind the medial malleolus and divides into the medial and lateral plantar arteries
- Supplies the posterior compartment structures of the lower leg

## Peroneal artery

- Arises near the origin of the posterior tibial artery and descends behind the fibula
- Numerous perforating branches supply the lateral compartment of the leg before ending at the ankle

## 3.2 Pathology of peripheral vascular disease

### In a nutshell ...

- PVD describes occlusive vascular disease in the limbs. Lower limb PVD is much more common than upper limb PVD
- Atherosclerosis with thrombosis is the most common cause of PVD, with vasculitides, connective tissue diseases and thromboembolic disease occurring less frequently
- Peripheral vascular disease is more extensive in patients with diabetes
- In people aged 50–75 years, 30% of the UK population has detectable occlusive disease, with about 15% being symptomatic

# Atherosclerosis

 **In a nutshell ...**

In the western world, complications of atherosclerosis cause more deaths per year than any other pathological process. Atherosclerosis is less common in the Far East and Africa where vasculitis is more common.

The most important risk factors are **smoking**, **hypertension**, **diabetes** and **hyperlipidaemia**.

A plaque initially develops as a fatty streak. There are two main hypotheses as to how it progresses: the injury hypothesis and the macrophage hypothesis.

A plaque comprises a fibrous cap, intraintimal core and basal region.

Complications include **thrombosis** and **embolism**.

Sequelae include vessel stenosis or occlusion.

**Risk factors for atherosclerosis**
- Smoking
- Hypertension
- Diabetes
- Male sex
- Hypercholesterolaemia
- Hypertriglyceridaemia
- High-fat diet
- Family history
- Obesity
- Old age
- Homocystinaemia

## Definition of atherosclerosis

- Focal intimal accumulation of lipids and fibrous tissue associated with smooth muscle proliferation
- Develops as a plaque beneath the endothelium
- In large and medium-sized arteries

## Development of atherosclerosis

The initial lesion is a fatty streak composed of a collection of lipids. Macroscopically these are seen as small raised dots on the endothelial surface of the blood vessel. These dots coalesce over time to form streaks. Such lesions have been recognised in children as young as 1 year. There are two main theories concerning the development of atherosclerosis: the response to injury hypothesis and the macrophage hypothesis.

**Response to injury hypothesis:** intimal damage may lead to monocyte and platelet adherence to endothelium, and migration into the vessel intima. Hypertension, shear stress, turbulent flow and chemical damage (eg nicotine and hyperlipidaemia) have all been implicated in causing intimal damage. Once inside the intima, localised inflammation and disruption of the endothelium encourage further platelet adhesion, leading to the release of thromboxane and platelet-derived growth factor (PDGF). This promotes smooth-muscle migration into the developing plaque. Inside the intima, monocytes become macrophages, able to scavenge molecules such as lipid to become foam cells.

**Macrophage hypothesis:** lipids (especially modified lipids such as oxidised low-density lipoprotein [LDL], increased by smoking) collect within macrophages derived from blood monocytes beneath the overlying endothelium. They may break down at the plaque base, leading to the formation of a lipid-rich pool, and secretion of cytokines and toxic metabolites propagate the disease process.

---

**Structure of atherosclerotic plaques**
- Superficial fibrous cap
- Intraintimal area with accumulations of lipids, smooth-muscle cells and macrophages/foam cells
- Basal zone with lipid accumulations and tissue necrosis

---

## Complications of atherosclerotic plaques

### Thrombosis

A thrombus is a solid mass of blood constituents formed within the vasculature (it is NOT a blood clot). Layers of platelets, fibrin and red blood cells will adhere in any area with prothrombotic properties. Predisposition to thrombus formation occurs when any of the changes described in Virchow's triad occur, namely:
- Alterations in the intima of the vessel (eg plaque thrombosis, endothelial damage)
- Altered blood flow (eg turbulence, stasis)
- Altered blood constituents (eg hypercholesterolaemia, smoking)

In arteries thrombosis is usually secondary to atheroma, whereas in veins it is usually secondary to venous stasis. Plaque thrombosis occurs after injury to the cap. This is either a deep injury, where the plaque fissures, or superficial erosion of the surface of the plaque. Either injury predisposes to thrombus formation, in addition to the presence of risk factors and alterations in blood flow caused by the atheromatous plaque itself.

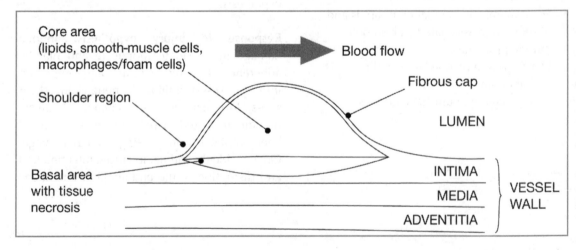

**Figure 9.6 The structure of an atherosclerotic plaque**

## Embolism

An embolus is a mass of material within the vasculature that can become trapped within small-calibre vessels and block the lumen. Most emboli are derived from thrombus, although they can also arise from tumour, amniotic fluid, fat or gas. Clinical effects depend on the region supplied by the blocked vessel, and whether it has a sufficient collateral vascular supply. The most common venous embolic phenomena arise from the leg veins, causing pulmonary emboli. Systemic arterial emboli may cause stroke, ischaemic bowel and renal infarcts, along with ischaemic limbs.

### Sources of arterial embolism

- Left ventricle (intraventricular thrombus after atrial fibrillation [AF], recent MI, cardiomyopathy)
- Heart valves (infective endocarditis)
- Aneurysm embolus
- Atherosclerotic plaque embolus
- Tumour embolus
- Paradoxical embolus

## Pathological consequences of atherosclerosis

- Vessel occlusion (slow occlusion by disease versus rapid occlusion by thrombus, eg MI)
- Vessel stenosis causing ischaemia (eg angina, limb claudication)
- Plaque thrombosis or haemorrhage (increases size of plaque, therefore see acute-on-chronic changes: stable-to-unstable angina, acute-on-chronic limb ischaemia)
- Embolisation of plaque or thrombotic material

## Vasculitides

The vasculitides include all inflammatory disorders of blood vessels. Often these are multisystem disorders with a predilection for highly vascular areas such as the skin, kidney, synovium or eye. They are probably due to a variety of pathological inflammatory processes (such as immune complex deposition or complement activation) that damage blood vessels, leading to thrombosis and resulting in ischaemia and infarction. Of the many disorders involving blood vessels, Buerger's disease, giant-cell arteritis and Takayasu's arteritis are most likely to be seen in vascular surgical practice.

### Buerger's disease (thromboangiitis obliterans)

- Progressive obliteration of distal arteries in young men who smoke heavily
- Most common in South Asian people and Ashkenazi Jews (associated with HLA-B5 and anticollagen antibodies in about 50%)
- Medium-sized arteries show transmural inflammation, intimal proliferation and thrombosis, with surrounding deposition of collagen
- Affects upper and lower limbs

Management includes smoking cessation, sympathectomy (relieves associated arterial spasm), antibiotics, foot care and analgesia. Prostaglandin infusions have been used to overcome acute ischaemia and allow collateral channels to open. Serial amputations (including upper limbs) are often required.

### Giant-cell arteritis

- Granulomatous chronic inflammatory process affecting elastic or muscular arteries

- Classically seen in superficial temporal or cranial arteries
- May present with headache and temporal tenderness (artery and overlying skin thickened and tender with decreased pulsation), jaw claudication, blindness
- Biopsy may not confirm diagnosis in 40% (small sample area, steroid treatment commenced, early stage of disease)
- Management with steroid is usually effective

### Takayasu's arteritis (pulseless disease)

- Inflammatory infiltrate affecting branches of the aortic arch
- Young or middle-aged women (commonly of Asian or Middle Eastern origin)
- Associated with pain, malaise and elevated ESR
- Presents with hypertension or ischaemic symptoms of the upper limb

## 3.3   Acute limb ischaemia

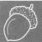

**In a nutshell ...**

This is a surgical emergency.
**Symptoms**
Pain, pallor, paraesthesia, perishingly cold, paralysis, pulseless.
**Management**
Includes symptom relief and restoration of arterial continuity:

- Thrombolysis
- Embolectomy
- Arterial bypass
- Reperfusion

It may be necessary to perform fasciotomies to prevent compartment syndrome.

## Causes of acute limb ischaemia

- Arterial embolus
- Acute thrombosis (or acute-on-chronic)
- Trauma
- Aortic dissection
- Thrombosed popliteal aneurysm
- Intra-arterial injection (iatrogenic or drug abuse)

## Symptoms of acute limb ischaemia

The mechanism of the pain is unknown but possibly related to anoxia, acidosis, and metabolite and substance P accumulation. Acute limb ischaemia can occur in the upper or lower limb. Symptoms vary with speed of occlusion and extent of collateral circulation. The usual presentation is with loss of pulses (eg radial in upper limb or femoral/popliteal/foot pulses in lower limb). The loss of pulses can be confirmed with a hand-held Doppler if unsure, along with the clinical recognition of these six **P**s, which are late signs:

- **P**ain
- **P**allor
- **P**araesthesia
- **P**erishingly cold
- **P**aralysis
- **P**ulseless

## Management of acute limb ischaemia

Acute limb ischaemia is a surgical emergency and must be resolved within 4–6 hours to prevent complications from tissue ischaemia. In acute-on-chronic ischaemia the limb may remain viable for longer, depending on collateral supply.

Note: nerve conduction disappears after 15–30 min of acute ischaemia; permanent muscle damage occurs after few hours, with the EHL being the last muscle to recover on revascularisation. Skin will tolerate ischaemia for up to 48 hours.

> **Principles of management of acute limb ischaemia**
> - Resuscitation (oxygen and intravenous fluids)
> - Immediate anticoagulation (5000 units heparin intravenously)
> - Analgesia
> - Restore arterial continuity
> - Identify and correct any underlying source of embolus

If the diagnosis is in doubt, or if arterial reconstruction may be needed, arteriography can be performed. Arterial embolism usually causes a sharp cut-off at the upper end of the occlusion, with poor collaterals.

## Thrombolysis

Thrombolysis may be performed if the limb is not too acutely ischaemic, allowing sufficient time for clot dissolution. It is the preferred choice for acute-on-chronic ischaemia. Tissue plasminogen activator (tPA), urokinase or streptokinase is introduced through a catheter inserted under fluoroscopic control, directly into the clot. Clot dispersal can be monitored by serial arteriography.

Complications of thrombolysis
- Puncture site haemorrhage/false aneurysm
- Retroperitoneal haemorrhage
- Stroke
- Gastrointestinal bleeding
- Anaphylaxis

## Contraindications of thrombolysis
- Extreme old age
- Recent surgery
- Peptic ulceration
- Recent stroke
- Bleeding tendencies

### Embolectomy
See Op box on page 757.

# Complications of acute limb ischaemia

## Reperfusion injury

Reperfusion injury describes the body's response after restoration of arterial continuity, due to release of high concentrations of products of metabolism (eg potassium, lactate, myoglobin) back into the general circulation. This can cause local and systemic effects.

After reperfusion, local tissue swelling occurs. This is due to osmotically active fragments produced by tissue necrosis and an increase in membrane permeability brought about by hypoxia. If unrelieved this swelling can cause further ischaemia and ultimately contractures (eg Volkmann's ischaemic contracture following upper limb ischaemia). This can be prevented by timely fasciotomy.

Systemically, reperfusion can cause rhabdomyolysis and renal failure. It may also cause pulmonary oedema/ARDS, myocardial dysfunction and clotting disorders.

## Compartment syndrome

### The anatomy of the muscle compartments in the limbs

The lower leg is divided into three compartments by the tibia and fibula, interosseous membrane and intermuscular septa; the posterior compartment has two components. These divisions become especially important after reperfusion of an ischaemic limb, and knowledge of the actions of the muscles and innervation of nerves within each compartment is essential in diagnosis of compartment syndrome.

### Lateral (peroneal) compartment
- Bounded by anterior and posterior intermuscular septa and peroneal surface of fibula
- Contains peroneus longus and brevis and superior peroneal nerve

### Anterior (extensor) compartment
- Bounded by medial tibial surface, interosseous membrane and anterior intermuscular septum
- Contains EHL, EDL, tibialis anterior muscle, peroneus, anterior tibial vessels and deep peroneal nerve

### Posterior compartment
- Bounded by posterior intermuscular septum and interosseous membrane
- In **deep compartment:** FHL, FDL, popliteus, tibialis posterior muscle, posterior tibial artery, tibial nerve
- In **superficial compartment:** gastrocnemius, soleus, plantaris, short saphenous vein (SSV) and sural nerve

### Injuries causing compartment syndrome
Fractures, crush injury, revascularisation, bleeding, burns or just severe shock. Prophylactic fasciotomies are indicated after some fracture fixations and revascularisation procedures, or in marked crush or vascular injuries.

### Pathology of compartment syndrome
The limbs are encircled with layers of deep fascia that divide the muscle groups into compartments. Tissue swelling within the compartment causes an increase in the intracompartmental pressure. When this pressure rises above the normal tissue perfusion pressure of the capillary bed (5–10 mmHg), the circulation to the tissues essentially ceases and they become ischaemic. Thus there may still be a palpable pulse on examination.

---

**Symptoms and signs of compartment syndrome**

**Early symptoms and signs**
- Pain out of proportion to the condition or injury
- Pain on stretching of the muscle group in the affected compartment
- Absent distal pulse

**Late symptoms and signs**
- Paralysis
- Weakness and tenderness
- Pale, cold limb
- Sensory loss

---

**Op box: Embolectomy (commonly femoral or brachial)**

**Indications**

Identification of embolus as a cause of limb ischaemia (usually after urgent angiography or duplex US). For acutely ischaemic upper limbs surgical exploration may be undertaken diagnostically. Bear in mind that the embolus may impact at the site of pre-existing occlusive disease in the lower limb.

**Preop**

Analgesia and resuscitation. Anticoagulation (intravenous heparin). Consent with intraoperative hazards and postoperative complications in mind. General, regional, or local anaesthetic for femoral embolectomy. Brachial embolectomy may be performed under local anaesthesia.

**Patient positioning**

Supine. Arm extended on arm board for brachial embolectomy.

**Incision**

- Femoral: longitudinal incision in groin below inguinal ligament and over femoral artery
- Brachial: transverse incision below the skin crease at the elbow

**Procedure**

- Femoral or brachial artery is identified and dissected free
- Vascular slings are placed proximally and distally to obtain control
- Patient is heparinised (eg 5000 units intravenous bolus)
- Vascular clamp applied proximally and distally and a transverse arteriotomy is performed
- Fogarty embolectomy balloon catheter (of appropriate balloon size) is passed distally, the balloon inflated and the catheter withdrawn slowly (drawing embolus out of the artery) – this is repeated proximally and distally until flow is restored (bear in mind that, once clear of embolus, control of the artery is vital)
- Arteriotomy is closed with non-absorbable sutures (eg fine Prolene)

**Intraoperative hazards**

Over-inflation of the Fogarty catheter inside the artery can cause damage to sections of artery and intimal stripping – this causes a very prothrombotic state and the artery is likely to thrombose postoperatively.

**Closure**

Close the wound in layers with absorbable sutures.

**Postop**

Continue formal anticoagulation; regular observations of limb perfusion must be performed (pulses, capillary refill, temperature, colour); re-exploration may be indicated if thrombosis occurs; always look for the source of the underlying embolus for definitive management.

**Complications**

Haemorrhage, postoperative thrombosis, limb loss.

**CHAPTER 9**

## Measurement of compartment pressures

Compartment pressure measurement may be misleading. Compartment syndrome is a clinical diagnosis.

Compartment pressures can be measured using a green needle connected to a pressure transducer. Prepare the skin with antiseptic solution (Betadine/chlorhexidine). Flush the needle through to ensure a continuous column of fluid to the transducer. Zero the transducer with the needle held at the level of the patient's leg and advance the needle perpendicularly through the skin and superficial fascia into the muscle compartment. Repeat the process for all compartments of the affected limb.

Pressures exceeding 30 mmHg may require surgical intervention in the form of fasciotomy.

### Managing compartment syndrome

If compartment syndrome is suspected clinically then plaster immobilisation and any bandaging must be removed immediately. Compartment pressures should be measured if there is doubt about the diagnosis, and, if elevated by >30 mmHg (or lower if diastolic BP is low), urgent fasciotomy must be performed.

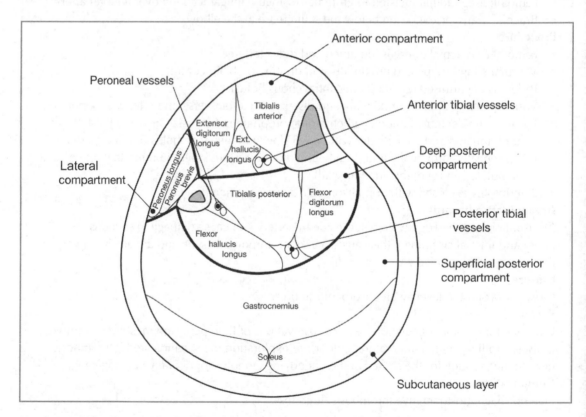

**Figure 9.7 The compartments of the lower limb**

## Procedure: Doing a fasciotomy

Once the diagnosis of compartment syndrome has been made there should be as little delay as possible in performing a fasciotomy. The trend is moving away from accident-room fasciotomies because the facilities are better in theatre, but every few minutes could cost the patient viable muscle.

- Confirm elevated compartment pressures if possible preoperatively, but not if it creates delay.
- The usual fasciotomy is a two-incision, four-compartment fasciotomy.
- The anterior and lateral compartments are decompressed through a lateral incision just anterior to the fibula and the skin is undermined anteriorly and posteriorly to expose these two compartments.
- The incision on the medial side of the leg opens the superficial posterior compartment and through this the deeper compartment is released.
- The fascia is divided usually via long, medial and lateral incisions, to allow tissue expansion and prevent ischaemia.
- All compartments of an affected limb should be fully opened (eg four-compartment fasciotomy in the lower limb).
- The visible muscles can be covered with sterile dressings and inspected regularly for perfusion.
- Necrotic tissue should be debrided at a later date.
- The fasciotomies can be closed later as an elective procedure and skin grafts can be used.

The sequelae of compartment syndrome
- Muscle wasting and nerve injury in the affected compartment
- Foot drop if the lateral compartment is affected (superficial peroneal nerve)

Compartment syndrome can also occur in the upper limb, especially the volar forearm, and the buttocks. Abdominal compartment syndrome is a different entity caused by swelling of abdominal contents post-laparotomy.

## Long-term management of acute limb ischaemia

Following the restoration of arterial flow to the limb, investigations are performed to identify the underlying cause of embolism:
- Echocardiography to assess left ventricular and heart valves
- Ultrasonography (especially abdominal aorta and popliteal arteries)
- Arteriography to look for other sources of emboli

Long-term anticoagulation is also required, initially with heparin and later with warfarin.

## 3.4 Chronic lower limb ischaemia

### In a nutshell ...

Chronic lower limb ischaemia is usually caused by atherosclerosis, often secondary to smoking or diabetes. The most common sites of arterial occlusive disease affecting the lower limb are:
- Aortic bifurcation
- Common iliac artery bifurcation
- Adductor hiatus (superficial femoral artery)
- Trifurcation disease
- Small-vessel disease

Patients present with pain ranging from intermittent claudication through to rest pain, and skin changes ranging from superficial ulceration to gangrene. Non-limb- or life-threatening peripheral arterial disease is best treated conservatively whereas radiological and surgical interventions are usually reserved for cases of failed medical management.

## Sites of arterial occlusive disease

### Aortoiliac occlusive disease

The abdominal aorta may become stenosed or even occluded due to atherosclerotic disease. Occlusion may occur gradually with development of collateral circulation to the lower limbs. Collateral circulation develops from the thoracic aorta via the IMA, intercostals, lumbar arteries, SMA and gonadal arteries.

Acute abdominal aortic occlusion presents dramatically with sudden ischaemia of the lower limbs and gastrointestinal tract. It may also involve the renal arteries if the level of disease is sufficiently high. It may be due to thrombosis during a low-flow state in a stenotic aorta, saddle embolus from the heart or aortic dissection.

### Infrainguinal arterial occlusive disease

Infrainguinal arterial occlusive disease also results from atherosclerosis. Common sites include the level of the adductor hiatus in the superficial femoral artery and at the trifurcation. Over time, a collateral circulation may develop (aided by exercise) to supply the lower limb.

Acute-on-chronic ischaemia may occur due to thrombosis on a ruptured plaque or impaction of an embolus at a site of narrowing.

## Symptoms of chronic lower limb ischaemia

- **Intermittent claudication (IC)** is the cramping pain experienced on exercise due to muscle ischaemia. It is due to occlusion or stenosis in the relevant proximal arteries. Calf claudication is the most common and usually starts after a consistent walking distance (called the claudication distance), and is relieved by rest. Note that the patient does not have to sit down to relieve the pain (a symptom of spinal stenosis) and once the pain has gone the patient can usually walk the same distance again before the pain recurs
- **Critical ischaemia** implies that without intervention limb loss may be imminent. The ABPI is usually <0.4
- **Rest pain** is severe, intractable, cramping pain, usually experienced at the extremities, due to critical ischaemia. Nocturnal rest pain is classically relieved by hanging the foot over the side of the bed (as dependency of the limb increases blood supply). For this reason

these patients often sleep upright in a chair
- **Ulceration** is tissue loss due to critical ischaemia. It typically occurs at the extremities. Arterial ulcers are classically described as being punched-out with sloughy, unhealthy bases
- **Gangrene** is tissue necrosis due to critical ischaemia. **Dry gangrene** is due to gradual interruption of the arterial supply to the tissues with black discoloration of the skin caused by staining by free haemoglobin from damaged capillaries. It is insensate, cold and hard, and does not smell. It occurs from distal to proximal. Untreated, gangrenous parts may demarcate (mummify) and auto-amputate. **Wet gangrene** describes ischaemic necrosis associated with infection by putrefactive organisms. It smells and you will see skin blebs. It requires emergency debridement and broad-spectrum antibiotics. **Gas gangrene** is usually due to clostridial infection. There will be crepitus and septicaemia from toxin release
- **Leriche syndrome** describes buttock, thigh and calf claudication with erectile dysfunction, and proximal muscle wasting due to distal aortic or proximal iliac stenosis or occlusion

## Examination of the ischaemic leg

### What to ask about
- Claudication and rest pain (onset and relieving factors)
- Painful or painless ulceration
- Risk factors for atherosclerotic disease (smoking, hypertension, diabetes, hyperlipidaemia, family history)

### What to look for
- **Changes associated with ischaemia:** the ischaemic leg is typically pale but a severely ischaemic leg may be red ('sunset foot')

due to acute inflammation and cellulitis secondary to tissue ischaemia, or bluish purple (cyanosis). The leg may be hairless with shiny skin. Individual toes may show the purple–black hue of a gangrenous digit; this may be hard, well demarcated and painless ('dry gangrene') or infected, soft and moist with surrounding painful, cellulitic tissue ('wet gangrene'). Ulceration may be present (ischaemic/neuropathic)
- **Venous guttering:** in a severely ischaemic foot the veins are collapsed and look like pale blue gutters in the subcutaneous tissue. In a normal circulation the veins never have time to empty fully because the arteries keep refilling them, even if the leg is elevated. Venous guttering on raising the leg 10–15° above the horizontal is a sign of significant ischaemia

---

**Differential diagnosis of chronic leg pain**
- **Arterial**
  PVD (atherosclerosis)
  Popliteal entrapment syndrome
  Vasculitis
- **Venous**
  Venous claudication
  Chronic venous insufficiency
  Post-phlebitic syndrome
- **Neurological**
  Spinal stenosis
  Lumbar radiculopathy
  Peripheral neuropathy
  Reflex sympathetic dystrophy
- **Orthopaedic**
  Chronic compartment syndrome
  Plantar fasciitis
- **Rheumatological**
  Arthritis (osteoarthritis, rheumatoid arthritis)
  Gout

---

## What to palpate

Palpate all peripheral pulses, starting with the aorta and working downwards. Compare right with left but bear in mind that disease may be bilateral. Test for delayed capillary refill in the feet. Feel for reduced temperature.

## How to carry out Buerger's test

In this bedside test for ischaemia, raise the patient's leg slowly to 90°, keeping it straight. The foot should remain pink until 90° if there is no vascular compromise. If the foot goes pale at 50° this indicates severe ischaemia, and at 25° it indicates critical ischaemia. This is Buerger's angle. In the second part of Buerger's test, sit the patient up and ask him or her to swing their legs over the edge of the bed. If the legs become engorged and red, Buerger's test is positive. The red colour occurs because sudden additional hypoxia causes a degree of vasodilatation and blood flows back more quickly under the influence of gravity (reactive hyperaemia).

# Conservative management of chronic lower limb ischaemia

Non-limb- or life-threatening peripheral arterial disease is best treated 'conservatively', whereas radiological and surgical interventions are usually reserved for cases of failed medical management.

## Conservative management of intermittent claudication

Intermittent claudication is usually managed by correction of risk factors. Walking to the limit of claudication often improves symptoms by improving cardiac performance, and by encouraging the development of a collateral circulation. Patients with claudication have a high incidence of concurrent cardiovascular and neurovascular disease and a high mortality rate due to MI and stroke.

Patients should:
- Stop smoking
- Exercise
- Improve their diet (low-fat)
- Lose weight

Management includes:
- Antiplatelet agents (aspirin, clopidogrel, dipyridamole)
- Aggressive BP management in patients with hypertension
- Aggressive blood sugar control in patients with diabetes
- Management of hypercholesterolaemia/ hyperlipidaemia with lipid-lowering drugs (statins)

Interventional radiological procedures (eg angioplasty, stenting) or surgery is not usually indicated for intermittent claudication and is reserved for critical ischaemia. However, it is occasionally offered for severe lifestyle-limiting symptoms despite adequate medical management.

## Conservative management of chronic critical ischaemia

Chronic critical ischaemia requires active limb revascularisation to prevent limb loss. However, concurrent conservative strategies for improving blood flow are also required:
- Stop smoking
- Optimise cardiac output
- Treat infections
- Anticoagulation (aspirin)

Investigation is then performed to identify the site/level of the arterial stenosis or occlusion (see Section 1.2).

## Non-surgical interventions for PVD

- **Angioplasty:** a balloon catheter is introduced over a guidewire passed through the stenosis or occlusion under fluoroscopic control. The balloon is then inflated across the stenosis or occlusion to dilate this section of the artery. This technique is good for short occlusions and works better for proximal than for distal disease
- **Stenting:** arterial stents are expandable metal prostheses that are placed across stenoses or occlusions to maintain arterial patency. They are usually balloon-expandable and introduced under fluoroscopic control, combined with angioplasty. Primary arterial stenting is now the mainstay of treatment for most symptomatic arterial stenoses and short occlusions that fail to respond to medical management. Stenting is also indicated for failed angioplasty, and for correction of intimal arterial defects
- **Lumbar sympathectomy:** used if arterial reconstruction is not feasible. This is usually chemical (phenol, translumbar injection with radiographic control), but it can be surgical. Blockade of the lumbar sympathetic chain improves blood supply to skin, with some relief of rest pain and numbness/tingling associated with chronic ischaemia
- **Drug therapy:** vasodilators can provide some increase in blood supply to the limb, especially in combination with antiplatelet therapy (aspirin), nifedipine, iloprost and pentoxifylline

## Surgery for PVD

These procedures can be divided into:

1. **Anatomical procedures** restore vascular continuity through the replacement of the diseased region (eg femoropopliteal bypass, femorodistal bypass)
2. **Extra-anatomical procedures** restore vascular continuity by diverting blood from other unrelated areas to the diseased region (and are also therefore useful as a salvage procedure if there is infection present), eg axillo-bifemoral and femorofemoral crossover grafts

Vascular grafts can be autologous or prosthetic:

- **Autologous:** the long saphenous vein (LSV) can be harvested and used in the reverse direction (flow not impeded by vein cusps) or used in situ after destruction of the vein cusps. Composite vein grafts are fashioned by end-to-end anastomosis of sections of arm vein to achieve desired length
- **Prosthetic:** Dacron or PTFE grafts are tubes of prosthetic material. They may be woven or plasticised and may be supported by an external scaffolding to prevent compression (eg during movement of limbs). They have a much lower patency rate than autologous grafts

|  | Advantages | Disadvantages |
|---|---|---|
| *Vein grafts* | Better patency rates (75–90% at 5 years) | May not be there (previous surgery including CABG, VV stripping, etc) |
|  | Respond better to angioplasty if required | Insufficient width or length |
|  | More resistant to infection Less neointimal hyperplasia at the anastomosis Easier to suture | Points of compression (eg knee joint) may compromise flow in certain positions |
| *Prosthetic grafts* | Limitless supply | Lower patency rates (60% at 5 years) |
|  | External scaffolding prevents compression and compromised flow | Higher rates of neointimal neoplasia More expensive |

**Principles of femoropopliteal and femorodistal bypass grafting**

## Indications

Chronic lower limb ischaemia with incapacitating claudication or critical ischaemia; may also be performed for acutely ischaemic limb (acute-on-chronic thrombosis, occluded popliteal aneurysm, etc).

## Preop

**Elective:** angiogram to assess inflow and run-off and plan sites for anastomosis; any lesions compromising inflow may be corrected with angioplasty prior to the procedure. Duplex marking of the long saphenous vein.

**Emergency:** analgesia and resuscitation; anticoagulation (intravenous heparin); urgent angiogram to assess cause, underlying disease and plan surgery.

General or regional anaesthetic. Consent with intraoperative hazards and postoperative complications in mind.

## Patient positioning

Supine. Prep and drape groin and leg.

## Incision

Longitudinal incision in groin below inguinal ligament and over common femoral artery (or alternative site of inflow) for proximal anastomosis.

Longitudinal incision at level of above- or below-knee popliteal artery (or alternative site of outflow such as crural vessels for femorodistal) for distal anastomosis.

Short longitudinal incisions over course of long saphenous vein for harvesting.

## Procedure

- Femoral and popliteal or crural arteries are identified and dissected free
- Vascular slings are placed proximally and distally to obtain control
- Vein graft is harvested and all tributaries ligated
- Patient is systemically heparinised and the vessels clamped proximally and distally
- A longitudinal arteriotomy is performed and the proximal anastomosis is sutured using non-absorbable suture (fine Prolene) and then tested for leaks
- The graft is tunnelled under the skin and muscle and the distal anastomosis is sutured and tested for leaks
- Intraoperative angiography or operative Doppler (op-Dop) testing confirms adequate flow rates through the graft

## Intraoperative hazards

Excessive undermining of skin flaps during vein harvesting predisposes the patient to flap breakdown and necrosis.

## Closure

Close the wound in layers with absorbable sutures.

**continued opposite**

**Postop**

Continue formal anticoagulation; regular observations of limb perfusion must be performed (pulses, capillary refill, temperature, colour) postoperatively; re-exploration may be indicated if thrombosis of the graft occurs.

**Complications**

- General to all patients with arteriopathy (risk of MI, stroke, renal failure)
- Risk of haemorrhage and infection
- Risk of graft failure (early; late) and worsening of symptoms
- Risk of limb loss

 **Principles of aorto-bifemoral, axillo-bifemoral and femorofemoral crossover grafts**

**Aorto-bifemoral bypass graft**

**Indication:** occlusive or stenotic aortoiliac disease not amenable to angioplasty or stenting.

**Procedure:** a bifurcated, prosthetic graft is anastomosed proximally to the aorta, and distally to the iliac or femoral vessels. Graft patency rates are excellent. Operative mortality rate is approximately 5%.

**Axillo-bifemoral grafting**

**Indication:** aortic or bilateral iliac occlusion or stenoses not amenable to angioplasty or stenting, in the presence of a hostile abdomen, or in a patient not fit for major abdominal surgery.

**Procedure:** a long graft is anastomosed proximally to the axillary artery as it passes under pectoralis major, and distally to the femoral arteries. Patency rates are less good than aorto-bifemoral grafting for this procedure but it is useful in high-risk cases with otherwise untreatable critical ischaemia.

**Femorofemoral crossover graft**

**Indication:** unilateral iliac occlusive disease not amenable to angioplasty or stenting

**Procedure:** a prosthetic vascular graft is anastomosed from one femoral artery, tunnelled subcutaneously and anastomosed to the other to restore flow. Mortality and patency rates are excellent. The procedure does not require general anaesthesia.

## Causes of graft failure

- **Early causes** (eg after 1 month): commonly technical failure (low flow state due to poor inflow or insufficient run-off)
- **Mid-term causes** (eg after 1 year): commonly neointimal hyperplasia causing stenosis in the graft
- **Late causes** (eg after 2–5 years): commonly atheromatous disease progression (in inflow or run-off)

### Early complications

- Haemorrhage
- Graft thrombosis
- Wound infection
- Swollen leg (reperfusion or DVT)
- Lymphatic fistula

### Late complications

- Graft thrombosis
- False aneurysm
- Graft infection

## 3.5 Amputations of ischaemic lower limbs

### Indications for amputation

The main indications for amputation are indicated by these three **D**s:
- **D**ying (eg vascular disease, gangrene)
- **D**angerous (eg tumour, severe infection)
- **D**amned nuisance (eg useless, painful limb after trauma, neurological damage)

In the UK the most common reason for amputation is PVD, but worldwide the main indication is trauma.

### Indications for amputation in the UK

- Vascular disease and diabetes (80%)
- Trauma (10%)
- Tumour and other reasons (10%)

## Levels of amputation

The level for amputation needs to be selected carefully. It needs to be proximal enough for good healing, but more distal amputations have better long-term outcome and rehabilitation. A correctly functioning knee joint should be preserved whenever possible. In below-knee amputations, ideally, 15 cm of bone below the knee should be conserved. However, a shorter stump is preferable to an above-knee amputation.

Upper limb amputations are much rarer than lower limb amputations and the principles are slightly different. The aims of maintaining length and function by carrying out minimal debridement are paramount. Loss of function is more disabling and less amenable to prosthetics than lower limb loss.

---

**The ideal stump**
- Heals by primary intention
- Is freely mobile
- Has good soft tissue cover over the bone end
- Has a conical shape
- Has a mobile joint above the amputation level
- Does not transmit pressure through the scar

---

## Levels of lower limb amputation (proximal to distal)

- **Hip disarticulation:** used mainly for soft tissue/bony malignancy in the upper thigh. Very rarely used for vascular disease
- **Above knee:** involves taking a bone section 25–30 cm below the greater trochanter, leaving 12 cm above the knee joint for the knee mechanism. This creates equal anterior and posterior semicircular skin flaps
- **Supracondylar (Gritti–Stokes):** involves supracondylar femoral division. The patella is fixed to the end of the femur with wire sutures. It is useful if more length is required than can be obtained from above-knee amputation, such as in bilateral amputees, to aid changing position in bed, etc. It is unpopular because there is a tendency for non-union of the patella to the femur, and it is difficult to fit a prosthesis
- **Through-knee:** quick to perform and is relatively atraumatic. However, there is poor healing in ischaemic disease. It is difficult to fit a prosthesis due to the bulbous stump
- **Below-knee:** the most popular level in severe ischaemia (can be done in 80%). Oximetry, thermography and arteriography can be used to help gauge the likelihood of success, but are not standard practice. The best guide to success is clinical judgement and flap bleeding at the time of surgery. The two most widely used methods are the long posterior flap (Burgess), using the posterior calf muscles to cover the bone ends 15 cm below the tibial tuberosity, and the skew flap (Kingsley Robinson) which is more popular and gives a better stump shape. There is little difference in healing rates
- **Syme's:** rarely used in vascular disease. The heel is disarticulated, and the malleoli excised and covered with a long posterior skin flap; 30% require revision at a higher level
- **Trans-metatarsal:** useful in diabetic gangrene of the forefoot. It requires no prosthesis. Individual rays can be amputated, and left to heal by secondary intention
- **Toes:** used in cases of trauma or diabetic infective gangrene in the presence of a good blood supply only

## Principles of surgery for amputation

Amputations for PVD and neoplasia tend to be more radical than those for trauma or diabetes in the absence of PVD. In PVD the healing of the distal stumps tends to be compromised by poor blood supply. In neoplastic disease good clearance is a priority.

As a general rule, the total length of flaps will need to be at least 1.5 times the diameter of the leg at the level of the bone section.

During surgery a tourniquet may be applied to provide a bloodless field in trauma or neoplasia, but not in cases where there is PVD.

## Postoperative management of amputation

- Analgesia
- Care of the unaffected limb
- Physiotherapy: to prevent flexion contractures and to build up muscle power and coordination
- Mobilisation

The patient should be mobilised as soon as possible, ideally after 5–7 days.

## Complications of amputations

### Early complications

Haemorrhage and haematoma formation

Infection (high stumps may have faecal contamination and develop gas gangrene)

Wound dehiscence

Ischaemia and gangrene of flaps

DVT and PE

### Late complications

Pain: phantom limb, amputation neuroma, causalgia (intractable burning pain due to sympathetic nerve growth down somatic nerves), scar pain due to adherence to bone, jacitation (sudden jumping of limb)

Chronic infection: osteitis, sinus formation

Ulceration of the stump

## Prostheses for lower limbs

Patients are more likely to walk on a prosthetic limb if they are younger, medically fit and well motivated. Early mobilisation is achieved using a POMAID (a temporary pneumatically attached prosthesis for early mobilisation). After this various types of prosthesis are available.

Sleeves and suction devices are best for below-knee amputation. They are more comfortable.

Straps are more likely to be used after above-knee amputation. They are less comfortable.

Various devices, spacers and fillers are available for transmetatarsal and toe amputations.

# 3.6 The diabetic foot

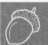 **In a nutshell ...**

The diabetic foot presents particular surgical problems due to a combination of:

- Atherosclerosis
- Peripheral neuropathy
- Impaired tissue metabolism
- Infection

## Atherosclerosis

- Accelerated in people with diabetes (thought to be due to intimal damage by hyperglycaemia)
- Typically trifurcation and distal small-vessel disease
- Large-vessel disease also occurs earlier and is more severe in people with diabetes
- May calcify and lead to incompressible vessels (palpable pulses and falsely high ABPI >1.0)
- Associated with arteriolar constriction and increased ischaemia

## Peripheral neuropathy

- Motor nerves: distortion of small muscles (clawing of toes and subluxation of joints) causes abnormal weight bearing and trauma
- Sensory nerves: glove-and-stocking paraesthesiae; unawareness of injury
- Autonomic nerves: disruption of vascular control and sweating (causing dryness of the skin and fissuring)

## Impaired tissue metabolism
- Due to hyperglycaemia
- Glycosylation of tissues renders them stiff and less pliable

## Infection
- Glucose-rich environment favours infection
- Generalised immune compromise

# Examination of the diabetic foot

**Features of diabetes in the leg and foot**
- **Ischaemic ulcers:** the heel, malleoli, head of fifth metatarsal, tips of toes, between the toes and the ball of the foot are typical sites for ischaemic ulceration. An ischaemic ulcer typically looks like a poorly healed wound or a punched-out lesion and has no surrounding callus. It may have associated wet or dry gangrene.
- **Neuropathic ulcers:** these are commonly seen on the soles of the feet. A neuropathic ulcer typically looks like a punched-out lesion surrounded by a ridge of hard calloused skin. A punched-out or vertical edge to an ulcer follows rapid death and sloughing of a full thickness of skin without successful attempts at self-repair, and is therefore seen in both neuropathic and ischaemic ulcers.
- **Charcot's joint:** painless, disorganised joint due to decreased sensation.
- **Loss of foot arches:** due to peripheral neuropathy.
- **Shiny hairless leg:** said to be typical but is non-specific.
- **Amputated toes:** small-vessel disease often leads to loss of digits by either surgery or auto-amputation of a gangrenous digit.
- **Necrobiosis lipoidica diabeticorum:** erythematous plaques over shins with a waxy appearance and brown pigmentation – can scar, become scaly or ulcerate.
- **Infections:** such as paronychia due to poor circulation.

# Management of the diabetic foot

All patients require education in foot care and good blood glucose control. They should wear accommodative footwear (soft leather or trainers) and skin and nail care should be performed by professionals. They require regular clinical examination and should seek early medical attention for trauma or ulceration.

Superficial ulceration requires good wound care and determination of underlying pathology. Neuropathic ulcers may require debridement and off-loading of pressure. Ischaemic ulcers require revascularisation.

Deep ulceration is often associated with deep tissue infection (and may include osteomyelitis). These ulcers require debridement to a base of healthy tissue and culture-specific antibiotics, and may require partial amputation. Ischaemic limbs will require revascularisation to enable healing.

# SECTION 4

# Carotid artery disease

## 4.1  Carotid anatomy

**In a nutshell ...**

Common carotid artery
External carotid artery
Internal carotid artery
The circle of Willis (see Chapter 6,
Neurosurgery – elective)

### Common carotid artery

- Arises from brachiocephalic trunk on right; arch of the aorta on left
- Ascends within the carotid sheath along with the internal jugular veins (laterally), vagus nerves (between and posterior to artery and vein) and ansa cervicalis, from a point posterolateral to the sternoclavicular joint
- Ends at the upper border of thyroid cartilage (C4)
- Divides (under cover of sternomastoid) into internal and external carotid arteries

### External carotid artery

- Arises from common carotid artery
- Supplies face, oral and nasal cavities, exterior of head and neck, inner surface of cranial cavity
- Spirals over internal carotid to lie laterally at level of C2
- Crossed by facial vein and hypoglossal nerve
- Gives off superior thyroid and posterior auricular branches before entering parotid gland between superficial and deep lobes (where it divides into terminal branches)

**Branches of the external carotid artery**
*Three branches from the front*
Superior thyroid
Lingual
Facial
*One deep medial branch*
Ascending pharyngeal
*Two branches from behind*
Occipital
Posterior auricular
*Two terminal branches*
Superficial temporal
Maxillary

## Internal carotid artery

- Arises from common carotid artery and continues within the carotid sheath to enter the skull via the carotid canal
- Usually no branches in the neck
- Supplies contents of cranial and orbital cavity (supplemented by vertebrobasilar system)
- Just above the carotid bifurcation there is a slight bulge in the internal carotid artery (ICA). This is the **carotid sinus**: it contains baroreceptors and is supplied by the glossopharyngeal nerve (stimulation causes bradycardia and hypotension)

- Behind the carotid bifurcation lies the **carotid body**, which contains chemoreceptors for oxygen, $CO_2$ and pH regulation

## Circle of Willis

This is the anatomical arrangement of the intracranial arteries (see Chapter 6, Neurosurgery – elective. It is supplied by both ICAs and the basilar artery, which forms from the vertebral arteries. It is important because complete occlusion of one ICA in the circle of Willis does not normally cause symptoms due to adequate collateral flow. However, the circle of Willis is only complete in about 50% of individuals.

# 4.2 Physiology of the cerebral circulation

 **In a nutshell ...**

The brain:
- Has a very high $O_2$ requirement
- Receives a very high proportion of the cardiac output (13%)
- Has a high blood supply volume per unit weight of tissue (55 ml/min per 100 g)
- Is intolerant of ischaemia and protects itself by a phenomenon called **autoregulation** (preferentially preserving its blood supply at BP of 60–160 mmHg)

Autoregulation occurs via **myogenic** or **metabolic** mechanisms.

Measurement of cerebral blood flow is important during surgery on the carotid artery and can be done using the Fick principle.

## Regulation of the cerebral circulation

The brain receives 13% of the cardiac output, ie 750 ml/min of blood. In addition, the brain has a large blood supply per unit weight of tissue, ie 55 ml/min per 100 g (100 ml/min per 100 g for grey matter) and it is very intolerant of ischaemia.

It has a number of methods by which it regulates constant blood supply despite inconsistent supply to other body parts (autoregulation). This **autoregulation** is extremely effective for mean BPs of 60–160 mmHg. BP <60 mmHg causes syncope and BP >160 mmHg causes brain oedema (because the blood–brain barrier permeability increases). The sympathetic nerve supply to cerebral vessels has little effect, allowing local factors to predominate.

Autoregulation is achieved by two mechanisms:

1. **Myogenic mechanisms:** these maintain perfusion over wide pressure range; increased pressure causes increased wall tension (Laplace) leading to smooth muscle contraction in vessel walls (constriction)

2. **Metabolic mechanisms:** cerebral vessels are very sensitive to changes in $PaCO_2$: increases cause marked vasodilatation locally and decreases cause vasoconstriction (dizzy sensation when hyperventilating). Changes of as little as 1 mmHg $CO_2$ can cause a change in cerebral blood flow of up to 5%

Any ischaemia affecting the medulla leads to an increase in systemic BP to improve supply, by alteration in outflow from the medullary centres. The carotid baroreceptors and chemoreceptors ensure that blood supply to the brain is one of the main determinants of systemic BP.

## Measurement of cerebral blood flow

### The Fick principle

This is used to calculate the blood flow to an organ by applying the law of conservation of mass. If the blood flowing into an organ contains a marker of known concentration and some of this marker diffuses into the organ, then its concentration in the blood leaving the organ will be lower. Remember:

$$Quantity = Concentration \times Volume$$

Therefore the quantity of marker entering the organ per unit time depends on the concentration of marker and volume per unit time (ie flow).

The quantity of marker leaving the organ per unit time depends on the blood concentration and the same blood flow:

As:

$$Flow\ in = \frac{Quantity_{in}}{Concentration_{in}}$$

And:

$$Flow\ out = \frac{Quantity_{out}}{Concentration_{out}}$$

Then:

$$Flow\ to\ organ = \frac{(Quantity_{in} - Quantity_{out})}{(Concentration_{in} - Concentration_{out})}$$

Note that $Concentration_{in} - Concentration_{out}$ is the quantity of marker taken up by the brain per unit time. Nitrous oxide can be used as a marker to calculate cerebral blood flow.

### Positron emission tomography

Positron emission tomography (PET) is a nuclear medicine technique whereby radiochemicals (produced in a cyclotron) are injected intravenously. These substances emit positrons that interact with the body to produce photons. The patient passes through a ring of detectors that receive the photons and create an image. The images reflect physiology rather than anatomical detail and can be used to assess metabolism, eg in tumours.

## 4.3 Carotid artery stenosis

### In a nutshell ...

- Stroke accounts for 10% of deaths in the UK, often due to thrombosis or emboli
- 15% of strokes are caused by carotid artery disease
- Current guidelines indicate that patients with symptomatic non-occluded carotid stenosis of 70% or more should be considered for endarterectomy because they have a 20–30% risk of stroke if left untreated
- Carotid angioplasty and endovascular stenting are emerging as an alternative

### Pathology of carotid artery stenosis

Stroke accounts for 10% of deaths in the UK. Causes of stroke include:

- Thrombosis (53%)
- Emboli (31%)
- Intracerebral haemorrhage (10%)
- Subarachnoid haemorrhage (6%)

Atherosclerosis at the carotid bifurcation is a common and potentially treatable cause of stroke. Carotid atheroma may cause symptoms by causing stenosis, limiting flow or embolisation. The effect of carotid atheroma depends on the degree of stenosis, the presence of collaterals (contralateral carotid and vertebro-basilar via the circle of Willis) and the nature of the plaque. The carotid bifurcation is commonly involved and shearing forces in the blood flow of this region cause the plaque to fracture and expose its thrombogenic core, promoting platelet aggregation.

### Presentation of carotid disease

**Symptoms of carotid disease**
- **Asymptomatic** carotid stenosis (a bruit may be audible on auscultation)
- **Amaurosis fugax:** transient blindness due to temporary retinal artery occlusion
- **Reversible ischaemic neurological deficit (RIND):** reversible defect >24 hours but <30 days
- **Transient ischaemic attack (TIA):** focal neurological deficit resolving within 24 hours (may or may not have CT-detectable brain changes)
- **Stroke:** focal neurological deficit secondary to a vascular event not resolving within 24 hours

Clinical presentation depends on arterial territory involved:

- Carotid territory: contralateral hemiparesis, dysphasia if dominant hemisphere
- Vertebrobasilar territory: vertigo, diplopia, blurred vision (occipital cortex), loss of consciousness, facial involvement, cerebellar signs

### Indications for treatment of carotid stenosis

Approximately 15% of strokes are caused by carotid disease. In patients with carotid stenosis, two large trials have assessed the benefit from surgical intervention compared to best medical management in carotid stenosis.

**Rationale for carotid intervention**
- European Carotid Surgery Trial (ECST)
- North American Symptomatic Carotid Endarterectomy Trial (NASCET)

These two large trials randomised patients with ipsilateral symptomatic stenoses (amaurosis fugax, TIA, stroke) within the previous 6 months to surgery or best medical management (control hypertension, antiplatelet therapy, modify risks). Carotid stenosis was assessed by angiography. The result suggested the following:

- Carotid endarterectomy should be offered to patients with ipsilateral stenoses >70% that have caused symptoms in the previous 6 months; the risk of having a subsequent stroke if there is a >70% stenosis in the carotid artery is 20–30%
- Urgent surgery can be performed for crescendo TIAs and it may also be performed for stroke-in-evolution to aid reperfusion of the watershed area around the damage
- Intervention for asymptomatic carotid stenosis is controversial; it is suggested that 20 carotid interventions may be needed to prevent a single stroke in these patients (number needed to treat or NNT)
- There is no indication for carotid intervention in patients with occluded carotid arteries at present

# Investigating carotid disease

## In a nutshell ...

Consider and exclude alternative causes for symptoms of focal cerebral ischaemia:
- **Embolism:** carotid stenosis, atrial fibrillation, endocarditis
- **Hypercoagulation states:** antithrombin III, protein C, protein S, factor V Leiden
- **Vasculitis:** autoantibodies (systemic lupus erthematosus [SLE], antiphospholipid syndrome)
- **Space-occupying lesion:** metastasis from tumours (common in smokers, eg lung)

Imaging investigations include:
- **Doppler US:** duplex of carotid artery, temporal transcranial ultrasonography
- **CT scan** of brain (areas of infarct) and carotid vessels
- **Arteriography:** arch aortogram, MRA, CTA

## Duplex Doppler ultrasonography

This is the gold standard screening test for assessing degree of carotid stenosis. It combines grey-scale ultrasonography to visualise stenosis with Doppler ultrasonography, which, by measuring velocity in the artery, allows direct measurement of the degree of stenosis.

| Advantages and disadvantages of Duplex Doppler US | |
| --- | --- |
| **Advantages of Duplex Doppler US** | **Disadvantages of Duplex Doppler US** |
| Non-invasive | Operator-dependent |
| Quick and easy | Poor views in calcified vessels |
| Gives information on nature of | May confuse velocities in ECA and ICA |
| stenosis and plaque morphology | Not good for very tight stenoses |
|  | May miss proximal or high lesions |

## CT scans

Enhanced CT head scanning may be used to exclude other intracranial pathology and may show cerebral infarcts (but it is better at showing haemorrhage).

Reconstructed three-dimensional CT angiograms can be used to visualise intracranial and extracranial arteries.

## Arteriography

### IADSA

- May use arch flush or selective carotid catheterisation
- Gives accurate anatomical visualisation of arterial lumen
- Good for confirming duplex findings (especially with tight stenoses and intracranial disease)
- Invasive (can precipitate cerebral infarction by causing embolisation or arterial spasm)
- Needs to be done in two planes
- Risk of TIA (2–3%) and stroke (about 0.1%) during procedure

## Transcranial Doppler

This is Doppler US performed through a 'window' of thin temporal bone to visualise middle cerebral artery blood flow. It is good for intraoperative monitoring of cerebral blood flow.

## MR angiography

This is a non-invasive technique that allows three-dimensional visualisation of intracranial and extracranial carotid arteries. It is sometimes used as an alternative to IADSA.

## Other investigations of carotid disease

These give further information on cerebral blood flow but are not generally used as primary diagnostic tests:

- Near-infrared spectroscopy
- Carbon dioxide reactivity studies

# Carotid endarterectomy

 ## Op box: Carotid endarterectomy

### Indications
Symptomatic ipsilateral carotid stenosis of >70%.

### Preop
Carefully document any existing neurological deficits while the patient is awake (especially cranial nerves and any deficits due to previous stroke). The procedure may be undertaken under general or local anaesthetic.

### Positioning
The patient is placed supine on the operating table with 30° head up, and the head tilted to the opposite side.

### Incision
A longitudinal incision at the anterior border of the sternomastoid.

### Procedure
- Deepen the incision through the platysma
- Identify the internal jugular vein at the anterior border of the sternomastoid; dissect the internal jugular vein free and retract it to expose the common carotid artery
- Continue the dissection proximally and distally to dissect out the common, internal and external carotid arteries
- Once the artery is dissected out, administer 5000 units heparin iv and allow sufficient circulation time
- Clamp arteries and perform longitudinal arteriotomy; at this stage it may be necessary to place a shunt to maintain cerebral perfusion
- Carefully remove the plaque, ensuring that a good endpoint is achieved distally
- Close the arteriotomy either directly or with a patch (Dacron or vein)

### Intraoperative hazards
Damage to cranial nerves: cutaneous branch of V (upper end of incision, below jaw), and mandibular branch of VII, IX, X, XII (especially due to retractors at the upper end of the wound).

### Closure
Place a small drain. Re-oppose other overlying tissues including platysma and skin, usually with a continuous suture.

### Postop
Postoperative evaluation of neurological function is performed regularly postoperatively and compared with preoperative function.

continued opposite

**Complications**

Complication and death rates are related to the presenting symptom (CVA > TIA > amaurosis fugax > asymptomatic) and to the presence of contralateral carotid disease:

- **Bleeding:** primary, reactionary or secondary
- **Haematoma:** may cause respiratory embarrassment
- **Cranial nerve injuries:** seen in 15% patients: cranial nerves V (cutaneous branches), VII (mandibular branch), IX, X, XII
- **TIA:** risk is 3–5% for symptomatic stenoses
- **CVA:** risk 1–2% and may be due to embolisation of debris at surgery or thrombosis of the surgical site (endarterectomy can cause the endothelium to be prothrombotic). Greatest risk is under anaesthetic and within the first 24 hours
- **Reperfusion syndrome (rare):** occurs >24 hours later and is due to loss of cerebral autoregulation and dramatic increases in cerebral blood flow causing oedema and raised intracranial pressure
- **Death:** 1–2% risk (MI is most common cause of death after carotid endarterectomy)

## Options for intraoperative patient monitoring

- Transcranial Doppler
- Near-infrared spectroscopy (transcranial $PCO_2$ monitoring)
- Local anaesthetic (LA) carotid endarterectomy with awake monitoring – the patient's neurological function can be continuously monitored during the procedure (conscious level, appropriate responses, speech, contralateral motor function, eg by squeezing a squeaky toy on command) and may eliminate the requirement for placement of a shunt (risks of dislodging embolus during placement)
- EEG
- Stump pressure measurements

## Carotid angioplasty and stenting

Early results with carotid angioplasty and stenting were encouraging. This is a less invasive procedure that avoids complications of open surgery, but it has not yet been fully evaluated in clinical trials. One potential hazard is dislodging of soft thrombus, causing microemboli. To prevent this, angioplasty catheters with cerebral protection devices have been designed so that any dislodged thrombus can be caught and prevented from going downstream to the brain. Recent results of randomised studies have shown open carotid endarterectomy to have better results than carotid angioplasty and stenting.

**CHAPTER 9**

## 4.4 Other carotid pathology

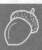

**In a nutshell ...**

- Carotid body tumours
- Carotid artery dissection
- Carotid artery aneurysms
- Fibromuscular dysplasia (FMD)

### Carotid body tumours (chemodectoma)

These are composed of paraganglionic cells of neural crest origin. They present equally in males and females, usually affecting people in their 50s but can occur at any age.

They present as masses in the neck adjacent to the hyoid bone anterior to sternomastoid. They are relatively smooth, compressible and pulsatile (but not classically expansile) due to their vascular component. Their high vascularity gives them a red–brown appearance, hence the description of 'potato tumours'. They may be mobile horizontally, but not vertically, and they often have a bruit. Size decreases with compression. About 5% are malignant, and this percentage increases with size. They are occasionally bilateral and easily diagnosed on CT. Angiography classically shows splaying of the carotid bifurcation by a vascular mass (the wine-glass sign). The preferred method of excision is dissection of the tumour off the vessel in the subadventitial plane. In elderly patients or in recurrent malignant tumours radiotherapy may be beneficial.

### Carotid artery dissection

Dissection of the carotid artery results from FMD, trauma or surgery, and presents with marked neurology. It is initially treated with systemic anticoagulation (unless due to trauma) to prevent thrombus formation and if it fails to settle it can be surgically repaired using an interpositional vein graft.

### Carotid artery aneurysms

Carotid aneurysms are rare and are caused by:
- Degenerative disease (atheroma)
- FMD
- Postoperative false aneurysm
- Mycotic aneurysm
- Trauma

They may present with a pulsatile mass, pain, Horner syndrome, cranial nerve dysfunction (compression) and cerebral ischaemia. They can be treated with interpositional grafting or ligation.

### Fibromuscular dysplasia

A rare condition affecting long unbranching arteries such as the carotid. It occurs bilaterally in 50% cases and is thought to have hormonal, mechanical and genetic aetiology. It looks like a string of beads on angiography with segmental stenosis and dilatation. Treatment is via progressive angioplasty.

# SECTION 5

# Vascular disorders of the upper limb

## In a nutshell ...

Vascular disorders of the upper limb encompass a wide variety of pathologies. Although atherosclerotic disease of the upper limb arteries is relatively rare, ischaemic symptoms can manifest from pathology such as emboli and aneurysmal disease, or more commonly vasospastic disorders, vasculitides and connective tissue disease. Assessment of the upper limb is much the same as in the lower limb, with particular attention to comparing sides, and use of duplex scanning and angiography for imaging disease.

## 5.1 Anatomy of upper limb arteries and veins

### In a nutshell ...

- Thoracic inlet
- Subclavian artery
- Axillary artery
- Brachial artery
- Ulnar artery
- Radial artery
- Upper limb veins

### Thoracic inlet

This is termed the thoracic *inlet* by anatomists but the thoracic *outlet* by surgeons!

- It is the root of the neck, above the apex of the lungs
- Its borders are:
  - Laterally: the inner border of the first rib
  - Medially: the anterior lip of the upper surface of the first vertebral body
  - Anteriorly: the suprasternal notch
- Its plane is obliquely disposed downwards and forwards (low injuries entering the neck can therefore damage structures in this area and then pass intrathoracically)

- It contains the subclavian artery and vein (as they pass over the top of the first rib and under the clavicle), the brachial plexus (as it emerges around the subclavian artery) and the phrenic nerve (between subclavian artery and vein)

## Subclavian artery

This arises on the left directly from the aorta, and on the right from the brachiocephalic trunk. It lies on the lateral border of scalenus anterior:

- Surface marking is a line arching upwards from sternoclavicular joint to 2 cm above middle of the clavicle
- The first part has three branches:
  - Vertebral artery
  - Internal thoracic (mammary) artery
  - Thyrocervical trunk (transverse cervical, suprascapular, inferior thyroid)
- The third part gives off the costocervical trunk (superior intercostal and deep cervical) and dorsal scapular artery, and this becomes the axillary artery at the outer border of the first rib

## Axillary artery

This is the continuation of the third part of the subclavian artery at the outer border of the first rib. It becomes the brachial artery at the lower border of teres major. It is closely related to the brachial plexus (cords); both are enclosed in the fascial axillary sheath.

It is divided into three parts by the pectoralis minor muscle; the main branches of each part are:

- First part: superior thoracic
- Second part: thoracoacromial, lateral thoracic

- Third part: subscapular, anterior and posterior circumflex humeral

## Brachial artery

This provides the main blood supply to the upper limb:

- It is a continuation of axillary artery at the lower border of teres major
- It descends in the anterior compartment of the arm dividing into the radial and ulnar arteries at the neck of the radius
- Profunda branch supplies the posterior compartment
- Median nerve initially lies laterally but then crosses anteriorly to lie medial to the artery in the antecubital fossa

## Ulnar artery

This passes medially and inferiorly in the anterior compartment of the forearm, running deep to flexor carpi ulnaris:

- It lies lateral to the ulnar nerve
- It ends by forming the superficial palmar arch with the superficial branch of the radial artery

Note: Allen's test assesses the relative contributions of the radial and ulnar arteries to the blood supply of the hand. Both arteries are occluded at the wrist: the patient makes a fist and the hand goes pale. One artery is released in turn and reperfusion of the hand assessed. It is useful for assessment before arteriovenous (AV) fistula formation, and gives information about the dominant blood supply to the hand.

The upper part gives off the common interosseous artery, which divides into anterior and posterior branches.

## Radial artery

Passes downwards and laterally under brachioradialis, emerging on its medial side near the wrist:

- Distally it lies on the radius, covered only by skin and fascia (its pulsation is felt here)
- Winds laterally before entering the palm between the two heads of the first dorsal interosseous muscle
- Supplies neighbouring muscles and ends as the deep palmar arch

## Upper limb veins

The veins of the upper limb, similar to the lower limb, consist of a deep and a superficial system. Knowledge of their course is of surgical importance for two reasons: first, for venous harvesting for graft formation and, second, for the formation of AV fistulas as a means of vascular access (see Section 5.7). There are a couple of common variations in the venous anatomy in the elbow region.

## Cephalic vein

- On radial side of arm
- Runs in groove between deltoid and pectoralis major muscles
- Pierces clavipectoral fascia and enters axillary vein

## Basilic vein

- Ulnar side of arm
- Arises from medial side of dorsal venous arch of the hand

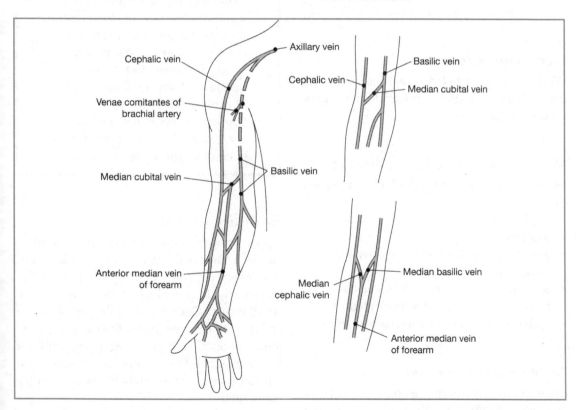

**Figure 9.8 The superficial veins of the upper limb**

### Axillary vein

- Formed by union of brachial and basilic veins
- Continues at the first rib as the subclavian vein
- Its tributaries correspond to the artery but it also receives the cephalic vein

## 5.2 Atherosclerotic disease of the upper limb

### In a nutshell ...

- Occlusive (atherosclerotic) disease
- Subclavian steal syndrome
- Aneurysmal disease
- Embolic disease

### Occlusive disease

When it occurs, atherosclerotic disease of the upper limb is usually confined to the larger vessels (eg subclavian artery).

### Management of occlusive disease

Occlusive disease of the upper limb is managed by:

- Angioplasty
- Stenting
- Bypass grafting (carotid to subclavian, axillary to axillary artery)
- Subclavian transposition (subclavian is divided at origin and re-implanted end-to-side on the common carotid artery)

### Aneurysmal disease

Upper body aneurysms account for 1% of peripheral aneurysms. They usually require surgical management:

- Either intrathoracic (causing Horner syndrome or venous congestion)
- Or extrathoracic (secondary to atherosclerosis, trauma, eg line placement, fibrous bands, cervical rib)

A complication of radial arterial line insertion is the development of a false radial artery aneurysm at the site of puncture. Occurs more frequently in patients with clotting disorders of any cause.

### Subclavian steal syndrome
- Caused by stenosis in the subclavian artery, proximal to the origin of the vertebral artery
- Any increase in demand for blood to the arm (eg cleaning windows!) causes reverse flow of blood from the cerebral circulation, through the vertebral artery, to supply the subclavian artery post-stenosis because the stenosis limits the blood flow obtainable from the aorta
- Loss of blood from the cerebral circulation may cause dizziness, loss of consciousness, ataxia, visual loss

### Embolic disease

Upper limb emboli usually arise from a cardiac source and lodge in the brachial artery. Paradoxical embolus from the venous system can give rise to upper limb emboli (via a cardiac septal defect). Occasionally a shower of smaller emboli may enter the upper limb causing small areas of distal ischaemia (eg digits). Splinter haemorrhages from infective endocarditis represent tiny, infected emboli passing into the upper limb.

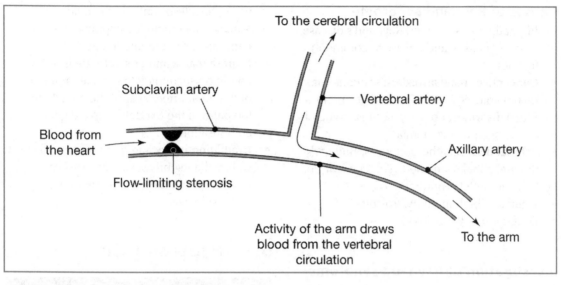

To the cerebral circulation

Subclavian artery

Vertebral artery

Blood from
the heart

Axillary artery

Flow-limiting stenosis

Activity of the arm draws
blood from the vertebral
circulation

To the arm

**Figure 9.9 Subclavian steal syndrome**

## Management of upper limb emboli

Upper limb emboli are managed by:

- Analgesia and resuscitation
- Anticoagulation (intravenous heparin); this sometimes enables conservative management of the limb
- Identification of embolus as cause of upper limb ischaemia (angiography/duplex or direct surgical exploration)
- Brachial embolectomy under LA (general if appropriate or necessary) using Fogarty catheter ± on-table angiograms or radiological intervention if required
- Postoperative anticoagulation
- Identification of source of embolus

## 5.3 Raynaud syndrome

### In a nutshell ...

This is characterised by episodic extreme digital vasospasm, often precipitated by cold. It is more common in females. May occur in the hands and feet.

There are three clinical phases:

1. Digital blanching due to arterial spasm (digits go white)
2. Cyanosis/pain due to stagnant anoxia (digits go blue)
3. Reactive hyperaemia due to accumulation of vasoactive metabolites (digits go red)

This may progress to ulceration, gangrene and digital amputation.

### Causes of Raynaud syndrome

- **Idiopathic:** this is called **Raynaud's disease** (primary cause), and it is more common in females
- **Connective tissue disorders:** scleroderma, rheumatoid, SLE, PAN (panarteritis nodosa)
- **Blood disorders:** cold agglutinins, cryoglobulinaemia, polycythaemia
- **Arterial disease:** atherosclerosis, Buerger's disease, subclavian aneurysm, cervical rib, thoracic outlet syndrome
- **Trauma:** vibration injury, frostbite
- **Drugs:** ergot, β blockers

### Investigation of Raynaud syndrome

This is aimed at ascertaining the underlying cause:

- Bloods: FBC, ESR, rheumatoid and autoantibodies screen
- Chest radiograph for cervical rib
- Duplex for arterial component
- CT/MR for thoracic outlet syndrome or subclavian aneurysm

### Treatment of idiopathic Raynaud syndrome

This is aimed at symptom control:

- Conservative: gloves, hand-warming devices, smoking cessation
- Drugs: nifedipine, prostacyclin
- Surgery: consider sympathectomy in extreme cases

### Other vasospastic disorders

- **Vibration white finger** occurs with prolonged exposure to high-frequency vibrating tools, which causes arterial vasospasm (especially in the cold). Management includes stopping exposure, hand warmers and nifedipine
- **Hypothenar hammer syndrome** is a rare condition secondary to repeated trauma of the ulnar artery against the hamate in the palm of the hand. It causes digital embolisation
- **Irradiation injury** after radiotherapy to chest wall/axilla (eg breast cancer). This can cause vessel rupture, thrombosis, stenosis and atherosclerosis

## 5.4 Hyperhidrosis

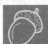

### In a nutshell ...

This is excessive sweating that can occur anywhere, but is most common and distressing in the palms, axillae and feet. It is classified with vascular disorders because treatment (sympathectomy) was traditionally performed by vascular surgeons for non-reconstructable critical ischaemia.

### Aetiology of hyperhidrosis

Aetiology is either primary (childhood, adolescence, familial) or secondary (hyperthyroid, phaeochromocytoma, hypothalamic tumours).

### Treatment of hyperhidrosis

Treatment can be surgical or conservative.

## Non-surgical management of hyperhidrosis

- Topical ammonium chloride
- Iontophoresis (electric current to incapacitate sweat glands)
- Botulinum toxin or Botox (decreases sympathetic activity)

## Surgical management of hyperhidrosis

- Skin excision
- Sympathectomy

---

**Examples of treatments for hyperhidrosis**

**Palmar hyperhidrosis** is treated by thoracoscopic sympathectomy or Botox.
**Axillary hyperhidrosis** is best treated by subcutaneous Botox.
**Plantar hyperhidrosis** is treated by chemical lumbar sympathectomy.
**Thoracoscopic sympathectomy** is performed by inserting a laparoscope into the pleural space via the axilla, deflating the lung, then obliterating the second, third and fourth sympathetic ganglia with diathermy or surgery, avoiding the stellate ganglion.
Complications of thoracoscopic sympathectomy include:

- Horner syndrome (ptosis, meiosis, anhidrosis due to stellate ganglion damage)
- Haemothorax
- Pneumothorax
- Compensatory hyperhidrosis

---

## 5.5 Thoracic outlet syndrome

 **In a nutshell ...**

This occurs when there is compression of the subclavian vessels or branches of the brachial plexus as they pass from the thorax into the arm. It occurs in 0.4% of the population; 70% are bilateral and 60% are symptomatic.

### Causes of thoracic outlet syndrome

- Cervical rib
- Abnormal muscle insertions or muscle hypertrophy
- Fibrous band
- Callus from old clavicular fracture
- Neck trauma
- Malignancy

### Symptoms and signs of thoracic outlet syndrome

- Arterial (ischaemic arm/hand): emboli
- Venous (swollen, warm, tender arm)
- Neurological (pain, paraesthesiae, weakness, wasting) (most common)

### Differential diagnosis of thoracic outlet syndrome

- Carpal tunnel syndrome
- Cervical spondylosis
- Raynaud syndrome
- Upper limb atherosclerotic disease
- Subclavian aneurysm

- Reflex sympathetic dystrophy
- TIA/stroke
- Trauma (whiplash injury)

## Examination and investigation of thoracic outlet syndrome

- Bilateral brachial BP measurement
- Roos' test: abduction and external rotation of the arm may precipitate symptoms
- Reduced or absent pulses
- Chest radiograph and thoracic outlet views (note: cervical rib may not be visible on radiograph)
- Cervical spine radiograph
- Nerve conduction studies
- Duplex ultrasonography
- Angiography (conventional, MRA or CTA)

## Treatment of thoracic outlet syndrome

- Physiotherapy
- Surgical decompression: resection of first part of first rib or divide anterior scalene muscle

## 5.6 Upper limb venous occlusion

### In a nutshell ...

This is less common than lower limb DVT. It may also cause PE.

## Presentation of upper limb venous occlusion

- Less common than lower limb DVT
- May also cause PE
- Can occur at any level in the venous drainage of the upper limb (common in the axillary/subclavian veins but can extend)
- Presents as painful, swollen, tender, warm upper limb
- Look for symptoms and signs of underlying cause

## Risk factors and causes

- Thoracic outlet syndrome
- Obstructive apical lung lesions
- Hypercoagulable states (congenital or underlying malignancy)
- Trauma
- Prolonged limb elevation with exercise (eg painting a ceiling)

## Treatment of upper limb venous occlusion

Upper limb venous occlusion is treated as for lower limb DVT:

- Anticoagulate
- Identify and treat underlying cause

# 5.7 Arteriovenous malformations and vascular access surgery

## In a nutshell ...

An AV fistula is an abnormal connection between arterial and venous systems. AV malformations consist of a huge spectrum of congenital and acquired vascular abnormalities. They have been placed in the upper limb section for convenience, although they can affect the legs and other parts of the body as well as the upper limbs.

**Congenital fistulas**
- Cirsoid
- Parkes–Weber syndrome
- Klippel–Trenaunay syndrome

**Acquired fistulas**
- Traumatic
- Surgical

## Congenital fistulas

These are rare, seen in approximately 1 per million live births. They are most commonly seen in the head/neck or extremities. Although present from birth they often enlarge during puberty or pregnancy. They may be **localised** or **multiple**.

## Localised fistulas (cirsoid aneurysm)

These appear as soft pulsatile swellings that are unsightly and may cause aching pain. The overlying skin/mucosa can ulcerate, with brisk haemorrhage. There is often a palpable thrill and machinery murmur present, which may be abolished by compressing the main feeding vessel. Investigation includes CT and selective arteriography. Those that arise during pregnancy should be treated expectantly because many regress after delivery. Treatment may be by embolisation or occlusion of the feeding vessel combined with excision. Direct injections of sclerosants have not been effective.

## Multiple fistulas (Parkes–Weber syndrome)

These usually present with an overall enlargement in limb size. There may be dilated superficial veins with ulceration and high-output cardiac failure may develop. The limb is hot with increased width and length associated with bone overgrowth. Differential diagnoses include Klippel–Trenaunay syndrome, local gigantism and lymphoedema. Arteriography characteristically shows rapid blushing through the abnormal communications with early arrival of dye in the veins. Individual fistulas are not visualised unless they are very large.

In the absence of heart failure or severe deformity management is usually expectant in early life. Later, ligation of the feeding vessels or injection of microspheres/embolisation may reduce the inflow. Amputation may be required in exceptional circumstances.

## Klippel–Trenaunay syndrome

These are congenital varicose veins and characteristic large naevi. There is bone and soft tissue hypertrophy in the affected limb, and there are often deep venous abnormalities. They affect the leg and buttocks.

## Acquired fistulas

These may result from accidental trauma (traumatic AV fistula) or be surgically created for renal haemodialysis.

### Traumatic AV fistulas

These usually follow simultaneous adjacent arterial and venous injury with a common haematoma. They take days to form, and there is usually a thrill and a bruit. Adjoining veins may become dilated and arterialised, eventually leading to venous hypertension, and possibly ulceration. Limb hypertrophy and lengthening may occur. If blood flow through the distal artery is sufficiently decreased distal ischaemia may occur. A fistula between larger vessels may be sufficient to create a left-to-right shunt, leading to heart failure if severe. Methods for closure include application of Duplex-directed pressure, insertion of a covered stent or surgical closure.

### AV fistulas for haemodialysis

These are usually created for long-term dialysis access and once formed can remain patent indefinitely. The connection of the artery to a vein results in a dilated vein, which is suitable for repeated cannulation and can deliver a high flow of blood for dialysis. The ideal site, as described by Brescia, is the radiocephalic fistula in the forearm, but other sites may be used.

The general rule in fistula formation is that the most distal site on the non-dominant arm is used. The procedure can be carried out under LA by side-to-side anastomosis of the radial artery and cephalic vein, although some surgeons ligate the distal vein or perform an end-to-side anastomosis to prevent the possibility of distal venous hypertension. Postoperatively, maintaining a warm limb and adequate hydration are necessary for successful fistula formation.

Expected patency rates are 60–90% at 1 year and 60–75% at 5 years. Generally, fistulas are not closed after a renal transplantation because they may subsequently be required again, although many thrombose spontaneously after transplantation. Indications for fistula closure are cosmetic, large flows leading to heart failure, and occasionally sepsis or distal embolisation.

## 6.1 Venous anatomy of the lower limb

**In a nutshell ...**

The venous system consists of the deep and superficial veins.

**Deep veins**
- Posterior tibial
- Anterior tibial
- Peroneal
- Soleal
- Gastrocnemius
- Popliteal
- Superficial femoral vein
- Deep (profunda) femoral vein
- Iliac veins

**Superficial veins**
- Long saphenous
- Short saphenous

### Deep veins

These accompany the arteries:
- Three paired stem veins: posterior tibial, anterior tibial and peroneal veins
- Two muscular veins: soleal vein and gastrocnemius vein

All join and form the popliteal vein in the popliteal fossa, where the short saphenous vein (a superficial vein) also joins the deep venous system.
- Popliteal vein becomes the superficial femoral vein and accompanies the superficial femoral artery
- This is joined by the profunda femoral vein and long saphenous vein (another superficial vein) at the saphenofemoral junction, and then becomes the iliac vein

Venous anatomy is very variable, and the deep veins are often multiple. Lower limb occlusive venous pathology is covered in Neurosurgery, Chapter 6. Upper limb venous occlusion is covered in Section 5.6 of this chapter.

## Superficial veins

These systems lie in the subcutaneous tissue and are involved in thermoregulation. They are responsible for becoming varicose veins. In the lower limb there are two main veins and their tributaries.

### Long saphenous vein (LSV)

This is the longest vein in the body. It runs from anterior to the medial malleolus (site for venous cut-down), along the medial side of the leg, and terminates at the saphenofemoral junction, just medial to the femoral pulse (surface marking 2.5 cm below and lateral to pubic tubercle or one fingerbreadth medial to the femoral artery in the groin crease).

It connects to the deep venous system at the:
- Saphenofemoral junction
- Mid-thigh perforator
- Medial calf perforators (usually three or four)

### Short saphenous vein (SSV)

This commences behind the lateral malleolus and runs along the posterolateral side of the calf to pierce the deep fascia and joins the popliteal vein in the popliteal fossa. It usually communicates with the deep (soleal and gastrocnemius) veins and the long saphenous system.

## 6.2 Physiology of lower limb veins

### In a nutshell ...

Venous return is maintained by the following:
- Heart (maintains a pressure gradient through the circulation)
- Calf muscle pump
- Venous valves
- Venomotor tone
- Respiratory movements

Venous return is impeded by gravity, which encourages peripheral pooling in dependent limbs.

## Venous return

### Venomotor tone

Venomotor tone is maintained by smooth muscle within the vein wall (under control of the sympathetic nervous system). On assuming an upright position, the decreased cardiac output due to dependant pooling leads to an increase in sympathetic discharge (which increases venous tone to reduce the capacitance of the system and increase venous return).

### Respiratory movements

Changes in intrathoracic pressure with inspiration and expiration influence venous return. When intrathoracic pressure decreases, venous return increases. When intrathoracic pressure increases, venous return decreases (as in the Valsalva manoeuvre) which in turn decreases cardiac output.

There are six points of communication between the deep and superficial venous systems:

- Long saphenous (saphenofemoral junction)
- Short saphenous (saphenopopliteal junction)
- Mid-thigh perforating veins
- Medial calf communicating veins (posterior tibial to posterior arch veins)
- Gastrocnemius communicating veins (short saphenous to muscle)
- Lateral calf communicating veins (short saphenous to peroneal)

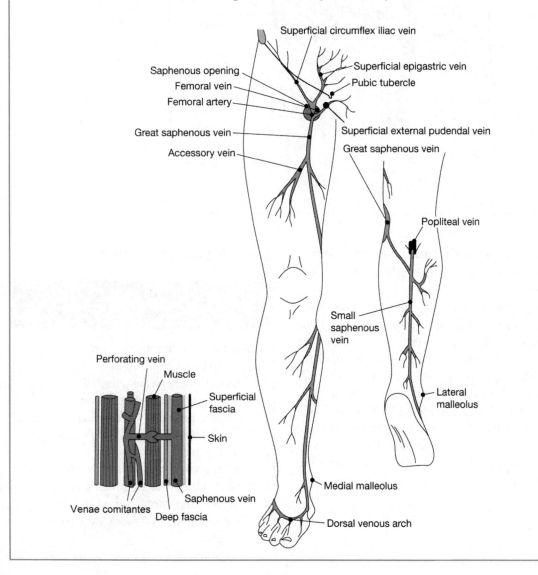

**Figure 9.10 Superficial lower limb venous anatomy**

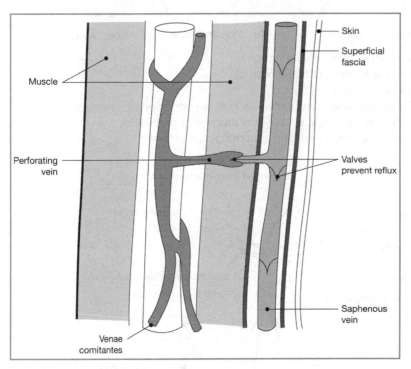

Muscle

Perforating vein

Venae comitantes

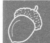

Skin

Superficial fascia

Valves prevent reflux

Saphenous vein

**Figure 9.11 The venous pump**

## Muscular activity and the calf pump

With an upright posture blood should pool in the distal venous system (which can occur with prolonged standing). However, deep veins have valves that prevent reverse flow in the column of blood within the veins. Also, as the calf muscles contract blood is forced upwards resulting in lower pressure in the deep veins during relaxation of muscular activity (this draws blood from superficial to deep veins via the communicating vessels, along the pressure gradient generated. These also have valves to ensure unidirectional flow. The flow is shown in Figure 12.11.

## 6.3 Varicose veins

### In a nutshell ...

Varicose veins are dilated, tortuous, elongated superficial veins.
- Occur in 2% of the population (increasing incidence with age)
- May be **primary** or **secondary** (due to an obstructed system, eg DVT, pelvic malignancy)
- Most common in the long saphenous system but may occur in the short saphenous distribution, or may be recurrent (after previous varicose vein surgery)

## Primary varicose veins

These form due to gravitational venous pooling and vein wall laxity causing venous dilatation and valve leakage. In long saphenous varicose veins this usually starts at the saphenofemoral junction, causing more pooling and dilatation in the proximal segment of the vein and leakage at the next valve. Eventually all the valves leak and there is a continuous column of blood below the heart, leading to increased venous pressure in the superficial veins of the legs (which may cause leg oedema and tissue damage, in turn leading to complications of varicose veins).

## Secondary varicose veins

If the deep venous system outflow is obstructed (eg DVT, pelvic malignancy) or deep or communicating venous valves are incompetent (eg post-phlebitic), then blood may be forced from the deep to the superficial system, resulting in increased superficial venous pressure and varicose veins. This can also be caused by a congenital absence or abnormality of the venous valves and, rarely, by severe tricuspid incompetence causing pulsatile varicosities!

This is significant because secondary varicose veins caused by an absent or poorly functioning deep venous system should not be surgically disconnected because this would leave no alternative effective path of venous return. Secondary varicose veins are associated with symptoms of chronic venous insufficiency.

## Symptoms of varicose veins

- Asymptomatic
- Cosmetic
- Ache
- Itch
- Ankle swelling
- Bleeding

- Thrombophlebitis (painful inflamed thrombosed superficial varicosities)
- Skin discoloration (haemosiderosis)
- Varicose eczema
- Lipodermatosclerosis (induration/inflammation in skin)
- Ulceration

---

**Risk factors for varicose veins**

- Age (peak 50–60)
- Female
- Obesity
- Pregnancy
- Occupations involving long periods of standing
- Family history
- Pelvic malignancy
- Previous DVT

---

## Examination of varicose veins

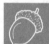 **In a nutshell ...**

**Inspect**
- Determine whether likely to be primary or secondary (include full exam for potential secondary causes)
- Determine site of incompetence:
  - Tap test
  - Cough test
  - Tourniquet test
  - Perthe's test
  - Hand-held Doppler tests

**Formal investigation for sites of incompetence using Duplex scanning**

This is performed initially with the patient **standing**. Inspect for ankle swelling, haemosiderosis, varicose eczema, lipodermatosclerosis and ulceration. Note the distribution and severity of varicosities. Palpate the veins for superficial thrombophlebitis and palpable perforating veins, and examine the popliteal fossa and groin for varices. A **saphena varix** is a compressible swelling due to a dilated varix at the saphenofemoral junction (which disappears on lying down).

Sites of incompetence used to be determined by several clinical tests. All these tests have been shown to be unreliable and have been superseded by ultrasound assessment:

- **Tap test:** palpate the proximal portion of the vein while tapping distally. If you feel an impulse it suggests that a column of blood exists between the point of tapping and the vein being palpated
- **Cough test:** the standing patient is asked to cough while you palpate the saphenofemoral junction. A positive cough impulse indicates saphenofemoral junction incompetence. This test is very unreliable
- **Tourniquet test:** the patient is placed in the supine position with the leg elevated and the veins emptied by manual 'sweeping'. A tourniquet is then placed on the mid-thigh and the patient is asked to stand. If veins below the tourniquet do not refill, assume that the site of incompetence is above the tourniquet (when the tourniquet is released these veins will then be seen to fill). The test can be repeated with the tourniquet at different levels to ascertain sites of incompetence. This test is more reliable than the cough test but less reliable than hand-held Doppler. If done with pressure from a hand or tourniquet on the saphenofemoral junction, this is the **Trendelenberg test**

- **Perthe's test:** once you have controlled the varicose veins by blocking off the superficial venous system with a tourniquet, venous drainage of the leg is carried out exclusively by the deep venous system (as if the patient had surgical disconnection of the saphenofemoral junction). Ask patients to go up and down on their toes, increasing arterial blood supply and activating the calf pump. If deep veins are patent this reduces venous engorgement of the limb. If the deep system is not patent or the valves are incompetent the opposite occurs. With the deep system incapable of draining the leg and the superficial system temporarily disconnected, the increased blood supply into the exercising leg has nowhere to drain, and patients experience a bursting pain of venous engorgement. This test shows why it is so important to check the patency of the deep venous system before carrying out varicose vein surgery. If the presenting complaint of venous insufficiency and engorgement of superficial veins is secondary to a non-functioning deep venous system (eg after a DVT), then stripping the superficial system on which the patient relies will only make it worse
- **Hand-held Doppler:** place the hand-held Doppler probe over the site of incompetence to be assessed (eg saphenofemoral junction) in the standing patient. The vein or leg is then compressed sharply below the probe, and a 'whoosh' is heard as the blood passes the hand-held Doppler. If the site to be assessed is incompetent, a second 'whoosh' is heard as blood passes back through an incompetent section of vein

Finally perform a full examination of the patient, paying special attention to the abdomen and pelvis, looking for secondary causes of varicose veins. Formal investigations of the sites of incompetence may be performed using duplex scanning or venography.

## Investigation of varicose veins

- Hand-held Doppler (as described above)
- Duplex Doppler US (see Section 1)
- Venography (see Section 1)

## Management of varicose veins

**In a nutshell ...**

Management options include:
- Conservative measures
- Compression stockings
- Sclerotherapy
- Endovenous laser therapy (EVLT)
- Endoluminal radiofrequency ablation (RFA)
- Foam injection
- Surgery

Varicose veins may be treated to relieve symptoms (ache, itch) or to prevent complications (bleeding, ulceration). Management is conservative or surgical. Take care when considering treatment of varicose veins for cosmetic reasons because the benefits of surgery might be outweighed by complications. Cosmetic surgery is not funded by the NHS.

- **Conservative measures** are a good option for uncomplicated, asymptomatic varicose veins

- **Compression stockings** press the veins, augment venous return, and thus reduce symptoms and complications; they are a good option in elderly people and those not fit enough for surgery, although stockings are often not well tolerated by younger patients
- **Sclerotherapy** involves injection of a 'sclerosant' (eg sodium tetradecyl sulphate [Fibro-Vein]) via a fine needle directly into the vein followed by compression bandaging. The sclerosant irritates the venous intima, causing inflammation and ultimately luminal obliteration. It works well for small varicosities (but not large veins or in the presence of significant venous incompetence)
- **Surgery** aims to disconnect the incompetent superficial system from the venous circulation
- **Other treatment modalities** include endovenous laser, endoluminal radiofrequency ablation and foam injection. These therapies act by damaging the venous endothelium, which is then compressed by occlusive bandaging of the treated limb. The damaged endothelium adheres and occludes the lumen of the vessels

## Surgery for varicose veins

**In a nutshell ...**

Surgical options:
- Open surgery with junction ligation and stripping of vein ± stab avulsions
- EVLT
- Radiofrequency ablation
- Foam ablation

Be aware of common anatomical variations (failure to deal with these leads to recurrence).

## Open surgery

Preoperative formal duplex skin marking is used to identify sites of incompetent perforators and the saphenopopliteal junction (SPJ) to aid identification during surgery. Preoperative marking of varicosities with the patient standing is imperative.

---

 **Op box: Junction ligation and stripping of varicose veins (LSV, SSV)**

**Indications**
Symptomatic varicose veins (exclude patients with a non-functioning deep venous system).

**Preop**
ALWAYS carefully mark all varicosities on the skin with the patient standing, immediately preoperatively and ask them to identify any troublesome varicosities (as they will be much less visible when the patient is asleep and supine). Perforators and the SPJ should be marked on the skin under formal duplex guidance. May be performed under GA, LA or regional anaesthetic. Women taking the oral contraceptive pill (OCP) should stop and use alternative contraception for 4 weeks before the procedure (increased risk of DVT).

**Positioning**
Supine position with 15° head-down tilt (supine for LSV; prone or lateral for SSV).

**Incision**
LSV: make groin crease incision just medial to the femoral pulse (note that in obese patients the saphenofemoral junction [SFJ] may be above the groin crease).
SSV: transverse incision in the skin crease of the popliteal fossa (at the level of the marked SPJ)

**Procedure – LSV**
Dissect out and carefully identify the SFJ before any vein is divided. Identify and divide tributaries beyond secondary branch points:
- Superficial circumflex iliac
- Superficial inferior epigastric
- Superficial external pudendal
- Posteromedial thigh branch (prevents medial thigh recurrence)
- Deep external pudendal (directly off common femoral vein)

Beware – these tributaries are very variable. Ligate SFJ flush to the common femoral vein – do not narrow the lumen of the common femoral and make sure that the ligature does not slip!
Strip LSV, with an endoluminal stripper, from groin to knee.
Avulse below-knee varicosities.

**Procedure – SSV**
Dissect out and carefully identify the SPJ before any vein is divided.
Divide and ligate any small tributaries leading into the SSV/SPJ.
Ligate the SPJ.
Avulse below-knee varicosities.

**continued opposite**

**Intraoperative hazards**

LSV: damage to the saphenous nerve (sensory loss) which runs with the vein below the level of the knee (do not advance endoluminal stripper lower than 1 handbreadth below knee).

SSV: damage to the common peroneal nerve (results in foot drop) or sural nerve (sensory loss).

**Closure**

Close the wound in layers with absorbable sutures.

Stab avulsions can be closed with Steri-Strips.

Apply compression bandages.

**Postoperative instructions**

Often done as a day case and so standard day-case procedures apply.

Compression bandaging remains in place for 24 hours

Replaced with thigh-length graduated compression stockings (wear day and night for 1 week; can then be removed at night).

Sit with feet elevated and encourage regular short exercise.

**Complications**

- Bruising and leg swelling
- Bleeding
- Infection
- Nerve damage (long saphenous – saphenous nerve; short saphenous – sural nerve)
- DVT

**Anatomical variation** is common and can be identified on duplex scanning. Variants include:

- Double saphenous veins
- Major thigh tributaries, including the accessory vein (joins long saphenous at mid-thigh)
- Major tributaries joining the superficial external iliac and superficial external pudendal veins

Risk factors and causes of varicose vein recurrence:

- **Recanalisation**
  - Failure to identify all tributaries at the initial operation (even small vessels can dilate)
  - Leaving segments of the saphenous vein in situ (especially in the thigh)
- **Neovascularisation** around the SFJ or SPJ

## Endovenous laser therapy

A guidewire is inserted into the LSV under ultrasound control, and the vein is cannulated. A laser probe is then advanced to the SFJ under ultrasound control, and slowly withdrawn, heating the endothelium and causing the vein to close to a fibrous thread. Tumescent cooling fluid is injected around the vein to prevent damage to surrounding tissues. Early trials show this technique to be as effective as conventional surgery, but with earlier mobilisation. It can be performed under LA or GA, and combined with tributary vein avulsion surgery. It can also be used for short saphenous varicose veins.

## Radiofrequency ablation

This technique is similar to EVLT except that the energy is provided by a radiofrequency ablation catheter. It works at a slightly lower temperature than EVLT. Results are equivalent.

### Foam sclerotherapy

For this treatment, a foam sclerosant is injected under ultrasound control directly into truncal varicosities. Results have been promising, but the technique has not become widely used due to a small incidence of neurological complications. It does not require GA.

## 6.4   Leg ulcers

> ### In a nutshell ...
>
> - An ulcer is a break in continuity of an epithelial surface
> - Ulcers are common and an expensive cause of morbidity
> - Although not all have vascular aetiology, leg ulcers often present to vascular clinics

### Causes of leg ulcers

- Venous (varicose veins, post-phlebitic, gravitational)
- Arterial (atherosclerosis)
- Neuropathic (diabetic, CVA, spina bifida, pressure sores)
- Trauma (plaster of Paris, injections, burns)
- Allergic
- Vasculitic and vasospastic (rheumatoid, SLE, PAN, scleroderma, Raynaud syndrome)
- Malignancy (basal cell carcinoma [BCC], squamous cell carcinoma [SCC], malignant melanoma, skin metastases, Marjolin's ulcer – SCC change in previous venous ulcer)
- Infective (TB, HIV)
- Artefactual (patient-induced or iatrogenic)
- Malnutrition (scurvy, ulcerative colitis)
- Lymphatic (infection, trauma)

### Associated factors contributing to leg ulcers

- Gravitational stasis
- Immobility
- Obesity
- Malnutrition
- Steroids

In practice, most ulcers are of mixed aetiology.

## Pathology of venous ulceration

Raised superficial venous pressure may be due to primary varicose veins, congenital valvular aplasia or deep venous incompetence. This is marked in the post-thrombotic limb. After significant DVT the thrombus becomes organised and the vessel may partially or totally recanalise. Thrombus irreversibly damages the valves in the deep venous system, leading to incompetence. Chronic venous insufficiency secondary to venous hypertension causes increased hydrostatic pressure from valve dysfunction and blood travelling from the deep to the superficial venous systems.

Venous hypertension has several effects:
- Restricts arterial replenishment of capillary blood
- AV shunt formation
- Dilation of venules causes leakage of plasma proteins into the tissues (lipodermatosclerosis is a term given to the combined skin and subcutaneous tissue changes of chronic venous hypertension: a progressive sclerosis of the skin and subcutaneous fat by fibrin deposition, tissue death and scarring – it results in a constricted appearance around the lower leg [oedema above and atrophy below] which resembles an inverted bottle, hence the term 'beer-bottle leg')
- Red blood cells (RBCs) are forced out into the tissues, resulting in pigmentation of the skin due to haemosiderin deposition

Together, these changes lead to the clinical picture of raised superficial venous pressure with ankle swelling, haemosiderosis, varicose eczema, lipodermatosclerosis and ultimately ulceration.

There are two main theories of ulcer formation:
1. Leucocyte trapping theory: raised venous pressure causes increased capillary pressure with fibrin exudation, white blood cell entrapment, congestion and thrombosis
2. Fibrin cuff theory: leaking from capillaries causes fibrin cuffing around the vessel with reduced nutrient and oxygen diffusion

## Examination of leg ulcers

First remove all dressings, applications and debris.

- Position, eg gaiter area (venous), sole of foot (arterial or neuropathic)
- Size
- Shape
- Edge – sloping, punched out, undermined, rolled, everted
- Base – slough, granulation tissue, tendon, bone
- Depth
- Discharge – serous, sanguineous, purulent
- Colour
- Temperature
- Tenderness
- Fixity
- Surrounding tissues:
  - Arteries/veins (including ABPI)
  - Nerves
  - Bones/joints
- Regional lymph nodes
- General examination

## Investigation of leg ulcers

- Duplex Doppler US (arterial and venous)
- Blood tests (FBC, ESR, sugar, autoantibodies)
- Swab (microbiology)
- Biopsy (malignant change, other aetiologies)
- Arteriography/venography (if indicated)

## Management of venous leg ulcers

Compression is most usually achieved with stockings or bandaging. Various regimens are described (three-layer, four-layer, paste). All aim to provide high external pressure at the ankle, graduating down to lower pressure in the upper calf, thus augmenting venous return and allowing ulcer healing. The progress of healing is monitored regularly. Non-healing ulcers require further assessment to exclude other aetiologies (eg Marjolin's change, vasculitis), and antibiotics if infected. If still not healing consider excision and split-skin graft or pinch-skin grafts.

Full compression (eg four-layer bandaging) can be applied for pure venous ulcers (ABPI >0.9). When there is an arterial component (ABPI 0.7–0.9) modified or lighter compression is required. An ABPI <0.7 requires correction of the underlying arterial abnormality. Four-layer compression bandaging consists of cotton wool (inner layer), crepe, elastic bandage and a cohesive bandage.

When the ulcer is healed, further management is required to maintain healing. This may be long-term compression stockings, or superficial venous surgery (long saphenous or short saphenous varicose veins) to correct the underlying venous abnormality.

## 6.5   Lymphoedema

### In a nutshell ...

**Lymphoedema** is an accumulation of tissue fluid in the extracellular compartment resulting from failure of the lymphatic system to transport fluid via the lymphatic vessels and lymph nodes. It is most common in the lower limb (80%) but may occur in the upper limb or scrotum. In contrast, **oedema** is an accumulation of tissue fluid in patients in whom a lymphatic abnormality has not been confirmed (eg cardiac/renal/nutritional).

### The lymphatics

The lymphatic system maintains a flow of lymph fluid of approximately 2–2.5 l/day, maintained by contractility of lymphatic channels and their patency. Lymph nodes absorb water and electrolytes from the lymphatic fluid.

### Causes of lymphoedema

#### Primary causes

- Congenital, idiopathic (Milroy's disease, lymphoedema praecox or tarda)

#### Secondary causes

- Following groin or axillary surgery
- Post-radiotherapy
- Due to malignancy
- Infection (eg filariasis caused by *Wuchereria bancrofti*)
- Lymphadenectomy
- Chronic inflammation

### Pathology of lymphoedema

**Primary lymphoedema** occurs due to a developmental lymphatic abnormality; 20% have a family history of swollen legs. This can be lymphatic channel aplasia, hypoplasia or hyperplasia. **Secondary lymphoedema** follows destruction or obstruction of the lymphatic channels by surgery, radiotherapy, malignancy or filariasis. This results in reduced lymphatic drainage, leading to limb swelling. The swelling may be initiated by an infective episode (eg cellulitis) or by minor limb trauma. Initially the oedema is pitting but over time fibrosis occurs, leading to the classic clinical picture of non-pitting oedema.

### Differential diagnosis of lymphoedema

Other causes of leg swelling
- Venous or post-phlebitic oedema
- Cardiac failure
- Hepatic insufficiency (hypoproteinaemia)
- Renal failure
- Gravitational or stasis oedema
- Congenital giant limb (including vascular abnormalities, see Section 5)

### Investigation of lymphoedema

The clinical diagnosis is usually obvious, but when doubt exists (especially in early primary lymphoedema) it can be confirmed by **lympho-scintigraphy**. A radioactive tracer is injected subcutaneously into the foot, and its progress is monitored with a gamma camera as it progresses to the proximal lymphatics and beyond. Delayed transit confirms the diagnosis.

More detailed anatomy can be elicited, eg before consideration of lymphatic reconstruction, by **lymphangiography**. A radio-opaque dye is

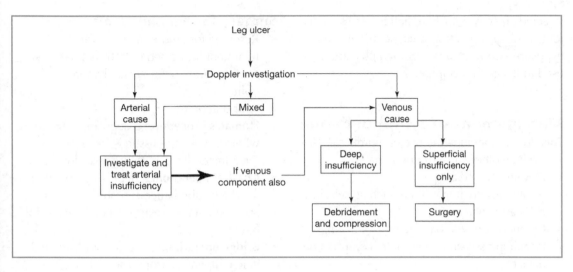

**Figure 9.12 The management of lower limb ulceration**

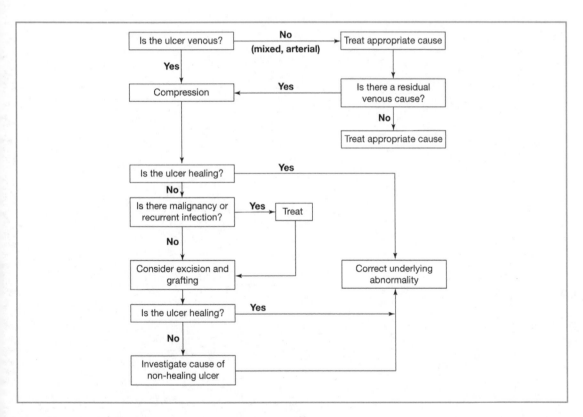

**Figure 9.13 Algorithm for venous ulcer management**

injected directly into lymphatic vessels of the foot using an operating microscope and direct exposure. Conventional radiographs are then used to image the lymphatics.

## Management of lymphoedema
This does not include the use of diuretics!
- Exclude other causes of oedema
- Elevate affected area
- Antibiotics (treat infections such as cellulitis early and aggressively)
- Compression with bandaging or stockings
- Lymphopress (serial pneumatic compression device)
- Surgery

## Surgery for lymphoedema
- Reserved for failure of conservative treatment (indicated in <10% of patients)
- Must be done before distal lymphatics obliterate
- Poor outcome
- **Homan's procedure:** a debulking operation where a wedge of tissue is removed from the affected limb, with primary closure
- **Charles' operation:** a debulking operation in which subcutaneous tissue is excised. Split-skin grafts are applied to the exposed fascia
- **Bridge operation:** a bypass for obstructed iliac lymphatics, from bisected inguinal nodes to an isolated small-bowel pedicle

# List of Abbreviations

| | |
|---|---|
| 5-HIAA | 5-hydroxyindole acetic acid |
| A&E | accident and emergency (department) |
| AAA | abdominal artery aneurysm |
| ABGs | arterial blood gases |
| ACE | antegrade colonic enema |
| ACh | acetylcholine |
| ACL | anterior cruciate ligament |
| ACTH | adrenocorticotropic hormone |
| ADH | antidiuretic hormone (vasopressin) |
| AF | atrial fibrillation |
| AFB/s | acid-fast bacillus/bacilli |
| AFP | alphafetoprotein |
| AIDS | acquired immunodeficiency syndrome |
| ALL | anterior longitudinal ligament |
| ALP | alkaline phosphatase |
| ALT | alanine aminotransferase |
| ANP | atrial natriuretic peptide |
| AP | anteroposterior |
| APBI | ankle–brachial pressure index |
| APC | argon plasma coagulation |
| APKD | adult polycystic kidney disease |
| APL | abductor pollicis longus |
| APTT | activated partial thromboplastin time |
| ARDS | adult respiratory distress syndrome |
| ARF | acute renal failure |
| ARM | anorectal malformation |
| ASD | atrial septal defect |
| ASIS | anterior superior iliac spine |
| AST | aspartate aminotransferase |
| ATLS | advanced trauma life support |
| ATN | acute tubular necrosis |
| ATP | adenosine triphosphate |
| AV | arteriovenous |
| AVM | arteriovenous malformation |
| AVN | atrioventricular node; avascular necrosis |
| BAL | bronchoalveolar lavage |
| BCC | basal cell carcinoma |
| BIH | benign intercranial hypertension |
| BM | blood glucose monitoring; bone marrow |
| BMI | body mass index |
| BP | blood pressure |
| BPH | benign prostatic hyperplasia |
| BXO | balanitis xerotica obliterans |
| CABG | coronary artery bypass graft |
| CAH | congenital adrenal hyperplasia |
| CAPD | continuous ambulant peritoneal dialysis |
| CBD | common bile duct |
| CCK | cholecystokinin |
| CEA | carcinoembryonic antigen |
| CF | cystic fibrosis |
| CIS | carcinoma in situ |
| CJD | Creutzfeldt-Jacob disease |
| CK | creatine kinase |
| CLO | *Campylobacter*-like organism |
| CMC | carpometacarpal (joint) |
| CMV | cytomegalovirus |
| CNS | central nervous system |
| CO | carbon monoxide; cardiac output |
| COPD | chronic obstructive pulmonary disease |
| COX | cyclo-oxygenase |
| CPAP | continuous positive-pressure airway pressure (ventilation) |
| CPB | cardiopulmonary bypass |
| CPEX | cardiopulmonary exercise testing |
| CPPS | chronic pelvic pain syndrome |
| CREST | **c**alcinosis, **R**aynauld's, **o**esophageal dysfunction, **s**clerodactyly, **t**elangectasia |
| CRF | chronic renal failure |
| CRH | corticotropin-releasing factor |
| CRP | C-reactive protein |
| CSF | cerebrospinal fluid |
| CT | computed tomography |
| CTC | CT colonography |
| CTEV | congenital talipes equinovarus |
| CVA | cerebrovascular accident |
| CVP | central venous pressure |

| | | | |
|---|---|---|---|
| CXR | chest X-ray | FNH | focal nodular hyperplasia |
| DCIS | ductal carcinoma in situ | FOB | faecal occult blood |
| DDH | developmental dysplasia of the hip | FSH | follicle-stimulating hormone |
| DEXA | dual-energy X-ray absorptiometry | FVC | forced vital capacity |
| DHCC | dihydroxycholecalciferol | GA | general anaesthesia |
| DHS | dynamic hip screw | GALT | gut-associated lymphoid tissue |
| DI | diabetes insipidus | GCS | Glasgow Coma Scale |
| DIC | disseminated intravascular coagulation | GFR | glomerular filtration rate |
| | | GGT | gamma-glutamyltransferase |
| DIP | distal interpharyngeal (joint) | GH | growth hormone |
| DMSA | dimercaptosuccinic acid | GI | gastrointestinal |
| DPG | 2,3 diphosphoglycerate | GIST | gastrointestinal stromal tumour |
| DPL | diagnostic peritoneal lavage | GnRH | gonadotropin-releasing hormone |
| DRE | digital rectal examination | GOR(D) | gastro-eosophageal reflux (disease) |
| DU | duodenal ulcer | GRP | gastrin-releasing hormone |
| DVT | deep vein thrombosis | HCC | hepatocellular carcinoma |
| EBV | Epstein–Barr virus | hCG | human chorionic gonadotropin |
| ECA | external carotid artery | HDU | high-dependency unit |
| ECG | electrocardiogram | HER-2 | human epidermal growth factor receptor-2 |
| ECU | extensor carpi ulnaris | | |
| EDL | extensor digitorum longus | HiB | Haemophilus influenzae type B |
| EHL | extensor hallucis longus | HIV | human immunodeficiency virus |
| ELISA | enzyme-linked immunosorbent assay | HLA | human leucocyte antigen |
| ELN | external laryngeal nerve | HNPCC | hereditary non-polyposis colon cancer |
| EMD | electro-mechanical dissociation | | |
| EMG | electromyogram | HOCM | hypertrophic obstructive cardiomyopathy |
| EMLA | eutectic mixture of local anaesthetic | | |
| ENT | ear, nose and throat (department) | HPV | human papillomavirus |
| EPB | extensor pollicis brevis | HR | heart rate |
| ER | (o)estrogen receptor | HRT | hormone replacement therapy |
| ERCP | endoscopic retrograde cholangiopancreatography | HSP | heat-shock protein |
| | | HSV | herpes simplex virus |
| ESR | erythrocyte sedimentation rate | HTLV-1 | human T-cell lymphotropic virus 1 |
| ESWL | extracorporeal shockwave lithotripsy | HUS | haemolytic uraemic syndrome |
| EUA | examination under anaesthetic | IARC | International Agency for Research on Cancer |
| EVLT | endovenous laser therapy | | |
| FAP | familial adenomatous polyposis | IBD | inflammatory bowel disease |
| FBC | full blood count | IBS | irritable bowel syndrome |
| FCU | flexor carpi ulnaris | ICA | internal carotid artery |
| FDL | flexor digitorum longus | ICAM | intercellular adhesion molecule |
| FDP | flexor digitorum profundus | ICP | intracranial pressure |
| FDS | flexor digitorum superficialis | IDDM | insulin-dependant diabetes mellitus |
| $FEV_1$ | forced expiratory volume in 1 second | IFN | interferon |
| FHL | flexor hallucis longus | IGF | insulin-like growth factor |
| FMD | fibromuscular dysplasia | IHD | ischaemic heart disease |
| FNA/C | fine-needle aspiration / cytology | IL | interleukin |

| | | | |
|---|---|---|---|
| IMA | inferior mesenteric artery | MTP | metatarsophalangeal (joint) |
| INR | international normalised ratio | NF | neurofibromatosis |
| INSS | international neuroblastoma staging system | NG | nasogastric |
| | | NHL | non-Hodgkin lymphoma |
| IPSS | International Prostate Symptom Score | NICE | National institute for Health and Clinical Excellence |
| ISC | intermittent self-catheterisation | | |
| ITP | idiopathic thrombocytopenic purpura | NODAT | new-onset diabetes after transplantation |
| ITU | intensive therapy unit | | |
| IUCD | intrauterine contraceptive device | NPI | Nottingham Prognostic Index (for breast cancer prognosis) |
| IV | intravenous | | |
| IVC | inferior vena cava | NSAID | non-steroidal anti-inflammatory drug |
| IVU | intravenous urography | NSCLC | non-small-cell lung carcinoma |
| JVP | jugular venous pressure (or pulse) | OA | osteoarthritis |
| KUB | kidneys, ureters, bladder | OCP | oral contraceptive pill |
| LA | local anaesthetic | OGD | oesophagogastroduodenoscopy |
| LAD | left anterior descending artery | ORIF | open reduction plus internal fixation |
| LCIS | lobular carcinoma in situ | PA | pulmonary artery |
| LDH | lactate dehydrogenase | $PaCO_2$ | partial pressure of carbon dioxide (arterial) |
| LFTs | liver function tests | | |
| LH | luteinising hormone | PAN | polyarteritis nodosa |
| LHRH | luteinising hormone-releasing hormone | $PaO_2$ | partial pressure of oxygen (arterial) |
| | | PAS | para-aminosalicylic acid |
| LIF | left iliac fossa | PBC | primary biliary cirrhosis |
| LIMA | left internal mammary artery | PCA | patient-controlled analgesia |
| LMP | last menstrual period | PCI | percutaneous coronary intervention |
| LMWH | low-molecular-weight heparin | PCL | posterior cruciate ligament |
| LP | lumbar puncture | PCNL | percutaneous nephrolithotomy |
| LSV | long saphenous vein | PCP | *Pneumocystis carinii* pneumonia |
| LUTS | lower urinary tract symptoms | PDA | patent ductus arteriosus |
| MAC | *Mycobacterium avium* complex | PE | pulmonary embolism |
| MALT | mucosa-associated lymphoid tissue | PEG | percutaneous endoscopic gastrostomy |
| MAP | mean arterial pressure | | |
| MC&S | microscopy, culture and sensitivity | PEJ | percutaneous endoscopic jejunostomy |
| MCP | metacarpophalangeal (joint) | | |
| MDT | multidisciplinary team | PET | positron-emission tomography |
| MEN | multiple endocrine neoplasia | PFTs | pulmonary function tests |
| MI | myocardial infarction | PG | prostaglandin |
| MIBG | meta-iodobenzylguanidine | PID | pelvic inflammatory disease |
| MRCP | magnetic resonance cholangiopancreatography | PIP | proximal interpharyngeal (joint) |
| | | PLL | posterior longitudinal ligament |
| MRI | magnetic resonance imaging | PPI | proton pump inhibitor |
| MRSA | methicillin-resistant *Staphylococcus aureus* | PSA | prostate-specific antigen |
| | | PSC | primary sclerosing cholangitis |
| MRTB | multidrug-resistant TB | PSIS | posterior superior iliac spine |
| MS | multiple sclerosis | PT | prothrombin time |
| MSU | mid-stream urine | PTFE | polytetrafluoroethylene |

| | | | |
|---|---|---|---|
| PTH | parathyroid hormone | TIPSS | transjugular intrahepatic portosystemic shunt |
| PTHC | percutaneous trans-hepatic cholangiography | TKR | total knee replacement |
| PTLD | post-transplant lymphoproliferative disorder | TME | total mesorectal excision |
| | | TNM | tumour, node, metastasis |
| PV | plasma viscosity | TOE | transoesophageal echocardiography |
| PVD | peripheral vascular disease | TPHA | *Treponema pallidum* haemagglutination assay |
| RA | rheumatoid arthritis | | |
| RBC | red blood cell | TPN | total parenteral nutrition |
| RIF | right iliac fossa | TRAM | transverse rectus abdominis myocutaneous (flap) |
| RLN | recurrent laryngeal nerve | | |
| RLQ | right lower quadrant | TRH | thyrotropin-releasing hormone |
| RPE | retinal pigment epithelium | TRUS | transrectal ultrasound |
| RPLND | retroperitoneal lymph node dissection | TSH | thyroid-stimulating hormone |
| RTA | road traffic accident | TT | thrombin time |
| RUQ | right upper quadrant | TTP | thrombotic thrombocytopenic purpura |
| SAH | subarachnoid haemorrhage | | |
| SBE | subacute bacterial endocarditis | TURBT | transurethral resection of bladder tumour |
| SBP | systolic blood pressure | | |
| SCC | squamous cell carcinoma | TURP | transurethral resection of prostate |
| SEPS | subfascial endoscopic perforator surgery | TWOC | trial without catheter |
| | | U&Es | urea and electrolytes |
| SERM | selective (o)estrogen receptor modulator | UC | ulcerative colitis |
| | | UGI | upper gastrointestinal |
| SFA | superior femoral artery | UICC | Union Internationale Contre le Cancre |
| SLE | systemic lupus erythematosus | | |
| SMA | superior mesenteric artery | US(S) | ultrasound (scan) |
| SPJ | saphenopopliteal junction | UTI | urinary tract infection |
| SSV | short saphenous vein | VATS | video-assisted thoracic surgery |
| SUFE | slipped upper femoral epiphysis | VC | vital capacity |
| SVC | superior vena cava | VEGF | vascular endothelial growth factor |
| TAPP | transabdominal preperitoneal (hernia repair approach) | VF | ventricular fibrillation |
| | | VIP | vasoactive intestinal peptide |
| TART | transanal resection of tumour | VP | ventriculoperitoneal |
| TB | tuberculosis | VSD | ventricular septal defect |
| TBG | thyroid-binding globulin | VT | ventricular tachycardia |
| TBNA | transbronchial needle aspiration | VUJ | vesicoureteric junction |
| Tc | technetium | VUR | vesicoureteric reflux |
| TCC | transitional cell carcinoma | VV | varicose vein |
| TEP | transabdominal extraperitoneal (hernia repair approach) | VVF | vesicovaginal fistula |
| | | WAGR | Wilms tumour, aniridia, genitourinary abnormalities, learning difficulties |
| (T)EVAR | (thoracic) endovascular AAA repair | | |
| TFTs | thyroid function tests | WBC | white blood cells |
| THC | trans-hepatic cholangiography | WCC | white cell count |
| THR | total hip replacement | ZN | Ziehl–Neelsen (stain) |
| TIA | transient ischaemic attack | | |

# Bibliography

## Books

Anderson JE (1978) *Grant's Atlas of Anatomy* (7th edition). Baltimore, MD: Lippincott Williams and Wilkins.

Bauby JD (1997) *The Diving Bell and the Butterfly*. New York, NY: Alfred A Knopf.

Barr ML, Kiernan JA (1988) *The Human Nervous System: An Anatomical Viewpoint* (5th edition). Baltimore, MD: Lippincott Williams and Wilkins.

Berne RM, Levy MN (eds) (1998) *Physiology: International Edition* (2nd edition). London: Mosby.

Browse N (1997) *The Symptoms and Signs of Surgical Disease* (3rd edition). London: Arnold.

Burnand K et al. (1992) *The New Aird's Companion in Surgical Studies* (3rd edition). London: Churchill Livingstone.

Cooke RS, Madehavan N, Woolf N (2001) STEP™. London: Royal College of Surgeons of England.

Corson JD, Williamson RCN (2000) *Surgery*. London: Mosby.

Dixon JM (2009) *Companion to Specialist Surgical Practice: Breast Surgery*. Saunders (Elsevier Publishing).

Dykes MI (2002) *Crash Course: Anatomy* (2nd edition). London: Mosby.

Ellis H (2002) *Clinical Anatomy*. Oxford: Blackwell Science.

Faiz O, Moffat D (2002) *Anatomy at a Glance*. Oxford: Blackwell.

Farr RF, Allisy-Roberts PJ (1988) *Physics for Medical Imaging*. London: WB Saunders.

General Medical Council (2011) *Good Medical Practice*.

Greenberg MS (2001) *Handbook of Neurosurgery* (5th edition). New York, NY:

Kirklin JW, Barratt-Boyes BG, Kouchoukos NT (eds) (2003) *Cardiac Surgery*. London: Churchill Livingstone.

Kleihues P, Cavenee WK (eds) (2000) *WHO Classification of Tumours of the Nervous System*. Lyon: IARC Press.

Martin E, (1990) *Concise Medical Dictionary*. NY: Oxford Press

Matta BF, Menon DK, Turner JM (eds) (2000) *Textbook of Neuroanasthesia and Critical Care*. Cambridge: Greenwich Medical Media.

McMinn RMH (1994) *Last's Anatomy, Regional and Applied* (9th edition). London: Churchill Livingstone.

McRae R (1996) *Clinical Orthopaedic Examination*. London: Churchill Livingstone.

McRae R (2002) *Practical Fracture Management* (4th edition). London: Churchill Livingstone.

Pallis C, Harley DH (1996) *ABC of Brainstem Death* (2nd edition). London: BMJ Publishing Group.

Raftery AT (ed) (2000) *Applied Basic Science for Basic Surgical Training*. London: Churchill Livingstone.

Snell RS (1986) *Clinical Anatomy for Medical Students* (3rd edition). USA: Little, Brown and Company.

Snell RS (2000) *Clinical Anatomy for Medical Students* (6th edition). Baltimore, MD: Lippincott Williams and Wilkins.

Thieme. Jones D (1999) *ABC of Colorectal Diseases*. London: BMJ Books.

## Peer reviewed publications

Anand SS, Wells PS, Hunt D, et al. (1998) 'Does this patient have deep vein thrombosis?' *Journal of the American Medical Association*, 279(14): 1094–1099.

Beral V (2003) 'Million Women Health Study' *Lancet*, 362: 419–427.

Calder SJ (1998) 'Fractures of the hip' *Surgery*, 16(11): 253–258.

Chesser TJS, Leslie IJ (1998) 'Forearm fractures' *Surgery*, 16(11): 241–248.

Crossman A, D'Agostiono Jr H, Geraci S (2002) 'Timing of coronary artery bypass graft surgery following acute myocardial infarction: A critical literature review' (book review) *Journal of Clinical Cardiology*, 25: 406–410.

Cuthbertson DP (1932) 'Observations on the disturbance of metabolism produced by injury to the limbs'. *Quarterly Journal of Medicine*, 1: 233–246.

Elefteriades J (2002) 'Natural history of thoracic aortic aneurysms' *Annals of Thoracic Surgery,* 74: S1877–S1880.

Kenealy J (1999) 'Cutaneous malignant melanoma' *Surgery,* 17(3): 68–72.

Vahedi et al., DECIMAL, DESTINY, and HAMLET investigators Early decompressive surgery in malignant infarction of the middle cerebral artery: a pooled analysis of three randomised controlled trials. *Lancet Neurol.* 2007 Mar; 6(3):215-22.

Filardo et al., Surgery for small asymptomatic abdominal aortic aneurysms. *Cochrane Database Syst Rev.* 2012 Mar 14;3: CD001835.

Bruls et al., Timing of carotid endarterectomy: a comprehensive review. *Acta Chir Belg.* 2012 Jan; 112(1):3-7.

Allum et al., Guidelines for the management of oesophageal and gastric cancer. *Gut.* 2011 Nov; 60(11):1449-72.

Hallissey et al., The second British Stomach Cancer Group trial of adjuvant radiotherapy or chemotherapy in resectable gastric cancer: five-year follow-up. *The Lancet,* 343(8909):1309-1312

Matuschek et al., The role of neoadjuvant and adjuvant treatment for adenocarcinoma of the upper gastrointestinal tract. *European Journal of Medicine Res.* 2011 Jun 21; 16(6):265-74.

Sjöström et al., Effects of bariatric surgery on mortality in Swedish obese subjects. *New England Journal of Medicine* 2007 Aug 23;357(8):741-52.

Li et al., Laparoscopic Roux-en-Y Gastric Bypass vs. Laparoscopic Sleeve Gastrectomy for Morbid Obesity and Diabetes Mellitus: A Meta-Analysis of Sixteen Recent Studies. *Hepatogastroenterology.* 2012 Aug 22; 60(121).

Gorenoi et al., Laparoscopic vs. Open appendectomy: systematic review of medical efficacy and health economic analysis. *GMS Health Technology Assessment* 2007 Jan 29;2: Doc22.

Sauerland et al., Laparoscopic vs conventional appendectomy--a meta-analysis of randomised controlled trials. *Langenbecks Archive of Surgery* 1998 Aug;383(3-4):289-95.

Libby et al., The impact of population-based faecal occult blood test screening on colorectal cancer mortality: a matched cohort study *British Journal of Cancer.*2012 Jul 10; 107(2):255-9

Gray et al., Adjuvant chemotherapy versus observation in patients with colorectal cancer: a randomised study. *Quasar Collaborative Group,Lancet.* 2007 Dec 15;370(9604):2020-9.

AXIS collaborators, James et al., Randomized clinical trial of adjuvant radiotherapy and 5-fluorouracil infusion in colorectal cancer (AXIS). *British Journal of Surgery.* 2003 Oct; 90(10):1200-12.

Atkin et al., Once-only flexible sigmoidoscopy screening in prevention of colorectal cancer: a multicentre randomised controlled trial. *The Lancet,*Volume 375, Issue 9726, Pages 1624 – 1633

Reyes AT *et al.* (1995) 'Technique for harvesting the radial artery as a coronary artery bypass graft' *Annals of Thoracic Surgery* 59(1): 118–126.

Wilson JMG, Junger G (1968) 'Principles and practice of screening for disease' *Public Health Papers,* 34. Geneva: World Health Organisation.

**Websites:**

www.sign.ac.uk (last accessed Sept 2012)

www.cancerscreening.nhs.uk (Last accessed Sept 2012)

www.euroscore.org (Last accessed Sept 2012)

www.nice.org.uk (Last accessed Sept 2012)

www.the-ia.org.uk (The Ileostomy and Internal Pouch Support Group) (Last accessed Sept 2012)

# Index